FUNDAMENTALS of NEUROIMAGING

FUNDAMENTALS of NEUROIMAGING

William W. Woodruff, M.D.
Clinical Assistant Professor
Department of Radiology
Jefferson Medical College
Thomas Jefferson University
Philadelphia, Pennsylvania
Associate, Division of Special Imaging
Clinical Supervisor, MRI
Department of Radiology
Geisinger Medical Center
Danville, Pennsylvania

W.B. SAUNDERS COMPANY
A Division of Harcourt Brace & Company
Philadelphia London Toronto Montreal Sydney Tokyo

W.B. SAUNDERS COMPANY
A Division of
Harcourt Brace & Company

The Curtis Center
Independence Square West
Philadelphia, Pennsylvania 19106

Library of Congress Cataloging-in-Publication Data

Woodruff, William W.
Fundamentals of neuroimaging / William W. Woodruff.

p. cm

ISBN 0–7216–3717–5

1. Central nervous system—Imaging. I. Title.
[DNLM: 1. Diagnostic Imaging. 2. Nervous System Diseases—diagnosis. WL 141 W893f]

RC349.D52W66 1993

616.8′04754—dc20

DNLM/DLC 92-13388

FUNDAMENTALS OF NEUROIMAGING ISBN 0–7216–3717–5

Printed in the United States of America.

Last digit is the print number: 9 8 7 6 5 4 3 2

DEDICATION

With love to Michele and our daughters,
Alex and Mary,
for their inimitable support and patience.

PREFACE

The goal of the author is to purvey a basic yet detailed neuroimaging textbook useful to residents, fellows, and practitioners in the imaging and clinical fields of the neurosciences. To maintain a practical perspective, attempts to describe minute details of arcane diseases have been abandoned in order to emphasize common manifestations of common disease processes. With few exceptions, material presented here is representative of that encountered daily on an active neuroimaging service.

The strengths, weaknesses, and indications for the use of commonly utilized radiographic modalities are assessed in regard to evaluation of specific disease processes. It is hoped that the reader will learn the most efficacious application of these imaging tools. The physics of planar imaging is not reviewed, as this is adroitly covered and widely available in multiple sources. As planar imaging has supplanted angiography in the evaluation of intracranial mass lesions, angiography is presented only in terms of primary vasculopathic conditions.

Region-specific anatomy is presented in sufficient detail to afford the reader an understanding of normal radiographic anatomy. Illustrations and planar images corroborate the anatomic prose. Discussion of pathology is presented in terms of a location approach. Multiple representative images are available to underscore the radiographic appearance of diseases that affect the central nervous system.

Where applicable, differential diagnoses are presented in tables. Emphasis is placed on the distinguishing radiographic and/or clinical features of these lesions.

WILLIAM W. WOODRUFF, M.D.

ACKNOWLEDGMENTS

This project is a collage of contributions from multiple, talented individuals at Geisinger Medical Center (GMC), Danville, Pennsylvania. Britain Roth, Director of Learning Resources, graciously offered the services of Medical Photography at GMC. I am indebted to Joseph Mentrikoski, Director of Medical Photography, and his associates, Diane Blue, Nathan Jeffery, Jackie Fetterman, Cathy Diggan, John Shaibley, Peggy Herman, Nancy Heddens, and Florence Beaver, for their superb, timely photographic support.

Special Projects–Word Processing, GMC, under the direction of Pam Shultz and Lisa Kanour, contributed enormously to this work. Janice Schlegel, Ruth Klock, Vickie Shaffer, Sue Brady, and Vicki Boudman consistently produced quality material under adverse conditions, often working late into the night and early morning to meet deadlines.

The creative input of medical illustrator Lisa Peñalver has been nonpareil. Despite a relocation to Fairbanks, Alaska, Lisa's transformation of ideas into detailed, high-quality illustrations proves that a picture is indeed worth a thousand words.

I gratefully acknowledge contributions of the technical staff of the Department of Special Imaging, GMC. The Magnetic Resonance Facility, under the direction of Mary Sedor-Edmeads, is staffed by Gretchen Oman, Inez Neitz, Sherry Herr, Chris Brady, Joyce Flagg, Robin Edwards, Barry Kremser, and Lew Tersavige. The Computed Tomography Section, under the direction of Ron Deutzer, is staffed by Lynn Wolff, John Harris, Louise Albright, Mike Fountain, Brenda Jones, and Dave Gregory. The Angiography Section is staffed by Michael Fluck, Karen Benner, and Dale Albright.

For my introduction to neuroradiology, a special thanks to J. Robert Kirkwood, M.D., of Baystate Medical Center, Springfield, Massachusetts. My subsequent experience at Duke University Medical Center, Durham, North Carolina, proved invaluable. It is there that I met, among others, E. Ralph Heinz, M.D., a talented neuroradiologist and gracious human being.

I am deeply indebted to Lisette Bralow, Editor-in-Chief of Medical Books at W. B. Saunders Company. Lisette provided the opportunity, knowledge, and experienced staff support to complete this task.

Finally, with compassion, I would like to acknowledge the many patients and their families who suffer with and endure the tragedies of these diseases.

WILLIAM W. WOODRUFF, M.D.

CONTENTS

1

THE SKULL

The current shift in emphasis on planar imaging has eclipsed the utility of the plain film examination of the skull. Rarely do skull x-rays add significant information in the neurodiagnostic evaluation of patients with central nervous system (CNS) disease. Nonetheless, some CNS diseases express abnormalities that may be detected on skull films. In general, these diseases affect the density of the skull, form detectable intracranial calcification, or cause remodeling of the skull secondary to local destruction or increased intracranial pressure. Following a review of the normal anatomy of the skull, the more common of these disease processes will be presented.

The skull consists of 20 bones, 14 of which

form the face and the remainder of which form the cranial vault.[1] The skull can be divided into anterior, middle, and posterior cranial fossae (Fig. 1–1). The floor of the anterior fossa is formed by the frontal and ethmoid bones, terminating posteriorly in the lesser wing of the sphenoid. The floor of the middle cranial fossa is formed by the greater wing of the sphenoid, terminating posteriorly in the petrous portion of the temporal bone. The floor of the posterior fossa is formed by the occipital bone and the dorsal surface of the petrous portion of the temporal bone.

The inner and outer tables are composed of dense compact cortical bone. The cancellous diploë is juxtaposed between the inner and outer tables. The bones of the cranial vault are separated by fibrous sutures. The sutures represent the region of most active bone formation. They fuse by the late second decade of life, after the growth of the vault has ceased.

NORMAL RADIOGRAPHIC ANATOMY

Lateral View (Fig. 1–2)

Sutures

The coronal suture separates the frontal bone anteriorly from the parietal bones posteriorly. The coronal suture terminates inferiorly at the greater wing of the sphenoid bone, forming the pterion. The lambdoid suture separates the parietal bones anteriorly from the occipital bone posteriorly. The lambdoid suture descends laterally from the midline junction with the sagittal suture at the lambda (posterior fontanelle). The lambdoid suture terminates at the mastoid portion of the temporal bone, where it continues as the occipitomastoid suture inferiorly and the parietomastoid suture superiorly. The parietomastoid suture continues anteriorly as the squamosal suture to meet the greater wing of the sphenoid bone.

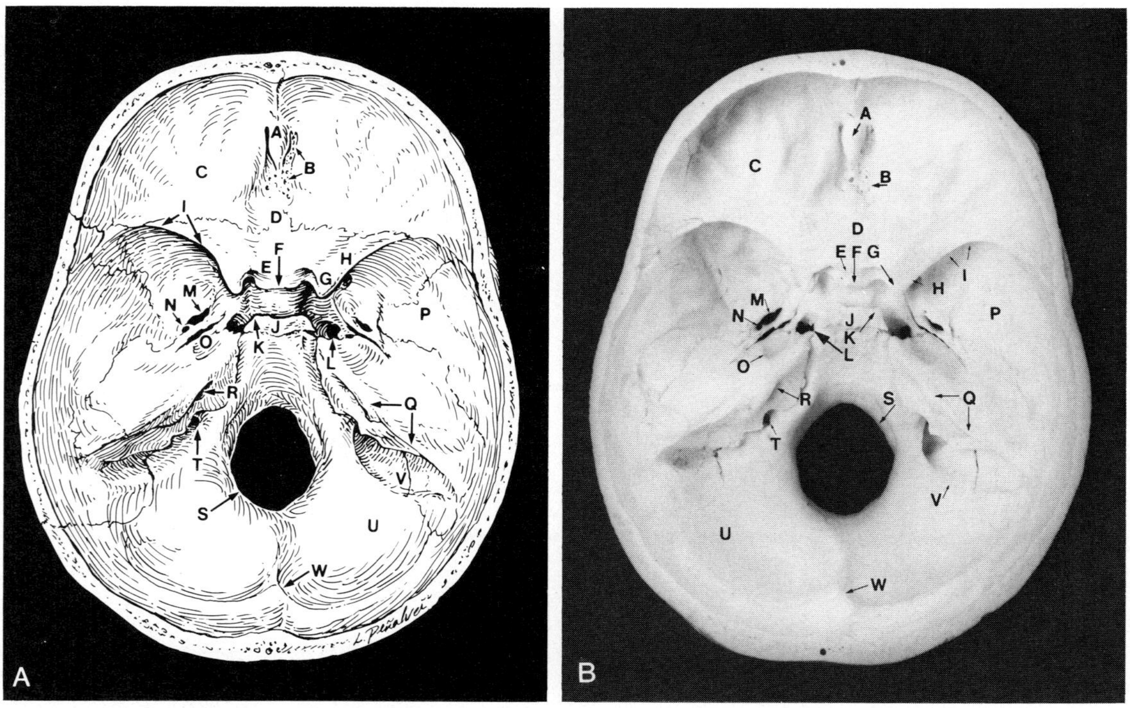

Figure 1–1. Cephalad view of open skull.

A, Drawing.

B, Photograph: *(A)* Crista galli, *(B)* cribriform plate, *(C)* floor of anterior cranial fossa, *(D)* planum sphenoidale, *(E)* limbus sphenoidale, *(F)* tuberculum sella, *(G)* anterior clinoid, *(H)* lesser wing of sphenoid, *(I)* sphenoid ridge, *(J)* dorsum sella, *(K)* posterior clinoid, *(L)* bony canal for precavernous carotid, *(M)* foramen ovale, *(N)* foramen spinosum, *(O)* depression for Meckel's cave, *(P)* floor of middle cranial fossa, *(Q)* petrous ridge, *(R)* internal auditory canal, *(S)* foramen magnum, *(T)* jugular foramen, *(U)* floor of posterior fossa, *(V)* sigmoid sinus, *(W)* torcular herophili.

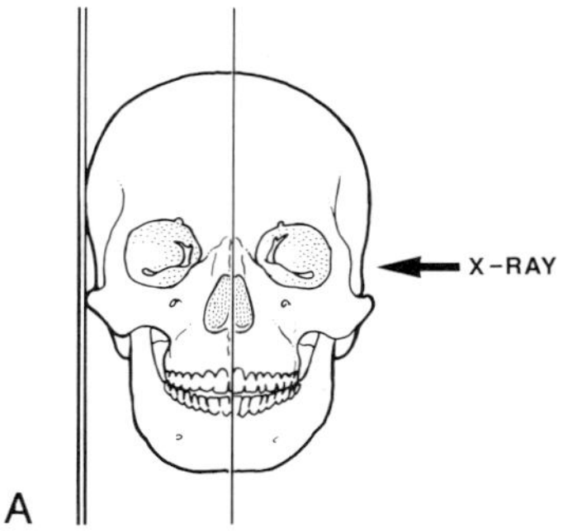

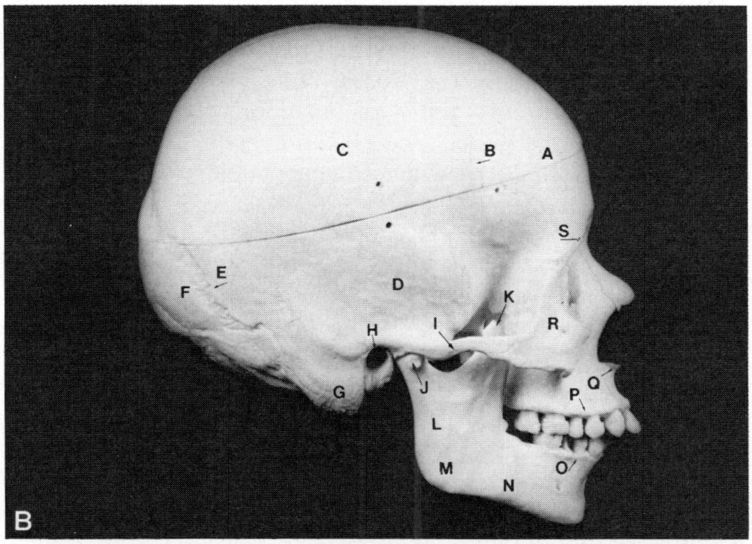

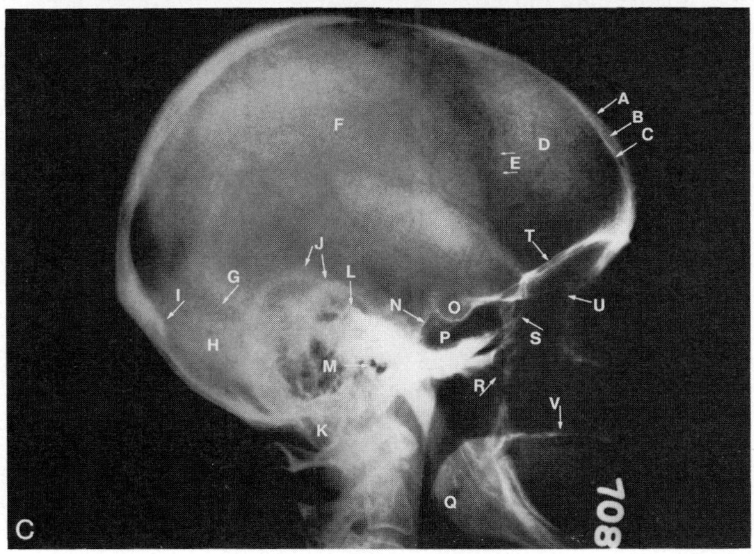

Figure 1–2. Lateral view of skull.

A, Positioning: With the side of interest adjacent to the cassette, the central beam is directed perpendicular to the film.

B, *(A)* Frontal bone, *(B)* coronal suture, *(C)* parietal bone, *(D)* squamosal portion of temporal bone, *(E)* lambdoid suture, *(F)* occipital bone, *(G)* mastoid tip, *(H)* external auditory canal, *(I)* zygomatic arch, *(J)* mandibular condyle, *(K)* coronoid process of mandible, *(L)* ramus of mandible, *(M)* angle of mandible, *(N)* body of mandible, *(O)* inferior alveolar ridge, *(P)* superior alveolar ridge, *(Q)* inferior nasal spine, *(R)* zygoma, *(S)* nasion.

C, *(A)* Outer table, *(B)* diploic space, *(C)* inner table, *(D)* frontal bone, *(E)* coronal suture, *(F)* parietal bone, *(G)* lambdoid suture, *(H)* occipital bone, *(I)* torcular herophili, *(J)* cartilaginous external ear, *(K)* mastoid, *(L)* petrous ridge, *(M)* external auditory canal, *(N)* clivus, *(O)* sella turcica, *(P)* sphenoid sinus, *(Q)* angle of mandible, *(R)* pterygopalatine fossa, *(S)* greater wing of sphenoid, *(T)* orbital roof, *(U)* cribriform plate, *(V)* hard palate.

Calvarium

Frontal Bone

The frontal bone develops from two separate ossification centers separated by the metopic suture. The metopic suture persists in 15% of normal adults. The glabella is the midline smooth elevation above the orbit. The frontal sinuses appear variable, enlarging the diploë, until they are fully developed by the late teenage years. With the exception of the small midline ethmoid bone, the frontal bone also forms the anterior two thirds of the floor of the anterior cranial fossa. The posterior floor is composed of the lesser wing of the sphenoid bone.

The orbital roof is the highest elevation in the floor of the anterior fossa and may be visualized as a separate line above the midline valley of the anterior fossa, the cribriform plate of the ethmoid bone. The crista galli is the anterior-most cephalad projection from the cribriform plate. It serves as an attachment point to the anterior falx and is visualized as a focal convex upward ridge. The cribriform plate continues posteriorly into the planum sphenoidale and limbus.

Parietal Bone

This flat bone is generally featureless with the exception of shallow vascular grooves along the inner table from the middle meningeal artery and vein.

Occipital Bone

This, the thickest of the skull bones, constitutes the dorsal boundary of the posterior cranial fossa. The occipital bone forms the entire ring of the foramen magnum and the caudal two thirds of the clivus. The occipital condyles articulate with the lateral masses of C1 of the cervical spine. The internal occipital protuberance or torcular herophili is a focal thickening of the inner table that defines the confluence of the straight, sagittal, and transverse dural sinuses.

Temporal Bone

The temporal bone, the most complex bone of the calvarium, is discussed in more detail in Chapter 11. The thin squamosal portion demarcates the lateral-most aspect of the middle cranial fossa. The dense petrous portion of the temporal bone forms the ridge separating the middle and posterior cranial fossae. The external auditory canals may be visualized as 1-cm (in greatest linear dimension) circular lucencies within the inferior portion of the dense petrosal ridge. The mastoid air cells lie dorsally, in the caudal-most temporal bone. The extent of aeration of these air cells is variable. Finally, the 2.5-cm styloid process extends ventrocaudally from the base of the temporal bone to serve as an attachment for three muscles and the stylomandibular ligament.

Sphenoid Bone

The sphenoid bone lies in the central portion of the skull base. The greater wings of the sphenoid bone demarcate the medial floor and anterior boundary of the middle cranial fossa. The greater wings of the sphenoid bone are depicted as gently curving C-shaped linear densities on the lateral film. The lesser wings of the sphenoid form a ridge that separates the anterior and middle cranial fossae. The lesser wings terminate in the anterior clinoid processes. The aerated sphenoid sinus is identified inferior and anterior to the sella turcica. The degree of aeration of the sphenoid sinus is variable. The sphenoid bone comprises the cephalad-most third of the clivus, before joining the occipital bone at the spheno-occipital synchondrosis.

Face

The 14 bones of the face are largely superimposed on the lateral view. The hard palate can be identified as a horizontal linear density, separating the teeth and alveolar ridge of the oral cavity below from the gas-filled structures of the maxillary sinus and nasal cavity above. The hard palate terminates anteriorly as the inferior nasal spine. The anterior and posterior walls of the maxillary sinus can be traced. The triangular outline of the lateral-most extension of the maxillary sinus, the zygomatic recess, overlies the maxillary sinus on the lateral view. The teardrop-shaped pterygopalatine fossa is juxtaposed between the posterior wall of the maxillary sinus anteriorly and pterygoid plates posteriorly. The thin bony septa of the ethmoid air cells are above the maxillary sinus. The nasal bone and its junction point with the frontal bone, the nasion, can be identified.

Although not strictly considered part of the calvarium, the mandible may be identified on lateral film. The condyle, neck, ramus, angle, and body are clearly depicted.

Sella (Fig. 1–3)

This view is obtained with a collimated lateral central beam limited to the sella. The planum sphenoidale, the posterior midline extension from the cribriform plate, terminates in the limbus. A shallow depression, the chiasmatic sulcus, continues inferiorly to end in the horizontal bony bridge of the tuberculum sellae. The anterior wall, floor, and posterior wall of the sella form a continuum of cortical bone. The posterior wall terminates in the dorsum sellae. The anterior clinoid processes constitute the posterior-most extension of the medial portion of the lesser wings of the sphenoid bone. The posterior clinoids form the anterior-most extension of the dorsum sellae.

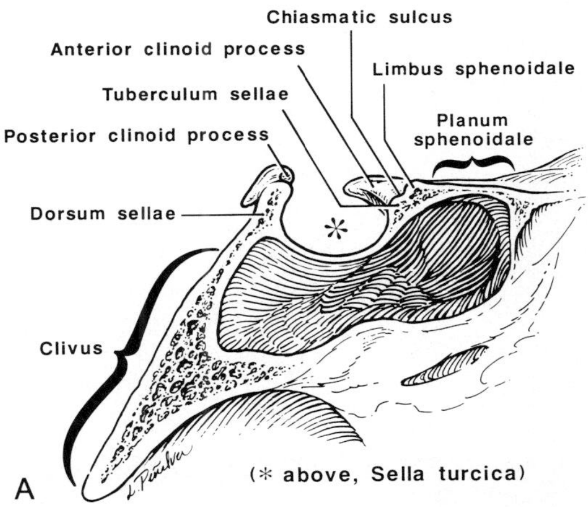

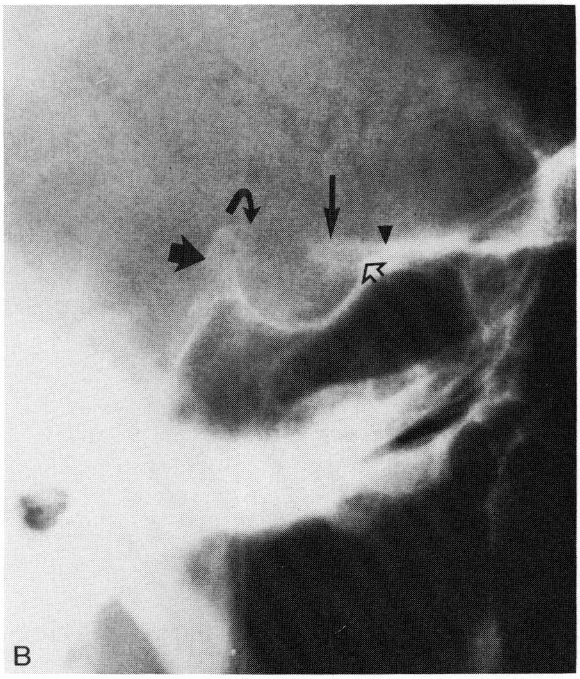

Figure 1–3. Lateral sella.
A, Drawing.
B, Radiograph. Coned-down lateral view—limbus *(black arrowhead),* tuberculum sellae *(open black arrow),* anterior clinoid *(thin black arrow),* posterior clinoid *(curved black arrow),* and dorsum sellae *(thick black arrow).*

Straight Posteroanterior View
(Fig. 1–4)

The straight posteroanterior (PA) view is obtained with the patient's head in an upright position, with the beam directed parallel to the orbitomeatal line and perpendicular to the film cassette.

The lambdoid suture projects medial to the more lateral coronal suture. The midline sagittal suture separates the parietal bones and extends from the coronal (bregma) to the lambdoid (lambda) sutures. The orbital roof is superimposed on the petrous ridge. The internal auditory canal is located within the midorbit. The cribriform plate and crista galli are identified midline in the anterior cranial fossa. The floor of the middle and posterior cranial fossae is superimposed on the petrous portion of the temporal bone. The medial and lateral walls of the maxillary sinus can be identified. The frontal sinus may project cephalad to the orbital roof. The nasal cavity, vomer, and middle and inferior turbinates are visualized. The innominate line represents the medial-most aspect of the temporal and infratemporal fossae. The innominate line projects over the lateral aspect of the orbit. The upper lateral rim of the orbit, composed of the zygomatic process of the frontal bone, can be visualized.

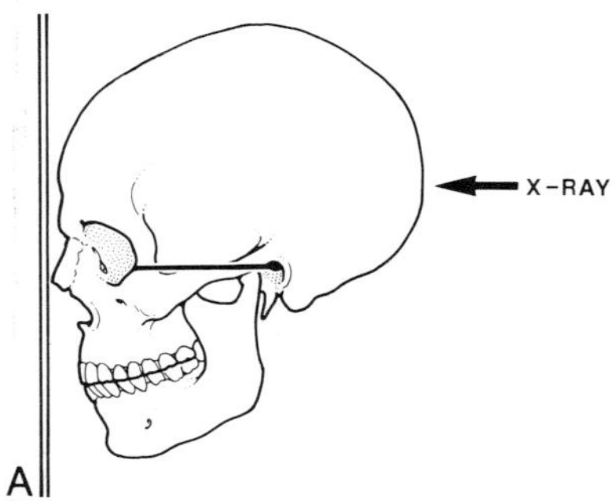

Figure 1–4. Straight posteroanterior (PA) view.

A, Positioning. In an upright position, the central beam is directed parallel to the orbitomeatal line and perpendicular to the film cassette.

B, *(A)* Parietal bone, *(B)* coronal suture, *(C)* frontal bone, *(D)* metopic suture, *(E)* superior orbital foramen, *(F)* superior orbital margin, *(G)* nasion, *(H)* nasal bones, *(I)* optic canal, *(J)* superior orbital fissure, *(K)* inferior orbital fissure, *(L)* inferior orbital margin, *(M)* inferior orbital foramen, *(N)* zygoma, *(O)* maxilla, *(P)* vomer, *(Q)* superior alveolar ridge, *(R)* inferior alveolar ridge, *(S)* mental foramen.

C, *(A)* Coronal suture, *(B)* lambdoid suture, *(C)* sagittal suture, *(D)* frontal sinus, *(E)* superior orbital margin, *(F)* petrous ridge, *(G)* internal auditory canal, *(H)* innominate line, *(I)* crista galli, *(J)* planum sphenoidale.

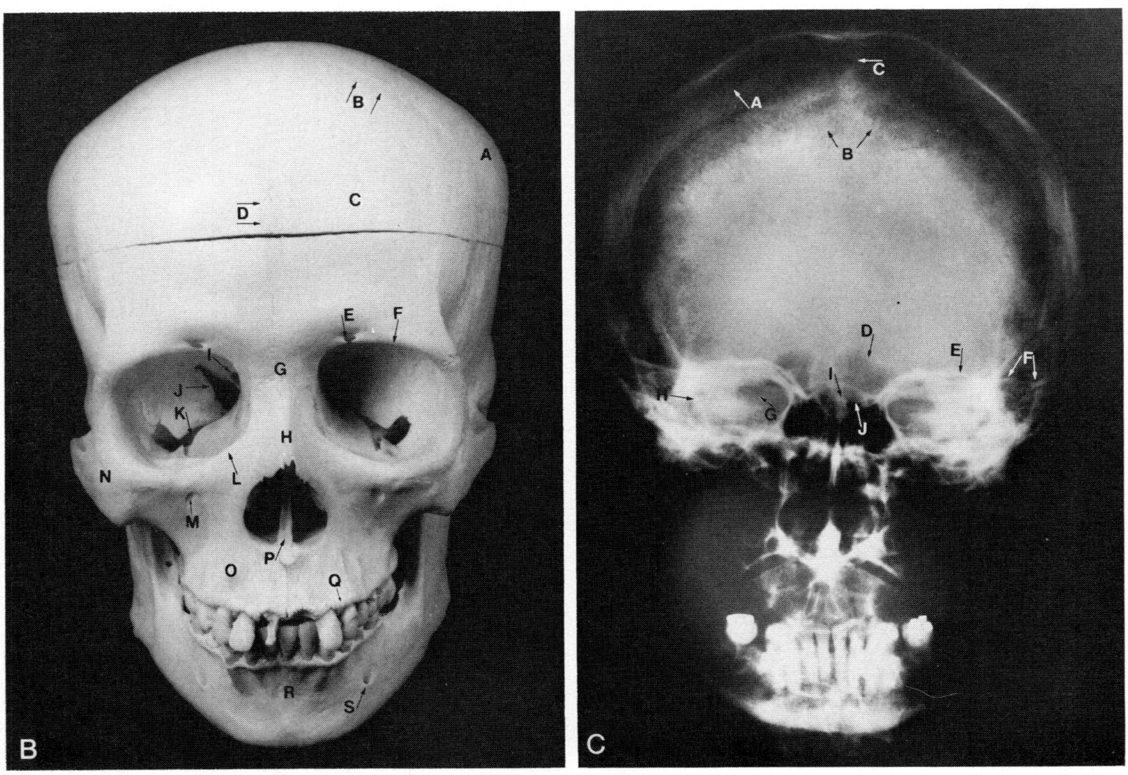

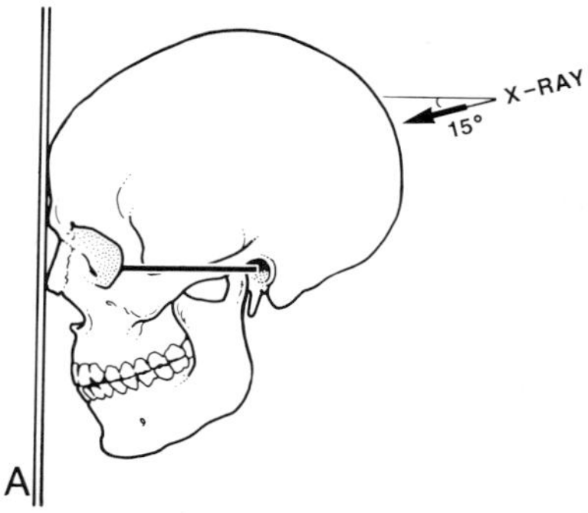

Figure 1–5. Caldwell view.

A, Positioning. In an upright position with the orbitomeatal line perpendicular to the film cassette, the central beam is directed 15 degrees caudal to the orbitomeatal line.

B, *(A)* Frontal bone, *(B)* superior orbital foramen, *(C)* superior orbital margin, *(D)* nasion, *(E)* zygomaticofrontal suture, *(F)* greater wing of sphenoid, *(G)* zygoma, *(H)* inferior orbital margin, *(I)* inferior orbital foramen, *(J)* maxilla, *(K)* vomer, *(L)* inferior turbinate, *(M)* mastoid tip, *(N)* body of mandible, *(O)* superior orbital fissure.

C, *(A)* Sagittal suture, *(B)* frontal sinus, *(C)* superior orbital margin, *(D)* lesser wing of sphenoid, *(E)* superior orbital fissure, *(F)* ethmoid sinus, *(G)* petrous ridge, *(H)* innominate line, *(I)* zygomaticofrontal suture, *(J)* floor of sella, *(K)* foramen rotundum, *(L)* vomer, *(M)* inferior turbinate, *(N)* mandibular ramus, *(O)* mandibular body, *(P)* arcuate eminence.

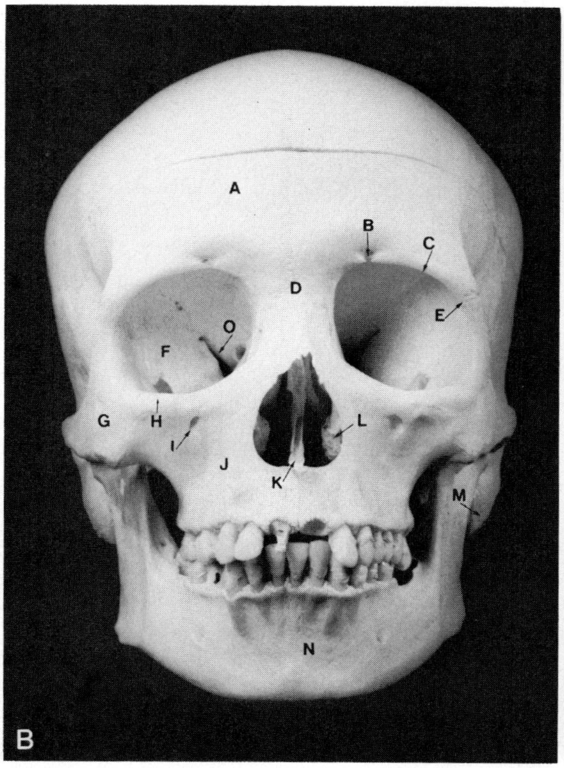

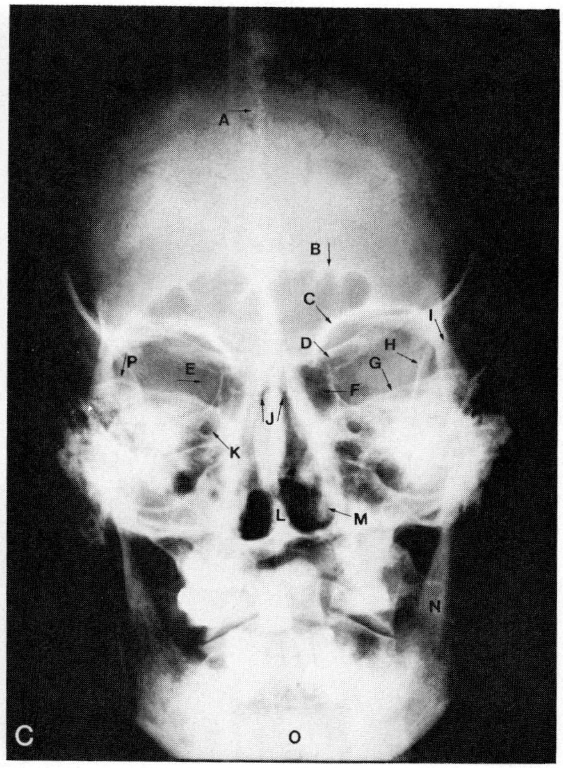

Caldwell View (Fig. 1–5)

For the Caldwell view, the position of the head is similar to that for the PA view. The beam is directed 15 degrees caudal to the orbitomeatal line. This view projects the orbit above the petrous portion of the temporal bone. The lesser and greater wings of the sphenoid are separated, revealing the superior orbital fissure. The foramen rotundum, conveying the maxillary division of the trigeminal nerve (V2), is projected as a circular lucency over the inferomedial orbit. The orbital rim including the superior orbital margin, the zygomatic process of the frontal bone, the zygoma, and the zygomaticofrontal suture can be identified. The innominate line projects clearly over the lateral third of the orbit. The floor of the anterior cranial fossa is projected inferior to the superior orbital rim. The septated frontal sinus projects a variable distance above the orbits. The ethmoid air cells straddle the medial orbital rims. The horizontal cribriform plate and vertically oriented crista galli are visualized at midline.

The floor of the sella bisects the vomer at the level of midorbit. Middle and inferior turbinates are identified along the lateral wall of the nasal cavity. The floor of the posterior fossa projects over the hard palate, extending laterally to the mastoid air cells. The upwardly convexed arcuate eminence of the petrous portion of the temporal bone is visualized along the midpetrous ridge.

Towne View (Fig. 1–6)

The Towne view is obtained with an anteroposterior (AP) beam angled approximately 35 degrees caudally with respect to the orbitomeatal line. The orbitomeatal line is perpendicular to the film cassette.

The occipital, parietal, and frontal bones are superimposed. The lambdoid suture lies within the coronal suture. The sagittal suture may be identified at midline, extending between the coronal and lambdoid sutures. The posterior clinoid processes and dorsum sellae project within the foramen magnum. The internal auditory canals are depicted as a focal concavity along the medial surface of the petrous portion of the temporal bones.

The facial bones and orbital structures are foreshortened and superimposed. The maxillary sinuses are triangular in this view. The inferior orbital fissure lies between the posterior superior wall of the maxillary sinus and the greater wing of the sphenoid.

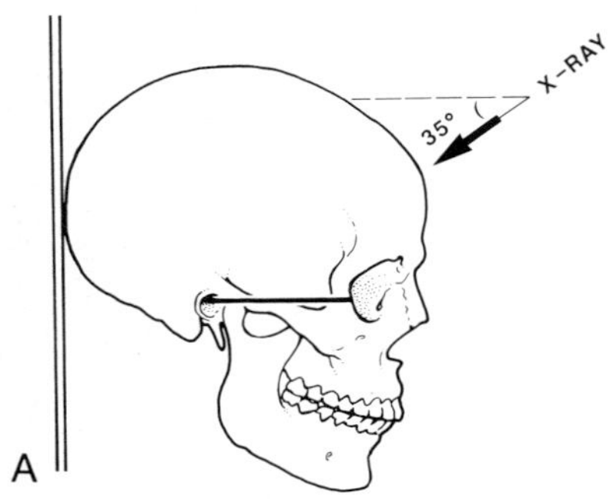

Figure 1–6. Towne view.

A, Positioning. In an upright position with the orbitomeatal line perpendicular to the film cassette, an anteroposterior (AP) central beam is directed 35 degrees caudal to the orbitomeatal line.

B, *(A)* Parietal bone, *(B)* lambdoid suture, *(C)* occipital bone, *(D)* torcular herophili, *(E)* course of transverse sinus, *(F)* foramen magnum, *(G)* dorsum sellae, *(H)* petrous ridge, *(I)* frontal bone, *(J)* zygomatic arch, *(K)* zygoma, *(L)* superior orbital margin, *(M)* inferior orbital fissure, *(N)* nasion, *(O)* lacrimal bone, *(P)* inferior orbital margin, *(Q)* maxilla.

C, *(A)* Sagittal suture, *(B)* lambdoid suture, *(C)* petrous ridge, *(D)* internal auditory canal, *(E)* posterior rim of the foramen magnum, *(F)* dorsum sellae, *(G)* inferior orbital fissure, *(H)* maxillary sinus.

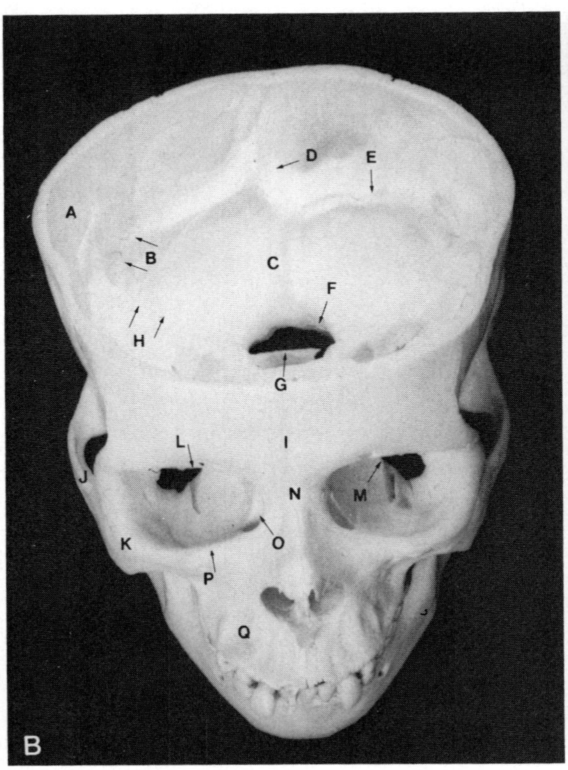

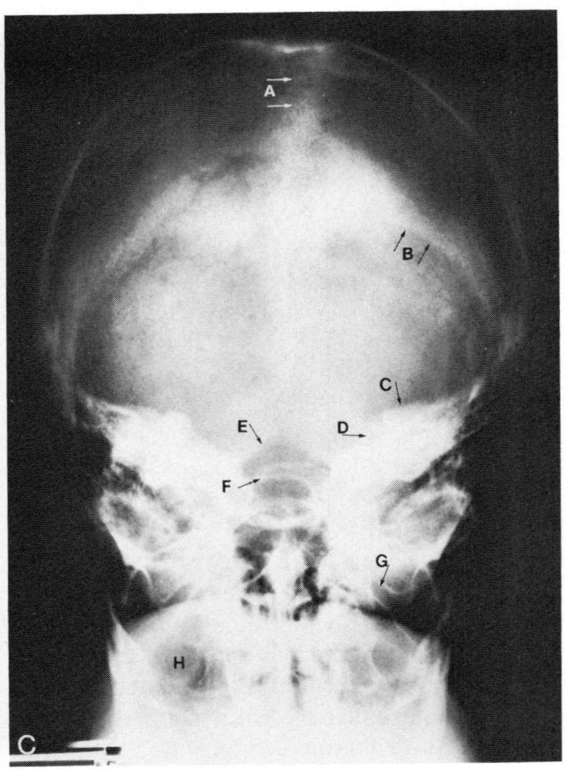

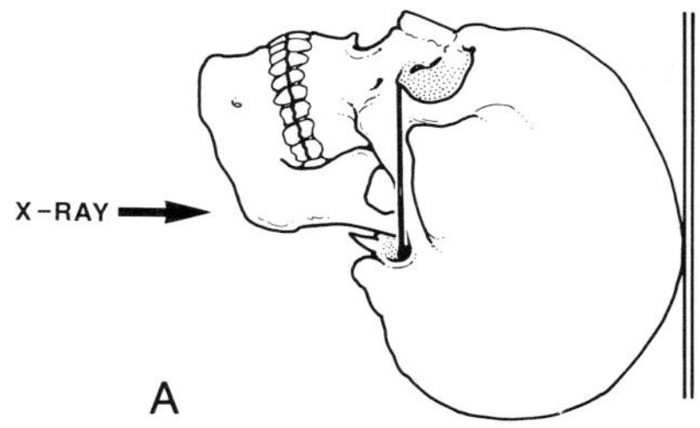

Figure 1–7. Submentovertex or basal view.

A, Positioning. With the vertex in contact with the film, a central beam is directed perpendicular to the infraorbitomeatal line and the film cassette.

B, *(A)* Body of mandible, *(B)* maxilla, *(C)* inferior orbital foramen, *(D)* zygomatic arch, *(E)* palatine bones of posterior hard palate, *(F)* medial pterygoid plate, *(G)* lateral pterygoid plate, *(H)* foramen lacerum, *(I)* foramen ovale, *(J)* foramen spinosum, *(K)* mandibular condyle, *(L)* carotid foramen, *(M)* caroticojugular spine, *(N)* pars nervosa, *(O)* jugular spine, *(P)* pars vascularis, *(Q)* occipital condyle, *(R)* stylomastoid foramen, *(S)* mastoid tip, *(T)* posterior rim of foramen magnum (opisthion).

C, *(A)* Body of mandible, *(B)* vomer, *(C)* lateral orbital wall, *(D)* lateral wall of maxillary sinus, *(E)* anterior wall of the middle cranial fossa (greater wing of sphenoid), (F) pterygopalatine fossa, *(G)* medial pterygoid plate, *(H)* lateral pterygoid plate, *(I)* foramen ovale, *(J)* foramen spinosum, *(K)* mandibular condyle, *(L)* anterior arch of C1, *(M)* odontoid, *(N)* foramen magnum.

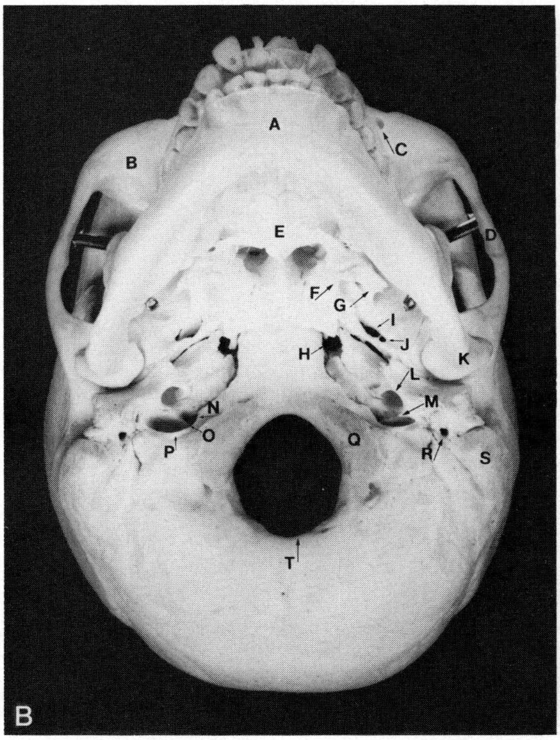

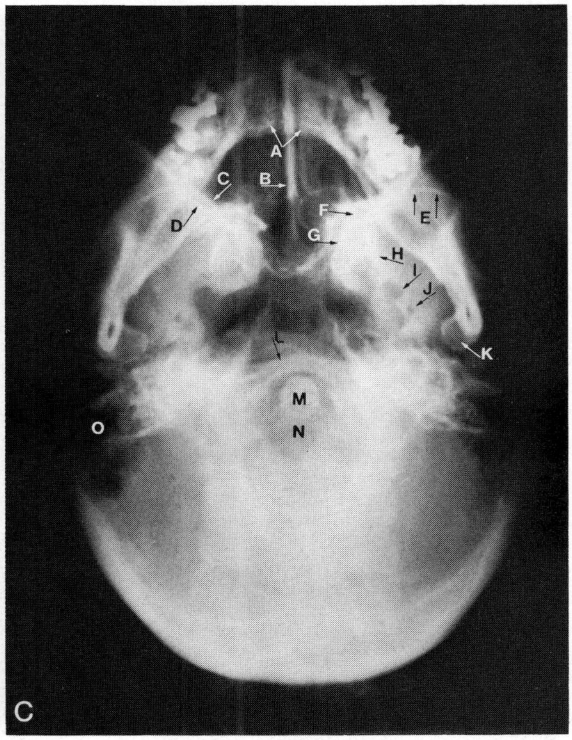

Basal (Submentovertex) View
(Fig. 1–7)

The film is located at the skull vertex positioned parallel to the infraorbitomeatal line. The beam is directed perpendicular to both.

Centrally, the odontoid appears circular, closely applied to the anterior arch of C1. The cervical spine is superimposed over the central half of the posterior fossa. The petrous portion of the temporal bone terminates laterally in the mastoid air cells.

The anterior border of the middle cranial fossa is composed of the greater wings of the sphenoid bone, which are depicted as convex anterior curvilinear densities. The foramen ovale, conveying the mandibular division of the trigeminal nerve (V3), and the smaller posterolateral foramen spinosum, conveying the middle meningeal artery, are visualized in the medial floor of the middle cranial fossa.

The C-shaped medial and lateral pterygoid plates are projected anterior and medial to the foramen ovale. The pterygoid fossa is located between the pterygoid plates. The posterior lateral wall of the maxillary sinus continues anteriorly and laterally as an S-shaped linear density. The straighter linear density partially superimposed over this is the lateral wall of the orbit. The pterygopalatine fossa is an oblong lucency juxtaposed between the pterygoid plates and the posterior maxillary sinus wall.

The sphenoid sinus lies medial to the pterygoid plates. The midline vomer is readily identified. The ethmoid air cells are superimposed over the nasal turbinates. Anteriorly, both are obscured by the mandible and the teeth.

Waters View (Fig. 1–8)

This view is obtained with the chin in contact with the film. The orbitomeatal line is directed at a 35-degree angle with respect to the film, and the PA beam is directed perpendicular to the film.

The maxillary and frontal sinuses are well visualized. The frontal sinuses are depicted above the superior orbital margin. This view depicts the petrous bone below the maxillary sinuses. The orbital margin including the zygoma, the zygomaticofrontal suture, and the zygomatic process of the frontal bone are well seen. The ethmoid and sphenoid sinuses are

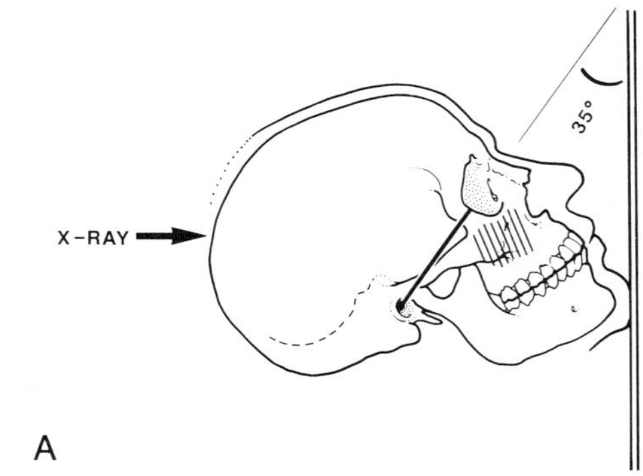

Figure 1–8. Waters view.

A, Positioning. With the orbitomeatal line directed 35 degrees caudad and the chin in contact with the film cassette, a central beam is directed perpendicular to the cassette.

B, *(A)* Frontal bone, *(B)* nasal bones, *(C)* superior orbital foramen, *(D)* superior orbital margin, *(E)* inferior orbital margin, *(F)* inferior orbital foramen, *(G)* maxilla, *(H)* zygoma, *(I)* zygomatic arch, *(J)* coronoid process of mandible, *(K)* body of mandible, *(L)* vomer.

C, *(A)* Frontal bone, *(B)* frontal sinus, *(C)* superior orbital margin, *(D)* nasal bones, *(E)* vomer, *(F)* innominate line, *(G)* inferior orbital margin, *(H)* inferior orbital foramen, *(I)* maxillary sinus, *(J)* lateral wall of maxillary sinus, *(K)* zygoma, *(L)* zygomatic arch, *(M)* coronoid process of mandible, *(N)* body of mandible, *(O)* odontoid.

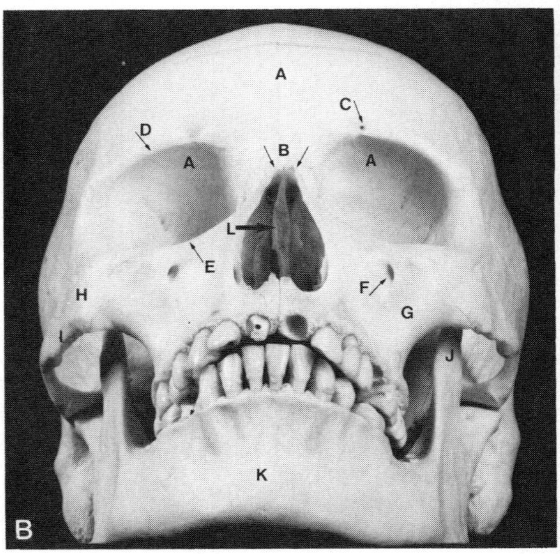

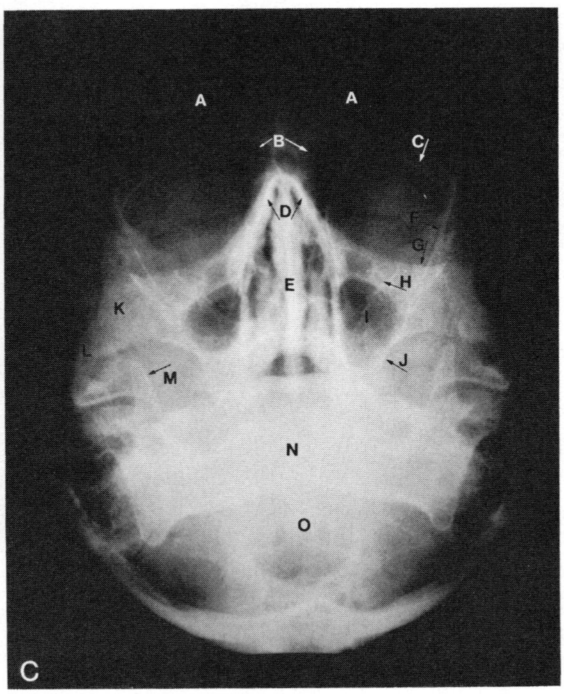

superimposed. The body, ramus, condyle, and coronoid process of the mandible are distorted, though well depicted.

INTRACRANIAL CALCIFICATIONS

Physiologic

Pineal. The pineal gland appears as an ovoid amorphic calcification on plain films in approximately 50% of adults.[2, 3] The incidence of calcification is thought to increase with age. The calcification should not exceed 10 mm in greatest linear dimension. It may appear punctate, peripheral, or amorphous. In nearly 20% of patients, the calcium detected on the lateral film will not be apparent on the frontal film. The position of the pineal should not vary more than 2.5 to 3 mm from midline on frontal films (Fig. 1–9).

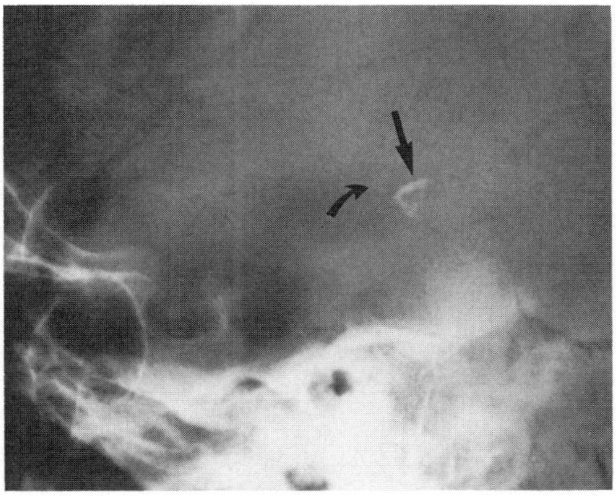

Figure 1–9. Pineal and choroid ("habenular") calcification (32-year-old male). Lateral film; a large amorphic pineal calcification *(straight arrow)* is located posterior to the C-shaped calcification of the tela choroidea of the third ventricle *(curved arrow)*.

Choroid. The choroid may calcify anywhere along its course within the lateral, third, or fourth ventricles. The two most common regions to calcify are the tela choroidea of the posterior third ventricle and the glomus of the choroid.

The most common site for choroid calcification is the posterior third ventricle. This midline reverse C–shaped calcification lies approximately 3 to 6 mm anterior to the pineal gland. It is present on lateral skull films in 50% of patients. It may be present in the absence of pineal calcification. This calcification has been referred to as the habenula, although at least one author[3] believes that the tela choroidea of the third ventricle and not the more posteriorly located habenular commissure is calcified (Figs. 1–9 and 1–10).

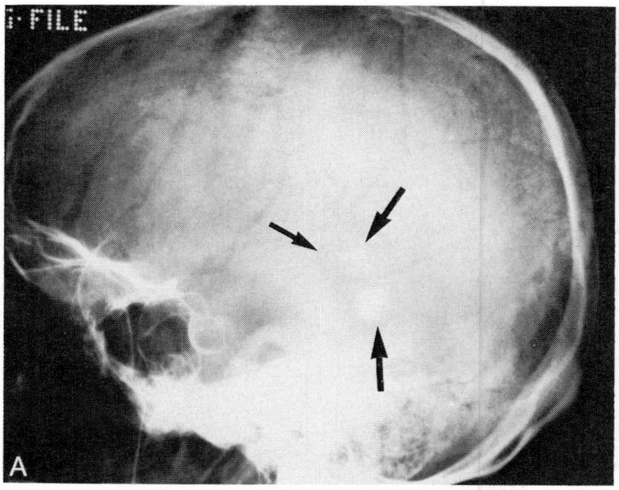

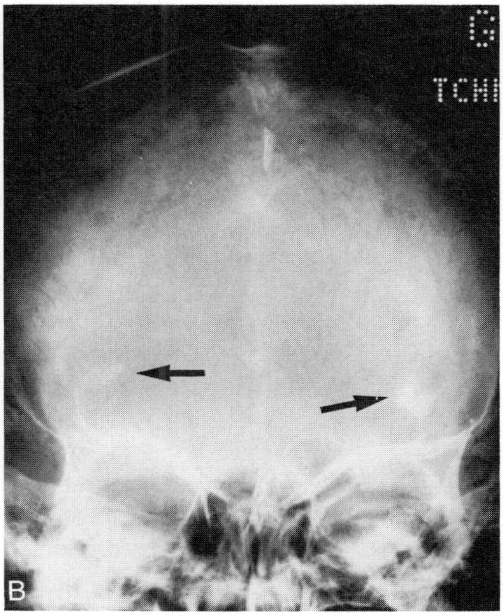

Figure 1–10. Choroid calcification (63-year-old female).

A, Lateral film. Homogeneous densities represent the glomus of the choroid *(large arrows)*. "Habenular" calcification is noted anteriorly *(small arrow)*.

B, Frontal film. There is marked asymmetry of the glomus calcification *(arrows)*.

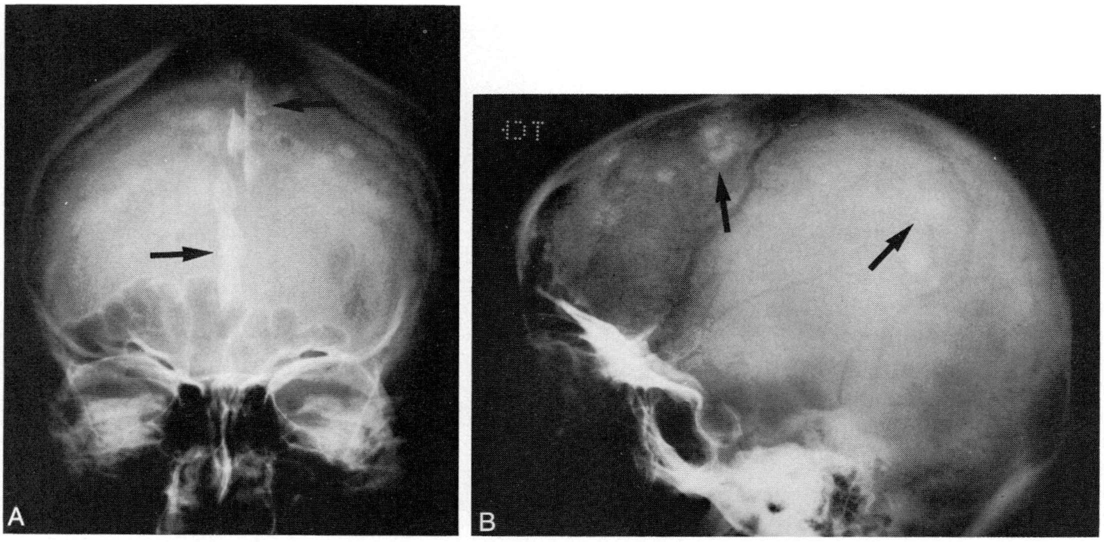

Figure 1–11. Dural calcification (61-year-old male).
A, Frontal film. Midline homogeneous calcifications *(arrows)* are present along the falx.
B, Lateral film. Note the oblong appearance of these densities *(arrows)*.

The second most common site for choroid calcification is the glomus. The glomus is a vascular fleshy enlargement of the choroid, located in the atrium of the lateral ventricles. The incidence of calcification increases with age and is present in approximately 10 to 20% of adults. The glomus usually lies 25 to 30 mm from the midline.[4] The calcification rarely exceeds 10 mm in greatest linear dimension. It has a variable appearance and may be asymmetric. The glomus may calcify around the periphery or appear as finely stippled calcification or a more coarse, "popcorn" nodular calcification (Fig. 1–10).

Dura. Any of the multiple dural surfaces may calcify. These calcifications are usually sharply marginated, are of uniform density, and may be single or multiple. The calcifications are usually flat, paralleling the dural surface. En face projections depict oblong, sharply marginated calcifications. The most common dural surfaces to calcify are the petroclinoid ligaments, falx cerebri, and tentorium (Fig. 1–11).

Arachnoid Granulations. The arachnoid or pacchionian granulations are located in a parasagittal position, are responsible for the transfer of cerebrospinal fluid (CSF) to the venous system, and infrequently calcify. These calcifications are usually multiple, 3 to 4 mm in greatest linear dimension, and of relatively homogeneous density (Fig. 1–12).

Basal Ganglia. The basal ganglia may calcify secondary to systemic disease or idiopathically. The lentiform nuclei are involved most commonly, and to a variable though symmetric degree. If the calcification is sufficiently dense to be identified on plain films, the nuclei usually appear punctate or thick and floccular.

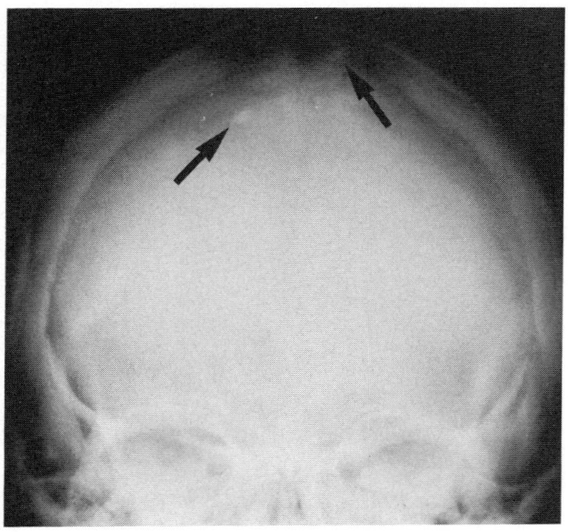

Figure 1–12. Arachnoid calcification (32-year-old female). Frontal film; small homogeneous densities *(arrows)* are located adjacent to the superior sagittal sinus.

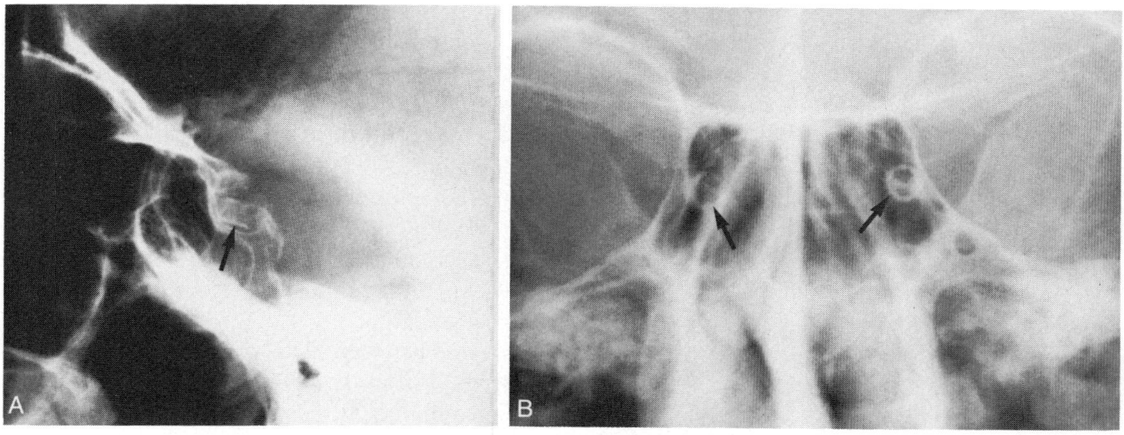

Figure 1–13. Carotid artery calcification (76-year-old female).
A, Lateral film. Linear, sigmoid-shaped calcifications *(arrow)* project over the sella.
B, Frontal film. Arcuate calcifications *(arrows)* are detected in a parasellar location.

Carotid Arteries. Atherosclerotic calcification of the wall of the cavernous internal carotid artery occurs frequently. On lateral films, parallel transverse linear densities project over the sella and cavernous sinus. On frontal films, parasellar rings project over the ethmoid air cells (Fig. 1–13).

Pathologic

Tuberous Sclerosis. This phacomatosis is described in more detail in Chapter 13. The plain film findings consist of multiple, irregularly shaped calcifications in the subependymal region. Basal ganglia and subcortical deposits may also occur. The calcifications are usually of bone density and less than 15 mm in greatest linear dimension. The calcifications have been reported to occur more frequently in affected patients with normal intellect.[5] Additionally, patchy areas of sclerosis have been reported in the frontal and parietal bones in these patients. These sclerotic regions may range from a few millimeters to a few centimeters in size.[6] The calcifications may not be manifest until after 2 years of age[2] (Fig. 1–14).

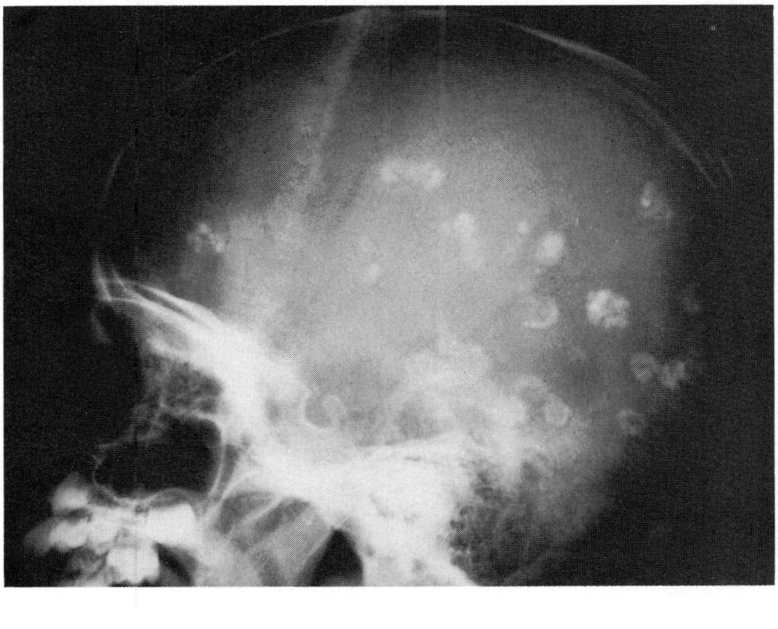

Figure 1–14. Tuberous sclerosis (9-year-old male). Lateral film; multiple irregular calcific densities overlie the course of the ventricular system and subcortical white matter.

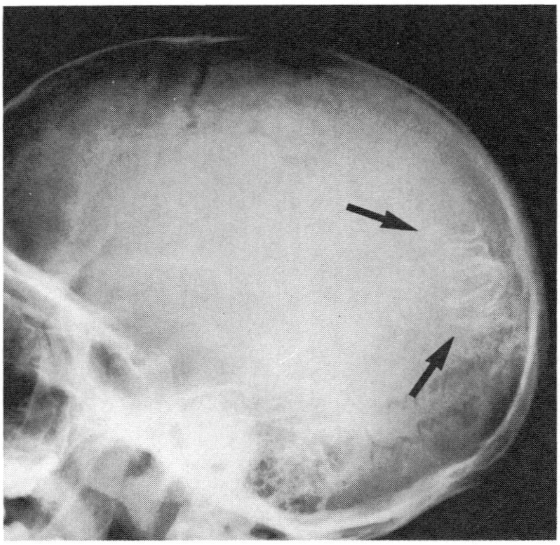

Figure 1–15. Sturge-Weber-Dimitri syndrome (14-year-old male). Lateral film; tram-track serpentine calcifications *(arrows)* are present in the occipital cortex.

Sturge-Weber-Dimitri Syndrome (Encephalotrigeminal Angiomatosis). This phacomatosis is described in more detail in Chapter 13. These patients present with a dermal nevus in the distribution of the trigeminal nerve. Patients may manifest variable degrees of mental retardation and may have seizures, hemiplegia, and/or glaucoma. Pathologically, venous angiomas of the leptomeninges exist. As a result, subjacent parenchymal degeneration and gliosis occur. Concentric layers of gray matter calcification are present. The calcifications on plain films are parallel, linear, and serpentine in appearance[2] (Fig. 1–15).

Cytomegalic Inclusion Disease. This in utero infection, caused by cytomegalovirus (CMV), is described in more detail in Chapter 8. Multiple calcifications may occur anywhere within the brain parenchyma. They may be nodular or curvilinear with a predisposition for the periventricular parenchyma. These calcifications are indistinguishable from those of toxoplasmosis.

Toxoplasmosis. This in utero infection is described in more detail in Chapter 8. A type of encephalitis, it results in widespread brain necrosis, with resultant dysmorphic calcification deposited throughout the parenchyma. Plain films demonstrate multiple nodular or curvilinear deposits of calcium throughout the brain (Fig. 1–16).

Craniopharyngioma. This entity, the most common cause of suprasellar calcification, is described in more detail in Chapter 10. Calcification occurs twice as frequently when the tumor occurs in children (80% of the cases) than when it occurs in adults. The pattern of calcification is variable but most often is curvilinear, occurring along all or a portion of the periphery of the tumor (Fig. 1–17).

Meningioma. Approximately 15% of meningiomas exhibit sufficient calcification to be detected on plain films. The calcification is usually of "cotton-wool" quality, resulting from the psammomatous calcification that occurs within the tumor matrix (Fig. 1–18). Me-

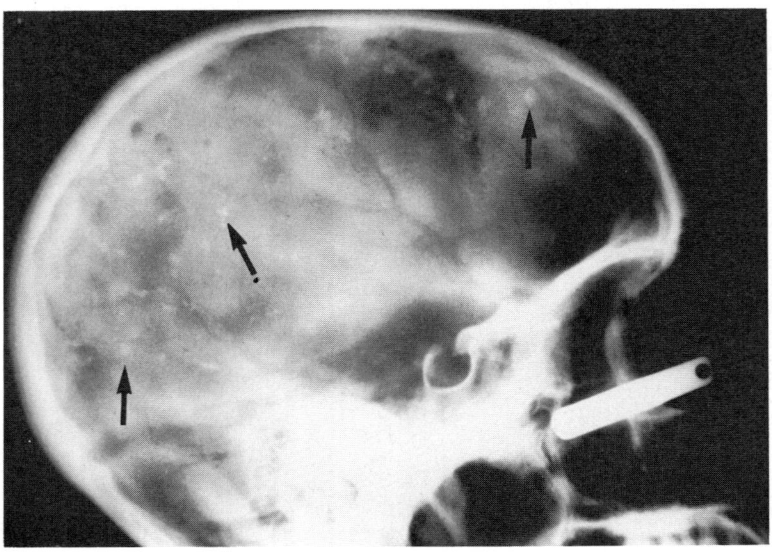

Figure 1–16. Toxoplasmosis (32-year-old female). Lateral film; multiple punctate calcifications *(arrows)* are scattered irregularly throughout the parenchyma.

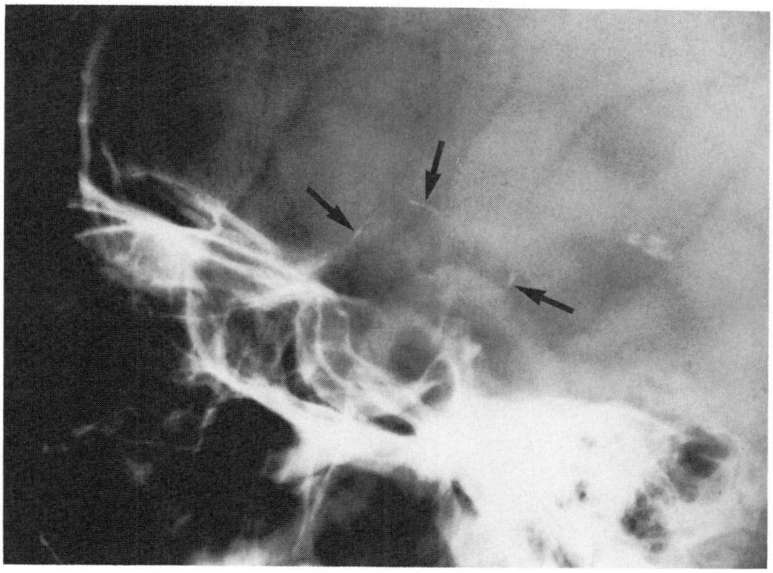

Figure 1–17. Craniopharyngioma (26-year-old female). Lateral film; a peripheral rim of linear calcification *(arrows)* is noted in the suprasellar cistern. Incidentally, the "habenula" and pineal are calcified.

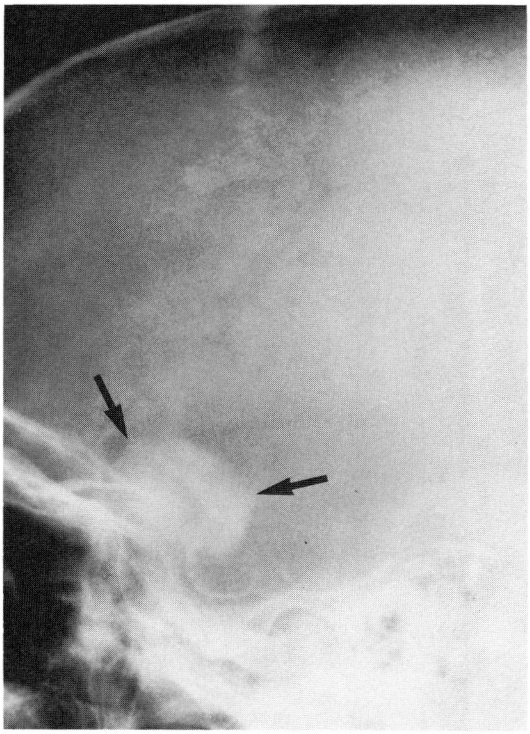

Figure 1–18. Meningioma (63-year-old female). Lateral film; the increased density of this lesion represents psammomatous calcification in this planum meningioma *(arrows)*.

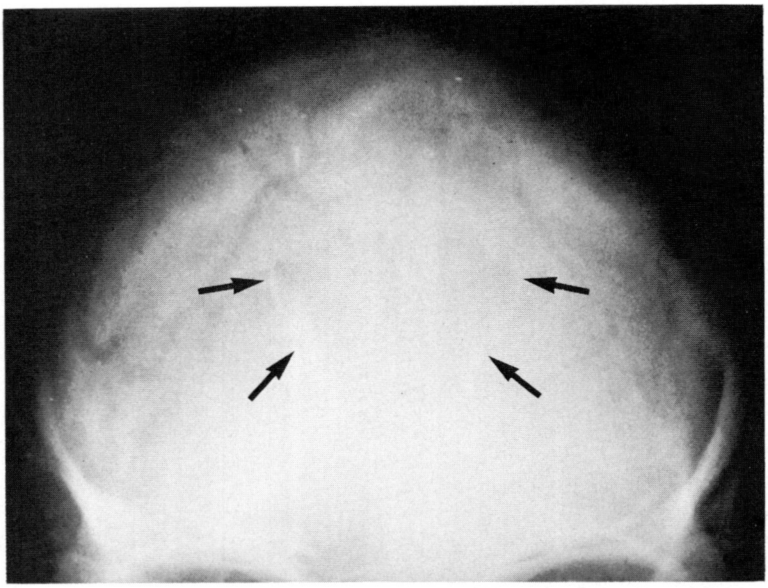

Figure 1–19. Lipoma (3-year-old female). Caldwell view; V-shaped calcification *(arrows)* centered at the midline marks the calcified periphery of this corpus callosum lipoma.

ningiomas are described in more detail in a later section.

Lipoma. Lipomas of the corpus callosum may calcify, usually at the periphery. Typically, a midline symmetric linear V-shaped appearance is detected on frontal films (Fig. 1–19).

Glioma. Although calcification may occur commonly in oligodendrogliomas, ependymomas, and low-grade astrocytomas, only 10 to 15% are visible on plain film examination. The calcification varies with respect to size, shape, and location, and it is usually present as a single cluster of finely stippled to coarsely nodular densities (Fig. 1–20).

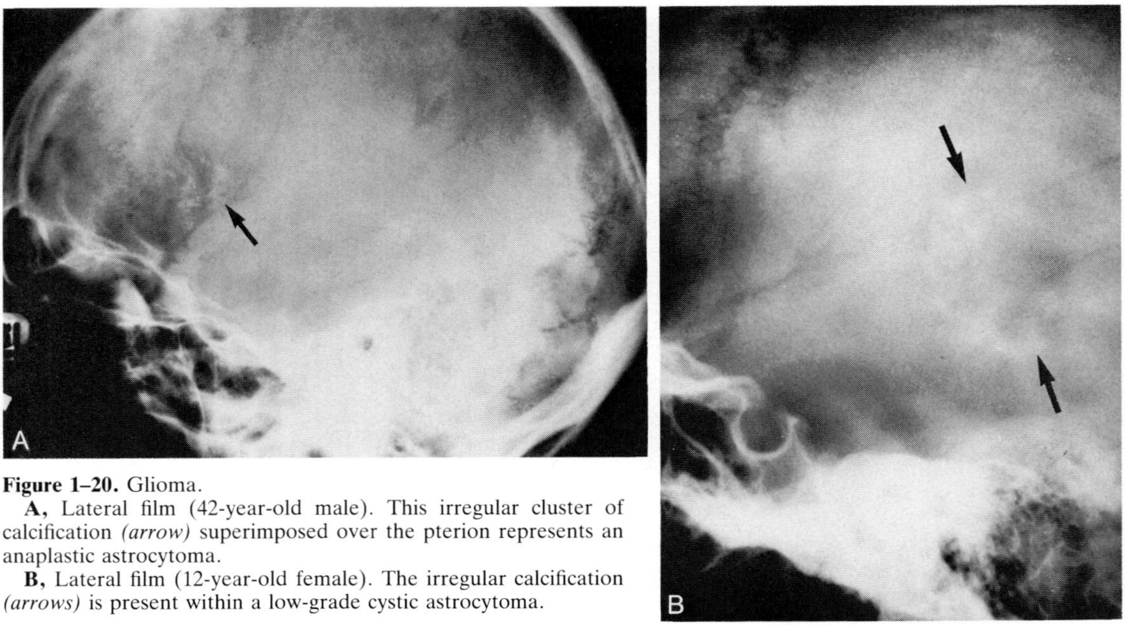

Figure 1–20. Glioma.

A, Lateral film (42-year-old male). This irregular cluster of calcification *(arrow)* superimposed over the pterion represents an anaplastic astrocytoma.

B, Lateral film (12-year-old female). The irregular calcification *(arrows)* is present within a low-grade cystic astrocytoma.

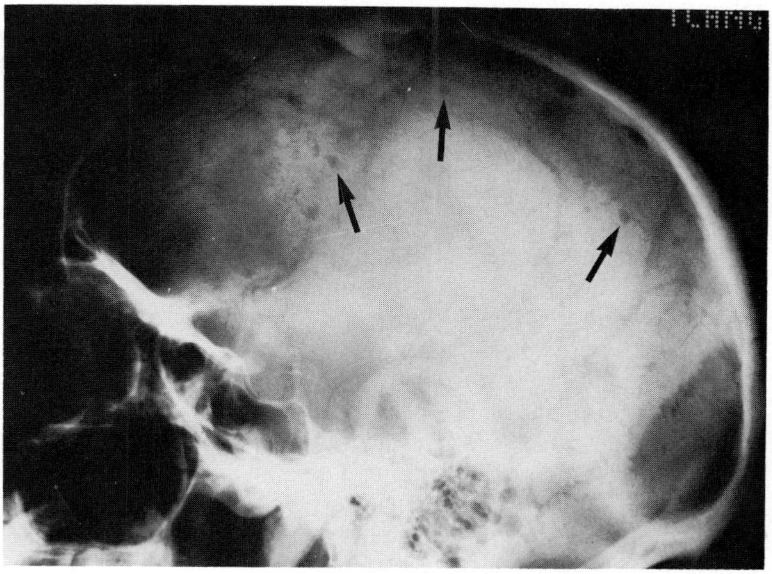

Figure 1–21. Venous lakes (48-year-old female). Lateral film; multiple well-circumscribed lucencies *(arrows)* are identified in a parasagittal location.

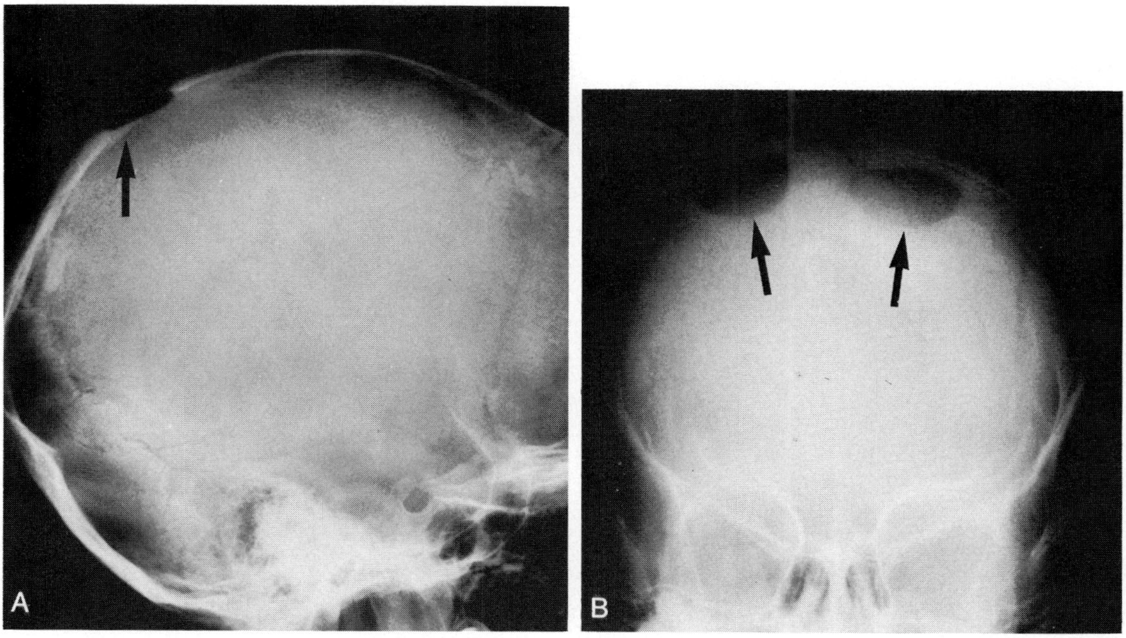

Figure 1–22. Parietal foramen (4-year-old female).

A, Lateral film. A well-circumscribed lucency *(arrow)* projects over the posterosuperior parietal bone.

B, Frontal film. The bilaterality of these well-circumscribed lucencies *(arrows)* and characteristic location confirm the diagnosis.

CONDITIONS AFFECTING BONE DENSITY

Decreased Density

Physiologic

Venous Lakes. These parasagittal shallow inner table depressions are located in the posterior frontal, parietal, and anterior occipital bones. Venous lakes are usually within 3 cm from midline and serve as a communication point between the superior sagittal sinus, cortical veins, and the pacchionian granulations. Often, linear depressions within the inner table representing cortical veins may terminate in these depressions (Fig. 1–21).

Parietal Foramen. These paired symmetric lucencies are located parasagittally in the posterior third of the parietal bone. Generally, these are a few millimeters in size and convey emissary veins; however, they may enlarge up to several centimeters in greatest dimension. Parietal foramina are always smoothly marginated and well circumscribed (Fig. 1–22).

Parietal Thinning. This condition usually involves the upper portion of the parietal bone and is most often bilateral. The outer table and diploë may be thin or absent. The inner table remains intact (Fig. 1–23).

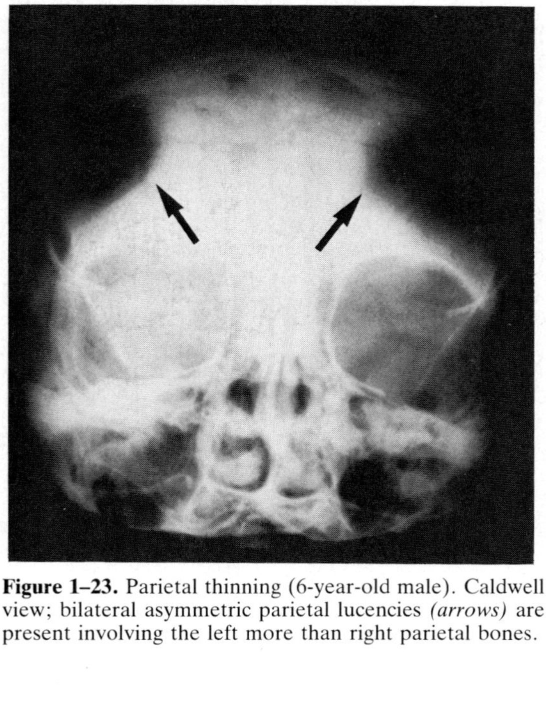

Figure 1–23. Parietal thinning (6-year-old male). Caldwell view; bilateral asymmetric parietal lucencies *(arrows)* are present involving the left more than right parietal bones.

Pathologic

Epidermoid. These benign ectodermal inclusion cysts of the diploë contain desquamated keratinized epithelium and cholesterol. The lesions are round, oval, or, less frequently, slightly lobulated, with sharply defined margins of sclerosis. Epidermoids are most commonly located adjacent to the coronal suture in the frontal or parietal bone or in the squamosal portion of the temporal bone.[7] In 50% of cases, the inner and outer tables are equally involved. The outer table may be involved alone in approximately one third of cases[7] (Fig. 1–24).

Hemangioma. These solitary regions of irregular lucency may be present anywhere within the calvarium. Radiating spicules of bone may be present in a sunburst pattern. The lesions vary in size from a few millimeters to a few centimeters and are relatively well circumscribed with areas of sclerosis. A palpable mass may be detected as the diploë expands (Fig. 1–25).

Eosinophilic Granuloma. This is the most benign form of the histiocytosis X group, which also includes Letterer-Siwe and Hand-Schüller-Christian disease. Proliferation of histiocytes produces bone lesions of similar appearance in this group of diseases. The lesions tend to be less numerous and sizable with eosinophilic granuloma.

The classic lesion is lytic, usually involving the outer table to a greater extent than the inner table, resulting in a beveled appearance. The lesions are usually sharply marginated without evidence of surrounding sclerosis. Mild sclerosis may, however, be detected as the lesion regresses (Fig. 1–26).

Multiple Myeloma. This is the most common primary malignancy of bone. These lesions affect the skull and long bones of adults. Multiple "punched-out," sharply delineated lesions without sclerosis are present. Sclerosis may, however, follow chemotherapy (Fig. 1–27).

Metastasis. Nearly all metastatic skull lesions are osteolytic, even in patients with blastic metastasis to other bones. The lesions are irregular in size and shape and are poorly marginated with uneven destruction of the diploë and inner and outer tables. Metastasis may be single or multiple (Fig. 1–28).

Text continued on page 23

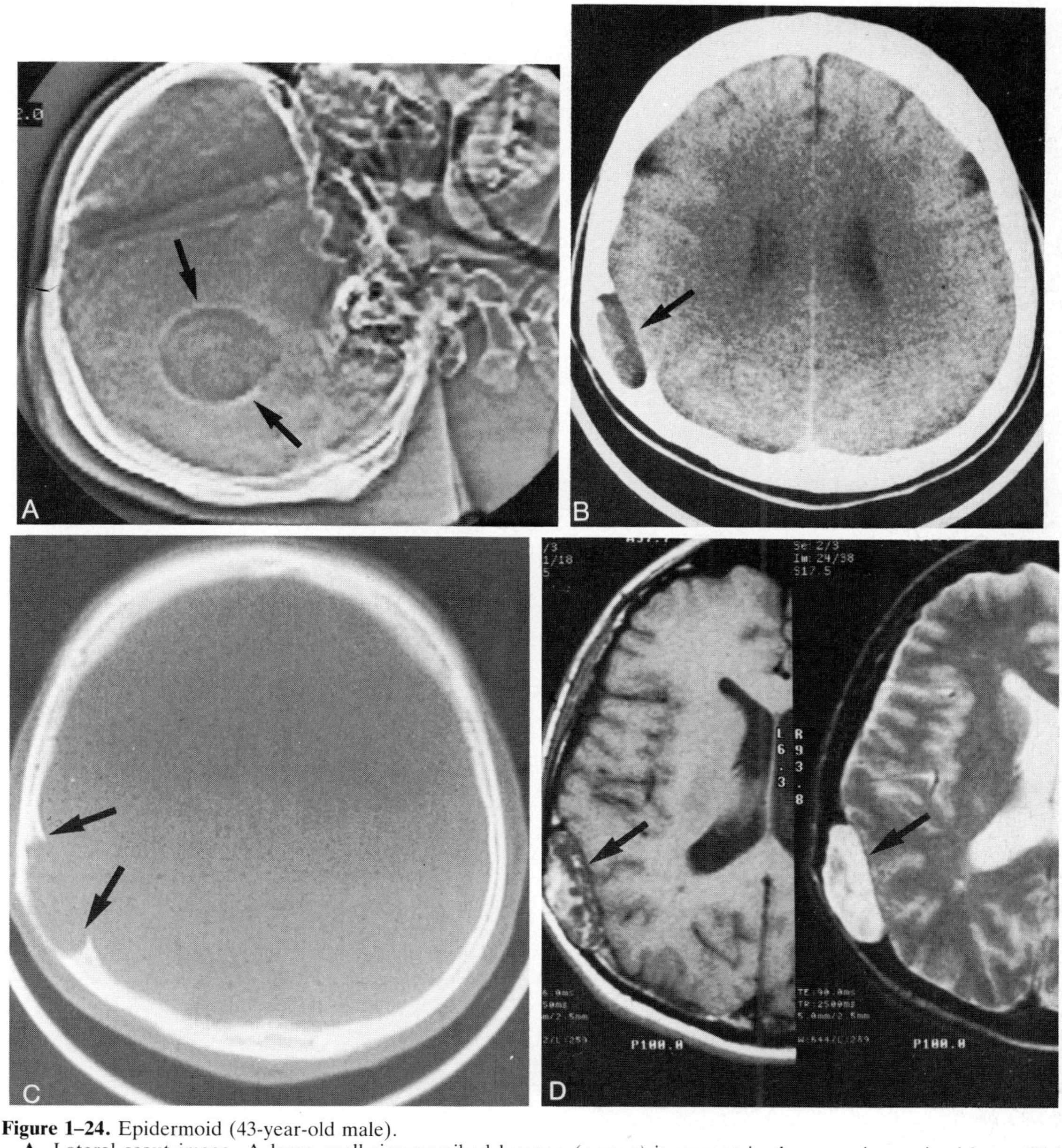

Figure 1–24. Epidermoid (43-year-old male).

A, Lateral scout image. A large, well-circumscribed lucency *(arrows)* is present in the posterior parietal bone. The lucency is surrounded by a thin rim of sclerotic bone.

B, Unenhanced computed tomography (CT). The lesion *(arrow)* is hypodense with respect to the adjacent brain parenchyma.

C, Bone windows. Benign scalloping of the skull *(arrows)* is noted.

D, T1 and T2 magnetic resonance imaging (MRI), respectively. The lesion *(arrows)* is heterogeneous on both spin echo sequences with regions of high-signal and low-signal intensity.

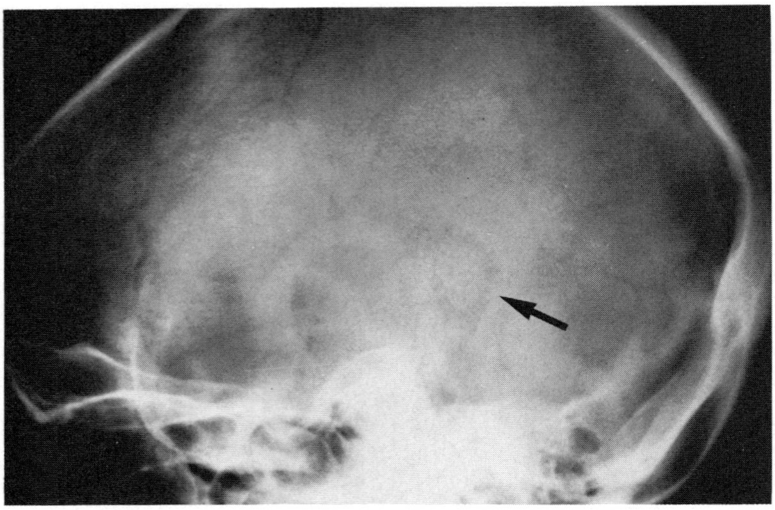

Figure 1–25. Hemangioma (12-year-old female). Lateral film; a solitary, irregular lucency *(arrow)* with radiating spicules of bone is present in the parietal bone.

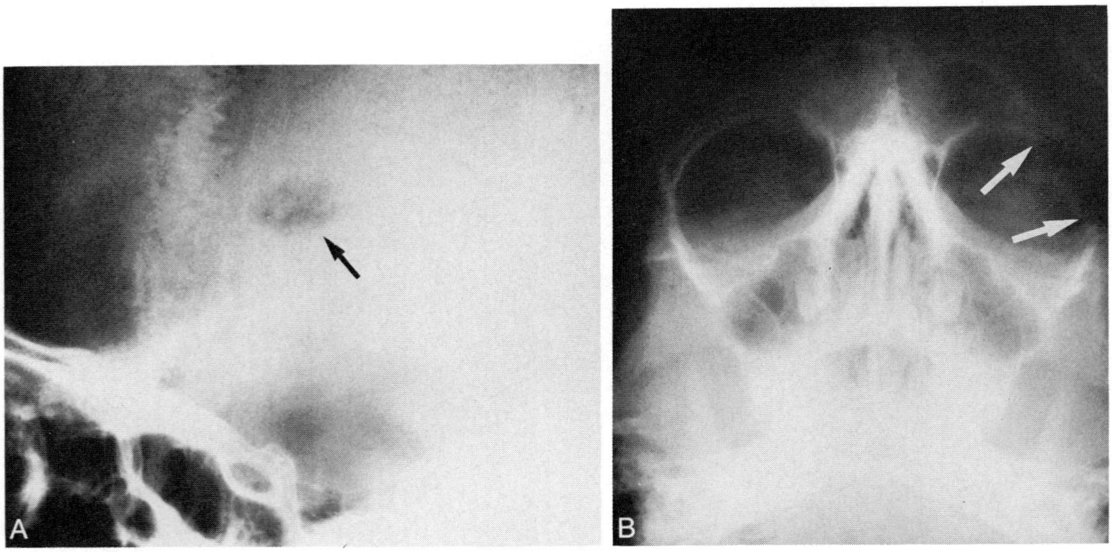

Figure 1–26. Histiocytosis.

A, Lateral film (22-year-old male). A solitary well-circumscribed lucency *(arrow)* is present in the parietal bone. There is no evidence of surrounding sclerosis in this patient with eosinophilic granuloma.

B, Waters view (7-year-old female). Lytic destructive changes of the zygomatic process of the frontal bone and zygoma *(arrows)* are detected in this patient with Hand-Schüller-Christian disease.

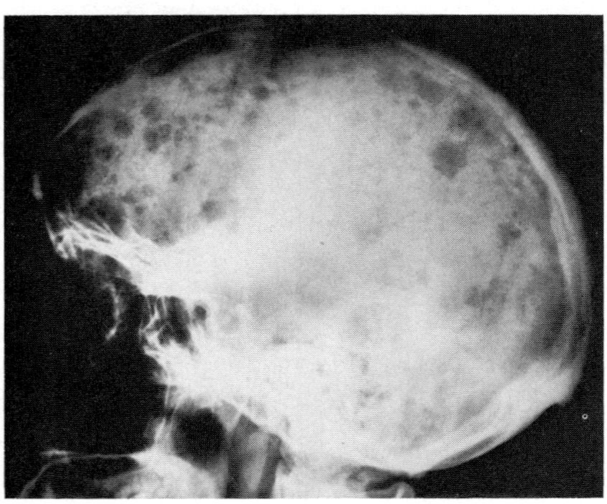

Figure 1–27. Multiple myeloma (55-year-old male). Lateral film; multiple, well-circumscribed "punched-out" lucencies are present involving the entire calvarium.

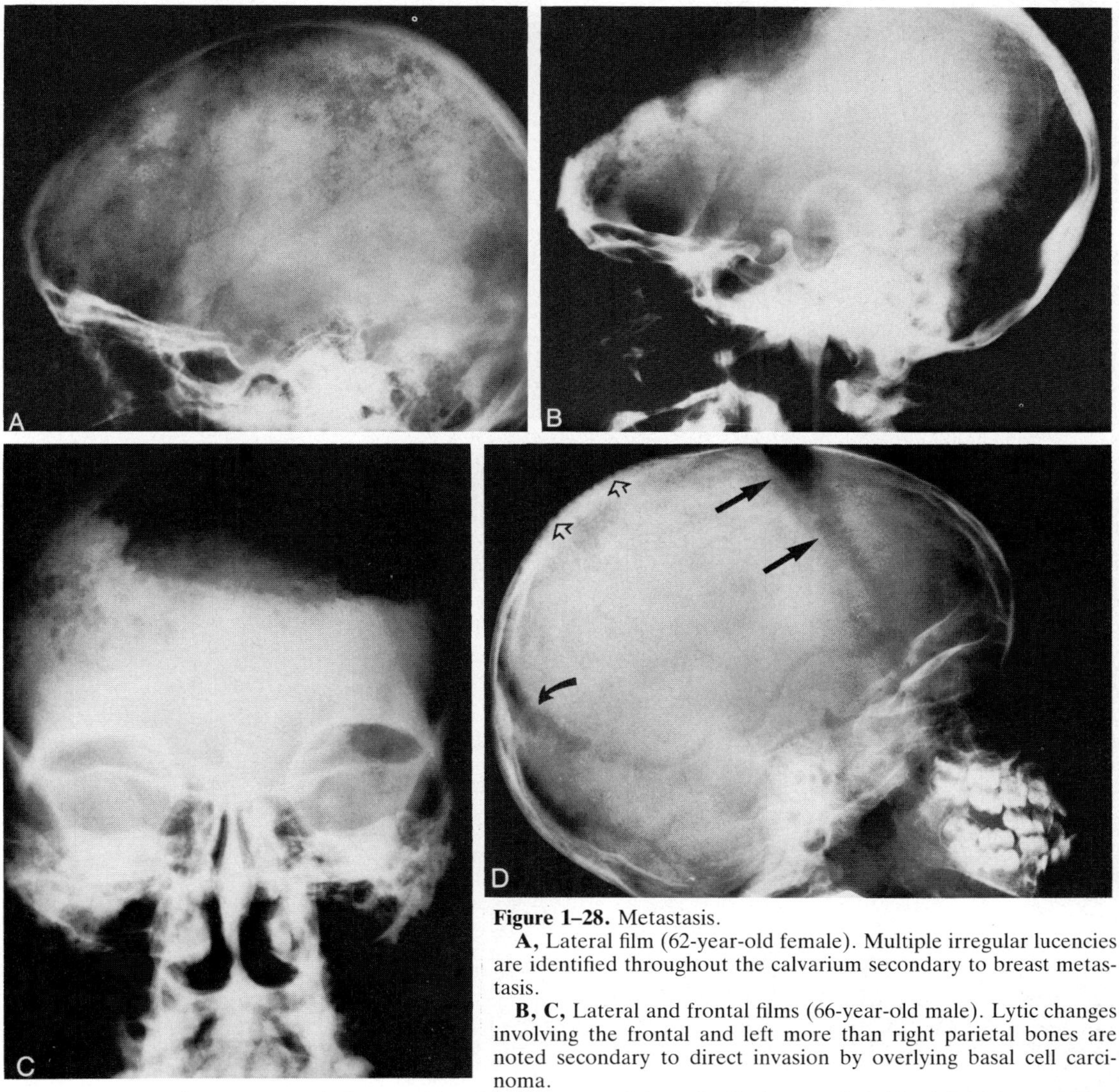

Figure 1–28. Metastasis.

A, Lateral film (62-year-old female). Multiple irregular lucencies are identified throughout the calvarium secondary to breast metastasis.

B, C, Lateral and frontal films (66-year-old male). Lytic changes involving the frontal and left more than right parietal bones are noted secondary to direct invasion by overlying basal cell carcinoma.

D, Lateral film (neuroblastoma) (2-year-old male). The coronal *(straight black arrows)* and lambdoid *(curved black arrow)* sutures are enlarged owing to bone resorption secondary to neuroblastoma. Cortical irregularities *(open black arrows)* also noted in the outer table of the parietal bone.

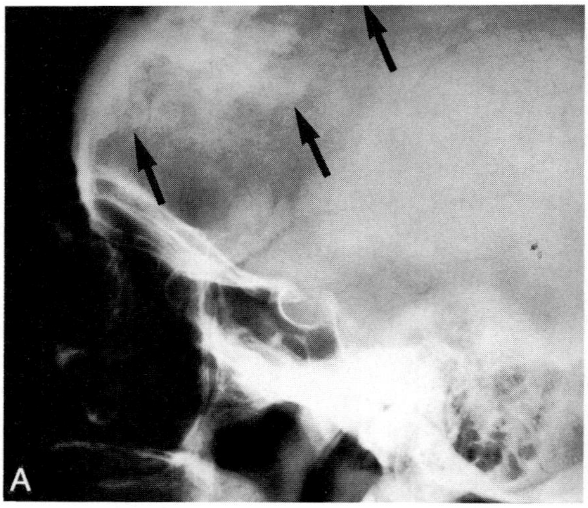

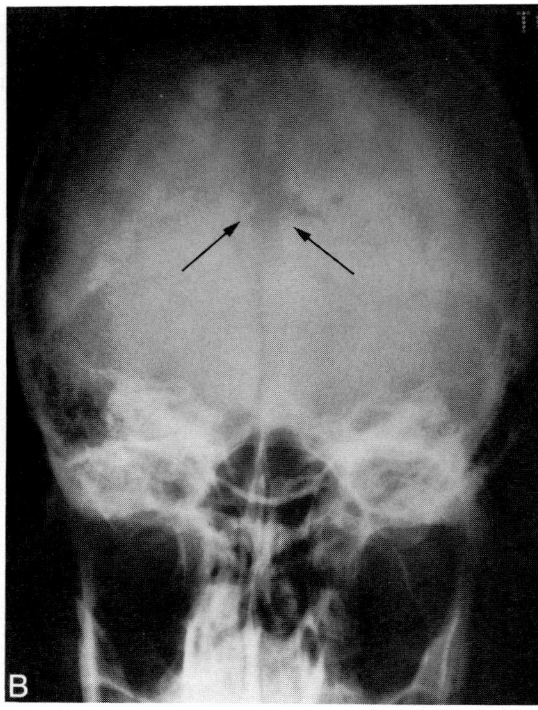

Figure 1–29. Hyperostosis frontalis (52-year-old female).

A, Lateral film. Homogeneous calcifications *(arrows)* extend from the inner table of the frontal bone.

B, Towne film. Sclerotic deposits involve the frontal bones bilaterally *(arrows)*, sparing the midline.

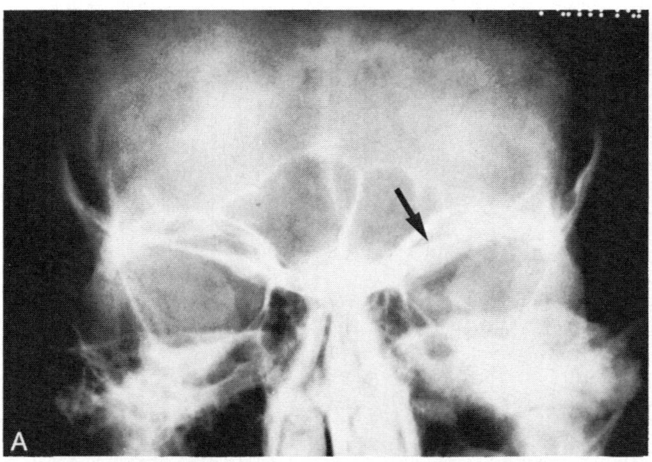

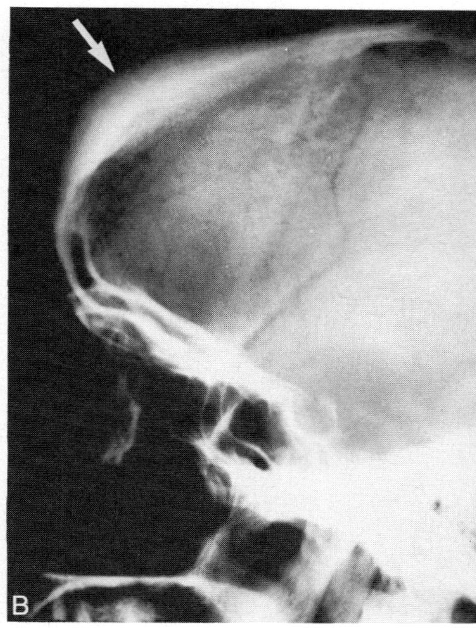

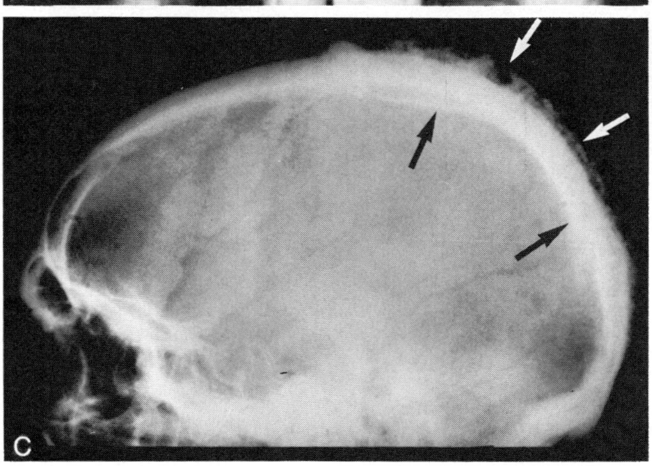

Figure 1–30. Meningioma.

A, Caldwell view (62-year-old female). Hyperostosis of the lesser wing of the sphenoid *(arrow)* is noted secondary to a meningioma of the floor of the anterior fossa.

B, Lateral film (49-year-old female). A midline frontal meningioma induces more hyperostosis of the outer *(arrow)* than of the inner table.

C, Lateral film (67-year-old female). An unusual "hair-on-end" hyperostosis *(white arrows)* is present secondary to an underlying parietal meningioma. Note the focal thickening of the calvarium *(black arrows)*.

Increased Density

Physiologic

Hyperostosis Frontalis Interna. This condition involves the diploë and inner table of the frontal bone with relative sparing of the outer table and midline. This condition occurs most frequently in middle-aged women. Plain films demonstrate a smooth, undulating region of increased density along the inner table of the frontal bone on lateral views. Frontal views demonstrate relative lucency overlying the expected position of the metopic suture (Fig. 1–29).

Pathologic

Meningioma. In addition to the tumor matrix calcification that may be detected on plain film examinations, meningiomas also induce secondary changes that may alter the appearance of the adjacent bone. Hyperostosis refers to the reactive bony changes of the inner table and diploë that frequently accompany meningiomas. As the bone gets thicker, it also becomes denser and the diploë less distinct. Bony destructive changes have also been noted, although much less frequently.

These dural base lesions receive arterial supply partly or totally from the external circulation. As a result, the vascular impressions along the inner table may become enlarged as the arteries hypertrophy to supply the tumor (Fig. 1–30).

Fibrous Dysplasia. Although this condition may be lytic, sclerotic, or mixed, most lesions that occur in the skull are sclerotic. The outer table is involved, with minimal changes occurring in the inner table. The sclerotic lesions take on a "ground-glass" appearance as the diploic space thickens. The lesions are irregularly shaped and may extend into and obliterate the paranasal sinuses or foramen of the skull base (Fig. 1–31).

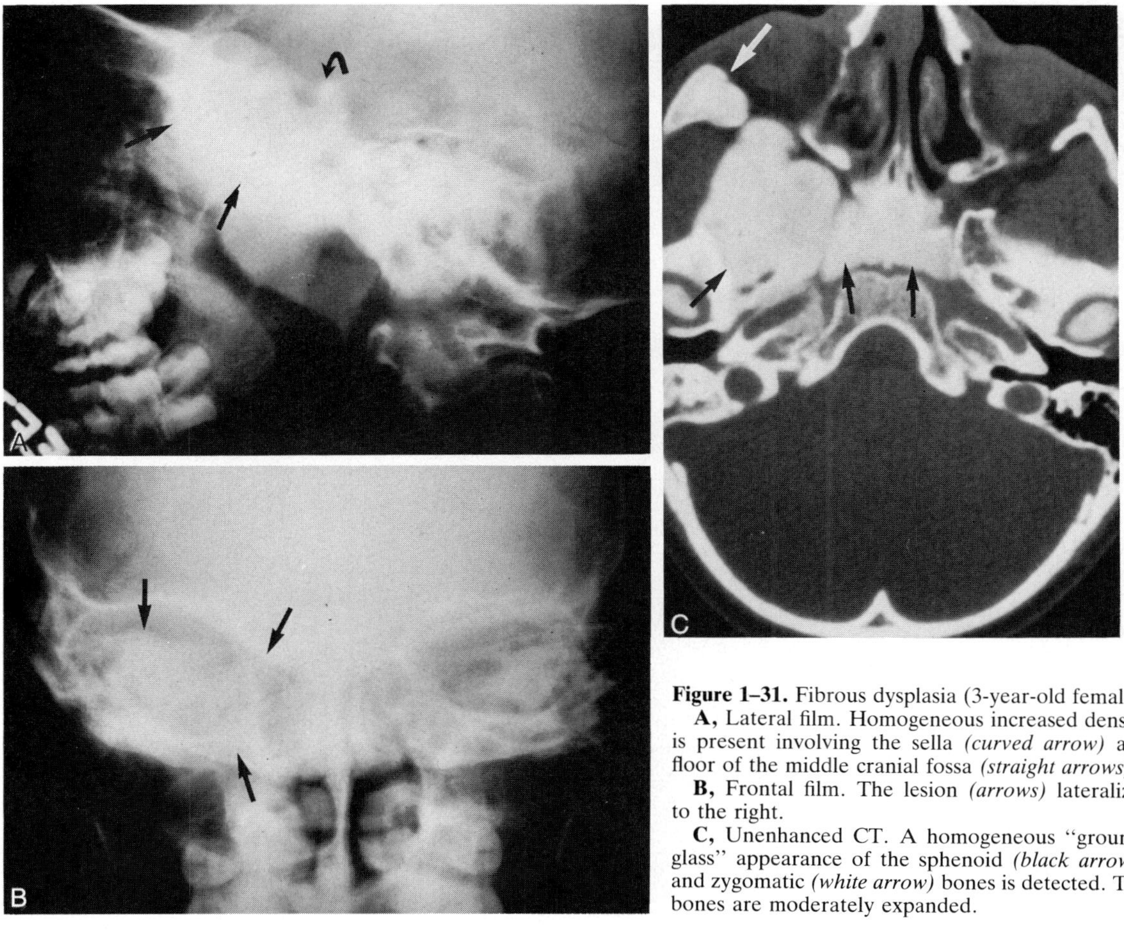

Figure 1–31. Fibrous dysplasia (3-year-old female).

A, Lateral film. Homogeneous increased density is present involving the sella *(curved arrow)* and floor of the middle cranial fossa *(straight arrows)*.

B, Frontal film. The lesion *(arrows)* lateralizes to the right.

C, Unenhanced CT. A homogeneous "ground-glass" appearance of the sphenoid *(black arrows)* and zygomatic *(white arrow)* bones is detected. The bones are moderately expanded.

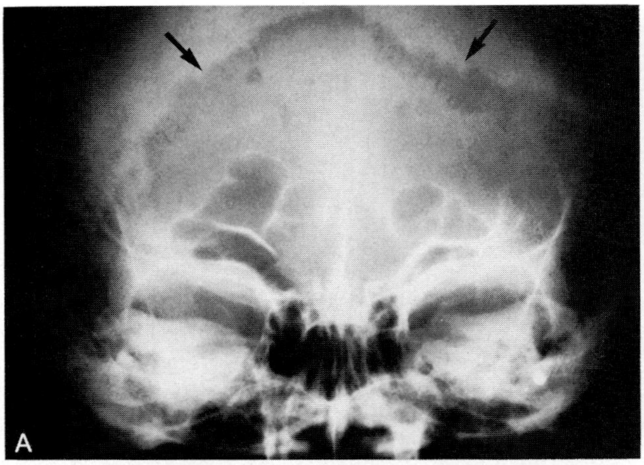

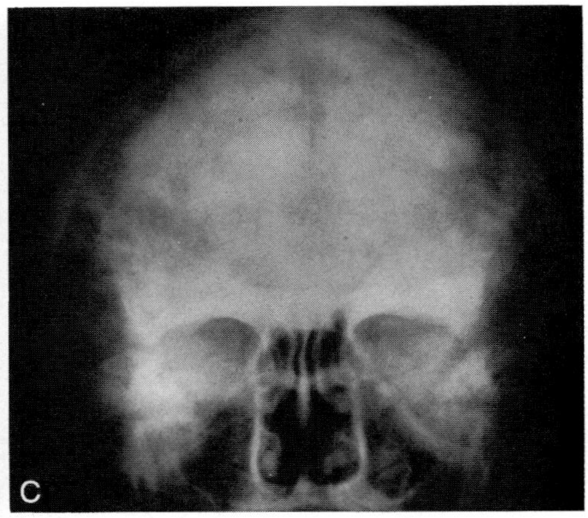

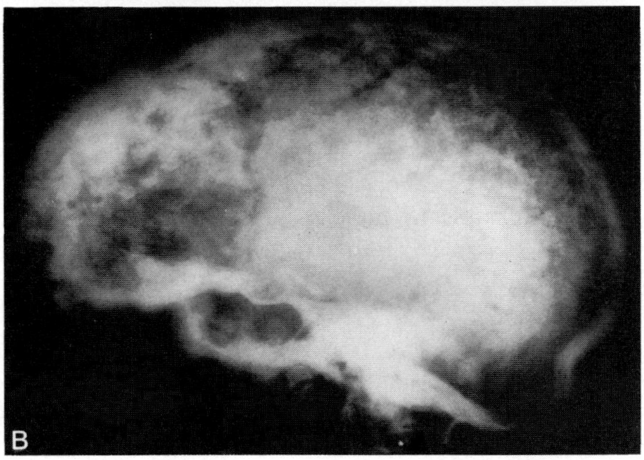

Figure 1–32. Paget's disease.

A, Frontal film (65-year-old male) (osteoporosis circumscripta). A geographic lucency *(arrows)* is noted involving a majority of the frontal bone.

B, C, Lateral and frontal films (81-year-old female) (sclerotic phase). There is marked thickening of the diploë and outer table. Platybasia is noted on the lateral film.

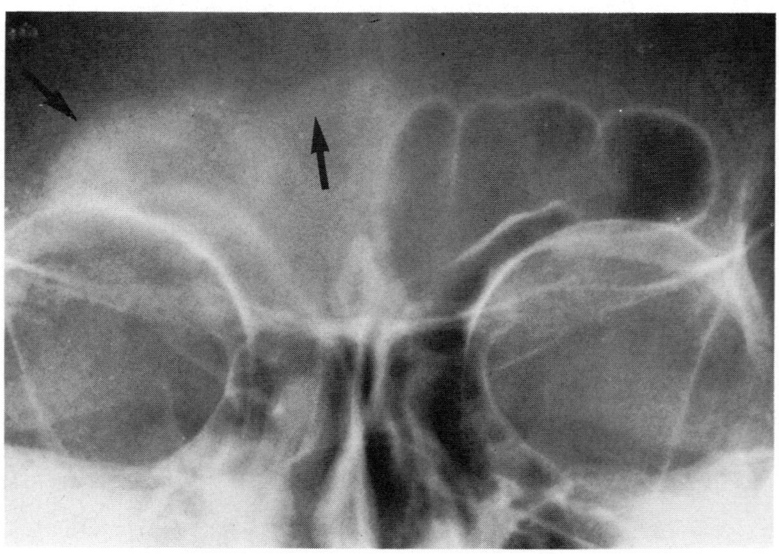

Figure 1–33. Osteomyelitis (48-year-old male). Caldwell view; there is diffuse bony sclerosis surrounding the right frontal sinuses *(arrows)* secondary to chronic osteomyelitis.

Mixed Density

Paget's Disease (Osteitis Deformans). This biphasic disorder may involve the adult skull. Initially, the osteolytic phase (osteoporosis circumscripta) begins in the frontal or occipital bones and extends toward the vertex. The outer table is involved, with relative sparing of the inner table.[8] A large, relatively well-marginated lesion of diminished density may be identified. The lytic phase of the disease is followed by a phase of recalcification that ultimately results in marked thickening and sclerosis of the diploë and outer table. As the bone of the skull thickens, the foramen at the skull base becomes progressively narrowed, compressing the exiting vessels and nerves. The skull softens, resulting in basilar invagination and possible compression of the cervical medullary junction (Fig. 1–32).

Osteomyelitis. Osteomyelitis may result from blood-borne transmission of a systemic infection or from direct inoculation during trauma. The bone may become infected as a result of direct spread from paranasal sinus or mastoid air cell infection. Initially, there may be resorption of the bone, periosteal reaction, and a prominent soft tissue mass. Once a significant amount of bone has been resorbed, an irregular lytic lesion may be detected. This lesion is usually poorly marginated. Sequestered islands of bone may be identified within the area of lucency.

Osteomyelitis may also induce sclerotic lesions. Sclerotic lesions may occur with chronic infection by low-virulence organisms or following treatment of an acute osteomyelitis. The regions of increased density are relatively poorly marginated (Fig. 1–33).

FRACTURES

Linear Fractures. These fractures are more common in the cranial vault. The fracture usually involves both the inner and outer tables, rendering the fracture line more lucent than the vascular impressions of the inner table. The fracture margins are usually well defined, lack sclerosis, and may traverse sutures and vascular impressions. The edges of the fracture may be separated or diastatic, rendering the fracture more apparent. In addition to a single linear lucency, the fracture may be comminuted (Fig. 1–34).

There is poor correlation between linear fractures and the underlying CNS sequelae. Frequently, the CNS is normal in the face of multiple skull fractures. Alternatively, life-threatening CNS injury may be sustained without evidence of skull fracture.

Depressed Fractures. In addition to diastasis of the calvarium, the fracture fragment(s) may be depressed for a variable distance. This may result in injury of the brain, its coverings, or the overlying vessels. Films obtained en face may show an irregular region of lucency with

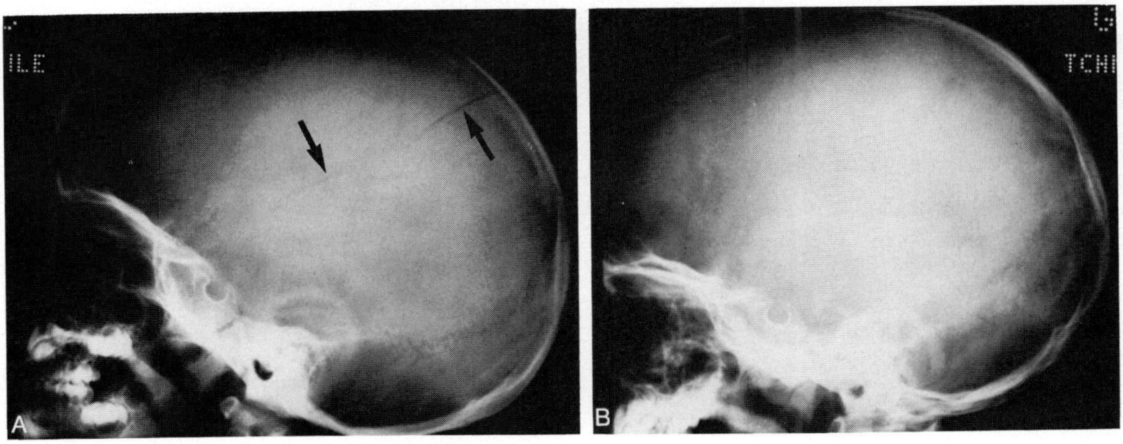

Figure 1–34. Linear fracture (3-year-old female).
A, Lateral film. A linear fracture *(arrows)* extends through the left parietal bone.
B, Lateral film. One year later, radiograph demonstrates no residual abnormality in this 4-year-old female.

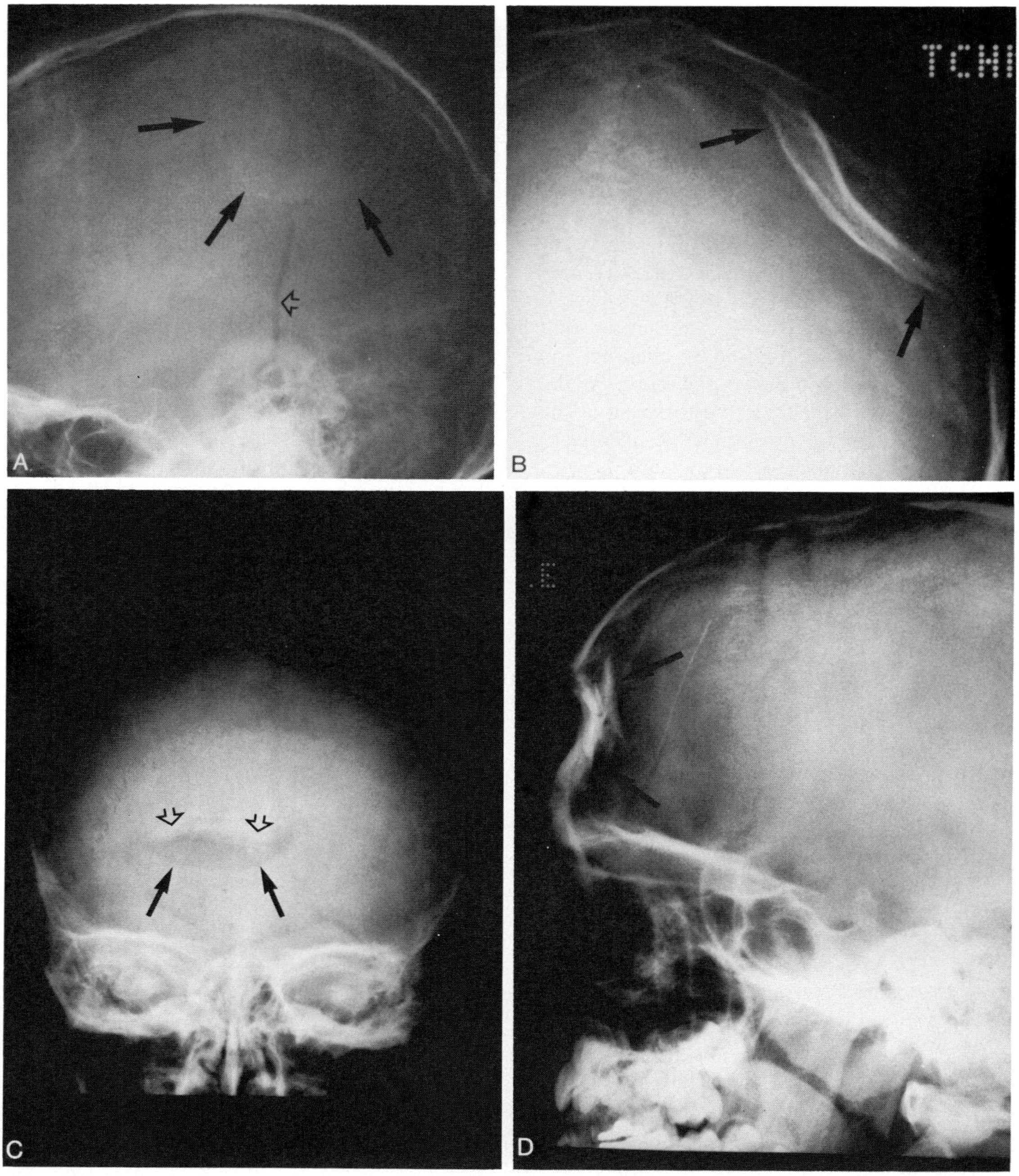

Figure 1–35. Depressed skull fractures.

A, Lateral film (18-year-old male). A linear lucency *(open arrow)* extends cephalad from the temporal bone ending in an irregular region of increased density *(arrows).*

B, Frontal film. A depressed skull fragment *(arrows)* is demonstrated on this orthogonal view.

C, Frontal film (17-year-old female). A well-circumscribed lucency *(black arrows)* is located just inferior to a poorly defined region of increased density *(open black arrows).*

D, Lateral film (8-year-old female). Fragments of a comminuted depressed skull fracture *(black arrows)* are noted, involving the frontal bone.

an adjacent region of density. These represent the diastasis and overlapping of the fragment with the host bone, respectively. Tangential views demonstrate the displaced fragment as well as the degree of displacement referrable to the host bone (Fig. 1–35).

Leptomeningeal Cyst. In general, linear fractures heal, often without evidence of prior injury. The healing process is much more accelerated in children than in adults. Rarely, in children, the meninges may herniate into a fracture cleft, transmitting CSF pulsation to the fracture margins. This results in pressure erosion of the margin and expansion of the fracture cleft—ergo, the "growing fracture" of childhood (Fig. 1–36).

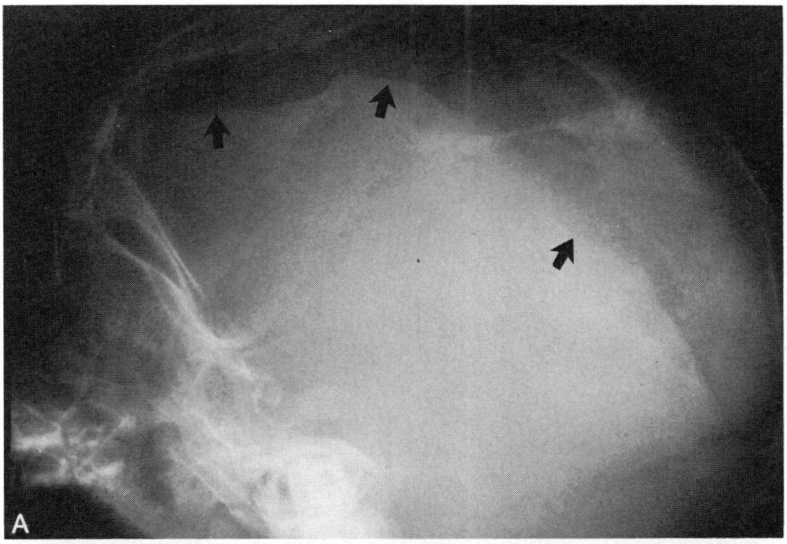

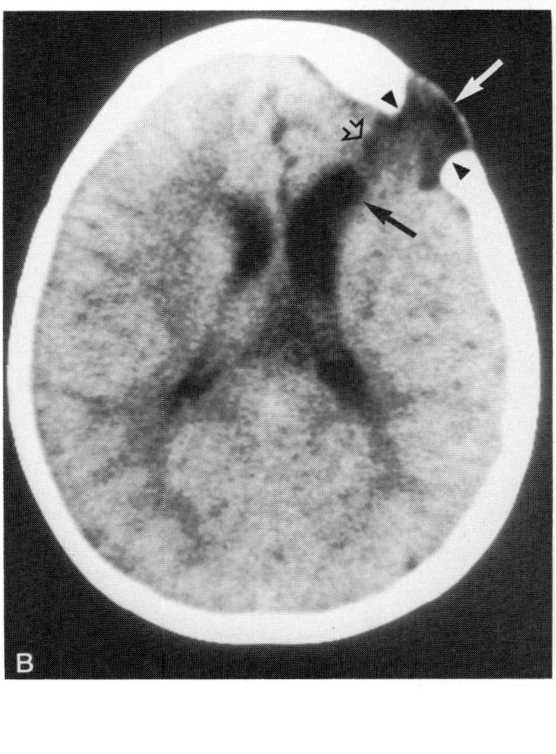

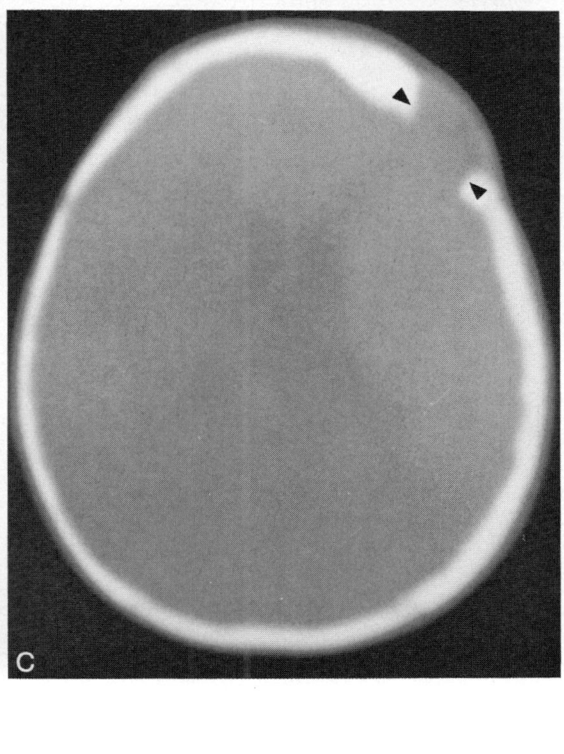

Figure 1–36. Leptomeningeal cyst (18-month-old male).

A, Lateral film. A well-circumscribed, benign-appearing lucency *(arrows)* is present involving the frontal and parietal bones.

B, Unenhanced CT. A hypodense cyst *(white arrow)* extends through the left frontal calvarial defect *(arrowheads)*. Encephalomalacic changes *(open arrow)* in the underlying parenchyma with commensurate enlargement of the frontal horn *(black arrow)* indicate parenchymal damage sustained at the time of the initial trauma 1 year earlier.

C, Bone windows. The margins of the calvarial defect *(arrowheads)* are smooth from chronic pressure erosion.

MISCELLANEOUS CONDITIONS AFFECTING THE SKULL

Increased Intracranial Pressure. The cranial vault responds predictably to increased pressure. The pressure may be the result of an intracranial mass or increased intracranial CSF (hydrocephalus). In young children, the response is sutural diastasis. The unfused sutures, the "weak link" in the cranial vault, will become diastatic in an attempt to accommodate the increased calvarial volume. In general, the suture should be less than 3 mm wide in a 2-year-old and less than 2 mm wide in a 3-year-old. Clinically, the anterior or posterior fontanelle, or both, may bulge as the patient develops megalencephaly (Fig. 1–37).

Once the sutures have fused (late teens), the changes of increased intracranial pressure are manifested about the sella turcica. Owing to either extension of the third ventricle into the sella or CSF pulsations through the diaphragma sellae, the increased CSF pressure is transmitted to the sella turcica. The cortex of the anterior wall of the dorsum is thinner than that of the floor of the sella. Increased intracranial pressure induces erosion of this cortex, producing a radiographically detectable indistinctness of the cortex. This is first manifested in the thinner anterior wall of the dorsum and later in the floor of the sella. Chronic increased intracranial pressure will continue to expand the sella at the expense of the dorsum and posterior clinoids (Fig. 1–38).

Prominent convolutional markings along the inner table of the calvarium may also be seen in increased intracranial pressure. Unfortunately, this may also occur to a lesser degree in normal patients and provides only suggestive evidence of increased intracranial pressure.

Craniosynostosis. This refers to premature fusion of one or more cranial sutures. As a result, growth ceases in the direction perpendicular to the long axis of the suture. Growth along the short axis of the suture continues, resulting in characteristic skull deformities. The bone adjacent to the fused suture becomes thickened, often resulting in a band of increased density parallel to the suture.

Sagittal Synostosis. The head elongates in an AP direction, resulting in dolichocephaly (Fig. 1–39).

Metopic Synostosis. This premature fusion of the suture separating the ossification centers of the frontal bone results in trigonocephaly.

Coronal Synostosis. Unilateral premature fusion of the coronal suture is the most common craniosynostosis and results in elongation

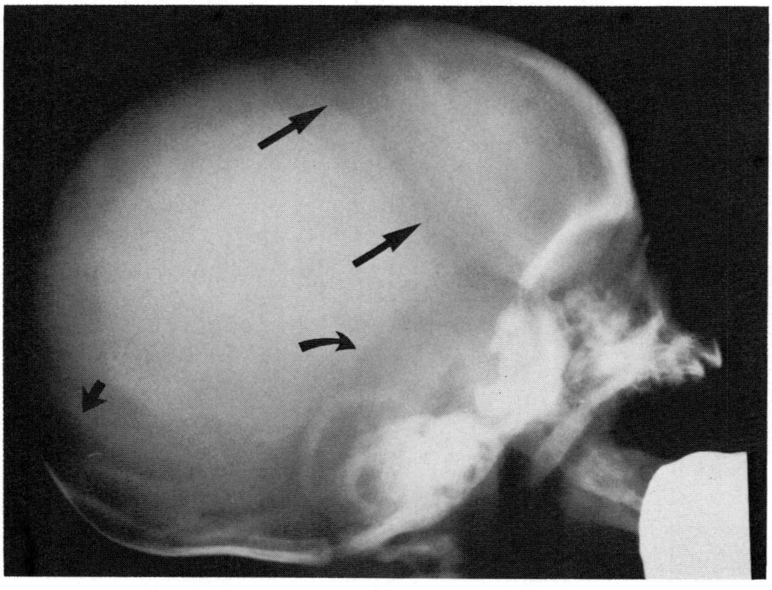

Figure 1–37. Increased intracranial pressure (3-month-old female). Lateral film; marked diastasis of the coronal *(long arrows)*, squamosal *(curved arrow)*, and lambdoid *(short arrow)* sutures is noted in this infant with congenital aqueductal stenosis.

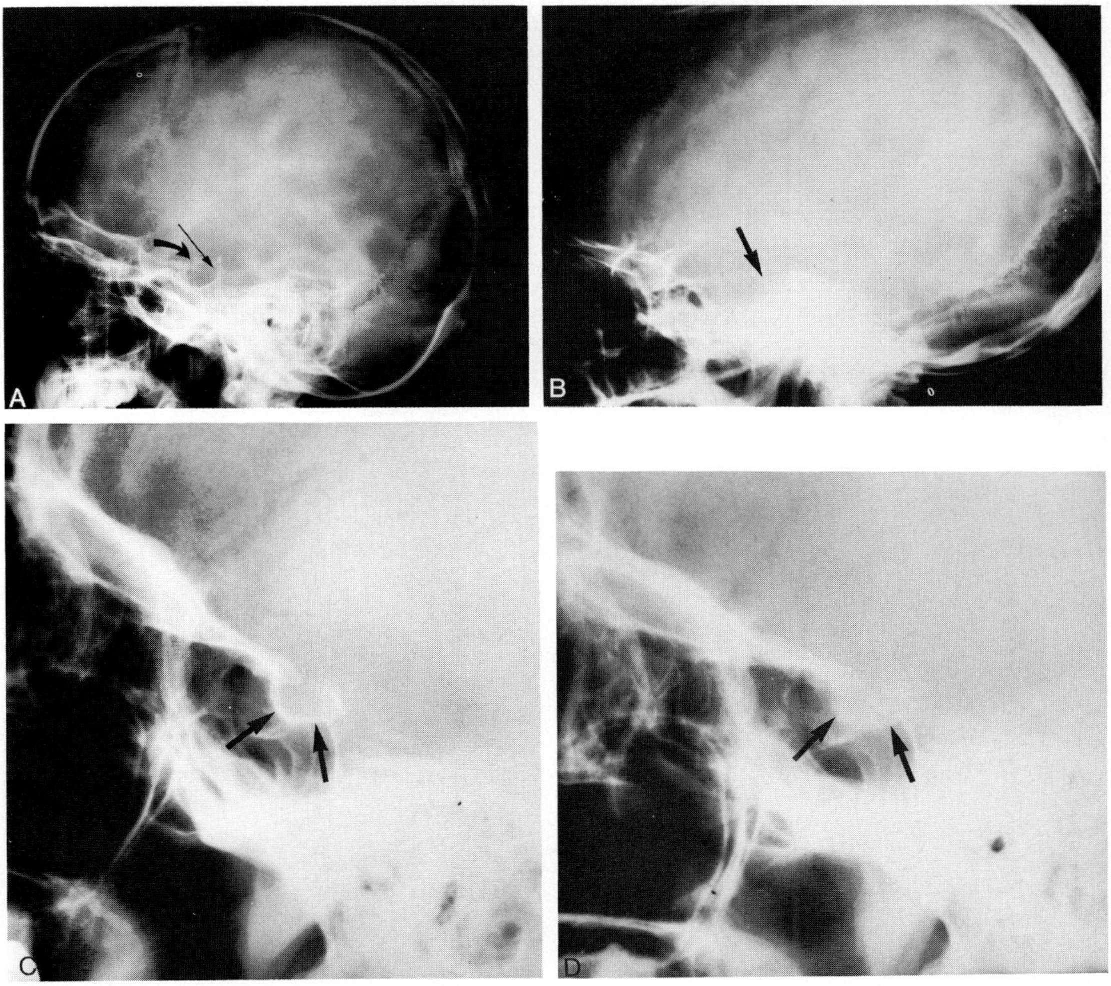

Figure 1–38. Increased intracranial pressure.

A, Lateral film (22-year-old male). Subtle loss of the cortex of the anterior dorsum sella *(arrow)* is noted reflecting the earliest changes of hydrocephalus. Incidental note is made of a sellar-suprasellar calcification *(curved arrow)* representing a craniopharyngioma.

B, Lateral film (27-year-old male). There is complete erosion of the dorsum sellae *(arrow)* secondary to chronic increased intracranial pressure in a patient with aqueductal stenosis.

C, Lateral film (38-year-old female). Normal-appearing sellar floor *(black arrows)* immediately after a subarachnoid hemorrhage.

D, Lateral film (18 months later). The floor of the sella *(arrows)* has become indistinct secondary to posthemorrhage communicating hydrocephalus.

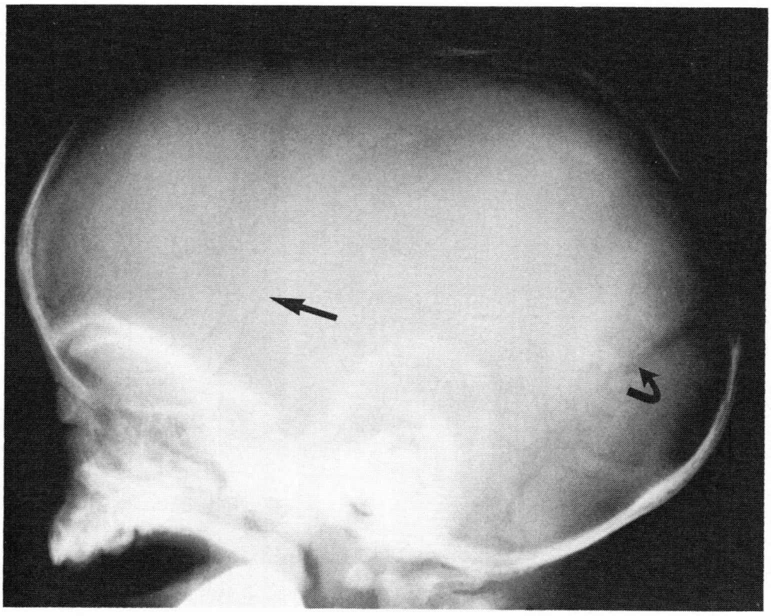

Figure 1–39. Sagittal suture synostosis (3-month-old female). Lateral film; note the marked dolichocephaly. Coronal *(straight arrow)* and lambdoid sutures *(curved arrow)* remain patent.

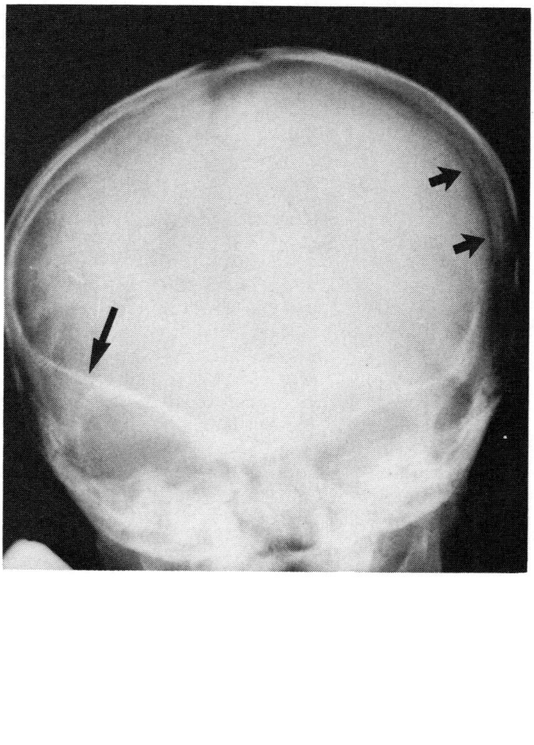

Figure 1–40. Unilateral coronal synostosis (4-month-old female). Caldwell view; the left coronal suture is patent *(short arrows)*. The right coronal suture is fused and inapparent. The orbital roof and greater wing of the sphenoid bone *(arrow)* are elevated (harlequin eye).

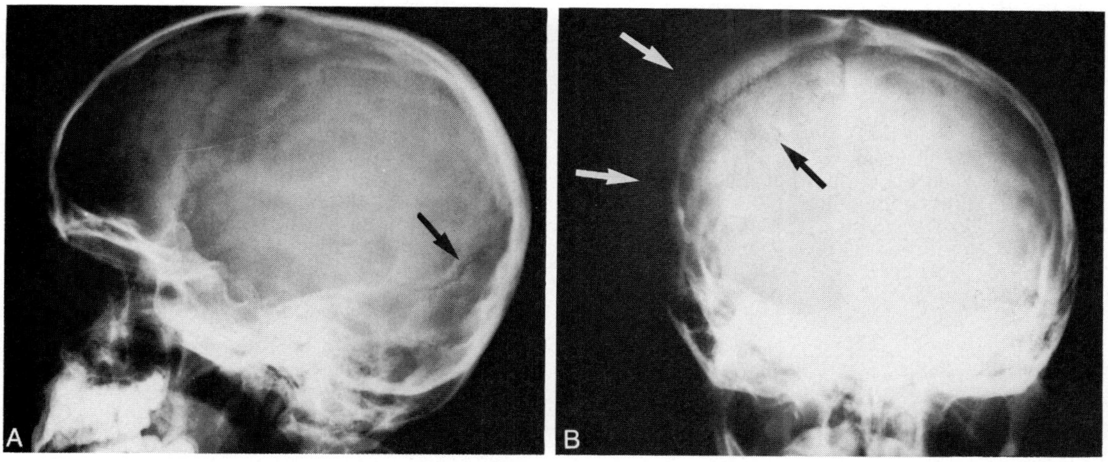

Figure 1–41. Unilateral lambdoid synostosis (12-year-old female).

A, Lateral film. A patent right lambdoid suture *(arrow)* is present. Deformity of the occiput is apparent.

B, Frontal film. The patent right lambdoid suture *(arrow)* is identified; however, its left-sided counterpart is absent. The distorted plagiocephalic skull *(white arrows)* is noted.

of the orbit and greater wing of the sphenoid bone, resulting in the "harlequin" eye as well as an oblique-shaped or plagiocephalic skull. Bilateral coronal synostosis leads to shortening of the skull and upward growth of the skull, resulting in turricephaly (Fig. 1–40).

Lambdoid Synostosis. As with coronal synostosis, this type of craniosynostosis may be unilateral or bilateral, leading to a plagiocephalic or turricephalic skull (Fig. 1–41).

Lückenschädel (Craniolacunia). This condition is seen almost exclusively in patients with Chiari II malformations with accompanying meningomyeloceles and is most likely secondary to disruption of mesenchymal development. Increased intracranial pressure is not thought to have any significant influence upon this condition. An irregular "honeycombed" appearance to the inner table is noted with alternating bony ridges and regions of circular or ovoid lucency. This condition usually reverts to normal by 1 year of age (Fig. 1–42).

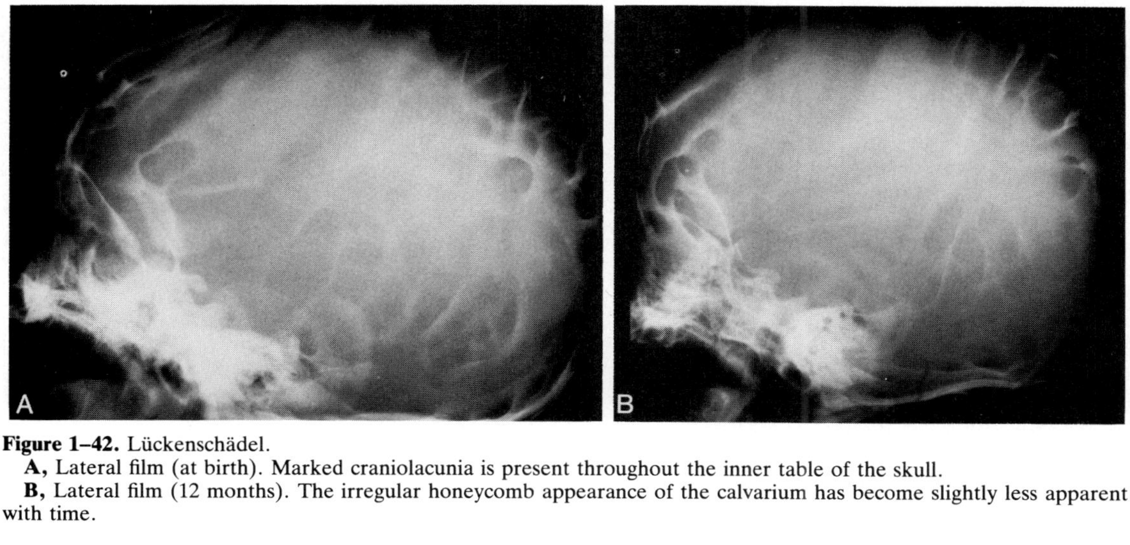

Figure 1–42. Lückenschädel.

A, Lateral film (at birth). Marked craniolacunia is present throughout the inner table of the skull.

B, Lateral film (12 months). The irregular honeycomb appearance of the calvarium has become slightly less apparent with time.

References

1. Warwick R, Williams PL: *Gray's Anatomy.* 35th ed. 1973; W.B. Saunders Co.; Philadelphia.
2. Taveras JM, Wood EH: *Diagnostic Neuroradiology.* 2nd ed. 1976; Williams & Wilkins Co.; Baltimore.
3. Kieffer SA, Gold LHA: Intracranial physiologic calcifications. Semin Roentgenol 1974; 9:151–162.
4. Yock DH: Skull, in Heinz ER, ed. *The Clinical Neurosciences.* 1984; Churchill Livingstone; New York.
5. Lagos JC, Holman LB, Gomez MR: Tuberous sclerosis: Neuroroentgenologic observations. AJR 1968; 104:171–175.
6. Greenfield GB: *Radiology of Bone Disease.* 3rd ed. 1980; J.B. Lippincott Co.; Philadelphia.
7. Currarino G, Rutledge JC: Temporoparietal dermoid cysts with intracranial extension. AJNR 1988; 9:385–387.
8. Thomas JE, Baker HL: Assessment of roentgenographic lucencies of the skull: A systematic approach. Neurology 1975; 25:99–106.

2

ANATOMY AND GENERAL APPROACH

ANATOMY

(Figs. 2–1 through 2–10)

The brain can be divided into three major components: the cerebral hemispheres, the brainstem, and the cerebellum. The bulk of the brain is composed of the cerebral hemispheres, which are derived from the prosencephalon. The hemispheres are structurally identical, separated by the falx cerebri, a dural extension that bisects the interhemispheric fissure. The hemispheres are attached and com-

Text continued on page 45

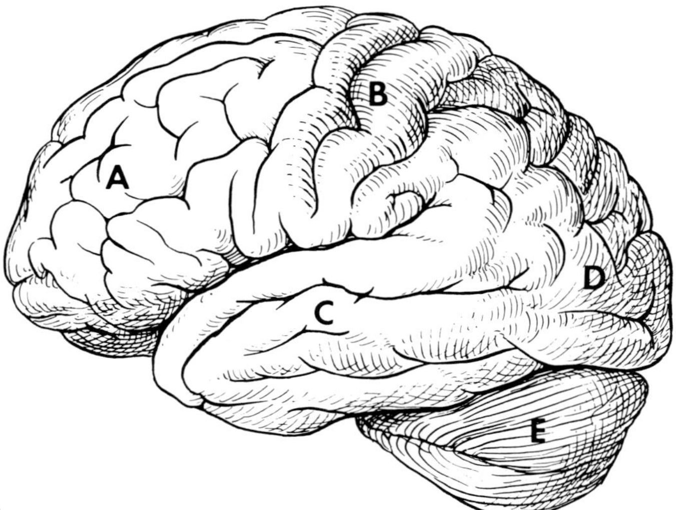

A

Figure 2–1. Gross anatomy.

A, Lateral view. (*A*) Frontal lobe, (*B*) parietal lobe, (*C*) temporal lobe, (*D*) occipital lobe, (*E*) cerebellum.

B, Base view. (*A*) Frontal lobe, (*B*) temporal lobe, (*C*) parietal lobe, (*D*) mesencephalon, (*E*) pons, (*F*) medulla, (*G*) cerebellum, (*H*) occipital lobe.

C, Vertex view. (*A*) Frontal lobe, (*B*) parietal lobe, (*C*) occipital lobe.

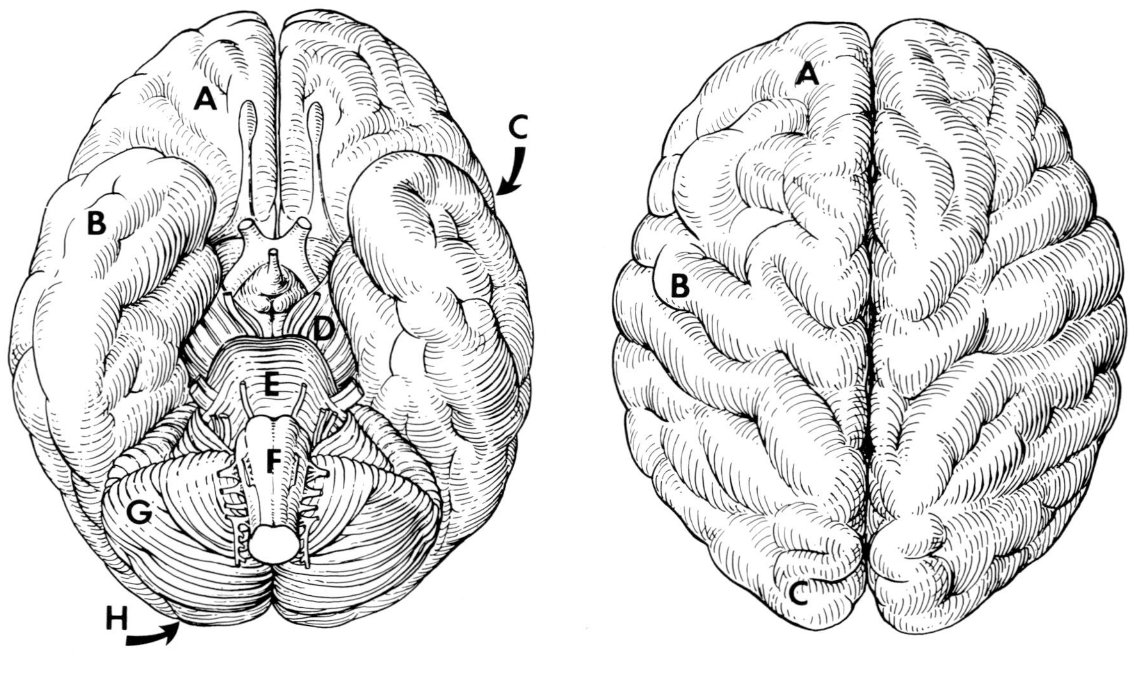

B

C

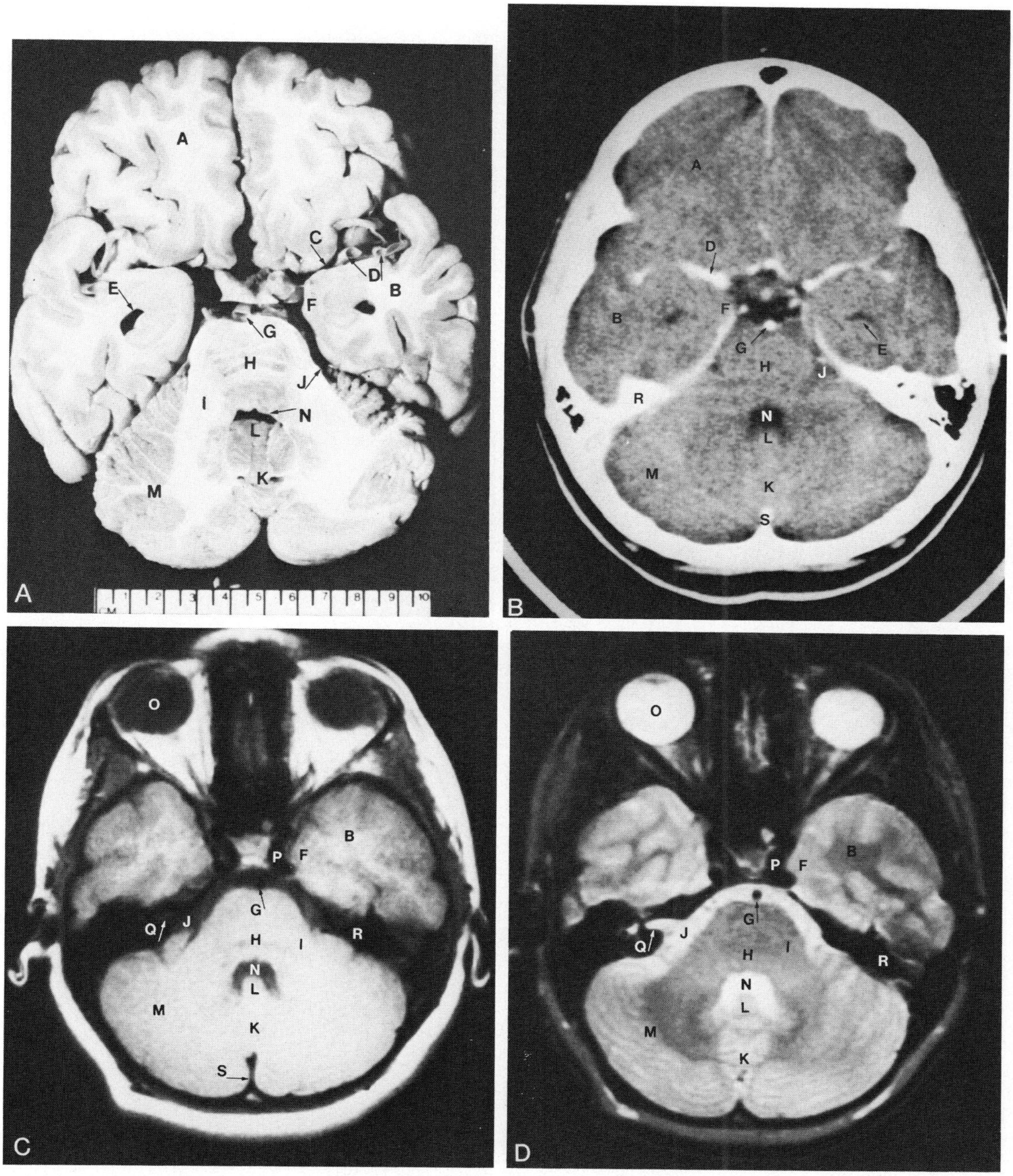

Figure 2–2. Axial anatomy. **A,** Gross. **B,** Enhanced computed tomography (CT). **C,** T1 magnetic resonance (MR). **D,** T2 MR. **A–D,** (*A*) Frontal lobe, (*B*) temporal lobe, (*C*) lateral cerebral fissure, (*D*) middle cerebral artery, (*E*) temporal horn, (*F*) uncus, (*G*) basilar artery, (*H*) pons, (*I*) cerebellar peduncle, (*J*) cerebellopontine angle, (*K*) vermis, (*L*) uvula of vermis, (*M*) cerebellar hemisphere, (*N*) fourth ventricle, (*O*) globe, (*P*) cavernous carotid artery, (*Q*) internal auditory canal, (*R*) petrous ridge, (*S*) falx cerebelli.

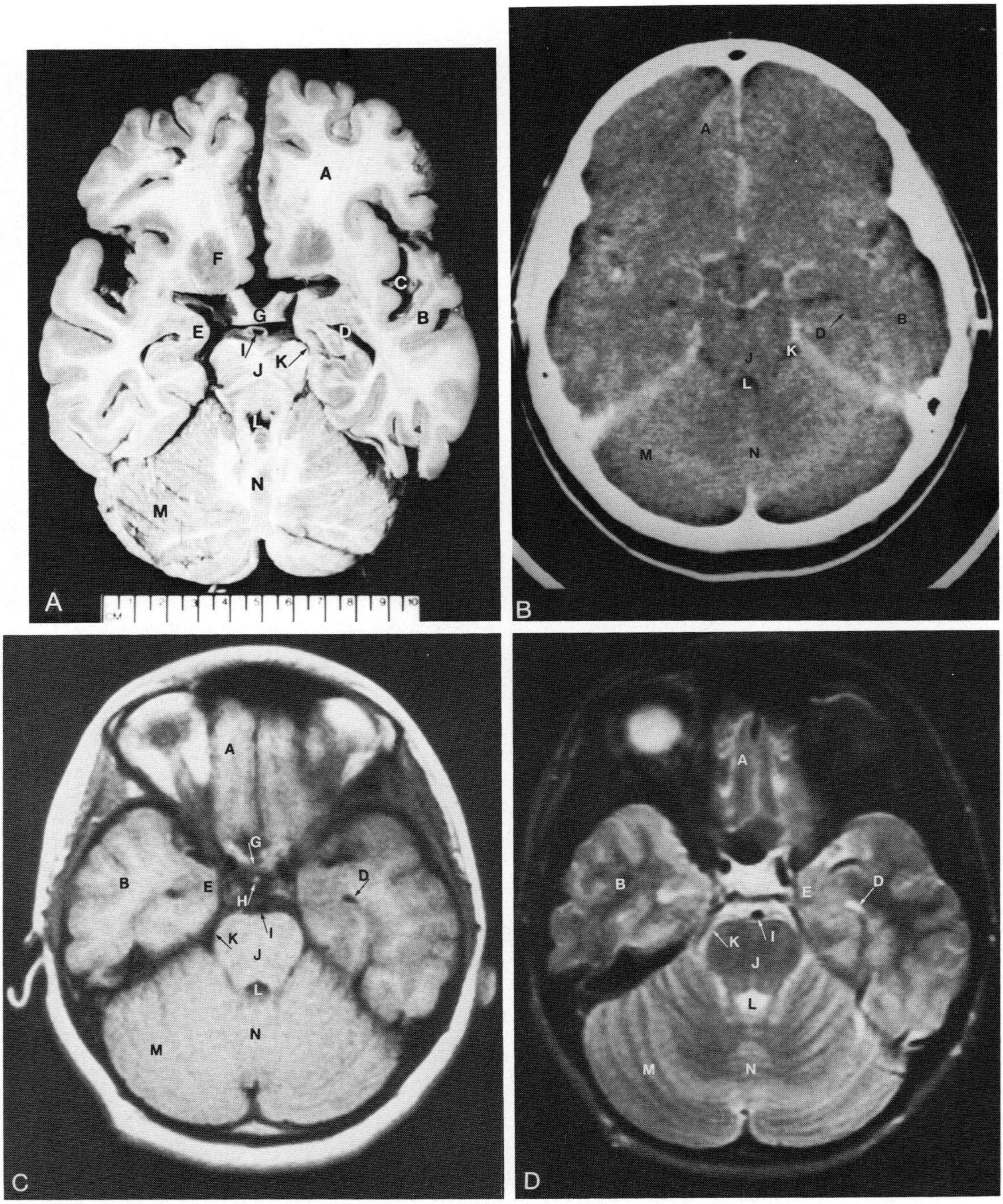

Figure 2–3. Axial anatomy. **A–D,** (*A*) Frontal lobe, (*B*) temporal lobe, (*C*) sylvian fissure, (*D*) temporal horn, (*E*) uncus, (*F*) base of caudate nucleus, (*G*) optic chiasm, (*H*) infundibulum, (*I*) basilar artery, (*J*) pons/mesencephalon, (*K*) ambient cistern, (*L*) superior fourth ventricle, (*M*) cerebellar hemisphere, (*N*) vermis.

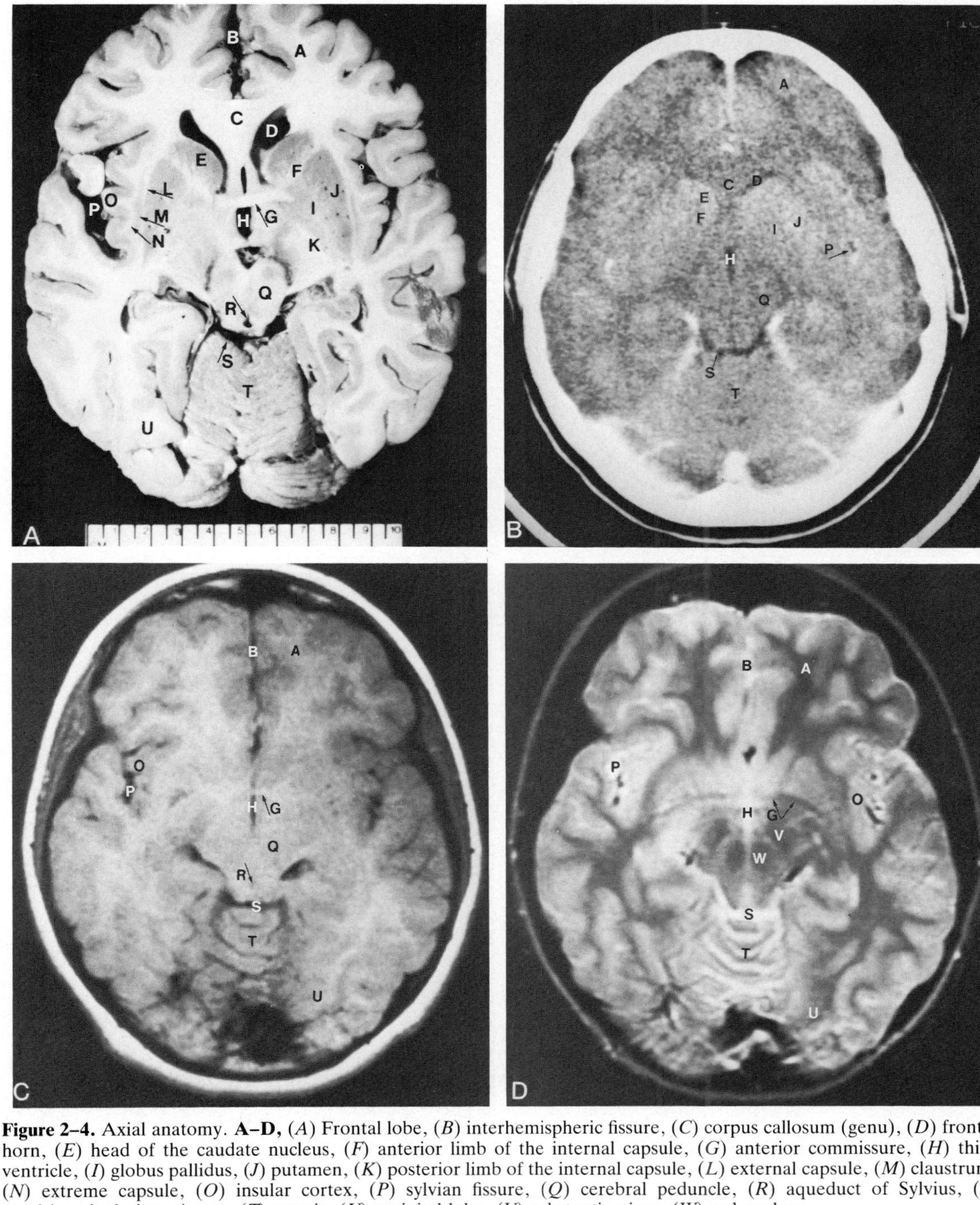

Figure 2–4. Axial anatomy. **A–D,** (*A*) Frontal lobe, (*B*) interhemispheric fissure, (*C*) corpus callosum (genu), (*D*) frontal horn, (*E*) head of the caudate nucleus, (*F*) anterior limb of the internal capsule, (*G*) anterior commissure, (*H*) third ventricle, (*I*) globus pallidus, (*J*) putamen, (*K*) posterior limb of the internal capsule, (*L*) external capsule, (*M*) claustrum, (*N*) extreme capsule, (*O*) insular cortex, (*P*) sylvian fissure, (*Q*) cerebral peduncle, (*R*) aqueduct of Sylvius, (*S*) quadrigeminal plate cistern, (*T*) vermis, (*U*) occipital lobe, (*V*) substantia nigra, (*W*) red nucleus.

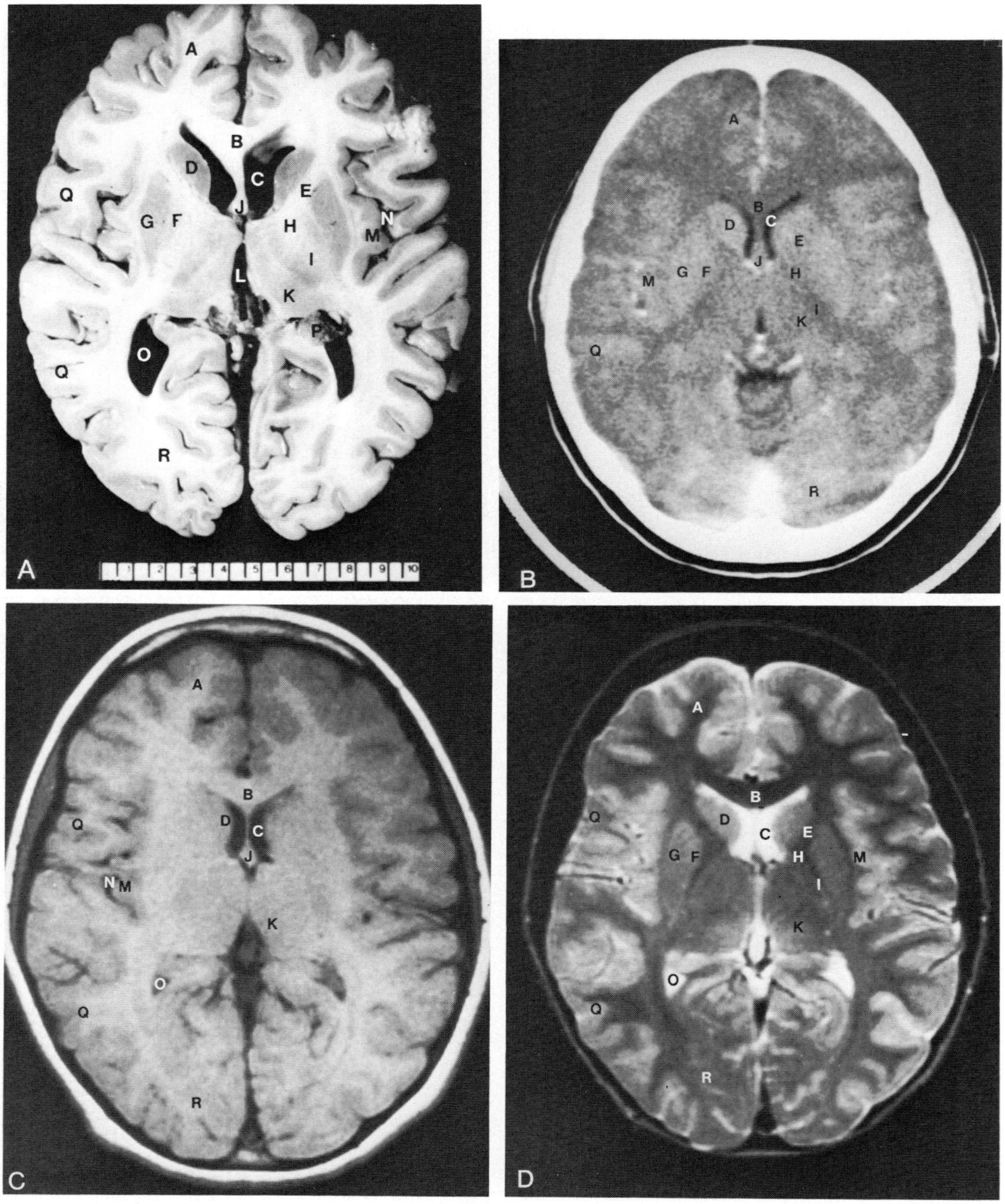

Figure 2–5. Axial anatomy. **A–D,** (*A*) Frontal lobe, (*B*) corpus callosum (genu), (*C*) frontal horn, (*D*) caudate nucleus, (*E*) anterior limb of internal capsule, (*F*) globus pallidus, (*G*) putamen, (*H*) genu of internal capsule, (*I*) posterior limb of internal capsule, (*J*) columns of fornix, (*K*) thalamus, (*L*) third ventricle, (*M*) insular cortex, (*N*) sylvian fissure, (*O*) atrium, (*P*) glomus of the choroid plexus, (*Q*) parietal lobe, (*R*) occipital lobe.

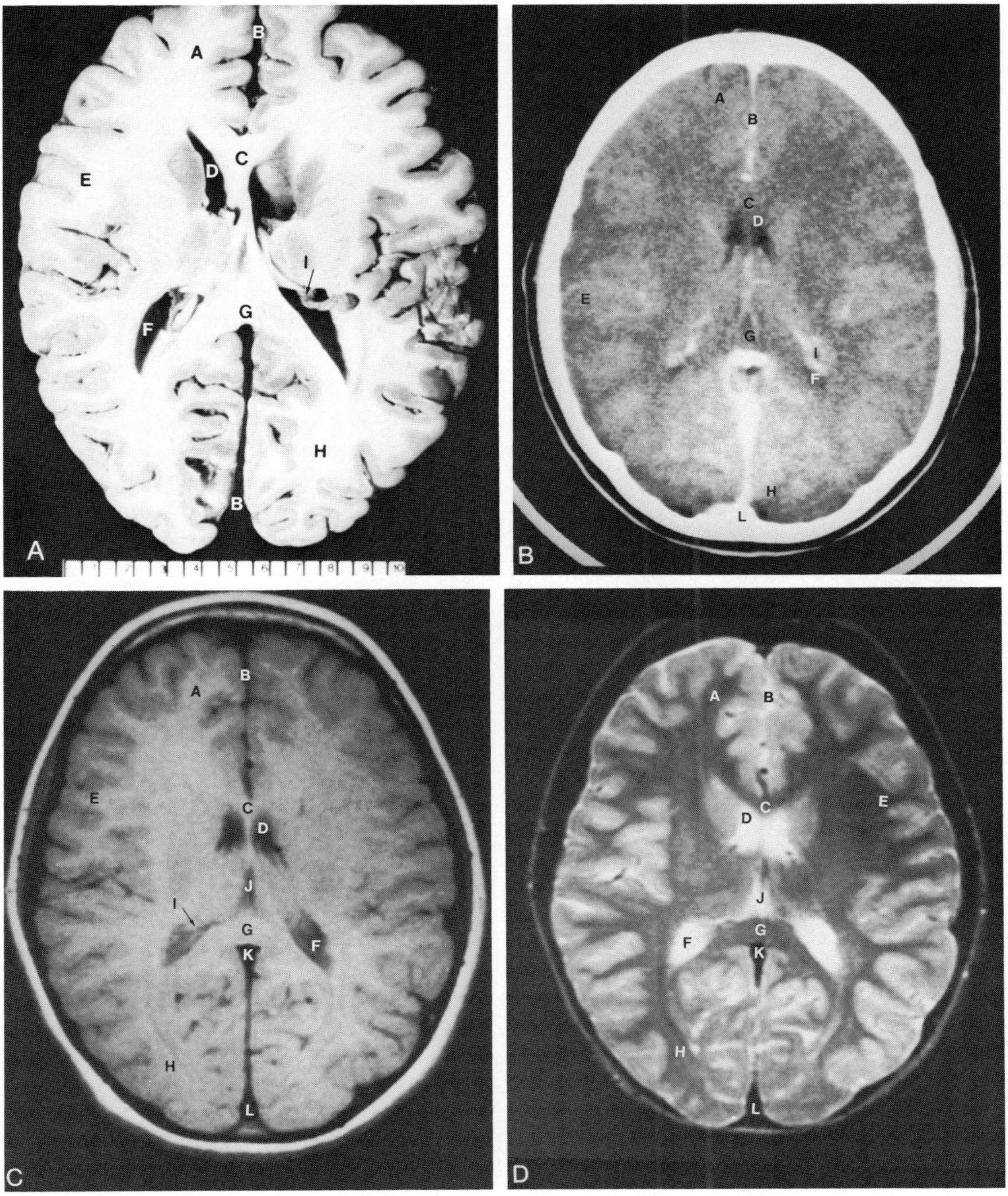

Figure 2–6. Axial anatomy. **A–D,** (*A*) Frontal lobe, (*B*) interhemispheric fissure, (*C*) corpus callosum (anterior body), (*D*) frontal horn, (*E*) parietal lobe, (*F*) atrium, (*G*) corpus callosum (splenium), (*H*) occipital lobe, (*I*) choroid plexus, (*J*) roof of third ventricle, (*K*) great vein of Galen, (*L*) superior sagittal sinus.

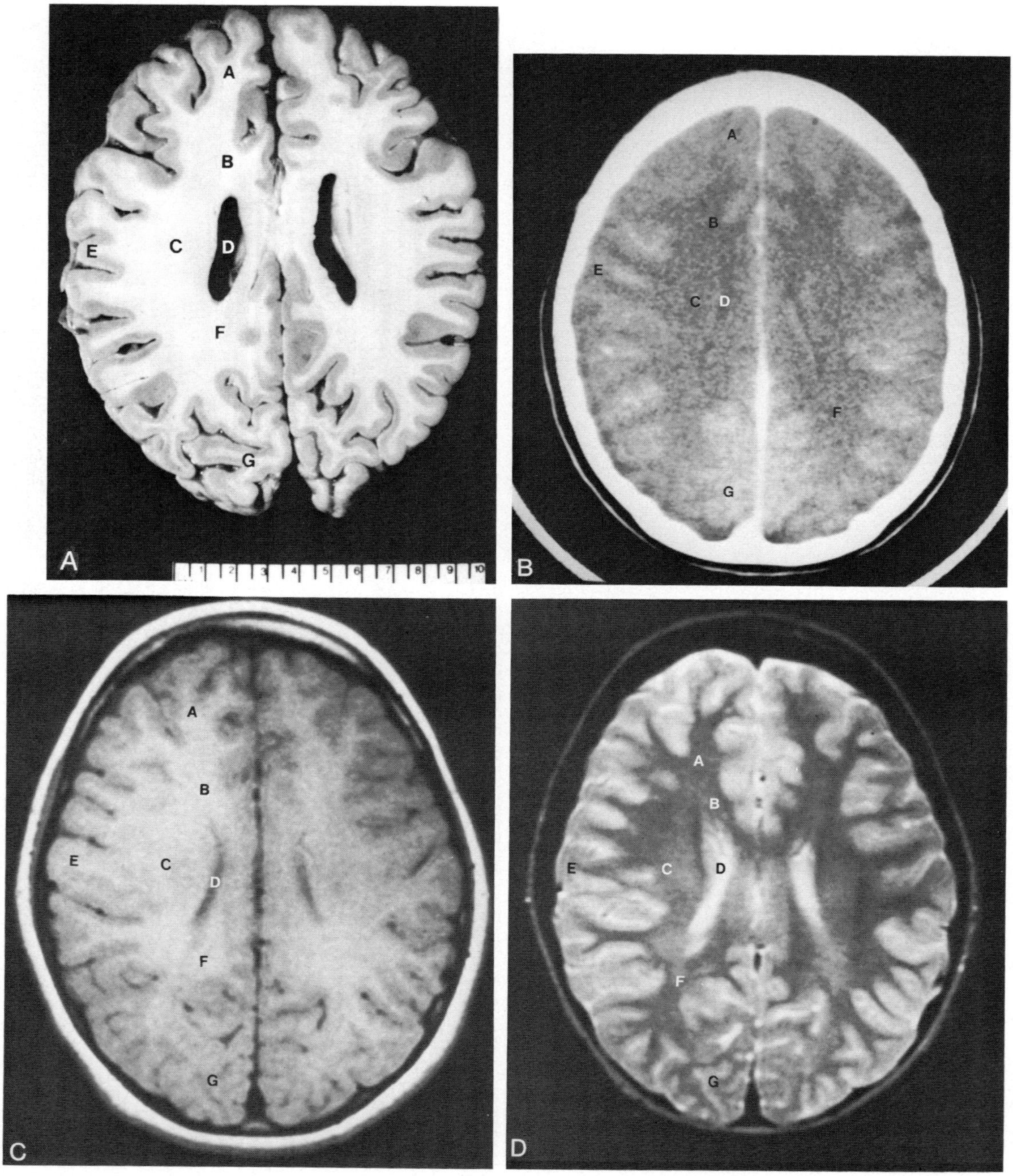

Figure 2–7. Axial anatomy. **A–D,** (*A*) Frontal lobe, (*B*) forceps minor, (*C*) centrum semiovale, (*D*) body of the lateral ventricle, (*E*) parietal lobe, (*F*) forceps major, (*G*) occipital lobe.

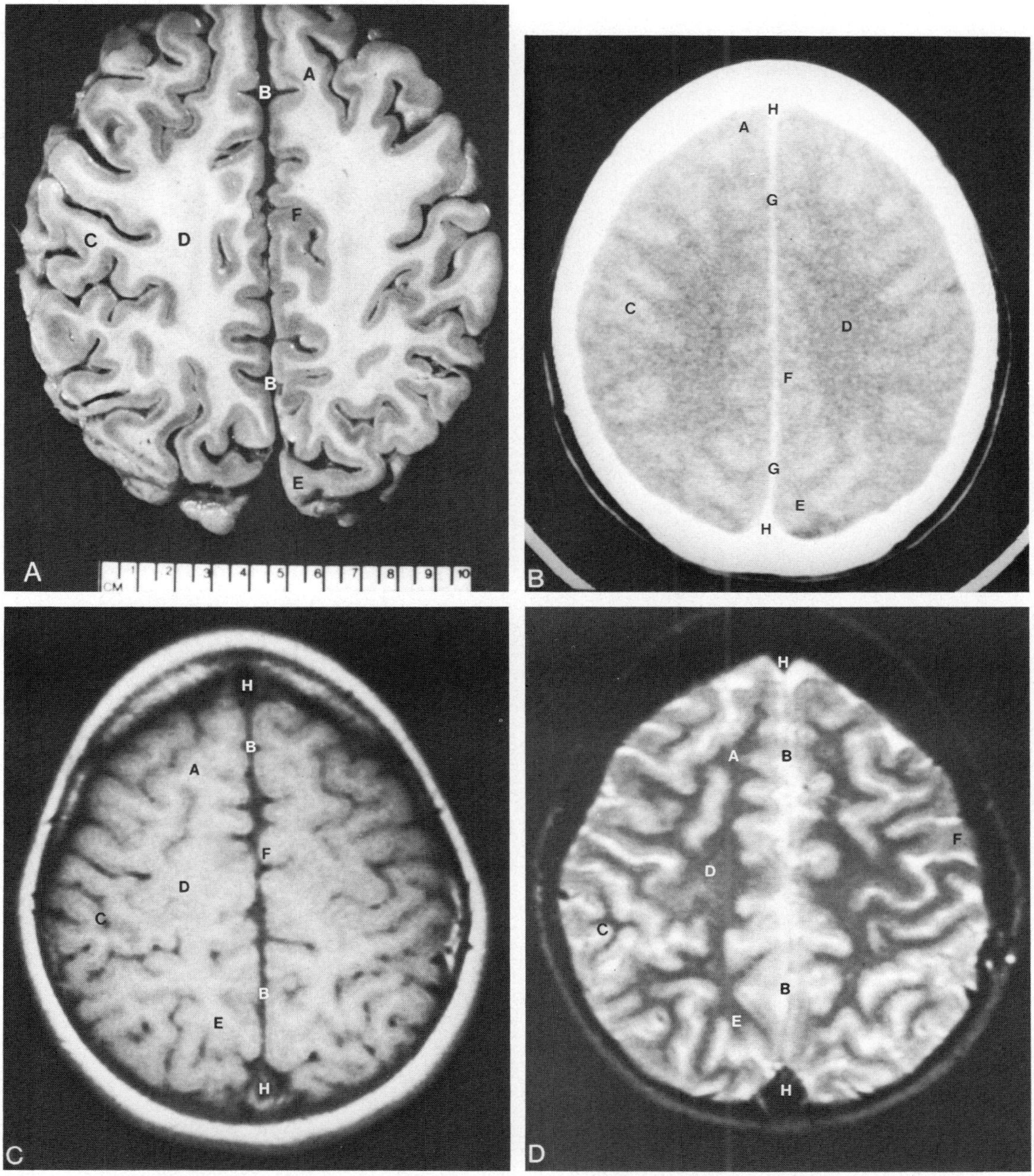

Figure 2–8. Axial anatomy. **A–D,** (*A*) Frontal lobe, (*B*) interhemispheric fissure, (*C*) parietal lobe, (*D*) centrum semiovale, (*E*) occipital lobe, (*F*) cortex, (*G*) falx cerebri, (*H*) superior sagittal sinus.

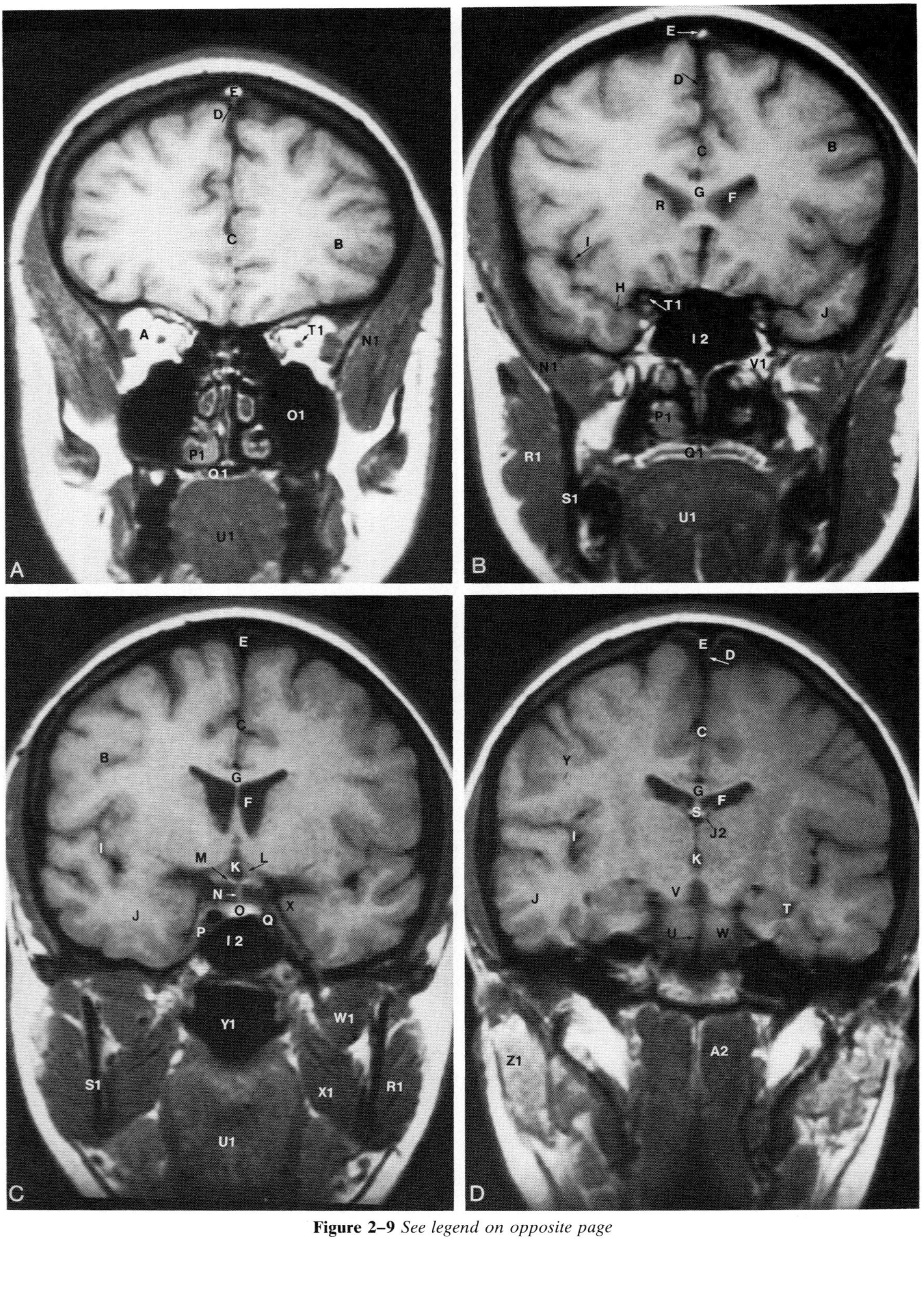

Figure 2–9 *See legend on opposite page*

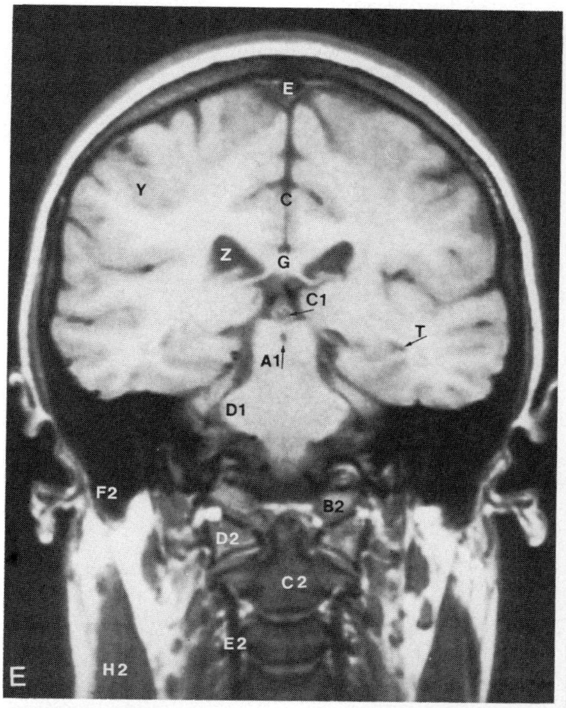

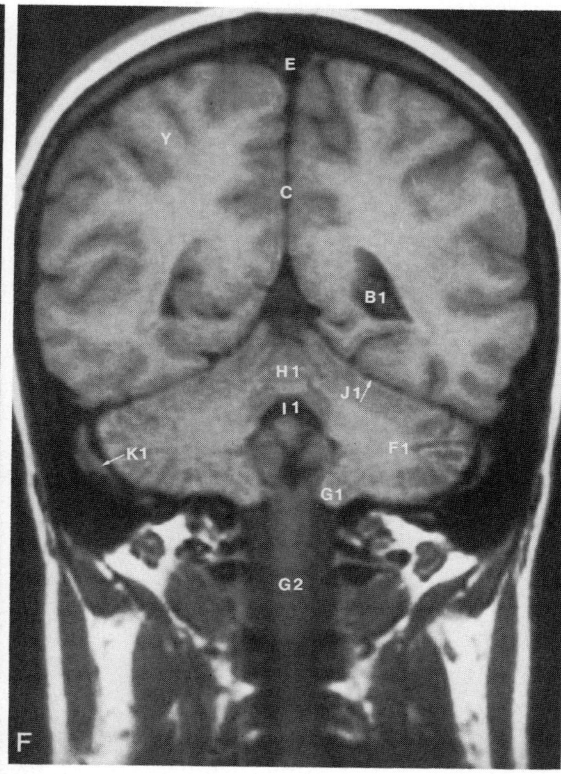

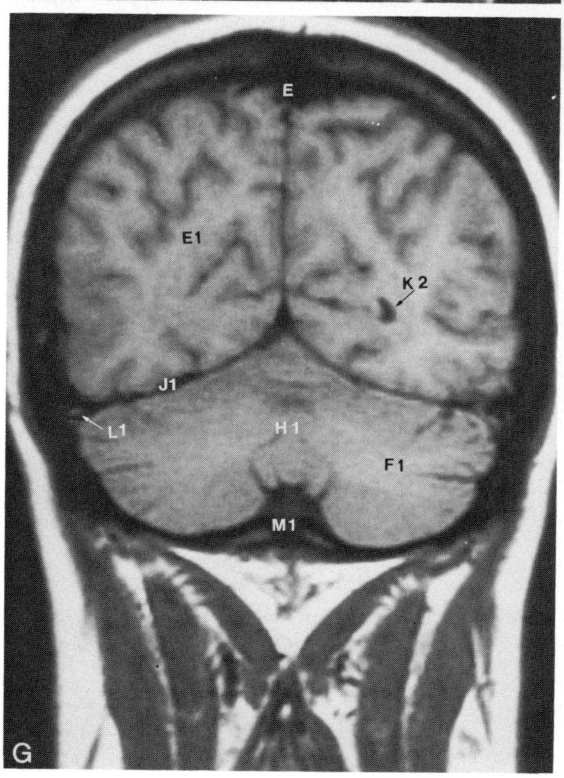

Figure 2–9. Coronal anatomy (T1 MR). **A–G** (anterior to posterior progression), (*A*) Orbit, (*B*) frontal lobe, (*C*) interhemispheric fissure, (*D*) falx cerebri, (*E*) superior sagittal sinus, (*F*) frontal horn, (*G*) corpus callosum, (*H*) lateral cerebral fissure, (*I*) sylvian fissure, (*J*) temporal lobe, (*K*) third ventricle, (*L*) hypothalamus, (*M*) optic chiasm, (*N*) infundibulum, (*O*) pituitary gland, (*P*) cavernous sinus, (*Q*) cavernous internal carotid artery, (*R*) caudate nucleus, (*S*) columns of fornix, (*T*) temporal horn, (*U*) basilar artery, (*V*) cerebral peduncle, (*W*) pons, (*X*) uncus, (*Y*) parietal lobe, (*Z*) body of lateral ventricle, (*A1*) aqueduct of Sylvius, (*B1*) atrium of the lateral ventricle, (*C1*) pineal gland, (*D1*) cerebellar peduncle, (*E1*) occipital lobe, (*F1*) cerebellar hemisphere, (*G1*) cerebellar tonsil, (*H1*) vermis, (*I1*) fourth ventricle, (*J1*) tentorium, (*K1*) sigmoid sinus, (*L1*) transverse sinus, (*M1*) cisterna magna, (*N1*) temporalis muscle, (*O1*) maxillary sinus, (*P1*) nasal turbinate, (*Q1*) hard palate, (*R1*) masseter muscle, (*S1*) mandible, (*T1*) optic nerve, (*U1*) tongue, (*V1*) pterygopalatine fossa, (*W1*) lateral pterygoid muscle, (*X1*) medial pterygoid muscle, (*Y1*) nasopharynx, (*Z1*) parotid gland, (*A2*) retropharyngeal soft tissue, (*B2*) occipital condyle, (*C2*) axis, (*D2*) atlas, (*E2*) vertebral artery, (*F2*) mastoid portion of the temporal bone, (*G2*) cervical cord, (*H2*) sternocleidomastoid muscle, (*I2*) sphenoid sinus, (*J2*) foramen of Monro, (*K2*) occipital horn.

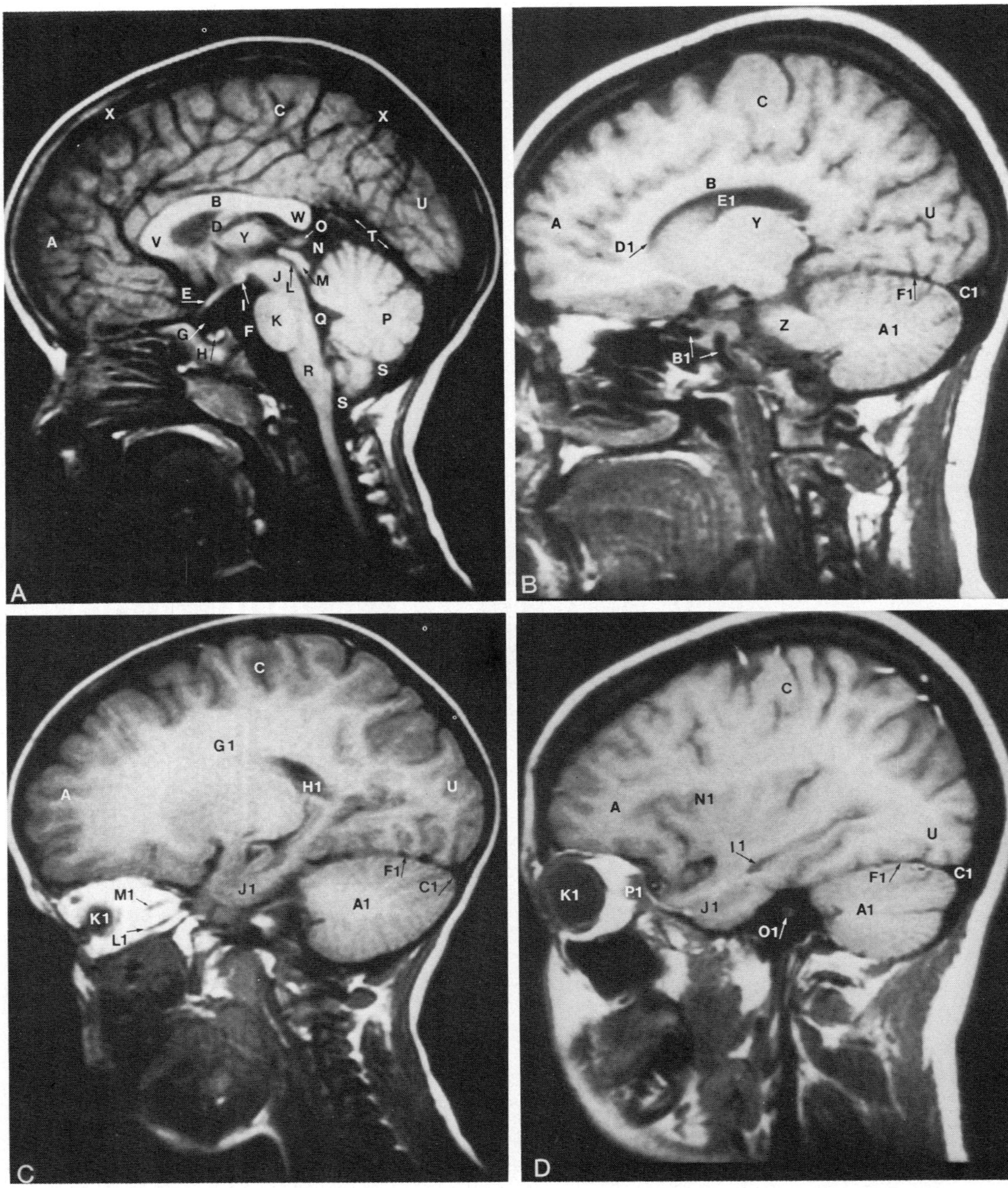

Figure 2–10. Parasagittal anatomy (T1 MR). **A–D** (medial to lateral progression), (*A*) Frontal lobe, (*B*) corpus callosum, (*C*) parietal lobe, (*D*) columns of fornix, (*E*) optic chiasm, (*F*) prepontine cistern, (*G*) suprasellar cistern, (*H*) pituitary gland, (*I*) mamillary body, (*J*) mesencephalon, (*K*) pons, (*L*) aqueduct of Sylvius, (*M*) tectal plate, (*N*) quadrigeminal plate cistern, (*O*) pineal gland, (*P*) vermis, (*Q*) fourth ventricle, (*R*) medulla, (*S*) cisterna magna, (*T*) straight sinus, (*U*) occipital lobe, (*V*) corpus callosum (genu), (*W*) corpus callosum (splenium), (*X*) superior sagittal sinus, (*Y*) thalamus, (*Z*) cerebellar peduncle, (*A1*) cerebellar hemisphere, (*B1*) cavernous internal carotid artery, (*C1*) transverse sinus, (*D1*) frontal horn, (*E1*) body of the lateral ventricle, (*F1*) tentorium, (*G1*) centrum semiovale, (*H1*) atrium of lateral ventricle, (*I1*) temporal horn, (*J1*) temporal lobe, (*K1*) globe, (*L1*) inferior rectus muscle, (*M1*) optic nerve, (*N1*) insular cortex, (*O1*) contents of internal auditory canal, (*P1*) lateral rectus muscle.

municate through a large white matter tract, the corpus callosum.[1]

The cerebral surface is markedly convoluted with deep sulci separating adjacent gyri. Specific gyri may be used to subdivide the brain into four major lobes. The lobes are designated frontal, temporal, parietal, and occipital, named for the overlying bone. The insular cortex is a deep invagination of the lateral cerebral surface that is covered by portions of the temporal lobe and the parietal operculum.

The gray matter is composed of neuronal cell bodies and is located primarily within the convoluted cortex. In addition, nuclear masses are located deep in the cerebral parenchyma adjacent to the lateral and third ventricles. These nuclear masses are denoted basal ganglia and are composed of the globus pallidus, putamen, caudate, and amygdaloid nuclear complex. The thalamus and portions of the hypothalamus also contain gray matter.

The cerebral white matter constitutes the core of the hemispheres. The white matter fibers are arranged into location-specific tracts that are projection, association, or commissural in nature. Projection fibers form the pathway of communication between the cortex and the target organ. They may be afferent or efferent. The corona radiata is the best example of projection fibers. These fibers converge, forming the internal capsule just cephalad to the midbrain. Association fibers connect cortical regions within the same hemisphere. The tracts may be short, connecting adjacent gyri, or long, interconnecting adjacent or remote lobes. Commissural fibers connect similar cortical regions between the hemispheres. The corpus callosum is the dominant commissural tract connecting each lobe of the brain with its counterpart. The anterior commissure is a small commissural tract connecting olfactory and inferior and medial temporal lobe gyri.

The ventricles are ependyma-lined cavities located deep within the parenchyma that contain the cerebrospinal fluid (CSF). CSF is produced largely by the choroid plexus. (This function is discussed in greater detail in Chapter 6.) There are four ventricles: the paired lateral ventricles and the midline third and fourth ventricles.

The brainstem consists of four major components: from cephalad to caudad, they are the diencephalon, the mesencephalon, the pons, and the medulla. The diencephalon is composed of the thalamic and juxtathalamic nuclei. The thalami form the lateral walls of the third ventricle. The mesencephalon, or midbrain, is the next most caudal component of the brainstem. The third and fourth cranial nerves arise from the mesencephalon. The aqueduct of Sylvius, which connects the third and fourth ventricles, resides within the dorsal midbrain and is covered by the tectal or quadrigeminal plate. The pons, origin of cranial nerves V through VII, forms a major component of the brainstem and is located in the midposterior fossa. The dorsal surface of the pons forms the floor of the fourth ventricle. The medulla, origin of cranial nerves VIII through XII, is the caudad-most component of the brainstem. The medulla tapers caudally as it merges with the cervical cord at the foramen magnum.

The cerebellum is positioned dorsal to the pons and medulla and occupies the majority of the posterior fossa. The cerebellum consists of the midline vermis and two lateral lobes or hemispheres. Like the cerebral hemispheres, the cerebellum consists of cortical gray matter and a white matter core with the deep gray matter nuclei. The cerebellum joins the lower three segments of the brainstem via paired white matter tracts designated the superior, middle, and inferior cerebellar peduncles.

The meninges are composed of the dura mater, arachnoid, and pia mater. The dura is the tough fibrous outermost layer that is also the periosteum of the inner table. The dura also extends centripetally to form the falx cerebri (bisecting the cerebral hemispheres in the interhemispheric fissure), the tentorium (separating the cerebral parenchyma above from the cerebellum in the posterior fossa), and a small falx cerebelli (located within the cisterna magna). The arachnoid is a thin lace-like membrane that bridges external surfaces of the brain. Deep to the arachnoid is the subarachnoid space within which the CSF circulates and the cortical vessels reside. The pia mater is the innermost membrane, which invests the cortical sulci and surrounds the vessels that penetrate the brain parenchyma.

GENERAL APPROACH TO DISTINGUISHING FEATURES

Planar imaging can be performed with computed tomography (CT) or magnetic resonance imaging (MRI). CT allows cross-sectional imaging over a relatively limited range of gantry movement and requires patient positioning to obtain coronal, oblique, or sagittal images. Computer-reformatted images may be obtained at the cost of spatial resolution. CT is a widely available technology and may be performed relatively quickly. CT excels in evaluation of patients with acute subarachnoid hemorrhage, patients with calcified intracranial lesions, and the acutely traumatized patient. Limitations of CT include use of ionizing radiation, image degradation from beam-hardening artifacts, and the frequent need for iodinated contrast. Tissue contrast in CT is inferior to that in MRI.

A screening brain CT examination at our institution consists of 5-mm contiguous axial images through the posterior fossa and 10-mm contiguous axial images through the supratentorial parenchyma. Iodinated intravenous contrast material is administered unless the patient is a trauma victim or is being evaluated for intracranial hemorrhage, infarct, or dementia.

The advantages of MRI include multiplanar image acquisition without the use of ionizing radiation. The increased tissue contrast and spatial resolution afforded by MRI permits earlier detection of most intracranial processes. The image is not degraded by beam-hardening artifacts, which limit the diagnostic utility of CT, particularly in the posterior fossa. MRI is uniquely sensitive to paramagnetic materials, which include hemoglobin degradation products.

The disadvantages of MRI include relative calcium insensitivity. MRI is generally less available than CT and more costly to perform. Ferromagnetic materials must remain outside the magnetic field. MRI is contraindicated in patients with cardiac pacemakers and certain metallic prostheses.

Our current screening brain MRI examination consists of parasagittal spin echo T1-weighted images using the following parameters: repetition time (TR) 300 to 500 msec, echo delay time (TE) 20 msec, field of view (FOV) 20 cm, matrix 256 × 192, excitations (Ex) 1, slice thickness 5 mm and slice gap 2 mm. Subsequently, axial spin density (SD) and T2-weighted images are obtained with a TR 3000 msec, TE 30 msec (SD) to 90 msec (T2), and FOV 24. Ex, slice thickness, and slice gap are constant. Finally, axial T1 images are obtained similar to the first sequence using a 24-cm FOV.

The decision to administer gadolinium is based on the appearance of the unenhanced scan. Gadolinium, like iodinated contrast, will demonstrate disruption of the blood-brain barrier (BBB), which accompanies most neoplasms, infarctions, infections, inflammation, and hematomas.

Based on radiographic characteristics, the etiology of an intracranial mass lesion may be apparent. Although a histologic diagnosis is not possible in many cases, certain morphologic features may corroborate a specific disease process. These radiographic findings are presented here.

Location

Successful localization of a lesion into the intra-axial or extra-axial compartment is the most helpful factor in arriving at a meaningful differential diagnosis. Intra-axial lesions arise from the brain parenchyma, are more common than extra-axial lesions, and usually signify a poorer prognosis. Extra-axial lesions arise extrinsic to the brain, often from the dura. It is not possible in every instance to compartmentalize a lesion, in which case both intra-axial and extra-axial processes should be considered within the differential diagnosis.

Several factors have been proposed to distinguish intra-axial from extra-axial masses[2] (Table 2–1; Fig. 2–11). Intra-axial lesions are usually surrounded by parenchyma and are

Table 2–1. PLANAR IMAGING CHARACTERISTICS THAT LOCALIZE MASS LESIONS

	Intra-axial	Extra-axial
Contiguous with dura	−	+*
Bony change	Uncommon	Common
Corticomedullary buckling	−	+
Displacement of cortical veins	Centrifugal	Centripetal
Adjacent cisterns	Effaced	Widened
Dural enhancement	−	+

*Only exception is intraventricular mass.

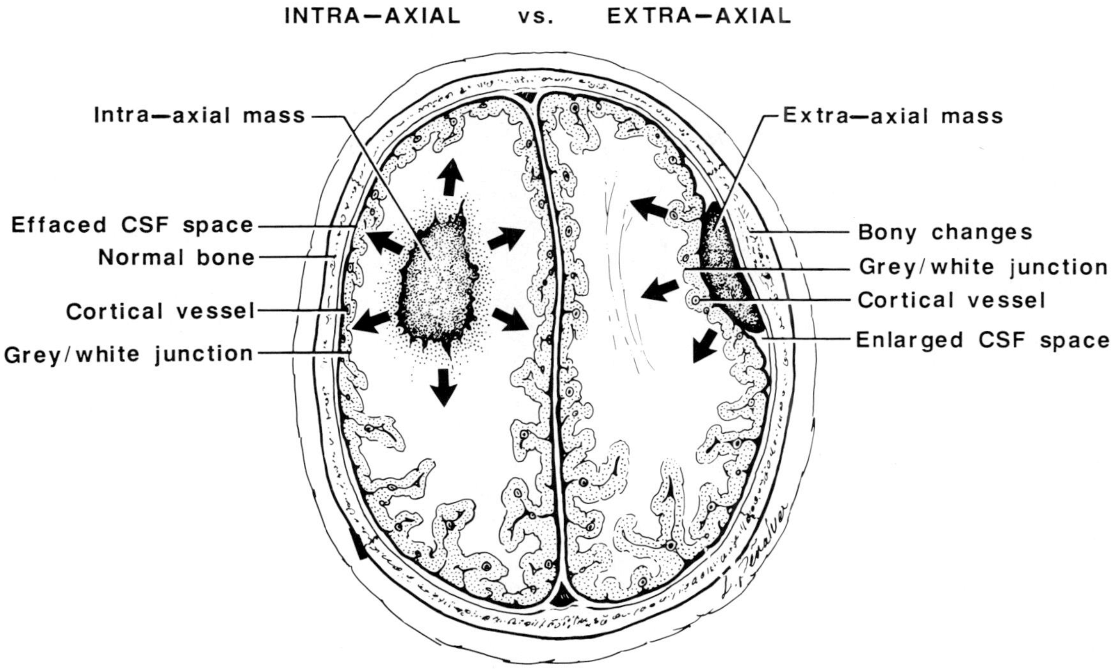

Figure 2–11. Intra-axial versus extra-axial: distinguishing radiographic characteristics.

often geographically removed from the ventricle or dural surface. The adjacent cisterns are compressed, and the corticomedullary junction and the cortical veins may be centrifugally displaced toward the inner table by the parenchymal mass (Fig. 2–12). Bony changes are rare with intra-axial lesions. Intra-axial mass lesions include glial neoplasm, parenchymal metastasis, abscess, hematoma, and infarction.

Extra-axial processes include meningioma,

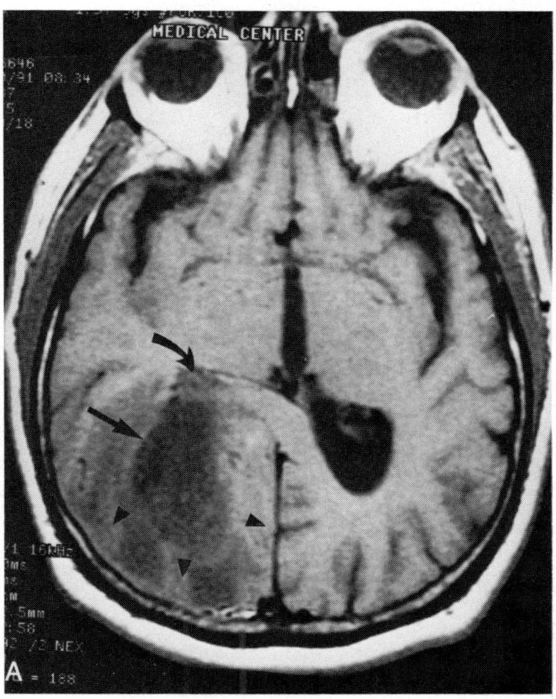

Figure 2–12. Intra-axial mass—glioblastoma multiforme (64-year-old male).

A, Axial T1. An ill-defined hypointensity (*arrow*) is present in the right occipital lobe. Displacement of the glomus of the choroid (*curved arrow*) and compression of the cortical sulci (*arrowheads*) indicate local mass effect.

Illustration continued on following page

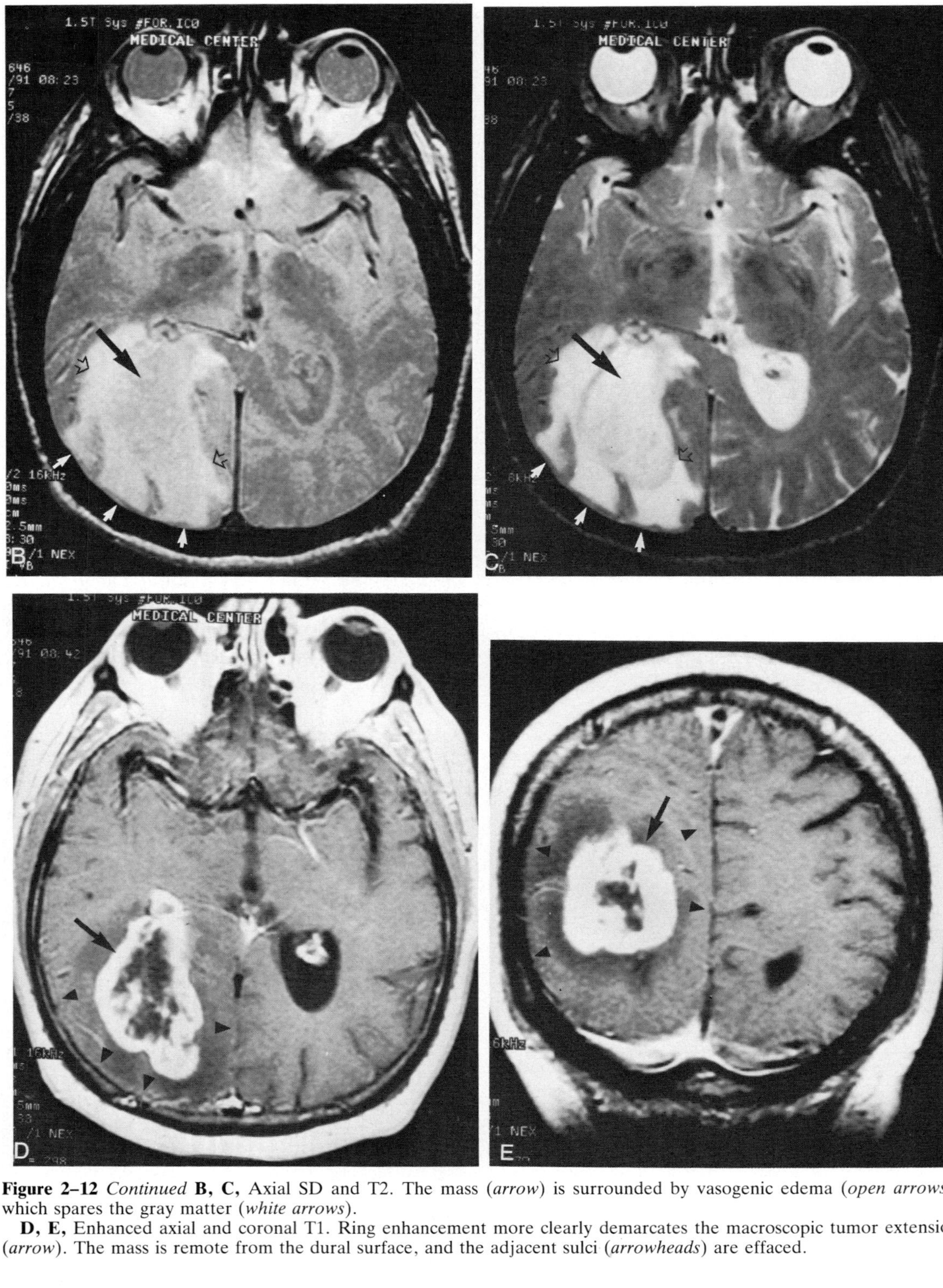

Figure 2–12 *Continued* **B, C,** Axial SD and T2. The mass (*arrow*) is surrounded by vasogenic edema (*open arrows*), which spares the gray matter (*white arrows*).

D, E, Enhanced axial and coronal T1. Ring enhancement more clearly demarcates the macroscopic tumor extension (*arrow*). The mass is remote from the dural surface, and the adjacent sulci (*arrowheads*) are effaced.

dermoid, epidermoid, arachnoid cyst, and subdural and epidural hematoma. Extra-axial lesions displace the brain from the inner table resulting in widening of the adjacent CSF space, and centripetal displacement of cortical vessels and the corticomedullary junction (corticomedullary buckling) (Fig. 2–13). Extra-axial lesions are in direct contact with the dura and may induce bony reactive changes, such as hyperostosis, erosion, and osteolysis. Extra-axial hemorrhages may be associated with skull fractures. Extra-axial processes may cross CSF cisterns and penetrate the dura. Reactive dural enhancement may corroborate an extra-axial process.

Mass Effect—Herniation

The volume of the mature calvarium is fixed. Intracranial masses grow at the expense of

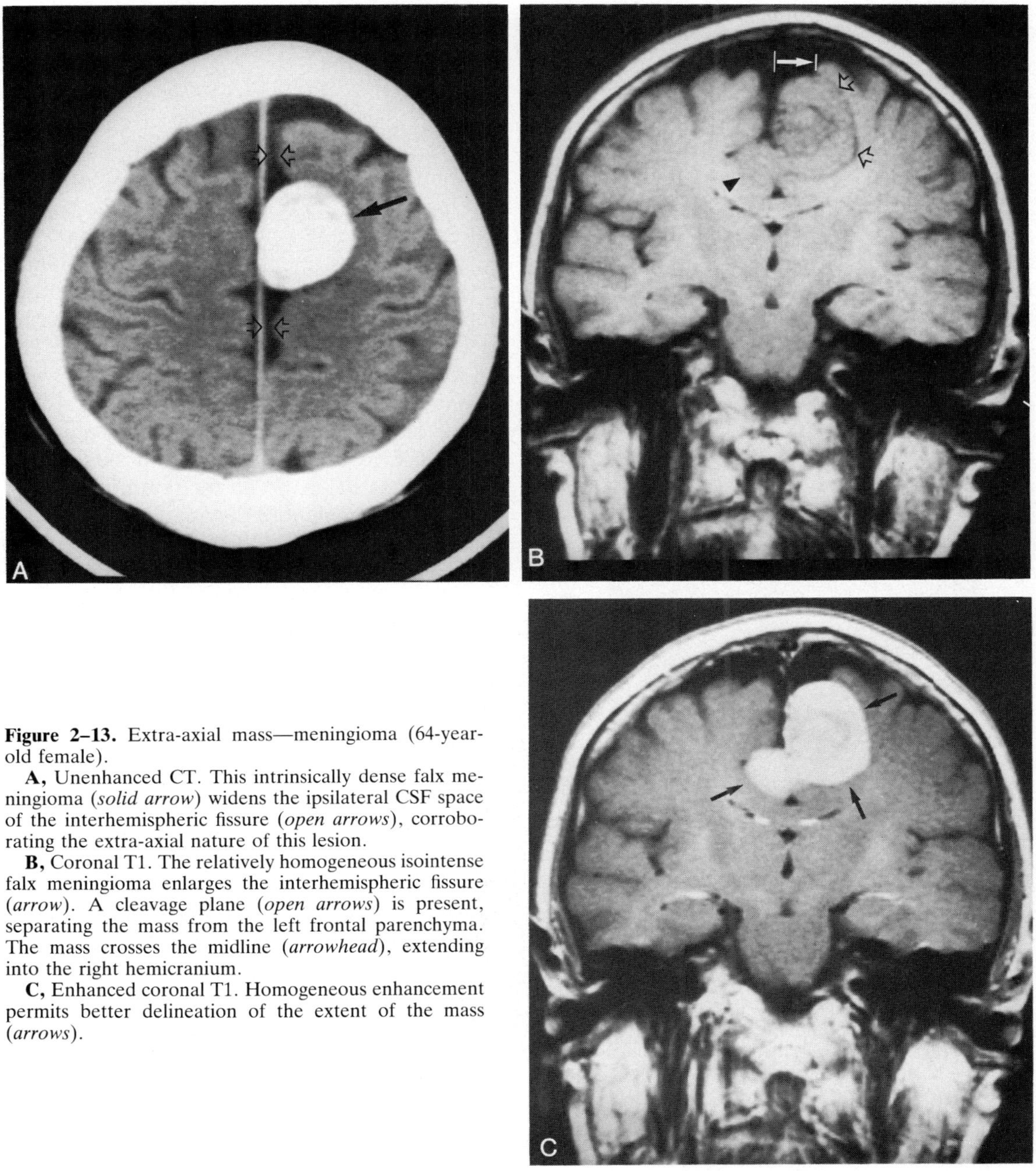

Figure 2–13. Extra-axial mass—meningioma (64-year-old female).

A, Unenhanced CT. This intrinsically dense falx meningioma (*solid arrow*) widens the ipsilateral CSF space of the interhemispheric fissure (*open arrows*), corroborating the extra-axial nature of this lesion.

B, Coronal T1. The relatively homogeneous isointense falx meningioma enlarges the interhemispheric fissure (*arrow*). A cleavage plane (*open arrows*) is present, separating the mass from the left frontal parenchyma. The mass crosses the midline (*arrowhead*), extending into the right hemicranium.

C, Enhanced coronal T1. Homogeneous enhancement permits better delineation of the extent of the mass (*arrows*).

normal structures. Displacement or herniation of the parenchyma from its normal position results from increasing mass effect. Parenchymal herniations occur in a predictable fashion about fixed dural or bony surfaces.

Subfalcial. Intracranial masses of sufficient size will displace the ipsilateral cerebral parenchyma beneath the falx. The body of the corpus callosum and lateral ventricle will herniate a variable distance into the contralateral hemicranium (Fig. 2–14). Progressive herniation will kink the contralateral foramen of Monro, resulting in trapping of the CSF within the contralateral ventricle. The CSF will continue to be produced by the choroid of the lateral ventricle. The resultant obstructive hydrocephalus will compound the effects of the mass and further elevate the intracranial pressure.

Transalar. The alae refer to the wings of the sphenoid bone as they make up the bony interface between the frontal and middle cranial fossa. Transalar herniation refers to the displacement of the temporal lobe into the anterior fossa by a middle cranial fossa mass lesion (Fig. 2–15). Alternatively, a frontal fossa lesion may displace the frontal lobe over the wings of the sphenoid into the middle fossa. Loss of the lateral cerebral fissure is a corroborative radiographic finding.

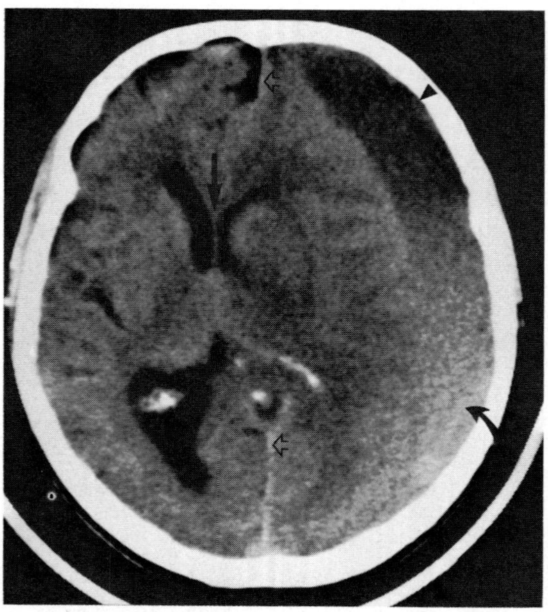

Figure 2–14. Subfalcial herniation—subdural hematoma (82-year-old male). Unenhanced CT; a left-to-right shift of midline structure (*straight solid arrow*) beneath the rigid falx (*open arrows*) signifies subfalcial herniation secondary to a subdural hematoma. The hyperdense cellular elements (*curved arrow*), which layer in the gravity-dependent portion of this collection, indicate that a rebleed has occurred in a chronic hematoma (*arrowhead*).

Uncal. The uncus is the medial-most temporal lobe, which also anatomically represents the lateral-most margin of the suprasellar cistern. An ipsilateral mass lesion will displace the uncus medially, resulting in commensurate deformity of the suprasellar cistern (Fig. 2–16). Progressive mass effect will result in effacement of the suprasellar cistern as the brain begins to herniate through the tentorium.

Transtentorial

Descending. Once a sizable supratentorial mass develops (whether acute or chronic), an ordered, predictable displacement of the brain substance occurs.[3] If a lateralizing mass is present, the brain is displaced into the contralateral calvarium (subfalcial herniation), the uncus migrates medially (uncal herniation), and the brain is displaced caudally through the tentorial incisura (Fig. 2–17). During this caudal migration, the brainstem is torqued and shifted to the side opposite the mass, with resultant enlargement of the ipsilateral ambient cistern. The suprasellar and interpeduncular cisterns become effaced and the cerebral parenchyma begins to fill the tentorial incisura with late effacement of the quadrigeminal plate cistern.

It is important to realize that the initial radiographic manifestations of descending transtentorial herniation occur anteriorly, involving the suprasellar cistern, and progress posteriorly with late effacement of the quadrigeminal plate cistern.

Downward displacement of the brainstem and parenchyma through the tentorial incisura may result in predictable complications. The posterior cerebral artery may become compressed by the free edge of the tentorium, resulting in infarction. Alternatively, cessation of arterial flow into the perforating arteries of the brainstem may precipitate brainstem hemorrhage known as a Duret's hemorrhage.

Ascending. Posterior fossa mass lesions result in displacement of the cerebellum and brainstem upward through the tentorial incisura or downward through the foramen magnum, or both.[4, 5] As the mass displaces the

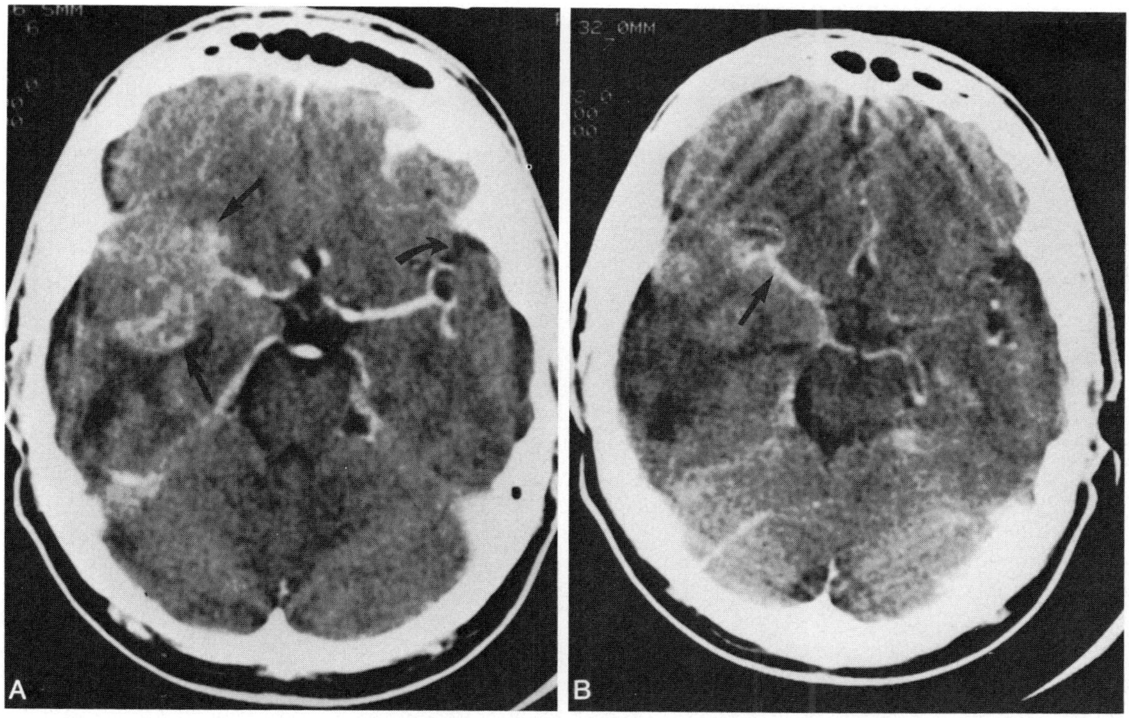

Figure 2–15. Transalar herniation—glioblastoma multiforme (56-year-old male).

A, Enhanced CT. An ill-defined infiltrative mass (*straight arrows*) enhances heterogeneously in the right temporal lobe. The mass obliterates the lateral cerebral fissure that is present on the contralateral side (*curved arrow*).

B, Enhanced CT. The middle cerebral artery (*arrow*) is displaced cephalad and anteriorly by the mass, which extends from the temporal toward the frontal lobe.

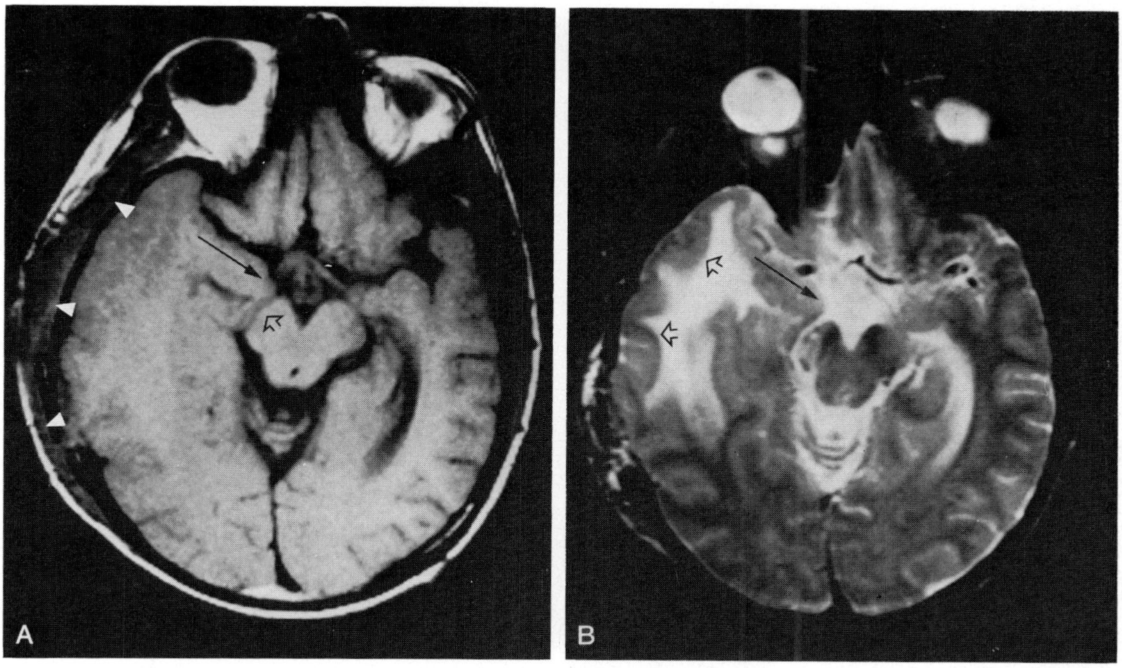

Figure 2–16. Uncal herniation—anaplastic astrocytoma (40-year-old male).

A, Axial T1. The uncus (*solid arrow*) is displaced medially, resulting in distortion of the suprasellar cistern. There is mild compression of the ipsilateral mesencephalon (*open arrow*). Prominence of extracranial soft tissues (*arrowheads*) is a result of recent surgical intervention.

B, Axial T2. Herniation of the uncus (*solid arrow*) is present. Vasogenic edema (*open arrows*) is present within the right temporal lobe.

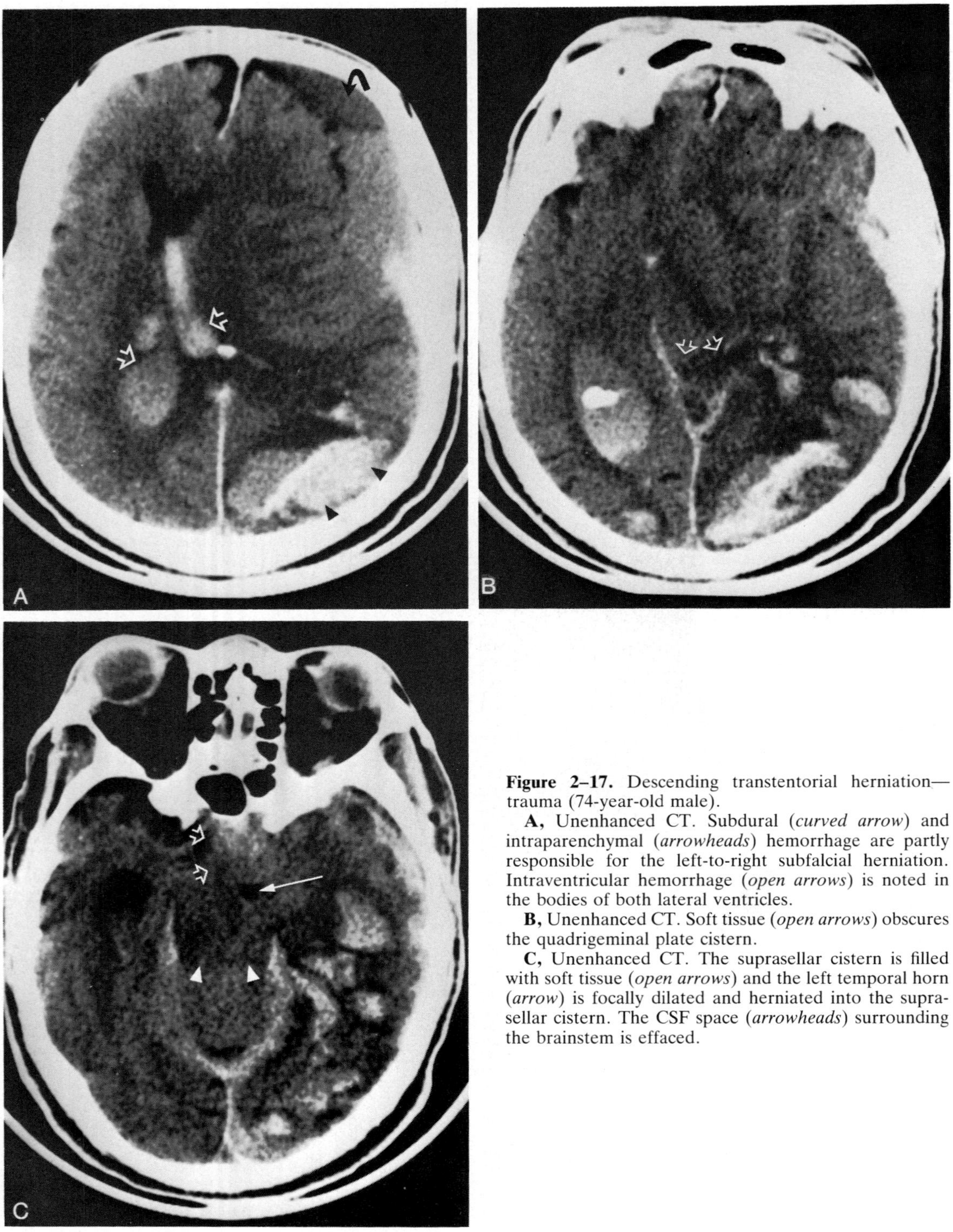

Figure 2–17. Descending transtentorial herniation—trauma (74-year-old male).

A, Unenhanced CT. Subdural (*curved arrow*) and intraparenchymal (*arrowheads*) hemorrhage are partly responsible for the left-to-right subfalcial herniation. Intraventricular hemorrhage (*open arrows*) is noted in the bodies of both lateral ventricles.

B, Unenhanced CT. Soft tissue (*open arrows*) obscures the quadrigeminal plate cistern.

C, Unenhanced CT. The suprasellar cistern is filled with soft tissue (*open arrows*) and the left temporal horn (*arrow*) is focally dilated and herniated into the suprasellar cistern. The CSF space (*arrowheads*) surrounding the brainstem is effaced.

brain superiorly through the incisura, progressive compression and flattening of the quadrigeminal plate is noted as the CSF space becomes obliterated (Fig. 2–18). Ultimately, the incisura is filled with soft tissue as the cerebellum and brainstem are displaced cephalad and obstructive hydrocephalus occurs. Downward displacement of the cerebellar tonsils and medulla through the foramen magnum may accompany this migration of parenchyma from the posterior fossa.

In contradistinction to descending herniation, the radiographic changes signifying ascending herniation occur posteriorly, involving the quadrigeminal plate cistern. The more anterior suprasellar cistern is rarely, if ever, effaced.

Intrinsic CT Density

Consideration of the intrinsic density of a lesion will be most helpful in developing an accurate differential diagnosis. Lesions, by virtue of their ability to absorb or attenuate x-ray photons, will be hypodense, isodense, or hyperdense to adjacent parenchyma (Table 2–2).

Hyperdense Lesions. These lesions possess high attenuation coefficients and thus greater Hounsfield units than does the adjacent brain. Lesions may be high density secondary to cellularity, hemorrhage, or calcification.

Cellularity. Neoplasms with high cellularity, particularly high nuclear-to-cytoplasmic ratio (lymphoma, meningioma), may be intrinsically dense (Fig. 2–19). Abscess capsules by virtue of cellularity and fibrous tissue will also appear high density. An isodense intra-axial lesion may appear hyperdense secondary to the low-density vasogenic edema that surrounds and envelops it.

Table 2–2. CT DENSITY

Moiety	Hounsfield Units
Bone	+1000
Calcification	+100
Acute blood	85
Tumor	30–60
Gray matter	35–40
White matter	25–30
CSF	0
Adipose	−100
Air	−1000

Hemorrhage. Acute hemorrhage measures approximately 85 Hounsfield units and may be secondary to multiple etiologies (Chapter 4) (Fig. 2–20). As the hemorrhage ages, breakdown and removal of cellular debris and hemoglobin products render the hemorrhage isodense to adjacent parenchyma.

Calcification. Certain intracranial processes will calcify at predictable rates. These include the primary intracranial neoplasms and vascular malformations (Fig. 2–21). Morphology and distribution of the calcification within a lesion may be lesion-specific.

Hypodense Lesions. Intracranial processes with low attenuation coefficients appear hypodense on CT, with Hounsfield units approaching or below 0. Hypodense lesions are those that contain fluid or fat.

Fluid. Arachnoid and porencephalic cysts appear hypodense on CT (Fig. 2–22). Cystic necrosis, a feature of higher-grade neoplasms, also appears hypodense on CT. Hounsfield units usually approach 0. The central abscess cavity may appear hypodense on CT. Chronic subdural hemorrhage will also appear hypodense as the cellular elements are lysed and the blood products destroyed (Fig. 2–23).

Adipose. Fat-containing lesions (lipoma, dermoid, teratoma) appear quite hypodense on CT, with Hounsfield units approximately −100. Lesions that contain lipoid or cholesterol material, such as epidermoids and craniopharyngiomas, also appear hypodense on CT, often with Hounsfield units equal to or slightly lower than those of CSF.

Signal Intensity on Spin Echo Sequences

By virtue of relaxation times and flow characteristics, lesions will appear high or low signal on spin echo sequences (Table 2–3). Long relaxation time correlates with low signal on T1 and high signal on T2. The converse is true of short relaxation times: tissues with short relaxation times appear high signal on T1 and low signal on T2.

T1-Weighted Short Relaxation Time (High Signal)

Adipose. Lipomas, dermoids, and teratomas will be in part or total high signal on T1-weighted images, depending on the contribu-

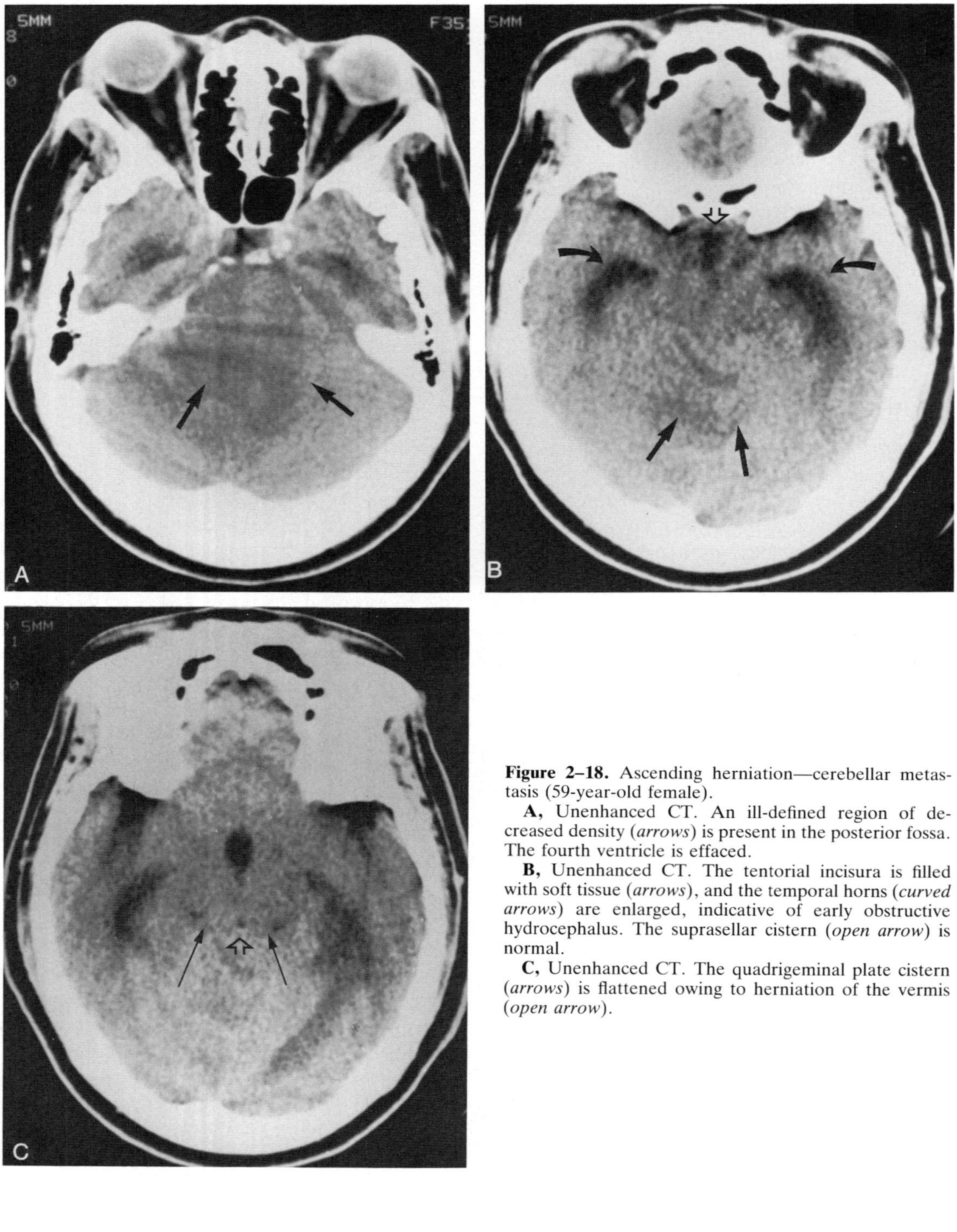

Figure 2–18. Ascending herniation—cerebellar metastasis (59-year-old female).

A, Unenhanced CT. An ill-defined region of decreased density (*arrows*) is present in the posterior fossa. The fourth ventricle is effaced.

B, Unenhanced CT. The tentorial incisura is filled with soft tissue (*arrows*), and the temporal horns (*curved arrows*) are enlarged, indicative of early obstructive hydrocephalus. The suprasellar cistern (*open arrow*) is normal.

C, Unenhanced CT. The quadrigeminal plate cistern (*arrows*) is flattened owing to herniation of the vermis (*open arrow*).

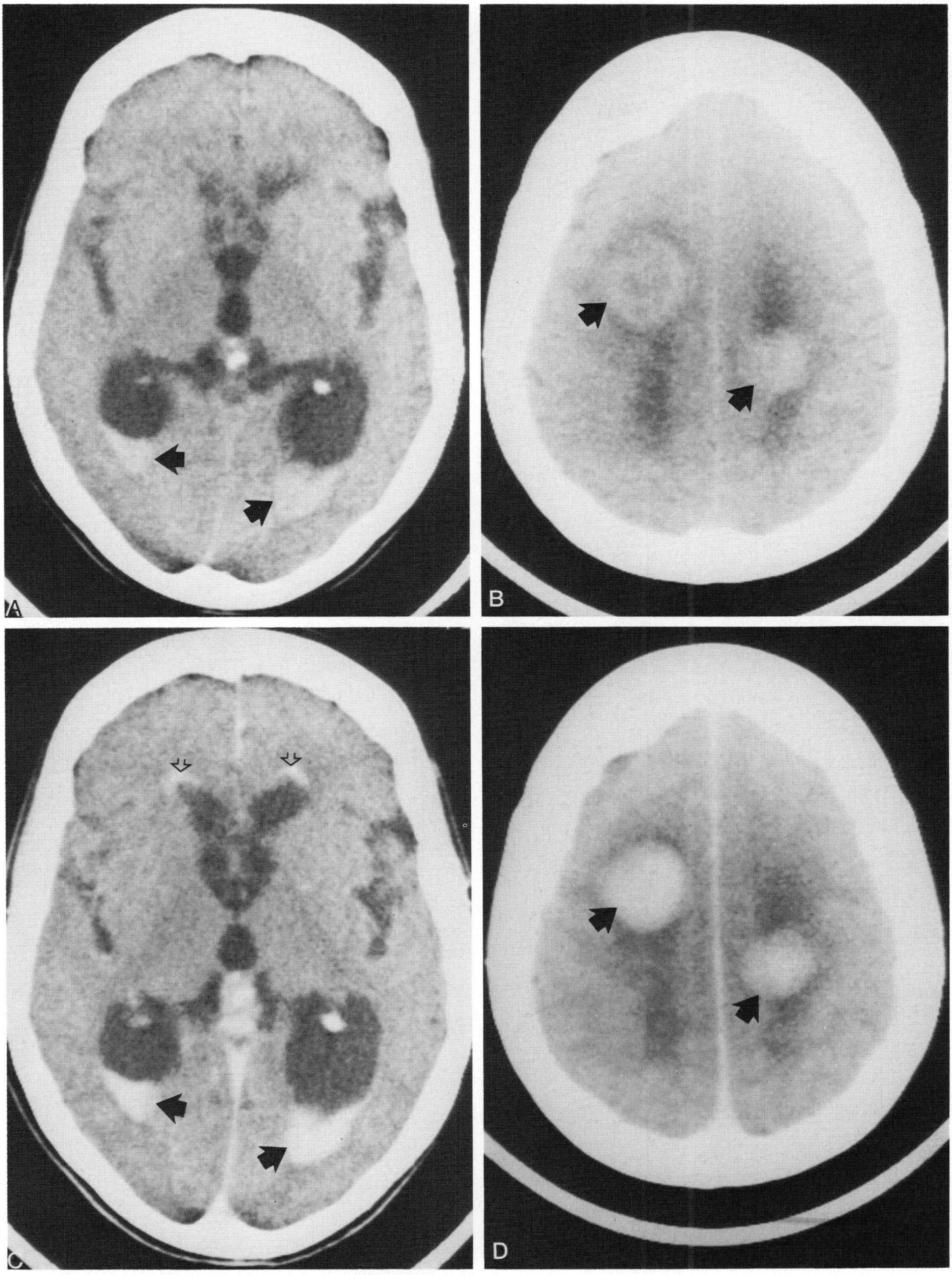

Figure 2–19. Hyperdense—lymphoma (72-year-old female).

A, Unenhanced CT. High-density material (*arrows*) fills the occipital horns.

B, Unenhanced CT. Biparietal high-density lesions (*arrows*) are present adjacent to the ventricular surface.

C, Enhanced CT. There is uniform enhancement of the tumor deposits in the occipital (*solid arrows*) and frontal horns (*open arrows*).

D, Enhanced CT. Uniform enhancement is also observed in the periventricular parietal lesions (*arrows*).

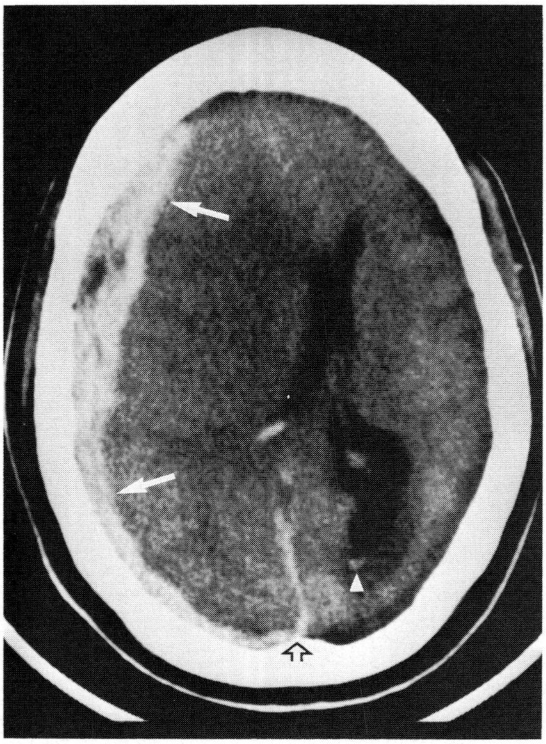

Figure 2–20. Hyperdense—subdural hematoma (57-year-old male). Acute subdural hematoma will present as a high-density, extra-axial mass (*arrows*), which may cross sutures but respects the midline falx (*open arrow*). Incidental note is made of intraventricular blood in the contralateral occipital horn (*arrowhead*).

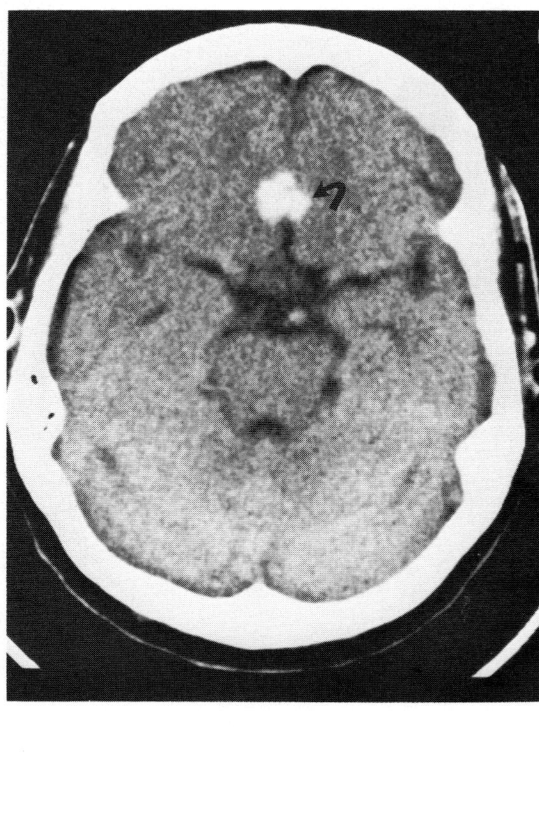

Figure 2–21. Hyperdense—meningioma (62-year-old female). Unenhanced CT; a globular, 1.5-cm (in greatest linear dimension) calcification (*arrow*) indicates the presence of a planum meningioma.

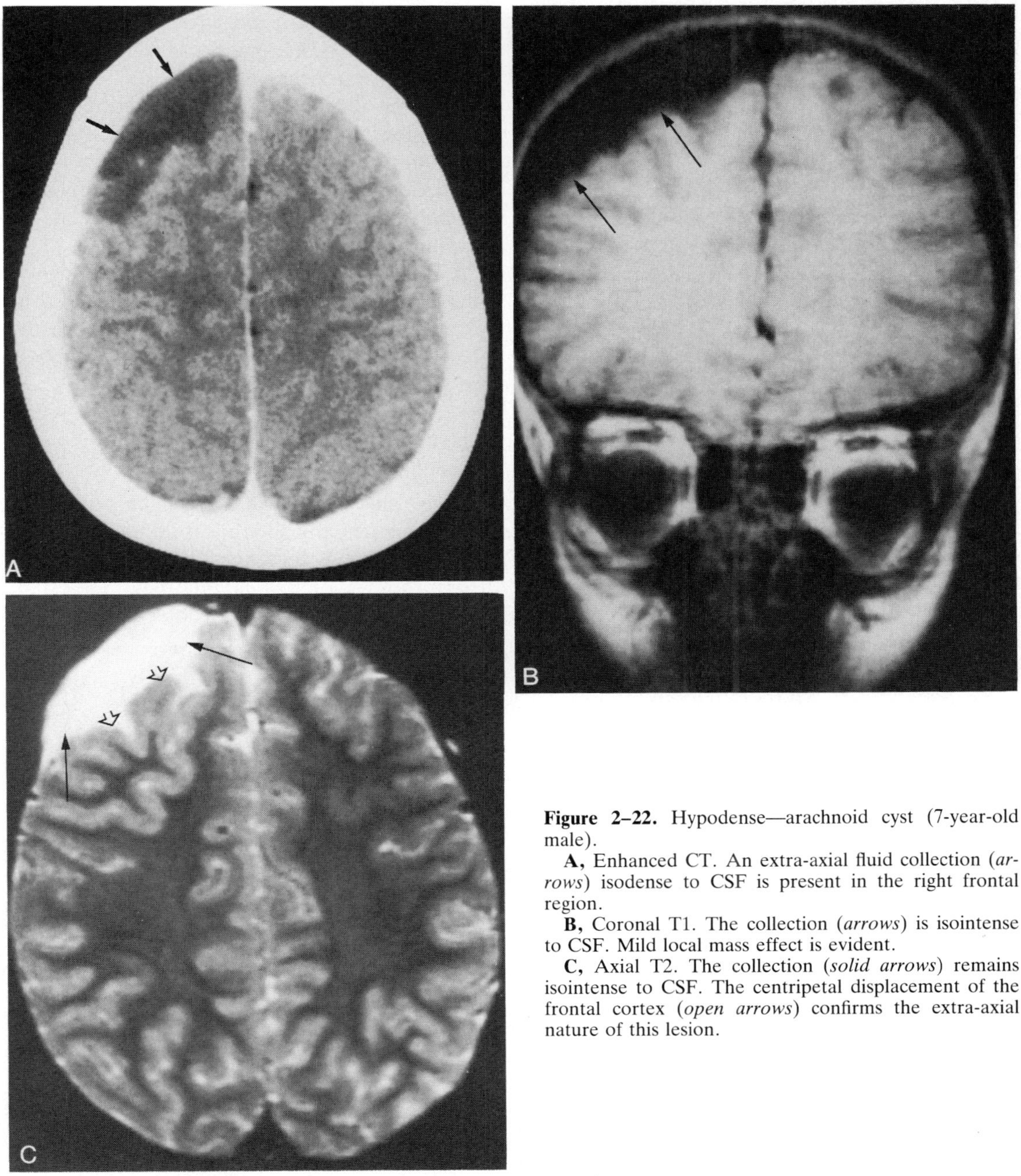

Figure 2–22. Hypodense—arachnoid cyst (7-year-old male).

A, Enhanced CT. An extra-axial fluid collection (*arrows*) isodense to CSF is present in the right frontal region.

B, Coronal T1. The collection (*arrows*) is isointense to CSF. Mild local mass effect is evident.

C, Axial T2. The collection (*solid arrows*) remains isointense to CSF. The centripetal displacement of the frontal cortex (*open arrows*) confirms the extra-axial nature of this lesion.

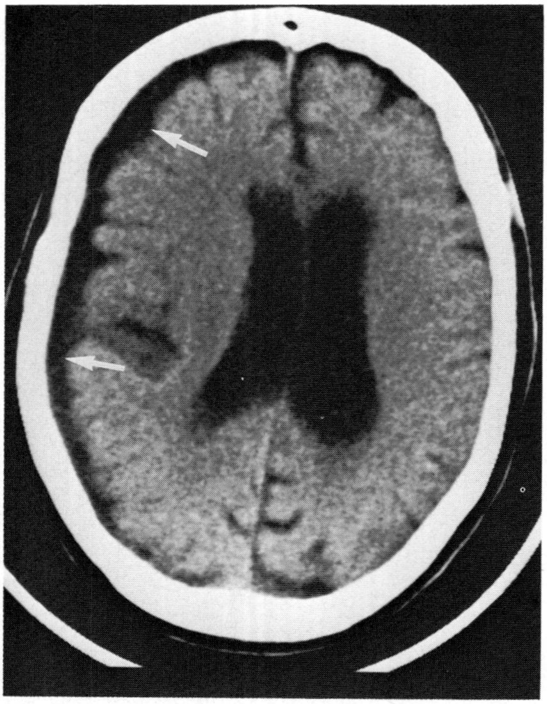

Figure 2–23. Hypodense—chronic subdural hematoma (61-year-old male). Unenhanced CT demonstrates an extra-axial fluid collection (*arrows*) isodense to CSF along the right hemicranium.

tion of other soft tissue components of the lesion (Fig. 2–24).

Methemoglobin. Methemoglobin in intracellular or extracellular state will be high signal on T1-weighted images, indicating a subacute to chronic hemorrhage[6] (Fig. 2–25*A*).

Flow. Flow-related enhancement or entrance phenomena with unsaturated protons yield high signal on T1-weighted images.[7] This occurs in predictable locations, often in cortical veins over the convexities, or on the first few slices of a spin echo sequence.

Protein. Proteinaceous fluid mixtures will be high signal on T1. The proteins slow the rapid random (brownian) motion of the water to coincide more closely with the electromagnetic frequency, expediting energy relase and promoting relaxation.

Contrast. Gadolinium possesses a magnetic moment many times greater than that of hydrogen protons. The effect is to enhance dramatically the relaxation of adjacent hydrogen protons.

Table 2–3. MRI SIGNAL INTENSITIES

T1	
Short Relaxation Time (High Signal)	***Long Relaxation Time (Low Signal)***
Adipose	Cortical bone
Methemoglobin	Air
Flow-related enhancement	Calcification
Proteinaceous fluid	CSF
Gadolinium	Edema
	High flow
T2	
Long Relaxation Time (High Signal)	***Short Relaxation Time (Low Signal)***
CSF	Cortical bone
Edema	Air
Extracellular methemoglobin	Calcification
Even echo rephasing	Deoxyhemoglobin
	Intracellular methemoglobin
	Hemosiderin-ferritin
	High flow

T1-Weighted Long Relaxation Time (Low Signal)

Bone and Air. Mobile hydrogen protons are not present to any significant degree in cortical bone or air. Accordingly, the signal emitted from these moieties is minimal. The signal intensity of bone marrow, however, is contin-

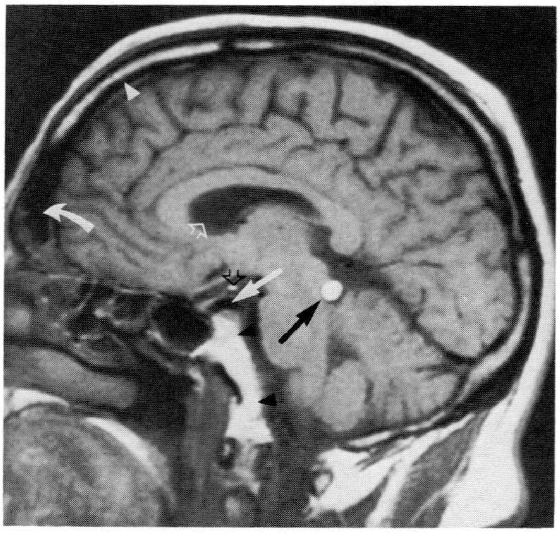

Figure 2–24. T1 signal characteristics—quadrigeminal plate lipoma (43-year-old female). Parasagittal T1; a solitary focus of high signal (*solid black arrow*) represents a quadrigeminal plate lipoma. High-signal lipoid material within the marrow of the clivus (*black arrowheads*) and posterior clinoid (*open black arrow*) is also noted. Foci of low signal include air in the frontal sinus (*curved white arrow*), vascular flow void in the cavernous carotid artery (*straight white arrow*), CSF in the lateral ventricle (*open white arrow*), and cortical bone (*white arrowhead*).

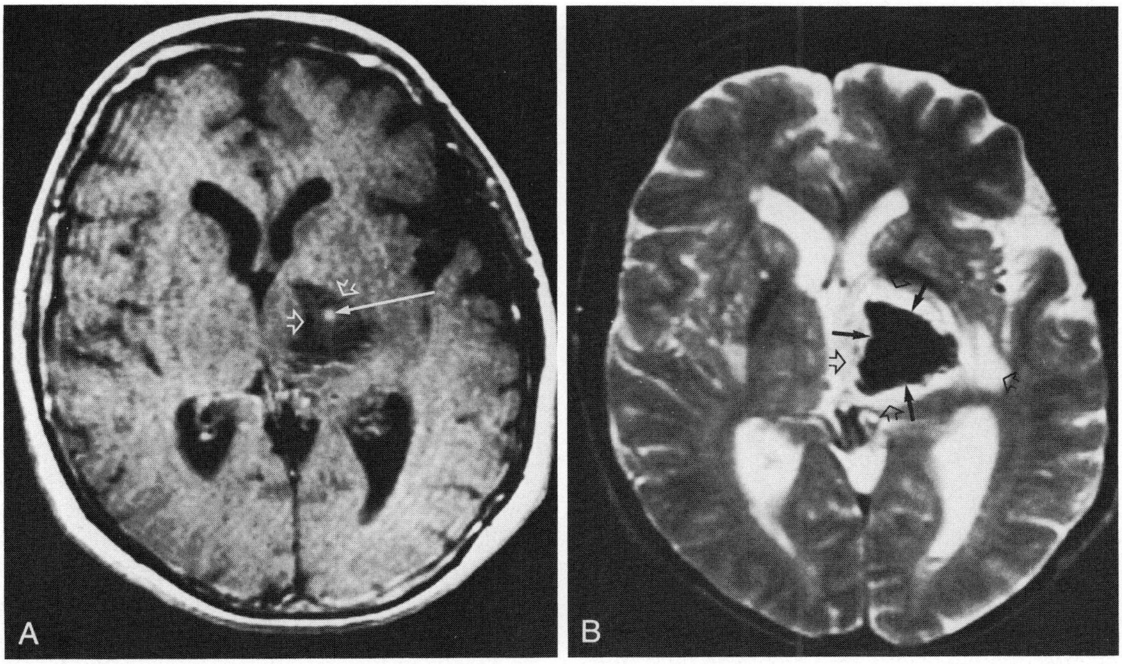

Figure 2–25. Signal characteristics—hypertensive hemorrhage (55-year-old male).

A, Axial T1. A triangular focus of diminished signal (*open arrows*) is present in the left anterior thalamus secondary to deoxyhemoglobin. A central punctate focus of high signal (*solid arrow*) indicates the presence of methemoglobin.

B, Axial T2. The deoxyhemoglobin and intracellular methemoglobin are uniformally low signal (*arrows*) on the T2 spin echo sequence. The surrounding high-signal material (*arrowhead*) represents vasogenic edema or serum or both.

gent on the amount of adipose tissue it contains.

Calcification. Spin echo MRI is relatively insensitive to calcification. Depending on the relationship of the voxel and the size of the calcification, the calcium may not be apparent or may appear as a region of diminished signal.

Fluid. Fluid within cysts or tumors will have diminished signal intensity, often comparable with that of CSF (see Fig. 2–22*B*).

High Flow. Because rapidly moving protons will not emit a signal, they appear as regions of signal void. This may be detected normally in the larger arteries and veins throughout the intracranial space. High-flow states in atypical locations may indicate the presence of highly vascular neoplasms or arteriovenous malformation.

T2-Weighted Long Relaxation Time (High Signal)

Fluid. Fluid present within benign porencephalic or arachnoid cysts and fluid within cystic neoplasms will be of high signal intensity (see Fig. 2–22*C*). Additionally, edema, regardless of etiology, will be high signal on T2-weighted images.

Extracellular Methemoglobin. This will be of high signal intensity on T2-weighted images and indicates the timing of a hemorrhage at least 2 to 4 weeks earlier.[6]

Even Echo Rephasing. Slow, laminar flow appears bright on the second echo of the spin echo sequence owing to the rephasing phenomena that occur.[8]

T2-Weighted Short Relaxation Time (Low Signal)

Bone, Air, Calcification. Lacking mobile hydrogen protons, these structures do not contribute significantly to the MRI signal.

Hemoglobin Degradation Products. Deoxyhemoglobin, intracellular methemoglobin, and hemosiderin-ferritin appear as diminished signal on T2-weighted images secondary to the paramagnetic effects (Fig. 2–25*B*). These products occur in acute, subacute, and chronic hemorrhages, respectively.[6]

High Flow. Signal from rapidly moving blood is negligible.

Multiplicity

Documentation of two or more intracranial lesions will refine the differential diagnosis in any given patient. Multiple lesions are most commonly blood-borne and usually include metastatic disease or infection/abscess (Figs. 2–26, 2–27). Synchronous high-grade gliomas occur in approximately 5% of patients with anaplastic astrocytomas or glioblastoma multiforme. Multiple lesions may be detected with central nervous system (CNS) lymphoma, particularly in the immunosuppressed population.

Pattern of Enhancement

The BBB is an organ-specific protective mechanism that isolates the brain from the systemic circulation. This barrier is found throughout the CNS, excluding the choroid plexus, hypophyseal portal system, pineal gland, area postrema, and falx. The tight junctions (zona occludens) of the endothelium are impervious to high-molecular-weight substances. As a result, iodine or gadolinium tagged to various carrier substances respects the BBB and is denied access to the cerebral parenchyma under normal conditions. Structures that lack a BBB will enhance with contrast.

Certain conditions may temporarily or permanently disrupt the BBB, rendering it ineffective in its task to protect the CNS. These conditions include, but are not limited to, infarction, infection, abscess, neoplasm, and trauma. In response to infarction, tumor, or infection, a vascular growth response (neovascularity) may be initiated. The vessels that develop will not contain a normal BBB. Commercially available iodine- or gadolinium-containing contrast substances have been designed to detect areas of incompetent or absent BBB. Imbibement of contrast into the parenchyma from the vascular system implicates BBB disruption. Although the pattern of enhancement is rarely lesion-specific, it may be helpful in arriving at a realistic differential diagnosis (Table 2–4).

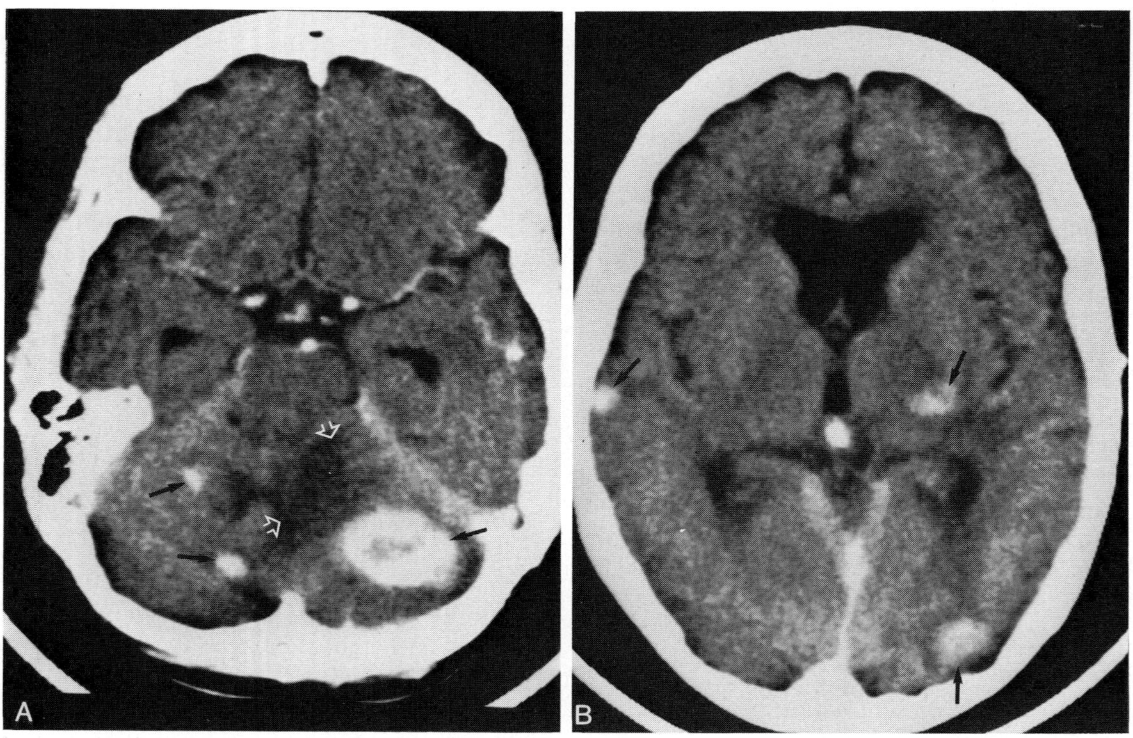

Figure 2–26. Multiplicity—breast metastasis (54-year-old female).

A, B, Enhanced CT. Multiple enhancing lesions (*solid arrows*) are noted within the posterior fossa and supratentorial parenchyma. Vasogenic edema (*open arrows*) accompanies the largest ring-enhancing lesion in the posterior fossa.

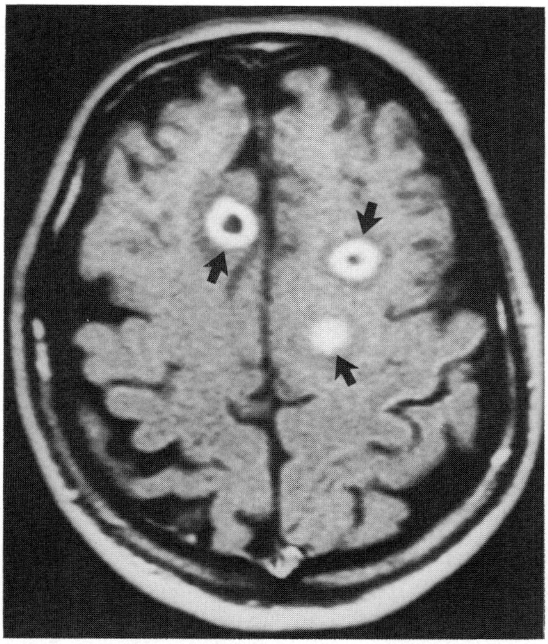

Figure 2–27. Multiplicity—abscess (46-year-old male). Enhanced axial T1; multiple ring-enhancing lesions (*arrows*) are present in the supratentorial parenchyma.

Finally, extra-axial lesions generally do not possess a BBB. These lesions have a blood-tumor interface that usually permits access to the contrast carrier molecule. Certain extra-axial tumors are avascular and thus do not enhance.

Nonenhancing. Some lesions, by virtue of relative benignancy (low-grade gliomas), may coexist without disruption of the BBB (Fig. 2–28). Typically, dermoids, epidermoids, and arachnoid cysts do not enhance significantly.

Table 2–4. ENHANCEMENT PATTERNS

Nonenhancing	Low-grade glioma Arachnoid cyst Epidermoid Cystic meningioma (rare)
Homogeneous	Low- to intermediate-grade glioma Lymphoma Meningioma Infarction (uncommon)
Ring	High-grade glioma Metastasis Abscess Resolving hematoma Infarction (uncommon)
Heterogeneous	High-grade glioma Infarction Cerebritis
Serpentine	Arteriovenous malformation Infarction Cerebritis

Homogeneous. Homogeneous enhancement may occur in any lesion but typically occurs in lymphomas, meningiomas, and intermediate-grade gliomas (Figs. 2–29, 2–30). Infarcts may rarely enhance homogeneously.

Ring. Ring enhancement can herald the presence of an abscess, resolving hematoma, or infarct (Fig. 2–31). High-grade primary neoplasms or metastasis may ring-enhance. Ring enhancement generally indicates necrosis, a common histologic finding in abscess, metastasis, or glioblastoma multiforme.

Heterogeneous. Heterogeneous enhancement occurs commonly in heterogeneous neoplasms, which will contain cystic and/or calcified moieties, or both. Any of the gliomas, particularly the oligodendrogliomas, ependymomas, and higher-grade astrocytomas (Fig. 2–32), may enhance in this fashion. Infarcts and cerebritis may also enhance heterogeneously.

Serpentine. Serpentine enhancement has been described most commonly with infarcts and arteriovenous malformations, but may occur also in cerebritis (Fig. 2–33).

Edema Pattern

Four major types of edema may occur.[9, 10] Although the radiographic appearance of these may overlap to some degree, the pathophysiologies of lesions are unique. As mentioned earlier, edema, regardless of location or etiology, is hypodense on CT. The MRI equivalent is of high signal intensity on T2-weighted spin echo images and has a subtle hypointensity relative to white matter on T1-weighted images.

Vasogenic. Vasogenic edema results from disruption of the BBB and osmosis of fluid from the systemic vascular pool into the extracellular space. Vasogenic edema is white matter edema. The fluid will infiltrate along the loose white matter matrix (association fibers), respecting the gray-white junction and certain, compactly arranged white matter tracts (commissural fibers).[11] The radiographic correlate is edema of the white matter, which outlines the gray-white junction, sparing the cortex. Attendant mass effect is present (Figs. 2–34, 2–35).

Ischemic. Ischemic edema results from inability to fuel the sodium-potassium cellular

Text continued on page 66

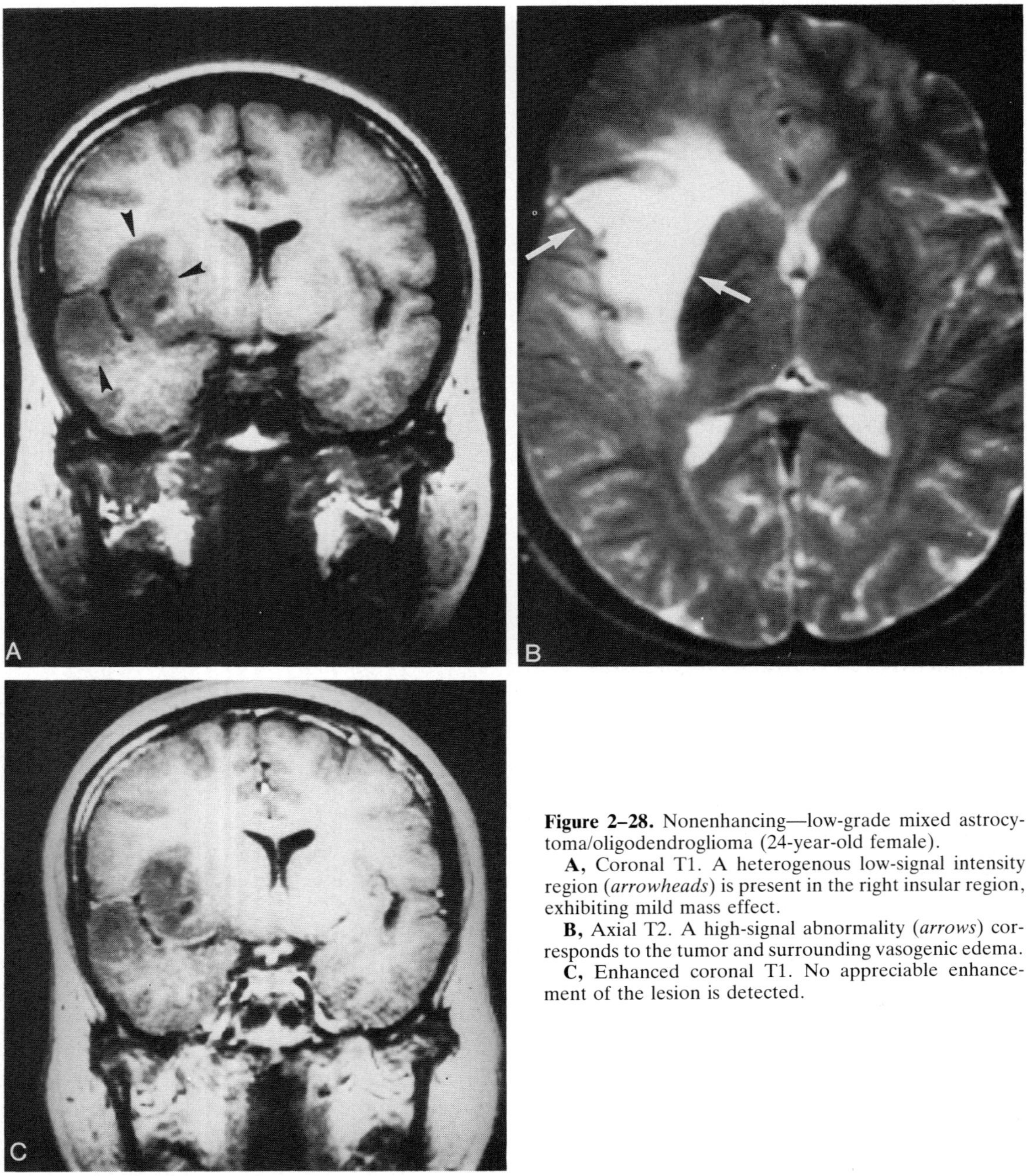

Figure 2–28. Nonenhancing—low-grade mixed astrocytoma/oligodendroglioma (24-year-old female).

A, Coronal T1. A heterogenous low-signal intensity region (*arrowheads*) is present in the right insular region, exhibiting mild mass effect.

B, Axial T2. A high-signal abnormality (*arrows*) corresponds to the tumor and surrounding vasogenic edema.

C, Enhanced coronal T1. No appreciable enhancement of the lesion is detected.

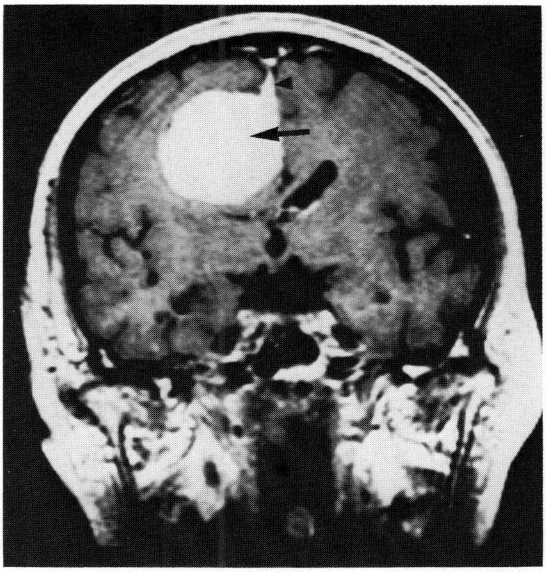

Figure 2–29. Homogeneous enhancement—meningioma (65-year-old female). Enhanced coronal T1; a homogeneously enhancing mass (*arrow*) arises from the falx. Adjacent dural enhancement (*arrowhead*), although not specific, corroborates the diagnosis of meningioma.

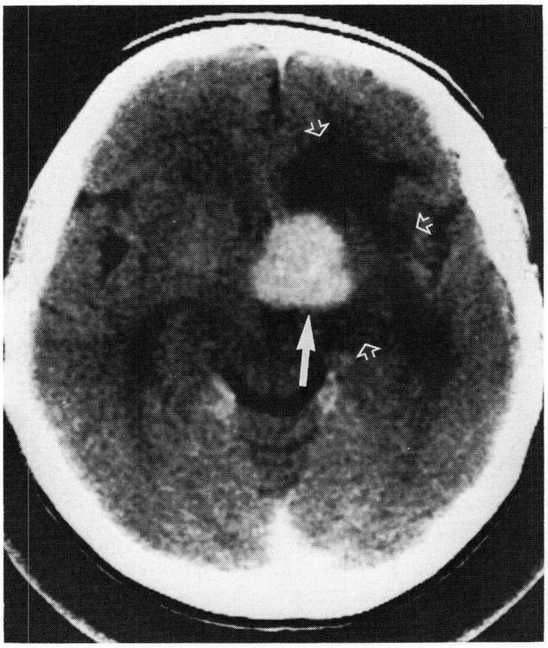

Figure 2–30. Homogeneous enhancement—lymphoma (40-year-old female). Enhanced CT; a solitary homogeneously enhancing hypothalamic lymphoma (*solid arrow*) is present with surrounding vasogenic edema (*open arrows*).

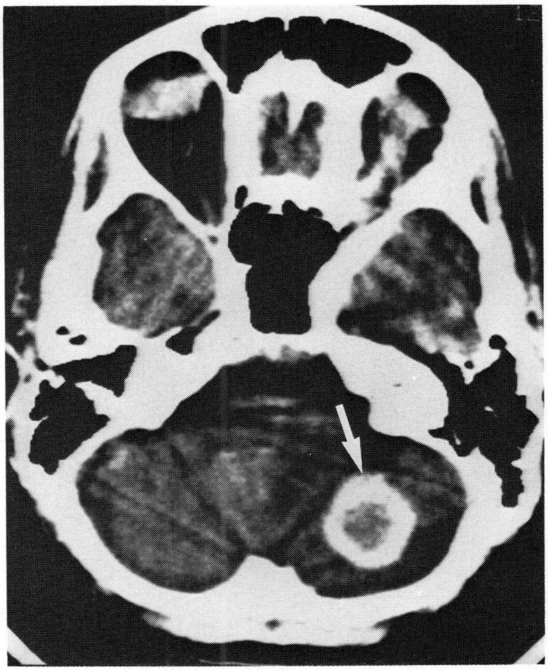

Figure 2–31. Ring enhancement—breast metastasis (54-year-old female). Enhanced CT; a solitary ring-enhancing lesion (*arrow*) is present in the left cerebellar hemisphere.

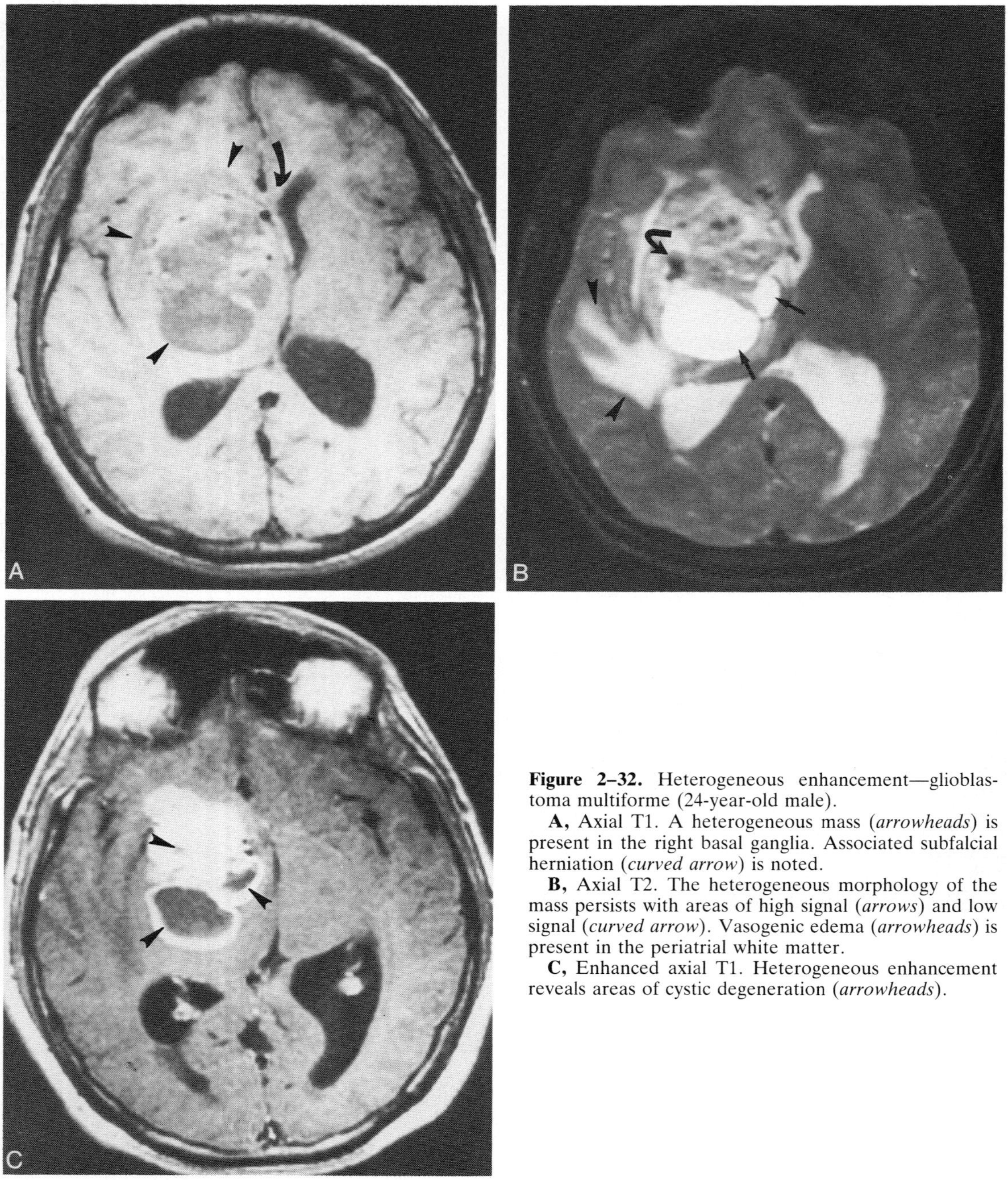

Figure 2–32. Heterogeneous enhancement—glioblastoma multiforme (24-year-old male).

A, Axial T1. A heterogeneous mass (*arrowheads*) is present in the right basal ganglia. Associated subfalcial herniation (*curved arrow*) is noted.

B, Axial T2. The heterogeneous morphology of the mass persists with areas of high signal (*arrows*) and low signal (*curved arrow*). Vasogenic edema (*arrowheads*) is present in the periatrial white matter.

C, Enhanced axial T1. Heterogeneous enhancement reveals areas of cystic degeneration (*arrowheads*).

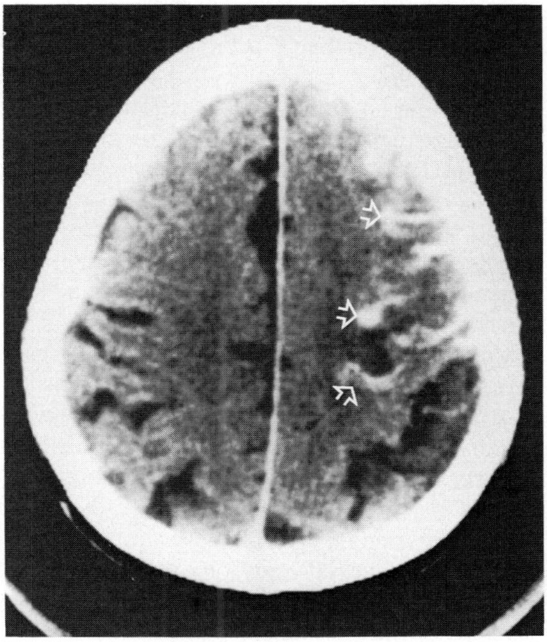

Figure 2–33. Serpentine enhancement—subacute infarct (75-year-old male). Enhanced CT; serpentine gyral enhancement (*open arrows*) is noted within the left middle cerebral artery distribution involving the parietal lobe.

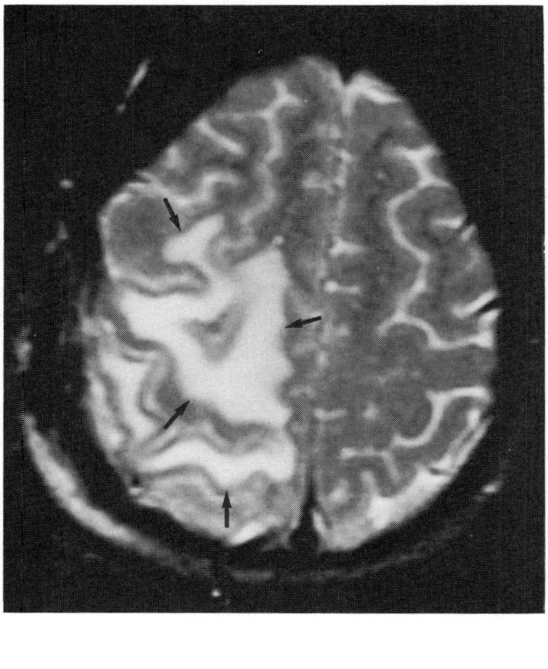

Figure 2–34. Vasogenic edema—anaplastic astrocytoma (40-year-old male). Axial T2; high-signal vasogenic edema (*arrows*) extends throughout the parietal vertex, sparing the cortical gray matter.

pump with oxygen. As a result, the sodium-potassium gradient is disrupted and sodium enters the cell with resultant osmosis of the extracellular water into the cell. The accumulation of intracellular fluid precipitates cellular swelling and further migration of water into the intracellular and extracellular spaces from the vascular system. Cross-sectional imaging initially reveals a subtle loss of the gray-white junction. The edema accumulates in both the gray and the white matter, often in a wedge shape with concomitant mass effect (Figs. 2–36, 2–37). Arterial infarcts generally conform to single-vessel distribution, respecting arterial border zones.

Cytotoxic. Cytotoxic edema results from a serious global anoxic-hypoxic episode, may be post-traumatic in origin,[12, 13] and in many ways is like ischemic edema. The fluid is intracellular and extracellular, but the edema is noted in a diffuse supratentorial distribution rather than respecting a single arterial distribution (Fig. 2–38). The "reversal sign" may be noted, in which the white matter becomes of greater density on CT than the gray matter. This pattern of edema heralds advanced irreversible brain damage.[14] The posterior fossa, for reasons not completely elucidated, remains normal, spared from this supratentorial event.

Periventricular Interstitial. Communicating or noncommunicating hydrocephalus may cause enlargement of the ventricles and elevation of the intraventricular pressure. This may result in stretching or tearing of the ventricular ependymal lining. The threshold of the ependyma to maintain fluid within the ventricular system is exceeded. Extracellular fluid accumulates within the periventricular white matter adjacent to the frontal horns and later along the bodies of the lateral ventricles. As a result, the margins of the frontal horns become indistinct as they merge imperceptibly with the hypodense periventricular white matter on CT. T2 MRI demonstrates confluent high signal extending a variable degree from the ventricular surface into the periventricular white matter. Spin density (long TR/short TE) will differentiate the high-signal periventricular edema from the lower-signal ventricular CSF (Fig. 2–39).

References

1. Carpenter MB, Sutin J: *Human Neuroanatomy,* 8th ed. 1983; Williams & Wilkins, Baltimore.
2. Curnes JT: MR imaging of peripheral intracranial neoplasms: Extraaxial versus intraaxial masses. J Comput Assist Tomogr 1987; 11:932–937.
3. Osborne AG: Diagnosis of descending transtentorial herniation by cranial computed tomography. Radiology 1977; 123:93–96.
4. Osborne AG, Heaston DK, Wing SD: Diagnosis of ascending transtentorial herniation by cranial computed tomography. AJR 1978; 130:755–760.
5. Hahn FJ, Witte RJ: CT signs of ascending transtentorial cerebellar herniation. J Comput Assist Tomogr 1989; 13:1091–1092.
6. Gomori JM, Grossman RI, Goldberg HI, et al: Intracranial hematomas: Imaging by high field MR. Radiology 1985; 157:87–93.
7. Bradley WG, Waluch V: Blood flow: Magnetic resonance imaging. Radiology 1985; 154:443–450.
8. Waluch V, Bradley WG: NMR even echo rephasing in slow laminar flow. J Comput Assist Tomogr 1984; 8:594–598.
9. Drayer BP, Rosenbaum AE: Brain edema defined by cranial computed tomography. J Comput Assist Tomogr 1979; 3:317–323.
10. Weisberg L, Greenberg J, Stazio A: Computed tomographic findings in brain swelling. Computerized Med Imaging and Graphics 1990; 14:263–268.
11. Cowley AR: Influence of fiber tracts on the CT appearance of cerebral edema: Anatomic-pathologic correlation. AJNR 1983; 4:915–925.
12. Zimmerman RA, Bilaniuk LT, Bruce D, et al: Computed tomography of pediatric head trauma: Acute general cerebral swelling. Radiology 1978; 126:403–408.
13. Lobato RD, Sarabia R, Cordobes F, et al: Post traumatic cerebral hemispheric swelling. J Neurosurg 1988; 68:417–423.
14. Han BK, Towbia RB, DeCouten-Myers G, et al: Reversal sign on CT: Effects of anoxic/ischemic cerebral injury in children. AJNR 1989; 10:1191–1198.

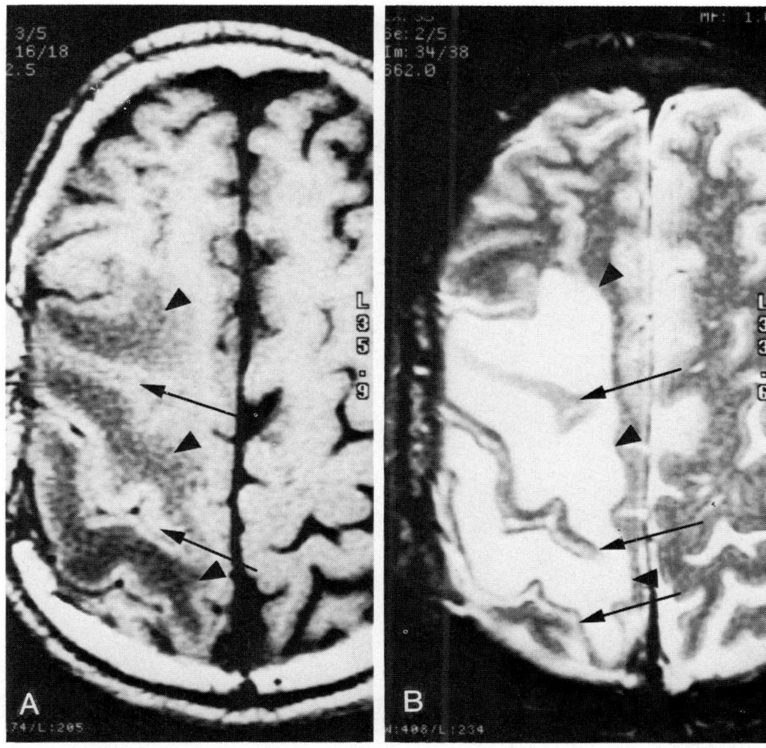

Figure 2–35. Vasogenic edema—anaplastic astrocytoma (54-year-old male).

A, Axial T1. The gray matter (*arrows*) of the right parietal lobe is preserved, and hypointense vasogenic edema (*arrowheads*) is present in the subadjacent white matter. The sulci are effaced, indicating mass effect.

B, Axial T2. The full extent of the vasogenic edema (*arrowheads*) is more conspicuous, silhouetting the preserved gray matter (*arrows*).

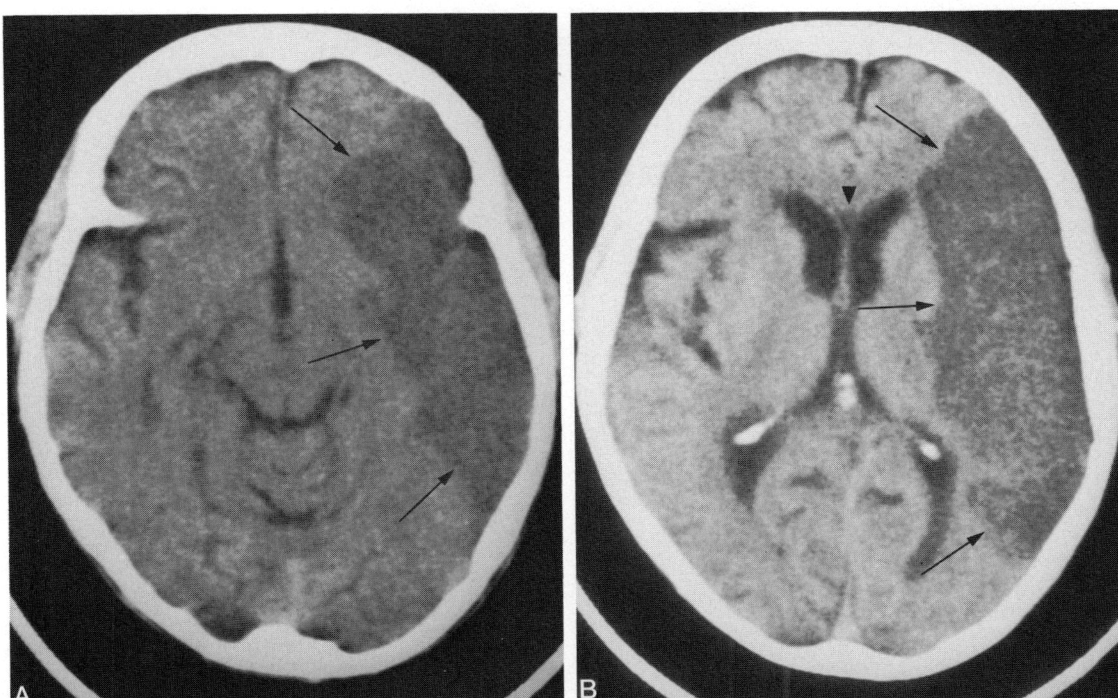

Figure 2–36. Ischemic edema—subacute infarct (62-year-old female).

A, Unenhanced CT. A wedge-shaped hypodensity (*arrows*) extends to the inner table, with loss of the gray-white junction.

B, Unenhanced CT. The ischemic edema (*arrows*) conforms to the middle cerebral artery distribution, involving the gray matter and the white matter. The cortical sulci are compressed, and there is slight subfalcial herniation (*arrowhead*) signifying a moderate degree of mass effect.

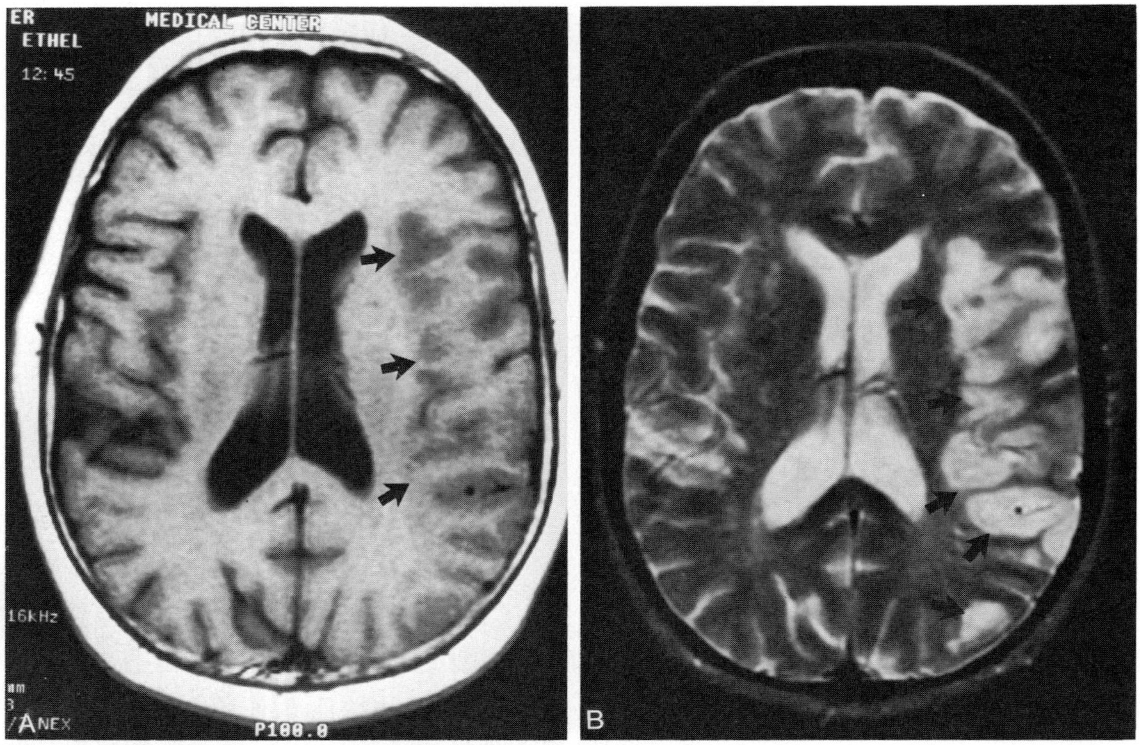

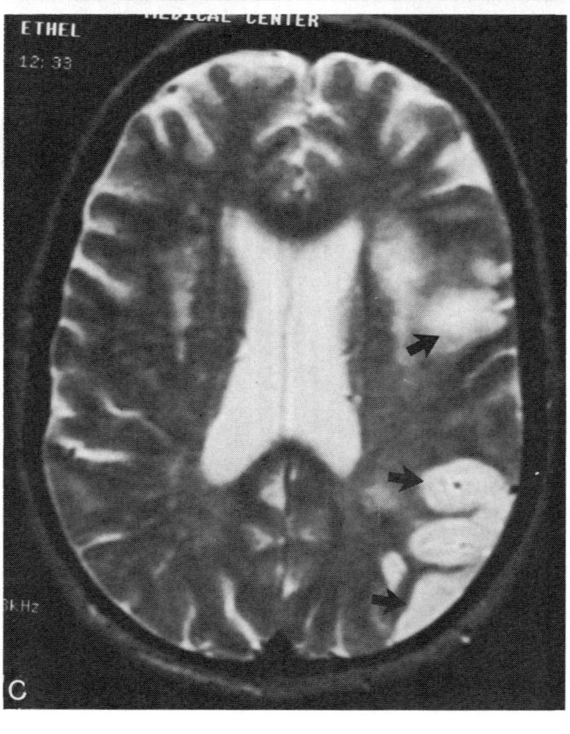

Figure 2–37. Ischemic edema—subacute infarction (71-year-old female).

A, Axial T1. Subtle decreased signal and local mass effect are present (*arrows*), effacing the sulci of the left sylvian fissure.

B, C, Axial T2. The cortical distribution and extent of the infarct (*arrows*) are more apparent on the long TR images.

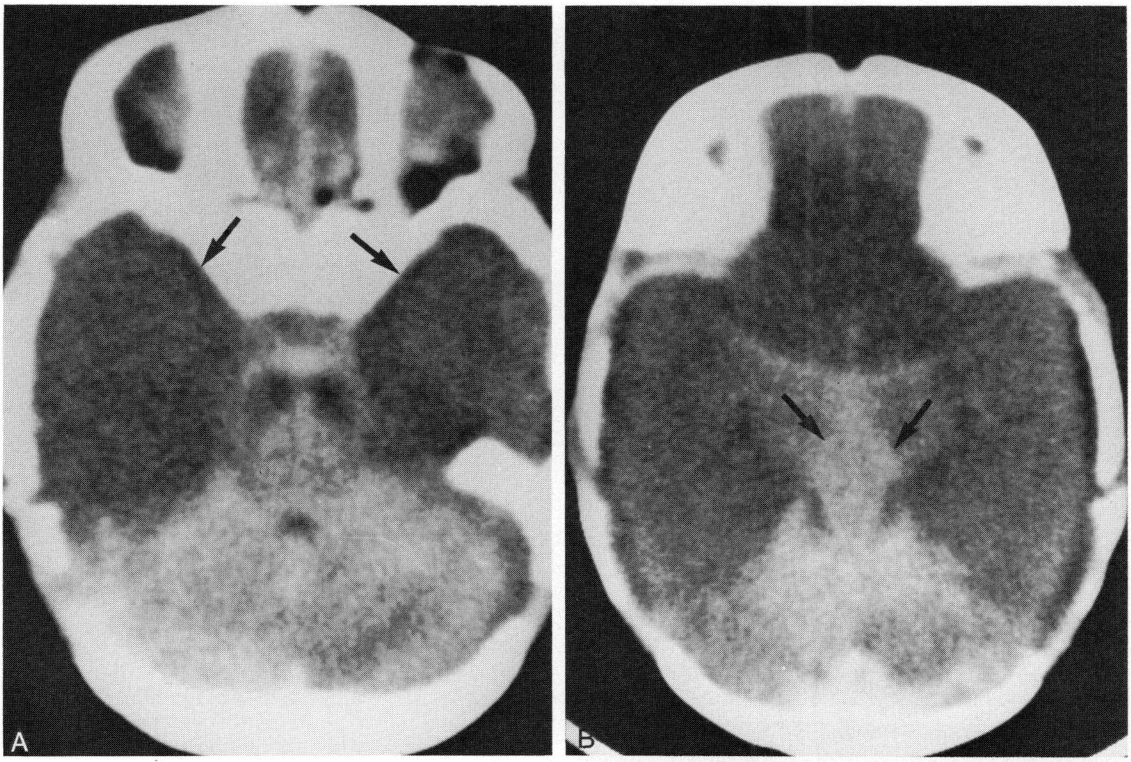

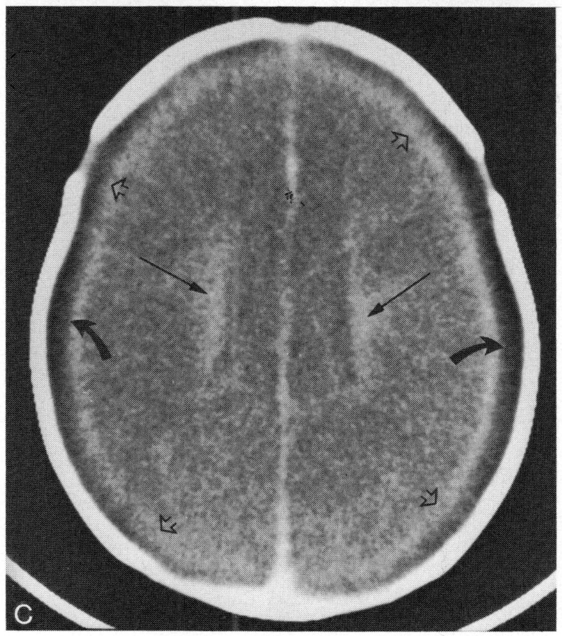

Figure 2–38. Cytotoxic edema—trauma (5-month-old female).

A, Unenhanced CT. The temporal lobes (*arrows*) are markedly hypodense compared with the normal-density cerebellum.

B, Unenhanced CT. This pattern persists with relative sparing of the brainstem (*arrows*).

C, Unenhanced CT. The deep white matter (*arrows*) is hyperdense, the gray-white junction (*open arrows*) is obscured, and bilateral subdural fluid collections (*curved arrow*) complicate this severe global ischemic process.

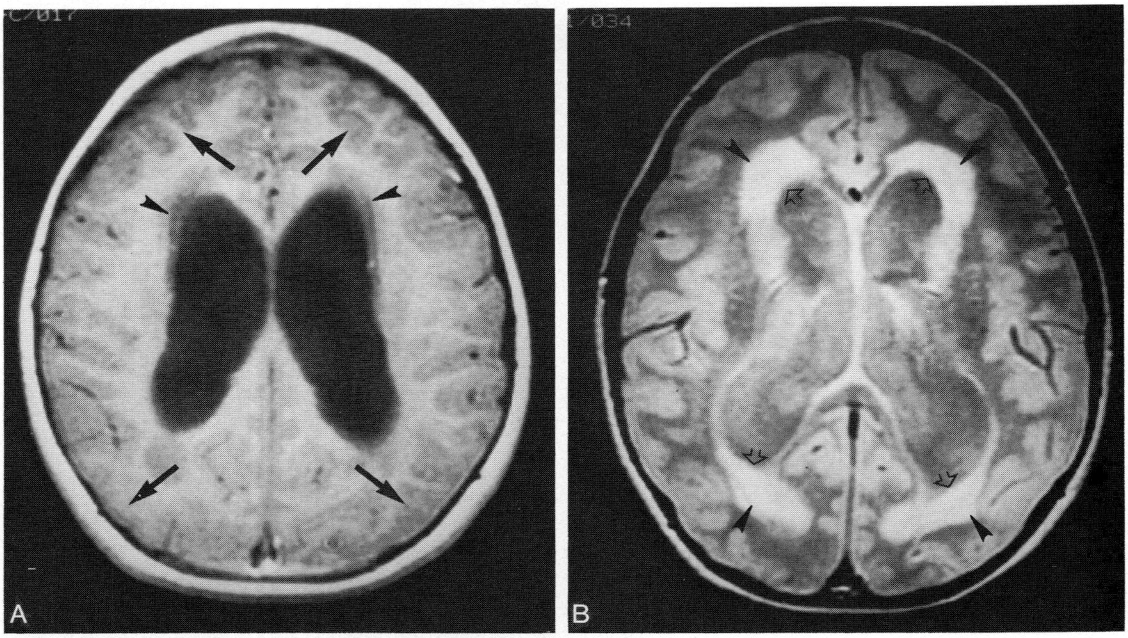

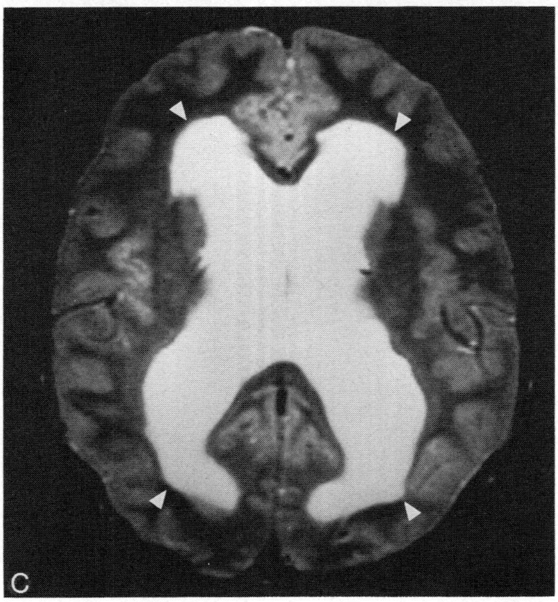

Figure 2–39. Periventricular interstitial edema—craniopharyngioma (8-year-old male).

A, Axial T1. The lateral ventricles are enlarged and the cortical sulci (*arrows*) effaced. Subtle foci of decreased attenuation (*arrowheads*) outline the anterior portions of the bodies of the lateral ventricles.

B, Axial SD. The periventricular interstitial edema is manifested as confluent foci of high signal (*arrowheads*) extending from the lateral ventricles (*open arrows*) into the periventricular white matter. The interface between the ventricular surface and edema is apparent on this imaging sequence.

C, Axial T2. The periventricular interstitial edema (*arrowheads*) is isointense to CSF and merges imperceptibly with the lateral ventricles.

3

INTRACRANIAL NEOPLASMS AND TUMORLIKE CONDITIONS

In this chapter, intracranial tumors and tumorlike conditions are presented using a biphasic approach. Based on histologic features, gliomas, lymphomas, gangliogliomas, and metastasis are discussed. Other lesions are presented using a location approach. Tumors that occur most commonly in the pediatric population or have radiographic features unique to the pediatric population are discussed in Chapter 13.

HISTOLOGIC APPROACH

Glioma

Glial cells form the matrix of the parenchyma and generally function as supportive cells for the neurons. A wide variety of glial cell neoplasms may occur, each of which may exhibit varying degrees of cellular atypia. Gliomas represent the most common primary malignancy of the central nervous system

(CNS); the most common type of glioma is the astrocytoma.

Astrocytoma

The astrocytic series encompasses a wide spectrum of neoplasms, ranging from relatively benign to highly malignant. Contingent on the presence or absence of necrosis, mitosis, and cellular atypia, tumors may be classified into low-grade and high-grade lesions. This histologic distinction of relative malignancy has significant prognostic implications. Certain radiographic findings are successful in classifying these tumors.

Low-Grade Astrocytomas

The astrocytes differ morphologically in different locations of the brain. Protoplasmic astrocytes are found in the middle layers of the cortex and basal ganglia. Fibrillary astrocytes reside in the superficial and deep layers of the cortex, as well as in the white matter. In response to non-neoplastic processes, fibrillary astrocytes may become "reactive" and in the process enlarge, resulting in gemistiocytic cells, or become thinned and elongated, resulting in pilocytic astrocytes. Any of these cells may give rise to cell line–specific astrocytomas.

The low-grade astrocytomas represent approximately 25% of all gliomas.[1] These lesions are slightly more common in men and generally occur between the ages of 25 and 45 years. On unenhanced computed tomography (CT), these lesions are of variable size and are generally homogeneous in density (Fig. 3–1). The tumors tend to be hypodense in approximately 50% of patients.[2] Focal areas of calcification occur in approximately 35% of cases.[2] Peritumoral edema may be absent or minimal. The absence of edema sometimes renders the margins of these lesions somewhat indistinct. Hemorrhage rarely occurs in low-grade gliomas. The tumor may enhance minimally or not at all following intravenous (IV) contrast administration.

The magnetic resonance imaging (MRI) correlate displays a lesion that is typically hypointense to surrounding parenchyma on T1 images and hyperintense to parenchyma on T2 images (Fig. 3–2). MRI is more sensitive than CT at detection of these lesions.[3]

The tumor is generally relatively well defined and appears homogeneous on MRI.[4] Peritumoral edema and contrast enhancement, although minimal, will be more conspicuous on MRI than on CT. Enhancement on MRI has been reported in approximately 16% of these lesions.[5]

Anaplastic Astrocytoma

In comparison with low-grade malignancies, anaplastic astrocytomas undergo increased mitotic rates, display more cellular atypia and nuclear pleomorphism, and promote vascular endothelial proliferation. These tumors usually occur more frequently in men than in women. The peak incidence is at 46 years.[6] Average survival following diagnosis is approximately 2 years.

On CT these lesions are more dense and heterogeneous than the low-grade astrocytomas. Because of the vascular endothelial proliferation, vasogenic edema and mass effect are more common in these lesions. Focal cystic areas may be identified within the tumor. These tumors enhance heterogeneously (Fig. 3–3).

MRI depicts a less well-defined lesion with moderate vasogenic edema and resultant mass effect. The lesion is more heterogeneous than its low-grade counterpart,[4] usually remaining low signal on T1 and high signal on T2 sequences.

Glioblastoma Multiforme

The histologic feature that distinguishes glioblastoma multiforme (GBM) from anaplastic astrocytomas is the presence of necrosis. This is the most common tumor of the astrocytic series. The peak incidence of GBM is at 50 to 60 years of age.[6] The lesion occurs more commonly in men. The average survival following diagnosis is less than 1 year.

The degree of heterogeneity, mass effect, and edema increase in these high-grade neoplasms.[2] Focal areas of calcification are less common in GBM. Contrast enhancement occurs in nearly every case and may be ringlike, revealing central areas of necrosis and cyst

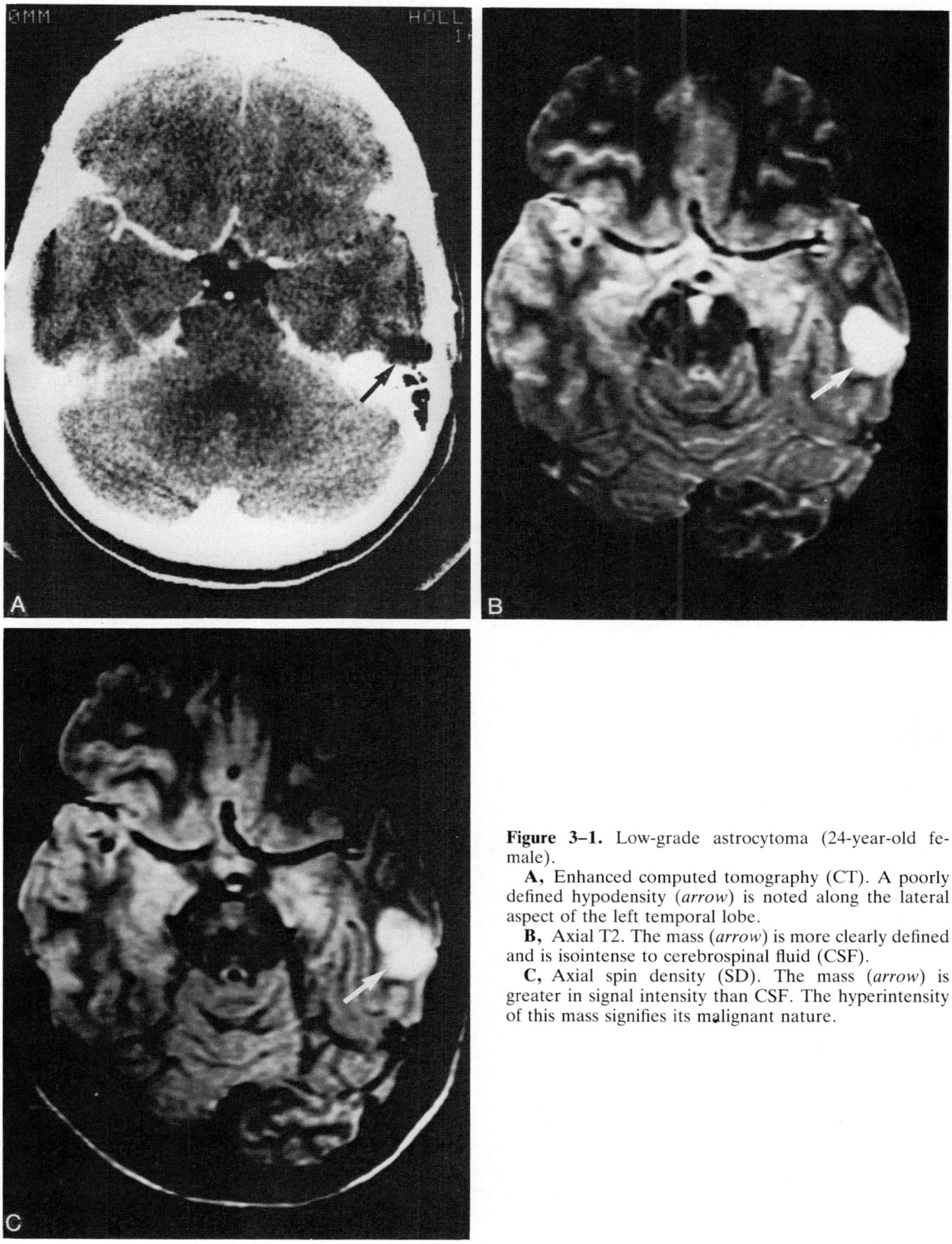

Figure 3–1. Low-grade astrocytoma (24-year-old female).

A, Enhanced computed tomography (CT). A poorly defined hypodensity (*arrow*) is noted along the lateral aspect of the left temporal lobe.

B, Axial T2. The mass (*arrow*) is more clearly defined and is isointense to cerebrospinal fluid (CSF).

C, Axial spin density (SD). The mass (*arrow*) is greater in signal intensity than CSF. The hyperintensity of this mass signifies its malignant nature.

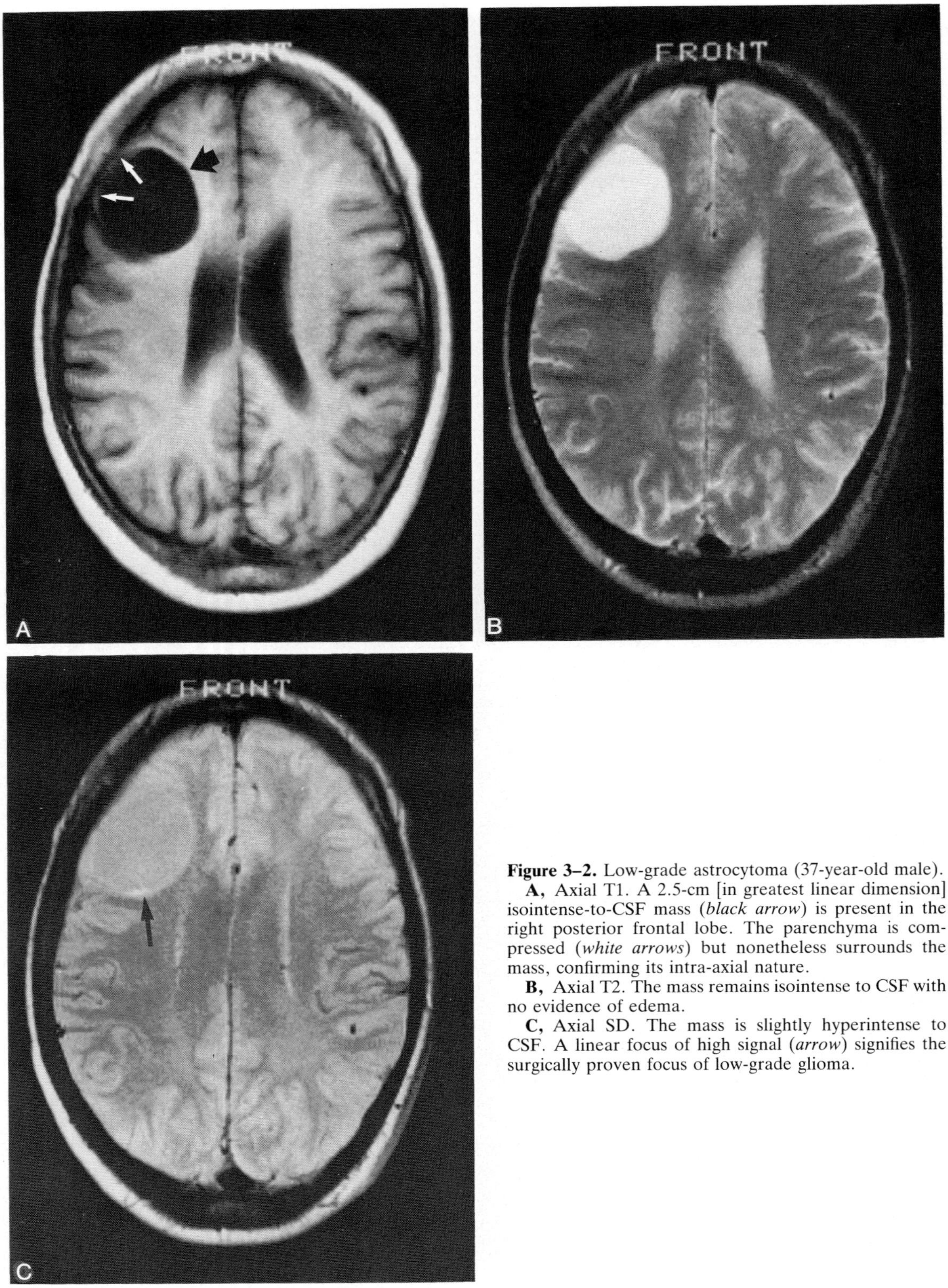

Figure 3–2. Low-grade astrocytoma (37-year-old male).

A, Axial T1. A 2.5-cm [in greatest linear dimension] isointense-to-CSF mass (*black arrow*) is present in the right posterior frontal lobe. The parenchyma is compressed (*white arrows*) but nonetheless surrounds the mass, confirming its intra-axial nature.

B, Axial T2. The mass remains isointense to CSF with no evidence of edema.

C, Axial SD. The mass is slightly hyperintense to CSF. A linear focus of high signal (*arrow*) signifies the surgically proven focus of low-grade glioma.

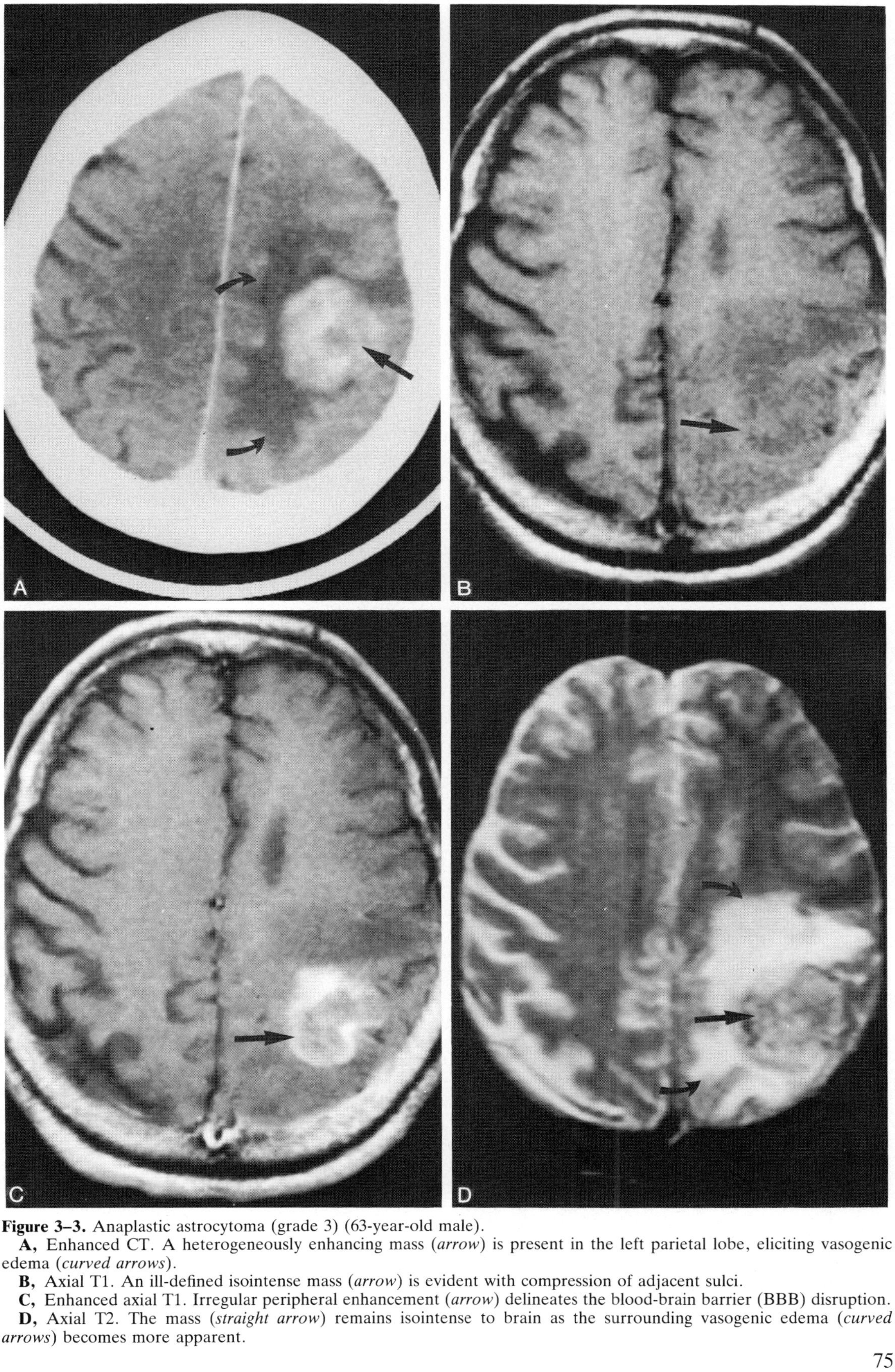

Figure 3–3. Anaplastic astrocytoma (grade 3) (63-year-old male).

A, Enhanced CT. A heterogeneously enhancing mass (*arrow*) is present in the left parietal lobe, eliciting vasogenic edema (*curved arrows*).

B, Axial T1. An ill-defined isointense mass (*arrow*) is evident with compression of adjacent sulci.

C, Enhanced axial T1. Irregular peripheral enhancement (*arrow*) delineates the blood-brain barrier (BBB) disruption.

D, Axial T2. The mass (*straight arrow*) remains isointense to brain as the surrounding vasogenic edema (*curved arrows*) becomes more apparent.

formation.[2] Like lymphomas, GBMs have a predilection to extend through the corpus callosum. The tumor is then called a "butterfly glioma" (Fig. 3–4).

MRI depicts a markedly heterogeneous lesion of mixed signal intensity on T1-weighted images (Fig. 3–5). Central areas of diminished signal are common, with more solid isointense material forming the periphery. Most often the tumor enhances heterogeneously. Synchronous tumors (two or more lesions at once) occur exclusively in anaplastic astrocytomas or GBM. Metachronous lesions (two or more lesions separated by time) more commonly occur in the higher-grade lesions, yet may occur in the lower-grade astrocytomas as well.[7]

Oligodendroglioma

The oligodendroglial cells are the support cells that produce and maintain the myelin that surrounds the neurons. Oligodendrogliomas represent 4 to 7% of all primary gliomas.[8, 9]

The neoplasms are relatively benign, slow-growing tumors that occur with equal prevalence in both sexes, at an average age of 35 years.[8] Patients usually present with seizures and headaches. The relative benignancy of this lesion explains a prolonged duration of symptoms (usually 15 years) before diagnosis is established. Although a frontal lobe predilection has been reported,[8] these lesions may occur throughout the supratentorial subcortical white matter.

Fifty percent of oligodendrogliomas are composed of a histologically "pure" cell population. In the remainder, mixed forms of the tumor exist, usually with varying amounts of astrocytic cells present.

Although calcification has been reported in up to 91%,[10] most series report a lower incidence (40%) of calcification.[8] The calcification may appear as clumps or flecks. The lesion will contain single or multiple cystic components in 20% of cases.

CT depicts an isodense-to-hypodense peripheral lesion that may contain calcification (Fig. 3–6). The degree of edema is variable though usually minimal. Hemorrhage into this tumor may also occur. The mixed form of oligodendroglioma carries the highest incidence of spontaneous hemorrhage of the glial series, at 29%.[6] Owing to the peripheral location and slow-growing nature of the lesion, erosion of the inner table has been reported in up to 17% of cases.[8] At least a mild degree

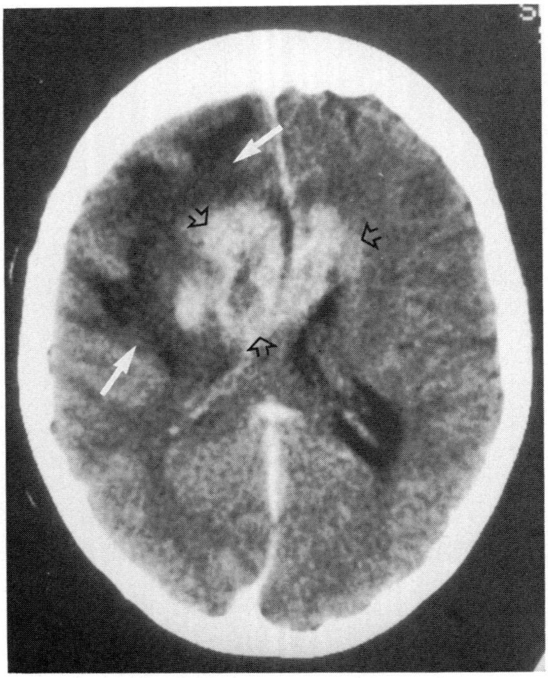

Figure 3–4. Butterfly glioma (64-year-old male). Enhanced CT; a heterogeneously enhancing mass (*open arrows*) crosses the genu of the corpus callosum. Vasogenic edema (*white arrows*) and mass effect are present.

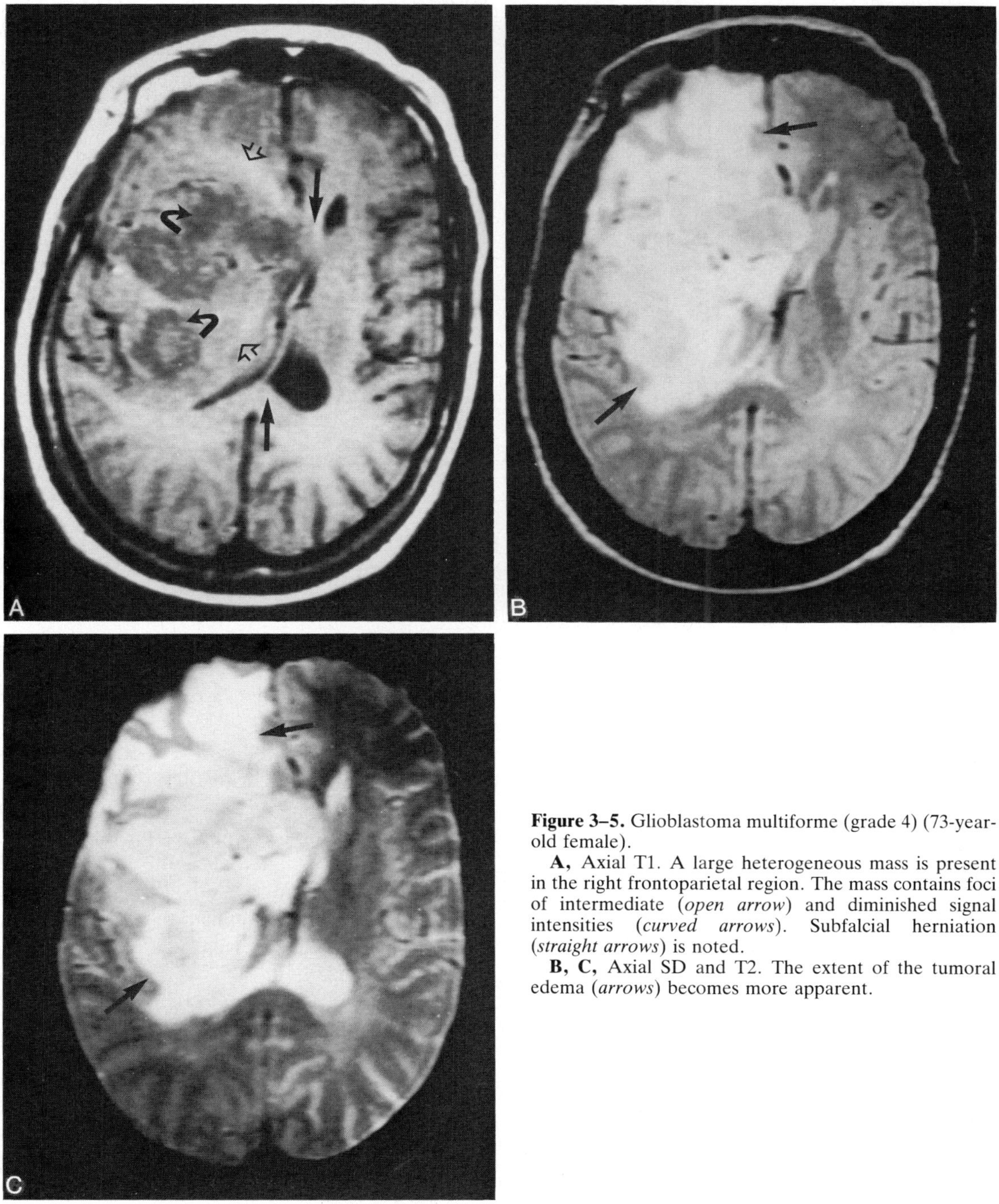

Figure 3–5. Glioblastoma multiforme (grade 4) (73-year-old female).

A, Axial T1. A large heterogeneous mass is present in the right frontoparietal region. The mass contains foci of intermediate (*open arrow*) and diminished signal intensities (*curved arrows*). Subfalcial herniation (*straight arrows*) is noted.

B, C, Axial SD and T2. The extent of the tumoral edema (*arrows*) becomes more apparent.

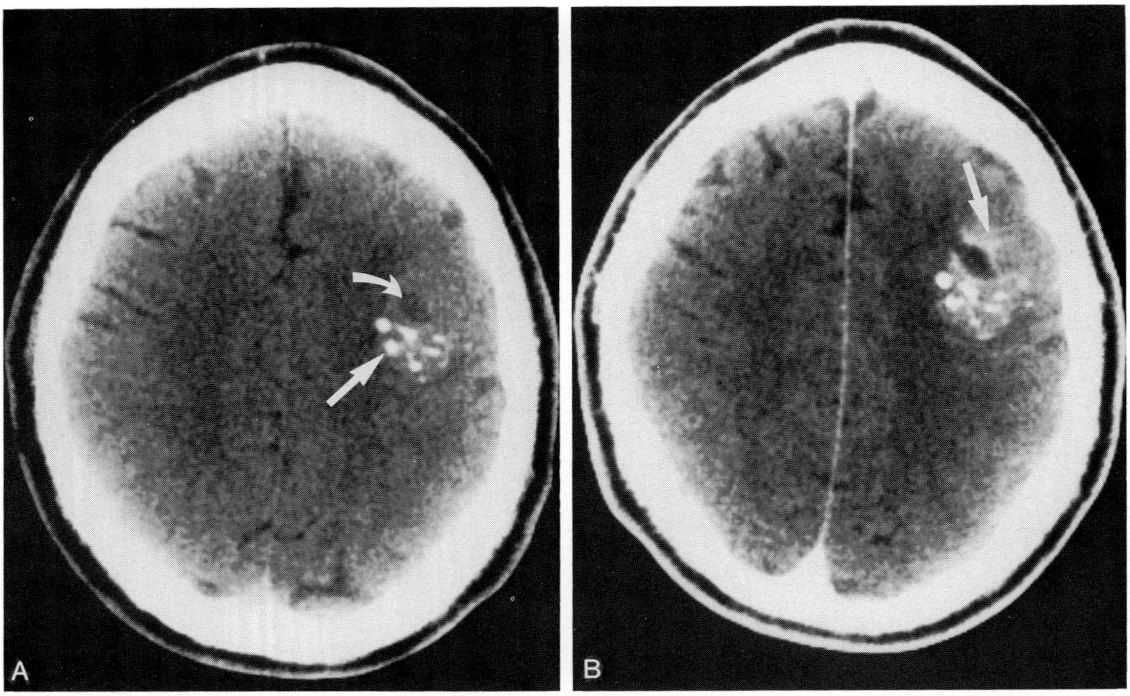

Figure 3–6. Oligodendroglioma (47-year-old male).
A, Unenhanced CT. A heterogeneous mass is located in the subcortical posterior left frontal lobe. The mass contains foci of calcification (*straight arrow*) and a focal cystic component (*curved arrow*).
B, Enhanced CT. The solid component of the tumor (*arrow*) enhances. Vasogenic edema is not a feature of this low-grade neoplasm.

of enhancement has been reported in 50% of these lesions.

MRI depicts the tumor as diminished signal on T1 and increased signal on T2 images (Fig. 3–7). The calcification may be inapparent or may appear as regions of diminished signal.[11] Cystic components of the tumor will have further diminished T1 and increased T2 signal intensity. The heterogeneous pattern of enhancement is more apparent on MRI than on CT.

Ependymoma

Ependymomas represent 0.3 to 6% of intracranial neoplasms. These tumors are most common in the posterior fossa in children, who almost invariably present with signs and symptoms of hydrocephalus. Posterior fossa ependymomas are described in more detail in Chapter 13. When ependymomas occur in adults, they are more frequently supratentorial in location and more commonly originate in the cerebral white matter (75 to 83%) than within the ventricular system.[12, 13]

The typical CT appearance of supratentorial ependymoma is that of a large parenchymal mass. The mass may exceed 4 cm in greatest linear dimension in 94% of cases[12] and is relatively heterogeneous with areas of cyst formation and diminished density in 56 to 83%.[12, 13] Tumor calcification has been reported in 30 to 50% of cases.[12, 13] Peritumoral edema is present in 30% and the margins of the tumor are well defined or moderately well defined in 75%.[12] Although hydrocephalus is a prevalent feature of the infratentorial lesion in children, hydrocephalus is present with only 50% of adult supratentorial tumors.[12] Enhancement will occur in nearly every lesion and is more likely to be heterogeneous or ringlike (Fig. 3–8).

The MRI signal characteristics of these lesions are nonspecific. Most commonly these lesions are hypointense on T1 and hyperintense on T2 images.[14] Cysts will appear isointense or hyperintense to cerebrospinal fluid (CSF) on T1 and T2 images. The calcification, if detectable, will appear as regions of relative signal void. Tumor delineation, spread, edema, and enhancement pattern are depicted more accurately on MRI than on CT.

Subependymoma

Subependymomas are slow-growing, relatively benign neoplasms composed of a mixture of astrocytes and ependymal cells. These tumors typically occur in the posterior fossa within or adjacent to the fourth ventricle.[15, 16] The tumor may displace the fourth ventricle anteriorly and superiorly and extend into the cerebellar vermis.[15] Less commonly, these lesions may occur adjacent to the third ventricle.[2]

The lesion is most frequently detected as an incidental finding at autopsy. If symptoms occur, they are usually related to the obstruction of CSF, with unsteadiness, vertigo, and vomiting.

The tumors are usually isodense to brain on CT,[15, 17] although cystic components have been described.[2] Calcification may occur in up to 50% of cases,[15] with homogeneous enhancement in 90%.[15] The tumor is relatively well-demarcated without evidence of infiltration. Hydrocephalus occurs in approximately 90% of clinically symptomatic patients.[15]

The MRI appearance of subependymoma is nonspecific. The tumor tends to be homogeneous and hyperintense to brain on T2 images. Calcification may be detected as areas of diminished signal. Cystic areas will have prolonged T1 and T2 relaxation times.

Lymphoma

Primary CNS lymphoma accounts for 0.2 to 2% of all primary CNS malignancies.[18, 19] Its incidence may be increasing, owing to an increase in the acquired immune deficiency syndrome (AIDS) and immunosuppressed patient populations.

Lymphoma has been reported to occur more commonly in men.[19–22] Although this lesion may occur at any age, it most frequently occurs in elderly patients between 50 and 65 years of age. Clinically, the patient may present with neurologic deficits including deterioration of intellect, decreased level of consciousness, and increased intracranial pressure or seizures.[21, 22] Headache, nausea, and vomiting also may be presenting features.[20]

Primary CNS lymphomas are usually non-Hodgkin's tumors and may be composed of one of 10 histologic types.[23] The most common variety is diffuse large-cell lymphoma. The radiographic characteristics of the histologic subtypes are not specific. The lesion may occur within the supratentorial or infratentorial parenchyma with a high incidence (75%) reported to be in contact with either the ependyma or the meninges.[23] The lesions commonly originate in the basal ganglia and periventricular white matter,[18] the subcortical white matter,[19] and the posterior fossa.[23]

The lesions are usually solitary and isodense-to-hyperdense to normal parenchyma on CT.[18–20, 22, 25] Enhancement occurs in nearly every case and is most commonly homogeneous,[19, 20, 22, 24, 25] although ring enhancement has been reported.[23] Edema is a variable feature and often not a prevalent characteristic of the tumor. Like GBM, lymphoma will extend through the corpus callosum to involve both hemispheres (Fig. 3–9).

MRI depicts a lesion isointense-to-hypointense to gray matter on T1 images. The lesion is hyperintense to gray matter on T2 images.[18] Peritumoral edema and enhancement are conspicuous on spin echo T2 and T1 sequences, respectively (Fig. 3–10).

Primary CNS lymphoma that occurs in AIDS patients may differ from that detected in non-AIDS patients.[18, 25, 26] The lesions tend to be multiple, to measure more than 2 cm in greatest linear dimension, to enhance in a homogeneous or ring fashion, and to be located more often in the temporal lobe and basal ganglia in AIDS patients.

Ganglioglioma

Gangliogliomas, tumors of children and young adults, account for less than 1% of all intracranial primary tumors. Histologically, these lesions are composed of two separate cell lines—glial cells and nerve cell elements—in varying proportions. If the nerve cells pre-

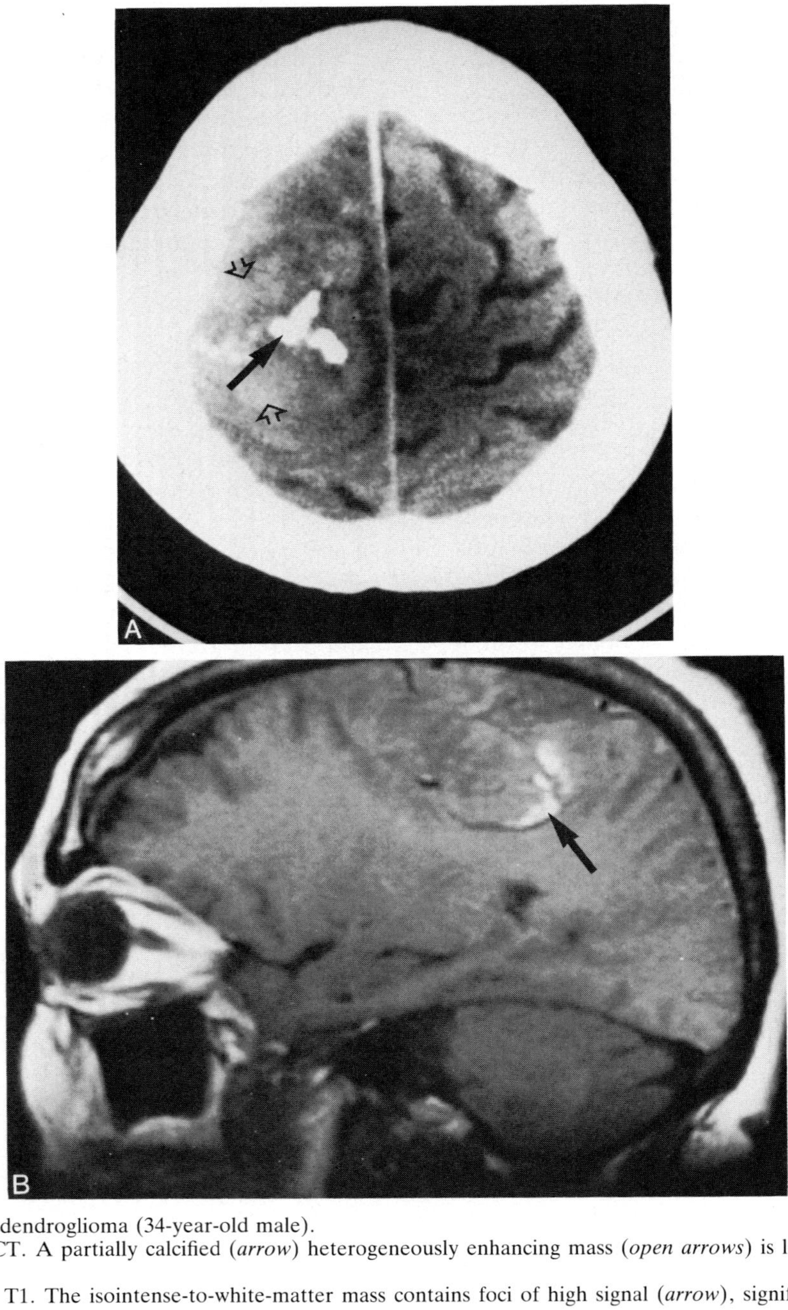

Figure 3–7. Oligodendroglioma (34-year-old male).

A, Enhanced CT. A partially calcified (*arrow*) heterogeneously enhancing mass (*open arrows*) is located in the right parietal region.

B, Parasagittal T1. The isointense-to-white-matter mass contains foci of high signal (*arrow*), signifying prior intratumoral hemorrhage.

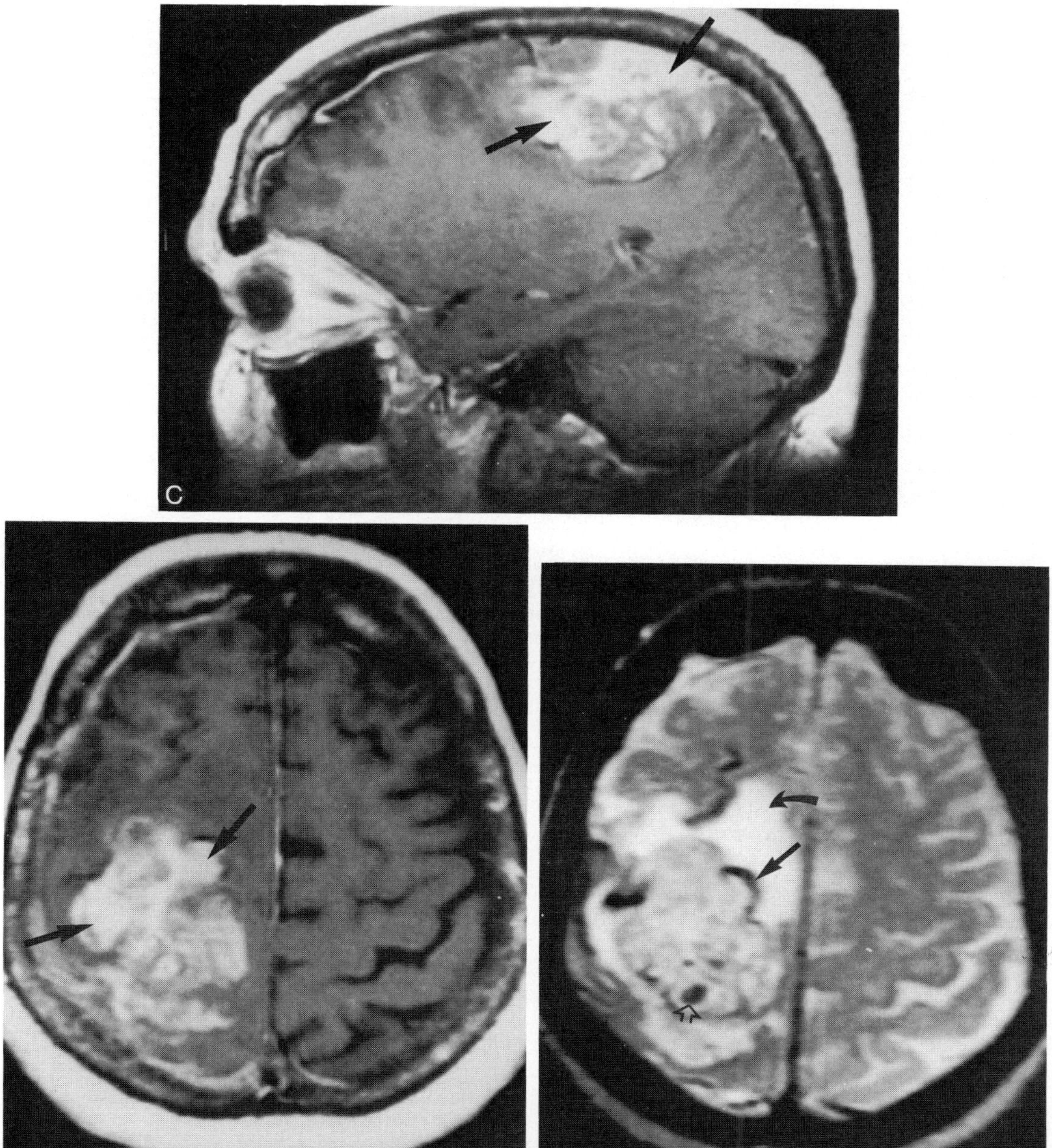

Figure 3–7 *Continued*

C, D, Enhanced parasagittal and axial T1. Heterogeneous enhancement (*arrows*) is observed within the tumor mass.

E, Axial T2. An incomplete hemosiderin ring (*straight arrow*) is present, with peripheral vasogenic edema (*curved arrow*). The mass is slightly hyperintense to brain. The focus of signal void (*open arrow*) may represent tumoral calcification or hemoglobin degradation products.

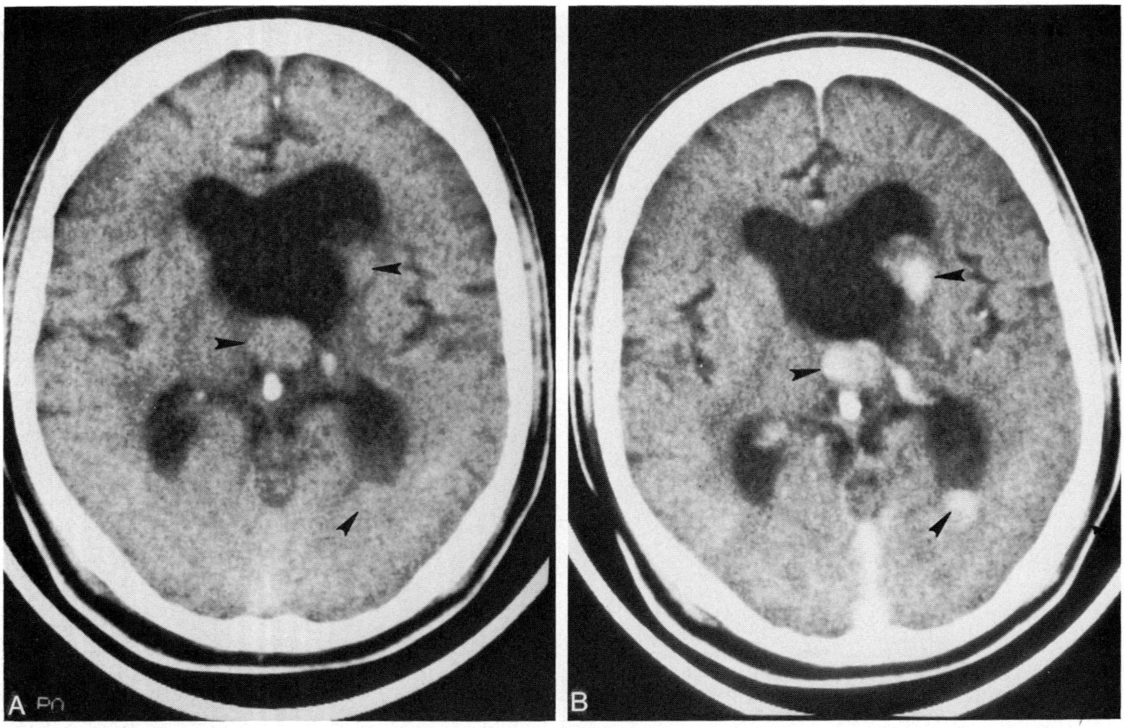

Figure 3–8. Ependymoma (37-year-old female).
A, Unenhanced CT. Multiple isodense-to-parenchyma, noncalcified intraventricular masses (*arrowheads*) are present.
B, Enhanced CT. The masses (*arrowheads*) become more apparent following administration of contrast.

dominate, the lesion is termed a ganglioneuroma; if the glial cells predominate, it is a ganglioglioma. The nonfocal long-standing symptoms that are reported in these patients corroborate the low-grade nature of these neoplasms. Patients most commonly present with a prolonged history of seizures.

Gangliogliomas may be solid or cystic in morphology. Solid tumors are more common and tend to occur in the temporal lobes and less commonly, in the basal ganglia.[27] Only 10% of the solid tumors contain calcification or small cystic areas detected on CT. Enhancement will occur to a variable degree in up to 80% of these patients (Fig. 3–11). The MRI characteristics of the solid tumors on T1 images are variable, with an equal number being hypointense, isointense, or hyperintense to brain. The lesion are usually high signal, referable to brain on T2 sequences (Fig. 3–12).

Cystic gangliogliomas may occur anywhere within the parenchyma but occur most commonly in the middle cranial fossa and the cerebellum. Calcification occurs more commonly in cystic (up to 63%) than in solid lesions.[27] Only 50% of the cystic lesions will enhance. The cystic component of the lesion is generally decreased signal on T1 images and increased signal on T2 images; however, there is some variability in the T2 signal characteristics of the lesion.[28] Edema is uncommon.

Metastasis

Metastases represent 20 to 30% of intracranial neoplasms. The metastatic deposits may involve the supratentorial or infratentorial parenchyma, leptomeninges, dura mater, or calvarium. Although nearly any primary tumor may metastasize to the brain, the most com-

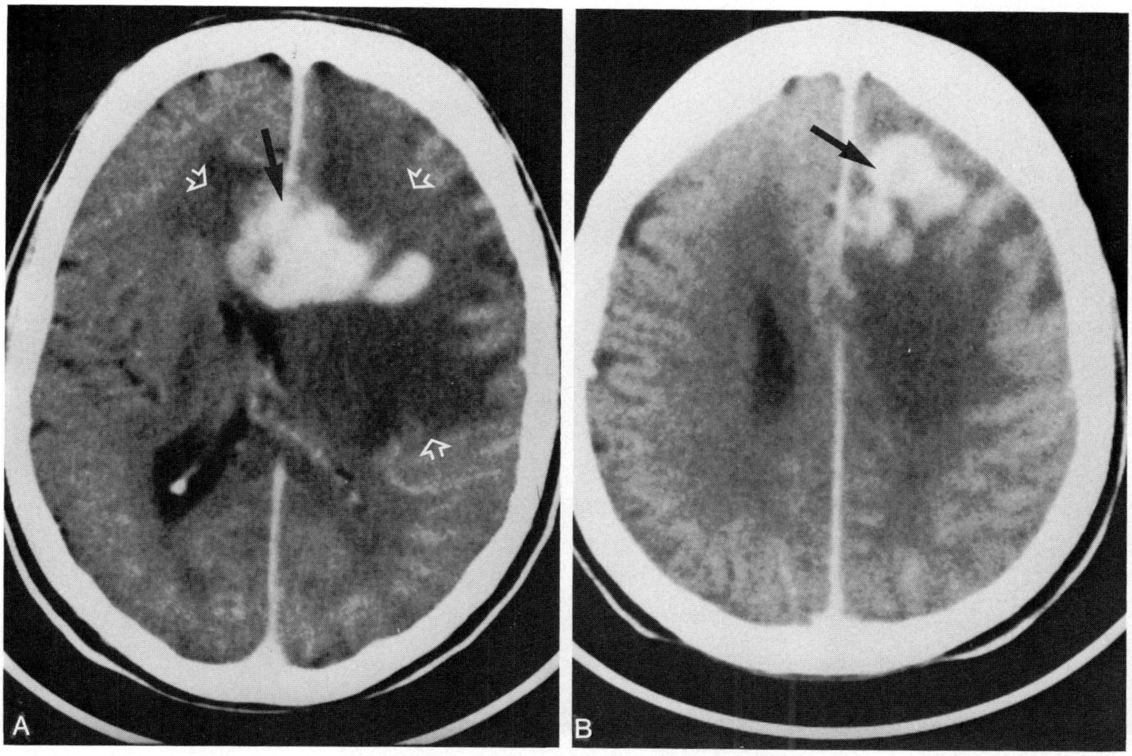

Figure 3–9. Primary central nervous system (CNS) lymphoma (63-year-old female).
A, Enhanced CT. Vasogenic edema (*open arrows*) surrounds an enhancing mass (*arrow*), which crosses midline.
B, Enhanced CT. The mass (*arrow*) extends cephalad to the superficial left frontal lobe.

mon ones encountered in the cerebral parenchyma are bronchogenic carcinoma, breast carcinoma, melanoma, and hypernephroma.

The lesions may be solitary or multiple and of various sizes. Metastases from a single primary tumor may be widely divergent in morphology. Metastatic lesions are usually associated with significant amounts of vasogenic edema and mass effect. Most metastatic lesions enhance to at least some degree. The most common pattern of enhancement is ring or nodular (Fig. 3–13). Rarely, some tumors will not enhance or produce any significant mass effect as the blood-brain barrier (BBB) remains intact.

Until recently, enhanced cranial CT was the method of choice in detecting intracranial metastasis. Lesion detection was improved by increasing loads of IV iodine and extending the time interval between contrast administration and scanning. The MRI evaluation of intracranial metastasis has yielded predictable results. Unenhanced MRI and enhanced CT were judged equal in lesion detection rate in two thirds of cases in one study.[29] Neither unenhanced MRI nor enhanced CT was clearly superior. MRI is more sensitive in demonstrating lesions located in the posterior fossa or close to a bony surface. Whenever CT was judged superior, it was related to the ability of contrast to demonstrate disruption in the BBB.

Gadolinium-enhanced MRI is the current modality of choice in evaluating intraparenchymal metastasis, surpassing unenhanced MRI[30] and double dose–delayed CT.[31] Enhanced MRI combines increased tissue sensitivity with ability to detect BBB disruption. The post-gadolinium T1-weighted sequence has been considered the most sensitive at lesion

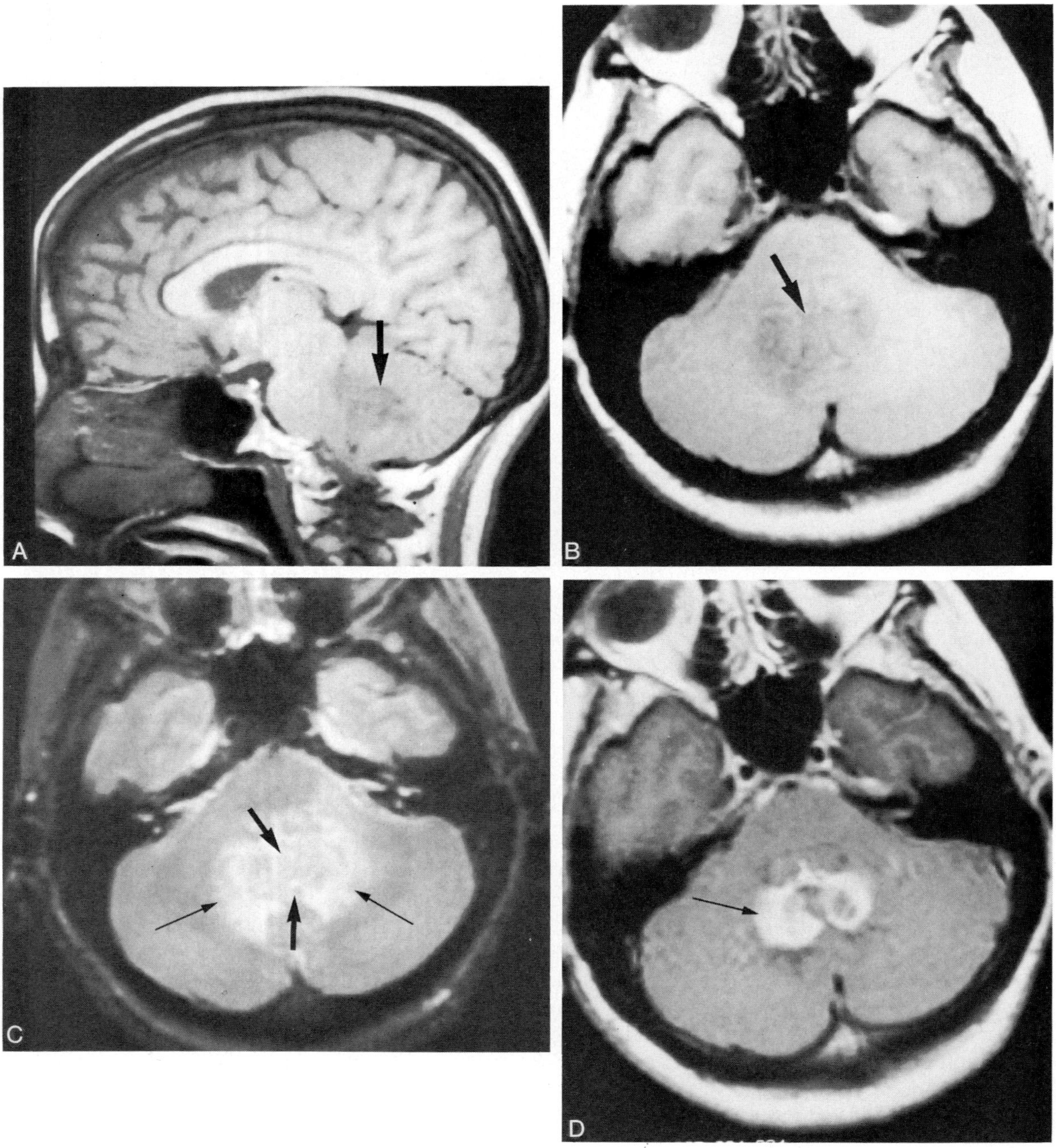

Figure 3–10. Lymphoma (62-year-old male).

A, B, Parasagittal and axial T1. A hypointense mass (*arrow*) fills the fourth ventricle.

C, Axial T2. Vasogenic edema (*long arrows*) surrounds the slightly hyperintense tumor mass (*short arrows*).

D, E, Enhanced axial T1. The midline posterior fossa mass (*long arrow*) enhances. Subependymal enhancement indicative of CSF metastases is noted in both frontal horns (*short arrows*).

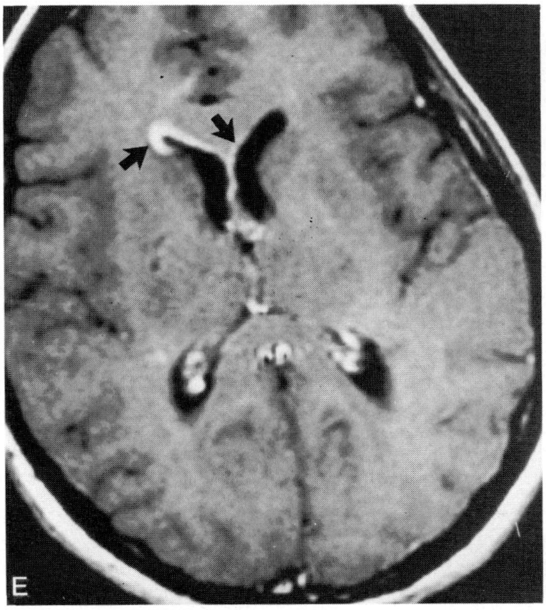

Figure 3–10 *Continued*

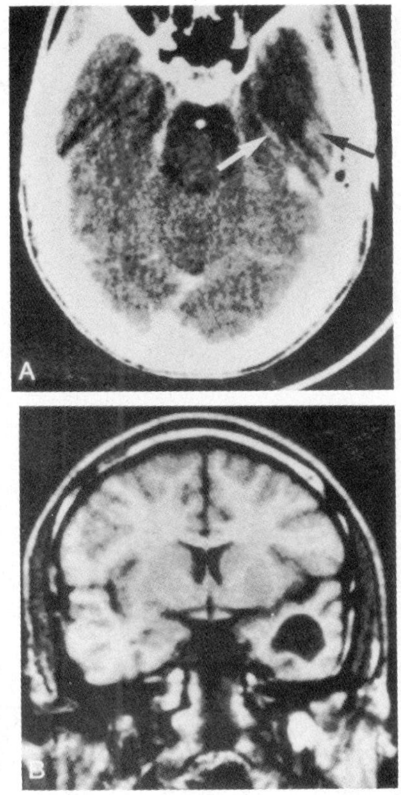

Figure 3–11. Ganglioglioma (21-year-old female).

A, Enhanced CT. A hypodense mass (*black arrow*) is present in the left temporal lobe. Subtle peripheral enhancement (*white arrow*) is detected.

B, Coronal T1. The mass is isointense to CSF. There is no significant mass effect. (M Castillo et al: Intracranial ganglioglioma: MR, CT, and clinical findings in 18 patients. AJNR 11:109–114, 1990, © by American Society of Neuroradiology, per Mary Giardina, January 16, 1992.)

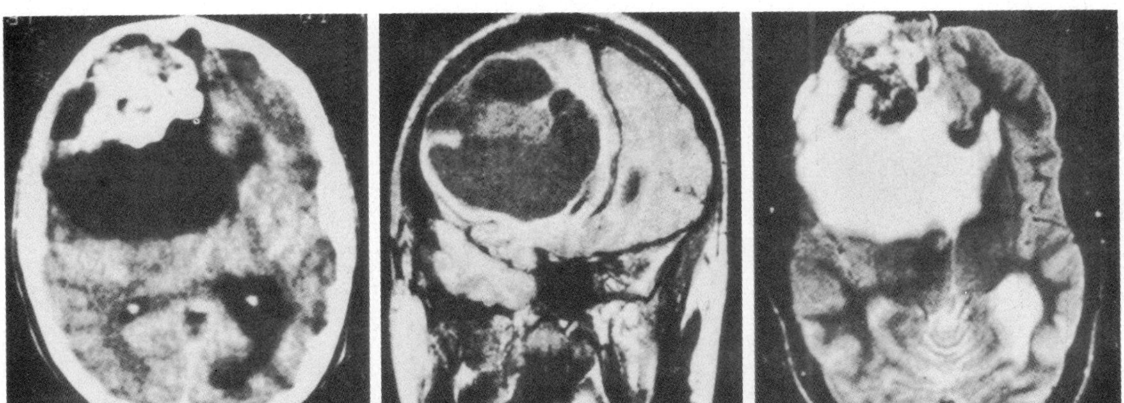

Figure 3–12. Ganglioglioma (17-year-old male).

A, Enhanced CT. A large cystic right frontal mass is present. The mass contains a large amorphic calcification. There is no appreciable enhancement.

B, Coronal T1. The lesion is heterogeneous with septa and regions of intermediate signal intensity.

C, Axial T2. The cystic moiety of the mass is isointense to CSF. The regions of signal void represent the dense amorphic calcification. (M Castillo et al: Intracranial ganglioglioma: MR, CT, and clinical findings in 18 patients. AJNR 11:109–114, 1990, © by American Society of Neuroradiology, per Mary Giardina, January 16, 1992.)

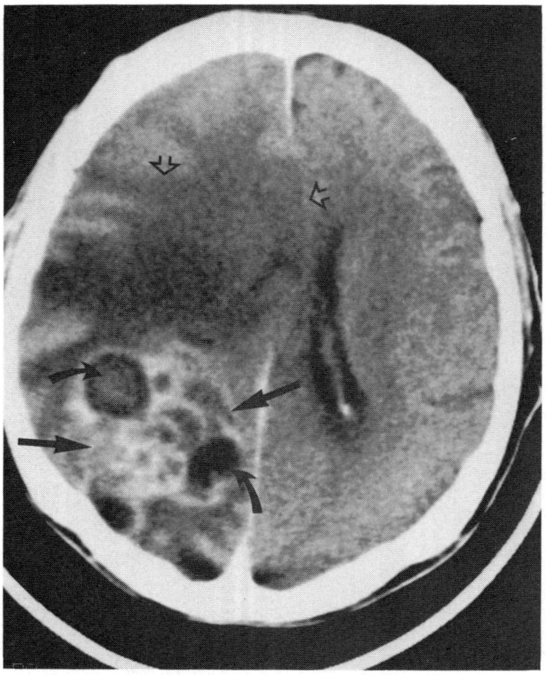

Figure 3–13. Metastasis—lung (61-year-old male). Enhanced CT; a heterogeneously enhancing mixed density mass (*arrows*) is present in the right parietal occipital region. Regions of cystic necrosis (*curved arrows*) are present. Extensive vasogenic edema (*open arrows*) accompanies the lesion.

detection[32] (Fig. 3–14). T1 images before gadolinium administration are useful to evaluate for bony lesions or metastases that may have hemorrhaged[32] (Fig. 3–15). In a small series of patients with parenchymal metastases,[33] the post-gadolinium T1 images were more sensitive than the pre-gadolinium T2 images at detecting small lesions (less than 10 mm in greatest linear dimension). Smaller lesions may not ordinarily promote a significant amount of vasogenic edema and therefore are less conspicious on the T2 sequences.

The leptomeninges or dura may serve as the site of seeding of metastatic disease (Fig. 3–16). Solitary metastases to the leptomeninges occur in less than 1% of all intracranial metastases. Alternatively, 6 to 18% of patients with CNS metastases may have involvement of the leptomeninges.[34] Breast carcinoma, small cell carcinoma, and lymphoma commonly seed the subarachnoid space, resulting in a carcinomatous leptomeningitis. Tumors that occur primarily within the CNS may also seed the CSF and result in leptomeningeal tumor. These tumors include the small round cell tumors, primitive neuroectodermal tumor (PNET) (medulloblastoma, pineoblastoma), germ cell

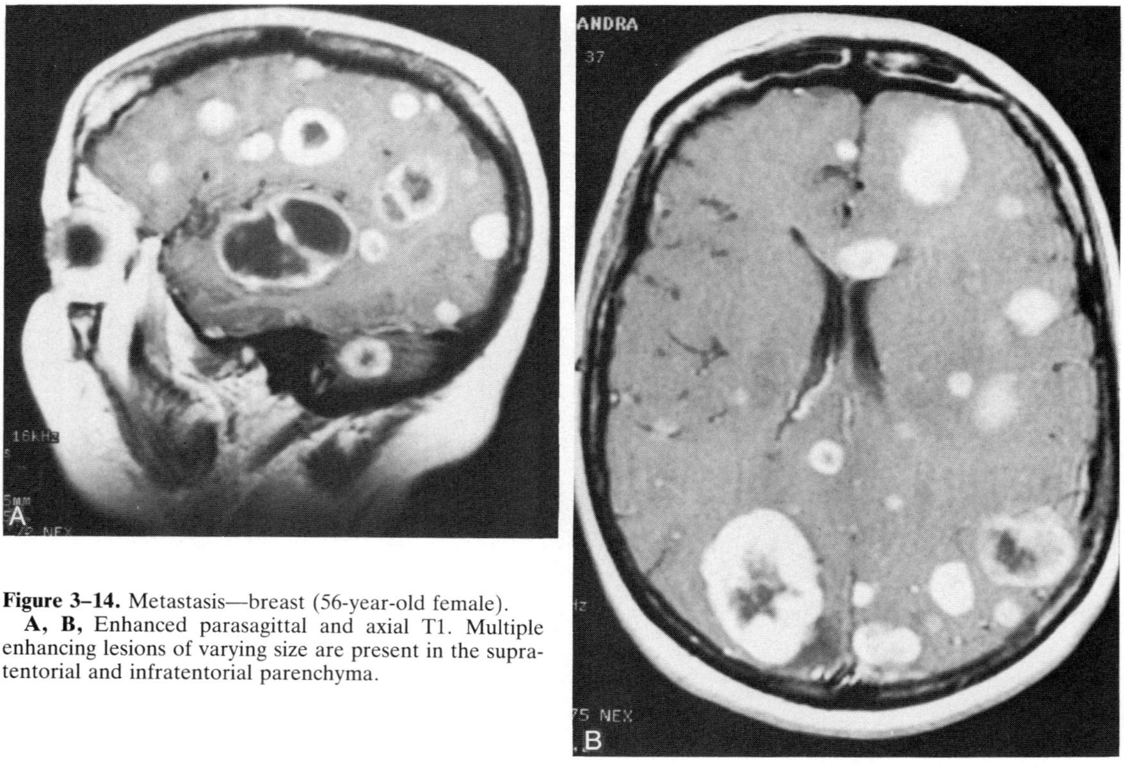

Figure 3–14. Metastasis—breast (56-year-old female).
A, B, Enhanced parasagittal and axial T1. Multiple enhancing lesions of varying size are present in the supratentorial and infratentorial parenchyma.

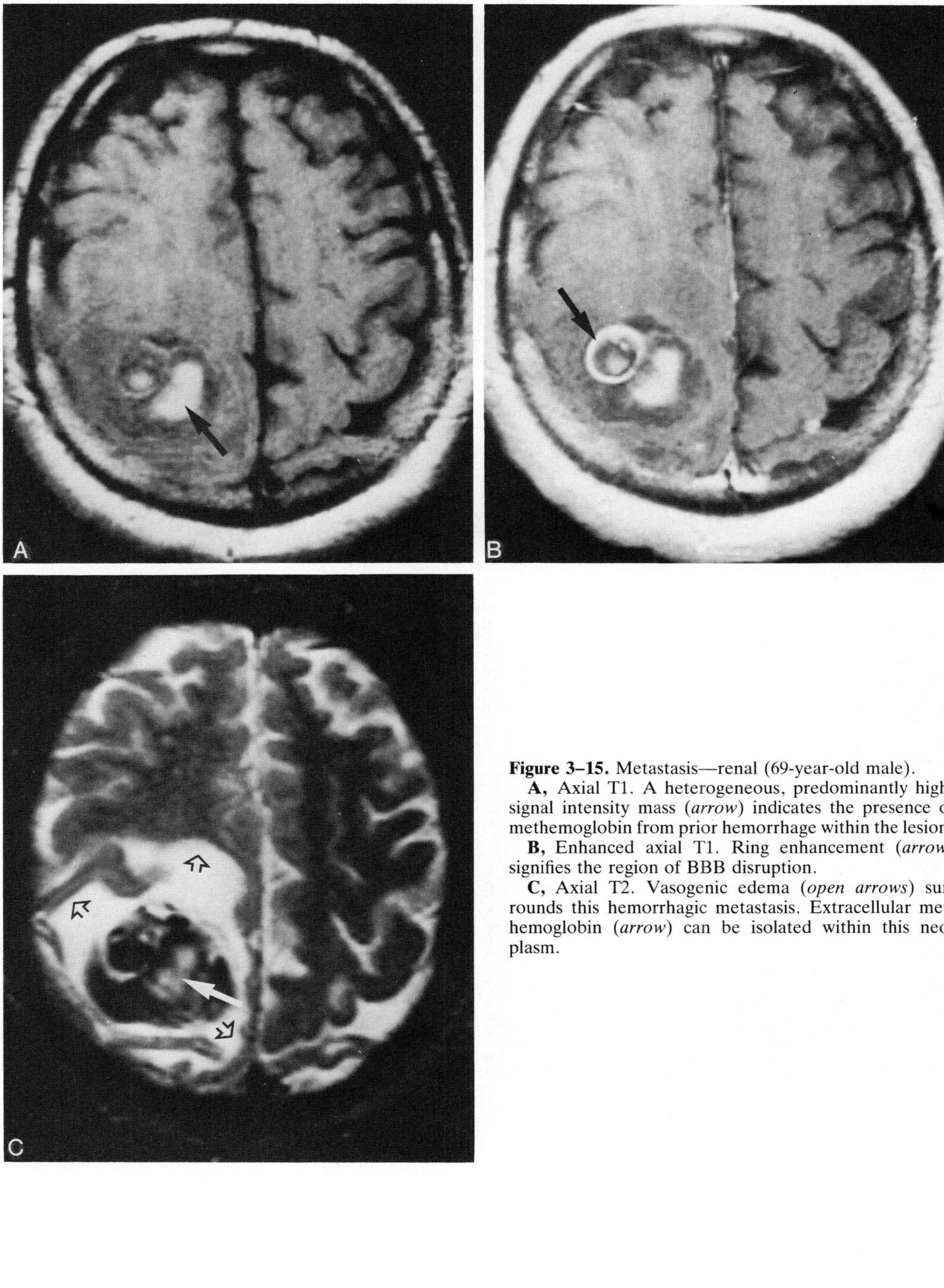

Figure 3–15. Metastasis—renal (69-year-old male).

A, Axial T1. A heterogeneous, predominantly high-signal intensity mass (*arrow*) indicates the presence of methemoglobin from prior hemorrhage within the lesion.

B, Enhanced axial T1. Ring enhancement (*arrow*) signifies the region of BBB disruption.

C, Axial T2. Vasogenic edema (*open arrows*) surrounds this hemorrhagic metastasis. Extracellular methemoglobin (*arrow*) can be isolated within this neoplasm.

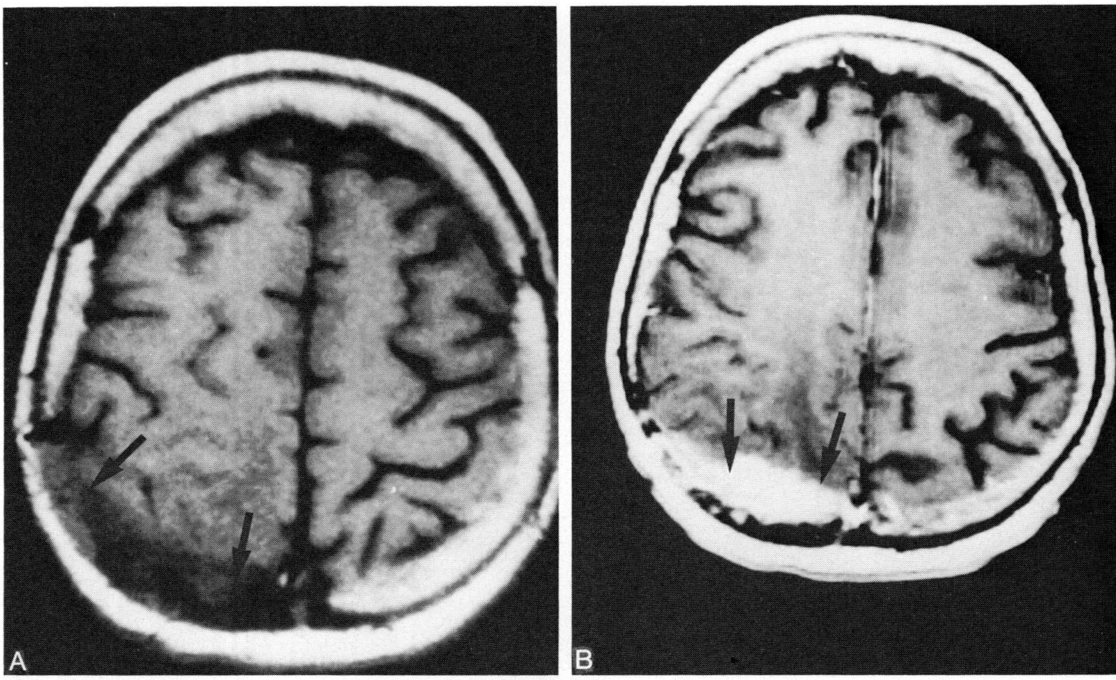

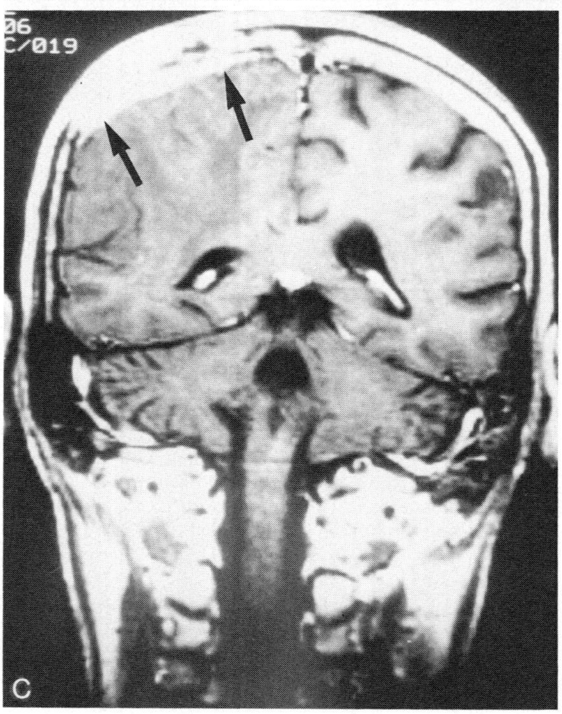

Figure 3–16. Metastasis—breast (65-year-old female).

A, Axial T1. Cortical sulci are locally effaced, and the marrow of the posterior right parietal bone (*arrows*) is replaced.

B, C, Enhanced axial and coronal T1. Homogeneous enhancement (*arrows*) signifies disruption of the inner and outer tables and infiltration of tumor into the extradural compartment.

neoplasms, ependymoma, leukemia, and any glioma that may have secondarily seeded the CSF during surgery. Tumor cells and attendant inflammation may interrupt CSF flow, resulting in communicating or noncommunicating hydrocephalus.

Radiographic manifestations of leptomeningeal tumor include effacement of the CSF spaces, sulcal-cisternal enhancement, communicating hydrocephalus, ependymal-subependymal enhancement, and thickened irregular tentorial enhancement.[35] Parenchymal metastases may be detected in up to 60% of patients with leptomeningeal tumor.[35] Owing to the proximity of the leptomeninges to cortical bone, gadolinium-enhanced MRI is more sensitive at detecting leptomeningeal disease than is enhanced CT.[36]

Although any CNS metastasis may hemorrhage, melanoma and choriocarcinoma do so at a rate significantly higher than that of other neoplasms. Bronchogenic carcinoma, as well as renal and thyroid cancers, also has a propensity to hemorrhage. Hemorrhages have been reported in between 50 and 100% of patients with melanoma. Melanoma is considered the third most common metastasis to the brain and the most likely to hemorrhage.[37] Acute hemorrhage appears as high density (approximately 80 to 90 Hounsfield units) on CT. Neoplastic hemorrhages may elicit more vasogenic edema than expected for the size and clinical timing of the hemorrhage. Contrast enhancement on CT may be difficult to detect when adjacent to high-density hemorrhage.

Hemorrhagic metastasis may be suspected on MRI if the normal time progression of hemoglobin degradation products is delayed or arrested, if there is an accumulation rather than resolution of edema, or if the hemosiderin ring is incomplete[38] (see Chapter 4). Gadolinium enhancement in the acute phase may indicate that a parenchymal hemorrhage may be secondary to metastatic disease. However, gadolinium enhancement normally occurs to some degree in the resolving hematoma.

Melanin is composed of paramagnetic materials that will alter the T1 and T2 relaxation times of these lesions[39] (Fig. 3–17). The melanin copolymers have a minimal influence on the signal intensity of melanoma metastasis when compared with the contribution of hemorrhage and hemoglobin breakdown products to the signal intensity.[40] Hemorrhagic melanoma is often intermediate to high signal on T1 and low signal on T2.

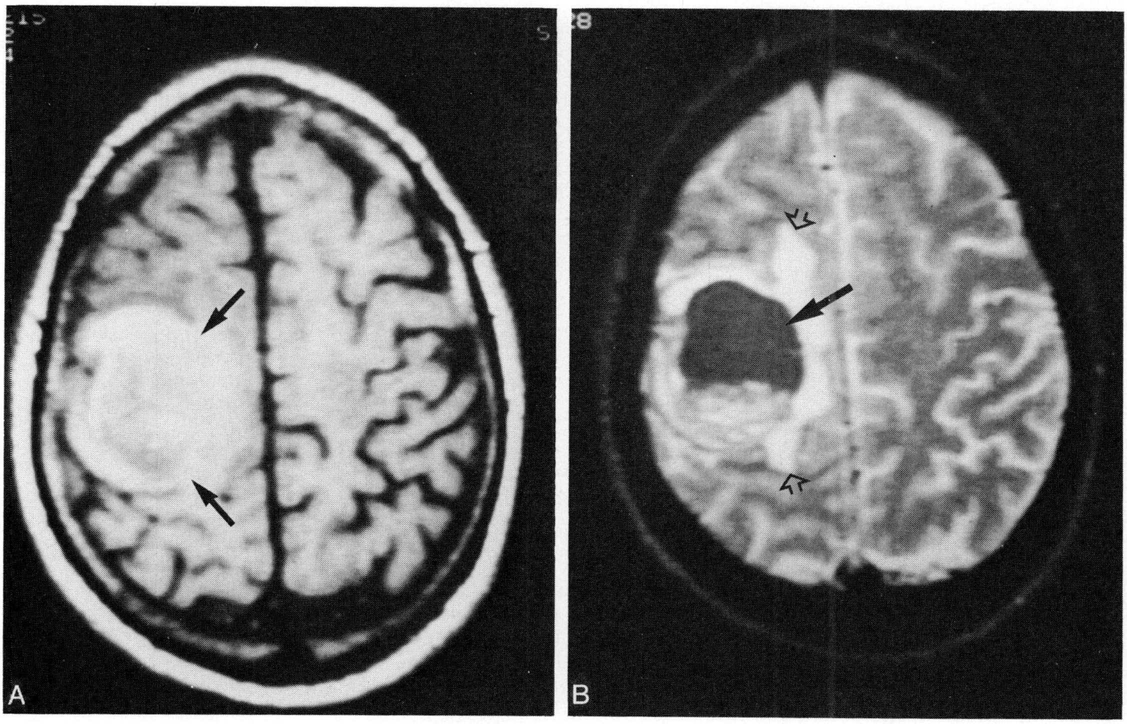

Figure 3–17. Metastasis—melanoma (69-year-old male).

A, Axial T1. An intrinsically high-signal mass (*arrows*) is present in the right parietal lobe. The high-signal mass may be due to methemoglobin, the paramagnetic copolymers of melanin, free radicals, or a combination thereof.

B, Axial T2. Vasogenic edema (*open arrows*) surrounds a heterogeneous, predominantly low-signal mass lesion (*arrow*). The low signal may be secondary to hemoglobin degradation products or melanin or both.

LOCATION APPROACH

Intraventricular Neoplasms

Some primary intracranial neoplasms occur exclusively within the ventricle; other neoplasms, though originating more commonly elsewhere, may also occur within the ventricle. Certain criteria are useful to corroborate intraventricular origin.[41] Determining the intraventricular location of a small lesion is usually not difficult if it is surrounded by CSF. Larger lesions may conform to the size and shape of the ventricle, may or may not engulf the choroid, or may cause local deformity of the ventricular wall. Patient age and tumor location are helpful in developing an accurate differential diagnosis[42] (Table 3–1).

Colloid Cyst

Colloid cysts are neuroepithelial cysts that arise from the folding of the primitive neuroepithelium, which forms the choroid plexus and ependyma. This congenital lesion grows slowly, presenting most frequently in middle-aged patients. These lesions represent less than 0.5% of all intracranial neoplasms and are almost exclusively located in the roof of the third ventricle. As the mass enlarges, it may occlude one or both foramina of Monro, resulting in obstructive hydrocephalus. The hydrocephalus uncommonly is intermittent. These lesions may be found less commonly in the lateral ventricles.[43]

The epithelial lining of the cyst continues to secrete materials that may be degraded into

Table 3–1. COMMON INTRAVENTRICULAR TUMORS

Entity	Location	Age (yr)	Planar Imaging Characteristics: *CT*	Planar Imaging Characteristics: *MRI*
Colloid cyst	3rd ventricle (anterior roof)	20–50	a. Hyperdense b. Enhancement: minimal to none c. ± Hydrocephalus	a. Heterogeneous b. T1: high signal in part or whole c. T2: low signal centrally, high signal peripherally
Subependymal giant cell astrocytoma	Lateral ventricle (near foramen of Monro)	5–30	a. Intrinsically dense b. Calcification: common (90%) c. Enhancement: homogeneous	a. T1: isointense to parenchyma b. T2: hyperintense to parenchyma c. Calcification: ↓ signal d. Enhancement: homogeneous
Astrocytoma	Frontal horn, 3rd ventricle	20–80	a. Hyperdense b. Calcification: 30% c. Enhancement: homogeneous	a. T1: isointense to hyperintense to parenchyma b. T2: hyperintense to parenchyma c. Enhancement: homogeneous
Ependymoma	Children, 4th ventricle; adults, lateral ventricle (body or atrium)	10–40	a. Hyperdense b. Calcification: 20–40% c. Enhancement: heterogeneous	a. T1: isointense to hyperintense to parenchyma b. T2: hyperintense to parenchyma c. Enhancement: heterogeneous
Choroid plexus papilloma	Children, lateral ventricle (atrium); adults, 4th ventricle	0–50	a. Hyperdense b. Calcification: 50% c. Enhancement: marked heterogeneous d. Hydrocephalus	a. T1: isointense to hyperintense to parenchyma b. T2: hyperintense to parenchyma c. Enhancement: heterogeneous
Meningioma	Lateral ventricle (atrium)	30–60	a. Well-circumscribed b. Hyperdense c. Calcification: 30–50% d. Enhancement: homogeneous	a. T1 and T2: isointense to parenchyma b. Enhancement: homogeneous

cholesterol. It is the contents of this cyst that account for the intrinsic high density, the most common CT appearance (Fig. 3–18). Less frequently, colloid cysts may be hypodense or isodense to parenchyma, with a central area of increased density.[43] The lesion may enhance along the periphery, but contrast enhancement is not a common feature of the lesion.

The MRI appearance of the colloid cyst is variable and heterogeneous.[43] Generally, the lesion partially or totally contains a region of increased signal intensity on T1 images (Fig. 3–19). The high T1 signal has been correlated with a high cholesterol content. A region of markedly diminished signal intensity within the central portion of the cyst may be present on T2-weighted sequences.

Subependymal Giant Cell Astrocytoma

This low-grade neoplasm arises from the giant, irregular astrocytes within the subependymal region, located along the lateral ventricle. The tumor projects into the ventricle adjacent to the foramen of Monro, frequently obstructing CSF flow from the ipsilateral lateral ventricle. Although most commonly associated with tuberous sclerosis (see Chapter 13), these lesions may occur in the absence of this phacomatosis.[44]

CT depicts an exophytic, soft tissue–density mass at the level of the foramen of Monro. The mass is relatively well circumscribed and partially calcified (90%),[42] and it enhances homogeneously (Fig. 3–20). Enhancement on CT may corroborate degeneration of a hamartoma into a giant cell astrocytoma.

MRI demonstrates a lesion that is isointense to parenchyma on T1 and hyperintense on T2. If large enough, the calcification may appear as a focus of decreased signal within the tumor. The lesion may be obscured partly by the high signal of the surrounding CSF on T2 images. Rarely, these lesions invade the parenchyma or promote vasogenic edema. Homogeneous enhancement is detected following administration of gadolinium.

Astrocytoma

Astrocytoma was the most common intraventricular mass lesion in one series, accounting for 21% of the total number of intraventricular tumors.[17] The lesions may be located anywhere throughout the supratentorial or infratentorial ventricular system and is most

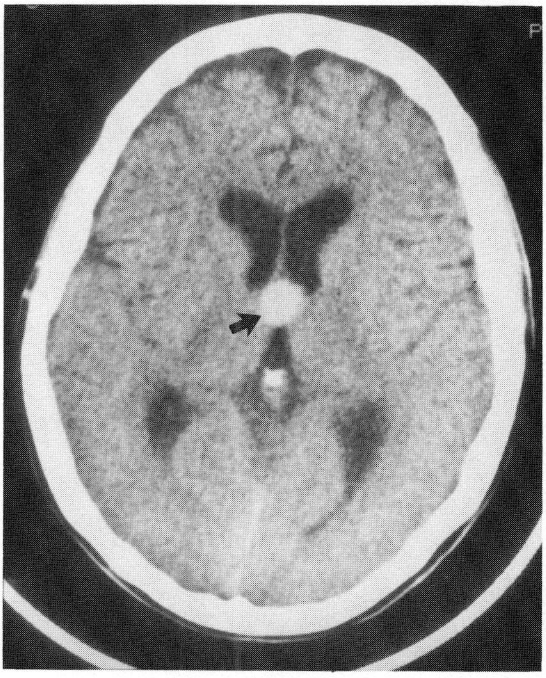

Figure 3–18. Colloid cyst (24-year-old female). Unenhanced CT; demonstrates an intrinsically dense, well-demarcated mass (*arrow*) in the superior third ventricle at the level of the foramen of Monro. There is no evidence of obstructive hydrocephalus.

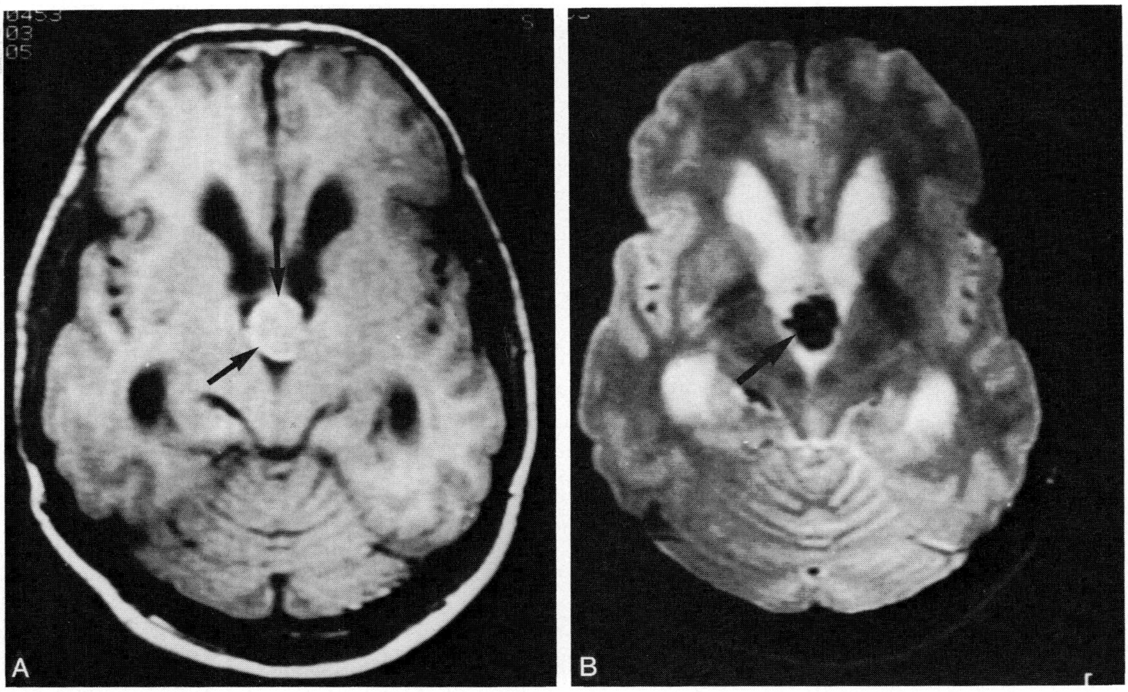

Figure 3–19. Colloid cyst (25-year-old male).

A, Axial T1. A mass of peripheral high signal (*arrows*) is present in the foramen of Monro. The central part of the cyst is isointense to white matter. Mild ventriculomegaly is noted.

B, Axial T2. The periphery of the cyst blends imperceptibly with the adjacent CSF, and the core of the lesion (*arrow*) is markedly hypointense.

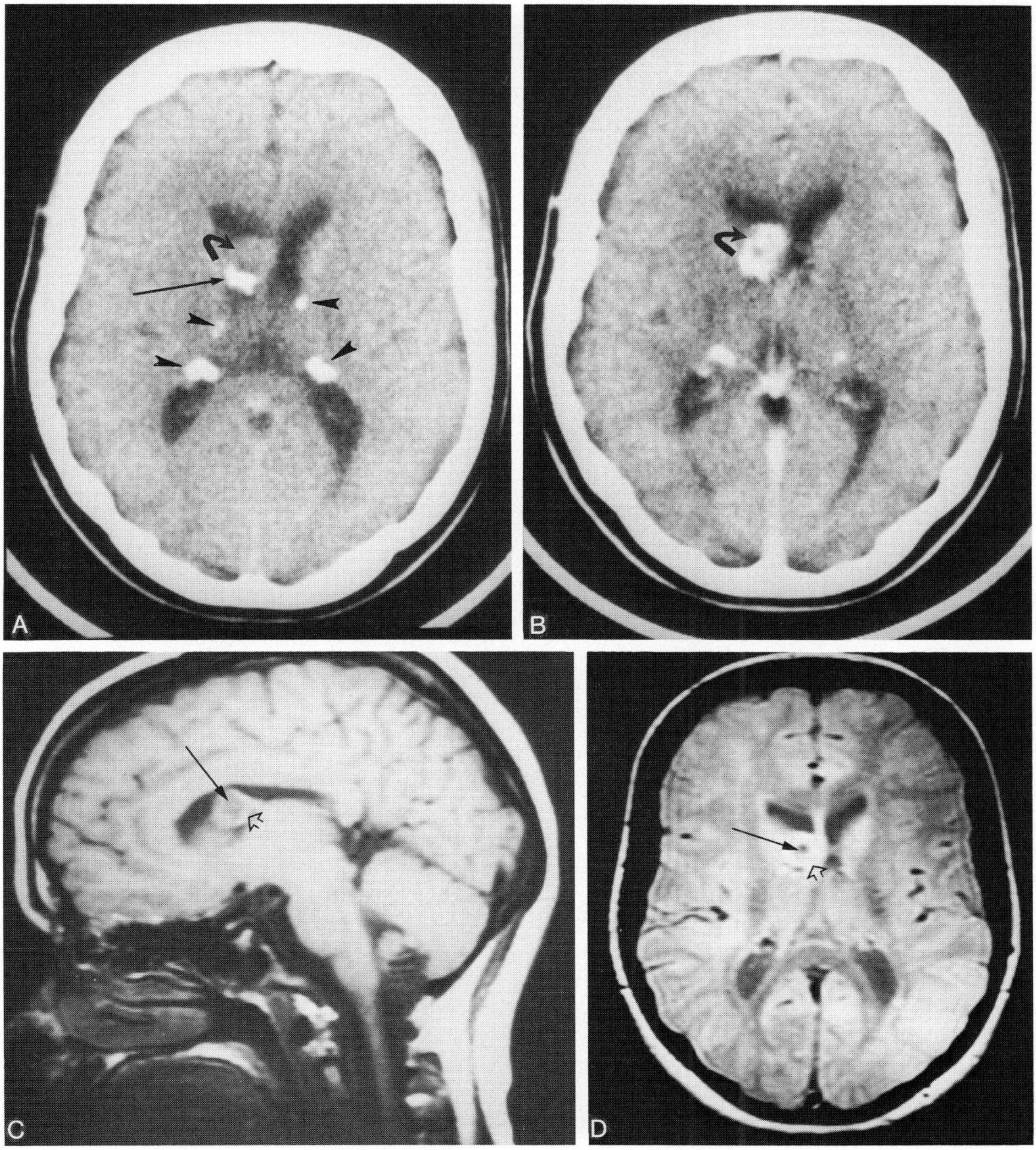

Figure 3–20. Giant cell astrocytoma (30-year-old male).

A, Unenhanced CT. A partially solid (*curved arrow*), partially calcified (*straight arrow*) mass is present in the frontal horn, adjacent to the foramen of Monro. Multiple periventricular calcifications (*arrowheads*) are present, confirming the diagnosis of tuberous sclerosis.

B, Enhanced CT. Enhancement corroborates the presence of malignant degeneration of a tuber into a giant cell astrocytoma (*curved arrow*).

C, Parasagittal T1. The mass is isointense to white matter (*arrowhead*) with a central region of diminished signal (*straight arrow*), which may be secondary to calcification.

D, Axial SD. The mass remains high signal (*open arrow*) along the periphery with a central region of diminished signal (*arrow*). There is no evidence of vasogenic edema.

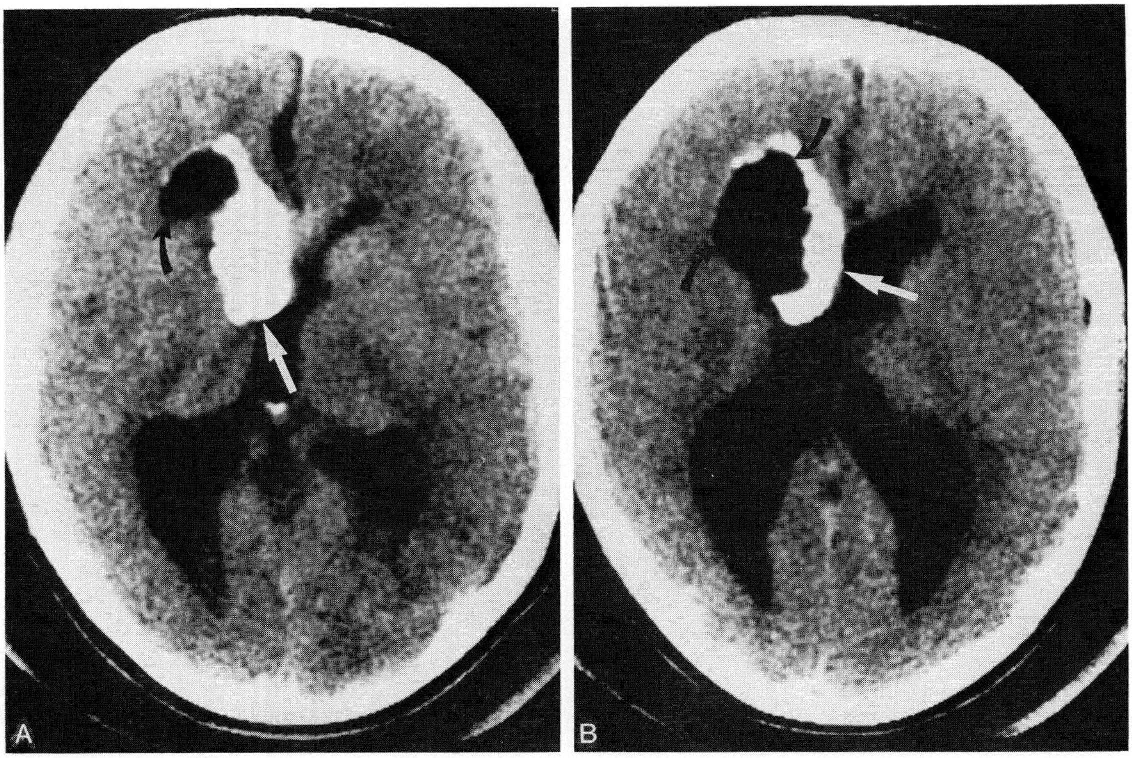

Figure 3–21. Low-grade astrocytoma (13-year-old male).
A, B, Unenhanced CT. A complex, partially calcified (*straight arrow*), partially cystic mass (*curved arrows*) is present within the right frontal horn. Only local mass effect is present with no evidence of vasogenic edema.

common in the frontal horns. The tumors likely arise in the periventricular white matter and secondarily extend into the ventricle.

The neoplasms are usually intrinsically hyperdense to brain (77%), partially calcified (31%), enhanced to some degree (86%), and associated with hydrocephalus (73%), most commonly at the level of the foramen of Monro[17] (Fig. 3–21).

Ependymoma

Ependymomas most frequently occur in the fourth ventricle in children (see Chapter 13). As mentioned, ependymomas that occur in adults most often involve the supratentorial parenchyma. When intraventricular ependymomas are encountered in adults, they typically occur in the body or the trigone of the lateral ventricle (see Fig. 3–8). The radiographic appearance of this lesion has been discussed.

Choroid Plexus Papilloma

These neoplasms represent less than 1% of all intracranial neoplasms and are derived from the epithelium covering the choroid plexus. These tumors may occur at any age, though most commonly they occur in children and young adults. They represent 42% of detected neonatal brain tumors in one series.[45] The most frequent site of origin is the fourth ventricle, followed by the lateral ventricles (left more often than right). The lesions tend to be supratentorial in children and infratentorial in adults.

This is the only neoplasm that increases the production of CSF, which has been documented at greater than four times normal.[46] Patients may present with a communicating hydrocephalus due to CSF overproduction.[17, 42, 46]

CT demonstrates an intraventricular mass, which may be quite large. The mass is usually hyperdense to parenchyma[42] and is partially calcified in greater than 50% of the cases. Small cysts, though not a prevalent feature, may be present. Marked enhancement with a lobulated contour may be detected (Fig. 3–22). Contrast enhancement renders the intratumoral cysts more conspicuous. Hydrocephalus is readily detected.

The MRI characteristics of choroid plexus papillomas are nonspecific. The intraventricular mass is isointense to parenchyma on T1 and hyperintense on T2. Calcium will diminish the signal intensity and cystic components will prolong the T1 and T2 relaxation times. Periventricular interstitial edema may accompany the hydrocephalus.

Meningioma

These lesions, which represent 5 to 20% of intracranial neoplasms, will be presented in more detail later in this chapter. Fewer than 2% of all meningiomas are intraventricular; the most common intraventricular location is the trigone of the lateral ventricle (left more often than right).

These lesions are commonly intrinsically dense on CT and isointense to parenchyma on MRI, are well marginated, contain focal calcification (44%), and enhance homogeneously[17] (Fig. 3–23). The ipsilateral temporal horn may be enlarged if the lesion is of sufficient size to prevent flow of CSF from the temporal horn to the atrium of the lateral ventricle.

Pineal Region Neoplasms

Pineal region tumors occur in children and young adults, most within the first three decades. Pineocytoma, however, may actually occur at a slightly older age (34 years).[47] Pineal region tumors represent less than 1% of intracranial neoplasms in adults, yet represent from 3 to 8% of intracranial neoplasms in children.[48] Patients may present with abnormal eye movements including Parinaud's syndrome (limitation of upward gaze resulting from compression of the tectal plate). If the lesion is large enough, it may displace the tectal plate sufficiently to occlude the aqueduct of Sylvius, resulting in obstructive hydrocephalus and increased intracranial pressure. Multiple, histologically divergent lesions may occur in the pineal region. These can successfully be classified into four major categories: germ cell tumors, glial tumors, pineal stem cell tumors, and meningiomas (Table 3–2). Although MRI is more sensitive than CT at detecting lesions of the pineal region, rarely are the signal characteristics sufficiently specific to render a histologic diagnosis.[49]

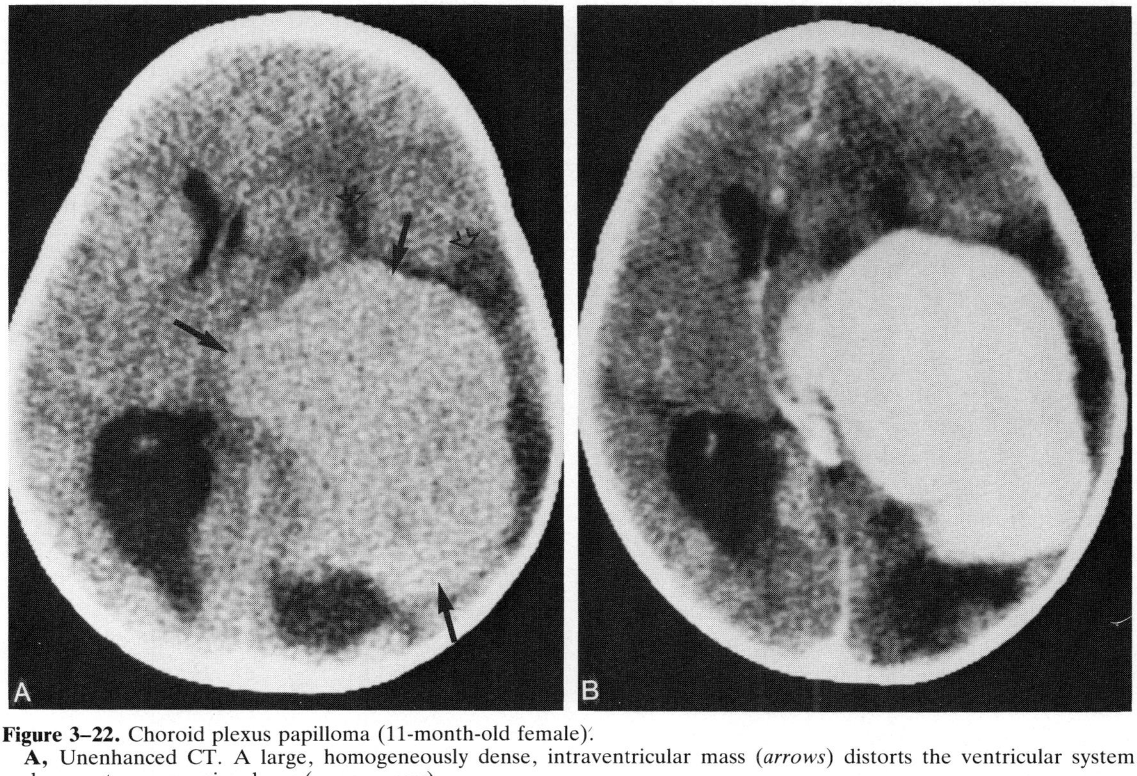

Figure 3–22. Choroid plexus papilloma (11-month-old female).

A, Unenhanced CT. A large, homogeneously dense, intraventricular mass (*arrows*) distorts the ventricular system and promotes vasogenic edema (*open arrows*).

B, Enhanced CT. The mass enhances homogeneously.

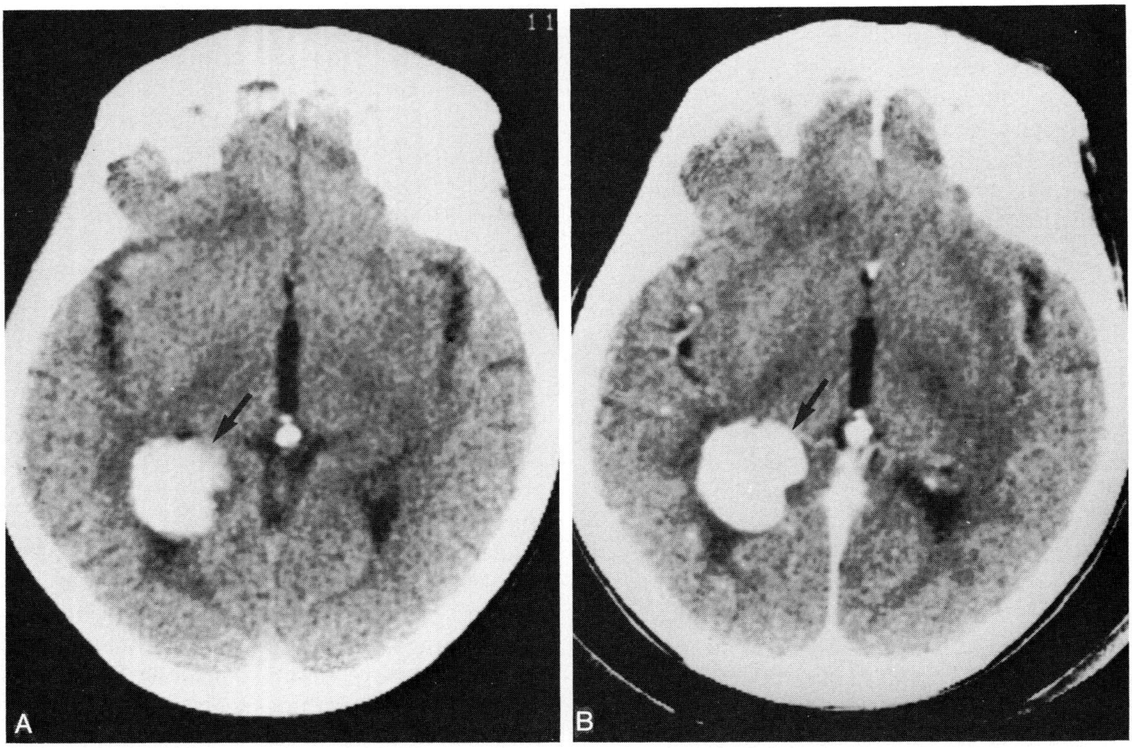

Figure 3–23. Meningioma (63-year-old female).
A, Unenhanced CT. A homogeneously dense mass (*arrow*) fills the atrium of the right lateral ventricle.
B, Enhanced CT. The mass (*arrow*) enhances homogeneously, producing a more distinct tumor-brain interface.

Germ Cell Neoplasms

The germ cell neoplasms are the most common group of tumors in the pineal region. Germinomas are the most common of the germ cell tumors to involve the pineal region, accounting for greater than 50% of all pineal region tumors.[44, 50]

Germinoma. Germinomas are suspected to arise from the primitive germ cells that migrate throughout the embryo during early fetal life. Germinomas occur almost exclusively in the pineal and parapineal regions or the suprasellar region. The pineal region is the most common location for intracranial germinomas in males. In females the most common location is the suprasellar region. The lesion presents between the second and third decades of life, occurring far more frequently in males. Male-to-female ratios range from 4:1[51] to 13:1.[47] Histologically, these tumors resemble testicular seminoma. Germinomas do not consistently produce any known serum or CSF tumor markers. Rarely, this lesion may produce beta–human chorionic gonadotropin (β-HCG), which may be elevated in the CSF and serum.

Radiograpically, these lesions are usually well-circumscribed, hyperdense, noncalcified masses that surround or abut the pineal gland.[47, 50, 51] The normal pineal gland will not exceed 10 mm in greatest linear dimension. The normal intrinsic pineal calcification may be engulfed by the tumor. In very rare instances, the tumor may produce a coarse, nodular calcification.[51] Homogeneous intense enhancement occurs in most cases (Fig. 3–24). Small cystic areas may be evident following contrast administration.[52] The MRI appearance is nonspecific. The tumor matrix is isointense to white matter on T1 and isointense to slightly hyperintense to white matter on T2 spin echo sequences[53, 54] (Fig. 3–25). The pineal gland calcification is usually not detected.

Teratoma. Intracranial teratomas occur most frequently in the pineal region. These tumors are found in men in the second to third decade of life. All three germ cell layers are found in this histologically divergent tumor.

Table 3–2. COMMON PINEAL REGION TUMORS

Cell Line	Age (yr)	Sex	Planar Imaging Characteristics: *CT*	Planar Imaging Characteristics: *MRI*	Remarks
Germ Cell					
Germinoma	10–30	Male:female 4–13:1	a. Isodense to hyperdense b. Enhancement: homogeneous c. Calcification: rare	a. T1: isointense to parenchyma b. T2: hyperintense to parenchyma c. Enhancement: homogeneous d. ± Small cysts	a. Most common pineal region tumor (50%) b. Intracranial germinoma in women more commonly suprasellar
Teratoma	10–30	Almost exclusively male	a. Heterogeneous: well-circumscribed b. Fat and calcification c. Solid tumor matrix enhances	a. Heterogeneous b. Fat: ↑ T1 c. Calcification: ↓ T1 and T2	a. Malignant variety produces AFP and β-HCG b. MRI appearance may be specific
Glial Cell					
Glioma	10–50	Male:female 1.5–5:1	a. Hypodense to parenchyma b. Enhancement: moderate c. Calcification: rare	a. T1: hypointense to isointense to parenchyma b. T2: isointense to hyperintense to parenchyma c. Enhancement: moderate, may reveal small cysts	a. May arise from pineal gland or extrinsic to gland b. Displaces pineal calcification anterior-superior
Pineal Stem Cell					
Pineocytoma	10–40	Male:female 1:1	a. Isodense to hyperdense to parenchyma b. Enhancement: homogeneous c. Calcification: common	a. T1: hypointense to isointense to parenchyma b. T2: hyperintense to parenchyma c. Enhancement: homogeneous	a. Calcified pineal region mass in female, most likely pineocytoma
Pineoblastomas	5–70	Male:female 1–4:1	a. Isodense to parenchyma b. Enhancement: marked heterogeneous c. Calcification: infrequent	a. T1: isointense to parenchyma b. T2: variable, usually hyperintense c. Enhancement: marked, heterogeneous	a. Histologically and biologically similar to PNET b. Invasive to adjacent parenchyma c. Dissemination through CSF
Meningioma	30–60	Male:female 1:2	a. Well-circumscribed b. Isodense to parenchyma c. Enhancement: homogeneous d. Dural attachment	a. T1 and T2: isointense to parenchyma b. Enhancement: homogeneous c. Dural enhancement	

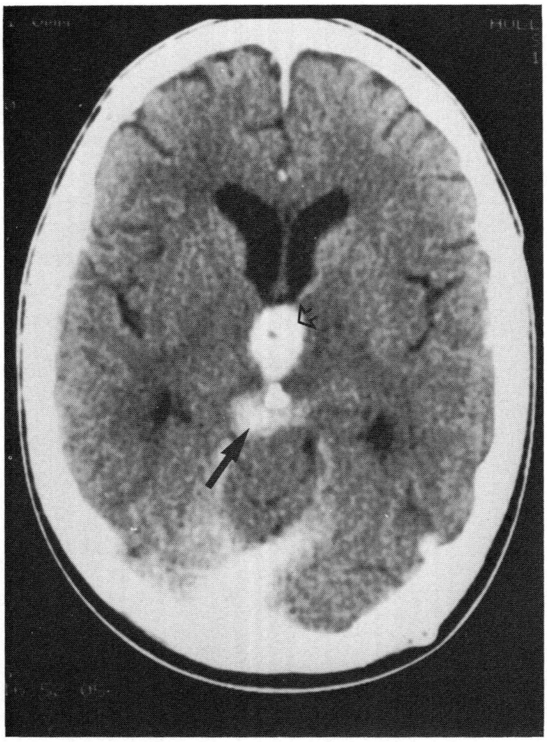

Figure 3–24. Pineal germinoma (26-year-old male). Enhanced CT; homogeneous enhancement in the pineal region (*arrow*) is present. Also, an enhancing mass (*open arrow*) is noted within the third ventricle, which indicates metastatic extension from the pineal region germinoma.

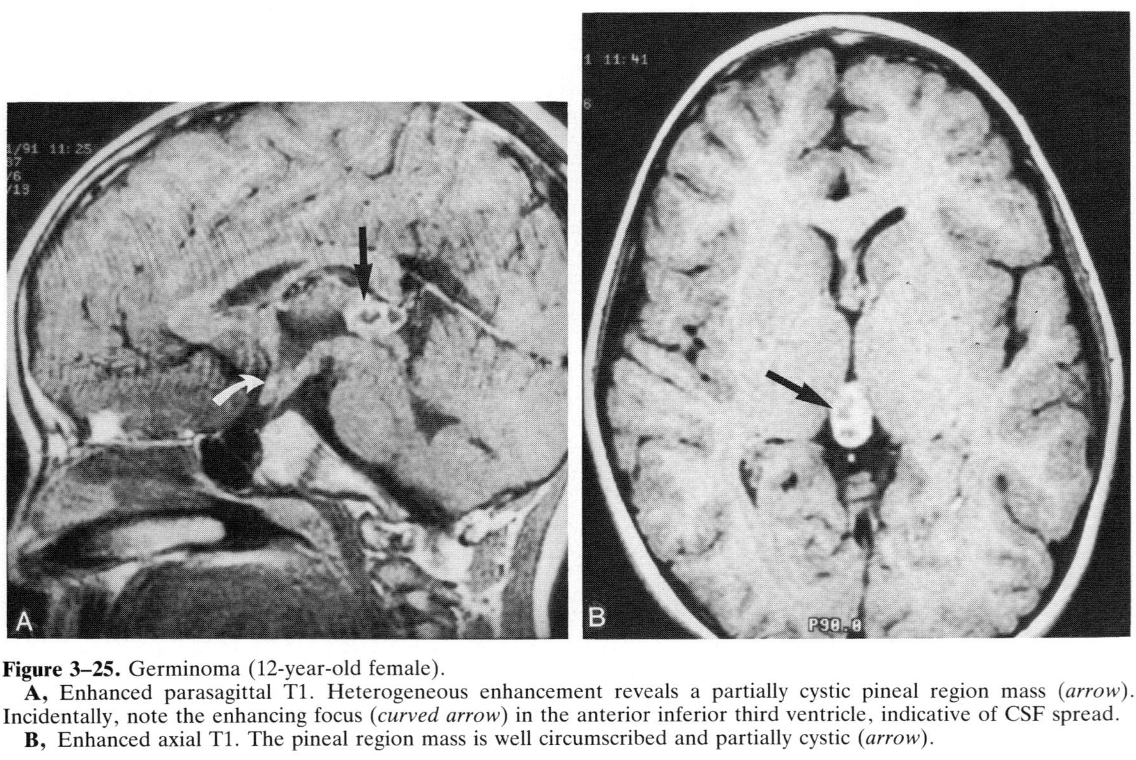

Figure 3–25. Germinoma (12-year-old female).

A, Enhanced parasagittal T1. Heterogeneous enhancement reveals a partially cystic pineal region mass (*arrow*). Incidentally, note the enhancing focus (*curved arrow*) in the anterior inferior third ventricle, indicative of CSF spread.

B, Enhanced axial T1. The pineal region mass is well circumscribed and partially cystic (*arrow*).

The lesions may be classified histologically as benign or malignant. The malignant tumor may produce elevated serum or CSF levels of alpha-fetoprotein (AFP) and β-HCG.[48]

Radiologically these tumors are usually well circumscribed with marked heterogeneous density from intratumoral calcium and fat. The tumor may enhance minimally or not at all.[51] Intratumoral cysts may become apparent on enhanced images.[52] The mass is also heterogeneous on MRI with areas of diminished signal secondary to calcification as well as increased T1 signal related to intratumoral fat. The MRI appearance of this lesion is usually specific.

Choriocarcinoma. This rare malignant infiltrative neoplasm is the only pineal region tumor to undergo spontaneous hemorrhage.[53] Serum and CSF levels of β-HCG, which are elevated in this condition, may be used to document effectiveness of treatment. The tumor is hyperdense on CT with calcification and will enhance homogeneously.[51] The MRI appearance is that of a heterogeneous infiltrative mass that is hyperintense to brain on T1- and T2-weighted spin echo imaging.[53]

Embryonal Cell Carcinoma. Embryonal cell carcinoma is a rare pineal region neoplasm that histologically resembles the embryonal cell carcinoma of the testes.[44] These lesions tend to be malignant, often with evidence of CSF metastasis. Serum and CSF levels of AFP and β-HCG are elevated.[48, 55] The lesion may be hyperdense, with marked enhancement. No demonstrable tumor calcification is present.[50, 51]

Endodermal Sinus Carcinoma. These rare yolk sac neoplasms are lesions of the pineal region. Elevated AFP levels may be detected in the serum and CSF.[48, 55] The lesion may be cystic, with abnormal calcification.[50] MRI depicts a round, isointense-to-brain lesion on T1, with heterogeneous signal intensity on T2 images.

Glial Neoplasms

Glial neoplasms may arise from the fibrillary astrocytes present in the pineal gland or may arise extrinsic to the gland from the tectal plate, mesencephalon, wall of the third ventricle, or adjacent temporal lobe. After germ cell tumors, glial tumors represent the second most common tumor encountered in the pineal region.[51] The glial cells are most frequently of the astrocytic series, in which varying grades of malignancy may be found.[50] Patients are usually in the second to sixth decade at time of diagnosis.

The tumors are usually hypodense and may be poorly marginated on CT[50, 51] (Fig. 3–26). The pineal calcification is usually of normal size and may be displaced anteriorly and superiorly. The tumor does not normally calcify unless irradiated. Pineal region astrocytomas may be cystic. The MRI signal characteristics are nonspecific. A round or ovoid tumor that is isointense to hypointense to brain on T1 and hyperintense to brain on T2 is often encountered. The degree of enhancement and extension into adjacent parenchyma increase with the degree of malignancy.

Pineal Stem Cell Neoplasms

Pineocytoma. Pineocytomas are low-grade neoplasms that originate from large cell pineocytes. These tumors represent less than 0.5% of all intracranial brain tumors and tend to occur at a slightly greater age (34 years) than other pineal region tumors.[47] This tumor generally occurs equally in both sexes[51]; however, some series report a female preponderance.[48]

Pineocytomas are generally well-circumscribed, noninvasive, slow-growing, isodense to hyperdense lesions that enhance in a homogeneous or nodular fashion[50, 51] (Fig. 3–27). Pineocytomas calcify at a higher rate than do germinomas.[50] The calcification often appears coarse and granular. A calcified pineal region mass in a woman is most likely to be a pineocytoma.[51] MRI is most useful at detecting the site of origin and extension into adjacent parenchyma, but the MRI signal characteristics are nonspecific.[56] The lesions often appear variable on T1 and high signal on T2.[52]

Pineoblastoma. Pineoblastomas arise from the small pineoblasts—primitive pineal stem cells. This highly malignant neoplasm is histologically similar to the small round cell tumors, retinoblastoma, medulloblastoma, and neuroblastoma.[44, 47, 57] These tumors occur at any age and are slightly more common in males. Pineoblastomas are invasive tumors that have a propensity to metastasize in the CSF spaces.

The tumor appears as a large, well-defined

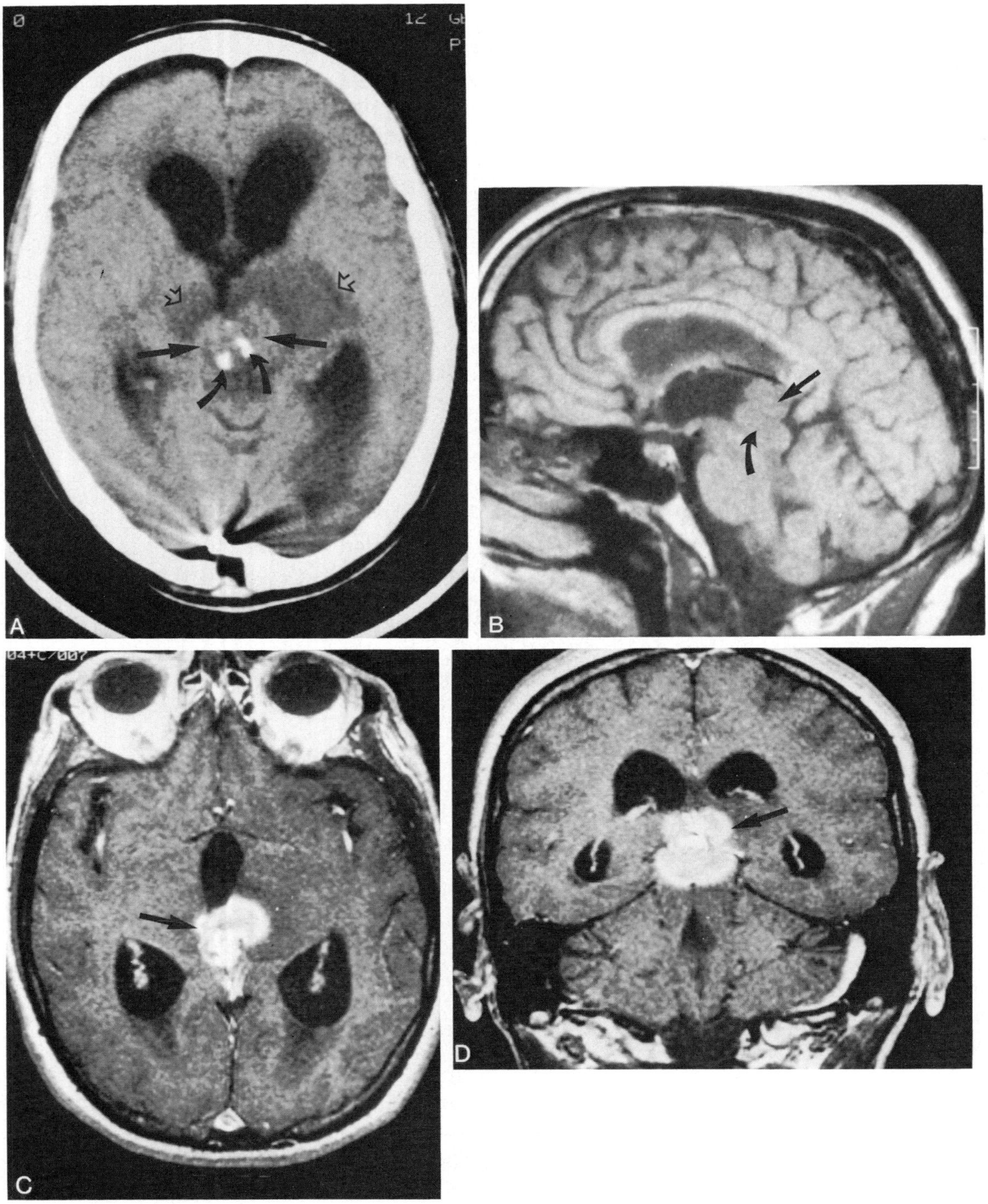

Figure 3–26. Pineal astrocytoma (55-year-old male).

A, Unenhanced CT. An isodense-to-brain mass (*arrows*) fills the pineal region. The tumor has produced nodular calcification (*curved arrows*). Vasogenic edema (*open arrows*) in the adjacent parenchyma is noted.

B, Parasagittal T1. The lobulated isointense mass (*arrow*) originated from the tectal plate (*curved arrow*).

C, D, Enhanced axial and coronal T1. The mass (*arrow*) enhances heterogeneously.

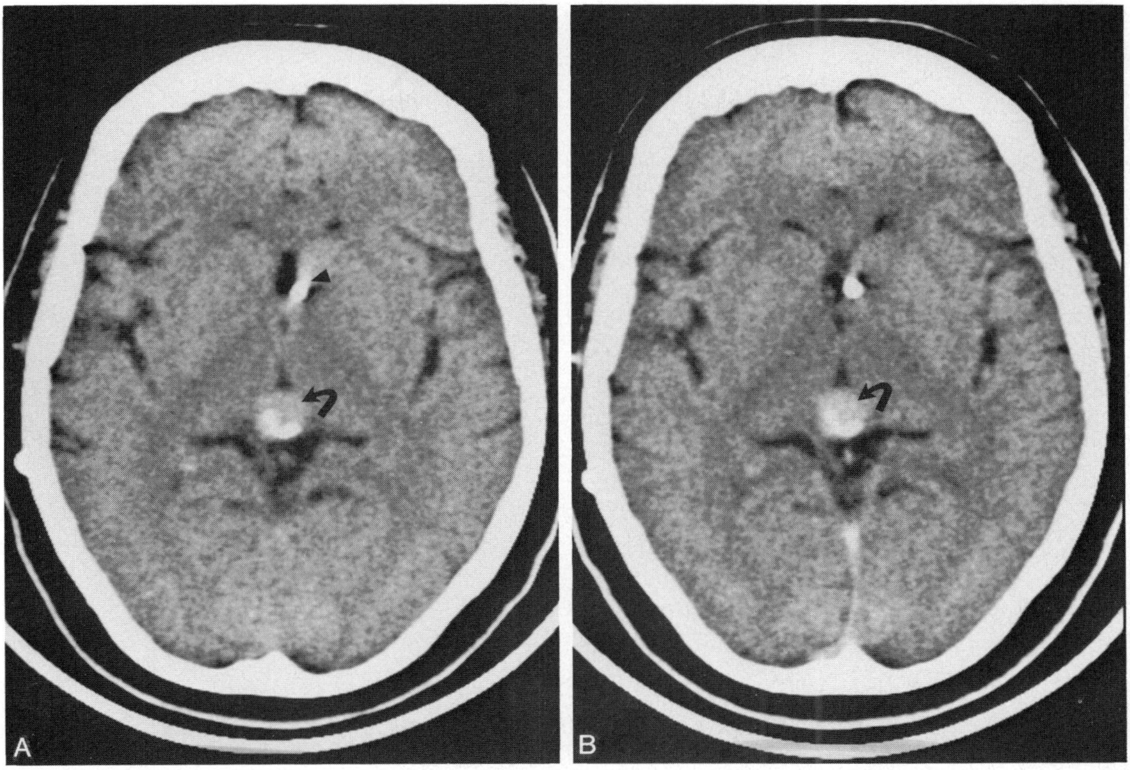

Figure 3–27. Pineocytoma (44-year-old female).

A, Unenhanced CT. A partially calcified pineal region mass (*curved arrow*) is present. The tip of a ventricular shunt tube (*arrowhead*) is adjacent to the left frontal horn.

B, Enhanced CT. The mass (*curved arrow*) enhances homogeneously following contrast administration.

mass without calcification. Enhancement is heterogeneous, often revealing a small central nidus of lucency (Fig. 3–28). These lucent foci are thought to represent areas of cystic degeneration.[51] Solid portions of the tumor are isointense to gray matter on T1 and usually hyperintense on T2-weighted spin echo sequences.

Meningioma

Although not a true lesion of the pineal gland, meningiomas that arise from the free edge of the tentorium or the velum interpositum may present as pineal region masses. (Meningiomas are discussed in more detail later in this chapter.)

Meningiomas are generally spherical hyperdense tumors that enhance homogeneously. Dural attachment may be demonstrated with coronal imaging[51] (Fig. 3–29). The classic MRI signal characteristics of this extra-axial neoplasm are that it is isointense to gray matter on T1 and isointense- to slightly hyperintense to gray matter on T2.[53]

Cerebellar Hemisphere

Intra-axial posterior fossa neoplasms are relatively common in children but less so in adults (Table 3–3). The most common primary cerebellar neoplasm in adults is hemangioblastoma; however, the most common cerebellar neoplasm in adults is the result of metastasis.

Hemangioblastoma. Hemangioblastomas are uncommon, relatively benign vascular endothelial origin neoplasms. These tumors represent less than 2.5% of primary intracranial neoplasms and account for 7% of intracranial neoplasms of the posterior fossa.[44] The neoplasm may occur at any age, frequently affecting young adults and children; the average age at diagnosis is 33 years. Polycythemia may be an accompanying feature of hemangioblastoma

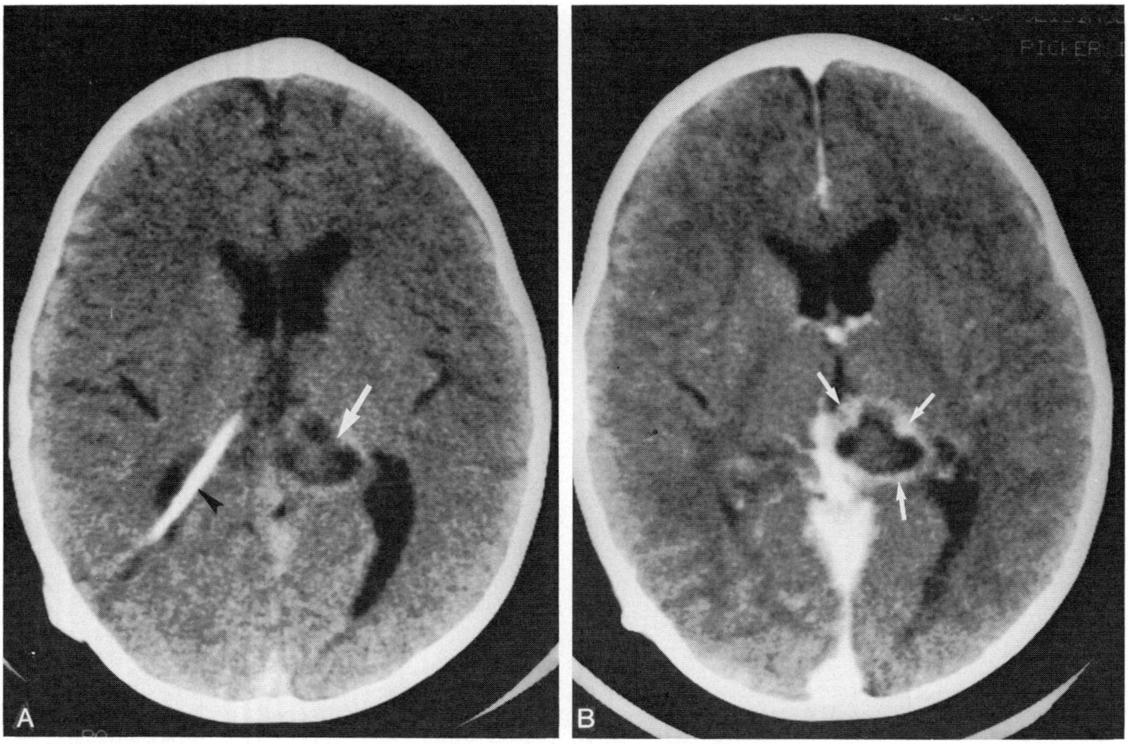

Figure 3–28. Pineoblastoma (8-year-old male).
A, Unenhanced CT. A hypodense mass (*arrow*) is present within the pineal region, extending into the adjacent parenchyma. A shunt tube (*arrowhead*) enters the right lateral ventricle.
B, Enhanced CT. Peripheral enhancement (*arrows*) more clearly defines the infiltrative margin of the mass.

Table 3–3. ADULT CEREBELLAR HEMISPHERIC TUMORS

Entity	Age (yr)	Planar Imaging Characteristics	
		CT	*MRI*
Hemangioblastoma	20–40	a. Cystic: enhancing mural nodule b. Solid: enhancing ± small cysts c. Minimal edema d. ± Multiple	a. Cyst isointense to CSF b. Solid: T1: isointense T2: hyperintense c. Solid tumor enhances vividly d. Minimal edema e. ± Multiple
Metastases	40–70	a. ± Multiple b. Marked enhancement, ring, variable c. Marked edema	a. T1: isointense b. T2: hyperintense c. ± Multiple d. Marked edema e. Marked enhancement
Glioma	<35	a. Cystic/solid b. Minimal edema c. Enhancement: moderate	a. Cystic: isointense to CSF on T1, T2; hyperintense SD b. Solid: T1: isointense T2: hyperintense c. Minimal edema d. Enhancement: moderate

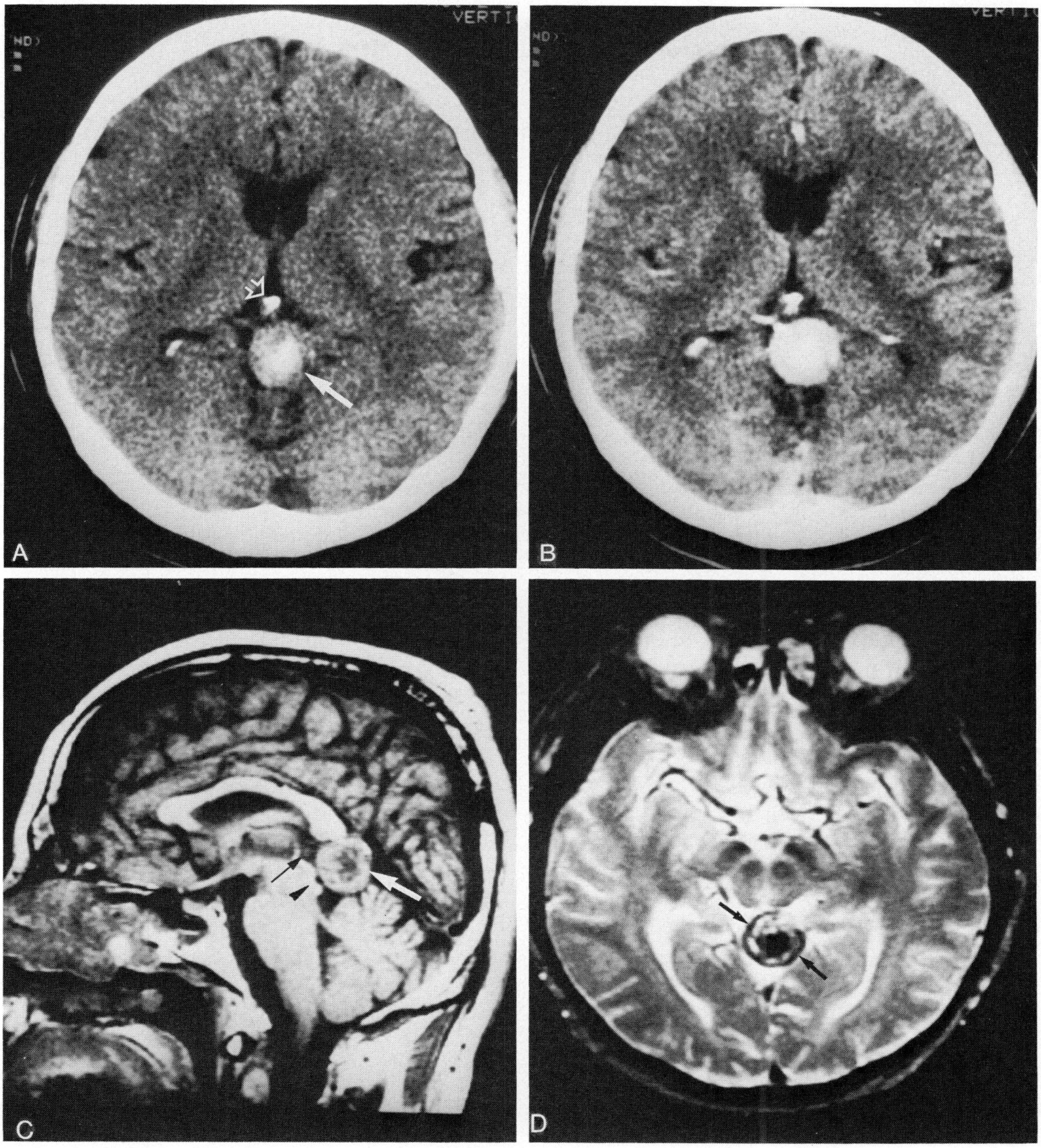

Figure 3–29. Pineal region meningioma (56-year-old male).

A, Unenhanced CT. Partially calcified 2-cm mass (*arrow*) is located within the pineal region. The calcified pineal gland (*open arrow*) can be detected anterior to the mass.

B, Enhanced CT. The mass enhances homogeneously, permitting better delineation of the lesion.

C, Parasagittal T1. The mass (*white arrow*) is heterogenous and fills the quadrigeminal plate and superior cerebellar cisterns but is extrinsic to the tectal plate (*arrowhead*) and the pineal gland (*black arrow*).

D, Axial T2. Markedly diminished signal (*arrows*) indicates probable calcification and possible remote hemorrhage.

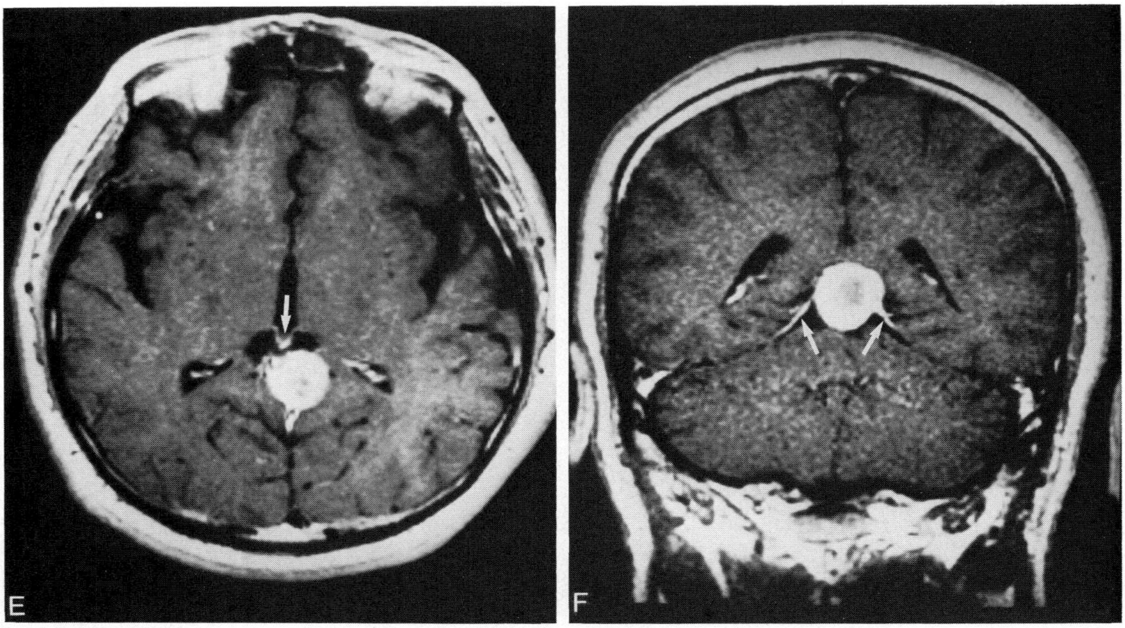

Figure 3–29 *Continued*
E, Enhanced axial T1. The mass enhances vividly and is clearly separate from the pineal gland (*arrow*).
F, Enhanced coronal T1. The dural attachment and enhancement (*arrows*) corroborate the meningeal origin of this lesion.

due to the erythropoietic factor isolated within the neoplasm. The tumor occurs most frequently in the cerebellar hemisphere, followed by the spinal cord and the medulla.[44] Less than 20% of patients with hemangioblastoma are associated with von Hippel–Lindau (VHL) disease. VHL disease, which includes multiple hemangiomas, angiomatosis of the retina, multiple renal and pancreatic cysts, and renal cell carcinomas, is discussed in more detail in Chapter 13.

The classic radiographic appearance of hemangioblastoma is that of a well-circumscribed cystic mass with an isodense to hyperdense mural nodule. The mural nodule enhances vividly following administration of contrast. These tumors do not calcify and generally do not promote significant vasogenic edema. The "classic" cystic appearance of this lesion is encountered less commonly than is the solid tumor morphology in some series.[58] The solid tumor may or may not contain small cysts. The solid tumor moiety enhances vividly.

Solid portions of the tumor on MRI are isointense to hypointense to brain on T1 images and hyperintense on T2 images; they may be heterogeneous. Cystic areas prolong both T1 and T2 relaxation times (Fig. 3–30). A secondary sign of hemangioblastoma is a serpentine signal void either within or incompletely surrounding the tumor (Fig. 3–31). The flow void is secondary to pathologic vessels that supply this tumor and have been detected in up to 72% of cases.[58] Spontaneous hemorrhage occurs in 5 to 10% of hemangioblastomas. Gadolinium-enhanced MRI is the most sensitive modality for lesion detection.

Metastasis. The common metastases have been discussed earlier in the chapter. Approximately 40% of CNS neoplasms involve the cerebellum. Common primary lesions that metastasize to the posterior fossa include those of the lung, breast, colon, and kidney and melanoma. Parenchymal hemispheric lesions may be solid or may have central areas of cystic necrosis. The tumors generally enhance, often in a peripheral, ring pattern (Fig. 3–32). Vasogenic edema, attendant mass effect, and noncommunicating hydrocephalus may complicate these posterior fossa lesions.

Glioma. Although posterior fossa gliomas occur most frequently in children, these neoplasms may also affect adults. The astrocytic series is the most prominent group of gliomas

Text continued on page 109

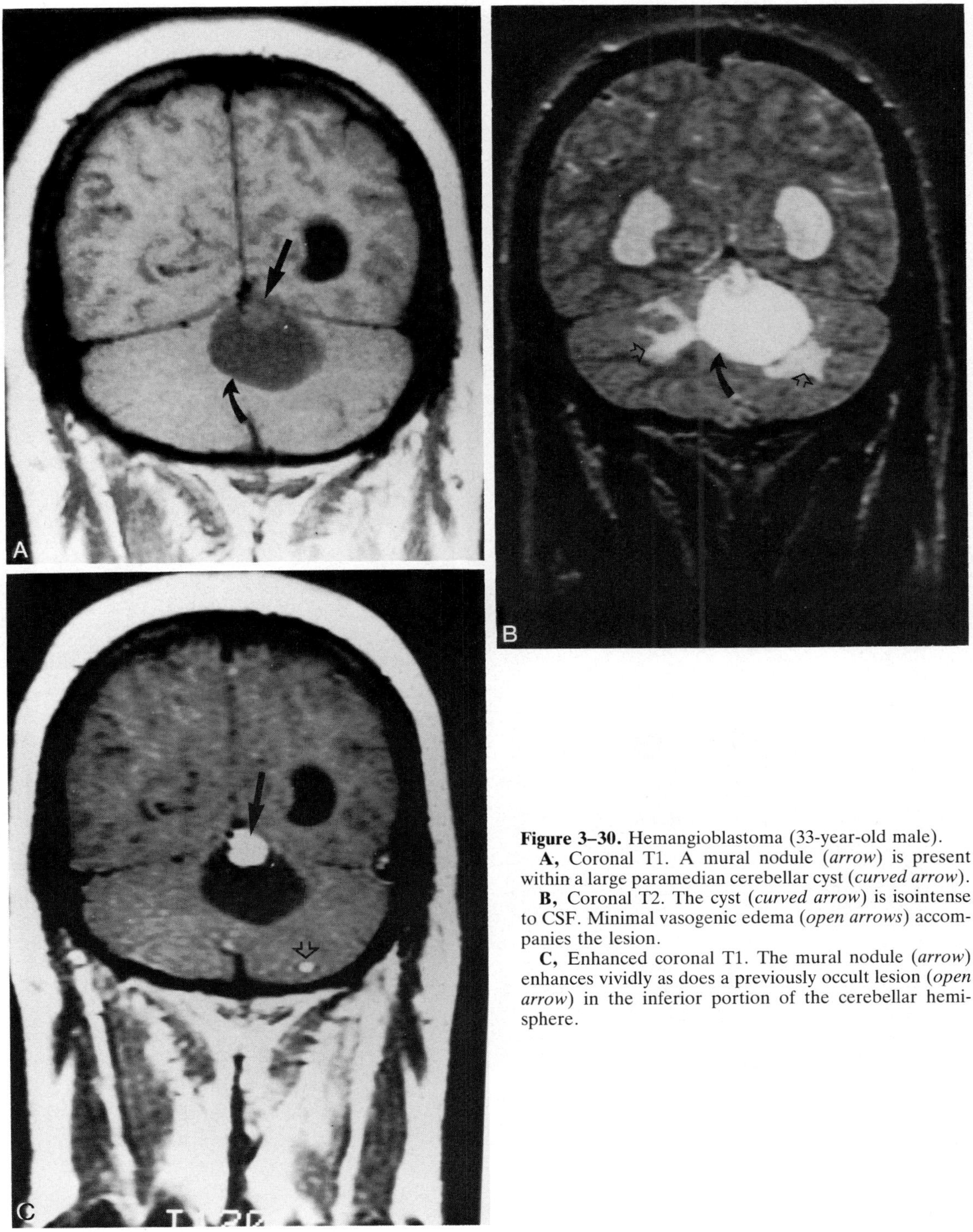

Figure 3–30. Hemangioblastoma (33-year-old male).

A, Coronal T1. A mural nodule (*arrow*) is present within a large paramedian cerebellar cyst (*curved arrow*).

B, Coronal T2. The cyst (*curved arrow*) is isointense to CSF. Minimal vasogenic edema (*open arrows*) accompanies the lesion.

C, Enhanced coronal T1. The mural nodule (*arrow*) enhances vividly as does a previously occult lesion (*open arrow*) in the inferior portion of the cerebellar hemisphere.

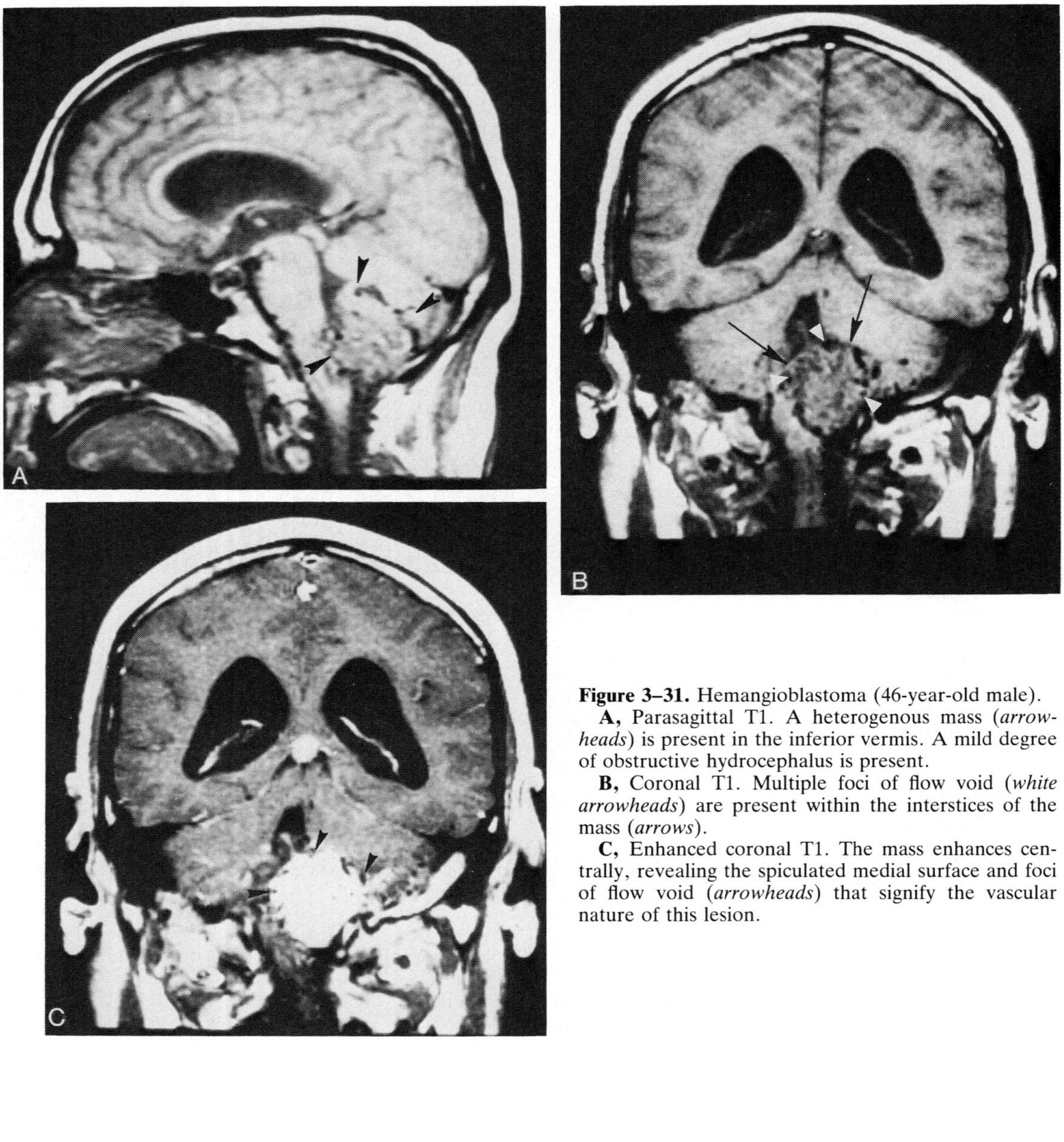

Figure 3–31. Hemangioblastoma (46-year-old male).

A, Parasagittal T1. A heterogenous mass (*arrowheads*) is present in the inferior vermis. A mild degree of obstructive hydrocephalus is present.

B, Coronal T1. Multiple foci of flow void (*white arrowheads*) are present within the interstices of the mass (*arrows*).

C, Enhanced coronal T1. The mass enhances centrally, revealing the spiculated medial surface and foci of flow void (*arrowheads*) that signify the vascular nature of this lesion.

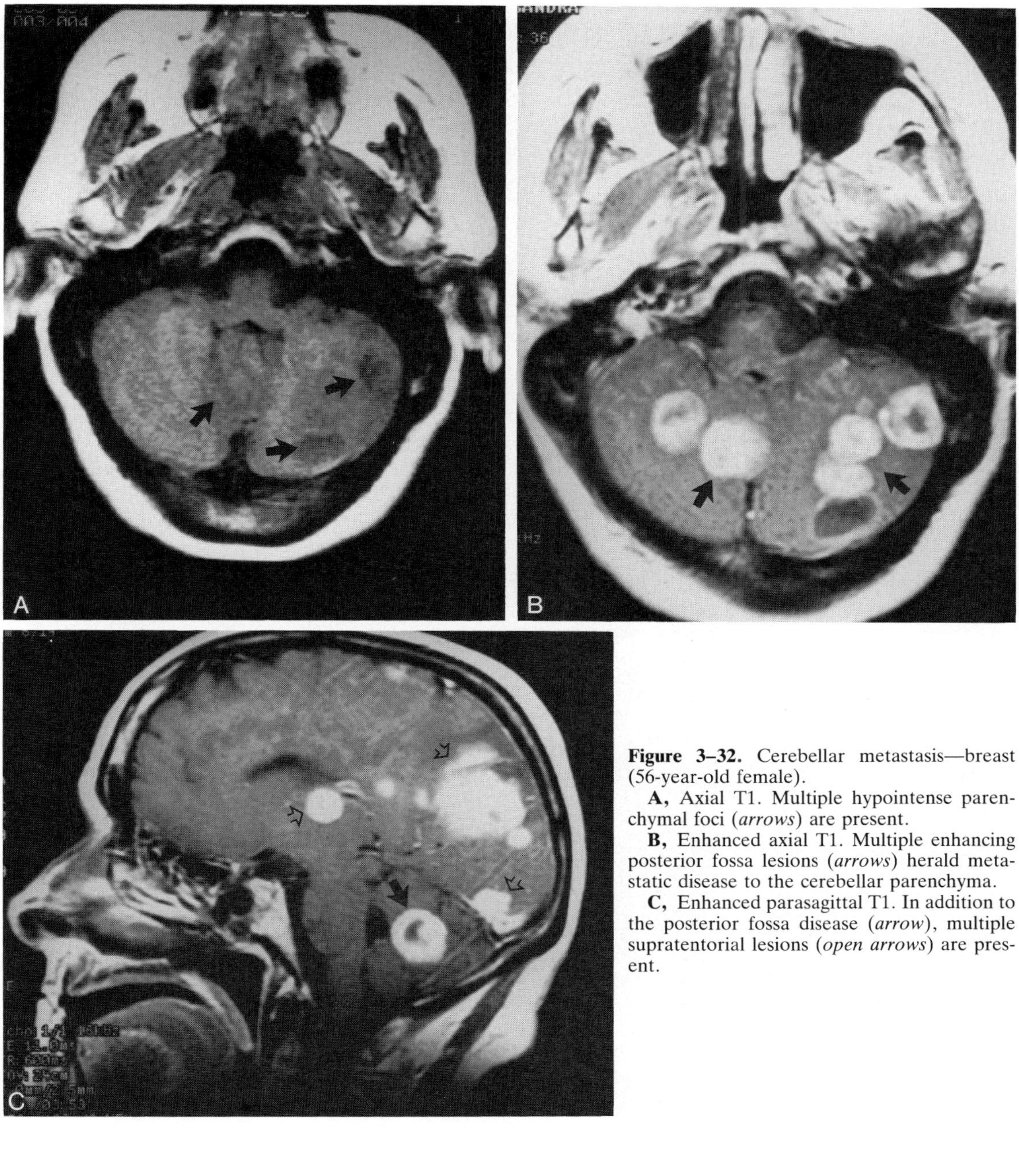

Figure 3–32. Cerebellar metastasis—breast (56-year-old female).

A, Axial T1. Multiple hypointense parenchymal foci (*arrows*) are present.

B, Enhanced axial T1. Multiple enhancing posterior fossa lesions (*arrows*) herald metastatic disease to the cerebellar parenchyma.

C, Enhanced parasagittal T1. In addition to the posterior fossa disease (*arrow*), multiple supratentorial lesions (*open arrows*) are present.

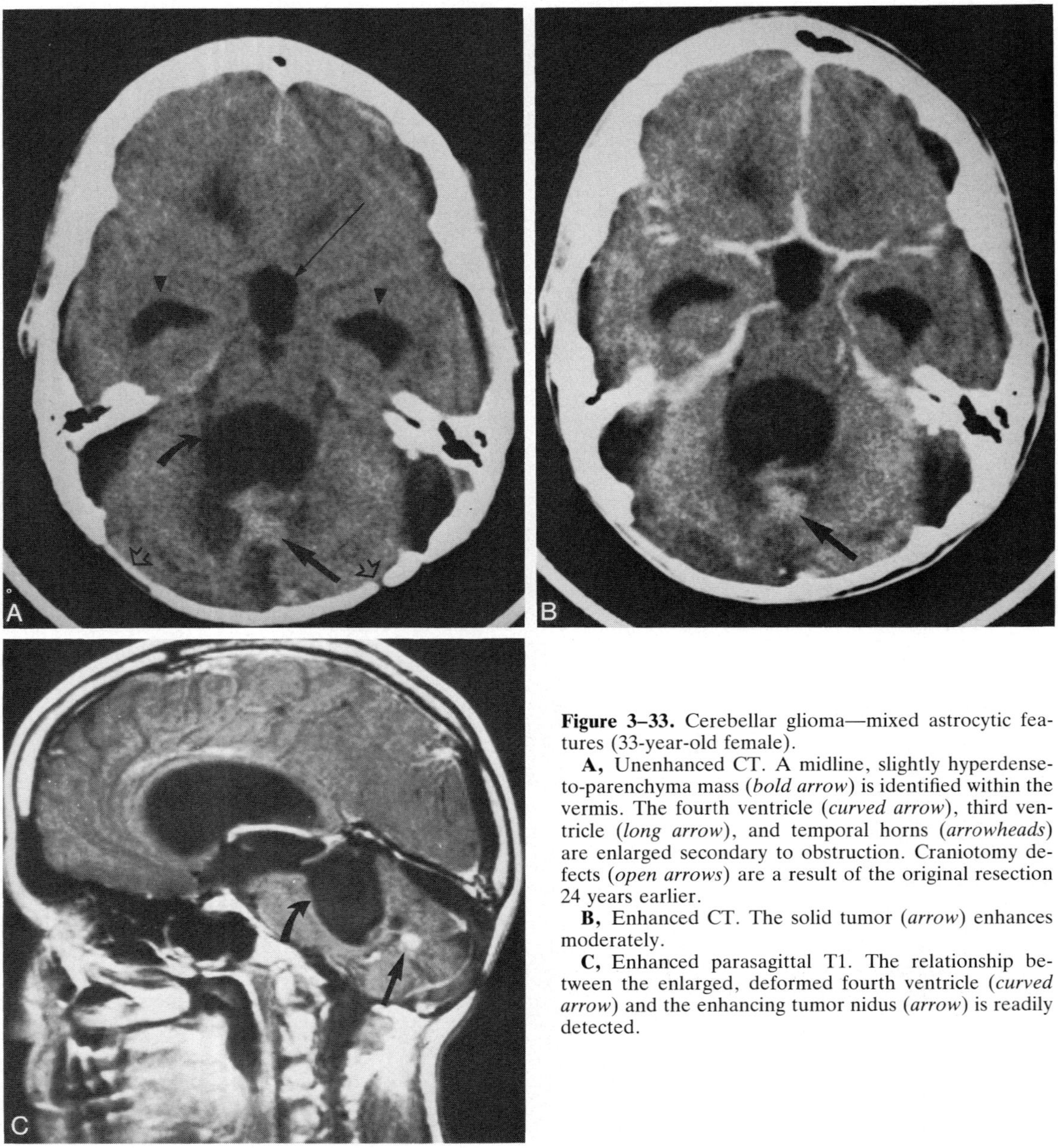

Figure 3–33. Cerebellar glioma—mixed astrocytic features (33-year-old female).

A, Unenhanced CT. A midline, slightly hyperdense-to-parenchyma mass (*bold arrow*) is identified within the vermis. The fourth ventricle (*curved arrow*), third ventricle (*long arrow*), and temporal horns (*arrowheads*) are enlarged secondary to obstruction. Craniotomy defects (*open arrows*) are a result of the original resection 24 years earlier.

B, Enhanced CT. The solid tumor (*arrow*) enhances moderately.

C, Enhanced parasagittal T1. The relationship between the enlarged, deformed fourth ventricle (*curved arrow*) and the enhancing tumor nidus (*arrow*) is readily detected.

to involve the posterior fossa parenchyma in adults. These lesions have characteristics similar to those of their low-grade supratentorial counterparts described previously (Fig. 3–33). The lesions may be solid, cystic, or both, and may arise within the vermis or, more commonly, from the cerebellar hemispheres.

Extra-axial Lesions (Table 3–4)

Meningioma

Meningiomas are the most common type of extra-axial neoplasm, accounting for nearly 20% of primary intracranial neoplasms.[44] Meningiomas arise from meningothelial cells. These cells are highly concentrated in the arachnoid villi, which explains the proclivity of these tumors to originate near dural sinuses. Meningiomas may arise in the parasagittal region, along the lateral convexities, the falx cerebri, the skull base, the sphenoid ridge, the floor of the anterior and middle cranial fossa, the tuberculum sella, the olfactory groove, the cerebellopontine angle, and less commonly within the ventricle.

Meningiomas occur at any age, though more commonly between the ages of 20 and 60 years, with a peak incidence at 45 years.[44] Intracranial meningiomas occur twice as frequently in females than in males. Intraspinal meningiomas occur four times more commonly in females.[44]

Based on microscopic criteria, meningiomas may be classified into six histologic variants including syncytial, fibroblastic, transitional, psammomatous, angioblastic, and sarcomatous.[44] It is possible to have two or more histologic variants located in different regions within a single tumor. With the exception of the angioblastic and sarcomatous neoplasms, these histologic variants all behave similarly. Meningiomas usually are slow growing and well circumscribed and tend to enlarge centrifugally, resulting in globular lesions. However, en plaque meningiomas will grow between the dura and the brain interface, resulting in a tortilla-shaped lesion. Invasion of the adjacent dura is common, but these lesions rarely invade the brain parenchyma. Angioblastic and sarcomatous meningiomas behave more malignantly, with rapid growth, invasion of the

Table 3–4. EXTRA-AXIAL LESIONS

Entity	Age (yr)	Sex	Location	Planar Imaging Characteristics: *CT*	Planar Imaging Characteristics: *MRI*
Meningioma	45	Male:female 1:2	a. Parasagittal b. Floor of middle and anterior fossae c. Tuberculum sella d. Olfactory groove e. Cerebellopontine angle	a. Intrinsically dense b. Calcification: 30% c. Homogeneously enhancing d. Hyperostosis	a. Isointense to parenchyma on T1 and T2 b. CSF cleavage plane c. Dural enhancement d. Edema variable
Epidermoid	30–40	Male:female 2:1	a. Cerebellopontine angle b. Parapituitary region c. Diploë of frontal or parietal bone d. Petrous apex	a. Isodense CSF b. No enhancement or edema c. Lobulated surface	a. Isointense to hyperintense to CSF on T1 and T2 (rarely high signal on T1) b. No enhancement or edema
Dermoid	10–25	Male:female 1–1.5:1	a. Midline posterior fossa; 4th ventricle b. 3rd ventricle, parasellar region	a. Heterogeneous fat/calcification b. No enhancement or edema	a. Heterogeneous: fat ↑ on T1; calcium ↓ on T1 and T2 b. No enhancement or edema
Arachnoid cyst	10–40	Males = Females	a. Middle fossa b. Posterior fossa c. Suprasellar region d. Quadrigeminal plate cistern e. Choroidal fissure	a. Isodense to CSF b. No enhancement or edema	a. Isointense to CSF on all spin echo sequences b. No enhancement or edema

underlying bone and brain, and a tendency to recur following surgery.

Meningiomas, regardless of histologic subtype, rarely metastasize extracranially. The proximity to the dural sinuses may play a role in the extracranial spread of these neoplasms. The lungs represent the most frequent site of distant metastasis. CSF metastasis is very rare.[59]

Meningiomas often induce hyperostosis, a local osteoblastic proliferation. This may be partly related to direct invasion of the inner table and medullary cavity or may be a reactive phenomenon to the meningioma and the secondary hypervascularity. The associated hyperostosis generally involves the adjacent bone, with thickening of the inner table and medullary cavity. Rarely, these lesions may be destructive with areas of osteolysis.

Meningiomas display extra-axial characteristics on CT. The tumor is usually clearly marginated and isodense to hyperdense to brain. Vasogenic edema in meningiomas varies; its presence and amount are related more to the site of origin than to tumor size. Tumors that arise parasagittally, along the convexities, or in the anterior frontal region are far more likely to be associated with vasogenic edema. Edema is not a predominant feature of subfrontal, parasellar, infratentorial, or intraventricular tumors.[59] Calcium is detectable on plain films in 15% of these patients. The rate of CT-detectable calcification in these tumors exceeds 30%.

As a rule, meningiomas enhance homogeneously. The tumor-brain interface and the rare, intratumoral cysts become more apparent following contrast administration (Fig. 3–34). The sarcomatous or angioblastic varieties may rarely display nonenhancing foci of necrosis (Fig. 3–35).

MRI accurately depicts the extra-axial nature of these lesions[60] (Fig. 3–36). The mass is usually isointense to hypointense to paren-

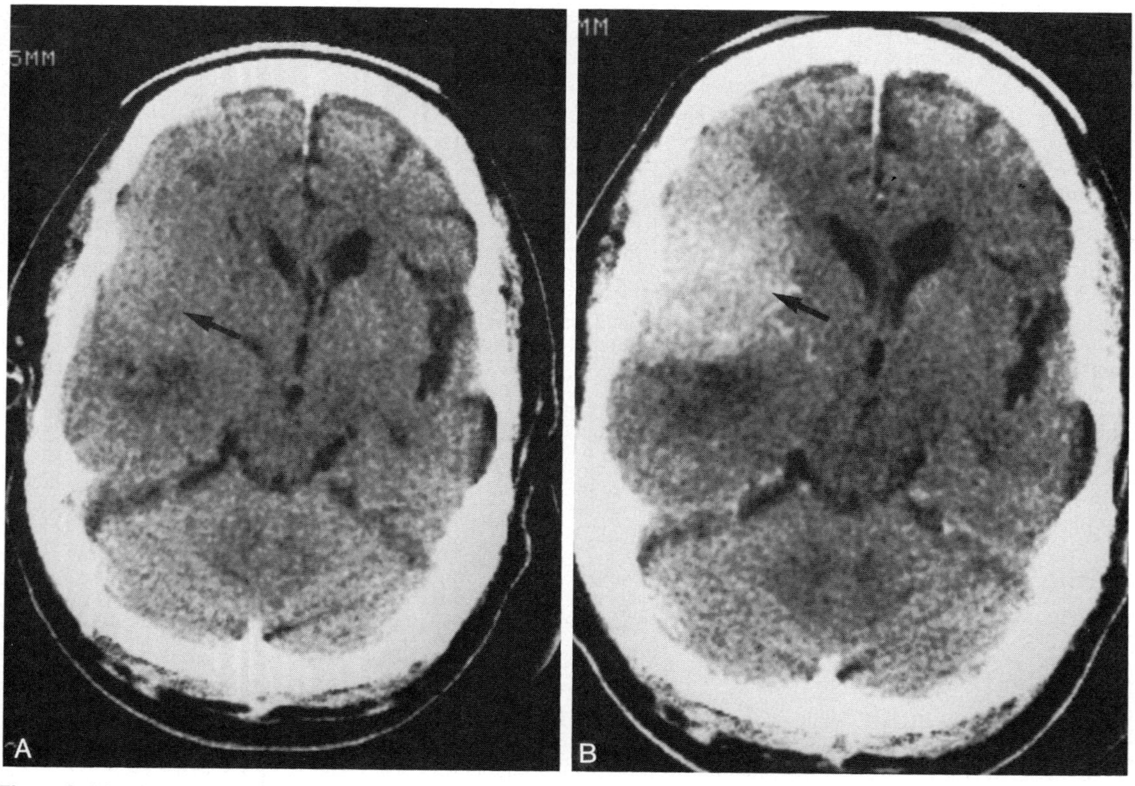

Figure 3–34. Meningioma (65-year-old male).
A, Unenhanced CT. An ill-defined high-density mass (*arrow*) effaces the right sylvian fissure.
B, Enhanced CT. The mass (*arrow*) enhances homogeneously. The relationship of the mass to the subjacent brain parenchyma becomes more apparent.

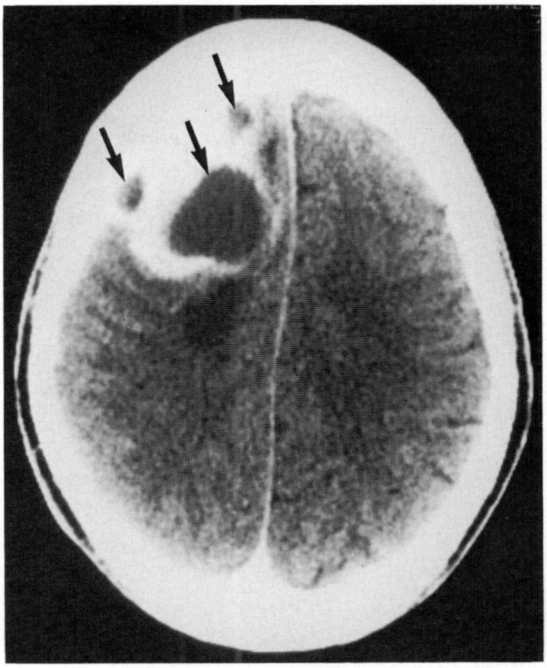

Figure 3–35. Meningioma—angioblastic (69-year-old male). A heterogeneously enhancing mass is present in the right frontal region. At least three regions of cystic necrosis (*arrows*) are located within the tumor matrix.

chyma on T1 images. The T2 appearance of these lesions is variable and may offer the ability to distinguish various histologic subtypes in some[61] but not all cases.[62] Lesions that are hypointense to cortex on T2 are often fibroblastic or transitional types. Syncytial or angioblastic variants are often hyperintense to cortex on T2. Specificity may be improved as secondary signs are evaluated. Presence of edema and cystic necrosis is more common with syncytial or angioblastic variance. Calcium is more common in the transitional or fibroblastic subtypes.

The tumor most commonly enhances homogeneously (Fig. 3–37). In a high percentage of cases (60 to 72%),[63, 64] a dural-based, linear region of enhancement extends away from the tumor. This linear enhancement tapers as it extends from the tumor margin and often enhances to a greater degree than the tumor itself. This dural enhancement most likely is due to proliferation of adjacent vascular connective tissue or, less likely, microscopic tumor invasion. The peritumoral dural enhancement is not necessarily specific for meningioma, as a small percentage (16%) of superficial malignant neoplasms may be associated with dural enhancement.[65] Dural enhancement has also been reported with sarcoidosis, lymphoma, leukemia,[66] and acoustic schwannomas.

Epidermoid

Epidermoid cysts are slow-growing ectodermal inclusion cysts that result from ectoderm trapped at the time of closure of the neural tube. These lesions are lined by stratified squamous epithelium and grow by way of desquamation of cells and debris into the cyst. The lesion may be cystic or solid with a high cholesterol or lipid concentration. Foci of calcification may be present rarely, scattered throughout the periphery of the lesion.

Epidermoids represent 0.3 to 1.8% of intracranial neoplasms.[67] These lesions may occur at any age, with a peak incidence in the fourth to fifth decade. Males are affected at twice the rate of females.[68] Epidermoids tend to spare the midline, occurring laterally. In decreasing order, the most frequent sites of involvement are the cerebellopontine angle, the parapituitary region, the diploë of the frontal and parietal bones, the spinal canal, and the petrous apex.

CT demonstrates a mass that is isodense to hypodense to CSF.[69] Epidermoid cysts may remain undetected if they do not produce

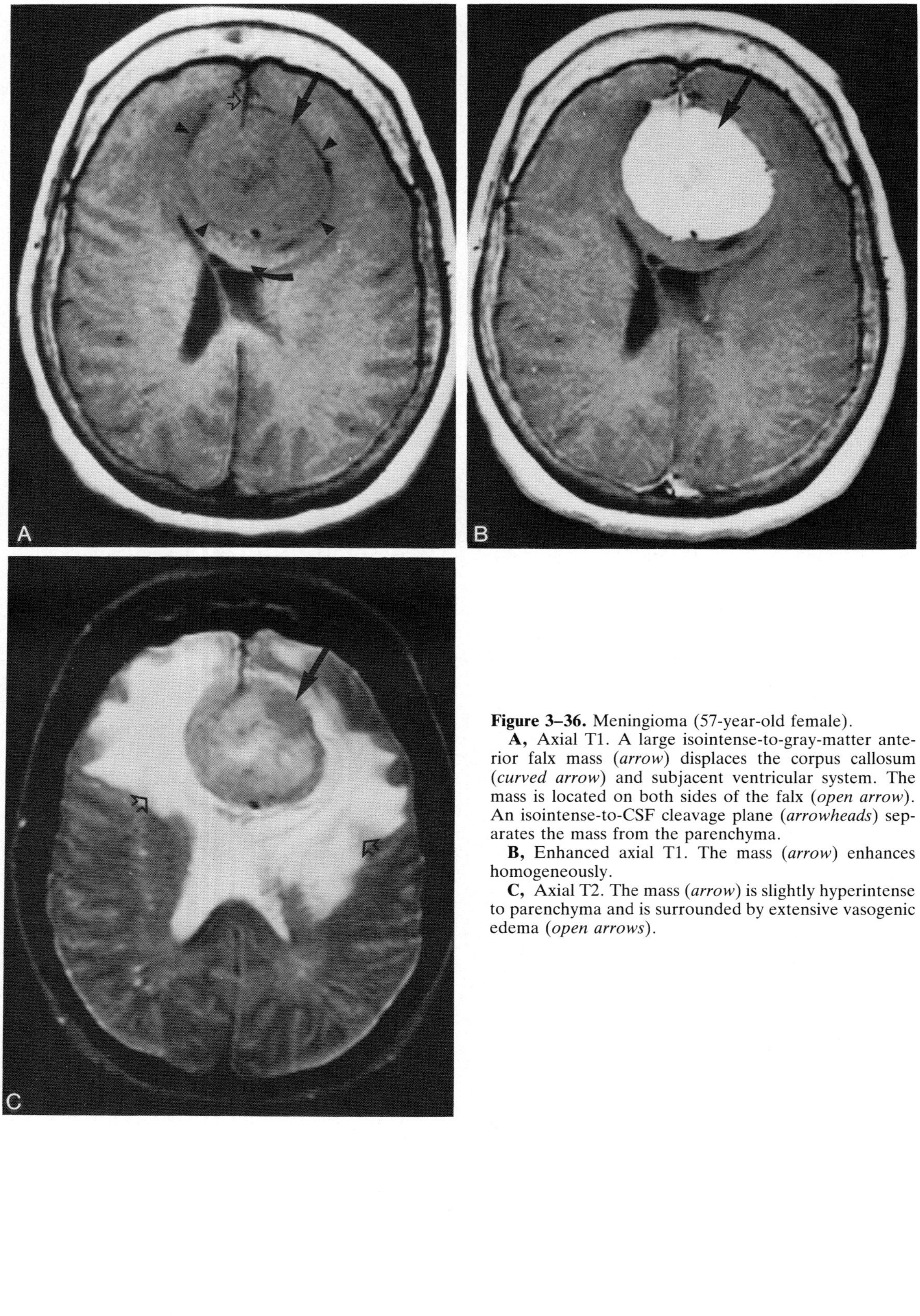

Figure 3–36. Meningioma (57-year-old female).

A, Axial T1. A large isointense-to-gray-matter anterior falx mass (*arrow*) displaces the corpus callosum (*curved arrow*) and subjacent ventricular system. The mass is located on both sides of the falx (*open arrow*). An isointense-to-CSF cleavage plane (*arrowheads*) separates the mass from the parenchyma.

B, Enhanced axial T1. The mass (*arrow*) enhances homogeneously.

C, Axial T2. The mass (*arrow*) is slightly hyperintense to parenchyma and is surrounded by extensive vasogenic edema (*open arrows*).

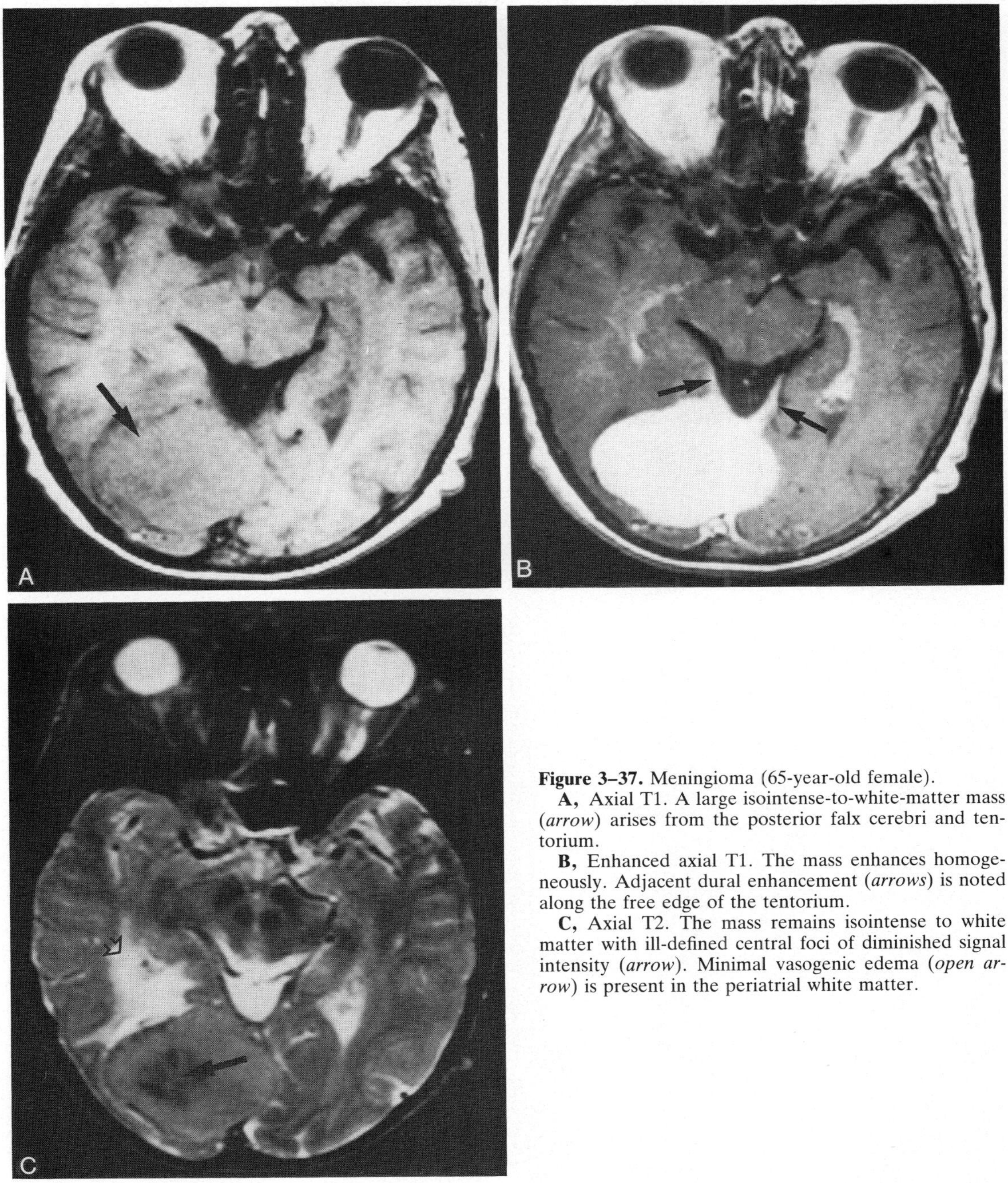

Figure 3–37. Meningioma (65-year-old female).

A, Axial T1. A large isointense-to-white-matter mass (*arrow*) arises from the posterior falx cerebri and tentorium.

B, Enhanced axial T1. The mass enhances homogeneously. Adjacent dural enhancement (*arrows*) is noted along the free edge of the tentorium.

C, Axial T2. The mass remains isointense to white matter with ill-defined central foci of diminished signal intensity (*arrow*). Minimal vasogenic edema (*open arrow*) is present in the periatrial white matter.

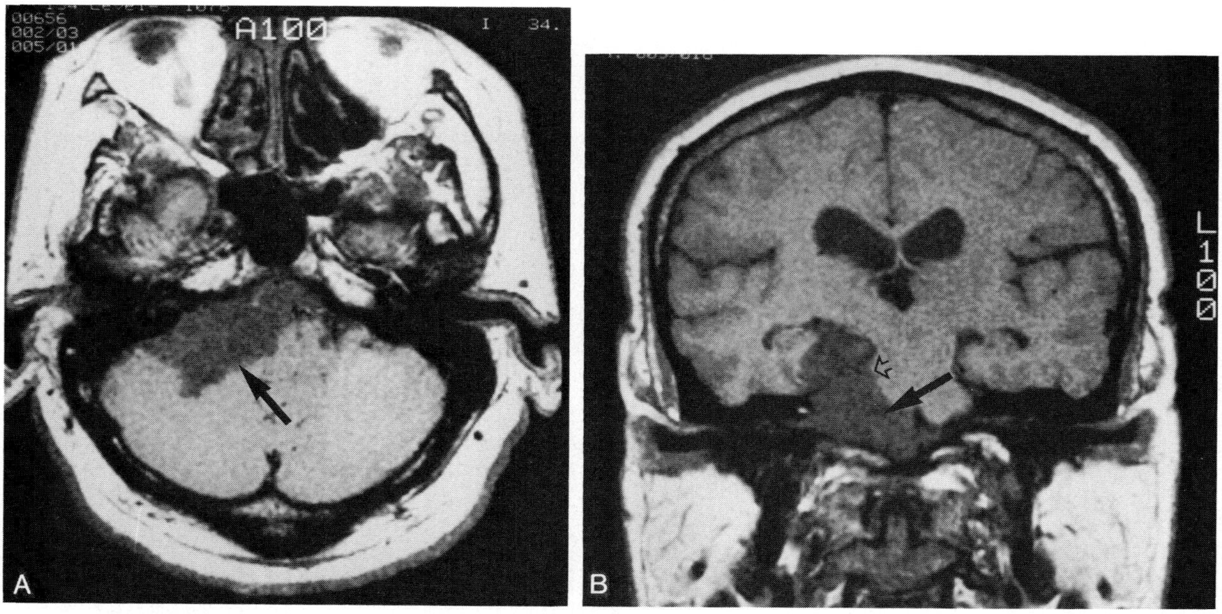

Figure 3–38. Epidermoid (50-year-old male).

A, B, Axial and coronal T1. A lobulated, slightly hyperintense-to-CSF mass (*arrow*) fills the right cerebellopontine angle (CPA), displacing the brainstem to the left. The mass extends through the tentorial incisura along the ambient cistern (*open arrow*).

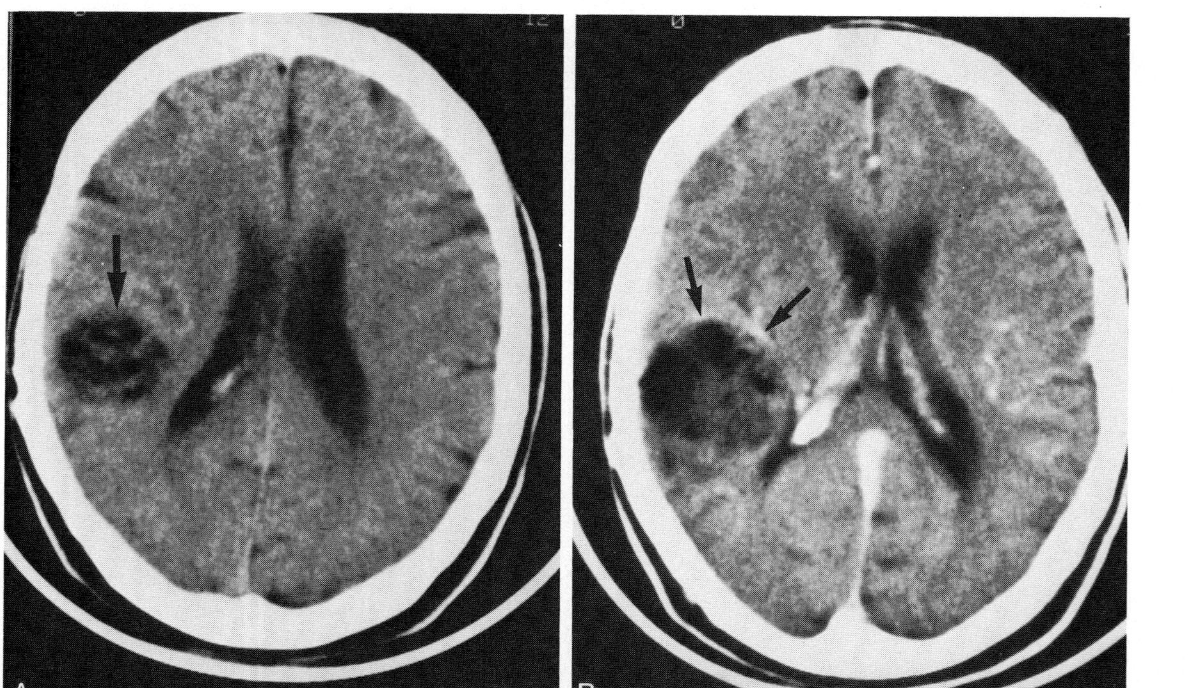

Figure 3–39. Dermoid (66-year-old male).

A, Unenhanced CT. A mixed-density mass (*arrow*) is identified arising from the right sylvian fissure. The mass contains regions of CSF density.

B, Enhanced CT at a more cephalad level. The tumor matrix does not enhance. There is a peripheral rim of enhancement (*arrows*) noted secondary to compression of the surrounding cortical vessels.

significant mass effect. Epidermoids rarely contain calcification and do not enhance following administration of contrast material. Intrathecal water-soluble contrast material may be used to silhouette the lobulated filling defect within the CSF cistern.

The MRI appearance of epidermoids is variable. The tumor may be isointense to CSF with relatively low signal on T1 and high signal on T2 images[68] (Fig. 3–38). Alternatively, lesions may be high signal intensity on T1 images.[70] Through carbon 13 MRI spectroscopy, lesions with high T1 signal are shown to have a high lipid content and are often cystic at surgery. Lesions with diminished T1 signal have minimal lipid content, contain trace cholesterol, and are more often solid at surgery. On spin-density images, these lesions may be surrounded by a rim of high signal, thought to represent trapped CSF between the tumor and adjacent brain.[68] Diffusion-weighted MRI has been used to distinguish epidermoids from extra-axial cysts.[71] Brownian motion within these extra-axial lesions can be measured and compared with water and oil phantoms. Molecular motion is greater in the CSF-containing cyst than in the epidermoid cyst, leading to a greater attenuation of signal in the former.

Dermoid

Dermoid cysts are inclusion cysts of ectodermal and mesodermal elements. The cyst is lined with stratified squamous cell epithelium and filled with hair follicles, sebaceous glands, and sweat glands. Like epidermoids, these are thought to arise during closure of the neural tube at 3 to 5 weeks of gestation.

Dermoids are predominantly midline tumors, found more commonly in the posterior fossa, in either the cisterna magna or the fourth ventricle. Supratentorial lesions may occur adjacent to the third ventricle in the parasellar region. These lesions are less common than epidermoids and generally present at a younger age.

Radiographically, these lesions are more heterogeneous than are epidermoids. Dermoids may be lower density than CSF secondary to the adipose tissue (Fig. 3–39). The solid tumor matrix may be isodense to parenchyma. Dermoids are more likely to contain calcium

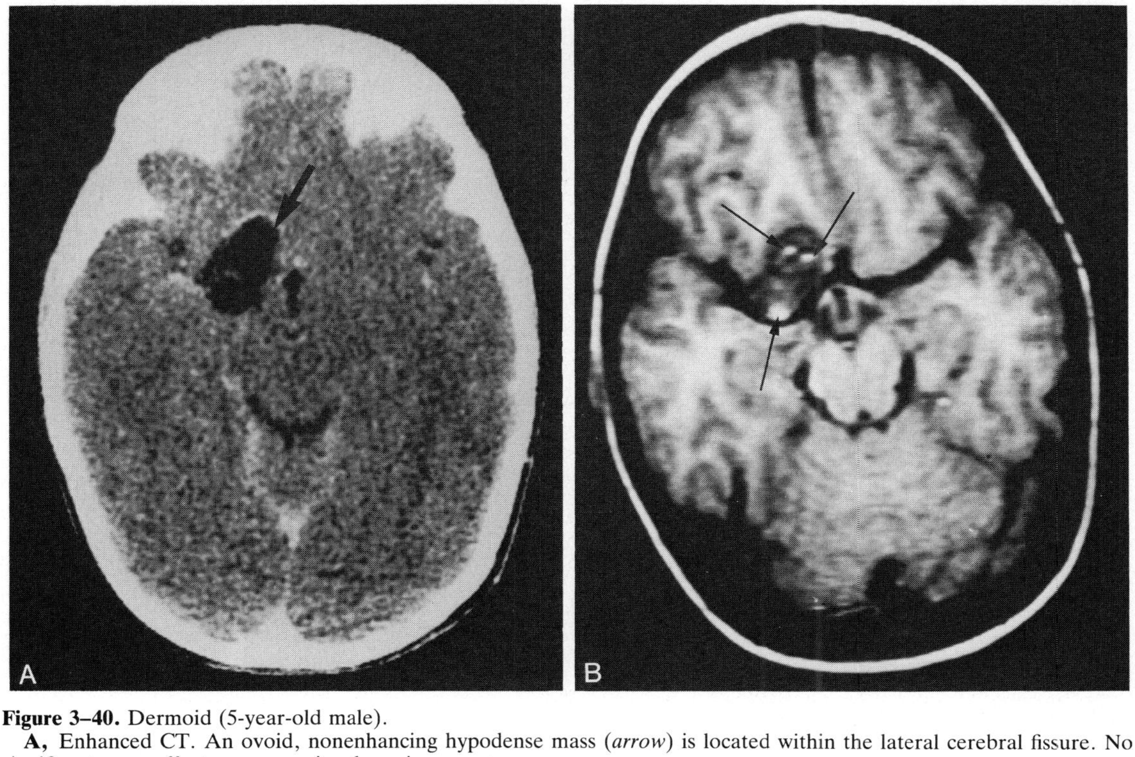

Figure 3–40. Dermoid (5-year-old male).

A, Enhanced CT. An ovoid, nonenhancing hypodense mass (*arrow*) is located within the lateral cerebral fissure. No significant mass effect or vasogenic edema is present.

B, Axial T1. The heterogeneous mass contains foci of high signal (*arrows*), representing fat.

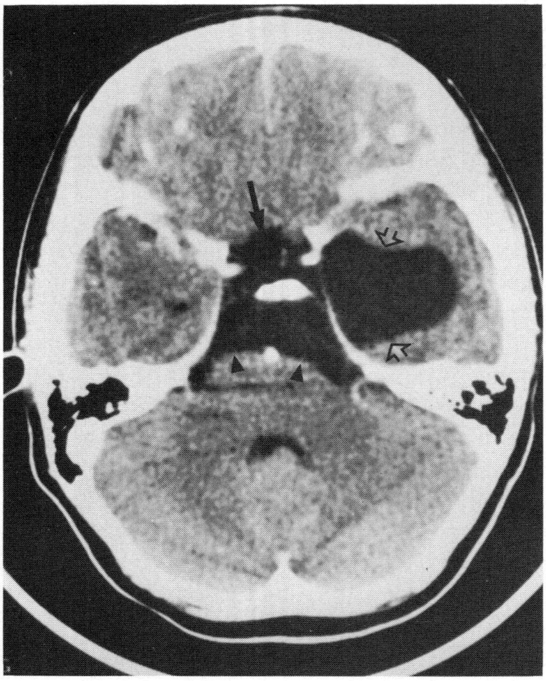

Figure 3–41. Arachnoid cyst (9-year-old female). Enhanced CT; a well-circumscribed, isodense-to-CSF mass extends into the suprasellar cistern (*arrow*), the left middle cranial fossa (*open arrows*), and the posterior fossa (*arrowheads*).

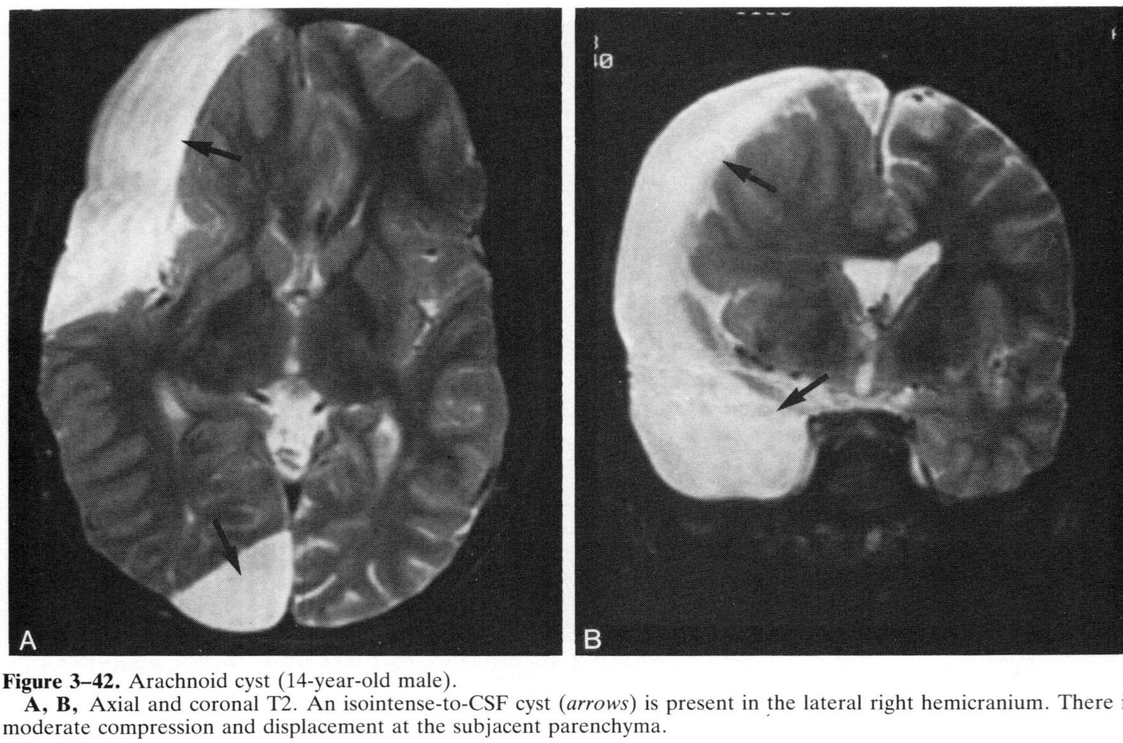

Figure 3–42. Arachnoid cyst (14-year-old male).

A, B, Axial and coronal T2. An isointense-to-CSF cyst (*arrows*) is present in the lateral right hemicranium. There is moderate compression and displacement at the subjacent parenchyma.

than are epidermoids. Although the lesion generally does not enhance, a thin rim of enhancement may be detected surrounding the lesion, which is thought to be secondary to compressed normal brain. Edema is rarely present.

MRI depicts an equally heterogeneous extra-axial mass. The adipose content of the lesion increases the T1 signal of this tumor (Fig. 3–40). Calcium may serve to diminish the T1 and T2 signal intensities. Rarely, the dermoid cyst may rupture, disseminating the fatty material through the CSF space.[72]

Arachnoid Cyst

These CSF-containing cysts represent less than 1% of intracranial masses. Arachnoid cysts most frequently are found in the middle cranial fossa, followed by the posterior fossa, suprasellar region, quadrigeminal plate, choroidal fissure, and frontal convexities, and within the ventricles.

The cysts may be stable or slowly progressive in size. Although most arachnoid cysts are asymptomatic, they may produce headaches, seizures, or focal deficits. Obstructive hydrocephalus may result if the lesion is strategically located along CSF pathways. Pituitary axis dysfunction may result from suprasellar arachnoid cysts.

Arachnoid cysts are isodense to CSF, smoothly marginated, nonenhancing lesions of variable size without associated edema (Fig. 3–41). MRI depicts a lesion that is isointense to CSF on all spin echo sequences (Fig. 3–42). The temporal lobe adjacent to the cranial fossa cyst may be small, perhaps an associated finding rather than one resulting from actual mass effect and compression of the temporal lobe.[73] Arachnoid cysts do not enhance following contrast administration.[74]

Peripheral, low-grade cystic astrocytomas may masquerade as arachnoid cysts. The low-grade tumor can be differentiated from arachnoid cysts on the long TR–short TE spin-density images, where the neoplasm will remain hyperintense to CSF (see Fig. 3–2).

References

1. Russell D, Rubinstein L. *Pathology of Tumors of the Nervous System,* 4th ed. London: Arnold, 1977.
2. Leeds NE, Elkin CM, Zimmerman RD: Gliomas of the brain. Semin Roentgenol 1984; 19:27–43.
3. Lee BCP, Kneeland JB, Cahill PT, et al: MR recognition of supratentorial tumors. AJNR 1984; 6:871–878.
4. Dean BL, Drayer BP, Bird CR, et al: Gliomas: Classification with MR imaging. Radiology 1990; 174:411–415.
5. Graif M, Bydder GM, Steiner RE, et al: Contrast-enhanced MR imaging of malignant brain tumors. AJNR 1985; 6:855–862.
6. Burger PC, Vogel FS, Green SB, et al: Glioblastoma multiforme and anaplastic astrocytoma. Cancer 1985; 56:1106–1111.
7. Tassel PV, Lee YY, Bruner JM: Synchronous and metachronous malignant gliomas: CT findings. AJNR 1988; 9:725–732.
8. Lee YY, Tassel PV: Intracranial oligodendroglioma: Imaging findings in 35 untreated cases. AJNR 1989; 10:119–127.
9. Zimmerman HM: The pathology of primary brain tumors. Semin Roentgenol 1984; 19:129–138.
10. Vonofakos D, Marcu H, Hacker H: Oligodendrogliomas: CT patterns with emphasis on features indicating malignancy. J Comput Assist Tomogr 1979; 3:783–788.
11. Holland BA, Kucharcyzk W, Brant-Zawadzki M, et al: MR imaging of calcified intracranial lesions. Radiology 1985; 157:353–356.
12. Armington WG, Osborn AG, Cubberley DA, et al: Supratentorial ependymoma: CT appearance. Radiology 1985; 157:367–372.
13. Swartz JD, Zimmerman RA, Bilaniuk LT: Computed tomography of intracranial ependymomas. Radiology 1982; 143:97–101.
14. Spoto GP, Press GA, Hesselink JR, et al: Intracranial ependymoma and subependymoma: MR manifestations. AJNR 1990; 11:83–91.
15. Jooma R, Torrens MJ, Bradshaw J, et al: Subependymomas of the fourth ventricle. J Neurosurg 1985; 62:508–512.
16. Gandolfi A, Brizzi RE, Tedeschi F, et al: Symptomatic subependymoma of the fourth ventricle. J Neurosurg 1981; 55:841–844.
17. Morrison G, Sobel DF, Kelley WM, et al: Intraventricular mass lesions. Radiology 1984; 153:435–442.
18. Schwaighofer BW, Hesselink JR, Press GA, et al: Primary intracranial CNS lymphoma: MR manifestations. AJNR 1989; 10:725–729.
19. Jack CR, Reese DF, Scheithauer BW: Radiographic findings in 32 cases of primary CNS lymphoma. AJR 1986; 146:271–276.
20. Kawakami Y, Trabuchi K, Ohnishi R, et al: Primary central nervous system lymphoma. J Neurosurg 1985; 62:522–527.
21. Henry JM, Heffner RR, Dillard SH, et al: Primary malignant lymphomas of the central nervous system. Cancer 1974; 34:1293–1302.
22. Jiddane M, Nicoli F, Diaz P, et al: Intracranial malignant lymphoma. J Neurosurg 1986; 65:592–599.
23. Jack CR, O'Neill BP, Banks PM, et al: Central nervous system lymphoma: Histologic types and CT appearance. Radiology 1988; 167:211–215.
24. Whelan MA, Kricheff II: Intracranial lymphoma. Semin Roentgenol 1984; 19:91–99.
25. Poon T, Matoso I, Tchertkoff V, et al: CT features of primary cerebral lymphoma in AIDS and non-AIDS patients. J Comput Assist Tomogr 1989; 13:6–9.

26. Goldstein JD, Zeifer B, Chao C, et al: CT appearance of primary CNS lymphoma in patients with acquired immunodeficiency syndrome. J Comput Assist Tomogr 1991; 15:39–44.
27. Castillo M, Davis PC, Takei Y, et al: Intracranial ganglioglioma: MR, CT and clinical findings in 18 patients. AJNR 1990; 11:109–114.
28. Tampieri D, Moumdjian R, Melanson D, et al: Intracerebral gangliogliomas in patients with partial complex seizures: CT and MR imaging findings. AJNR 1991; 12:749–755.
29. Sze G, Shin J, Krol G, et al: Intraparenchymal brain metastases: MR imaging versus contrast-enhanced CT. Radiology 1988; 168:187–194.
30. Russell EJ, Geremia GK, Johnson CE, et al: Multiple cerebral metastases: Detectability with Gd-DTPA-enhanced MR imaging. Radiology 1987; 165:609–617.
31. Davis PC, Hudgins PA, Peterman SB, et al: Diagnosis of cerebral metastases: Double-dose delayed CT vs. contrast-enhanced MR imaging. AJNR 1991; 12:293–300.
32. Sze G, Milano E, Johnson C, et al: Detection of brain metastases: Comparison of contrast-enhanced MR with unenhanced MR and enhanced CT. AJNR 1990; 11:785–791.
33. Healy ME, Hesselink JR, Press GA, et al: Increased detection of intracranial metastases with intravenous Gd-DTPA. Radiology 1987; 165:619–624.
34. Tyrrell RL, Bundschuh CV, Modic MT: Dural carcinomatosis: MR demonstration. J Comput Assist Tomogr 1987; 11:329–332.
35. Lee YY, Glass JP, Geoffray A, et al: Cranial computed tomographic abnormalities in leptomeningeal metastasis. AJNR 1984; 5:559–563.
36. Sze G, Soletsky S, Bronen R, et al: MR imaging of the cranial meninges with emphasis on contrast enhancement and meningeal carcinomatosis. AJNR 1989; 10:965–975.
37. Kondziolka D, Bernstein M, Resch L, et al: Significance of hemorrhage into brain tumors: Clinicopathological study. J Neurosurg 1987; 67:852–857.
38. Destian S, Sze G, Krol G, et al: MR imaging of hemorrhagic intracranial neoplasms. AJNR 1988; 9:1115–1122.
39. Atlas SW, Grossman RI, Gomori JM, et al: MR imaging of intracranial metastatic melanoma. J Comput Assist Tomogr 1987; 11:577–582.
40. Woodruff WW, Djang WT, McLendon RE, et al: Intracerebral malignant melanoma: High-field-strength MR imaging. Radiology 1987; 165:209–213.
41. Silver AJ, Ganti SR, Hilal SK: Computed tomography of tumors involving the atria of the lateral ventricles. Radiology 1982; 145:71–78.
42. Jelinek J, Smirniotopoulos JG, Parisi JE, et al: Lateral ventricular neoplasms of the brain: Differential diagnosis based on clinical, CT, and MR findings. AJNR 1990; 11:567–574.
43. Maeder PP, Holtas SL, Basibuyuk LN, et al: Colloid cysts of the third ventricle: Correlation of MR and CT findings with histology and chemical analysis. AJNR 1990; 11:575–581.
44. Rubenstein LJ: *Tumors of the Central Nervous System.* Armed Forces Institute of Pathology. Washington, DC, 1981.
45. Radkawski MA, Naidich TP, Tomita T, et al: Neonatal brain tumors: CT and MR findings. J Comput Assist Tomogr 1988; 12:10–20.
46. Eisenberg HM, McComb G, Lorenzo AV: Cerebrospinal fluid overproduction and hydrocephalus associated with choroid plexus papilloma. J Neurosurg 1974; 40:381–385.
47. Chang T, Teng MMH, Guo WY, et al: CT of pineal tumors and intracranial germ-cell tumors. AJNR 1989; 10:1039–1044.
48. Edwards MSB, Hudgins RJ, Wilson CB, et al: Pineal region tumors in children. J Neurosurg 1988; 68:689–697.
49. Müller-Forell W, Schroth G, Egan PJ: MR imaging in tumors of the pineal region. Neuroradiology 1988; 30:224–231.
50. Zimmerman RA, Bilaniuk LT, Wood JH, et al: Computed tomography of pineal, parapineal and histologically related tumors. Radiology 1980; 137:669–677.
51. Ganti SR, Hilal SK, Stein BM, et al: CT of pineal region tumors. AJNR 1986; 7:97–104.
52. Zee CS, Segall H, Apuzzo M, et al: MR imaging of pineal region neoplasms. J Comput Assist Tomogr 1991; 15:56–63.
53. Tien RD, Barkovich AJ, Edwards MSB: MR imaging of pineal tumors. AJNR 1990; 11:557–565.
54. Kilgore DP, Strothers CM, Starshak RJ, et al: Pineal germinoma: MR imaging. Radiology 1986; 158:435–438.
55. Allen JC, Nisselbaum J, Epstein F, et al: Alphafetoprotein and human chorionic gonadotropin determination in cerebrospinal fluid. J Neurosurg 1979; 51:368–374.
56. Nakagawa H, Iwasaki S, Kichikawa K, et al: MR imaging of pineocytoma: Report of two cases. AJNR 1990; 11:195–198.
57. Peyster RG, Ginsberg F, Hoover ED: Computed tomography of familial pineoblastoma. J Comput Assist Tomogr 1986; 10:32–33.
58. Lee SR, Sanches J, Mark AS, et al: Posterior fossa hemangioblastomas: MR imaging. Radiology 1989; 171:463–468.
59. Rosenbaum AE, Rosenbloom SB: Meningiomas revisited. Semin Roentgenol 1984; 19:8–26.
60. Curnes JT: MR imaging of peripheral intracranial neoplasms: Extraaxial vs. intraaxial masses. J Comput Assist Tomogr 1987; 11:932–937.
61. Elster AD, Challa VR, Gilbert TH, et al: Meningiomas: MR and histopathologic features. Radiology 1989; 170:857–862.
62. Demaerel P, Wilms G, Lammens M, et al: Intracranial meningiomas: Correlation between MR imaging and histology in 50 patients. J Comput Assist Tomogr 1991; 15:45–51.
63. Aoki S, Sasaki Y, Machida T, et al: Contrast-enhanced MR images in patients with meningioma: Importance of enhancement of the dura adjacent to the tumor. AJNR 1990; 11:935–938.
64. Goldsher D, Litt AN, Pinto RS, et al: Dural "tail" associated with meningiomas on Gd-DTPA-enhanced MR images: Characteristics, differential diagnostic value, and possible implications for treatment. Radiology 1990; 176:447–450.
65. Wilms G, Lammens M, Marchal G, et al: Prominent dural enhancement adjacent to nonmeningomatous malignant lesions on contrast enhanced MR images. AJNR 1991; 12:761–764.
66. Tien RD, Yang PJ, Chu PK: "Dural tail sign": A specific MR sign for meningioma? J Comput Assist Tomogr 1991; 15:64–66.
67. Yuh WTC, Barloon TJ, Jacoby CG, et al: MR of

fourth-ventricular epidermoid tumors. AJNR 1988; 9:794–796.
68. Tampieri D, Melanson D, Ethier R: MR imaging of epidermoid cysts. AJNR 1989; 10:351–356.
69. Vion-Dury J, Vincentelli F, Jiddane M, et al: MR imaging of epidermoid cysts. Neuroradiology 1987; 29:333–338.
70. Horowitz BL, Chari MV, James R, et al: MR of intracranial epidermoid tumors: Correlation of in vivo imaging with in vitro ^{13}C spectroscopy. AJNR 1990; 11:299–302.
71. Tsuruda JS, Chew WM, Moseley ME, et al: Diffusion-weighted MR imaging of the brain: Value of differentiating between extraaxial cysts and epidermoids. AJNR 1990; 11:925–931.
72. Smith AS, Benson JE, Blaser SI, et al: Diagnosis of ruptured intracranial dermoid cyst: Value of MR over CT. AJNR 1991; 12:175–180.
73. Robertson SJ, Wolpert SM, Runge VM: MR imaging of middle cranial fossa arachnoid cysts: Temporal lobe agenesis syndrome revisited. AJNR 1989; 10:1007–1010.
74. Sherman JL, Camponovo E, Citrin CM: MR imaging of CSF-like choroidal fissure and parenchymal cysts of the brain. AJNR 1990; 11:939–945.

4

INTRACRANIAL HEMORRHAGE

Intracranial hemorrhage (ICH) is often heralded by an acute presentation with devastating neurologic consequences, frequently in a previously healthy individual. ICH is commonly encountered and readily detected on neuroimaging studies. The most frequent cause of ICH is trauma, although multiple factors may predispose a patient to develop ICH. In addition to describing the location, size, and degree of mass effect, it is incumbent upon the radiologist to comment on the plausible etiology(ies) of ICH. Treatable causes of ICH should be identified early to permit formulation of an appropriate treatment plan.

The etiology of ICH may be accurately deduced given the patient's age, medical history, and the pattern of ICH. However, in certain circumstances, the ICH does not fall into the typical pattern and the history may be noncontributory. In these circumstances, corroborative studies such as magnetic resonance imaging (MRI), contrast-enhanced planar imaging, or angiography may be required to arrive at the correct diagnosis. The computed tomography (CT) and MRI appearance of ICH, patterns of hemorrhage, and specific etiologic factors are discussed here.

RADIOGRAPHIC EVALUATION

Computed Tomography

Appearance

Acute (Less Than 1 Week). Intracranial blood, by virtue of the protein moiety (globin), has a high attenuation coefficient and is accordingly high density on CT (80–90 Hounsfield units, or HU) (Fig. 4–1). The iron within the hemoglobin molecule is responsible for only 7 to 8% of the total attenuation, whereas calcium does not contribute significantly to the density observed on CT.[1] A linear relationship exists between the x-ray attenuation and the patient's hematocrit at the time of hemorrhage (Table 4–1).

The hemorrhage reaches its maximum attenuation in the first 2 to 4 hours, during which time clot formation and retraction occur. There is no evidence of contrast enhancement in the acute phase of the uncomplicated hematoma. Regardless of the cause of the intraparenchymal hemorrhage (IPH), vasogenic edema will surround the lesion, becoming greatest by 4 to 5 days. Accordingly, the degree of mass effect increases to a maximum at this point.

Subacute (1 Week to 1 Month). IPH will continue to decrease in attenuation, initially at the periphery and later in the central portion of the hemorrhage. The vasogenic edema surrounding the hemorrhage will begin to decrease and the margins of the hemorrhage become less distinct. Ring enhancement may be detected following intravenous (IV) contrast administration in this phase, secondary to breakdown in the blood-brain barrier (BBB) and perivascular infiltration.[2] At this stage, the enhancement may be altered by tightening the BBB with steroids.[3,4] After the first week there is a trend to diminish the amount, mass effect, edema, and attenuation of the IPH.

Chronic (Greater Than 1 Month). The trends established during the subacute phase persist; namely, the density, mass effect, edema, and contrast enhancement diminish. At some time late in the subacute or early in the chronic phase, the IPH becomes isodense to brain. As the mass effect resolves, the hemorrhage may be inapparent on the unenhanced examination. The enhancement detected early in the chronic phase is secondary to the vascularity of granulation tissue forming a collagenous capsule around the resolving hematoma and is not significantly altered by steroids. The chronic sequela of IPH may be a focal, nonenhancing encephalomalacic cavity that is isodense to cerebrospinal fluid (CSF).

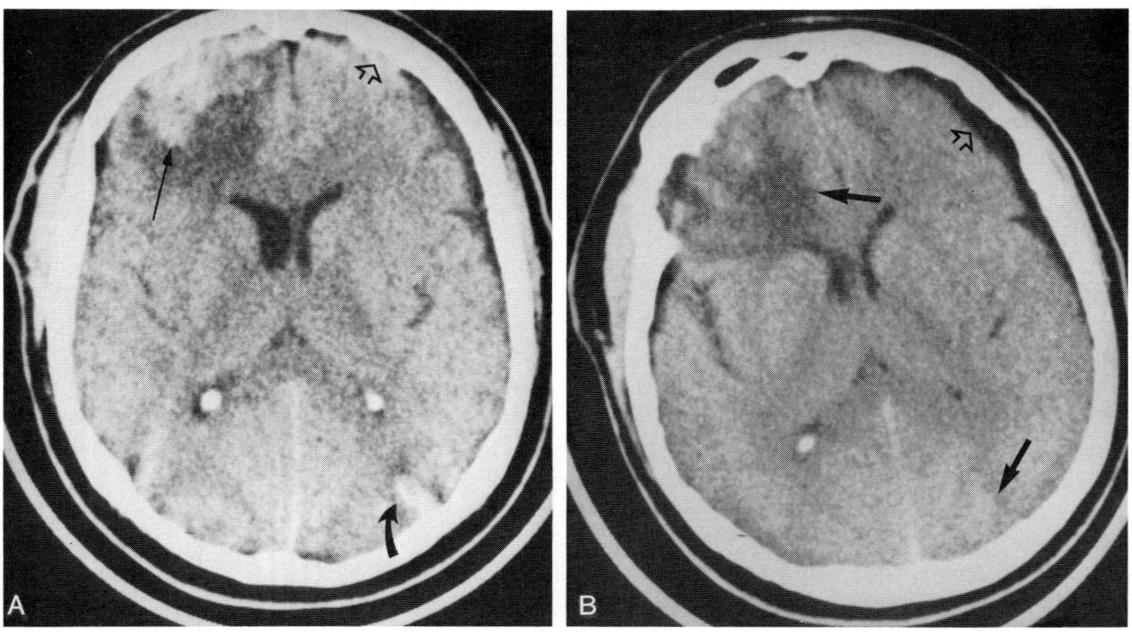

Figure 4–1. Computed tomography (CT) appearance of hemorrhage—motor vehicle accident (43-year-old male).

A, Unenhanced CT. Right frontal *(arrow)* and left parieto-occipital *(curved arrow)* hematomas are present. Both are surrounded by varying amounts of vasogenic edema. Incidentally, a chronic left subdural hematoma is present with evidence of loculated hyperdense acute rebleed *(open arrow)*.

B, Unenhanced CT (10 days later). The intraparenchymal hemorrhages have become nearly isodense to brain with minimal residual edema *(arrows)*. The left subdural hematoma *(open arrows)* has become homogeneously hypodense.

Table 4–1. CT APPEARANCE OF IPH

	Acute	Subacute	Chronic
Time frame	5–7 days	1 week–1 month	>1 month
Density	80–90 HU*	40–60 HU	0–20 HU
Edema	Maximum 4–5 days	↓ to normal	Absent
Mass effect	Maximum 4–5 days	↓ to normal	Atrophy, encephalomalacia
Enhancement	None	Heterogeneous or ring	Early, ring; late, none

*HU = Hounsfield units.

Role of Contrast

The use of IV contrast in the evaluation of acute ICH should be limited to specific situations. Diagnoses of neoplasm, arteriovenous malformation (AVM), or aneurysm may be confirmed by contrast administration. In the latter two conditions, the unenhanced CT examination alone is often sufficiently characteristic to confirm the diagnosis without contrast. Also, in the latter two conditions pancerebral angiography will likely be performed for preoperative planning.

Most importantly, when the patient's age and history do not correlate with the pattern of ICH, IV contrast administration may be useful. In these instances, any pathologic enhancement within or remote from the hemorrhagic focus may be helpful in arriving at the appropriate diagnosis.

Role of Angiography

Angiography should be performed in a select group of patients with ICH. Any patient with an atraumatic lobar hemorrhage with no known history of intracranial disease or bleeding diathesis should undergo diagnostic angiography.[5] In a 1987 study involving 67 patients with nontraumatic lobar hematomas, angiography was diagnostic in 43%.[5] The likelihood of a diagnostic angiogram increased to 77% when subarachnoid hemorrhage was present.

Magnetic Resonance Imaging

The marked sensitivity of MRI to the paramagnetic breakdown products of hemoglobin renders this an ideal tool to evaluate the age and etiology of ICH (Table 4–2).

Oxyhemoglobin

Under normal physiologic conditions, the majority of the red blood cells that compose a hematoma initially contain oxygenated hemoglobin from the arterial circulation. Iron is in the +2 valence state (ferrous). Two oxygen molecules occupy these electrons, yielding no available unpaired electrons. As a result, oxyhemoglobin is not paramagnetic.[6, 7]

The T1 and T2 signal characteristics of oxyhemoglobin are thus a function of the water content in the serum of the extravasated blood.[3] On short repetition time/echo delay time (TR/TE) spin echo sequences oxyhemoglobin is isointense to hypointense to white matter. The long TR/TE signal characteristics of oxyhemoglobin are slightly hyperintense to white matter. In practice, oxyhemoglobin is rarely detected owing to the relatively rapid conversion to deoxyhemoglobin.

Deoxyhemoglobin

Desaturation takes place within hours after red blood cells are sequestered from the circulation. The product of desaturation is deoxyhemoglobin, a water-soluble, paramagnetic substance.

Desaturation is the process whereby the oxygen molecules dissociate from the heme moiety of hemoglobin. The oxygen-hemoglobin dissociation curve portrays the affinity of hemoglobin for oxygen. Several factors are known to shift this curve to the right, thereby diminishing the affinity of hemoglobin for oxygen. The hematoma is a stagnant collection in which metabolic wastes accumulate. As lactic acid, carbon dioxide, and hydrogen ion concentrations increase, the oxygen-hemoglobin dissociation curve shifts to the right, further expediting desaturation, which results in increased deoxyhemoglobin concentration.[8]

The iron in deoxyhemoglobin remains in the ferrous (+2) valence state. Once oxygen is released from the iron atom, four unpaired electrons are present, rendering the compound

Table 4–2. MRI APPEARANCE OF IPH

	Oxyhemoglobin	Desaturation ⇌	*Deoxyhemoglobin*	Oxidation →	*Intracellular Methemoglobin*	Lysis →	*Extracellular Methemoglobin*	→	*Hemosiderin-Ferritin*
Paramagnetic	−		+		+		+		+
Fe Valence State	+2 (Ferrous)		+2 (Ferrous)		+3 (Ferric)		+3 (Ferric)		+3 (Ferric)
Unpaired Electrons	1		4		5		5		10,000
Relaxation Mechanism			T2-PRE		T2-PRE PEDD-PRE		PEDD-PRE		T2-PRE
Signal Intensity									
T1	→ ↓		→ ↓		↑		↑		→
T2	↑		↓ ↓		↓		↑		↓ ↓

T2-PRE = T2 proton relaxation enhancement.
PEDD-PRE = proton electron dipole-dipole proton relaxation enhancement.

paramagnetic.[9] Intracellular deoxyhemoglobin is heterogeneously distributed and, thus, displays heterogeneous magnetic susceptibility. (Magnetic susceptibility is an indication of how easily a substance may be magnetized. Unpaired electrons will align with and augment the applied magnetic field. Magnetic susceptibility is the ratio of additional field strength to the strength of the applied magnetic field.[3, 10]) The greater susceptibility within the cell than outside the cell results in magnetic field gradients across the cell membrane when an external magnetic field is applied. As the water protons diffuse through the varying magnetic fields, they tend to lose phase coherence, thus shortening the T2 relaxation time (Fig. 4–2). This has been called T2 proton relaxation enhancement (T2-PRE) by Gomori and coworkers.[7] The T2-PRE varies as a square function of the applied magnetic field and the magnetic susceptibility.[3] The effects of T2-PRE are also more apparent with longer inter-echo interval (TE). Deoxyhemoglobin is isointense to hypointense to parenchyma on T1 images and markedly hypointense on long TR/TE (T2-weighted) images.

Methemoglobin

Oxidation of deoxyhemoglobin to methemoglobin commences 3 to 5 days following hemorrhage. The iron atom is converted from the ferrous state (four unpaired electrons) to the ferric state (five unpaired electrons). In addition, structural changes occur within the globin that permit adjacent water protons to achieve sufficient proximity to the unpaired electrons to diminish the T1 and T2 relaxation times significantly (Fig. 4–3).

The oxidation of deoxyhemoglobin to methemoglobin is irreversible. The process usually begins in the periphery of the lesion and proceeds centripetally. The complete conversion to methemoglobin may take 3 weeks or more. Proton electron dipole-dipole proton relaxation enhancement (PEDD-PRE)[7] refers to selective T1 and T2 shortening that occurs secondary to the interaction of water protons and the unpaired electrons of the ferric iron. The unpaired electrons of methemoglobin are accessible to the water protons that must travel within 3 Å of the electrons. The unpaired electrons create fluctuations in the local magnetic field because of their large magnetic moment. (Magnetic moment refers to the magnetic properties of a dipolar nucleus to behave like a bar magnet when exposed to an applied magnetic field.) The magnetic moment of the unpaired electrons is more than 1000 times that produced by proton motion. The water protons therefore align more rapidly with the magnetic field and result in shortening of T1 and T2 relaxation times. Unlike with T2-PRE, this reaction is not field-dependent. Intracellular methemoglobin also possesses heterogeneous magnetic susceptibility, resulting in T2-PRE. Because of the simultaneous effects of PEDD-PRE and T2-PRE, MRI depicts intracellular methemoglobin as high signal on T1 and low signal on T2-weighted images (WIs).

Hemolysis occurs, resulting in release of methemoglobin. This diminishes the difference in the magnetic susceptibility between the intracellular and the extracellular environments, with commensurate decrease in the selective T2-PRE. The PEDD-PRE persists, resulting in a high-signal collection on T1, which is isointense on T2 WI. As the methemoglobin becomes diluted, it loses its PEDD enhancement. The spin density (SD) and T2 characteristics approach those of CSF. The MRI appearance of dilute extracellular methemoglobin is high signal on T1 and high signal on T2 WI.[11]

Hemosiderin-Ferritin

Degradation of methemoglobin liberates myriad ferric ions that are stored on hemosiderin and ferritin. These iron storage proteins are found adjacent to intraparenchymal hemorrhages. Each compound may contain an excess of 10,000 ferric ions.

Hemosiderin is an insoluble protein found within the lysosomes of reactive macrophages. Ferritin is a soluble protein found more widely distributed within glial cells or macrophages.[12] Heterogeneous magnetic susceptibility is in part secondary to sequestration by confining membranes. A T2-PRE is responsible for the markedly decreased T2 signal intensity, which may be so pronounced as to be apparent even on T1 images[3] (Fig. 4–4).

Edema

As mentioned in the preceding section on CT of hemorrhage, vasogenic edema accumulates around intraparenchymal hemorrhages.

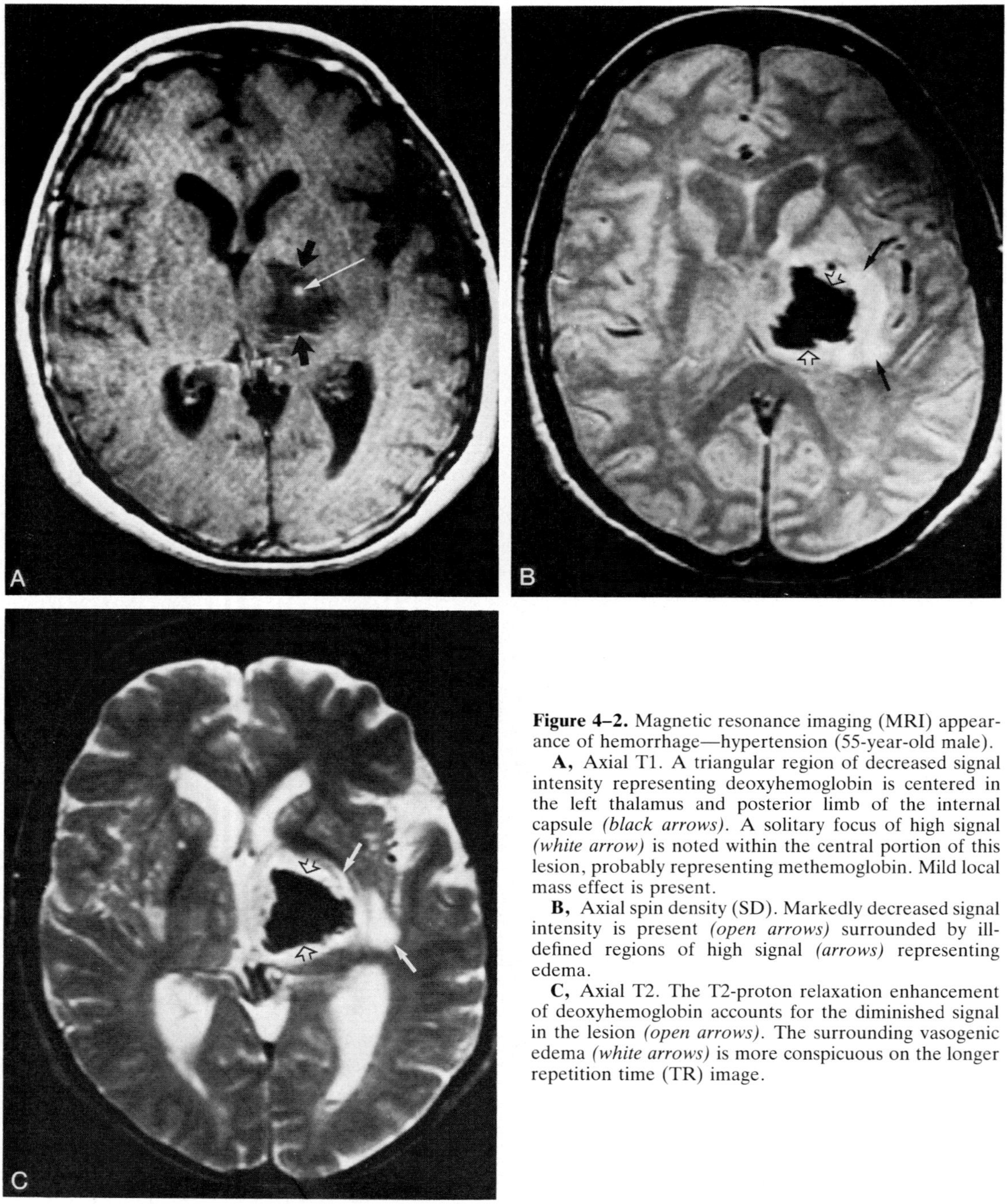

Figure 4–2. Magnetic resonance imaging (MRI) appearance of hemorrhage—hypertension (55-year-old male).

A, Axial T1. A triangular region of decreased signal intensity representing deoxyhemoglobin is centered in the left thalamus and posterior limb of the internal capsule *(black arrows)*. A solitary focus of high signal *(white arrow)* is noted within the central portion of this lesion, probably representing methemoglobin. Mild local mass effect is present.

B, Axial spin density (SD). Markedly decreased signal intensity is present *(open arrows)* surrounded by ill-defined regions of high signal *(arrows)* representing edema.

C, Axial T2. The T2-proton relaxation enhancement of deoxyhemoglobin accounts for the diminished signal in the lesion *(open arrows)*. The surrounding vasogenic edema *(white arrows)* is more conspicuous on the longer repetition time (TR) image.

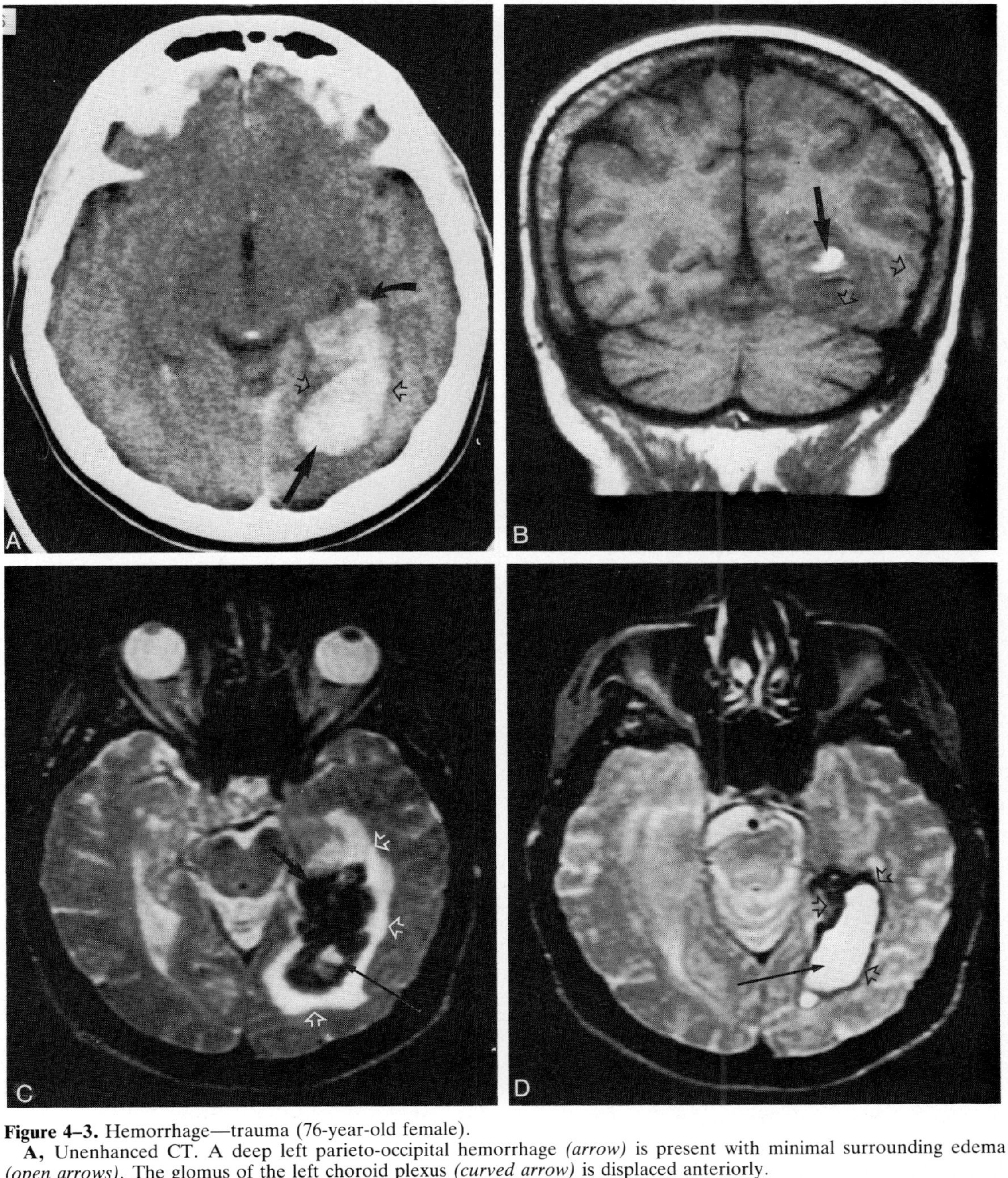

Figure 4–3. Hemorrhage—trauma (76-year-old female).

A, Unenhanced CT. A deep left parieto-occipital hemorrhage *(arrow)* is present with minimal surrounding edema *(open arrows)*. The glomus of the left choroid plexus *(curved arrow)* is displaced anteriorly.

B, Coronal T1. A solitary focus of high signal *(arrow)* representing methemoglobin is present centrally within the hemorrhage. A mild degree of local mass effect is present with effacement of the adjacent sulci *(open arrows)*.

C, Axial T2. High-signal edema *(open arrows)* surrounds an intraparenchymal collection of deoxyhemoglobin *(short arrow)*. Centrally a high-signal focus *(long arrow)* is present, which may represent serum or extracellular methemoglobin.

D, Axial T2 (2 months later). The vasogenic edema has resolved. Low-signal hemosiderin/ferritin *(open arrows)* surrounds the high-signal extracellular methemoglobin *(arrow)*.

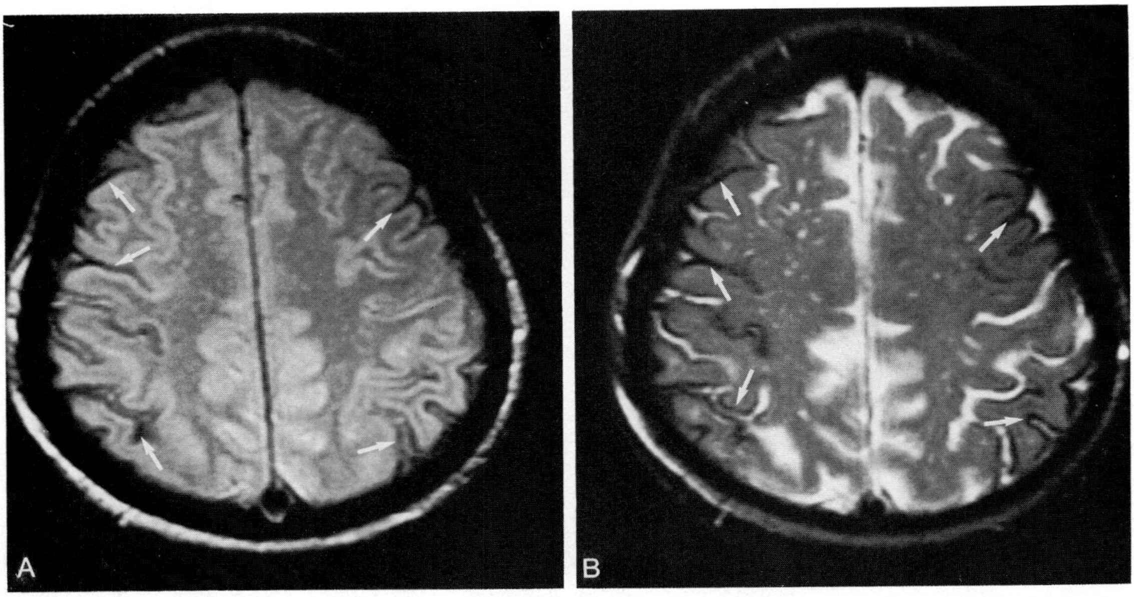

Figure 4–4. MRI appearance of chronic hemorrhage—superficial siderosis (60-year-old male with history of remote subarachnoid hemorrhage of undetermined etiology).

A, Axial SD. Linear foci of diminished signal intensity *(arrows)* are identified along the pial surface of multiple sulci.

B, Axial T2. Susceptibility effects render these areas of hemosiderin deposition even more conspicuous on the more heavily T2-weighted images *(arrows)*.

The point of maximum edema is 4 to 5 days following the bleed and should gradually resolve in 3 to 4 weeks. The edema will be high signal on T2 and low to intermediate signal on T1-weighted images.

LOCALIZATION

Extra-axial

Epidural

The dura mater is the periosteum of the bones that compose the cranial vault. Thus, prior to sutural fusion (late teens) the epidural space of the parietal bone and the epidural space of the frontal bone are separate, potential spaces. The sutures offer relative resistance to the extension of the epidural hemorrhage and often demarcate their anterior and posterior extension. Tethered by the attached dura, epidural hemorrhages are usually biconvex (Figs. 4–5 and 4–6). Extension across a dural sinus signifies an epidural collection. The subdural collection respects the dural sinuses, owing to division of the dura mater, which envelops the sinus.

Epidural hematomas (EDHs) are usually arterial and most frequently result from trauma. The middle meningeal artery enters the skull through the foramen spinosum, ascending between the dura and the bone before bifurcating along the squamosal portion of the temporal bone. Associated fractures have been reported in 91% of patients with epidural hematomas.[13] Skull fractures are much less common in the pediatric population. Trauma to the middle meningeal artery leads to arterial hemorrhage and stripping of the dura from the bone as the blood rapidly accumulates. Seventy-one percent of EDHs are temporoparietal in location.[13] Less commonly, EDHs may be venous in origin, secondary to trauma or coagulopathy (Fig. 4–7). Venous EDH occurs most commonly in the posterior fossa or adjacent to the occipital lobes.

Three CT stages of EDH have been described.[13] Acute epidural hematomas are composed in part of hypodense fresh, nonclotted blood. In the early stage, a swirled lucency in an otherwise dense clotted hemorrhage may be seen. Subacute EDHs are composed of clotted blood and are typically homogeneously dense. Chronic EDHs may be of mixed density or lucent with an enhancing membrane.

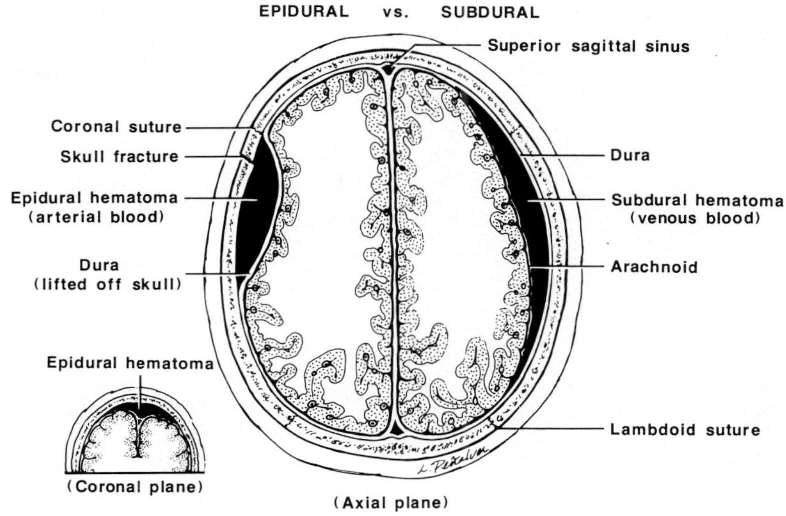

Figure 4–5. Hematoma: epidural versus subdural.

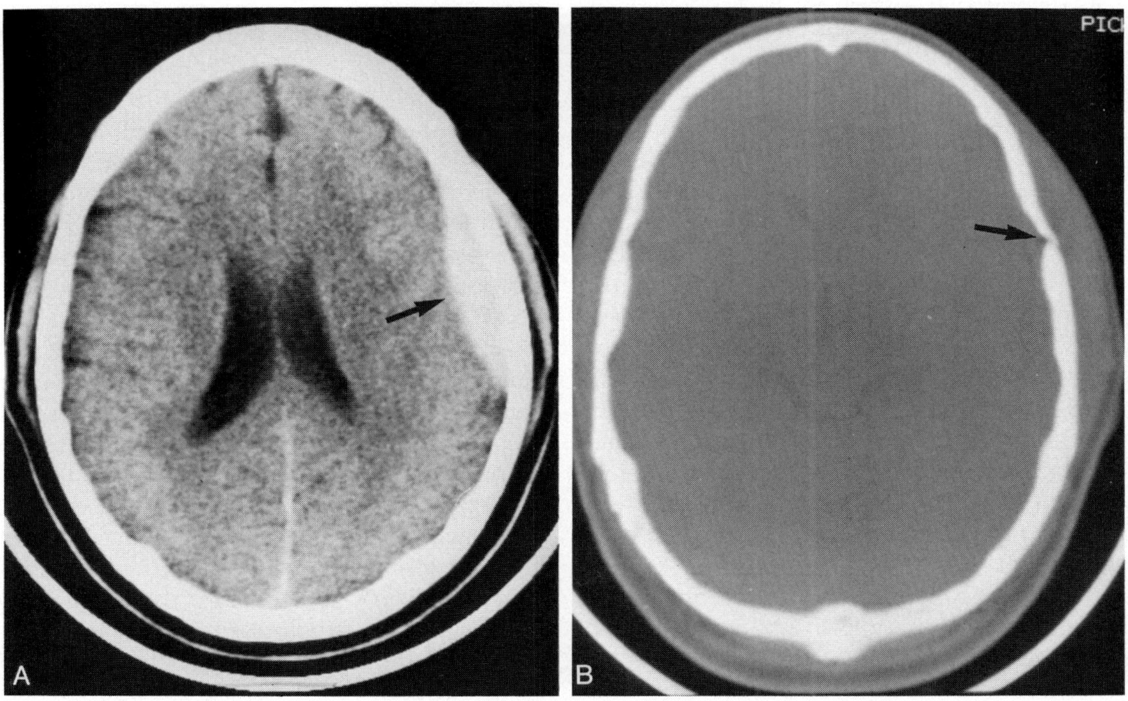

Figure 4–6. Epidural hematoma—motor vehicle accident (16-year-old male).

A, Unenhanced CT. A biconvex, hyperdense epidural collection *(arrow)* is present under the left parietal bone. Local mass effect is present.

B, Bone windows. A linear, minimally displaced fracture of the left parietal bone *(arrow)* is present.

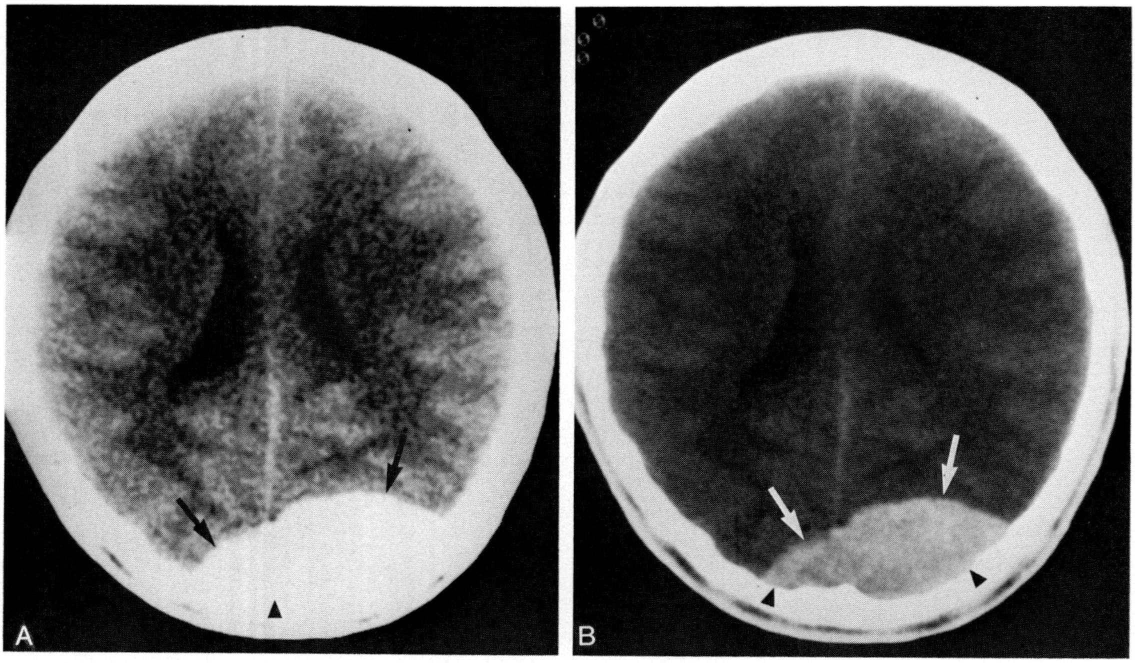

Figure 4–7. Venous epidural hematoma—bleeding diathesis (27-year-old male).
A, Unenhanced CT. An intrinsically dense lesion *(arrows)* crosses the expected insertion point of the falx *(arrowhead)*.
B, Unenhanced CT at wider windows. The epidural venous hemorrhage *(arrows)* can be differentiated from the inner table *(arrowheads)*.

Subdural

Subdural hemorrhages (SDHs) are located between the dura mater and the subjacent arachnoid membrane. These collections tend most often to conform to the shape of the brain, exhibiting concave inner margins (see Fig. 4–5). Less commonly, SDHs may be straight or even convex in appearance.[14] Convex inner margins may mimic EDHs and are often seen in the face of brisk, ongoing hemorrhage.[15] The subdural collection will freely cross cranial sutures but will not cross the midline insertion of the falx or the tentorial attachment.[5]

SDHs most often are the sequelae of trauma, but only rarely is there an associated skull fracture. Less commonly, coagulopathies, tumors,[16] or aneurysms may be responsible for SDHs. The acute SDH is hyperdense on CT (Fig. 4–8). Gradually, over 10 to 14 days, the hemorrhage becomes isodense to parenchyma. The subacute isodense SDH may be manifest only by attendant mass effect (Fig. 4–9). Absorption of blood products results in a hypodense collection on CT in the chronic state, within 1 month (Fig. 4–10). Rebleed into a chronic lesion is diagnosed when a fluid level is present. The high-density clot and hemoglobin reside in the gravity-dependent posterior portion of the collection. The chronic hemorrhage is less dense and layers over the acute material[17] (Fig. 4–11). Rebleeds are often signified by membranes that may appear within the fluid collections, often loculating small cavities of hemorrhage. These membranes are intrinsically dense and will frequently enhance.

Mixed-density acute SDHs have also been described. These mixed-density collections are theoretically attributable to extruded serum during the early phase of clot retraction or to CSF within the subdural space. Regardless of the cause, the mixed-density acute SDH tends to be larger, to be associated with greater subfalcial herniation, and to have a twofold-increased mortality when compared with the homogeneous hyperdense acute SDH.[18] The mixed-density SDH more frequently has a convex inner margin.

The MRI appearance of acute and subacute

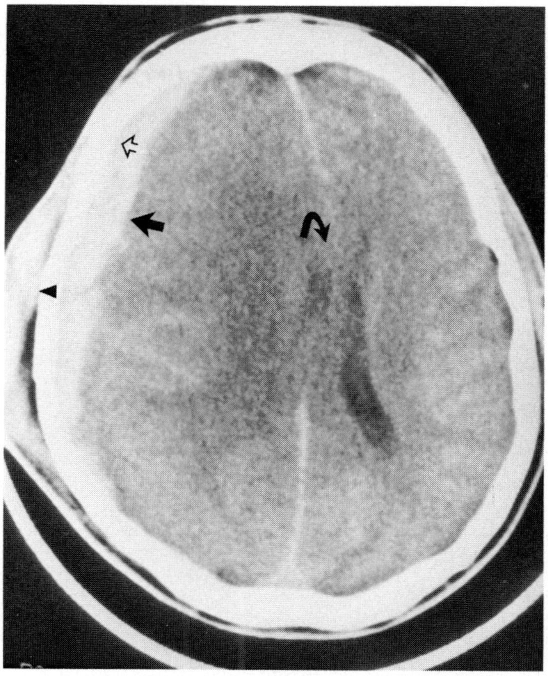

Figure 4–8. Subdural hematoma—motor vehicle accident (25-year-old male). Unenhanced CT; a hyperdense subdural hematoma *(arrow)* is present on the right. The hematoma is concave medially and layers over the brain surface, crossing the coronal suture *(open arrow)*. Subfalcial herniation *(curved arrow)* is present. Incidentally, marked extracranial soft tissue swelling *(arrowhead)* is present.

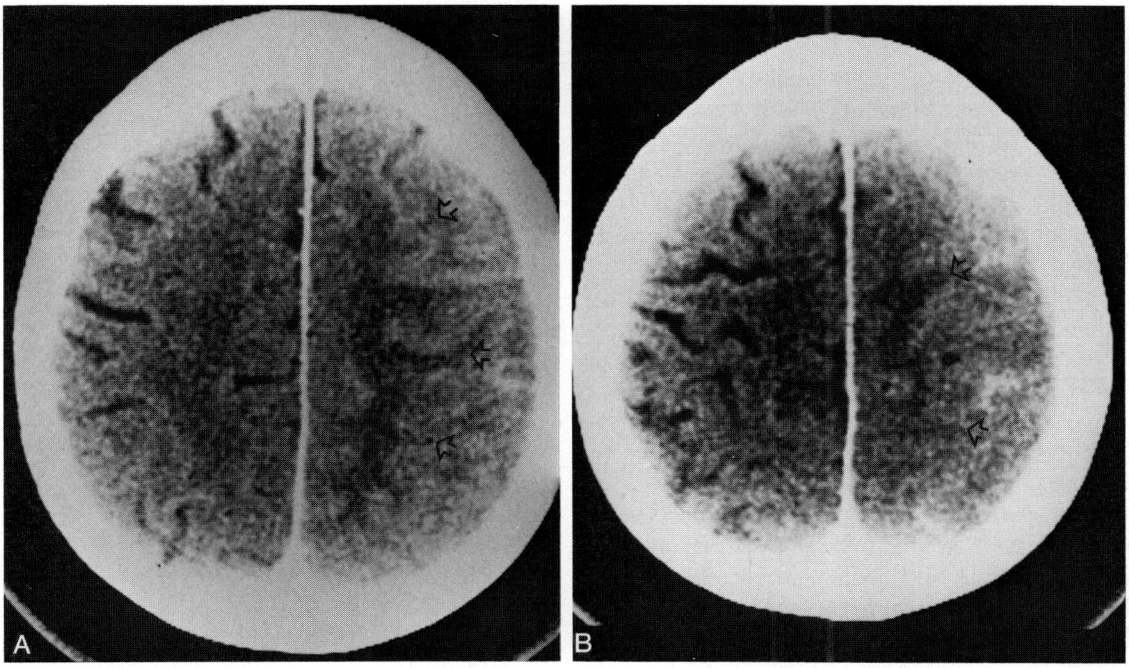

Figure 4–9. Isodense subdural hematoma (69-year-old male).

A, Enhanced CT performed 2 weeks after trauma. Cortical sulci along the inner table and interhemispheric fissure are effaced on the left. Also, the corticomedullary junction is displaced medially *(open arrows)*, indicating the presence of an extra-axial mass lesion.

B, Enhanced CT. Similar changes are noted at the vertex with effacement of the sulci and corticomedullary buckling *(open arrows)*.

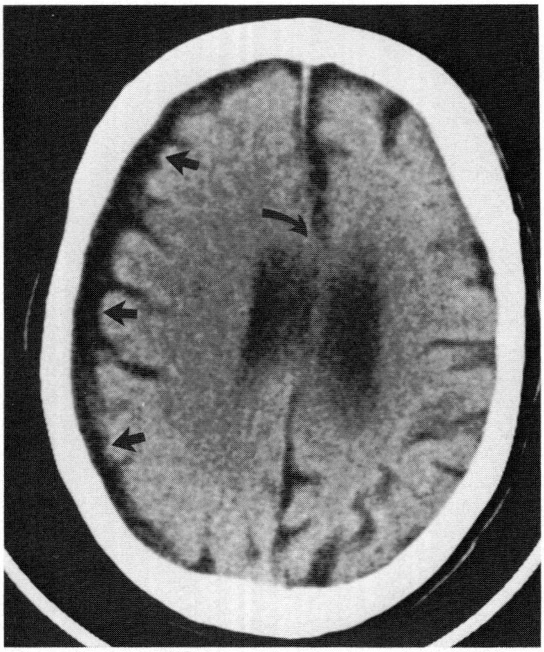

Figure 4–10. Chronic subdural hematoma (61-year-old male). Unenhanced CT; a hypodense subdural hematoma *(arrows)* is present over the lateral cortex of the right hemisphere. Slight right-to-left subfalcial herniation *(curved arrow)* is noted.

SDH is similar to that of acute and subacute IPH (Figs. 4–12 through 4–14). Probably because of the lack of BBB, the signal characteristics of chronic SDH may differ from those of chronic IPH.[19] Effective removal of methemoglobin and hemosiderin will prevent significant concentration of these substances within the collection and will alter the signal characteristics accordingly.

Acute SDHs are decreased signal on T2 WI secondary to the presence of deoxyhemoglobin. As deoxyhemoglobin is oxidized to methemoglobin, high signal appears on T1 WI around the periphery of the collection, later filling in completely. The T2-PRE effects seen with intracellular methemoglobin may not be noted in SDH, suggesting early cell lysis and homogeneous distribution of free methemoglobin.

Chronic hematomas become isointense on T1 WI and hyperintense on T2-weighted sequences. These differences reflect diminished concentrations of methemoglobin, which may be secondary to dilution, absorption, and/or degradation.[19] Rebleed in the presence of vascular membranes or loculated compartments within the subdural collection hampers the effective removal of hemosiderin-laden macrophages. Accordingly, the T2-PRE effects of the hemosiderin markedly decrease the T2 signal.

Subarachnoid

The most common cause of subarachnoid hemorrhage (SAH) is trauma, although the significance of such a hemorrhage in this setting is often overshadowed by coexistent life-threatening hemorrhages elsewhere in the body. Ruptured aneurysm is the next most common cause of SAH. Blood may also be present in the subarachnoid space with bleeding AVM, coagulopathy, or hemorrhagic infarct.

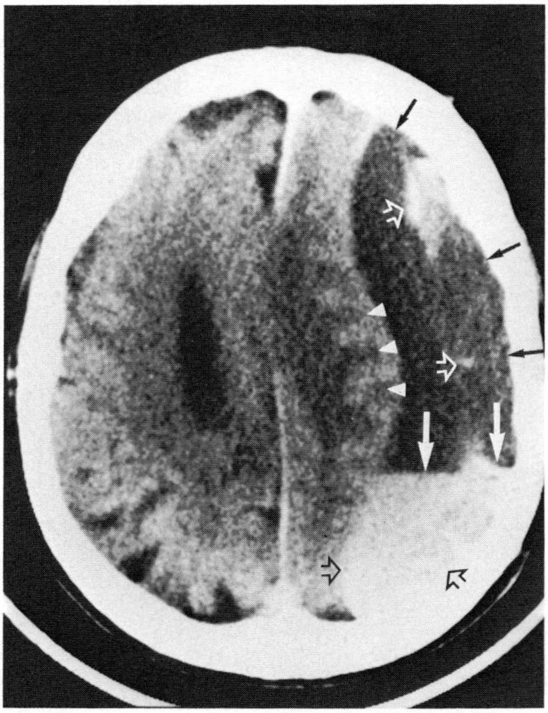

Figure 4–11. Subdural hematoma, acute-chronic (65-year-old male). Unenhanced CT; a fluid level *(solid white arrows)* indicates the acute *(open black arrows)* and chronic *(solid black arrows)* components of this subdural hemorrhage. Acute blood *(open white arrows)* also collects along the membrane of the hemorrhage. The extra-axial nature of the lesion is corroborated by the medial displacement of the gray-white junction *(arrowheads)*.

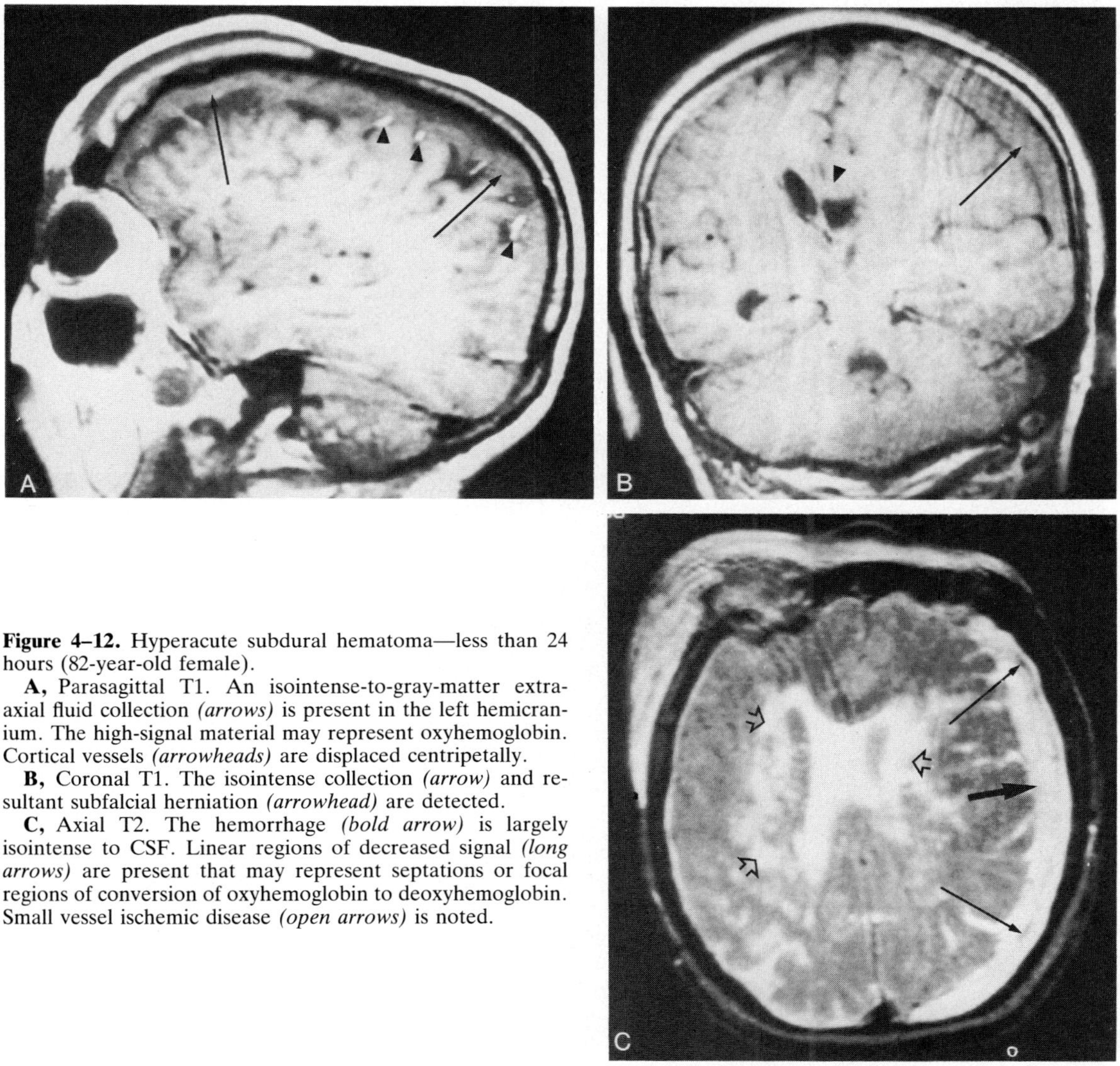

Figure 4–12. Hyperacute subdural hematoma—less than 24 hours (82-year-old female).

A, Parasagittal T1. An isointense-to-gray-matter extra-axial fluid collection *(arrows)* is present in the left hemicranium. The high-signal material may represent oxyhemoglobin. Cortical vessels *(arrowheads)* are displaced centripetally.

B, Coronal T1. The isointense collection *(arrow)* and resultant subfalcial herniation *(arrowhead)* are detected.

C, Axial T2. The hemorrhage *(bold arrow)* is largely isointense to CSF. Linear regions of decreased signal *(long arrows)* are present that may represent septations or focal regions of conversion of oxyhemoglobin to deoxyhemoglobin. Small vessel ischemic disease *(open arrows)* is noted.

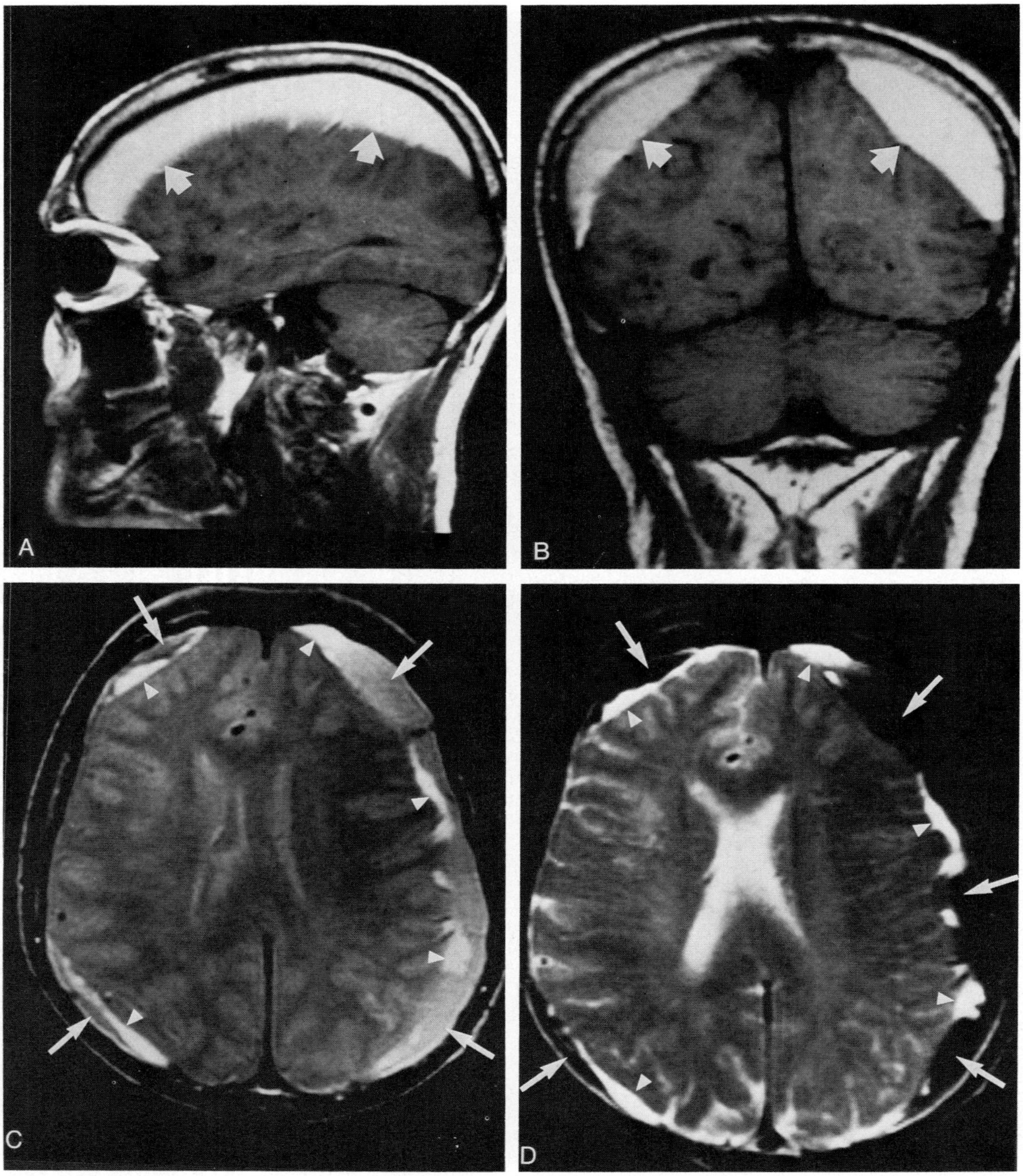

Figure 4–13. Bilateral subdural hematoma (79-year-old male).

A, Parasagittal T1. A rind of high signal representing methemoglobin *(arrows)* is present within the left subdural space.

B, Coronal T1. Bilateral subdural hemorrhages *(arrows)* are present.

C, D, Axial SD and T2. It is possible to distinguish the high-signal extracellular methemoglobin *(arrowheads)* from the low-signal intracellular methemoglobin or deoxyhemoglobin *(arrows)* in the bilateral subdural hemorrhagic collections.

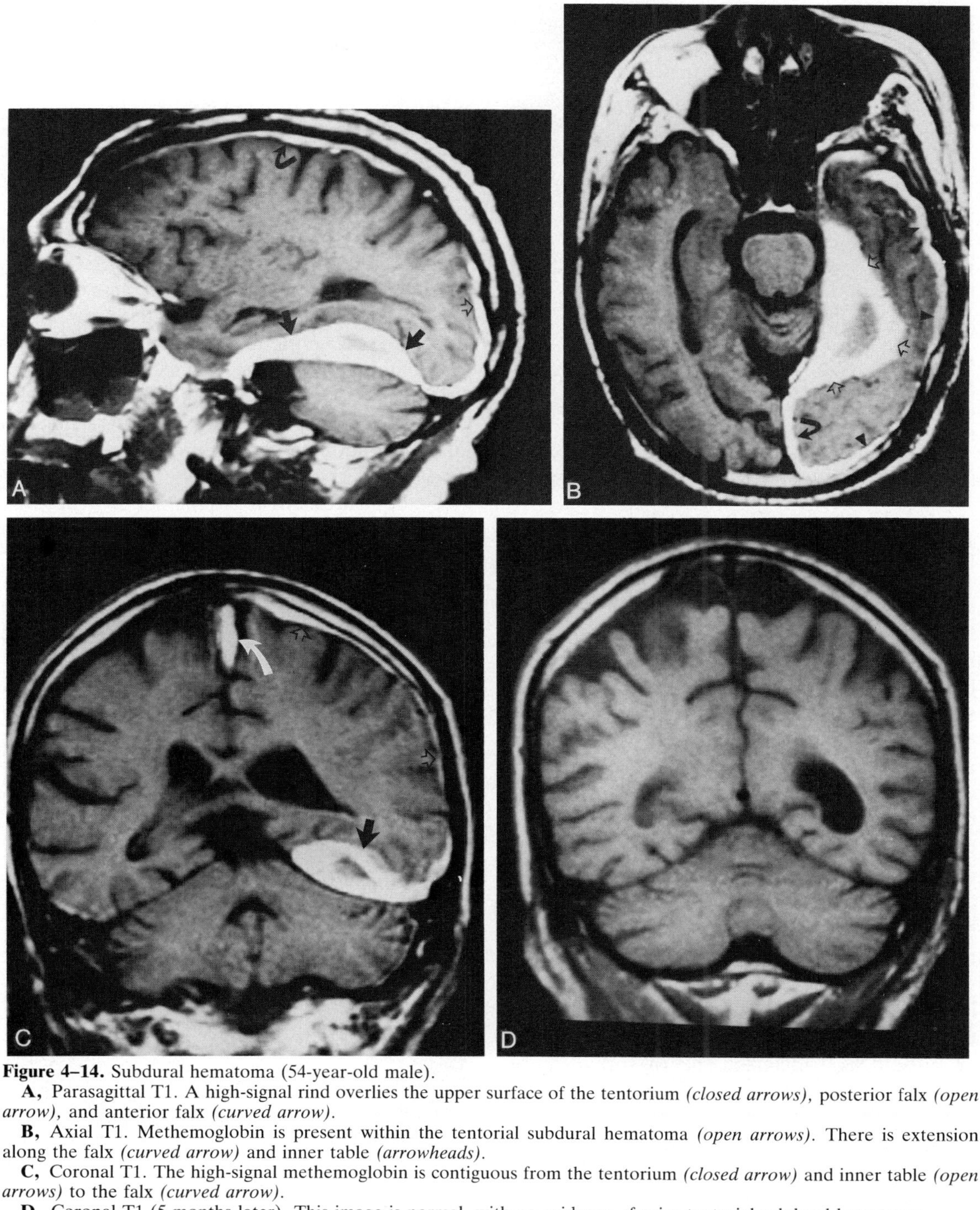

Figure 4–14. Subdural hematoma (54-year-old male).

A, Parasagittal T1. A high-signal rind overlies the upper surface of the tentorium *(closed arrows)*, posterior falx *(open arrow)*, and anterior falx *(curved arrow)*.

B, Axial T1. Methemoglobin is present within the tentorial subdural hematoma *(open arrows)*. There is extension along the falx *(curved arrow)* and inner table *(arrowheads)*.

C, Coronal T1. The high-signal methemoglobin is contiguous from the tentorium *(closed arrow)* and inner table *(open arrows)* to the falx *(curved arrow)*.

D, Coronal T1 (5 months later). This image is normal, with no evidence of prior tentorial subdural hematoma.

Illustration continued on following page

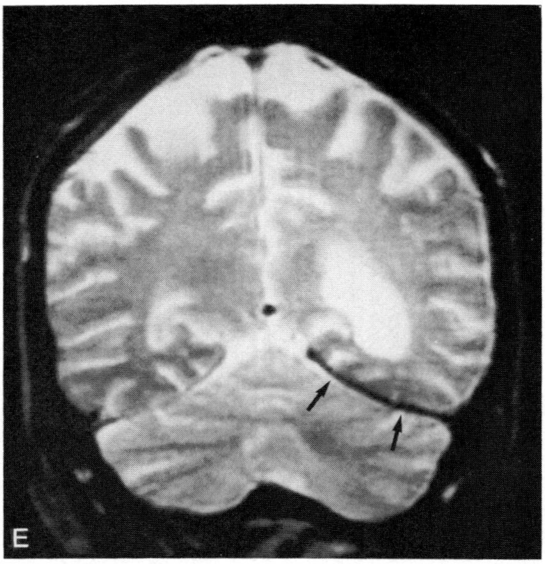

Figure 4–14 *Continued*
E, Coronal T2. A thin rim of low signal *(arrows)* is present along the left tentorial leaf, the result of hemosiderin or ferritin.

Once red blood cells enter the subarachnoid compartment, they are cleared via absorption, lysis, and/or phagocytosis. The majority are sequestered in the arachnoid villi and effectively cleared from the CSF into the vascular system. It is estimated that 50% and 90% of the red blood cells are cleared within 1 day and 1 week, respectively.[20] Red blood cells suspended in CSF also undergo lysis. Cell lysis begins within hours after hemorrhage and reaches a maximum in 5 to 7 days. Lysis releases oxyhemoglobin into the CSF as well as lesser amounts of hemoglobin, methemoglobin, iron, and heme pigments. Red blood cells may be phagocytized by CSF macrophages.

CT appearance of subarachnoid hemorrhage is that of a high-density collection within the CSF space (Fig. 4–15). The hemorrhage may be present as a localized clot or spread more diffusely throughout the CSF spaces. As the blood products are cleared, the CSF density will diminish, ultimately returning to normal.

MRI is relatively insensitive to SAH in the acute stage. This is partly due to the oxygen tension of CSF, which delays conversion of oxyhemoglobin to paramagnetic deoxyhemoglobin.[3] In vitro experiments[21] have demonstrated similar relaxation times between parenchyma and concentrated acute subarachnoid blood. As methemoglobin begins to accumulate, the T1 relaxation is shortened.[22] Diffusion and dilutional factors compromise the sensitivity of MRI to detect SAH. Anecdotally, MRI has detected focal clot in the subarachnoid space that was not detected by CT.[23]

Chronic or repetitive SAH may cause accumulation of hemosiderin-laden macrophages in the leptomeninges, subpial tissue, and the cranial nerves.[24] Generally, there are no associated clinical findings. However, a rare clinical condition known as superficial siderosis does exist. Clinical findings include hearing loss, cerebellar dysfunction, pyramidal tract signs, and progressive mental deterioration. Heterogeneous distribution of intracellular hemosiderin leads to a T2-PRE and field-dependent diminished signal on T2 WI. The distribution of this signal abnormality parallels the cortical gyri (see Fig. 4–4).

Complications of SAH include hydrocephalus and vasospasm with possible infarct. Hy-

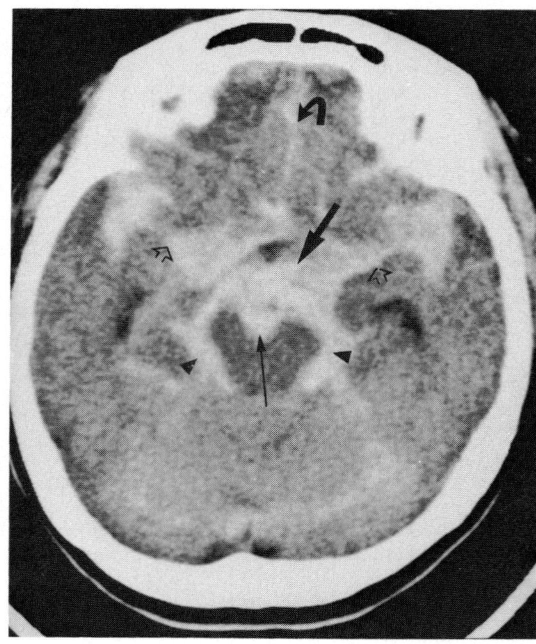

Figure 4–15. Subarachnoid hemorrhage—aneurysm (47-year-old female). Unenhanced CT; a large amount of high-density acute blood is present in the subarachnoid spaces of the basilar cisterns. The ambient *(arrowheads)*, interpeduncular *(thin arrow)*, and suprasellar cisterns *(bold arrow)* are filled with blood. The lateral cerebral fissures *(open arrows)* and interhemispheric fissures *(curved arrow)* also contain hemorrhage.

drocephalus is the result of disruption of CSF flow caused by red blood cells and various proteinaceous breakdown products. If these products reflux into the ventricular system, noncommunicating hydrocephalus may develop. Alternatively, these proteinaceous compounds may obstruct the pacchionian granulations, resulting in a communicating hydrocephalus (see Chapter 6).

Vasospasm and resultant ischemia occur in 25% of patients following aneurysm rupture.[25] In ischemic patients the likelihood of a favorable prognosis diminishes by 50% and mortality doubles to 40% compared with the nonischemic patient. Ischemia remains the leading cause of death and disability following SAH. The single most important predictor of cerebral ischemia, exceeding even clinical evaluation, is the presence of focal, thick collections of subarachnoid blood on CT.[25]

Intraventricular

Primary intraventricular hemorrhage (IVH) may result most commonly from trauma, coagulopathy, or subependymal vascular malformation. Hypertensive hemorrhages, by virtue of their proximity to the ventricular system, may also rupture secondarily into the ventricles. The parenchymal focus of the hypertensive hemorrhage may be inconspicuous (Fig. 4–16).

IVH may clot, forming a cast of the ventricular system, and result in outflow obstruction of CSF into subarachnoid spaces, with resultant noncommunicating hydrocephalus. Blood may also exit the ventricle and undergo the same physiologic breakdown and absorption as subarachnoid blood.

The acute hemorrhage is of high density (80 to 90 HU) on CT. As the breakdown and absorption of hemoglobin progress, the blood becomes less dense, proceeding to isodense to CSF.

In the acute stage, CT is more accurate than MRI in detection of IVH. After 2 to 3 days, deoxyhemoglobin accumulates, resulting in a T2-PRE and decreased signal on T2 images.

Subependymal siderosis results in subependymal deposition of hemosiderin-laden reactive macrophages. This condition may follow IVH and results in a T2-PRE.[24]

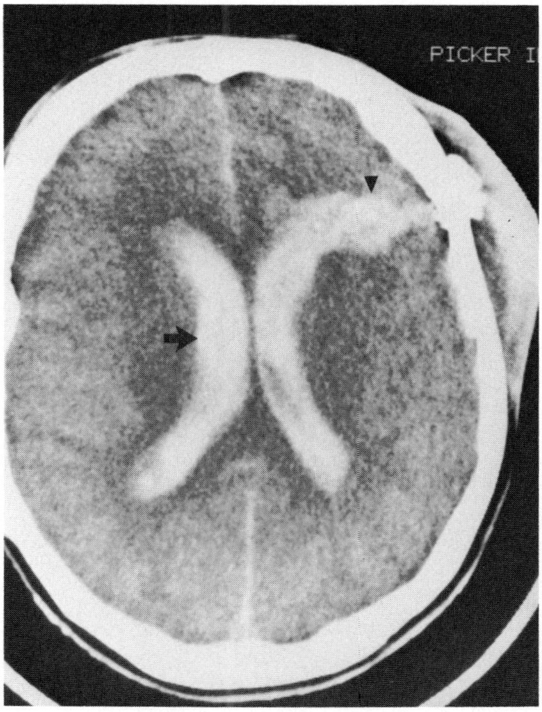

Figure 4–16. Intraventricular hemorrhage—gunshot wound (27-year-old male). Unenhanced CT; a large amount of blood *(arrow)* fills both lateral ventricles. Intraparenchymal hemorrhage *(arrowhead)* in the left frontal lobe indicates the trajectory of the bullet.

Intraparenchymal

Contusion

Contusion results from blunt trauma that, in effect, bruises or crushes the brain parenchyma. The brain may be affected at the site of impact (coup lesion) or opposite the site of impact (countrecoup lesion). The brain may be involved anywhere along its surface, most commonly where it can move against rigid structures such as the inner table, floor of the anterior fossa, sphenoid wings, petrous ridge, and falx (Fig. 4–17). The temporal, frontal, and parietal lobes are most frequently affected.

Contusions are usually confined to the gray matter with relative sparing of the underlying white matter. The crown of the gyrus absorbs the maximum impact and, in effect, protects the depths of the sulci. Accordingly, these injuries tend to extend quite superficially. The contusion may be bland with evidence of adjacent edema or may result in petechial hemorrhages.

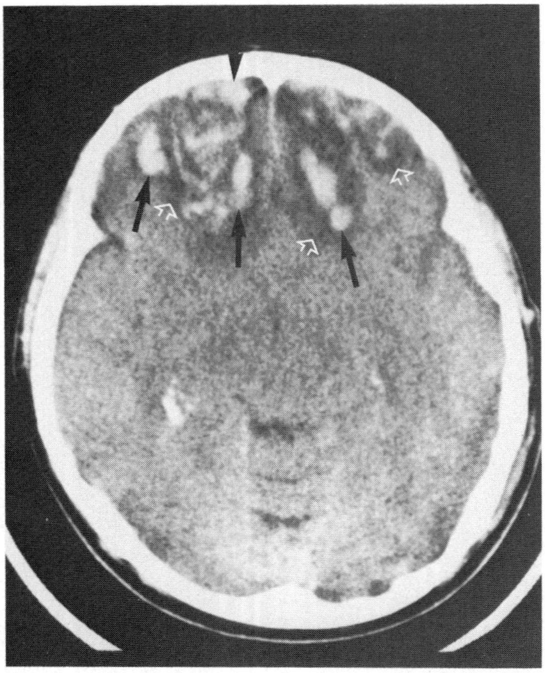

Figure 4–17. Contusion—motor vehicle accident (50-year-old male.) Unenhanced CT; small, irregular collections of blood *(arrows)* are present in the frontal and subfrontal gray matter and to a lesser degree in the white matter. Vasogenic edema *(open arrows)* in part surrounds these contusions.

Although CT is currently the modality of choice in evaluating patients with acute trauma, CT may be relatively insensitive to contusions.[26] Factors accounting for this include the following: (1) peripheral location of the injury subjects it to artifact from adjacent bone; (2) only a minimal petechial hemorrhage may be present, scattered diffusely over a wide area without a significant focal collection; (3) within hours, vasogenic edema may accumulate, diminishing the density of the contusion. In fact, edema may be the predominant feature of contusion with very little if any observable hemorrhage.

MRI is nearly twice as sensitive (98% versus 56%) at detecting contusion than CT.[23] This is particularly true in the face of bland or nonhemorrhagic contusion. The T2-weighted spin echo sequence is very sensitive to free water. MRI also excels in the subacute and chronic stages of hemorrhagic contusion, as it is sensitive to the paramagnetic breakdown products of hemoglobin as well as edema.

Hematoma

Multiple etiologies may be responsible for IPH including trauma, hypertension, infarct, AVM, tumor, coagulopathy, or amyloid angiopathy. Each are discussed in more detail in the following section. The macroscopic and microscopic appearances of hematoma differ little, regardless of the cause. A well-defined lesion composed of clotted red cells is noted displacing the parenchyma. The hematoma dissects along white matter fiber tracts, separating rather than destroying the parenchyma. A thin rim of partially necrotic parenchyma may surround the hematoma. As the perivascular inflammatory changes occur with disruption of the BBB and an attendant increase in edema, there is a commensurate increase in the degree of mass effect. The parenchymal reaction includes macrophages, fibroblasts, and vascular proliferation in attempts to encapsulate the hemorrhage with a dense collagenous capsule.[27] As the blood products are absorbed and the inflammatory reaction is diminished, the sequela may be a small encephalomalacic cavity. The CT and MRI appearances of IPH have been reviewed.

IPH may not be contained completely by the parenchyma. If sufficiently close to a CSF space, the hemorrhage may dissect through the parenchyma, rupturing into the ventricle or through the cortex into the subarachnoid space. Generally, the point of maximum hemorrhage will indicate the most likely location of the source.

ETIOLOGY OF HEMORRHAGE

Trauma

Trauma is the most common cause of ICH in our patient population. The location, quantity, and appearance of ICH secondary to trauma are markedly variable. IPH most frequently involves the temporal and frontal lobes. The hemorrhage may be multiple or solitary, deep or superficial, and ipsilateral (coup) or contralateral (contracoup) to the initiating force. Focal hematomas, petechial hemorrhage, or both may be present. Focal or diffuse cerebral swelling (cytotoxic edema) may accompany the hemorrhage.

Extra-axial hemorrhages occur most frequently as a result of trauma. Epidural, subdural, subarachnoid, and intraventricular hemorrhages may occur as isolated collections or in concert with one another (Fig. 4–18).

Diffuse axonal injury is a rare form of intracranial trauma. These shear injuries are the result of differential motion that occurs between the gray matter and the white matter. This differential motion is secondary to the difference in density of these moieties. The radiographic manifestations may be minimal in the face of severe clinical deterioration. Diffuse swelling, punctate subcortical hemorrhages, eccentric corpus callosal hemorrhages, and subarachnoid and punctate white matter hemorrhages adjacent to the third ventricle are the radiographic manifestations of shearing injury[28] (Fig. 4–19). Diffuse axonal rupture may be nonhemorrhagic and not visualized on CT. The initial clinical presentation is immediate onset of coma, lack of increased intracranial pressure, decerebrate posture, and often a persistent vegetative state.

CT is the most appropriate modality to evaluate the post-traumatic patient. Surgically significant disease (IPH, EDH, SDH) is readily detected by CT, and CT is also sensitive to SAH and fractures. CT is more readily available, more rapidly performed, and more "user-friendly" when multiple patient support devices are required. Clearly, MRI is more sensitive at detecting small (nonsurgical) EDHs, SDHs, and contusions because of the lack of bone artifact inherent with CT. MRI is also more sensitive than CT at detecting nonhemorrhagic conditions such as bland contusions[26] and hypothalamic and brainstem infarcts.[29] MRI should be used to evaluate coma and focal neurologic deficits in patients with "normal" head CT assessment.

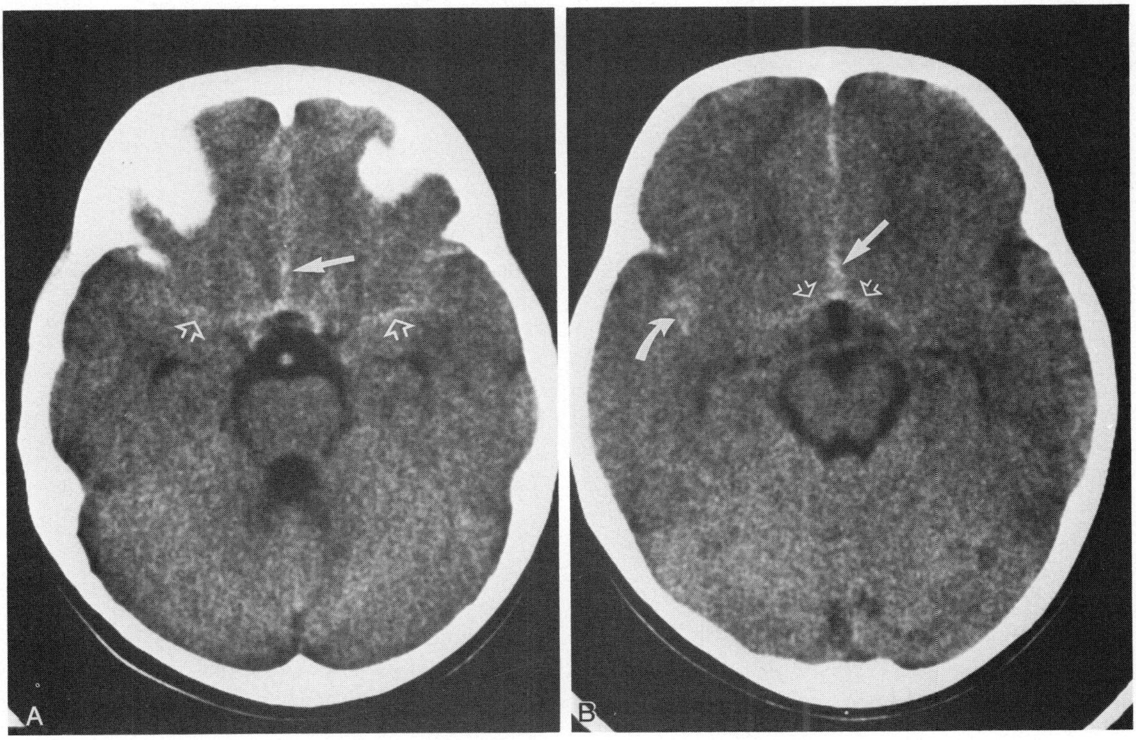

Figure 4–18. Trauma—subarachnoid hemorrhage (18-month-old male).

A, Unenhanced CT. High-density material representing acute blood is present within the interhemispheric fissure *(arrow)* and lateral cerebral fissures *(open arrows)*.

B, Unenhanced CT. The subarachnoid blood extends from the interhemispheric fissure *(arrow)* to the ventralmost suprasellar cistern *(open arrows)* and right sylvian fissure *(curved arrow)*.

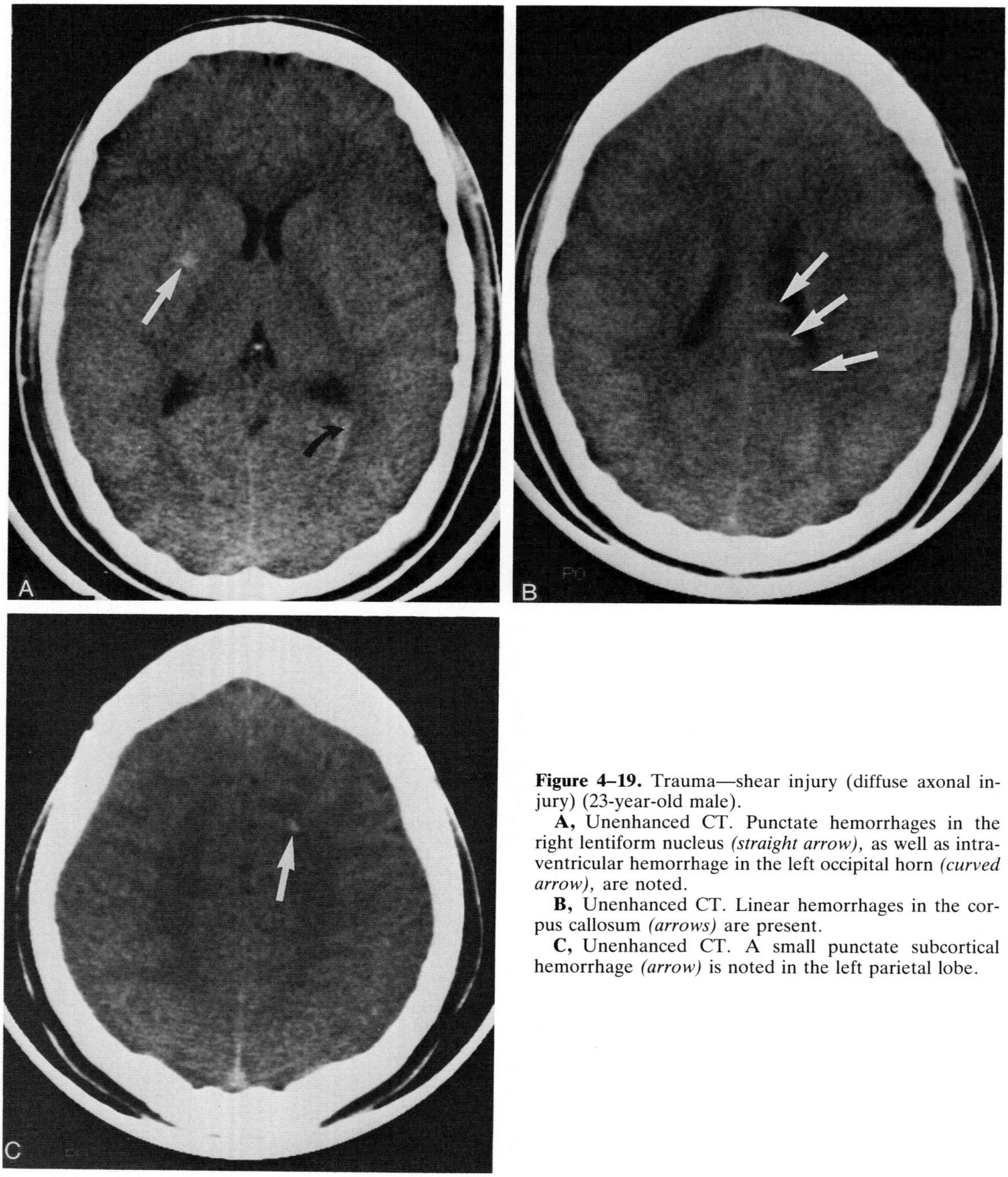

Figure 4–19. Trauma—shear injury (diffuse axonal injury) (23-year-old male).

A, Unenhanced CT. Punctate hemorrhages in the right lentiform nucleus *(straight arrow),* as well as intraventricular hemorrhage in the left occipital horn *(curved arrow),* are noted.

B, Unenhanced CT. Linear hemorrhages in the corpus callosum *(arrows)* are present.

C, Unenhanced CT. A small punctate subcortical hemorrhage *(arrow)* is noted in the left parietal lobe.

Hypertension

Hypertension is the most common cause of spontaneous IPH. Classic teaching attributes hypertensive hemorrhages to the rupture of microscopic aneurysms (Charcot-Bouchard) arising from perforating end arteries. Yet a recent histopathologic review[29a] of in excess of 2800 brain specimens, 95 of which had ICH, revealed only 5 Charcot-Bouchard aneurysms, none of which were associated with hemorrhage. This work led the authors to postulate: (1) Charcot-Bouchard aneurysms are rare, with a smaller frequency than ICH; (2) Charcot-Bouchard aneurysms are not the precursors to most ICH; (3) the "aneurysms" described by Charcot and Bouchard most likely represented tortuosity or benign ectasia, as both are difficult to distinguish from aneurysm on routine histologic examination. The most common locations for hypertensive hemorrhage are the basal ganglia (especially the putamen), the thalamus (Fig. 4–20), and, less frequently, the brainstem and dentate nucleus (Fig. 4–21). These hemorrhages are variable in size, are solitary, and may rupture into the ventricular system.

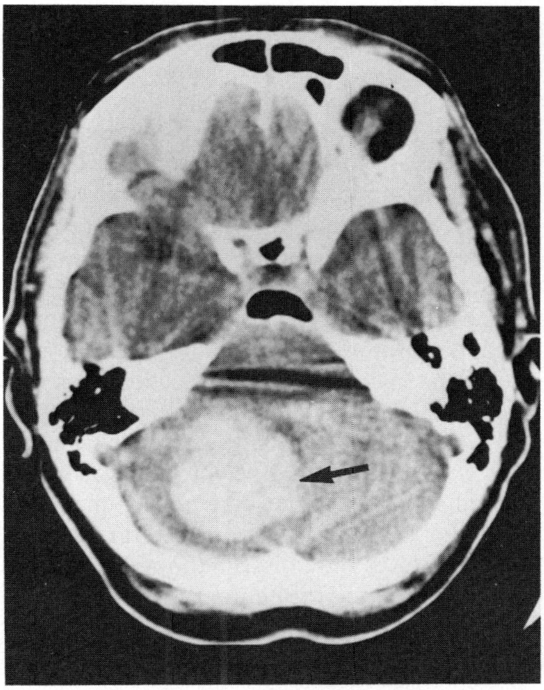

Figure 4–21. Hypertensive dentate nucleus hemorrhage (79-year-old female). Unenhanced CT; a large paramedian hemorrhage *(arrow)* is present within the right cerebellar hemisphere. Subsequent workup of this patient, who presented in hypertensive crisis, was negative.

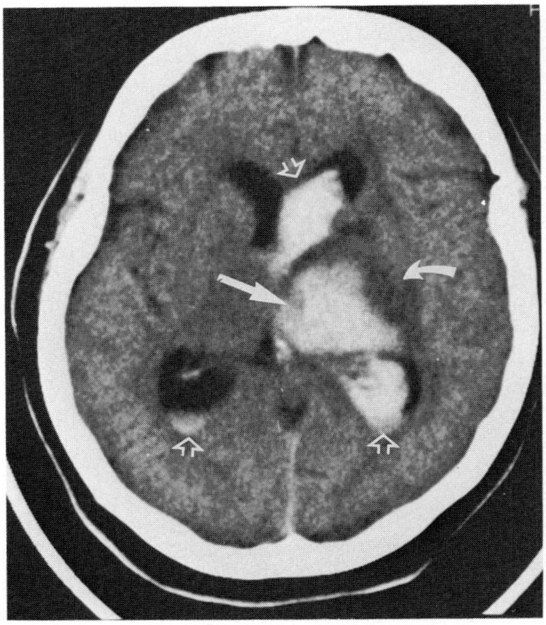

Figure 4–20. Hypertensive thalamic hemorrhage (74-year-old female). Unenhanced CT; a thalamic hypertensive hemorrhage *(arrow)* has extended into the ventricular system *(open arrows)*. A mild amount of vasogenic edema *(curved arrow)* surrounds the parenchymal focus.

Hypertensive hemorrhages in the frontal lobe usually occur below the frontal horns and tend to be larger than hematomas in normotensive patients and herald a more guarded prognosis.[30]

Aneurysm

Congenital and mycotic aneurysms most frequently hemorrhage. Congenital aneurysms occur in the anterior and posterior communicating arteries (33% each), the middle cerebral trifurcation (20%), and miscellaneous locations (posterior inferior cerebellar artery [PICA], basilar tip, and so on). Mycotic aneurysms are usually in peripheral branches of the anterior circulation. Aneurysmal rupture most frequently results in SAH. Typically, the amount of subarachnoid blood exceeds that seen with trauma.

Localization of the blood on CT may provide a clue to the location of the aneurysm and may tailor the subsequent angiographic evaluation. Anterior communicating artery aneurysms may rupture into the cistern of the lamina terminalis and may extend cephalad into the interhemispheric fissure or septum pellucidum (Fig. 4–22). If the jet is directed posteriorly-superiorly, the blood may gain access to the third ventricle through the lamina terminalis. If the jet is directed laterally, the blood may dissect into a frontal lobe.

Posterior communicating artery aneurysms rupture into the suprasellar cistern. The blood may enter the ipsilateral temporal horn through the mesotemporal lobe. Parenchymal blood may accumulate within the temporal lobe. Basilar tip aneurysm may rupture into the suprasellar and quadrigeminal plate cisterns and into the third ventricle (Fig. 4–23).

Middle cerebral artery aneurysms may rupture into the sylvian and/or lateral cerebral fissures. Blood may dissect through the temporal tip to enter the temporal horn (Fig. 4–24). Blood may also dissect through the external and extreme capsule and cephalad into the parietal lobe. These hemorrhages are usually more lateral than those seen with hypertension.

Mycotic aneurysms are the result of septic emboli, related to subacute bacterial endocarditis, IV drug use, or cardiac shunts. *Staphylococcus aureus* and *S. epidermidis* are the most common organisms responsible for the formation of mycotic aneurysms.[31] Owing to the minute size of the emboli, mycotic aneurysms tend to be located more peripherally than congenital aneurysms (Fig. 4–25). The organisms invade the wall, inciting inflammation and necrosis. The arterial wall weakens, leading to focal dilatation. The hemorrhages that result from rupture of these aneurysms tend to be intraparenchymal and are associated with a higher morbidity and mortality than are ruptured congenital aneurysms.

Atherosclerotic aneurysms tend not to bleed and are discussed in more detail in the next chapter.

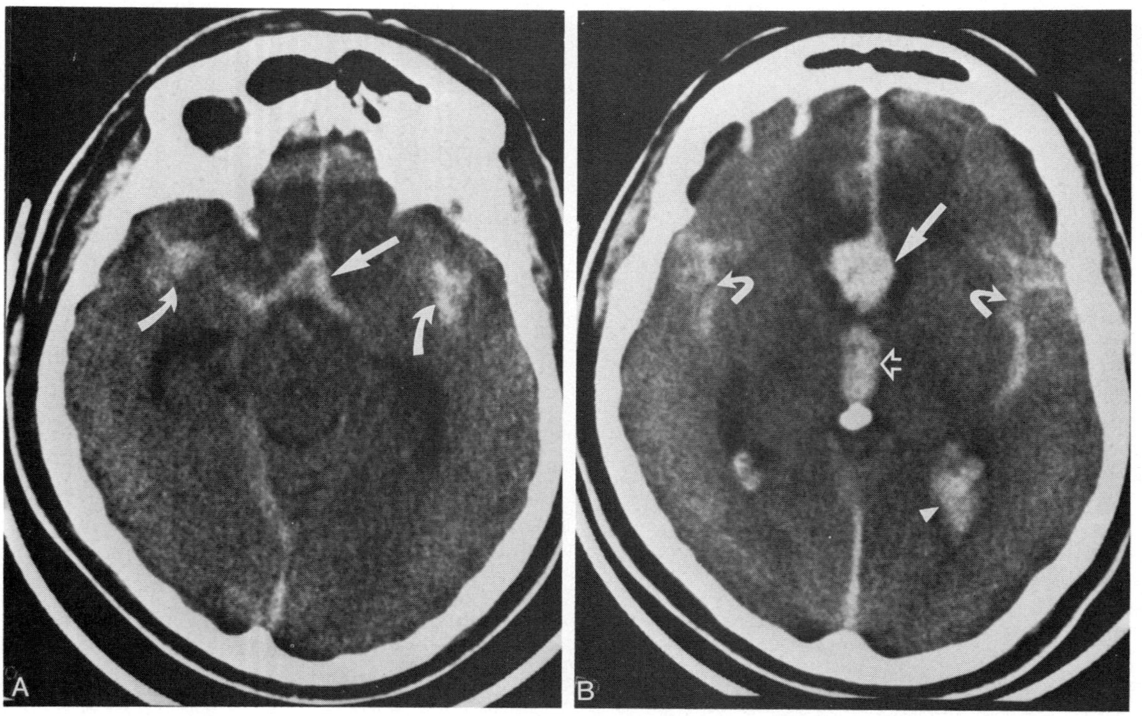

Figure 4–22. Anterior communicating artery aneurysm (48-year-old female).

A, Unenhanced CT. Subarachnoid blood is present in the anterior suprasellar cistern *(straight arrow)* and sylvian fissures bilaterally *(curved arrows).*

B, Unenhanced CT. A large clot *(straight arrow)* is located within the interhemispheric fissure, indicating that the most likely location for this aneurysm is the anterior communicating artery. Blood is also present in the posterior third ventricle *(open arrow),* left atrium *(arrowhead),* and sylvian fissures *(curved arrows).*

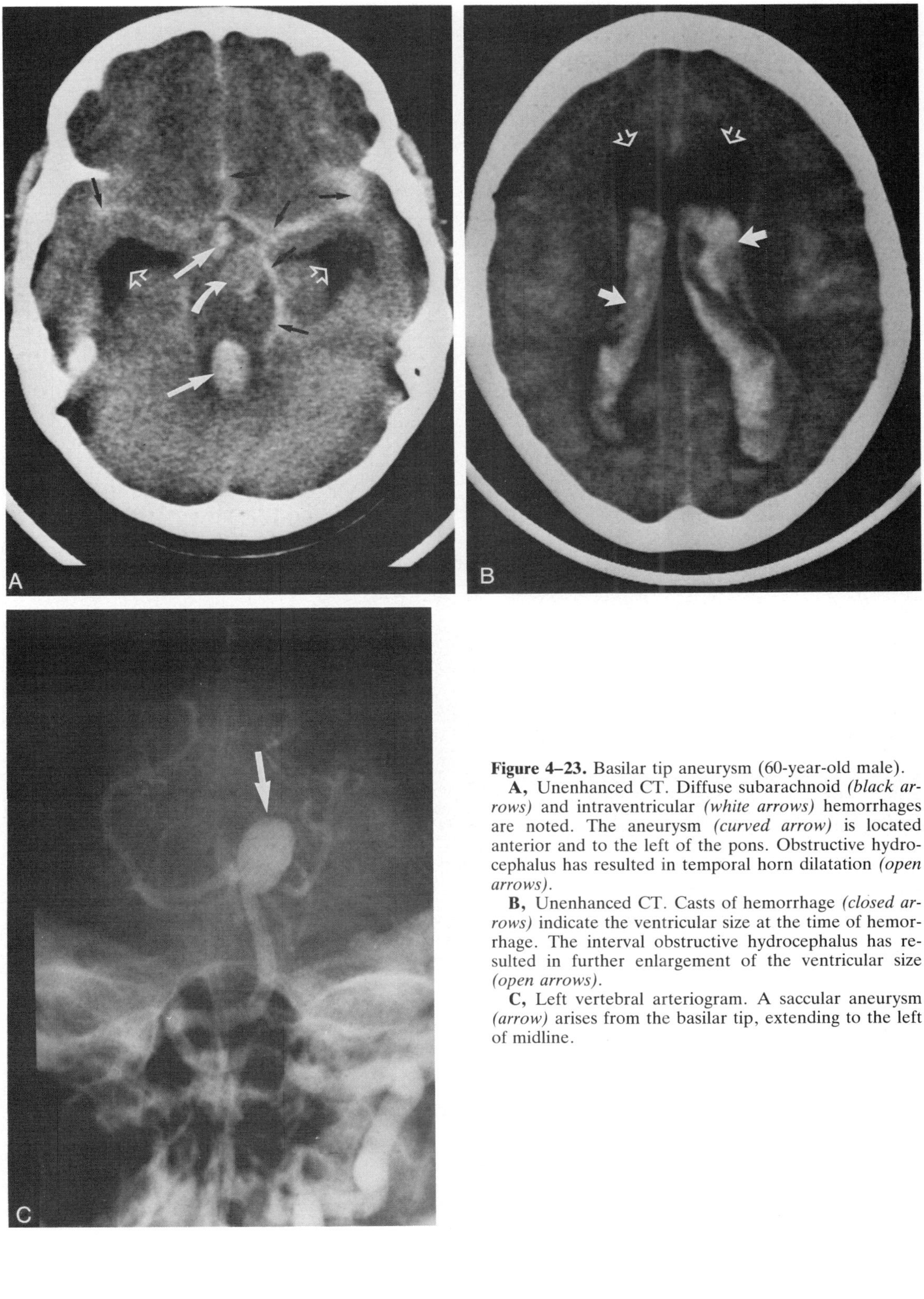

Figure 4–23. Basilar tip aneurysm (60-year-old male).

A, Unenhanced CT. Diffuse subarachnoid *(black arrows)* and intraventricular *(white arrows)* hemorrhages are noted. The aneurysm *(curved arrow)* is located anterior and to the left of the pons. Obstructive hydrocephalus has resulted in temporal horn dilatation *(open arrows)*.

B, Unenhanced CT. Casts of hemorrhage *(closed arrows)* indicate the ventricular size at the time of hemorrhage. The interval obstructive hydrocephalus has resulted in further enlargement of the ventricular size *(open arrows)*.

C, Left vertebral arteriogram. A saccular aneurysm *(arrow)* arises from the basilar tip, extending to the left of midline.

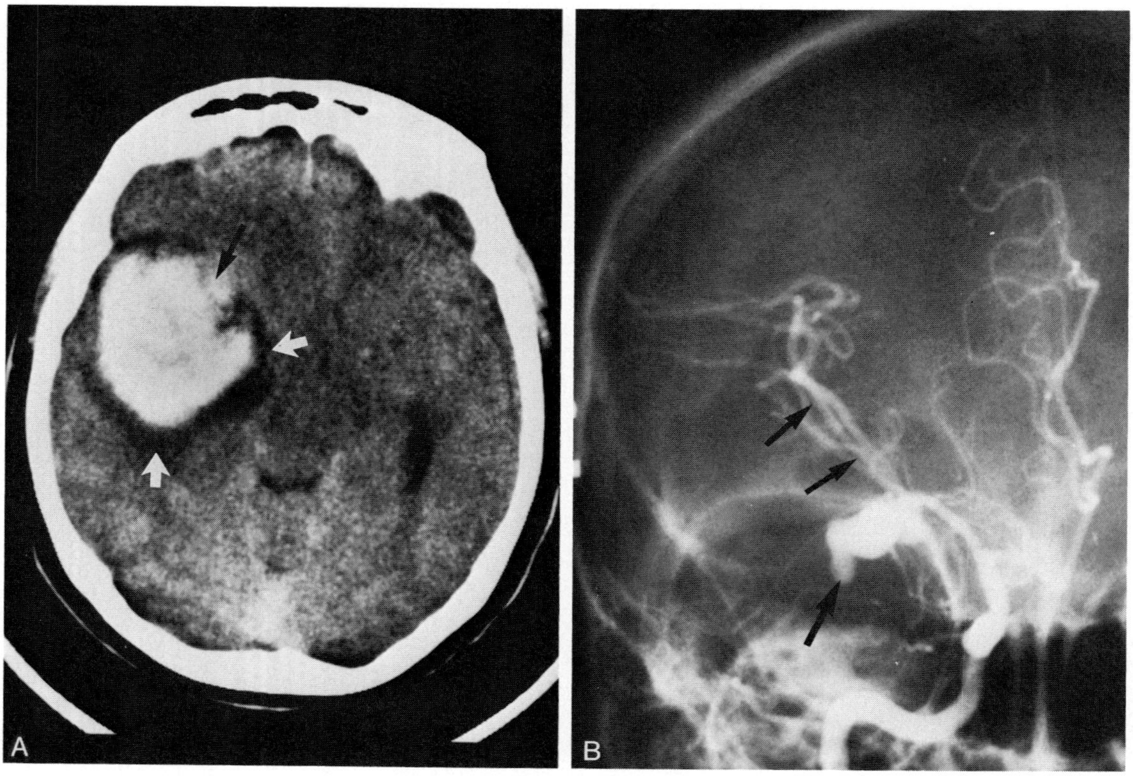

Figure 4–24. Right middle cerebral artery aneurysm (58-year-old female).

A, Axial CT. A 4-cm right frontotemporal hematoma *(black arrow)* surrounded by vasogenic edema *(white arrows)* is noted in the right middle cranial fossa.

B, Right common carotid arteriogram. A lobulated 1.7-cm (in greatest linear dimension) aneurysm *(large arrow)* is noted with avascular mass effect and displacement of the right middle cerebral artery *(small arrows)*.

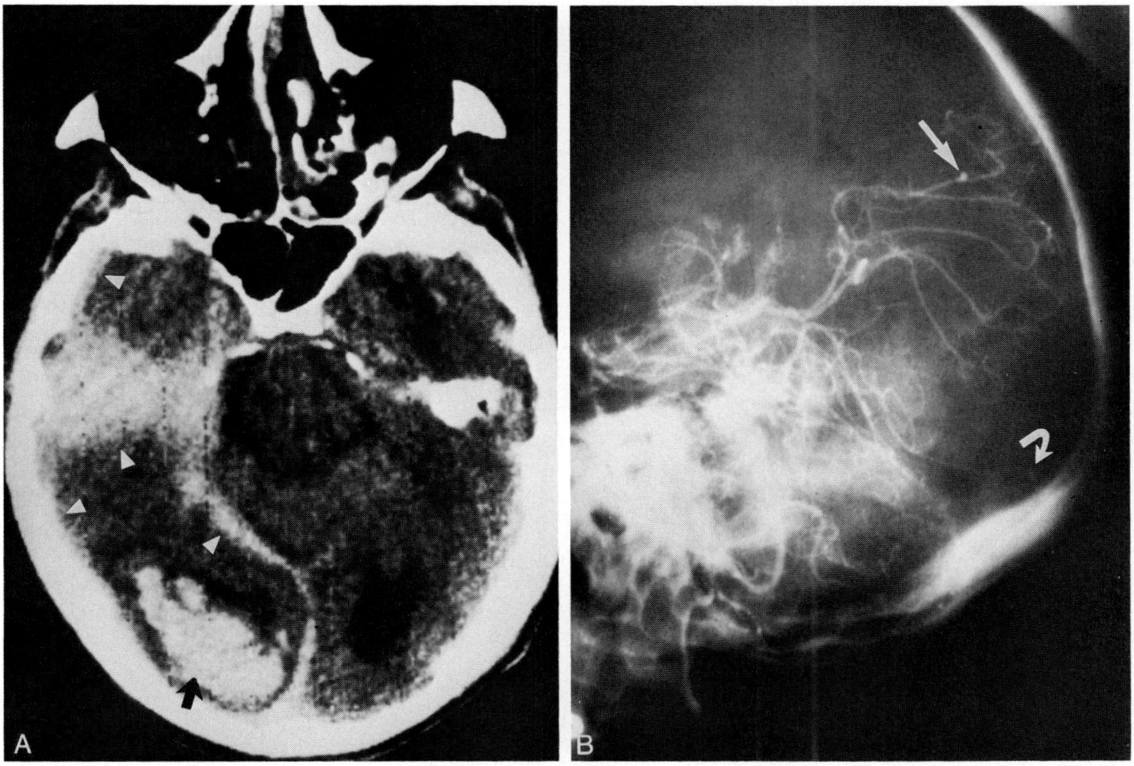

Figure 4–25. Mycotic aneurysm rupture—bacterial endocarditis (58-year-old male).

A, Unenhanced CT. Acute IPH *(arrow)* and SDH *(arrowheads)* are present.

B, Lateral left vertebral angiography. Two separate peripheral aneurysms are identified. The ruptured right calcarine artery aneurysm *(curved arrow)* is associated with avascular mass effect. A second, parieto-occipital artery aneurysm *(arrow)* is also noted.

Infarction

Arterial

Nearly 20% of all arterial infarcts are hemorrhagic. Hemorrhagic infarcts result from transient cessation of flow long enough to permit anoxic injury to the endothelial cells. Once flow is reinstituted the injured endothelial cells no longer possess the ability to contain the arterial systolic pressure. The result is exudation of blood from the damaged vessel into the surrounding parenchyma. Transient cessation of flow may be the result of embolus, prolonged hypotension with subsequent restoration of flow, occlusion with recruitment of collaterals, or temporary compression of the posterior cerebral artery (PCA) against the tentorium during descending transtentorial herniation.[3] The hemorrhages are petechial and usually restricted to the infarcted gray matter. Patients receiving anticoagulants may undergo diffuse bleeding with accumulation of sizable hematomas in the white and gray matter.

The initial CT examination may show a bland infarct with a wedge-shaped hypodensity respecting arterial border zones, extending to the cortex. A repeat CT in 2 to 3 days may show ill-defined gyral hyperdensity (Fig. 4–26). The accompanying ischemic edema may distort the margins of the hemorrhage and diminish the density of the collection, potentially rendering it isodense or only slightly hyperdense to normal parenchyma.

Three significant differences that affect the MRI characteristics exist between the hemorrhagic arterial infarct and the typical IPH. In attempts to alleviate the anoxic condition, multiple reperfusion processes are available to elevate the partial pressure of oxygen. This abundant oxygen delays the formation of deoxyhemoglobin. Consequently, the T2-PRE effects of deoxyhemoglobin may not be present in the early phase of hemorrhage.[6, 32] The second difference is the type and magnitude of edema that is present by the time hemorrhage becomes apparent; the edema is ischemic and found in greater amounts than that

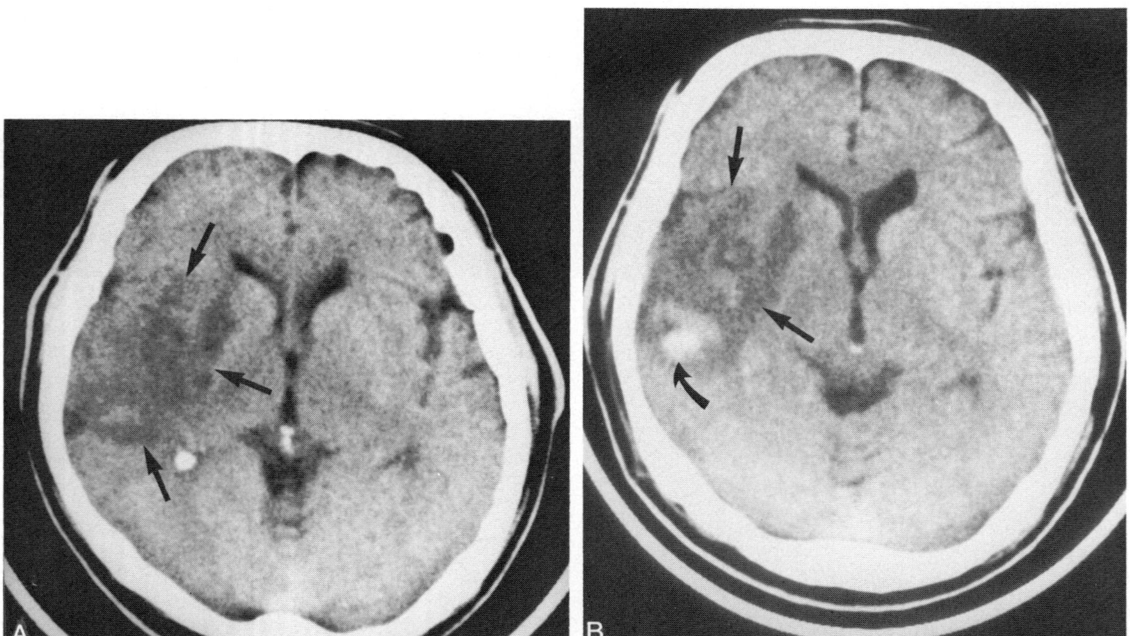

Figure 4–26. Hemorrhagic infarction (61-year-old male).

A, Unenhanced CT (24 hours post ictus). An ill-defined, wedged-shaped hypodensity *(arrows)* is present in the right middle cerebral artery (MCA) distribution.

B, Unenhanced CT (48 hours post ictus). Intraparenchymal hemorrhage *(curved arrow)* has developed in this infarction. The ischemic edema *(arrows)* has become better marginated in the 24-hour interval since the previous examination.

associated with a typical hematoma. Finally, the localization of the hemosiderin to the cortex in the chronic phase of infarction is atypical.

Venous

Venous infarcts result from inability to drain the venous blood properly along the appropriate pathways. The venous pressure becomes elevated, and ultimately the capillaries and venules rupture. Venous infarcts are frequently hemorrhagic, multiple, and superficial. Hemorrhagic infarcts occur in 20% of patients with sinus thrombosis, which may occur secondary to dehydration, infection, sepsis, malignancy, trauma, pregnancy, oral contraceptive use, and polycythemia. The superior sagittal sinus is the most common one to thrombose, followed by the transverse and sigmoid sinuses.

Sinus thrombosis can be detected with unenhanced CT examination as an intrinsically dense sinus "cord sign."[33] A "delta sign" is apparent following contrast administration.[34, 35] IV contrast material will not enter the thrombosed sinus. The delta-shaped enhancement of the dura that surrounds the sinus results in the "delta sign." The collateral pathways of flow will be enlarged. MRI is more sensitive than CT in the diagnosis of sinus thrombosis. Lack of flow void[6] and decreased signal on T2 secondary to deoxyhemoglobin[36] are noted in the acute state. Methemoglobin will render the sinus increased signal on T1 and T2[37, 38] in the subacute phase. The MRI pattern of chronic thrombosis is one of recanalization of the sinus and return to normal signal. Magnetic resonance angiography (MRA) using phase-contrast angiography has successfully demonstrated sinus occlusion.[39] Planar imaging demonstrates subcortical hemorrhage, which may be multiple and may not respect arterial territories (Fig. 4–27).

Vascular Malformation

Vascular malformations as a group are discussed in more detail in Chapter 5. From the standpoint of intracranial hemorrhage, focus will be on the high flow AVMs. AVMs are congenital anomalous communications between the arteries and veins. Lack of intervening capillaries permits a dramatic increase in flow through these lesions. From 80 to 90% of AVMs are supratentorial; their size may vary widely. Of all patients with AVM, 1.4 to 7% have associated aneurysms.[40, 41] When detected, the aneurysms are more often responsible for the hemorrhage than are the AVMs. Hemorrhage usually occurs in the second to fourth decades. Ruptured AVMs result in IPH in at least 50% of cases (Fig. 4–28). Less commonly, SAH and IVH may occur.

The vasospasm that may complicate SAH from aneurysm rupture is rarely seen with AVMs that hemorrhage into the subarachnoid space. This is in part related to the amount and location of the blood. Typically, AVMs are associated with minimal subarachnoid blood. Also, the location of the blood may be peripheral, remote from the vessels at the base of the brain.

Certain planar imaging characteristics may distinguish ICH secondary to AVM from that secondary to other causes. CT may depict an intrinsically dense draining vein that may enhance following contrast administration. Calcification within the lesion may be detected with CT. MRI will adroitly display the acute IPH and hemoglobin breakdown products. T1 images usually display serpentine channels of flow void. T2 images are variable, with flow void secondary to high flow, and high signal secondary to even echo rephasing and slow flow (see Chapter 5). MRI evidence of adjacent chronic hemorrhage may corroborate the diagnosis.

Neoplasm

Primary or secondary neoplasms account for 10 to 15% of IPHs. The propensity to hemorrhage may be related to neovascularity, vessel invasion, rate of tumor growth, necrosis, and infarction, and possibly may occur secondary to fibrinolysis (Fig. 4–29). Primary brain tumors hemorrhage infrequently at a rate of 0.8 to 5.4%.[42, 43] The most common intra-axial brain tumors to hemorrhage are mixed oligoastrocytoma, low-grade glioma, glioblastoma multiforme, and ependymoma.[3, 42] The common hemorrhagic metastases to the paren-

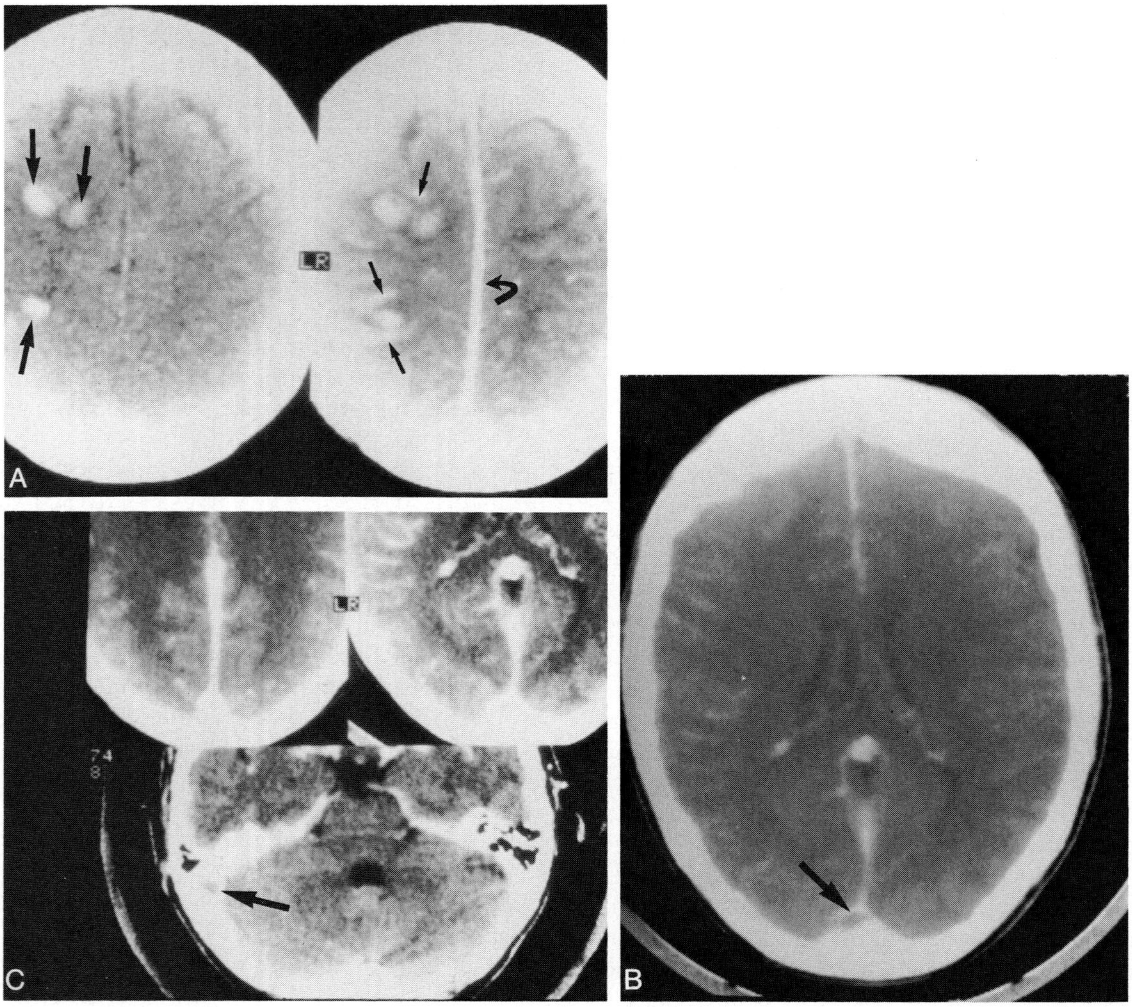

Figure 4–27. Hemorrhagic venous infarction (72-year-old female).

A, CT (left, unenhanced). Multiple parenchymal hemorrhages *(arrows)* are present in the right parietal lobe. Minimal local mass effect is present.

CT (right, enhanced). Minimal parenchymal enhancement *(arrows)* adjacent to the hemorrhagic foci is detected. The enhancing falx cerebri *(curved arrow)* is much thicker than normal owing to collateral venous flow.

B, Enhanced CT. The "delta" sign *(arrow)* is noted in the superior sagittal sinus.

C, Enhanced CT. The dural sinus thrombus has extended into the right transverse sinus *(arrow)*.

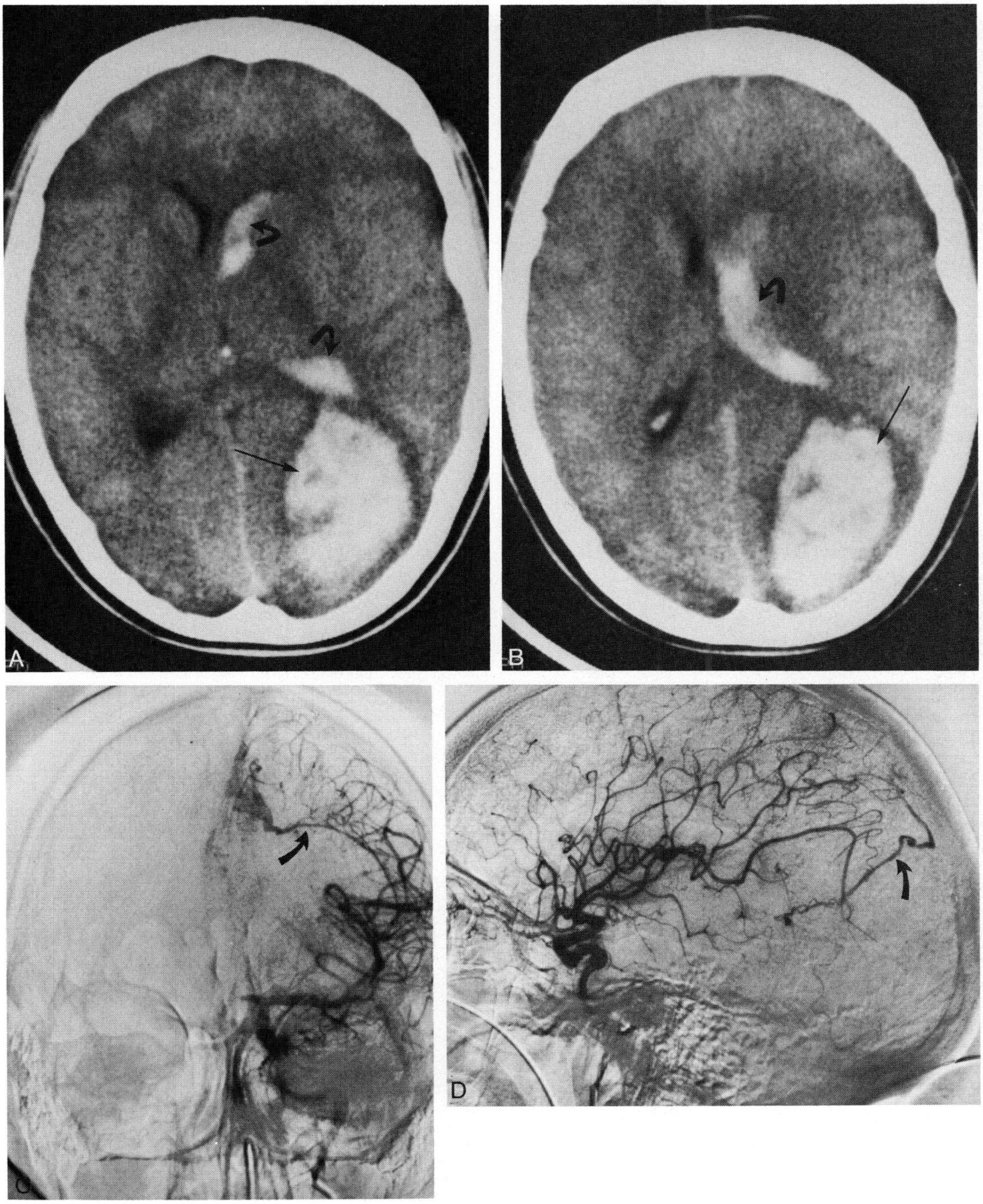

Figure 4–28. Arteriovenous malformation (AVM) (28-year-old female).

A, B, Unenhanced CT. A left occipital parenchymal hematoma *(arrow)* has dissected into the left lateral ventricle *(curved arrows)*.

C, D, Anteroposterior (AP) and lateral left internal carotid angiogram. Because of local hematoma and mass effect, only a portion of this AVM opacifies from the left angular artery *(curved arrow)*.

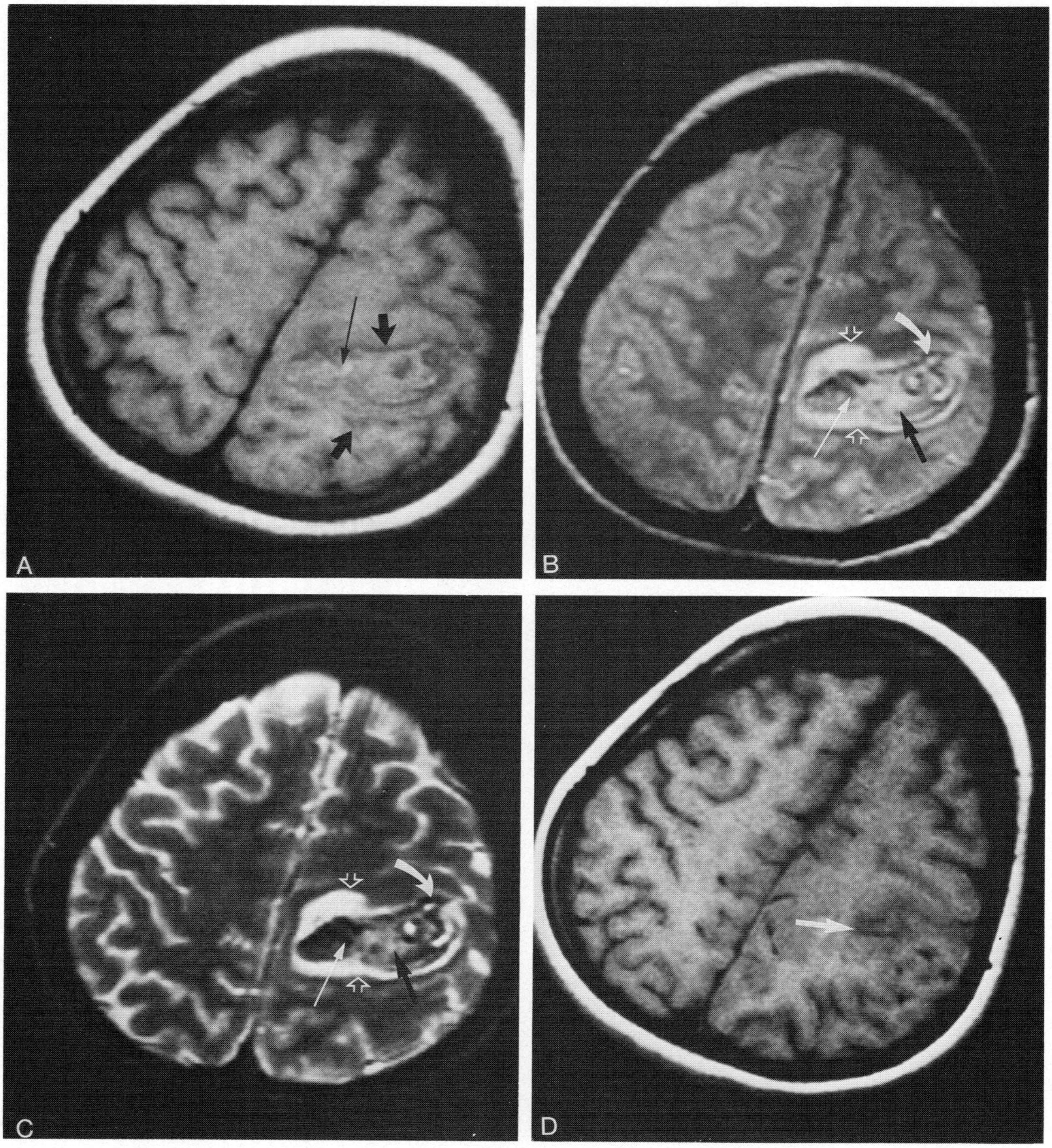

Figure 4–29. Choriocarcinoma metastasis (43-year-old female).

A, Axial T1. An ill-defined mass *(short arrows)* is present in the left parietal lobe. The mass contains foci of high signal *(long arrow)* representing methemoglobin.

B, C, Axial SD and T2. The mass is more complex than expected for a simple hemorrhage. Presumed foci of intracellular methemoglobin *(thin white arrow)* and an incomplete hemosiderin ring *(curved arrow)* are interspersed with a tumor *(black arrow)*. Vasogenic edema *(open arrows)* surrounds the lesion.

D, Axial T1. The mass is ill-defined with a horizontal band of diminished signal intensity *(arrow)*.

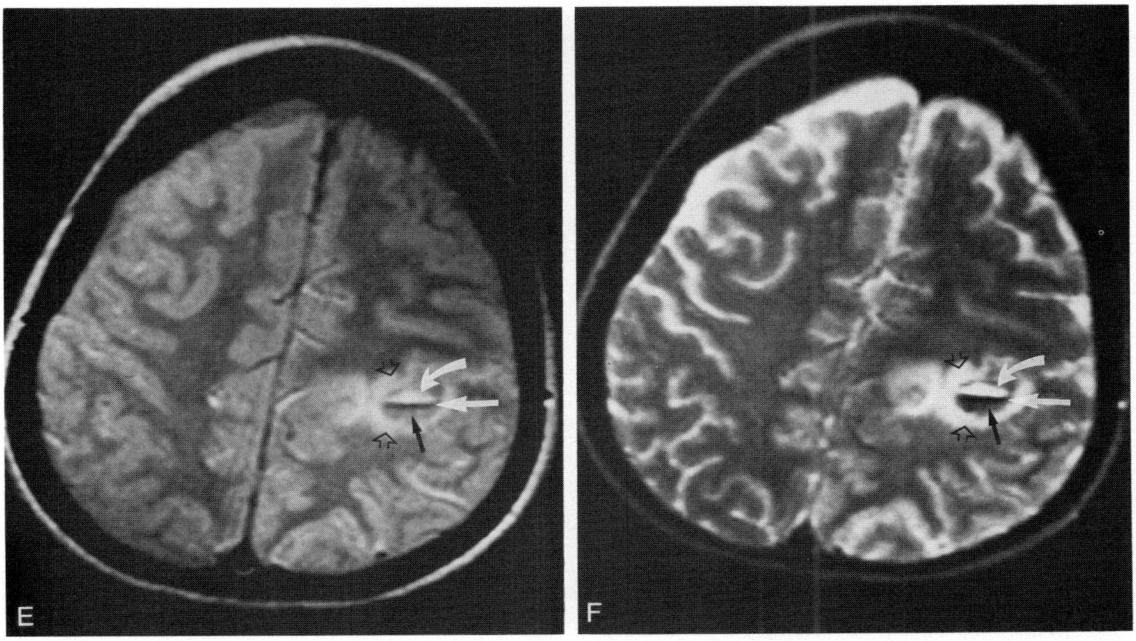

Figure 4–29 *Continued*
E, F, Axial SD and T2. A three-layered fluid collection is noted, consisting of high-signal serum or extracellular methemoglobin *(curved arrow),* deoxyhemoglobin or intracellular methemoglobin *(straight white arrow),* and tumor cells *(straight black arrow).* Vasogenic edema *(open arrows)* surrounds the lesion.

chyma are melanoma, bronchogenic carcinoma, and choriocarcinoma.[43] Less commonly, metastatic renal and thyroid have been implicated.

Multiplicity, excessive vasogenic edema, and early, irregular enhancement suggest the presence of neoplasm on planar imaging.[44] Sensitive to hemoglobin degradation products, MRI is particularly well suited in evaluating suspected neoplasm-related IPH. Delay in the evolution of IPH, presence of multiple stages of hemorrhage simultaneously, incomplete or absent hemosiderin ring, and pronounced, persistent vasogenic edema all corroborate a possible underlying neoplasm.[9, 45, 46]

Coagulopathy

Coagulopathy may result from a primary hematologic disorder or anticoagulant therapy. Regardless of the cause, coagulopathy may result in hemorrhage into any compartment. In the presence of coagulopathy, all the aforementioned conditions will hemorrhage at an increased rate. Accordingly, hemorrhages occur often in the basal ganglia in concert with hypertension. History of a primary coagulopathy or of warfarin (Coumadin) therapy will be most useful in assessing the cause of a specific hemorrhage.

Planar imaging may demarcate solitary or multiple hemorrhages in any location. These hemorrhages may have fluid levels that may indicate poor clotting mechanism[30, 46a] (Figs. 4–30, 4–31).

Amyloid Angiopathy

Amyloid angiopathy is a histologically established condition affecting patients greater than 60 years of age. This lesion is a function of senescence and results in deposition of amyloid in the adventitia and media of medium- and small-sized arteries and arterioles in the leptomeninges and cerebral cortex. As the deposits increase, the lumen narrows. The vessel walls may undergo fibrinoid degeneration and miliary aneurysm formation.[47] Resultant IPH may occur. The hemorrhages are usually lobar, located in supratentorial parenchyma with relative sparing of the cerebellum, brainstem, and basal ganglia.[48, 49]

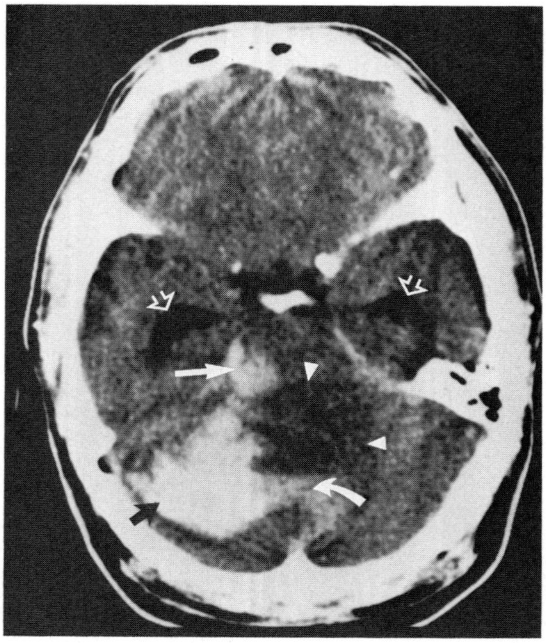

Figure 4–30. Coagulopathy (52-year-old male). Unenhanced CT; an irregular parenchymal hemorrhage *(black arrow)* is located within the right cerebellar hemisphere. The hemorrhage also extends into the upper pons *(straight white arrow)* and vermis *(curved white arrow)*. Vasogenic edema *(arrowheads)* incompletely surrounds the hemorrhage. The temporal horns *(open arrows)* are enlarged, indicating obstructive hydrocephalus.

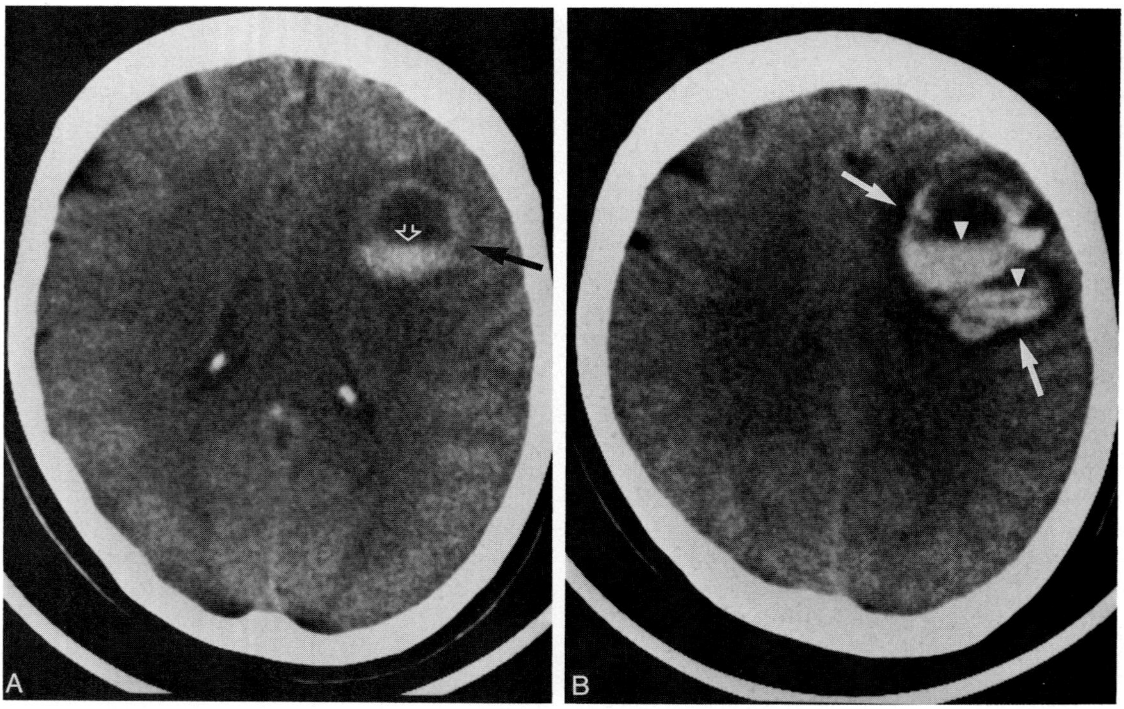

Figure 4–31. Coagulopathy—drug-induced thrombocytopenia (61-year-old female).

A, Unenhanced CT. A complex intraparenchymal hemorrhage *(arrow)* is present in the left anterior parietal lobe. A fluid level is present *(open arrow)*.

B, Unenhanced CT. The loculated hemorrhage contains at least two fluid levels *(arrowheads)*. Vasogenic edema *(solid arrows)* surrounds the hemorrhage.

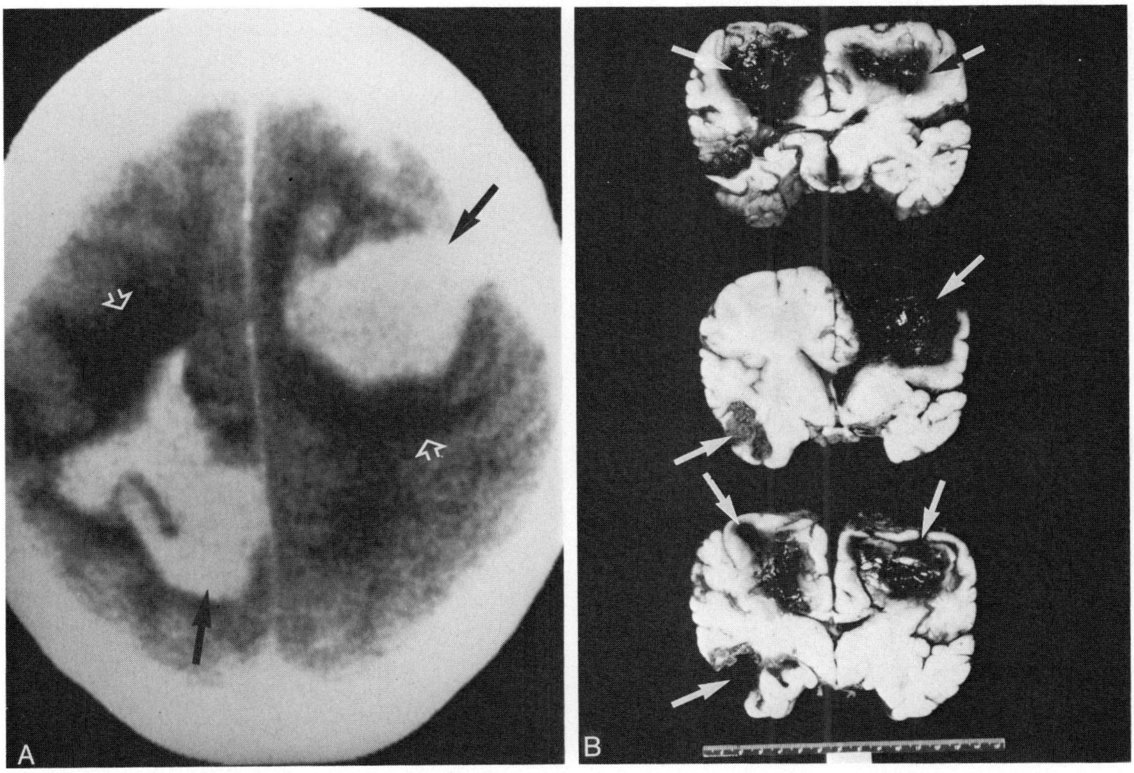

Figure 4–32. Amyloid angiopathy (83-year-old male).

A, Unenhanced CT. Two separate, large superficial hemorrhages *(arrows)* are present in the parietal vertices. A moderate amount of vasogenic edema *(open arrows)* and mass effect accompanies each lesion.

B, Coronal brain sections. Multiple intraparenchymal hemorrhages *(arrows)* of different ages are present throughout both hemispheres.

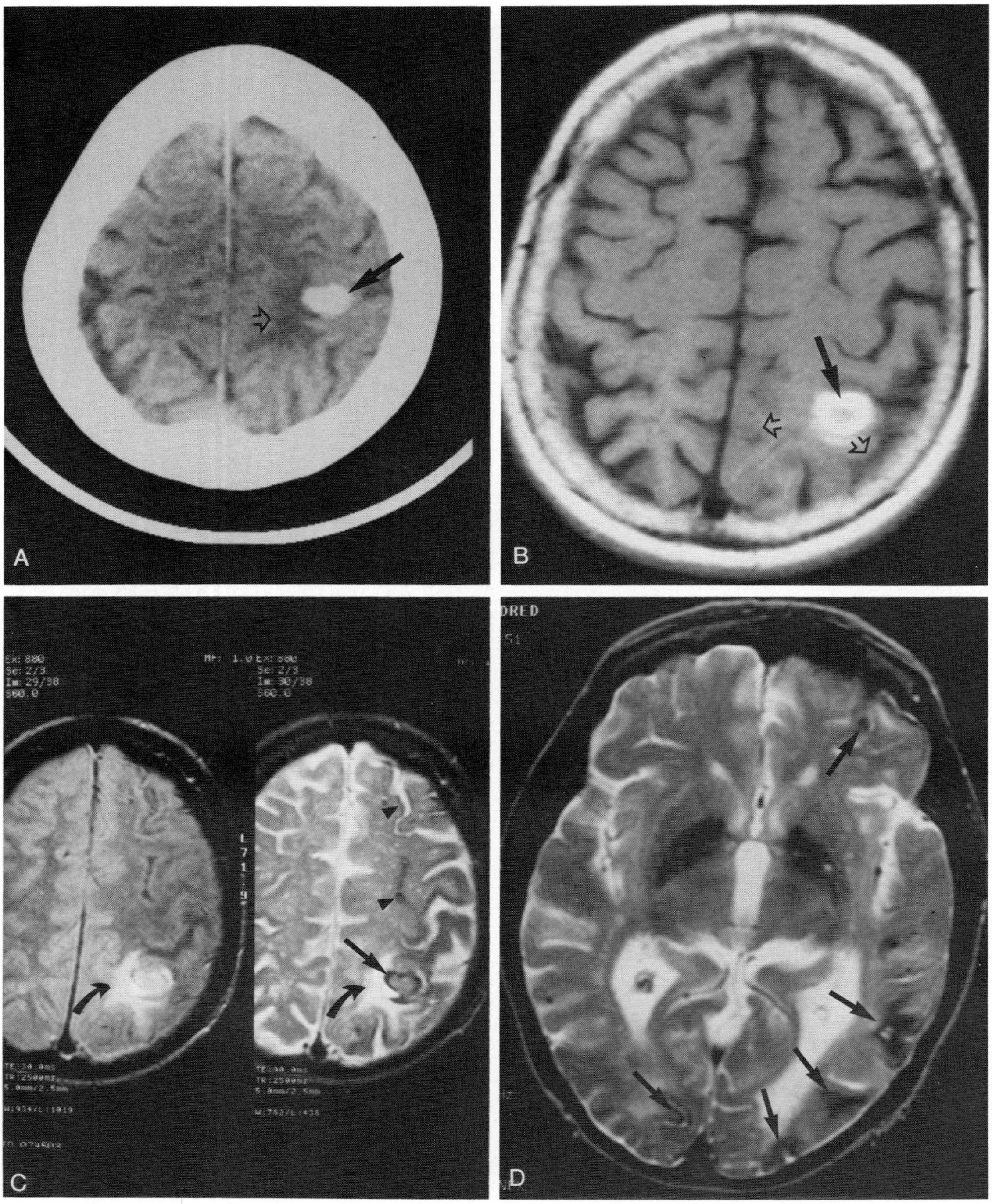

Figure 4–33. Amyloid angiopathy (75-year-old female).

A, Unenhanced CT. A left parietal subcortical hematoma *(arrow)* is present with minimal surrounding vasogenic edema *(open arrow)*.

B, Axial T1. Methemoglobin *(arrow)* is present in the periphery of the lesion. Sulcal effacement *(open arrows)* confirms mild local mass effect.

C, Axial SD and T2. Vasogenic edema *(curved arrow)* surrounds the medial portion of the lesion. Intracellular methemoglobin *(arrow)* is present within the hemorrhage. Note additional remote foci of diminished T2 signal *(arrowheads)*.

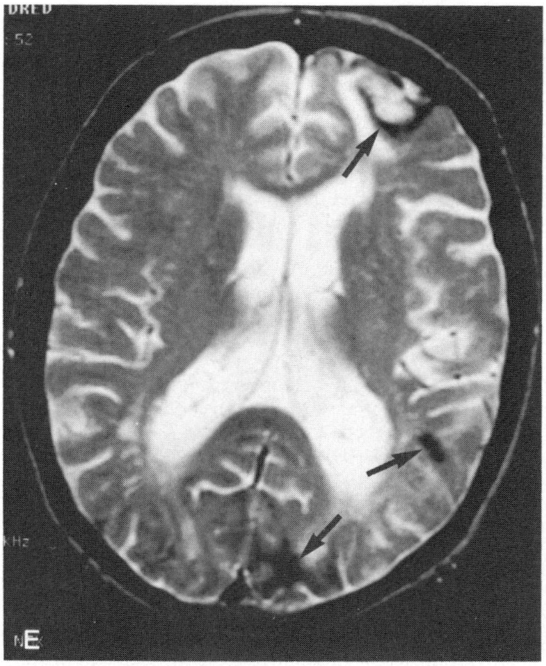

Figure 4–33 *Continued*
D, E Axial T2. Hemosiderin and ferritin deposits *(arrows)* are the sequela of multiple prior superficial parenchymal hemorrhages, common with amyloid angiopathy.

On planar imaging, the hemorrhages are often multiple, superficial, and poorly marginated, and are associated with variable amounts of vasogenic edema (Fig. 4–32). MRI findings in addition to IPH include high-signal abnormalities in the white matter indicative of small vessel hypoperfusion from vascular compromise.[49] MRI may also depict multiple superficial hemosiderin-ferritin deposits indicative of prior hemorrhage (Fig. 4–33).

Vasculitis

Drug-induced vasculitis is a rare cause of ICH. Sympathomimetics (amphetamines and cocaine) are most commonly implicated. A necrotizing angiitis is demonstrated. Cellular infiltrates and fibrinoid necrosis of the media and intima of the cerebral arterioles occur with formation of microaneurysms.[50] The hemorrhage may be intraparenchymal or subarachnoid in location.[51–53] Cerebral infarctions are also noted. In some studies,[52] there has been a high incidence of underlying structural anomalies, including AVMs and aneurysms, underscoring the need for pancerebral angiography in these patients. The mortality of ICH related to vasculitis approaches 50%. The hemorrhagic condition may be secondary to sympathomimetic stimulation (increased blood pressure, heart rate, and vasoconstriction), acute cardiac toxicity, or vasculitis.

References

1. New PJ, Aronow S: Attenuation measurements of whole blood and blood fractions in computed tomography. Radiology 1976; 121:635–640.
2. Zimmerman RD, Leeds NE, Naidich TP: Ring blush associated with intracerebral hematoma. Radiology 1977; 122:707–711.
3. Grossman RI, Bello JA: Neuroradiologic evaluation of intracranial hemorrhage; categorical course No. 705. RSNA 1990.
4. Laster DW, Moody DM, Ball MR: Resolving intracerebral hematoma: Alteration of the "ring sign" with steroids. AJR 1978; 130:935–939.
5. Loes DJ, Smoker WRK, Biller J, et al: Nontraumatic lobar intracerebral hemorrhage: CT/angiographic correlation. AJNR 1987; 8:1027–1030.
6. Grossman RI, Gomori JM, Goldberg HI, et al: MR imaging of hemorrhagic conditions of the head and neck. Radiographics 1988; 8:441–454.
7. Gomori JM, Grossman RI, Goldberg HI, et al: Intracranial hematomas: Imaging by high-field MR. Radiology 1985; 157:87–93.
8. Guyton AC: *Textbook of Medical Physiology,* 5th Ed, 1976. WB Saunders, Philadelphia.
9. Destian S, Sze G, Krol G, et al: MR imaging of hemorrhagic intracranial neoplasms. AJNR 1989; 9:1115–1122.
10. Gomori JM, Grossman RI: Mechanisms responsible for the MR appearance and evolution of intracranial hemorrhage. Radiographics 1988; 8:427–440.
11. Gomori JM, Grossman RI, Hackney DB, et al: Variable appearances of subacute intracranial hematomas on high-field spin-echo MR. AJNR 1987; 8:1019–1026.
12. Thulborn KR, Sorensen AG, Kowall NW, et al: The role of ferritin and hemosiderin in the MR appearance of cerebral hemorrhage: A histopathologic biochemical study in rats. AJNR 1990; 11:291–297.
13. Zimmerman RA, Bilaniuk LT: Computed tomographic staging of traumatic epidural bleeding. Radiology 1982; 144:809–812.
14. Forbes GS, Sheedy PF, Piepgras DG, et al: Computed tomography in the evaluation of subdural hematomas. Radiology 1978; 126:143–148.
15. Braun J, Borovich B, Guilburd JN, et al: Acute subdural hematoma mimicking epidural hematoma on CT. AJNR 1987; 8:171–173.
16. Wang AM, Chinwuba CE, O'Reilly GV, et al: Subdural hematoma in patients with brain tumor: CT evaluation. J Comput Assist Tomogr 1985; 9:511–513.
17. Kao MC: Sedimentation level in chronic subdural hematoma visible on computerized tomography. J Neurosurg 1983; 58:246–251.
18. Reed D, Robertson WD, Graeb DA, et al: Acute subdural hematomas: Atypical CT findings. AJNR 1986; 7:417–421.
19. Fobben ES, Grossman RI, Atlas SW, et al: MR

characteristics of subdural hematomas and hygromas at 1.5T. AJNR 1989; 10:687–693.
20. Hayman LA, Pagani JJ, Kirkpatrick JB, et al: Pathophysiology of acute intracerebral and subarachnoid hemorrhage: Applications to MR imaging. AJNR 1989; 10:457–461.
21. Chakeres DW, Bryan RN: Acute subarachnoid hemorrhage: In vitro comparison of magnetic resonance and computed tomography. AJNR 1986; 7:223–228.
22. Bradley WG, Schmidt PG: Effect of methemoglobin formation on the MR appearance of subarachnoid hemorrhage. Radiology 1985; 156:99–103.
23. Hackney DB, Lesnick JE, Zimmerman RA, et al: MR identification of bleeding site in subarachnoid hemorrhage with multiple intracranial aneurysms. J Comput Assist Tomogr 1986; 10:878–880.
24. Gomori JM, Grossman RI, Goldberg HI, et al: High-field spin-echo MR imaging of superficial and subependymal siderosis secondary to neonatal intraventricular hemorrhage. Neuroradiology 1987; 29:339–342.
25. Adams HP, Kassell NF, Torner JC, et al: Predicting cerebral ischemia after aneurysmal subarachnoid hemorrhage: Influences of clinical conditions, CT results and antifibrinolytic therapy. Neurology 1987; 37:1586–1591.
26. Hesselink JR, Dowd CF, Healy ME, et al: MR imaging of brain contusions. A comparative study with CT. AJNR 1988; 9:269–278.
27. Nelson JS: *Anderson's Pathology,* 9th ed. Kissane JM, Ed. CV Mosby, St Louis, 1990.
28. Zimmerman RA, Bilaniuk LT, Genneralli T: Computed tomography of shearing injuries of the cerebral white matter. Radiology 1978; 127:393–396.
29. Zimmerman RA, Bilaniuk LT, Hackney DB: Head injury: Early results of comparing CT and high-field MR. AJNR 1986; 7:757–764.
29a. Moody DM, Challa VR, Bell MA: Charcot-Bouchard aneurysms and brain hemorrhage: A 124-year old puzzle. Paper 140, presented at the 30th annual meeting of the American Society of Neuroradiology. St. Louis, MO, 1992.
30. Weisberg LA, Stazio A: Nontraumatic frontal lobe hemorrhage: Clinical-computed tomographic correlations. Neuroradiology 1988; 30:500–505.
31. Bohmfalk GL, Story JL, Wissinger JP, et al: Bacterial intracranial aneurysm. J Neurosurg 1978; 48:369–382.
32. Hecht-Leavitt C, Gomori JM, Grossman RI, et al: High-field MRI of hemorrhagic cortical infarction. AJNR 1986; 7:581–585.
33. Buonanno FS, Moody DM, Ball MR, et al: Computed cranial tomographic findings in cerebral sinovenous occlusion. J Comput Assist Tomogr 1978; 2:281–90.
34. Kim KS, Walczak TS: Computed tomography of deep cerebral venous thrombosis. J Comput Assist Tomogr 1986; 10:386–390.
35. Goldberg AL, Rosenbaum AE, Wang H, et al: Computed tomography of dural sinus thrombosis. J Comput Assist Tomogr 1986; 10:16–20.
36. Macchi PJ, Grossman RI, Gomori JM, et al: High field MR imaging of cerebral venous thrombosis. J Comput Assist Tomogr 1986; 10:10–15.
37. Snyder TC, Sachder HS: MR imaging of cerebral dural sinus thrombosis. J Comput Assist Tomogr 1986; 10:889–891.
38. Hulcelle PJ, Dooms GC, Mathurin P, et al: MR of unsuspected dural sinus thrombosis. Neuroradiology 1989; 21:217–221.
39. Rippe DJ, Boyko OB, Spritzer CE, et al: Demonstration of dural sinus occlusion by the use of MR angiography. AJNR 1990; 11:199–201.
40. Crawford PM, West CR, Chadwick DW, et al: Arteriovenous malformations of the brain: Natural history in unoperated patients. J Neuro Neurosurg Psychiatr 1986; 49:1–10.
41. Perret G, Nishioka H: Report on the cooperative study of intracranial aneurysms and subarachnoid hemorrhage. Section VI, Arteriovenous Malformations. J Neurosurg 1966; 25:467–490.
42. Kondziolka D, Bernstein M, Resch L, et al: Significance of hemorrhage into brain tumors: Clinicopathological study. J Neurosurg 1987; 67:852–857.
43. Mandybur TI: Intracranial hemorrhage caused by metastatic tumors. Neurology 1977, 27:650–655.
44. Sze G, Krol G, Olsen WL, et al: Hemorrhagic neoplasms: MR mimics of occult vascular malformations. AJNR 1987; 8:795–802.
45. Atlas SW, Grossman RI, Gomori JM, et al: Hemorrhagic intracranial malignant neoplasms: Spin-echo MR imaging. Radiology 1987; 164:71–77.
46. Barkovich AJ, Atlas SW: Magnetic resonance imaging of intracranial hemorrhage. Radiol Clin North Am 1988; 26:801–820.
46a. Pfleger MJ, Hardee EP, Hayman LA: Fluid/fluid levels in intracerebral hematoma: A sign of coagulopathy. Alternate Paper #9, presented at the 30th annual meeting of the American Society of Neuroradiology. St. Louis, MO, 1992.
47. Okazaki H, Reagan TJ, Campbell RJ: Clinicopathologic studies of primary cerebral amyloid angiopathy. Mayo Clin Proc 1979; 54:22–31.
48. Wagle WA, Smith TW, Weiner M: Intracerebral hemorrhage caused by cerebral amyloid angiopathy: Radiographic-pathologic correlation. AJNR 1984; 5:171–176.
49. Loes DJ, Biller J, Yuh WTC: Leukoencephalopathy in cerebral amyloid angiopathy: MR imaging in four cases. AJNR 1990; 11:485–488.
50. Yu YJ, Cooper DR, Wellenstein DE: Cerebral angitis and intracerebral hemorrhage associated with methamphetamine abuse. J Neurosurg 1983; 58:109–111.
51. Nalls G, Disher A, Daryabagi J: Subcortical cerebral hemorrhages associated with cocaine abuse: CT and MR findings. J Comput Assist Tomogr 1989; 13:1–5.
52. Jacobs IG, Roszler MH, Kelly JK, et al: Cocaine abuse: Neurovascular complications. Radiology 1989; 170:223–227.
53. Delaney P, Estes M: Intracranial hemorrhage with amphetamine abuse. Neurology 1980; 30:1125–1128.

5

VASCULAR LESIONS

VASCULAR MALFORMATIONS
- **High Flow**
  - Arteriovenous Malformation
  - Vein of Galen Aneurysm
- **Normal Flow**
  - Venous Angioma
- **Low Flow**
  - Cavernous Angioma
  - Capillary Telangiectasia

ANEURYSMS
- **Congenital**
- **Atherosclerotic**
- **Traumatic**
- **Mycotic**

VASCULAR MALFORMATIONS

Vascular malformations are congenital anomalies of the vascular system in which the normal communication between the arteries and veins is aberrant. The circulation time of the blood through the malformation may be altered. The vascular malformations are presented here, based on flow rates and using traditional classification scheme[1, 2] (Table 5–1).

High Flow

Arteriovenous Malformation

Arteriovenous malformation (AVM) is the most common type of vascular malformation. Male-to-female ratio has been reported to range from 1:1 to 2:1.[1, 3–5] Macroscopically, the lesion consists of a racemose network of dilated, tortuous, elongated vessels with characteristics common to both arteries and veins. There are no intervening capillaries between these vessels; hence, the high flow rate. The tangled mass varies markedly in size, from a few millimeters to several centimeters. Microscopically, the vessels lack muscle and elastic fibers. Regions of segmental dilatation may be apparent.[1] The vessels are often separated by intervening brain parenchyma, which may be gliotic.

Although AVMs may occur anywhere within the central nervous system (CNS), 80 to 90% are supratentorial,[6, 7] most often in the middle cerebral distribution. Aneurysms may coexist in 1.4 to 7% of cases.[5, 7] When present, the aneurysm is located on a feeding artery in up to 75% of cases.[7] In the general population, the incidence of aneurysm is 5.3 to 7 times greater than that of AVM.[5, 8]

The clinical presentation is contingent on the location and size of the AVM and on the presence of hemorrhage. Seizures occur most frequently, followed by progressive focal neurologic deficits[4, 5, 7, 9] and headache. The risk of a patient with an AVM developing epilepsy over 20 years is 18%; however, if the AVM is located in the temporal lobe, percentage of risk increases twofold, to 37%.[7] Patients may

Table 5–1. NEUROIMAGING FEATURES OF VASCULAR MALFORMATIONS

	Arteriovenous Malformation	Venous Angioma	Cavernous Angioma	Capillary Telangiectasia
CT Unenhanced	Irregular Hyperdense Calcification Atrophy	Solitary Dense Tubular structure	Solitary or multiple dense lesions—may contain calcification	Solitary density, pons
Enhanced	Serpentine enhancement Draining veins	Transcerebral vein and caput medusae	Minimal to no enhancement	Minimal to no enhancement
MRI T1	Multiple Tubular flow void	Solitary Tubular flow void	Focus of heterogeneous signal, multiple; no flow effects	Like cavernous angioma although solitary, pons
T2	Flow void or increased signal (EER)*	Flow void or increased signal (EER)	Complex heterogeneous (both ↑ and ↓) signal surrounded by rim of ↓ signal, multiple	Like cavernous angioma, solitary, pons
Angiography Technique Contrast	↑ as PRN	Normal amount†	↑ amount, prolonged injection	↑ amount, prolonged injection
Filming	4–6/sec	Standard‡	Delayed	Delayed
Vessels	1. Ipsilateral internal and external carotid 2. Contralateral common 3. Dominant vertebral	Ipsilateral Internal Circulation	Ipsilateral Internal Circulation	Dominant, vertebral
Findings Arterial	Hypertrophied arterial feeders, nidus, early venous	Normal	Normal	Normal
Venous	Multiple ectatic Early draining veins	Solitary transcerebral vein, caput medusae	Normal; may see late capillary blush	Normal

*EER = Even echo rephasing.
†Standard contrast for cut film angiography (dose may be decreased by 50% for digital angiography)
(60% Reno) injection: internal carotid artery (ICA) or dominant vertebral artery (6 ml sec/8 ml total)
(300 mg% Isovue) external carotid artery (ECA) (3 ml sec/6 ml total)
common carotid artery (CCA) (8 ml sec/12 ml total)
‡Standard filming sequence: 2/sec × 4, 1/sec × 6.

exhibit signs and symptoms of acute intracranial mass if hemorrhage occurs. Hemorrhage is most often intraparenchymal, although a subarachnoid or intraventricular component may be present.

The mean risk of rupture and hemorrhage is 2 to 3% per annum.[4, 10] The risk of rebleed is up to 6% for the first year after hemorrhage[10] and returns to 2 to 3% per annum afterward. The initial hemorrhage is most common between the second and fourth decades; it may be fatal in up to 29% of patients, with 23% of patients exhibiting long-term morbidity.[4] Although studies have reported a greater likelihood of hemorrhage in smaller lesions,[10] this has been refuted by others.[4] Presence of hypertension has no predictive value for hemorrhage.[4] Pregnant patients have increased incidence of hemorrhage, presumably secondary to hypervolemia.[7]

Computed tomography (CT) most often depicts a heterogeneous, mixed-density mass[9] that may contain focal calcification (Fig. 5–1). Although variable in size, AVMs average 3 cm in greatest linear dimension. There is usually no evidence of edema unless hemorrhage has occurred.

Mass effect is not evident unless the AVM is of significant size or hemorrhage has occurred. In absence of hemorrhage, the degree of mass effect is much less than expected for the size of the lesion. Although regional blood flow may be dramatically increased owing to arteriovenous (AV) shunting, the adjacent brain parenchyma may not be adequately perfused. As a result, atrophic changes may be identified adjacent to the AVM. Smaller AVMs may not be detected unless intravenous (IV) contrast material is administered. The lesion most often enhances heterogeneously and is poorly marginated.[9] Large enhanced serpentine draining veins may be detected.

Sensitivity to flow and to hemoglobin degradation products renders magnetic resonance

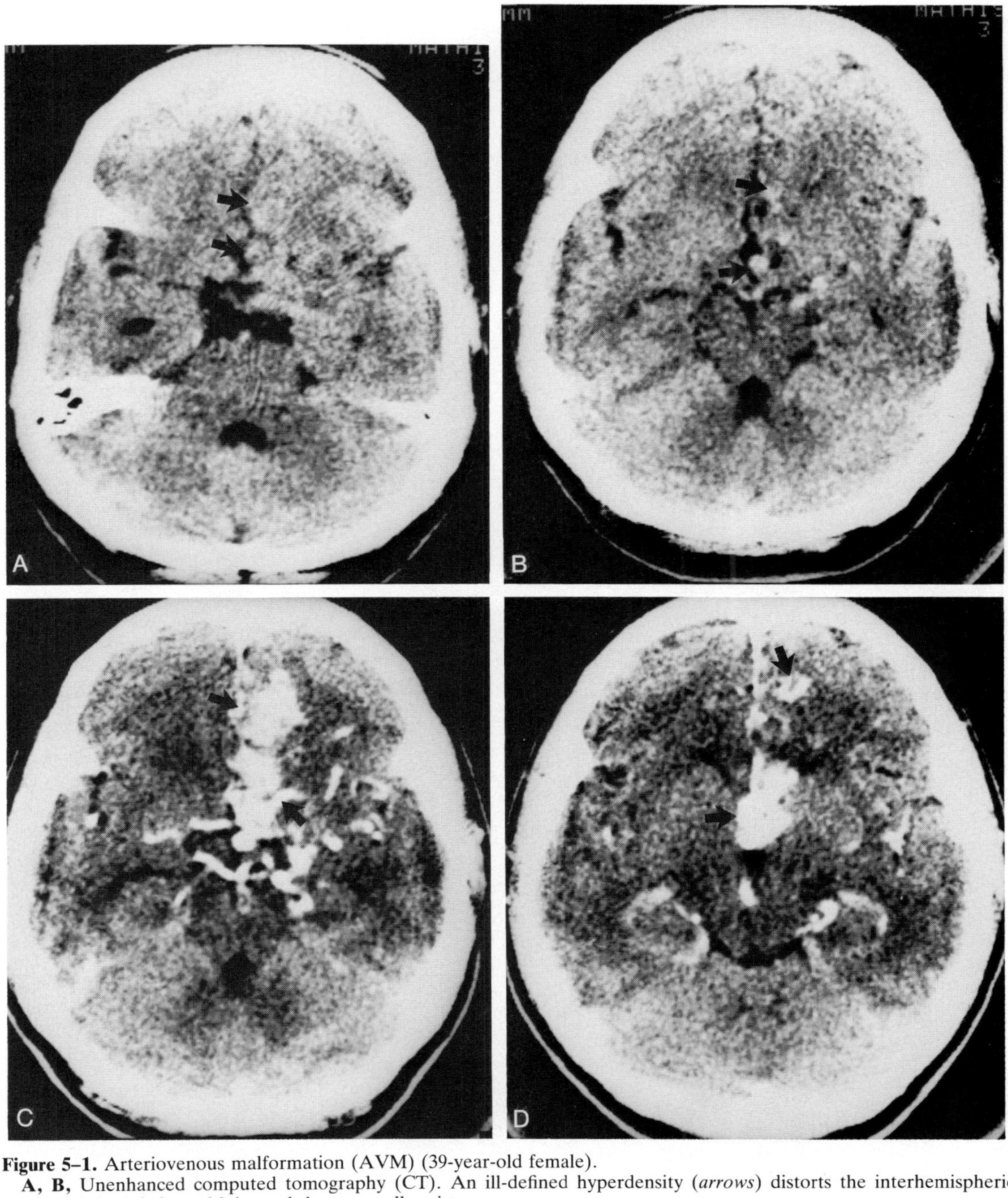

Figure 5–1. Arteriovenous malformation (AVM) (39-year-old female).

A, B, Unenhanced computed tomography (CT). An ill-defined hyperdensity (*arrows*) distorts the interhemispheric surface of the left frontal lobe and the suprasellar cistern.

C, D, Enhanced CT. Serpentine enhancement (*arrows*) confirms the diagnosis of AVM. Note the lack of edema or significant mass effect.

imaging (MRI) an ideal tool with which to study patients with AVMs. Signal void related to flow is frequently seen on T1 spin echo sequences[11–13] (Fig. 5–2). T2 spin echo sequences may display flow void from high flow, as well as high signal from even echo rephasing (EER) in slower-flowing moieties of the lesion.[8] MRI can detect the location of the AVM nidus, mass effect on parenchyma, major arterial feeders, and venous drainage.[13] Minor arterial feeders are more difficult to see because of their small size, multiplicity, and

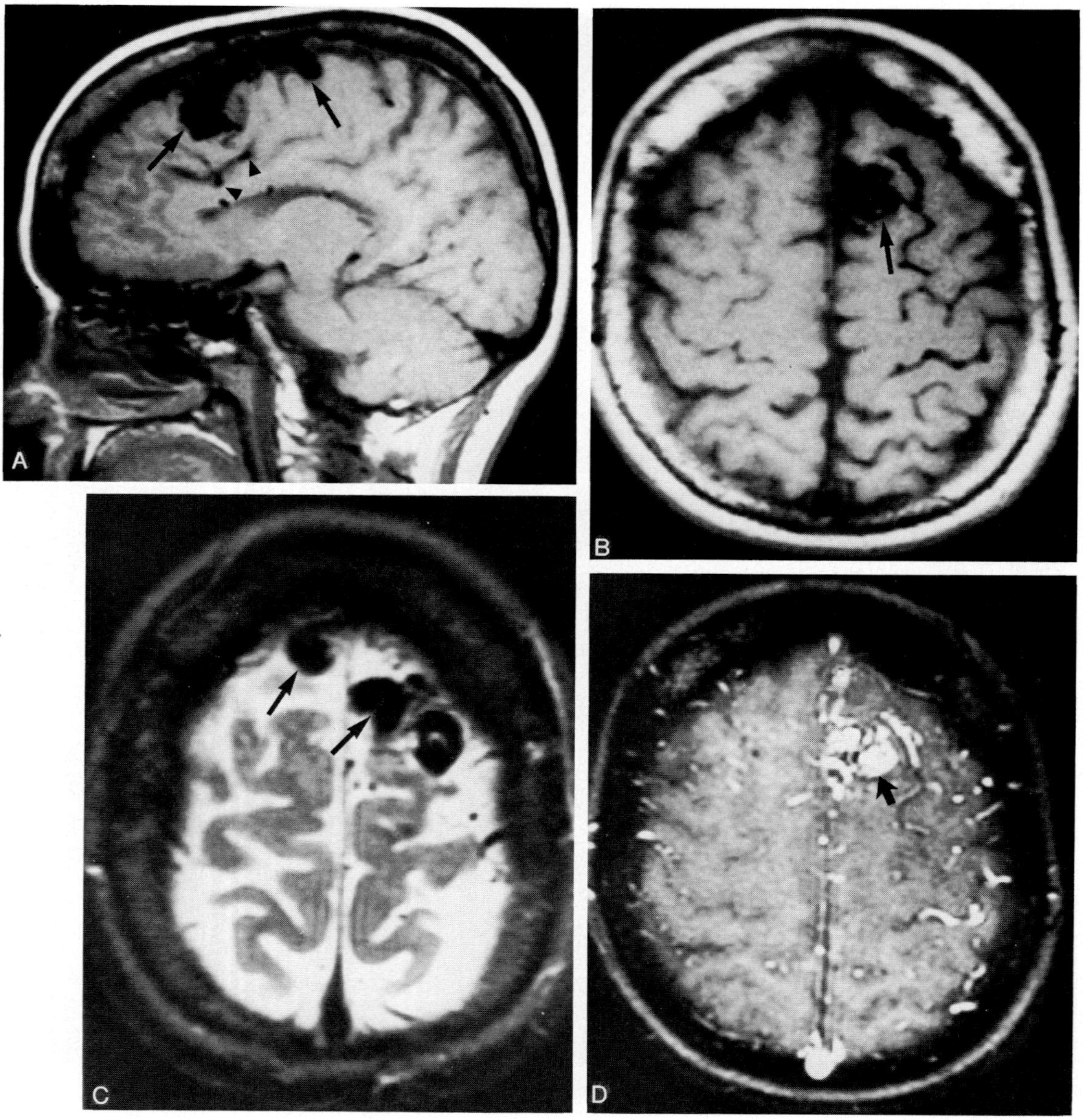

Figure 5–2. AVM (25-year-old female).

A, Parasagittal T1. An ectatic serpentine focus of signal void (*arrows*) is identified in the left paramedian frontoparietal region. Enlarged feeding arteries are present (*arrowheads*) proximal to the lesion.

B, Axial T1. The nidus of flow void (*arrow*) is noted.

C, Axial T2. Multiple foci of flow void (*arrows*) are present in the right and left paramedian frontoparietal region.

D, Axial multi-planar gradient–recalled (MPGR). High signal (*arrow*) is identified in the previous regions of flow void.

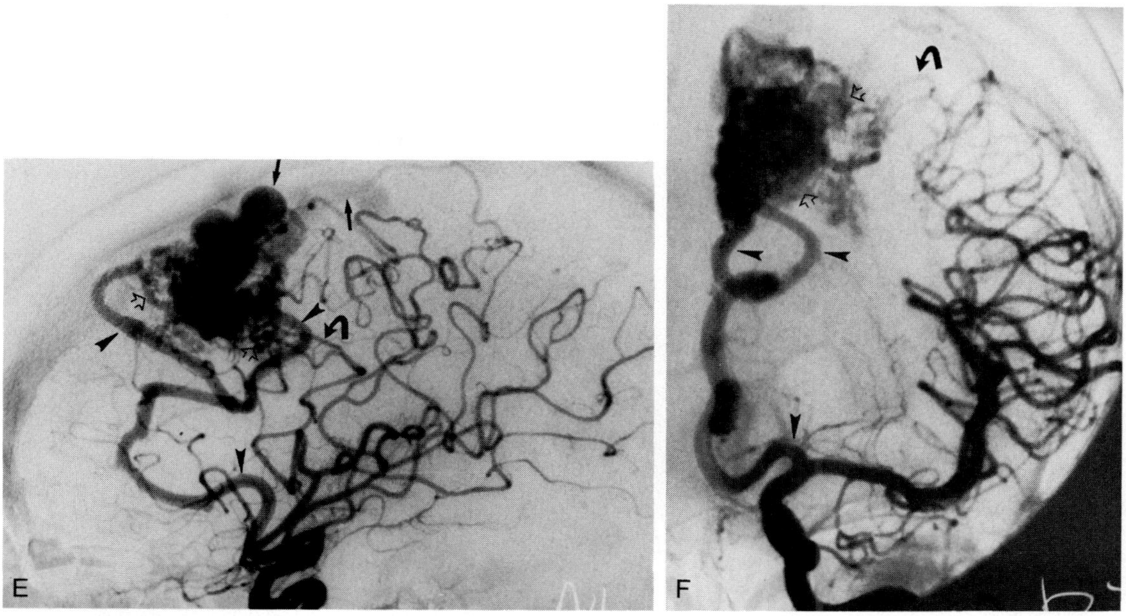

Figure 5–2 *Continued*
E, F, Lateral and anteroposterior (AP) internal carotid angiography (midarterial). Enlargement of the anterior cerebral artery and its tributaries (*arrowheads*) and early shunting into the nidus (*open arrows*) and draining veins (*arrows*) are identified. The anterior portion of the middle cerebral artery (*curved arrow*) also supplies the AVM.

overlap among vessels. MRI adroitly evaluates the presence of anoxia, edema, and gliosis in the parenchyma surrounding the lesion.

With gradient recalled acquisition techniques,[14] flow void perpendicular to the imaging plane may be rendered high signal, distinguishing it from calcification, air, or hemosiderin (Fig. 5–3). Turbulent flow, slow flow, or in-plane flow may appear intermediate signal on the gradient recalled acquisition techniques. At present, MRI may be used to supplement CT information but has not obviated the need for angiography for operative planning. Advances in magnetic resonance angiography (MRA) will continue to bridge this gap. Using three-dimensional (3-D) MRA, all feeding vessels have been detected in 70% of AVMs. Two-dimensional (2-D) MRA is optimal for the slow flow, venous side of the lesion.[13]

The angiographic evaluation of AVM should be tailored to evaluate arterial feeders, magnitude of shunt, and venous drainage pattern. AVMs may receive arterial supply from cerebral or cerebellar vessels (pial), from meningeal vessels (dural) (Fig. 5–4), or from both (mixed) (Fig. 5–5). Dural vessels supply 21% of supratentorial AVMs and 50% of infratentorial AVMs.[6] Accordingly, the ipsilateral external carotid artery should be evaluated in patients with superficial supratentorial AVMs. Most patients who present with AVMs are less than 40 years old and free of significant carotid bifurcation disease. Selective internal carotid artery (ICA) catheterization should be undertaken, the volume of contrast increased according to the estimated flow rate, and rapid-sequence (4 to 6 per second) magnification films in orthogonal planes obtained. Deep lesions, or those that cross the midline, should undergo similar evaluation of the contralateral side. If there is low suspicion for contralateral supply, a routine common carotid artery examination should be performed.

Workup of infratentorial AVMs should include magnification, high-volume, orthogonal rapid-filming techniques.

Vein of Galen Aneurysm

The term "aneurysm" in this case is a misnomer. This lesion represents an ectasia of the vein of Galen that is secondary to increased flow from an AV fistula. The posterior choroi-

Text continued on page 167

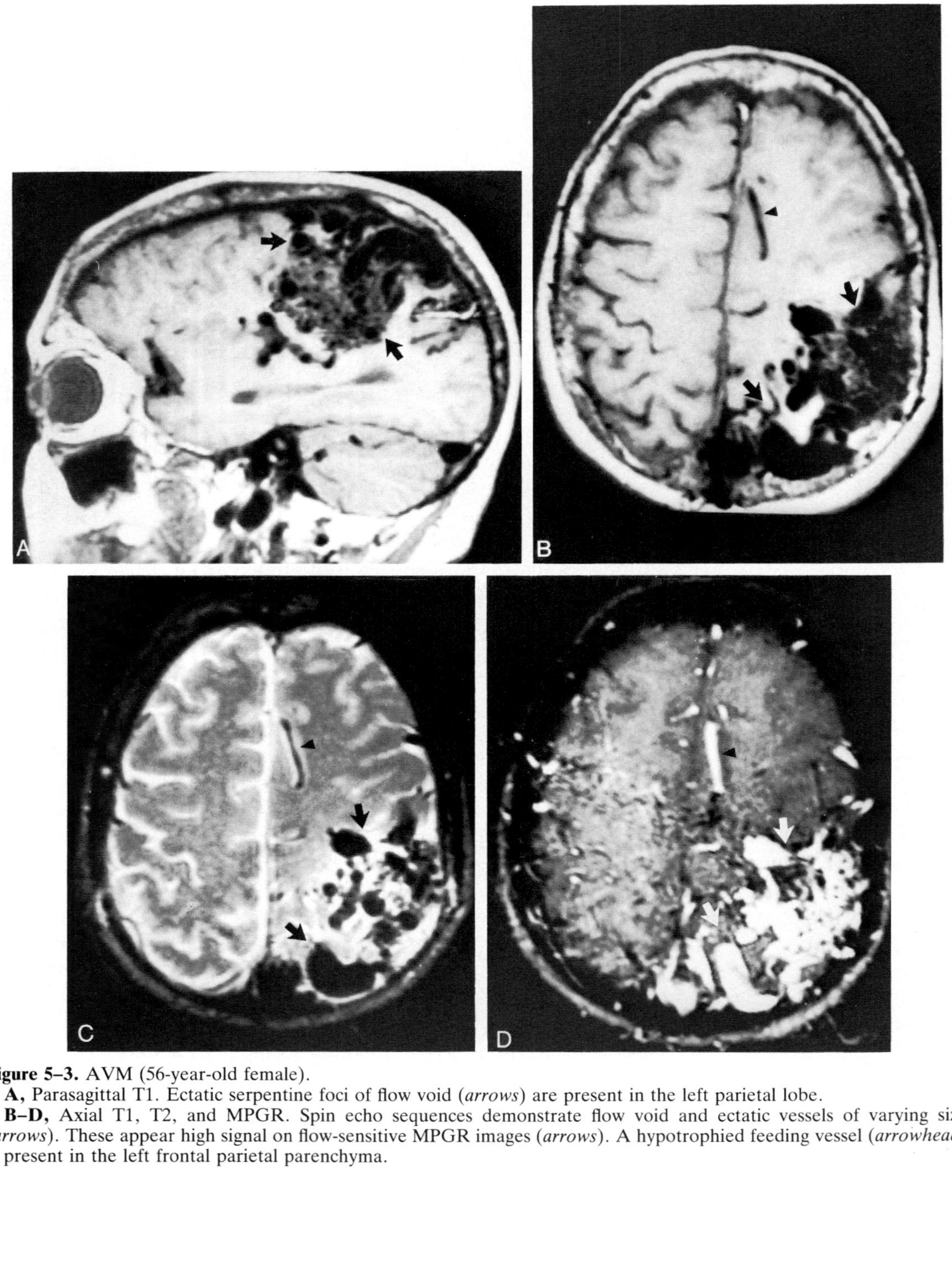

Figure 5–3. AVM (56-year-old female).

A, Parasagittal T1. Ectatic serpentine foci of flow void (*arrows*) are present in the left parietal lobe.

B–D, Axial T1, T2, and MPGR. Spin echo sequences demonstrate flow void and ectatic vessels of varying size (*arrows*). These appear high signal on flow-sensitive MPGR images (*arrows*). A hypotrophied feeding vessel (*arrowhead*) is present in the left frontal parietal parenchyma.

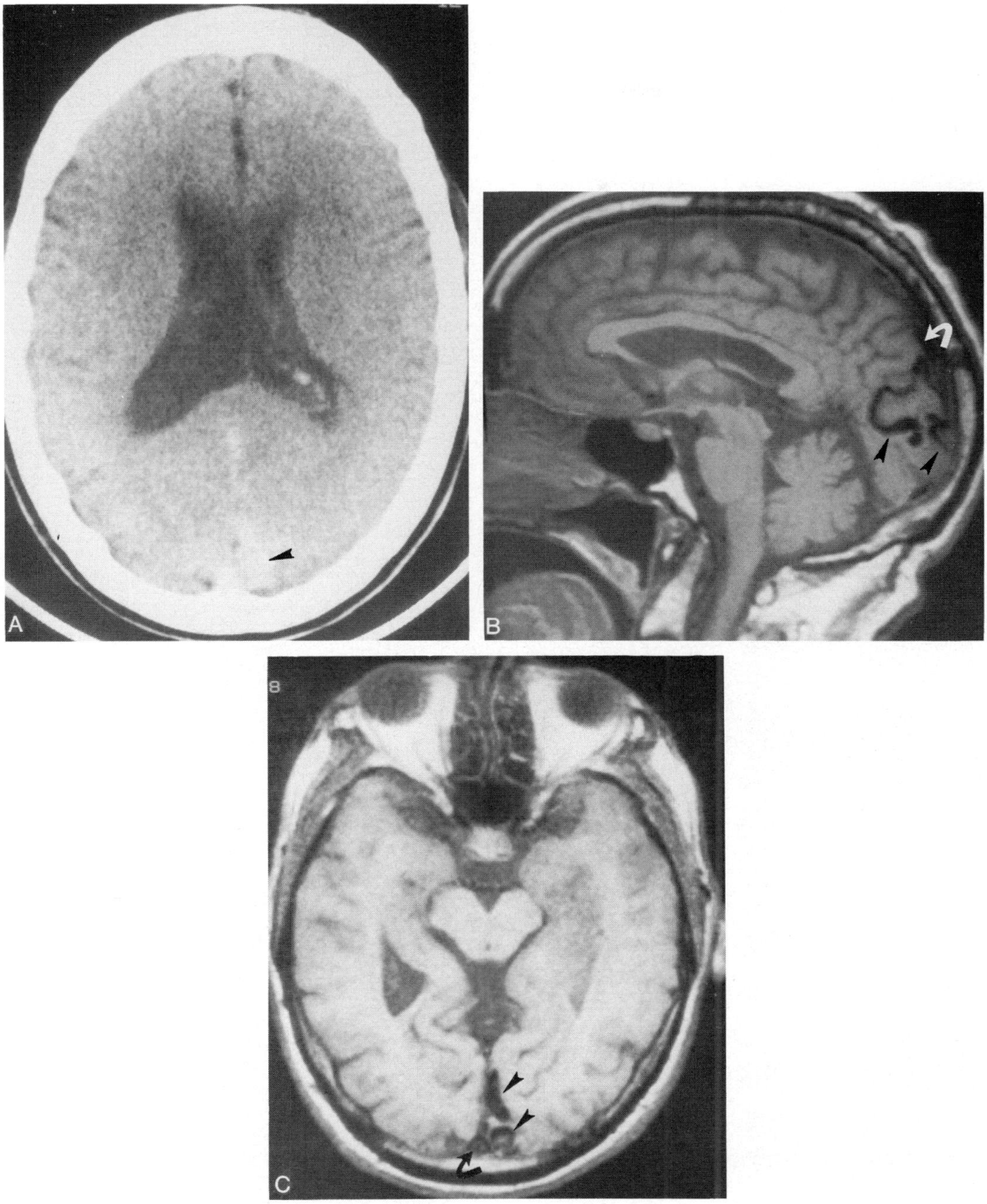

Figure 5–4. Dural AVM (67-year-old male).

A, Unenhanced CT. An ill-defined focus of increased attenuation (*arrowhead*) is present in the left paramedian occipital lobe.

B, Parasagittal T1. The serpentine focus of flow void (*arrowheads*) and its relationship to the superior sagittal sinus (*curved arrow*) are noted.

C, Axial T1. In addition to the superior sagittal sinus (*curved arrow*) a linear, ectatic focus of flow void (*arrowheads*) correlates with the CT findings.

Illustration continued on following page

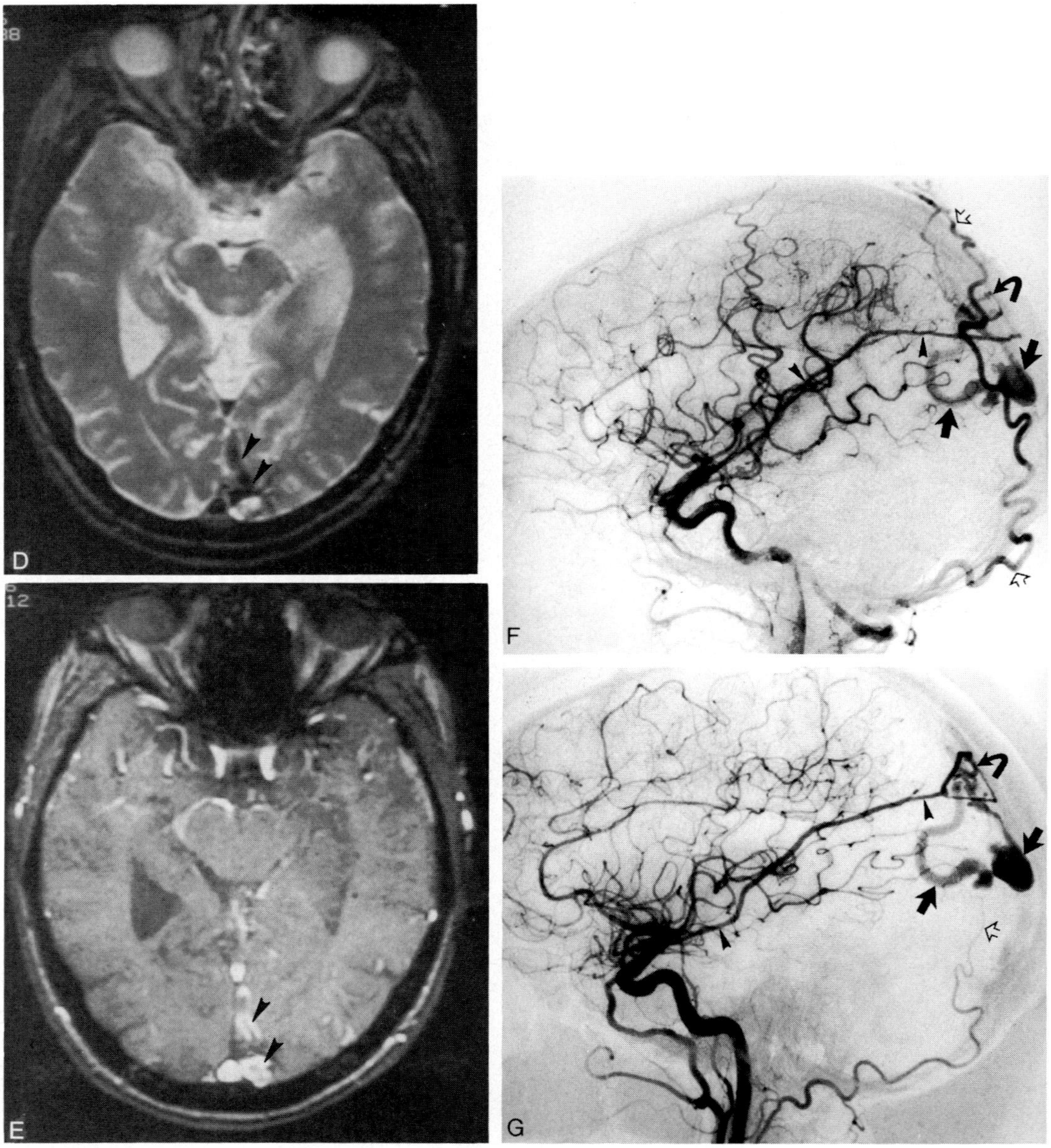

Figure 5–4 *Continued*

D, E, Axial T2 and MPGR. Flow characteristics are again demonstrated as signal void on T2 (*arrowheads*) and increased signal on gradient echo imaging (*arrowheads*).

F, G, Lateral right and left common carotid angiography (midarterial phase). A dural AVM (*curved arrow*) fills from both middle meningeal arteries (*arrowheads*) and the right-greater-than-left occipital arteries (*open arrow*). The venous side of this lesion (*solid arrows*) fills promptly, before draining into the superior sagittal sinus (not visualized).

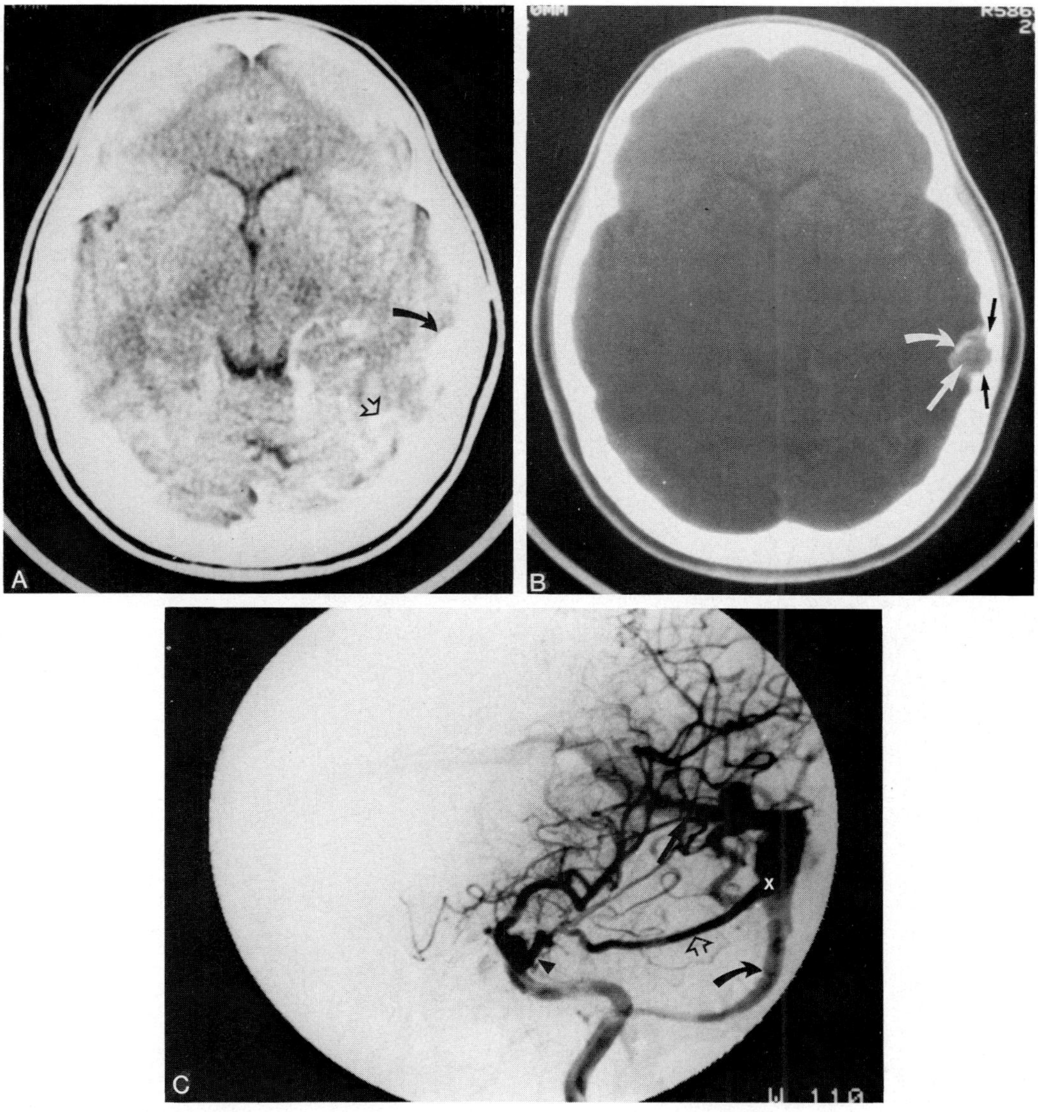

Figure 5–5. Mixed dural-pial AVM (24-year-old female).

A, Enhanced CT. An enhancing 1.5-cm focus (*curved arrow*) is located adjacent to the left parietal bone. Ill-defined serpentine foci of enhancement (*open arrow*) are suggestive of adjacent blood vessels.

B, Enhanced CT (wide windows). Erosion of the inner table is present (*black arrows*) and the mass (*straight white arrow*) is partially calcified (*curved white arrow*).

C, D, AP and lateral digital left internal carotid artery angiogram. The hypotrophied middle meningeal artery (*open arrow*) arises from the ophthalmic artery (*arrowhead*). Also, middle cerebral vessels supply the AVM (*long thin arrow*). Early venous shunting is present with opacification of the ipsilateral transverse (*solid arrow*) and sigmoid sinuses (*curved arrow*).

Illustration continued on following page

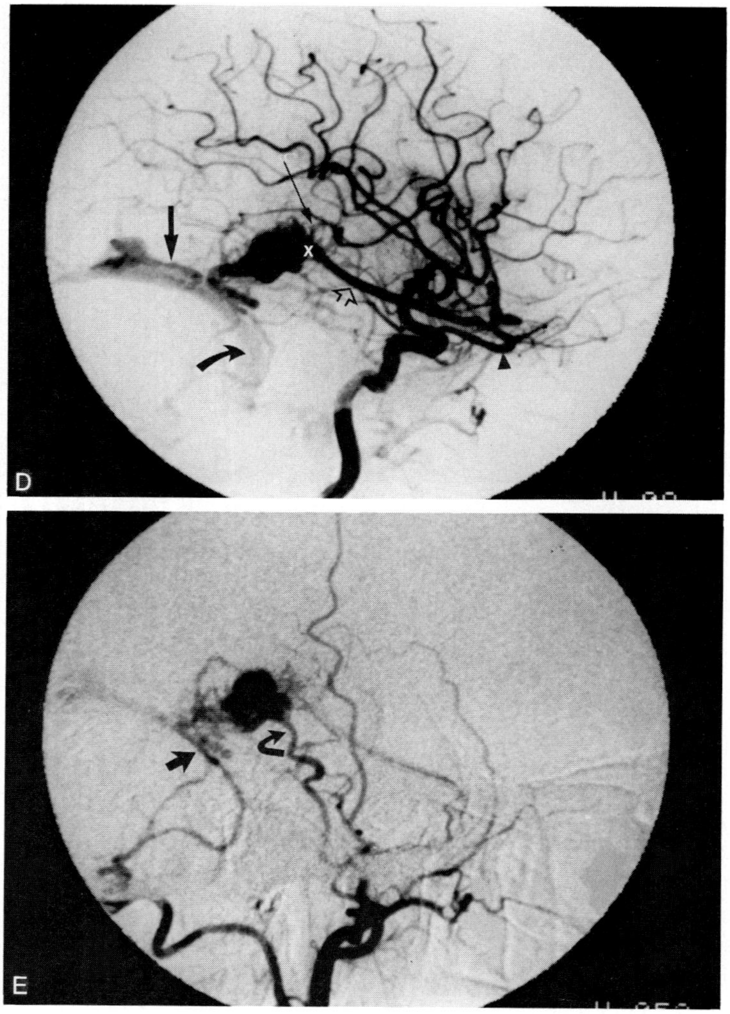

Figure 5–5 *Continued*
D, See legend on previous page.
E, Lateral digital left external carotid. Hypertrophied occipital (*arrow*) and superficial temporal (*curved arrow*) arteries supply the dural-based nidus.

dal arteries typically supply this lesion. A coexistent parenchymal AVM may be present. The lesion usually is brought to medical attention in the newborn to adolescent period. Four distinct clinical syndromes have been described in these patients.[15] The earlier the presentation, the greater the degree of AV shunting. Neonates with this lesion have intractable congestive heart failure owing to the marked degree of AV shunting. Patients may present with mild congestive heart failure or cardiomegaly in the 1- to 6-month period. Patients less than 1 year of age may present with hydrocephalus or cranial bruit or both. Patients who have a parenchymal nidus in addition to the fistula generally come to medical attention later, at approximately 15 months of age, whereas those with a direct fistula tend to do so by 4.2 months of age.[16] In adolescents, presenting signs and symptoms may include syncope, headache, or subarachnoid hemorrhage (SAH).

The prevalence of venous sinus anomalies in these patients has led some authors[16, 17] to hypothesize that the arterial changes seen in this condition may be a response to venous occlusive disease. Venous "obstacles" were identified in all patients evaluated by Lasjaunias and colleagues.[17] Observations were issued regarding the location of the obstruction in reference to the vein of Galen and the type of hydrocephalus encountered. The closer the obstruction to the vein of Galen, the greater the degree of ectasia, the greater the mass effect on the tectal plate, and the greater the likelihood of noncommunicating hydrocephalus. Distal venous occlusion at the skull base or jugulare foramen resulted in dilatation of the vein of Galen to a lesser degree and insignificant mass effect on the aqueduct. The hydrocephalus identified in these patients is secondary to diminished resorption of cerebrospinal fluid (CSF) at the pacchionian granulations and a communicating hydrocephalus due to the elevated venous pressure.

CT evaluation of a vein of Galen aneurysm depicts a midline, homogeneously dense mass of variable size in the location of the vein of Galen. The mass is smooth and well marginated, lacks edema, and enhances homogeneously (Fig. 5–6). Arterial feeders of various sizes that may fill the basilar cisterns and surround the brainstem may be apparent before and after administration of contrast material. The ventricles may be enlarged, with a pattern of communicating or noncommunicating hydrocephalus. Parenchymal calcification may be detected,[16] reflecting histologic changes commonly seen in these patients. The parenchyma is often abnormal secondary to intraventricular hemorrhage, hemorrhagic infarcts, or laminar or spongy necrosis.[18]

The MRI correlate is signal void on T1-weighted spin echo sequences. The T2-weighted spin echo appearance is more variable, reflecting areas of turbulent flow as well as stasis.[19] High flow will appear as signal void on T2, whereas turbulence or stasis may appear as higher signal. Gradient recalled acquisition will increase the signal of the ectatic vein of Galen. MRA may be a useful adjunct to evaluate these patients (Fig. 5–7); however, the ischemic or hemorrhagic conditions attendant with this lesion are more readily evaluated with MRI.

The approach to the angiographic workup of these lesions is similar to that of the previously described AVMs. Bilateral internal carotid arteries and at least one vertebral artery should be evaluated with rapid-film magnification techniques (Fig. 5–8). Digital angiography, using a limited contrast load, will permit complete angiographic evaluation of these patients. Care must be taken not to exceed the recommended contrast dose per kilogram of body weight.

Normal Flow

Venous Angioma

Venous angiomas may result from in utero maldevelopment or occlusion of the venous drainage of the supratentorial or infratentorial parenchyma. To accommodate the flow through the capillary bed, the medullary veins dilate and drain into a solitary transcerebral vein forming a characteristic caput medusae or hydra. The transparenchymal vein usually drains cortically, although it may drain into a subependymal vein in the wall of the lateral ventricle. Microscopic analysis demonstrates dilated, hyperplastic veins with single-layered

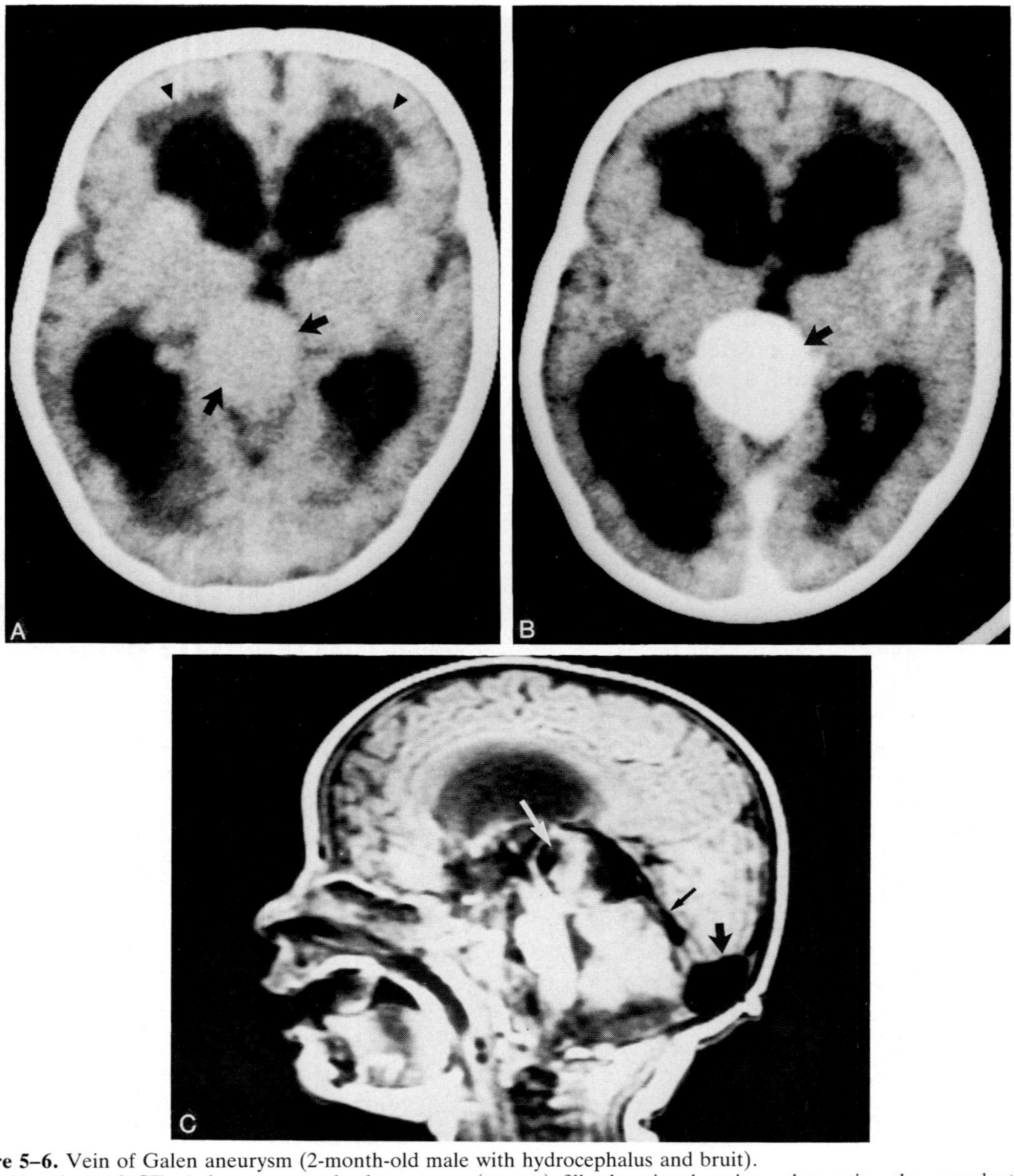

Figure 5–6. Vein of Galen aneurysm (2-month-old male with hydrocephalus and bruit).

A, Unenhanced CT. A homogeneously dense mass (*arrows*) fills the pineal region, obstructing the aqueduct and causing proximal ventricular dilation and periventricular interstitial edema (*arrowheads*).

B, Enhanced CT. The mass (*arrow*) enhances homogeneously.

C, Parasagittal T1. Heterogeneous signal indicates turbulent flow present within the vein of Galen (*white arrow*). The proximal straight sinus (*thin black arrow*) and the confluence of sinuses (*thick black arrow*) are markedly hypotrophied.

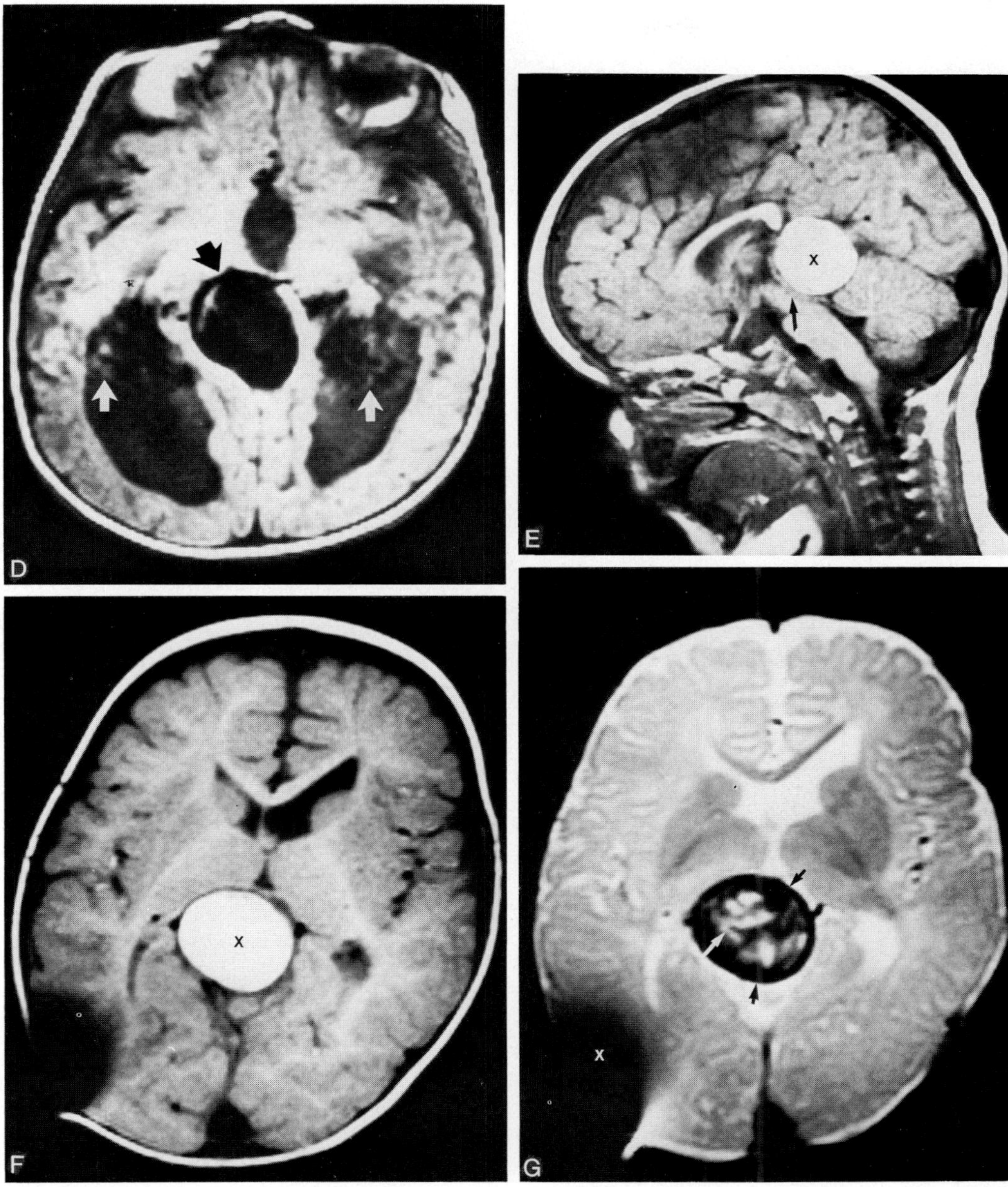

Figure 5–6 *Continued*

D, Axial T1. Flow void is present in the ectatic vein of Galen (*arrow*). Flow-related ghosting artifact is present in the phase-encoded direction (*white arrows*).

E, F, Parasagittal and axial T1 (6 months later, following spontaneous thrombosis). The vein of Galen (*X*) is now homogeneously increased signal secondary to presence of methemoglobin. The aqueduct remains compressed (*arrow*).

G, Axial T2. The signal is more heterogeneous, secondary to high-signal extracellular methemoglobin (*white arrow*) and low-signal intracellular methemoglobin (*black arrows*). There is no longer ghosting in the phase-encoded direction. Artifact from metal reservoir for shunt catheter is noted (*X*).

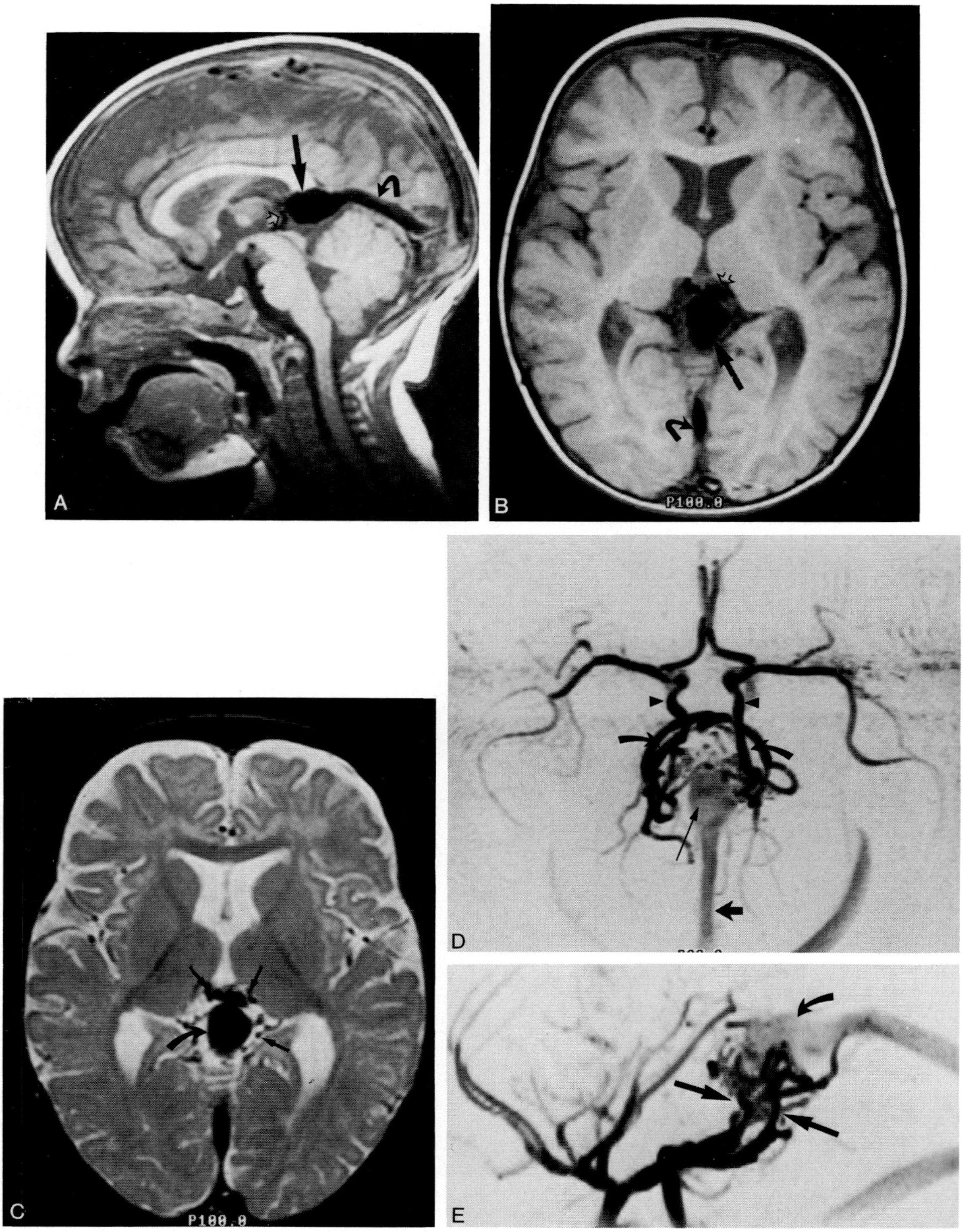

Figure 5–7. Vein of Galen aneurysm (16-month-old male).

A, B, Parasagittal and axial T1. The vein of Galen (*arrow*) is ectatic. The straight sinus (*curved arrow*) is enlarged. A serpentine flow void (*open arrow*) is located in the pineal region, presumably representing a posterior choroid feeder.

C, Axial T2. The ectatic vein of Galen (*curved arrow*) is surrounded by multiple hypertrophied vascular structures (*arrows*) of varying size.

D, Collapsed base view (three-dimensional phase-contrast MRA). The ectatic vein of Galen (*long arrow*) and straight sinus (*arrow*) are supplied by multiple feeders from the posterior cerebral arteries (*curved arrows*). The posterior communicating arteries (*arrowheads*) are markedly hypertrophied.

E, Lateral projection view (three-dimensional phase-contrast MRA). The ectatic posterior cerebral artery tributaries (*arrows*) supply the ectatic vein of Galen (*curved arrow*).

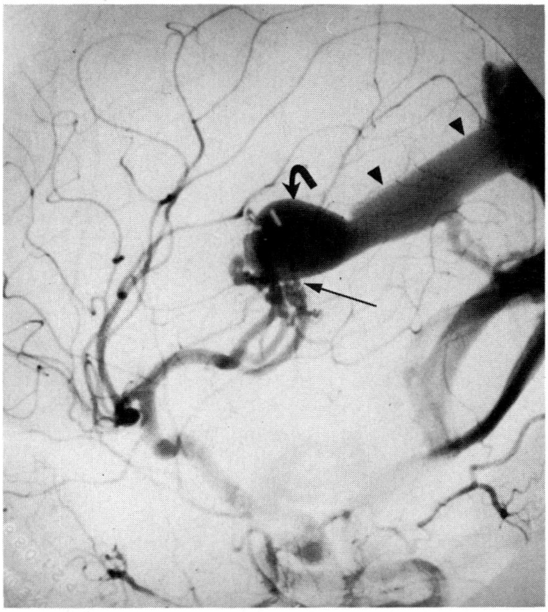

Figure 5–8. Vein of Galen aneurysm (2½-year-old male). Lateral left common angiography (postoperative); although the parenchymal nidus has been largely removed, the arteriovenous (AV) fistula (*straight arrow*) and residual ectasia of the vein of Galen (*curved arrow*) persist. The anomalous parieto-occipital sinus (*arrowheads*) is ectatic.

endothelial walls reinforced by collagen. The arterial component of this malformation is normal.[20] Normal intervening brain parenchyma may be present within the centripetally draining venules.

Venous angiomas may occur anywhere within the CNS and have been reported in the spinal cord.[2] These lesions are usually asymptomatic, discovered as an incidental finding on neuroimaging or autopsy. The likelihood of bleeding is remote, although anecdotally we have seen an intraparenchymal hemorrhage from a cerebellar venous angioma in a pregnant 24-year-old patient.

CT images obtained parallel to the transcerebral vein may demonstrate a linear region of increased attenuation extending from the parenchyma into the cortex. Images obtained perpendicular to the vessel may depict a punctate focus of increased attenuation that extends over several slices. Contrast will increase the attenuation of these lesions and will demonstrate converging medullary veins (Fig. 5–9). Generally, there is no evidence of mass effect, edema, or hemorrhage.[21]

MRI demonstrates signal void on T1-weighted images and variable foci of increased signal on T2-weighted images secondary to EER[22, 23] (Figs. 5–10, 5–11). Gradient recalled acquisition will render these lesions bright. Planar imaging characteristics are usually specific enough to produce the diagnosis without angiography.

Transit time between the arteries and veins is normal; there is no evidence of AV shunting. Also, there are no arterial phase abnormalities. The angiographic workup should include magnification films obtained at a standard filming sequence and injection rate. The venous side may opacify early and will stay opacified as long as do adjacent veins.[24]

Low Flow

Cavernous angiomas and capillary telangiectasias are the low-flow vascular malformations. Definitive distinction between these entities is based on histologic criteria. Nonetheless, certain imaging characteristics, including location and multiplicity, may be helpful to suggest the diagnosis. Both lesions may be inapparent on angiography and, as a result, are labeled "cryptic vascular malformations."

Cavernous Angioma

These well-defined masses of variable size may occur anywhere within the CNS. The malformation may be lobulated or mulberry-shaped with a honeycomb of blood-filled unequal caverns separated by irregular fibrous strands.[1, 25] Regions of thrombosis and calcification are present. The adjacent parenchyma is often gliotic and stained with hemosiderin. Microscopically, the cavernous angioma lacks a capsule. The vessels resemble capillaries without elastic tissue or muscle. There is no intervening brain parenchyma.

The diagnosis is usually made in the third to sixth decades. Patients present most frequently with seizures,[2] although rarely the lesion will rupture with severe intraparenchymal hemorrhage.[2] Cavernous angiomas may be multiple in 25 to 33% of patients.[1, 8] Men are affected more commonly than women.[1]

CT depicts a well-circumscribed region of increased density that may appear homogene-

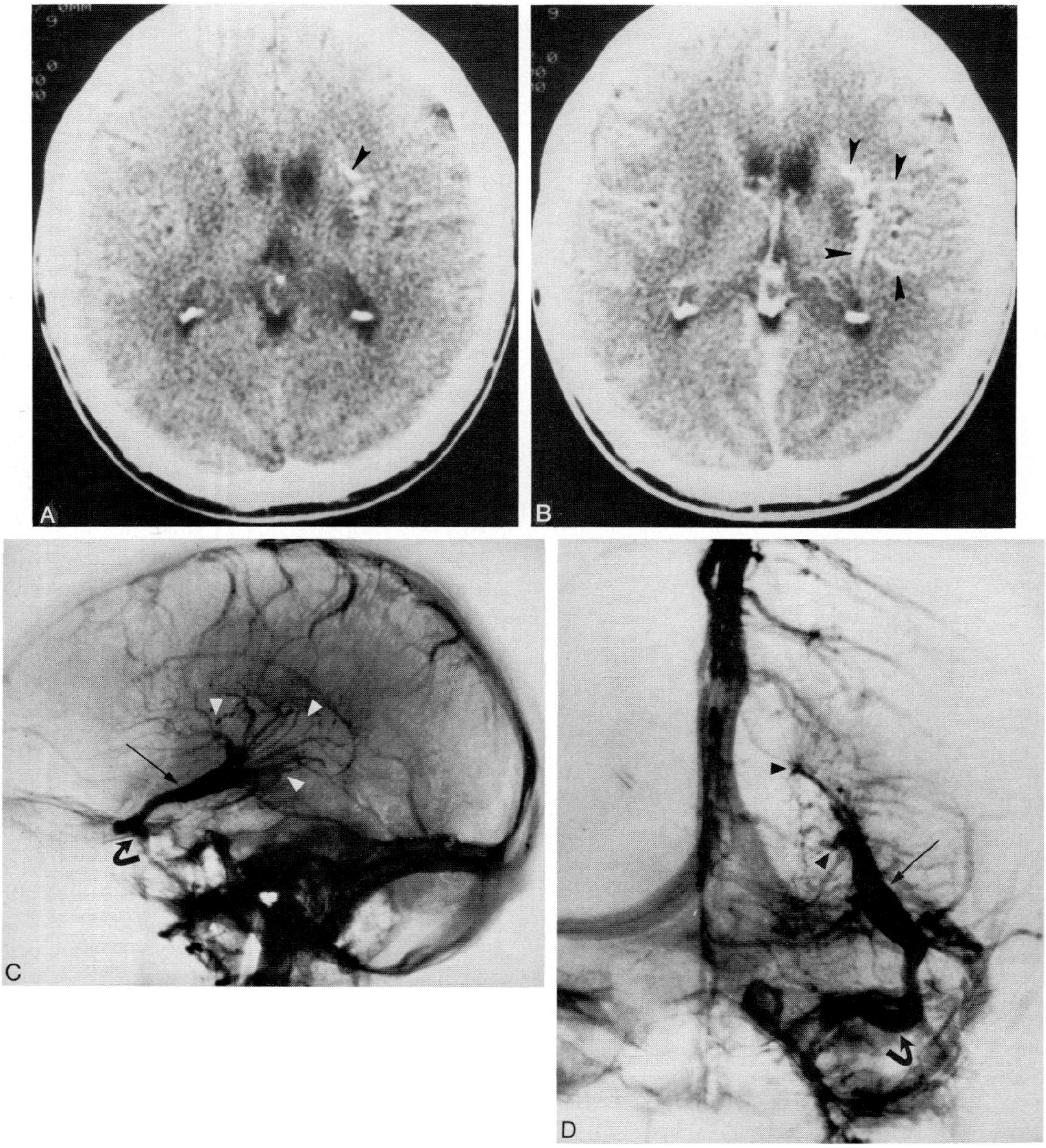

Figure 5–9. Venous angioma (48-year-old female).

A, Unenhanced CT. Floccular calcification (*arrowhead*) is present in the basal ganglia and internal capsule on the left.

B, Enhanced CT. Multiple linear foci of enhancement (*arrowheads*) radiate from the nidus of calcification.

C, D, Lateral and AP left internal carotid angiography, late venous phase. Multiple arborized feeding venules (*arrowheads*) drain into a solitary transcerebral vein (*straight arrow*), forming a hydra or caput medusae. There is subsequent drainage into the sphenoparietal sinus (*curved arrow*).

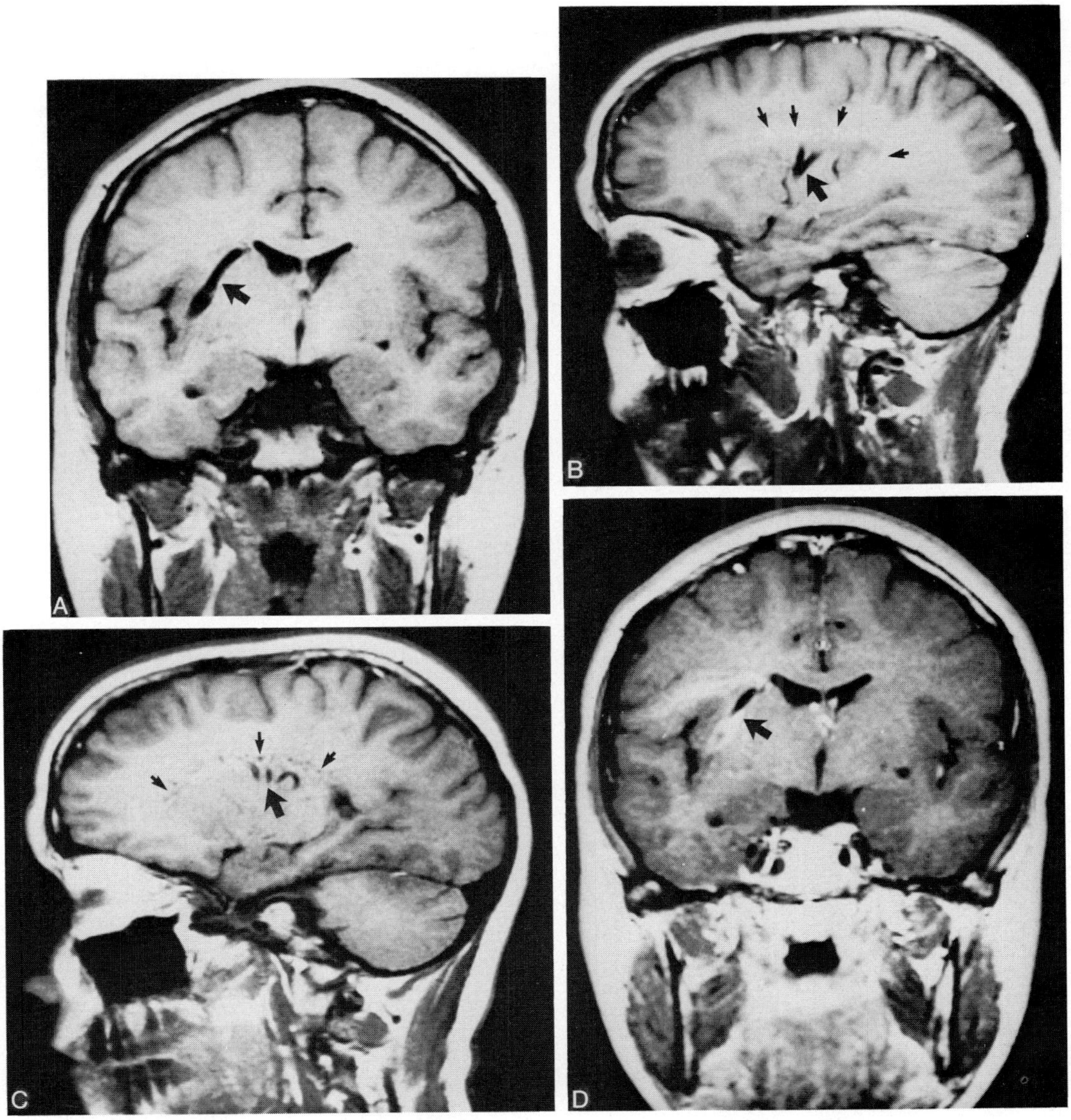

Figure 5–10. Venous angioma (24-year-old female).

A, Coronal T1. A solitary, linear focus of flow void (*arrow*) represents a large transcerebral vein. The vein drains from the ventricular surface to the cortex.

B, C, Parasagittal T1. The transcerebral vein (*large arrow*) is surrounded by punctate foci of increased signal (*small arrows*) secondary to entry phenomena on *B* and multiple foci of decreased signal (*small arrows*) secondary to flow on *C*.

D, Enhanced coronal T1. Decreased T1 relaxation time secondary to slow flow with gadolinium is detectable (*arrow*).

Illustration continued on following page

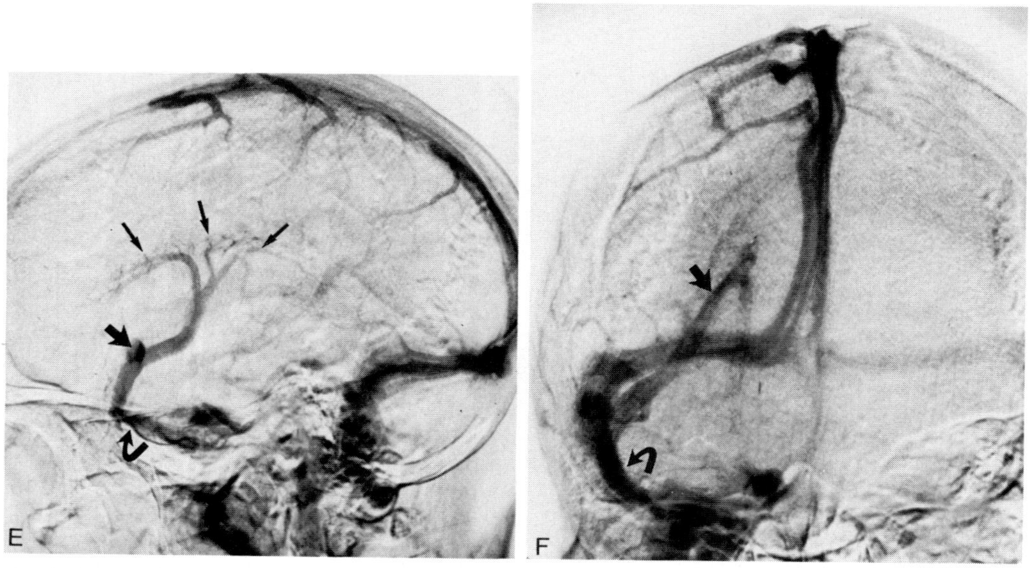

Figure 5–10 *Continued*

E, F, Lateral and AP right internal carotid angiography, venous phase. A solitary transcerebral vein (*large arrow*) is filled by multiple venules (*small arrows*) and drains into the sphenoparietal sinus (*curved arrow*). (The sphenoparietal sinus is superimposed over the sigmoid sinus on the AP film.)

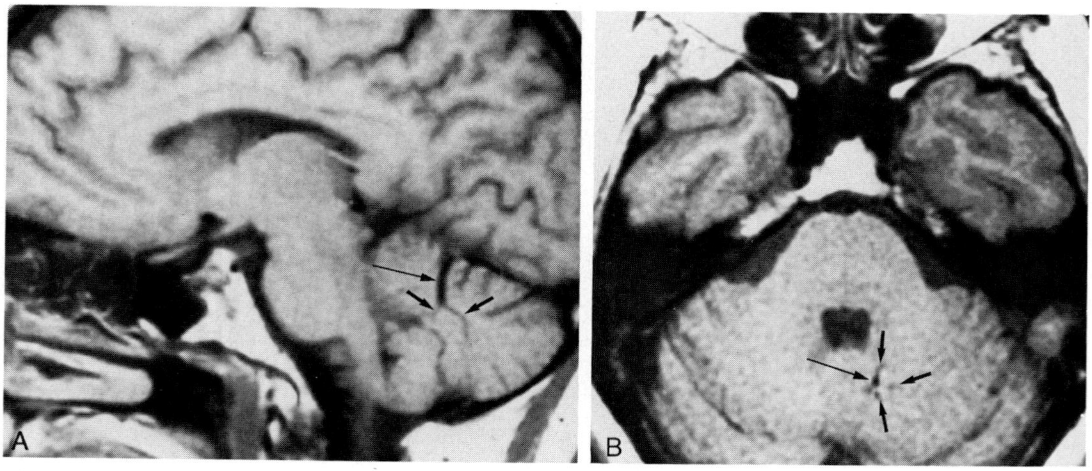

Figure 5–11. Venous angioma (42-year-old female).

A, Parasagittal T1. A solitary transcerebellar vein (*long arrow*) drains into the straight sinus. Multiple small venules (*small arrows*) drain the left cerebellar hemisphere.

B, Axial T1. A solitary focus of flow void (*long arrow*) represents the transcerebellar vein. Small venules are present (*small arrows*) surrounding the vein.

ous or mottled.[26] Dystrophic calcification and atrophy of the adjacent parenchyma may be detected (Fig. 5–12). Edema and mass effect, although uncommon, are seen only with acute or subacute hemorrhage. The lesion will enhance minimally following contrast administration. The intrinsic density of the lesion may obscure the enhancement. Small punctate calcified cavernous angiomas may be detected with CT only.[12]

MRI depicts a well-marginated mass of heterogeneous signal on T1 and T2 (Fig. 5–13).

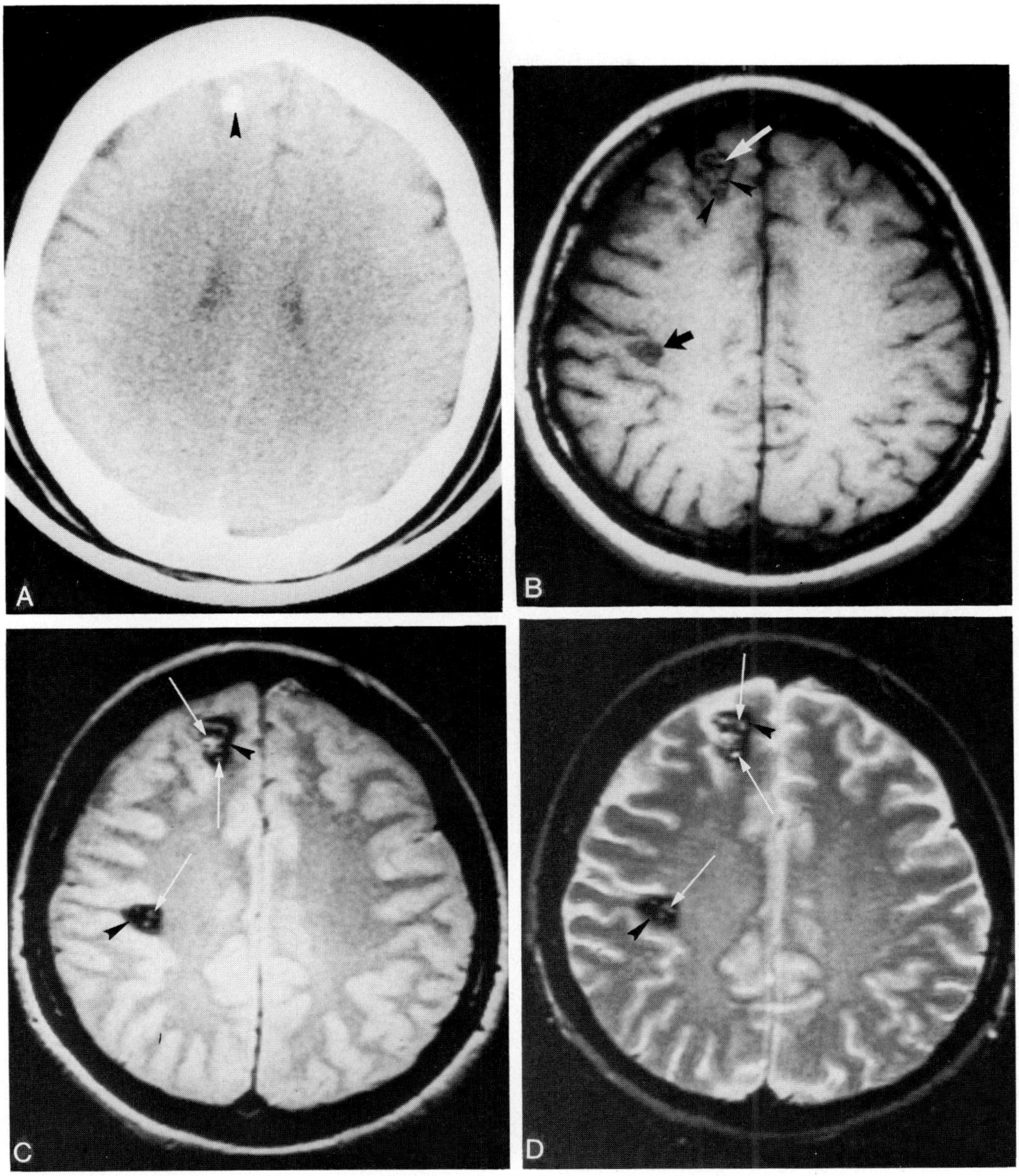

Figure 5–12. Cavernous angioma (49-year-old female).

A, Unenhanced CT. An 8-mm calcification (*arrowhead*) is located in the right paramedian frontoparietal region.

B, Axial T1. The mass is of heterogenous signal intensity with areas of high signal (*white arrow*) and areas of low signal (*arrowheads*). A second similar lesion (*black arrow*) is present in the ipsilateral parietal lobe.

C, D, Axial spin density (SD) and T2. The lesions contain a low-signal periphery (*arrowheads*) presumed to represent iron in hemosiderin and ferritin. A high-signal central portion of the lesion (*white arrows*) representing extracellular methemoglobin is noted. There is no evidence of mass effect or vasogenic edema.

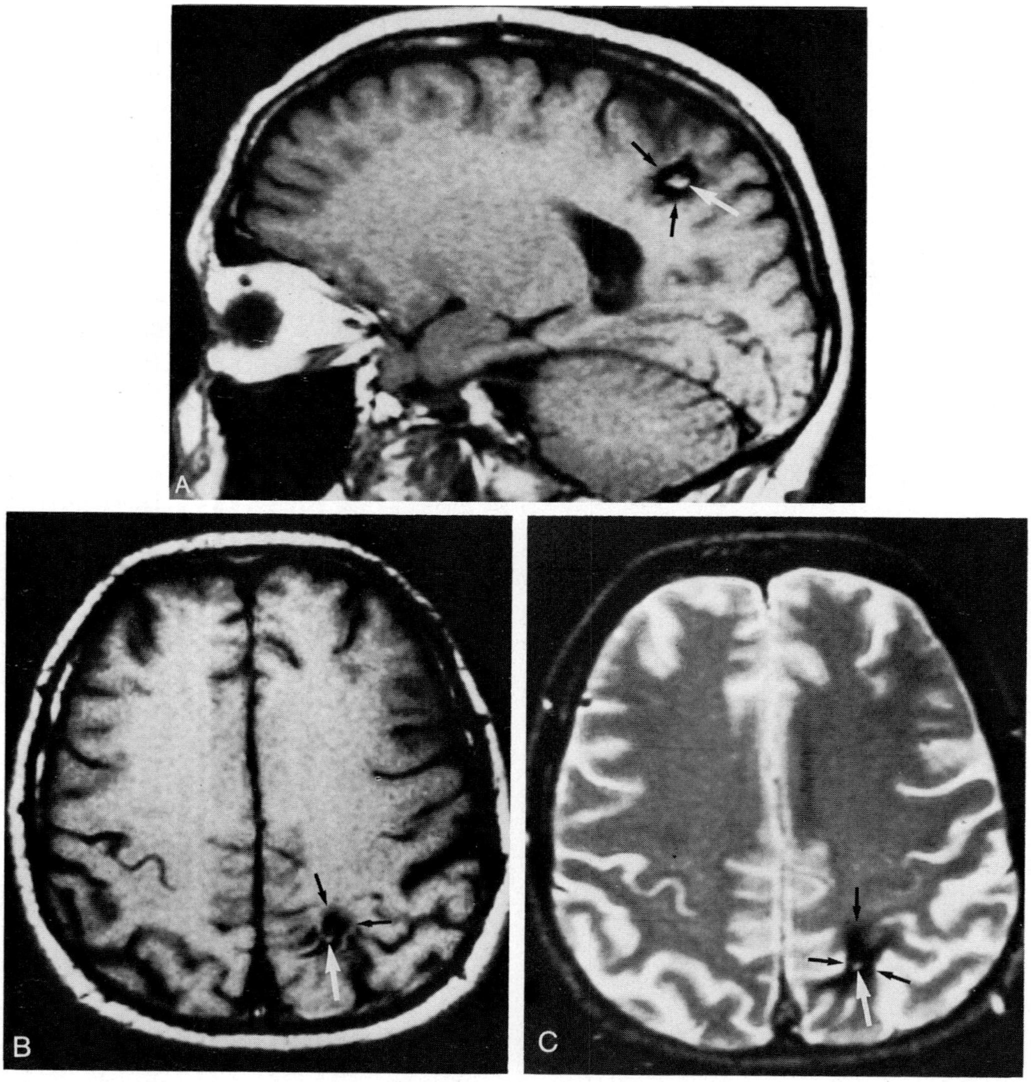

Figure 5–13. Cavernous angioma (42-year-old female).

A, B, Parasagittal and axial T1. A focus of increased signal representing methemoglobin (*white arrow*) is identified within the left posterior parietal lobe. This is surrounded by a region of diminished signal (*black arrows*) secondary to the T2 effects of hemosiderin.

C, Axial T2. The central focus of increased signal (*white arrow*) represents extracellular methemoglobin. The region of diminished signal surrounding this (*black arrows*) is due to hemosiderin and ferritin. There is no evidence of vasogenic edema.

The signal is the result of hemoglobin degradation products of various ages and the nonresorbable cavernous angioma nidus.[27] The blood flow through this lesion is negligible and does not contribute to the signal characteristics. Cavernous angioma may be differentiated from a resolving hematoma by absence of vasogenic edema (unless there has been recent hemorrhage) and the complexity of the matrix of the lesion. Typically the lesion is surrounded by low signal on T2, which is due to presence of hemosiderin or ferritin.

Absence of shunting and significant flow alters the angiographic approach to the slow-flow vascular malformations. Magnification subtraction technique or digital films of the cerebral circulation should be obtained using a prolonged injection[28] and delayed imaging in attempts to evaluate a focal blush. These lesions are most commonly angiographically occult. The vessels associated with this malformation are generally below the resolution capabilities of the current imaging equipment.

Capillary Telangiectasia

Capillary telangiectasias differ slightly from cavernous angiomas. On histologic perusal, intervening neural tissue is present within the interstices of this malformation.[1, 3] These lesions are almost always solitary and most frequently occur within the pons. The incidence of clinical hemorrhage is quite minimal. The lesions are incidental findings on neuroimaging examinations and autopsy.

CT,[29] MRI, and angiographic characteristics are identical to those of the cavernous angioma except for location and the solitary nature of the capillary telangiectasia (Fig. 5–14).

ANEURYSMS

Aneurysms are focal dilatations of the arterial walls that are of multifactorial origin. Clinical findings, age of presentation, location, and angiographic appearance are often specific for each category of aneurysm.

Congenital

Congenital aneurysms account for more than 80% of intracranial aneurysms. The pathophysiology of congenital aneurysms is not completely understood. Fibrous tissue defects in the intracranial arteries are present at birth in everyone. The exact mechanism that predisposes 5 to 7% of the population to form aneurysms remains elusive.[30] Microscopic evaluation demonstrates a focal endothelium-lined fibrous tissue–encapsulated aneurysm arising from the parent vessel at a point where the media and internal elastic membrane are absent.

Congenital or "berry" aneurysms occur slightly more frequently in women and are uncommon before puberty. It is generally agreed that 80 to 90% of congenital aneurysms arise from the internal carotid artery or its tributaries. Although each major series differs by 10 to 15%, anterior and posterior communicating artery aneurysms are roughly equal in prevalence, accounting for a total of 66% of these lesions. The middle cerebral artery trifurcation accounts for 15 to 20%, with remaining aneurysms arising from the basilar artery and its branches. Multiple aneurysms have been reported in 15 to 25% of cases.[30, 31]

SAH, with resultant extreme headache, meningismus, and photophobia, is the most common clinical presentation of ruptured aneurysm. Sixty-two percent of cases of the first SAH occur between 40 and 64 years of age, with a peak frequency between 50 and 54 years.[31] SAH is more common in women, with a 3:2 ratio; however, before the age of 40 SAH is more common in men. Nontraumatic SAH occurring in the second decade is equally likely to be related to AVM as it is to aneurysm. SAH in the fifth decade, however, is 25 times more likely to be related to aneurysm than to AVM.[31]

Overall mortality from the initial rupture approaches 55%.[32] If left untreated, patients who survive 6 months risk a 3.5% per annum risk of rebleed for the first decade following the initial hemorrhage. Mortality from the second bleed is 67%,[32] with a 2% per annum risk of fatal rebleed in the first decade after rupture. The presence of previous SAH predisposes patients to intraparenchymal and intraventricular hemorrhage from subsequent aneurysm rupture.[33] This may, in part, be related to the fibrin and fibrous adhesions that form around the aneurysm, preventing free access of blood to the subarachnoid space.

CT evaluation of nonruptured aneurysms depicts an isodense to slightly hyperdense cisternal defect that may be partially calcified[34] (Fig. 5–15). With the use of high-resolution enhanced CT, initial published detection rates of 78.6% for 7-mm aneurysms[34] have improved to 97.4% detection for 3-mm aneurysms.[35] The diameter of the vessels of the circle of Willis approaches 3 mm, so it is unlikely that the CT detection rate for smaller aneurysms will improve. Contrast-enhanced CT may detect homogeneous enhancement if the lumen of the aneurysm is patent. Thrombus will appear hypodense referable to the enhancing lumen and arterial wall (Fig. 5–16).

The CT appearance of hemorrhage secondary to aneurysmal rupture has been described in Chapter 4. The hemorrhages may accumulate locally in the adjacent cisterns, parenchyma, or ventricle, revealing the location of

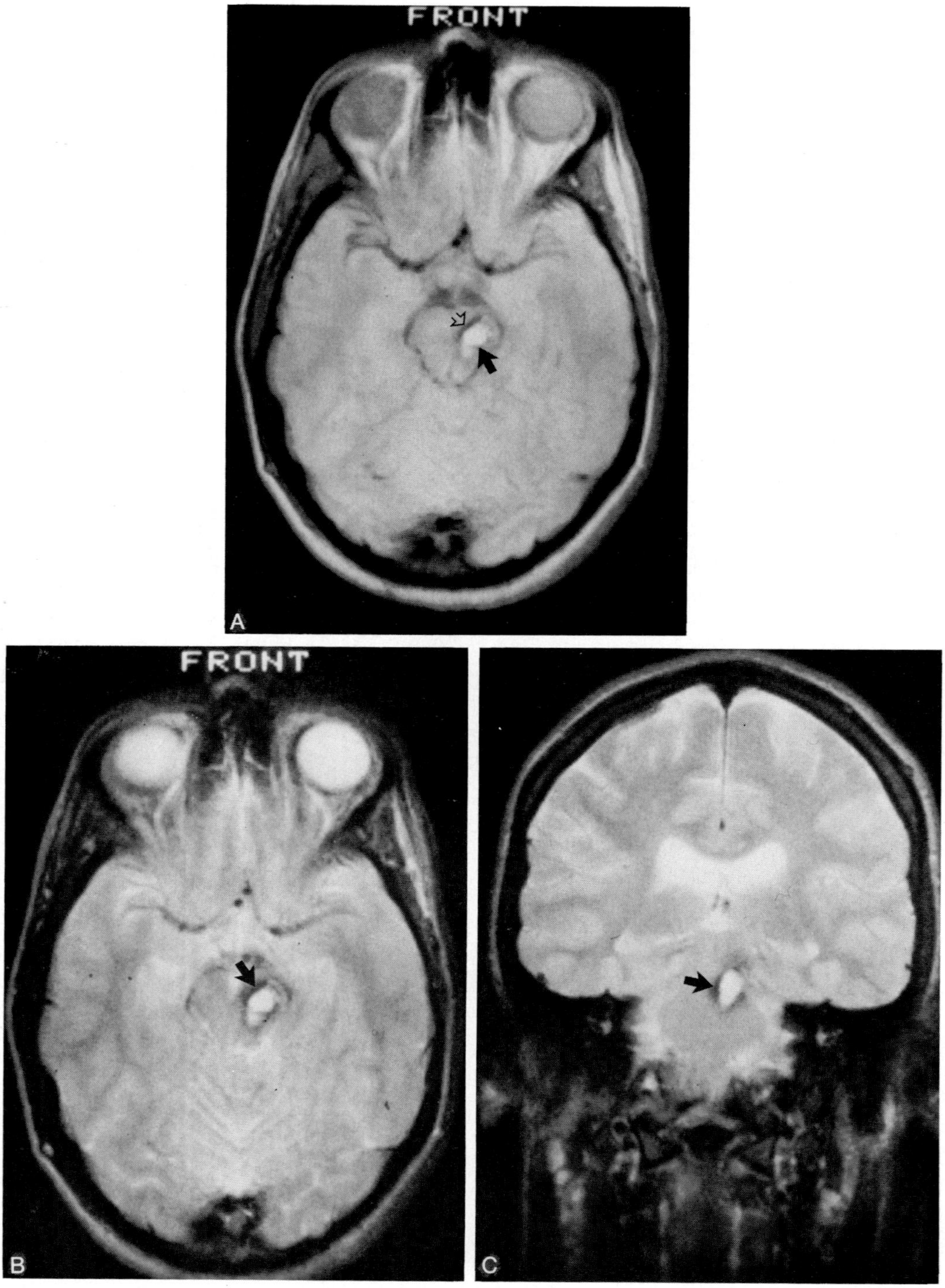

Figure 5–14. Capillary telangiectasia (42-year-old female).

A, Axial T1. A predominantly hyperintense focus (*arrow*) is present in the left lower mesencephalon. There is a rim of decreased signal (*open arrow*) along a portion of the periphery of the lesion.

B, C, Axial and coronal T2. The rim of diminished signal (*arrow*) is now more apparent. There is no evidence of vasogenic edema.

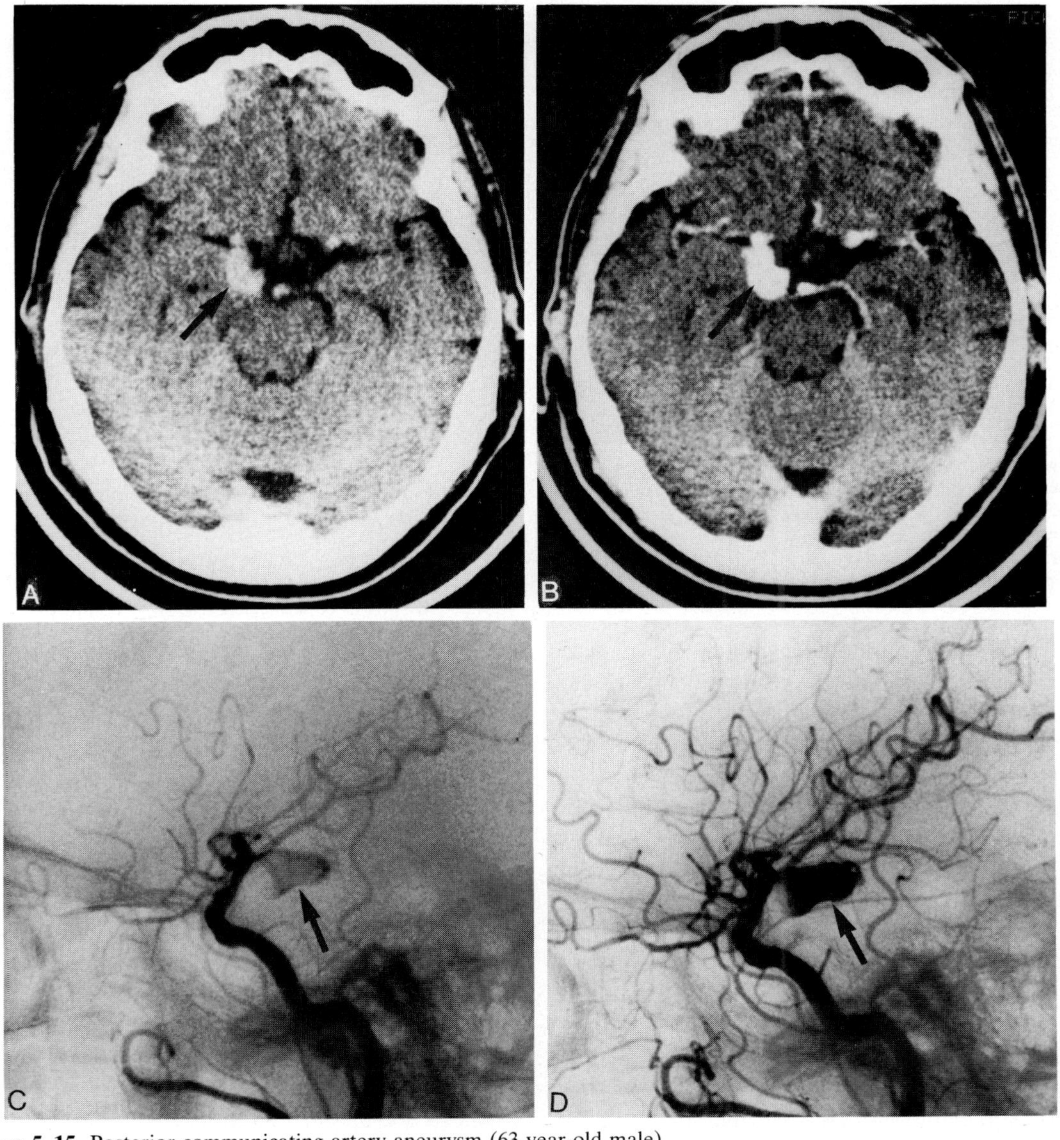

Figure 5–15. Posterior communicating artery aneurysm (63-year-old male).

A, Unenhanced CT. An intrinsically dense mass (*arrow*) distorts the right lateral aspect of the suprasellar cistern.

B, Enhanced CT. The mass (*arrow*) enhances homogeneously revealing its relationship with the circle of Willis.

C, D, Lateral right common carotid arteriography. The early and late arterial phase films demonstrate the typical jet effect of the aneurysm (*arrow*) filling with contrast.

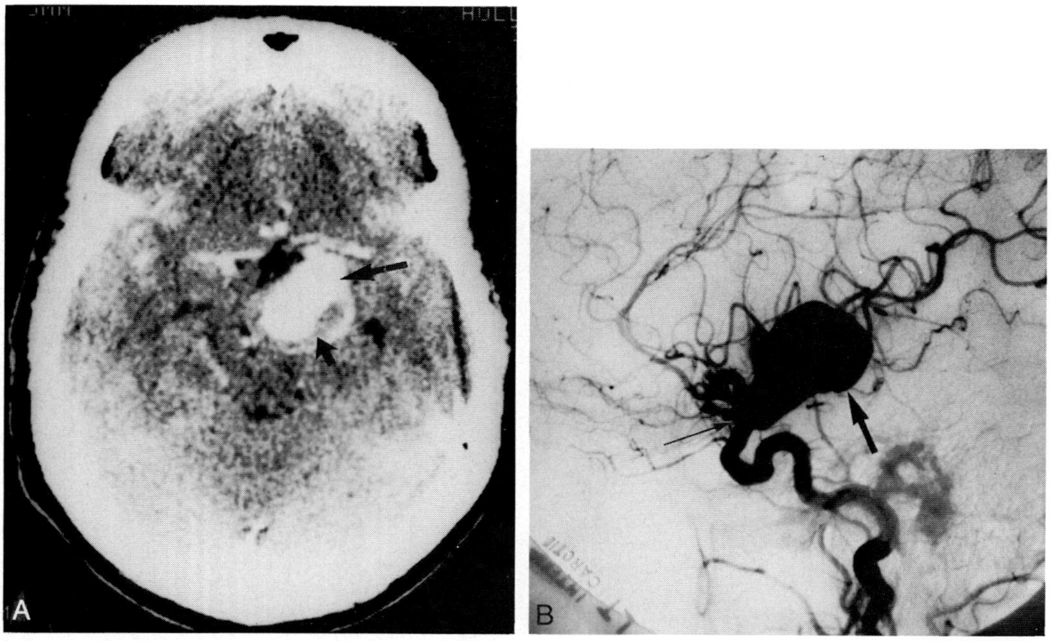

Figure 5–16. Giant aneurysm (44-year-old female).
A, Enhanced CT. A well-circumscribed mass is present in the left suprasellar region. The aneurysm in part enhances homogeneously (*long arrow*), representing a patent lumen. The thrombus (*short arrow*) does not enhance. There is no evidence of associated vasogenic edema.
B, Lateral left common carotid angiography. A large well-circumscribed aneurysm (*thick arrow*) extends from the supraclinoid carotid bifurcation (*thin arrow*).

the aneurysm. The aneurysm may be detected as a focus of relatively low density if surrounded by blood. The aneurysm may become more dense than adjacent hemorrhage if contrast material is administered.[36]

Flow within the aneurysm will exhibit flow void on T1- and T2-weighted spin echo sequences (Fig. 5–17). Thrombus, if present, will exhibit laminated foci of alternating high and low signal related to methemoglobin and hemosiderin, respectively.[37] MRA techniques currently allow sufficient definition of the circle of Willis to permit detection of 3- to 4-mm aneurysms.[38]

Angiographic evaluation of patients with suspected aneurysm rupture includes magnification and arterial phase filming. The goal of the angiographer is to locate the aneurysm, define its relationship to the parent vessel, evaluate for focal spasm, and evaluate the remainder of the anterior and posterior circulation for additional aneurysms. When possible, it is desirable to select the internal carotid artery to avoid overlapping external branches as well as to increase the likelihood of filling of the anterior and posterior communicating arteries. Selective ICA catheterization should not be performed in the aged population until a fluoroscopic evaluation of the carotid bifurcation has excluded significant atherosclerotic disease.

Atherosclerotic

Atherosclerosis results in scarring and loss of elasticity of arterial walls, which may result in fusiform irregular aneurysms.[30] These aneurysms are encountered most frequently in the basilar artery and in the posterior and middle cerebral arteries. It is quite rare for these lesions to rupture. Rather, the aneurysms present with local mass effect and compression of adjacent structures.

CT imaging demonstrates enlarged vessels in the adjacent cisterns, which may enhance homogeneously following contrast administration. MRI will depict the flow effects of the aneurysm. Arterial phase angiography demonstrates elongated, irregular regions of ectasia in the basilar, posterior, and middle cerebral arteries.

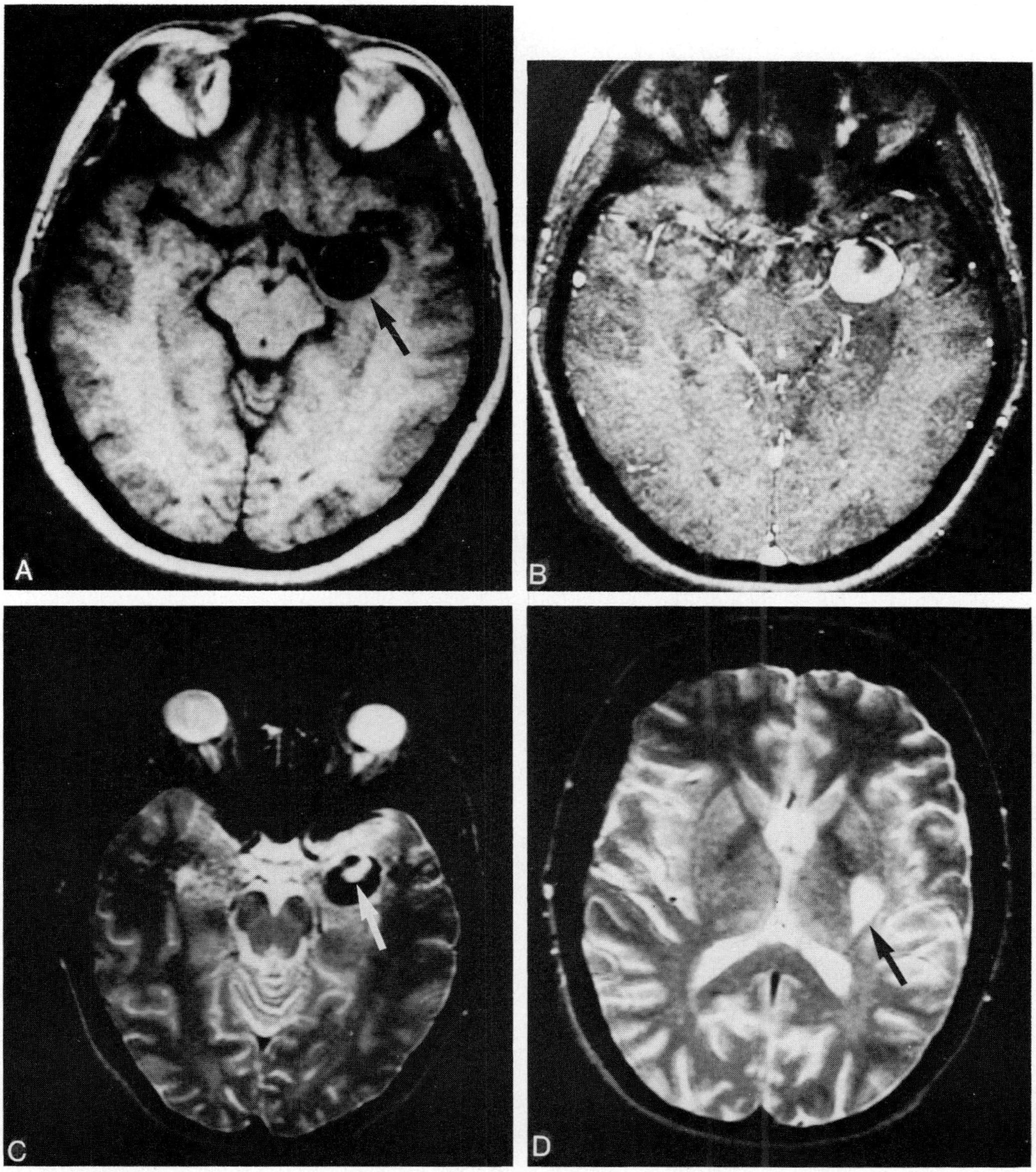

Figure 5–17. Middle cerebral artery (MCA) aneurysm (36-year-old female).

A, Axial T1. A circular region of flow void (*arrow*) is present in the left cerebral fissure.

B, Axial MPGR. High-signal flow is present in the lesion.

C, Axial T2. High signal (*arrow*) likely representing turbulence is identified within the aneurysm.

D, Axial T2. A wedge of ischemic edema (*arrow*) is present in the MCA perforator distribution. The infarct is secondary to mechanical compression or emboli from the aneurysm.

Illustration continued on following page

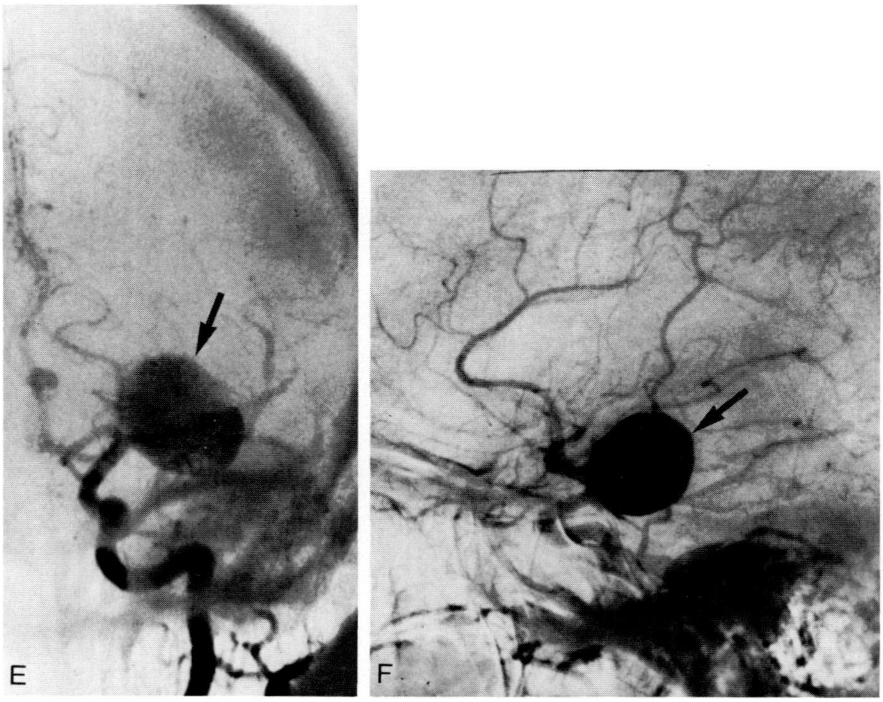

Figure 5–17 *Continued*

E, F, AP and lateral left common carotid angiography. A spherical smooth-walled aneurysm (*arrow*) fills from the proximal MCA.

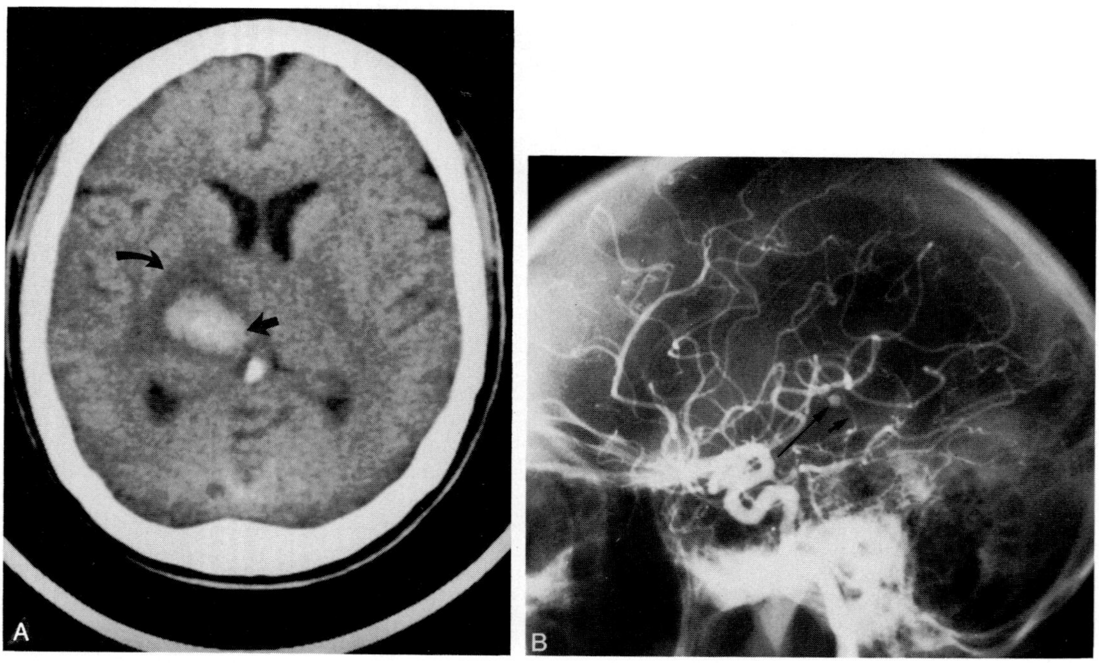

Figure 5–18. Mycotic aneurysm.

A, Unenhanced CT. A right thalamic hemorrhage (*arrow*) is present with minimal edema (*curved arrow*) and mass effect.

B, Lateral right internal carotid arteriogram. A small deep mycotic aneurysm (*long arrow*) arises from the right anterior choroidal artery (*short arrow*).

Traumatic

Trauma may result in the formation of an aneurysm or AV fistula. The aneurysm may result from penetrating injury; alternatively, a cortical vessel may be injured against the falx or a vessel may transiently herniate into a skull fracture, resulting in aneurysm formation.

Unlike congenital aneurysms, which are deep and juxtaposed to the circle of Willis, post-traumatic aneurysms are peripheral and usually cortical in location.

Mycotic

Before the term "mycotic" was refined to specify fungal processes, it was used to denote any infectious process. Mycotic aneurysms represent approximately 4 to 5% of all intracranial aneurysms.[39] Mycotic aneurysms most frequently are the result of infectious endocarditis, occurring in 3% of all patients admitted with bacterial endocarditis.[40] The organism invades the vasa vasorum of the arterial wall, resulting in inflammation and necrosis. The weakened mural segment expands focally. These aneurysms are frequently multiple and occur in distal branches of the anterior, the middle, or, less commonly, the posterior cerebral arteries. Mortality approaches 80% of patients with ruptured aneurysm.

Planar imaging readily demonstrates intracranial hemorrhage, which is associated with the ruptured mycotic aneurysm (Fig. 5–18). Angiographic evaluation includes magnification arterial filming to evaluate the presence of one or multiple peripheral aneurysms. The aneurysms are dynamic, often resolving after appropriate antibiotic therapy.

References

1. Russell DS, Rubinstein LJ: *Pathology of Tumors of the Nervous System*. 4th ed, 1977. Williams and Wilkins, Baltimore.
2. McCormick WF: The pathology of vascular ("arteriovenous") malformations. J Neurosurg 1966; 24:807–816.
3. Morris JH: The nervous system. *Robbins Pathologic Basis of Disease*. Cotran RS, Kumar V, Robbins SL (eds): 4th ed, 1989. WB Saunders, Philadelphia.
4. Brown RD, Wiebers DO, Forbes G, et al: The natural history of unruptured intracranial arteriovenous malformations. J Neurosurg 1988; 68:352–357.
5. Perret G, Nishioka H: Report on the cooperative study of intracranial aneurysms and subarachnoid hemorrhage. Section VI: Arteriovenous malformations. J Neurosurg 1966; 25:467–490.
6. Newton TH, Cronqvist S: Involvement of dural arteries in intracranial arteriovenous malformations. Radiology 1969; 93:1071–1078.
7. Crawford PM, West CR, Chadwick DW, et al: Arteriovenous malformations of the brain: Natural history in unoperated patients. J Neurol Neurosurg Psychiatry 1986; 49:1–10.
8. Atlas SW: Intracranial vascular malformations and aneurysm, current imaging applications. Radiol Clin North Am 1988; 26:821–837.
9. Terbrugge K, Scotti G, Ethier R, et al: Computed tomography in intracranial arteriovenous malformations. Radiology 1977; 122:703–705.
10. Graf CJ, Perret GE, Torner JC: Bleeding from cerebral arteriovenous malformations as part of their natural history. J Neurosurg 1983; 58:331–337.
11. Lee BCP, Herzberg L, Zimmerman RD, et al: MR imaging of cerebral vascular malformations. AJNR 1985; 6:863–870.
12. Kucharczyk W, Lemme-Pleghos L, Uske A, et al: Intracranial vascular malformations. Radiology 1985; 156:383–389.
13. Edelman RR, Wentz KU, Mattle HP, et al: Intracerebral arteriovenous malformations: Evaluation with selective MR angiography and venography. Radiology 1989; 173:831–837.
14. Needell WM, Maravilla KR: MR flow imaging in vascular malformations using gradient recalled acquisition. AJNR 1988; 9:637–642.
15. Amacher AL, Shillito J: The syndromes and surgical treatment of aneurysms of the great vein of Galen. J Neurosurg 1973; 39:89–98.
16. Seidenwurm D, Berenstein A, Hyman A, et al: Vein of Galen malformations: Correlation of clinical presentation. Arteriography and MR imaging. AJNR 1991; 12:347–354.
17. Lasjaunias P, Ter Brugge K, Lopez-Ibor L: The role of dural anomalies in vein of Galen aneurysms: Report of six cases and review of the literature. AJNR 1987; 8:185–192.
18. Norman MG, Becker LE: Cerebral damage in neonates resulting from arteriovenous malformations of the vein of Galen. J Neurol Neurosurg Psychiatry 1974; 37:252–258.
19. Roosen N, Schirmer M, Lins E, et al: MRI of an aneurysm of the vein of Galen. AJNR 1986; 7:733–735.
20. Cabanes J, Blasco R, Garcia M, et al: Cerebral venous angiomas. Surg Neurol 1979; 11:385–389.
21. Lotz PR, Quisling RG: CT of venous angiomas of the brain. AJNR 1983; 4:1124–1126.
22. Cammarata C, Han JS, Haaga JR, et al: Cerebral venous angiomas imaged by MR. Radiology 1985; 155:639–643.
23. Augustyn GT, Scott JA, Olson E, et al: Cerebral venous angiomas: MR imaging. Radiology 1985; 156:391–395.
24. Wendling LR, Moore JS, Kieffer SA, et al: Intracerebral venous angioma. Radiology 1976; 119:141–147.
25. Sigal R, Krief O, Houtteville JP, et al: Occult cerebrovascular malformations: Follow-up with MR imaging. Radiology 1990; 176:815–819.
26. Lemme-Plaghos L, Kucharczyk W, Brant-Zawadzki M, et al: MR imaging of angiographically occult vascular malformations. AJNR 1986; 7:217–222.

27. Gomori JM, Grossman RI, Goldberg HI, et al: Occult cerebral vascular malformations: High-field MR imaging. Radiology 1986; 158:707–713.
28. Numaguchi Y, Kishikawa T, Fukui M, et al: Prolonged injection angiography for diagnosing intracranial cavernous hemangiomas. Radiology 1979; 131:137–138.
29. Yeates AE, Enzmann D: Cryptic vascular malformations involving the brainstem. Radiology 1983; 146:71–75.
30. Nelson JS: Pathology of the nervous system. *Anderson's Pathology*. Kissane JM (ed): 9th ed, 1990. CV Mosby, St Louis.
31. Locksley HB: Report on the cooperative study of intracranial aneurysms and subarachnoid hemorrhage. Section V, Part 1: Natural history of subarachnoid hemorrhage, intracranial aneurysms and arteriovenous malformations. J Neurosurg 1966; 25:219–239.
32. Winn HR, Richardson AE, Jane JA: The long-term prognosis in untreated cerebral aneurysm. I. The incidence of late hemorrhage in cerebral aneurysm: A 10-year evaluation of 364 patients. Ann Neurol 1977; 1:358–370.
33. Crompton MR: Intracerebral hematoma complicating ruptured cerebral berry aneurysm. J Neurol Neurosurg Psychiatry 1962; 25:378–386.
34. Yamamoto Y, Asari S, Sunami N, et al: Computed angiotomography of unruptured cerebral aneurysms. J Comput Assist Tomogr 1986; 10:21–27.
35. Schmid UD, Steiger HJ, Huber P: Accuracy of high resolution computed tomography in direct diagnosis of cerebral aneurysms. Neuroradiology 1987; 29:152–159.
36. McCormack J, Peyster RG, Brodner RA, et al: CT visualization of ruptured berry aneurysm within hematoma: The flip-flop sign. J Comput Assist Tomogr 1986; 18:28–31.
37. Atlas SW, Grossman RI, Goldberg HI, et al: Partially thrombosed giant intracranial aneurysms: Correlation of MR and pathologic findings. Radiology 1987; 162:111–114.
38. Ross JS, Masaryk TJ, Modic MT, et al: Intracranial aneurysms: Evaluation by MR angiography. AJNR 1990; 11:449–456.
39. Bohmfalk GL, Story JL, Wissinger JP, et al: Bacterial intracranial aneurysms. J Neurosurg 1978; 48:369–382.
40. Moskowitz MA, Rosenbaum AE, Tyler HR: Angiographically monitored resolution of cerebral mycotic aneurysms. Neurology 1974; 24:1103–1108.

6

VENTRICULOMEGALY

NORMAL CEREBROSPINAL FLUID PHYSIOLOGY

Production

The cerebrospinal fluid (CSF), an ultrafiltrate of the blood plasma, is a clear, colorless solution containing small amounts of protein, glucose, and potassium, and relatively large amounts of sodium and chloride. The primary function of the CSF is to support the brain, insulating it from the inner table and dural surfaces when there are abrupt changes in the body's direction or speed. The CSF also removes waste products of neuronal metabolism, drugs, and other substances that may diffuse into the brain from the blood system.

The choroid plexus, which produces 70 to 80% of the CSF, is located in the temporal horns and bodies of the lateral ventricles, posterior third ventricle, and roof of the fourth ventricle (Fig. 6–1). Cuboidal epithelial cells of the choroid actively secrete sodium from the plasma into the CSF. Chloride follows passively, resulting in a greater osmotic pressure in the CSF than in the plasma. Water travels by osmosis from the plasma into the CSF. The remaining 20 to 30% of CSF is produced through diffusion across the meningeal surface over the convexities or intraventricularly through the ependymal surface lining the ventricles.

On average, 150 ml of CSF is present within the dura of the cranium and spine, 25% of which is within the ventricles. The choroid produces on average 800 ml daily, or approximately 0.5 ml per minute.[1]

Pathways

The CSF produced within the ventricles and subarachnoid space must travel to the arachnoid villi (pacchionian granulations) located within the dural sinuses, most commonly the superior sagittal sinus, to become absorbed. The CSF proceeds from the lateral ventricles through the foramen of Monro into the midline third ventricle. Flow is then directed through the aqueduct of Sylvius into the fourth ventricle. CSF may exit the fourth ventricle through the lateral foramina of Luschka or the midline foramen of Magendie. The CSF then enters the subarachnoid space around the lower brainstem (cisterna magna) (Fig. 6–2).

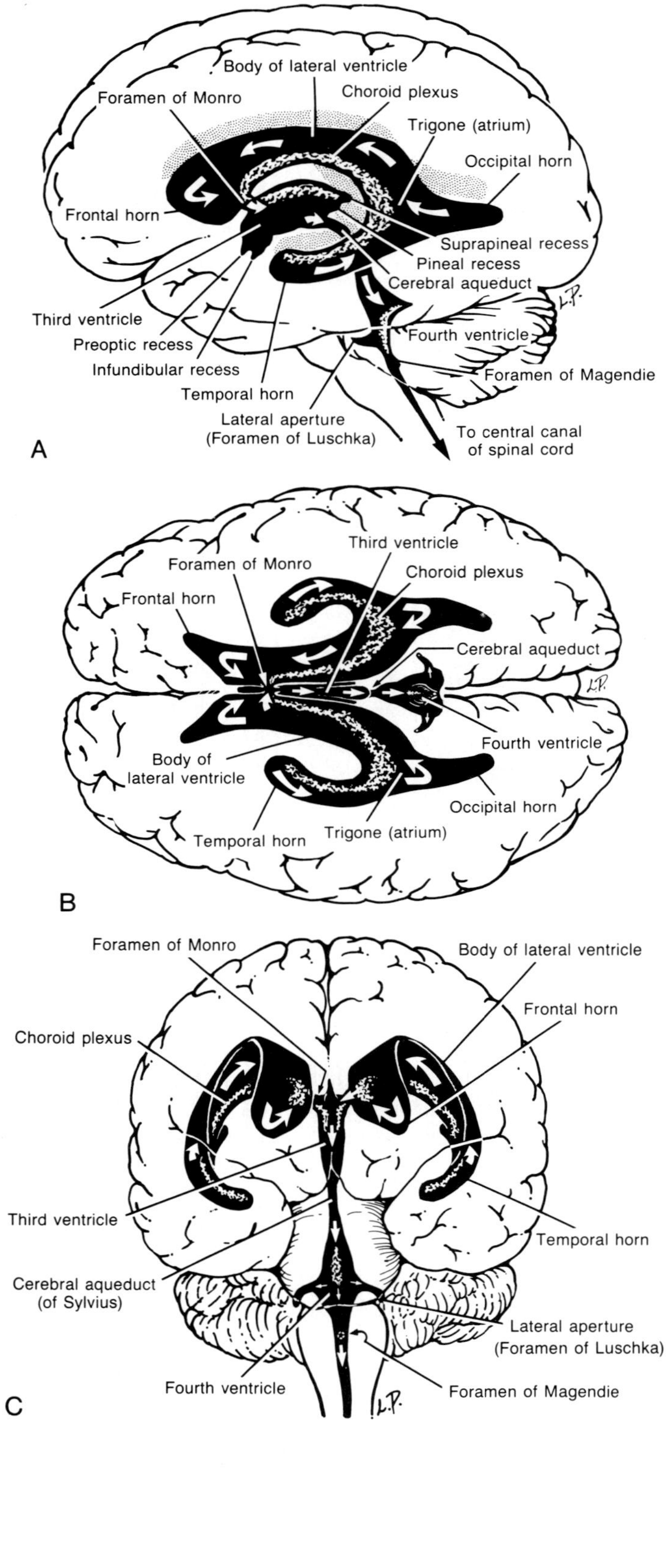

Figure 6–1. Ventricular system. **A,** Lateral perspective. **B,** Cephalad perspective. **C,** Frontal perspective.

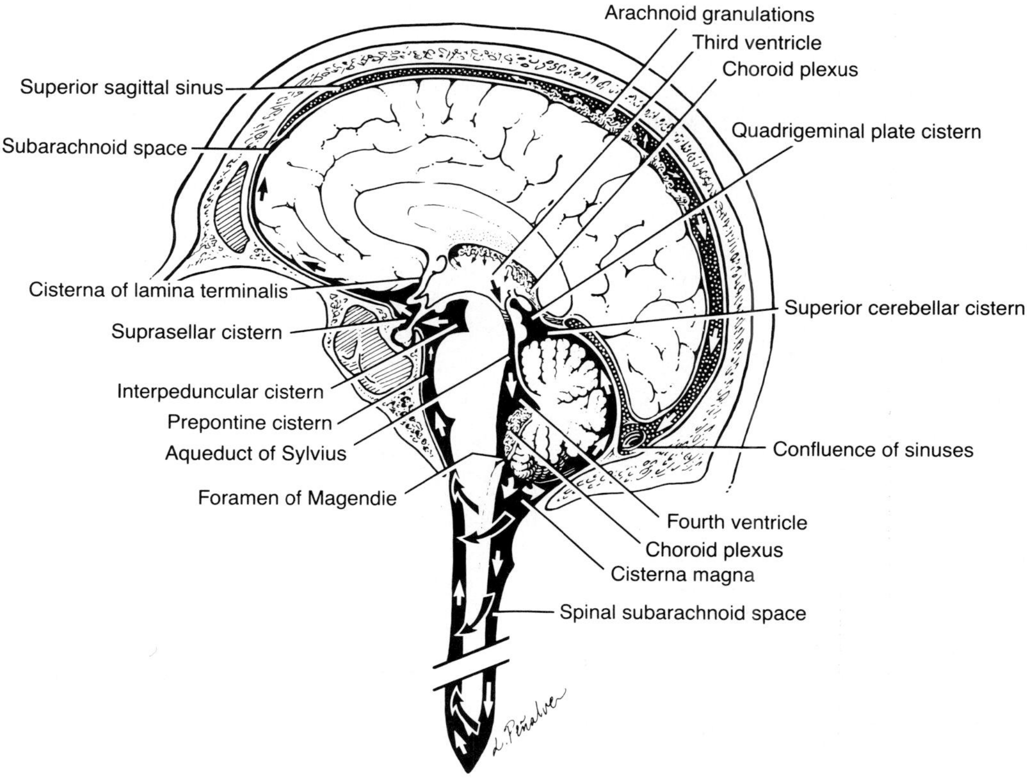

Figure 6–2. Cerebrospinal fluid (CSF) pathways. Lateral perspective.

The CSF may flow into the spinal canal to circulate around the cord or it may flow cephalad into the cistern surrounding the brainstem, through the tentorial incisura, and into the basilar cistern. The CSF continues cephalad over the convexities in the subarachnoid space to reach the pacchionian granulations at the level of the superior sagittal sinus.

Magnetic resonance imaging (MRI) is the most sensitive noninvasive modality for evaluating CSF flow. Early reports[2] demonstrated flow void on the spin echo MRI in the aqueduct and foramen of Magendie in normal patients. These represent regions in which the cross-sectional area of the CSF space is diminished; consequently CSF flow is increased. It was determined that using cardiac gating techniques, the CSF flow was intimately related to cardiac systole and diastole. The flow void was noted to increase when the systemic arterial pulse wave was transmitted to the brain. Gradient echo techniques are even more sensitive at detecting CSF flow than are gated spin echo.[3] More recent work[4] has demonstrated simultaneous flow void in the foramen of Monro and the aqueduct. Flow is directed craniocaudal in systole and caudocranial in diastole, with each phase of the cardiac cycle lasting an equal length of time. Systole in the subarachnoid spaces precedes that of the ventricles, permitting reflux of a minimal amount of CSF into the fourth ventricle. The fourth ventricle and cisterna magna serve as mixing chambers for the CSF, which enters the former in diastole and the latter in systole.

Absorption

In order to maintain a constant volume of CSF within the ventricles and subarachnoid spaces, CSF absorption must be commensurate with CSF production. Absorption occurs primarily at the arachnoid villi. These arborized structures have large surface areas that are markedly permeable. The arachnoid granulations project into the venous dural sinuses and are most numerous in the superior sagittal sinus (Fig. 6–3). CSF flow into the venous system is pressure-dependent, occurring when the CSF pressure is 3 to 6 cm of water greater than the venous pressure. The arachnoid villi function as one-way valves, permitting flow only from the CSF into the dural venous sinuses.

HYDROCEPHALUS

Hydrocephalus is a condition that exists when there is an excessive amount of CSF within the cranial vault. Hydrocephalus results from interruption of balance between CSF production and absorption. Excessive CSF production is rarely the cause of hydrocephalus. The most common etiology of excess CSF production is a choroid plexus papilloma (see Chapter 4).

Hydrocephalus most commonly results from inability to absorb CSF at the rate at which it is produced. The CSF flow to the arachnoid villi may be impeded, or the transfer of CSF into the venous system at the level of the arachnoid villi is inefficient.

Noncommunicating

In this condition the CSF produced by the choroid remains within the ventricular system, unable to enter or "communicate" with the subarachnoid space. Depending on the point of obstruction, all or a portion of the ventricular system may be distended. As the production of CSF is not pressure-dependent, the choroid will continue to secrete sodium, and water will continue to collect within the ventricular system via osmotic gradients despite the presence of a distal obstruction.

A mass lesion that obstructs the egress of CSF will distend the upstream, or proximal, ventricular system. The downstream, or distal, ventricular system may be of normal size. For example, a lesion at the level of the foramen of Monro will distend both lateral ventricles, whereas the third ventricle, aqueduct, and fourth ventricle will be normal. Alternatively, a mass lesion that obstructs the outlet of the fourth ventricle will distend the entire ventricular system.

As the ventricles become progressively more distended, the threshold of the ependyma to contain the CSF is exceeded. In addition the ependyma may be torn, stretched to the point of disruption. CSF will be pressure-driven into the periventricular white matter, resulting in periventricular interstitial edema. This occurs most commonly at the level of the frontal horns and atria of the lateral ventricles.

In planar imaging of the patient with hydrocephalus the strategy is twofold. Initially, the point of obstruction must be identified. The proximal ventricular system will be enlarged, usually with an abrupt transition point at the level of the mass (Fig. 6–4). The frontal horns will be enlarged and ballooned outward with a decrease in the frontal horn angle to less than 95 degrees. (The frontal horn angle refers to the angle created by the anterior margin of the frontal horns, at the level of the superior third ventricle.) The temporal horns are a very

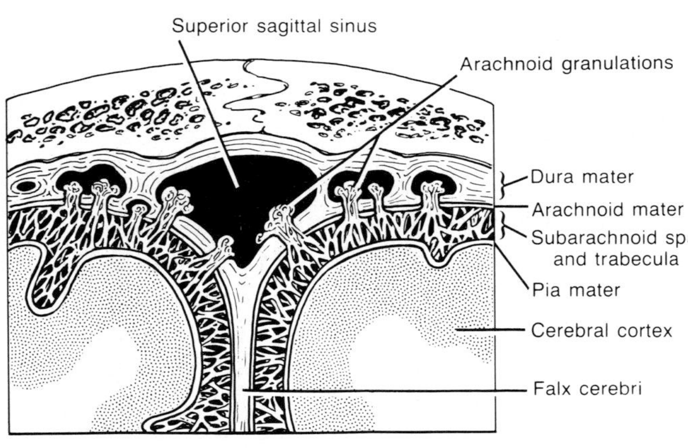

Figure 6–3. CSF absorption; arachnoid granulation. Coronal perspective.

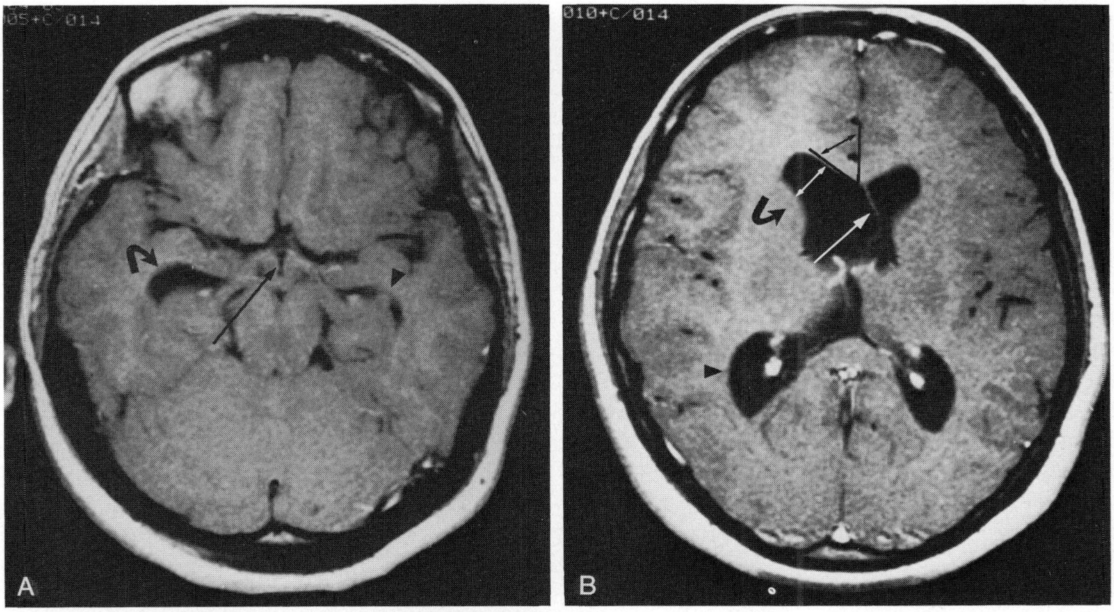

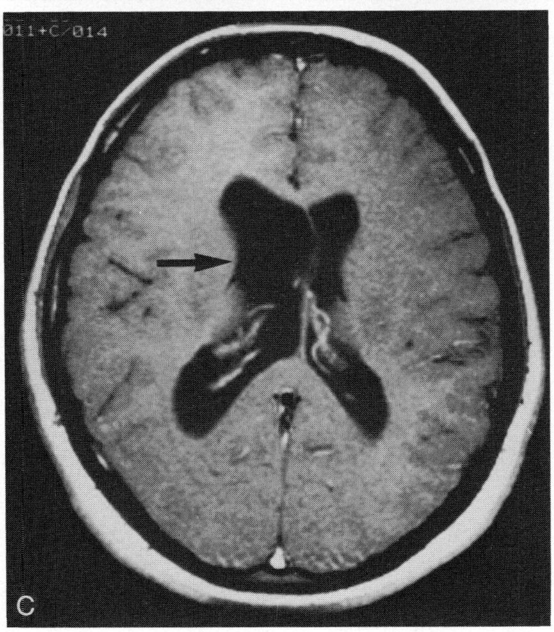

Figure 6–4. Unilateral noncommunicating hydrocephalus; subependymal cyst (37-year-old female).

A, Enhanced axial T1. The right temporal horn (*curved arrow*) is enlarged. The anterior inferior third ventricle (*arrow*) and left temporal horn (*arrowhead*) are normal.

B, Enhanced axial T1. The right frontal horn is enlarged (*white double-headed arrow*), decreasing the right frontal horn angle (*black double-headed arrow*) and laterally displacing the right head of the caudate (*curved arrow*). The septum pellucidum (*white arrow*) is deviated. The atrium of the right lateral ventricle (*arrowhead*) is slightly larger than that of the left.

C, Enhanced axial T1. The body of the right lateral ventricle (*arrow*) is significantly larger than that of the left.

sensitive indicator of hydrocephalus (Fig. 6–5). They are the first segment of the lateral ventricle to distend when acute hydrocephalus occurs. The temporal horns will enlarge in proportion to the remainder of the lateral ventricle in the hydrocephalic patient[5, 6] (Fig. 6–6). The cephalad surface of the corpus callosum will assume an upward convexity.[7] Owing to diffuse enlargement of the third ventricle, the mammillary bodies will be displaced caudally, diminishing the mammillopontine distance.[8] The walls of the anterior third ventricle may be convexed (Fig. 6–7). Periventricular interstitial edema will render the contour of the ventricular margin somewhat indistinct on CT and T1- and T2-weighted images. The spin density images depict the periventricular interstitial edema as hyperintense to CSF within the ventricle. To accommodate the increased ventricular volume, the brain parenchyma is compressed against the inner table, at the expense of the cortical subarachnoid space (Fig. 6–8). The cortical sulci may be completely effaced in the later stages.

The second task of the neuroimager is to identify the etiology of the obstruction. The mass may be within the ventricular system or more commonly it is extrinsic to the ventricle, causing significant compression of the ventricular system. Increased tissue contrast and multiplanar imaging capabilities will render MRI a more sensitive modality to accomplish this task. The common site-specific causes of noncommunicating hydrocephalus are listed in Table 6–1 and are discussed separately in appropriate chapters.

The plain film findings of hydrocephalus have been presented in Chapter 1. In infants and young children the sutures will separate, resulting in megalocephaly. Adult-onset hydrocephalus results in erosion of the dorsum sella and, more rarely and less predictably, prominence of convolutional markings.

Communicating

Communicating hydrocephalus indicates there is free egress or communication of CSF

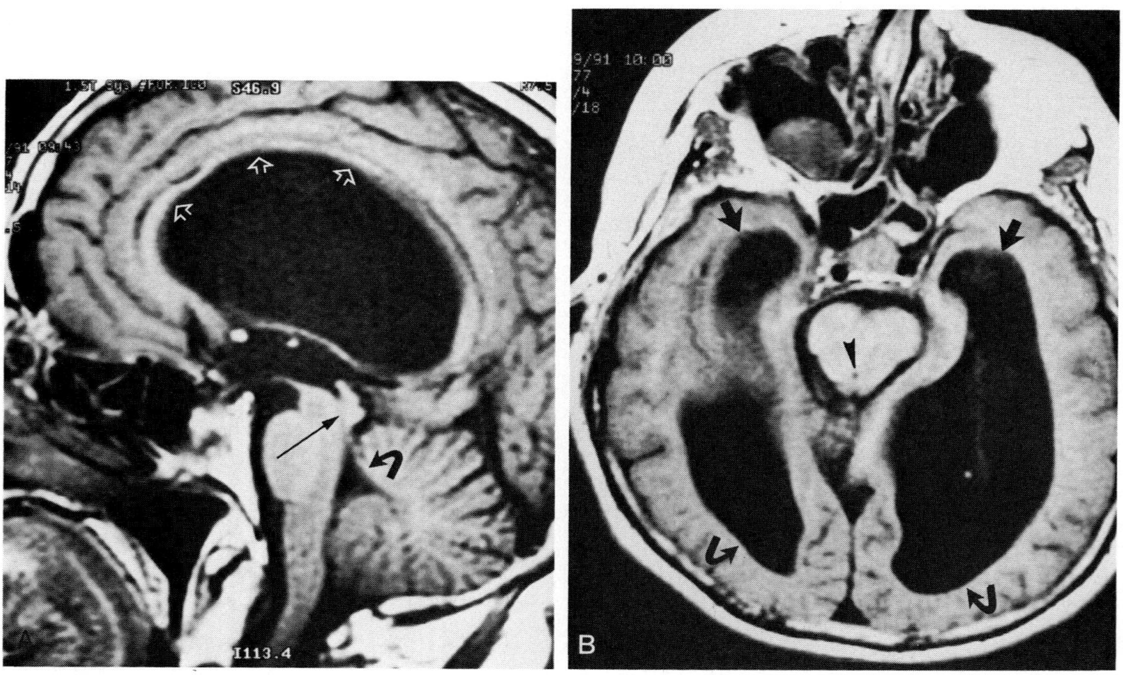

Figure 6–5. Noncommunicating hydrocephalus; chronic aqueductal stenosis (45-year-old female).

A, Parasagittal T1. The caudal aqueduct (*arrow*) is stenotic, the fourth ventricle (*curved arrow*) is at the lower limit of normal in size, and the corpus callosum (*open arrows*) is markedly bowed.

B, Axial T1. The temporal horns (*arrows*) and occipital horns (*curved arrows*) are dilated. The aqueduct (*arrowhead*) is attenuated.

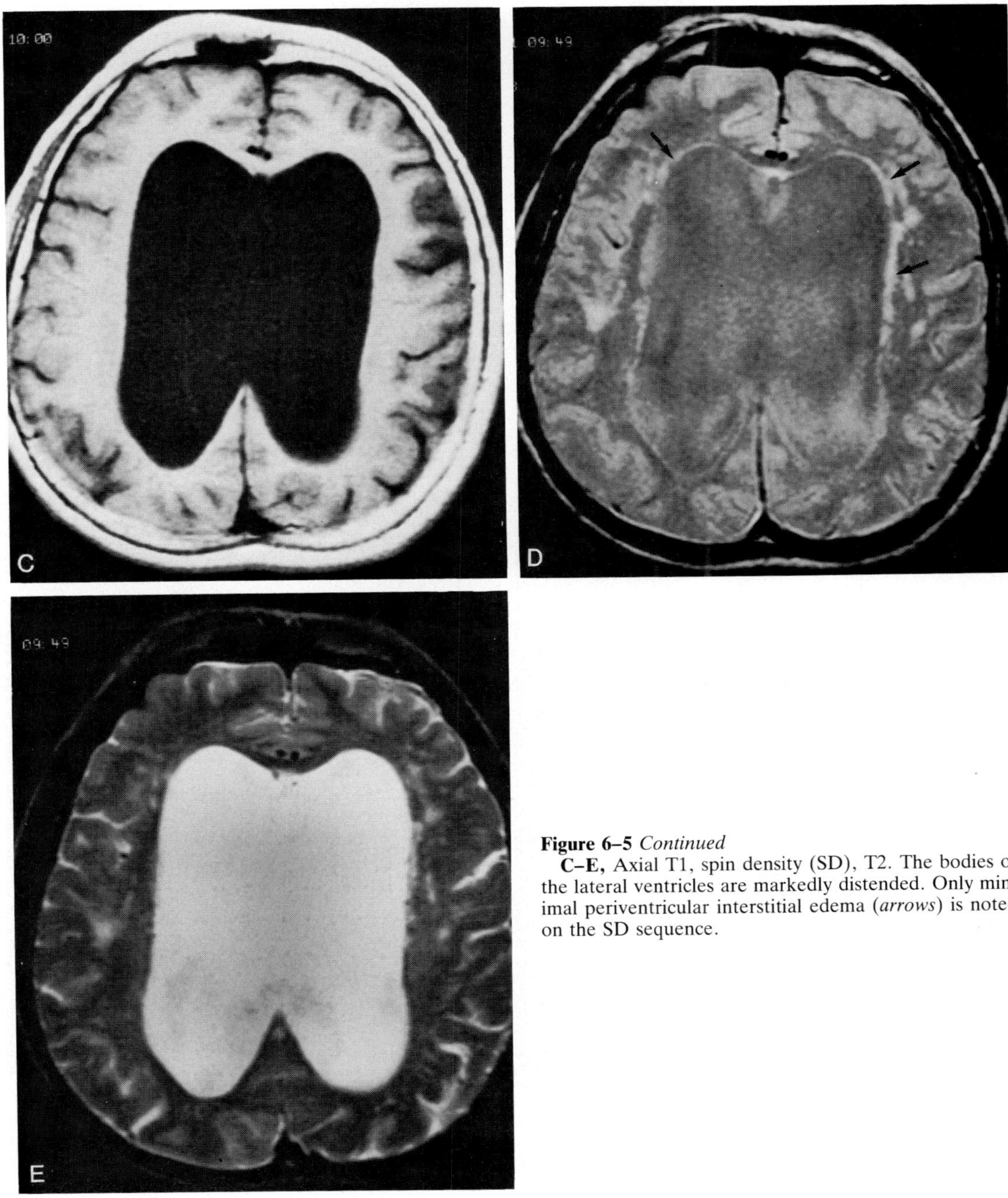

Figure 6–5 *Continued*
C–E, Axial T1, spin density (SD), T2. The bodies of the lateral ventricles are markedly distended. Only minimal periventricular interstitial edema (*arrows*) is noted on the SD sequence.

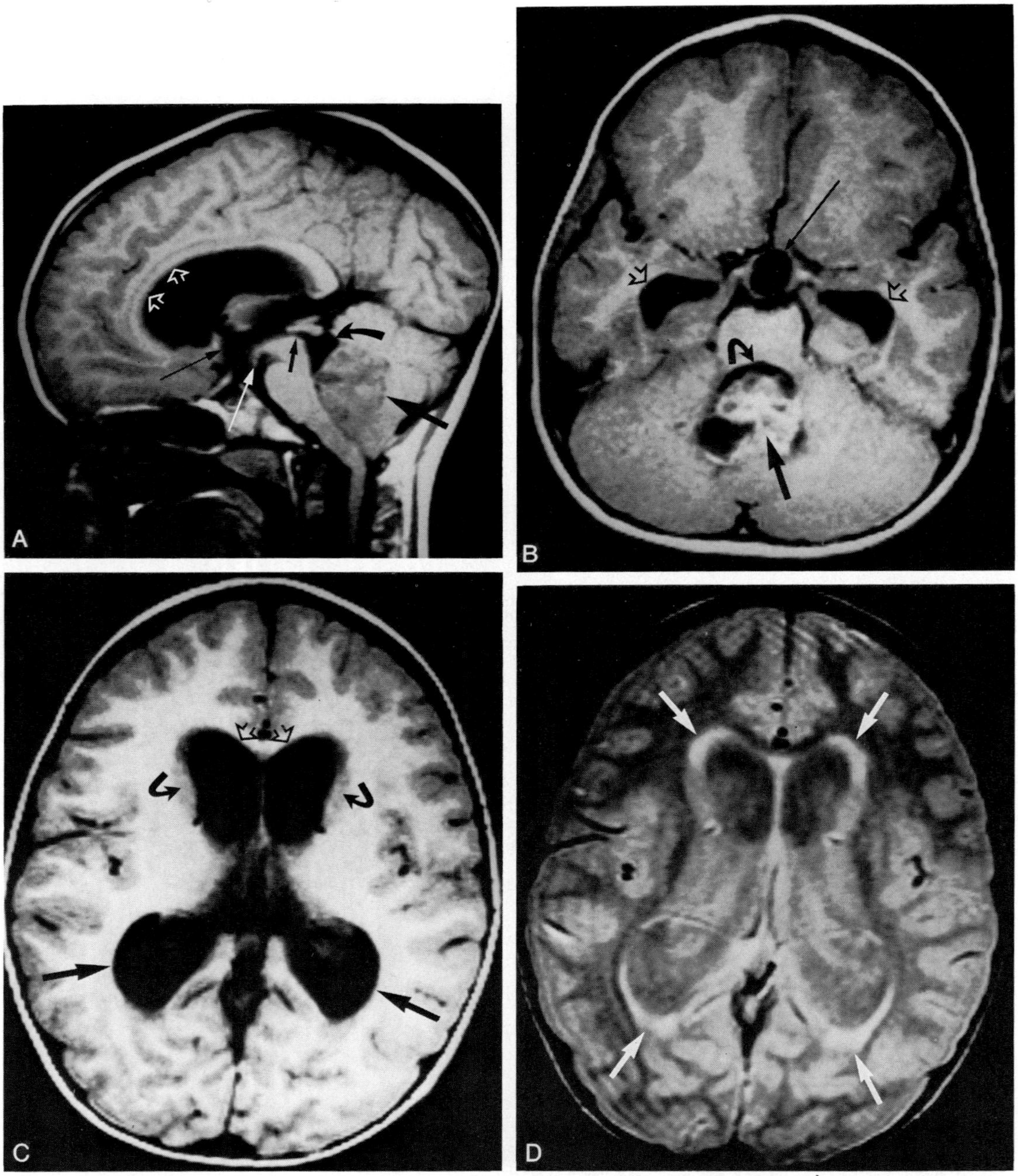

Figure 6–6. Noncommunicating hydrocephalus; primitive neuroectodermal tumor (PNET) (4-year-old female).

A, Parasagittal T1. A heterogeneous mass (*bold arrow*) fills the caudal fourth ventricle and has produced the following changes: (1) distention of the cephalad fourth ventricle (*curved arrow*), (2) distention of the aqueduct of Sylvius (*short arrow*), (3) distention of the third ventricle (*thin black arrow*), and (4) bowing of the corpus callosum (*open arrows*). The mammillary bodies (*thin white arrow*) are displaced caudally, effectively reducing the mammillopontine distance.

B, Enhanced axial T1. The enhancing mass (*arrow*) has distorted the fourth ventricle (*curved arrow*) and enlarged the temporal horns (*open arrows*) and third ventricle (*long arrow*). The lateral margins of the third ventricle are convexed.

C, Axial T1. The frontal horns (*open arrows*) and atria (*arrows*) of the lateral ventricles are distended. The heads of the caudate nuclei (*curved arrows*) are displaced laterally. The cortical sulci are attenuated.

D, Axial SD. High-signal periventricular interstitial edema (*arrows*) shrouds the lateral ventricular surface.

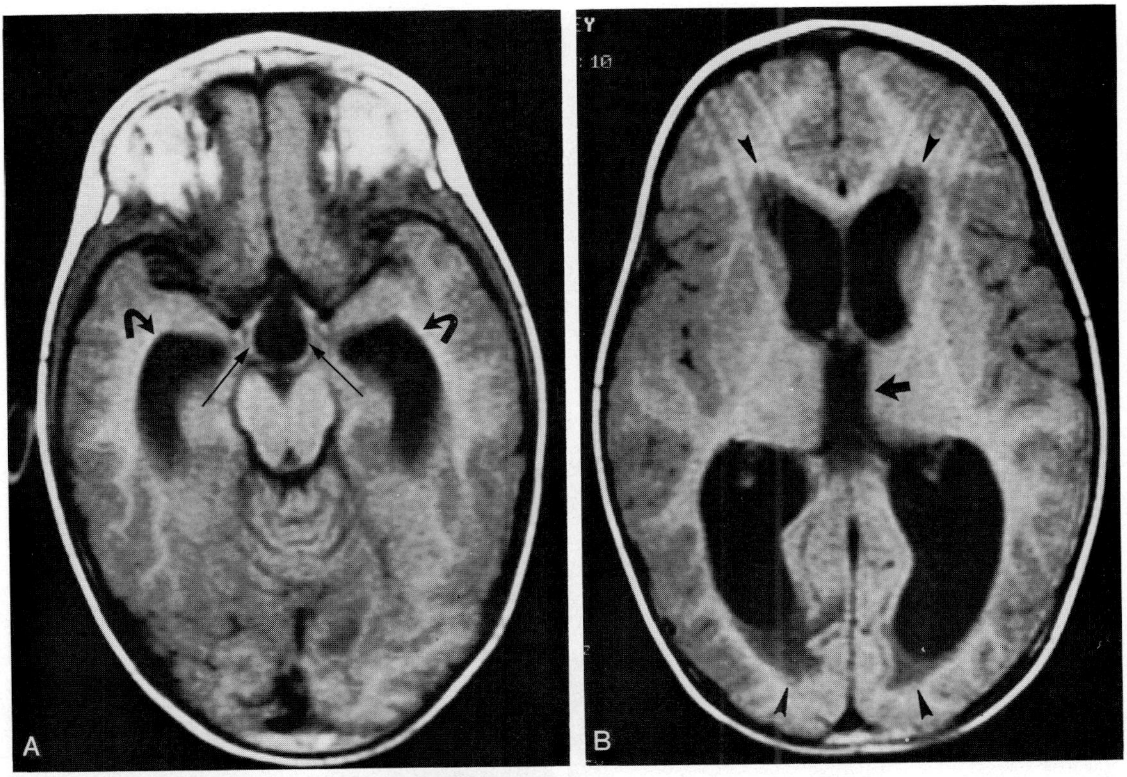

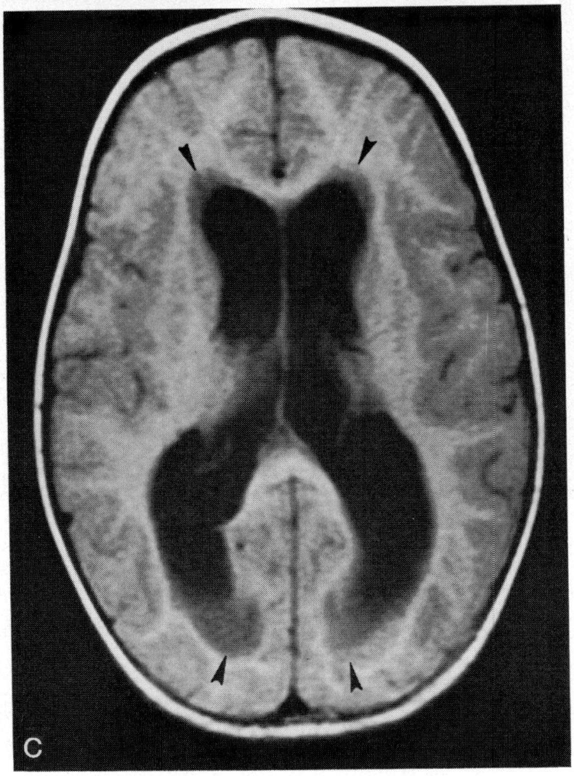

Figure 6–7. Noncommunicating hydrocephalus; aqueductal stenosis (6-year-old male).

A, Axial T1. The walls of the anterior third ventricle (*arrows*) are convexed. The temporal horns (*curved arrows*) are markedly distended.

B, C, Axial T1. The superior third (*arrow*) and lateral ventricles are enlarged. Periventricular interstitial edema (*arrowheads*) caps portions of the ventricular surface.

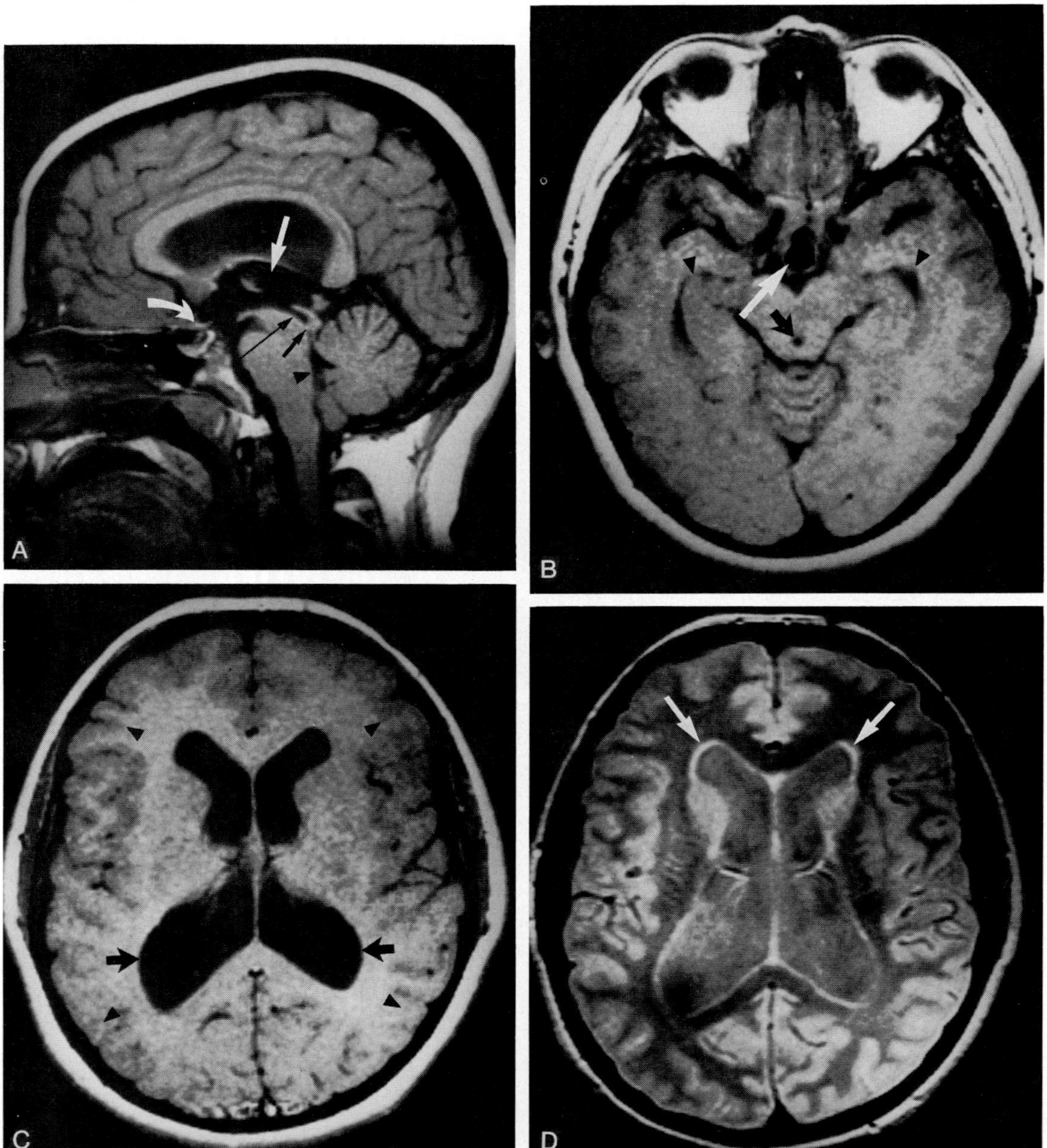

Figure 6–8. Noncommunicating hydrocephalus; chronic aqueductal stenosis (32-year-old male).

A, Parasagittal T1. A web or band (*short black arrow*) narrows the caudal aqueduct. The cephalad aqueduct (*long arrow*) is slightly prominent, as is the third ventricle (*white arrow*). The optic chiasm (*curved arrow*) is displaced caudally to the diaphragma sellae by the enlarged third ventricle. The fourth ventricle (*arrowhead*) is at the lower limit of normal in size.

B, Axial T1. The cephalad aqueduct (*black arrow*) is distended; the temporal horns (*arrowheads*) and third ventricle (*white arrow*) are mildly distended.

C, Axial T1. The lateral ventricles (*arrows*) are mildly enlarged. The cortical sulci (*arrowhead*) are effaced.

D, Axial SD. Only minimal periventricular interstitial edema (*arrows*) is present in the white matter near the frontal horns. Commonly, the amount of periventricular interstitial edema will decrease in amount with chronicity.

Table 6–1. COMMON CAUSES OF NONCOMMUNICATING HYDROCEPHALUS

Site of Obstruction	Adults	Children
A. Lateral Ventricle		
1. Trigone	Meningioma	Choroid plexus papilloma
2. Body	Glioma	PNET Glioma
B. Foramen of Monro/Anterior 3rd Ventricle	Colloid cyst Craniopharyngioma Macroadenoma Meningioma Subfalcial herniation	Craniopharyngioma Hypothalamic glioma Chiasmatic glioma Subfalcial herniation
C. Posterior 3rd Ventricle	Pineal germinoma Tentorial meningioma Glioma Pineocytoma	Pineal germinoma Pineoblastoma (PNET)
D. Aqueduct	Adult aqueductal stenosis Periaqueductal glioma or metastasis Ascending or descending transtentorial herniation	Aqueductal stenosis Vein of Galen aneurysm Ascending or descending transtentorial herniation
E. 4th Ventricle	Metastasis Cerebellar infarct Cerebellar hemorrhage Glioma Meningioma	Medulloblastoma (PNET) Cystic cerebellar astrocytoma Ependymoma Chiari II malformation Dandy-Walker malformation

PNET, primitive neuroectodermal tumor.

between the ventricular system and the subarachnoid space. However, CSF flow from the basilar cisterns to the arachnoid villi is obstructed or there is direct impairment of absorption at the level of the arachnoid villi. Obstruction of flow in the subarachnoid space may be the result of subarachnoid hemorrhage, meningitis, or tumor infiltration.

Communicating hydrocephalus may also be the result of impaired absorption at the arachnoid villi. This may also be caused by aforementioned hemorrhage, tumor, or inflammatory cells blocking the villi. Elevation of the venous pressure will decrease the pressure gradient responsible for CSF absorption. The venous pressure may be elevated with dural AVM, vein of Galen aneurysm, skull base tumor obstructing the venous outflow, or thrombosis of the dural sinuses.

On planar imaging, the pattern of ventriculomegaly may be similar for communicating and noncommunicating hydrocephalus (Table 6–2). The frontal horns are expanded. The frontal horn angle is acute and the temporal horns are proportionately enlarged to the remainder of the lateral ventricular system (Fig. 6–9). The third and fourth ventricles, as well as the juxtaposed aqueduct of Sylvius, may be enlarged. The third ventricle may be less distended and the amount of periventricular

Table 6–2. DISTINGUISHING FEATURES OF HYDROCEPHALUS

	Noncommunicating Hydrocephalus*	Communicating Hydrocephalus	Atrophy (Hydrocephalus Ex Vacuo)
Frontal Horns	+ +	+ +	+ +
Frontal Horn Angle	<95°	<95°	>95°
Temporal Horns	+ + Proportionate to body of lateral ventricle	+ Proportionate to body of lateral ventricle	– Less than body of lateral ventricle
Anterior 3rd Ventricle	+ + Convexed walls	+ Convex → parallel walls	+ Parallel walls
Aqueduct	+	+	±
4th Ventricle	+	±	+
Periventricular Interstitial Edema	+ +	+	–
Cortical Sulci	–	+	+ +

*Assumes distal 4th ventricular obstruction.

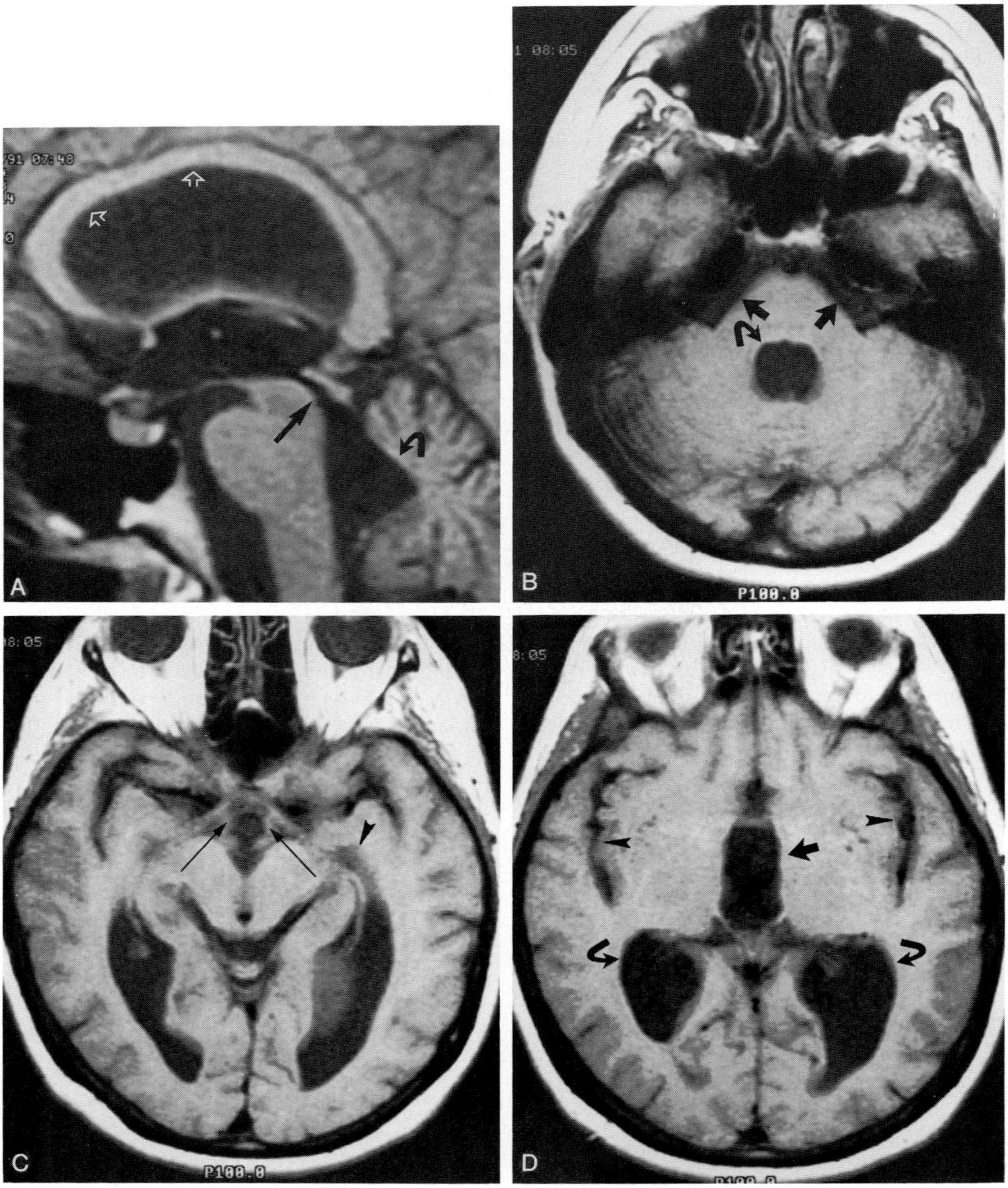

Figure 6–9. Communicating hydrocephalus (43-year-old male).

A, Parasagittal T1. The fourth ventricle (*curved arrow*) is distended, the aqueduct (*arrow*) is prominent, and the corpus callosum (*open arrows*) is bowed.

B, Axial T1. The fourth ventricle (*curved arrow*) and cerebellopontine angle cisterns (*arrows*) are enlarged.

C, Axial T1. The left temporal horn (*arrowhead*) is moderately enlarged. The walls of the anterior third ventricle (*arrows*) are slightly convex.

D, Axial T1. The third ventricle (*arrow*) and atria of the lateral ventricles (*curved arrows*) are prominent. The sylvian fissures (*arrowheads*) are moderately prominent.

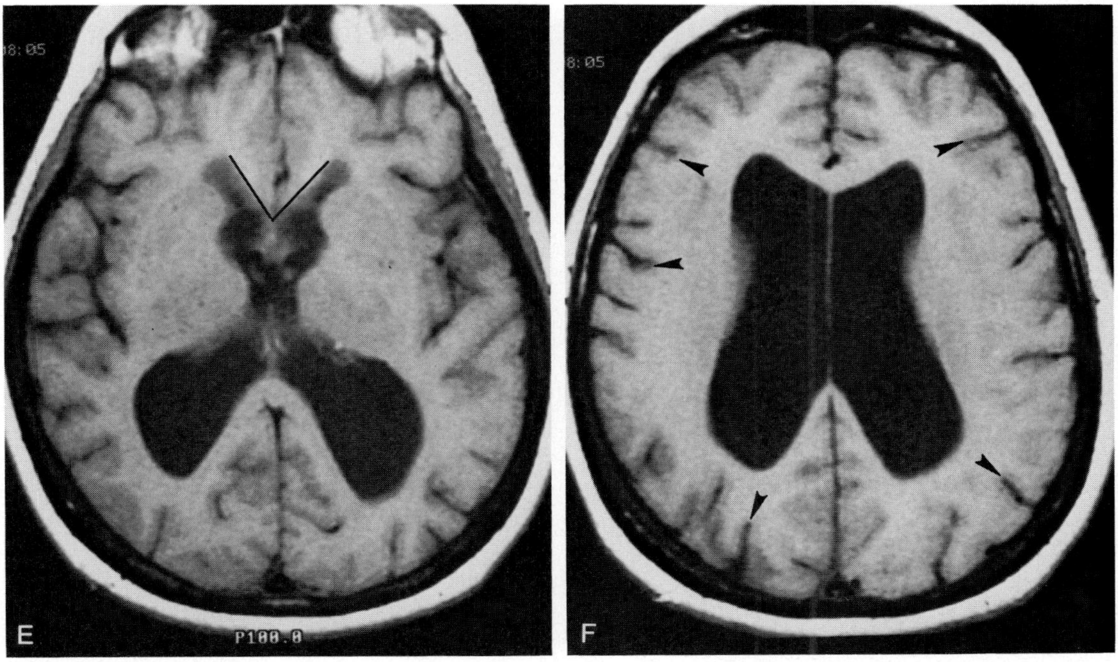

Figure 6–9 *Continued*
E, Axial T1. The frontal horn angle (*black lines*) is acute.
F, Axial T1. The cortical sulci (*arrowheads*) are present, though less prominent than the ventricular system.

interstitial edema may be less with communicating than with noncommunicating hydrocephalus.

The subarachnoid space upstream to the point of obstruction will be enlarged with effacement of the downstream subarachnoid space. For example, if the point of obstruction is at the level of the tentorium, the ventricles and CSF spaces of the posterior fossa will be enlarged and the supratentorial subarachnoid space and sulci may be attenuated.

Normal Pressure Hydrocephalus

This clinically diagnosed condition described by Hakim and Adams[9] consists of gait apraxia, dementia, and urinary incontinence. The gait disorder varies from careless slow, stiff-legged, shortened steps to total incapacity to stand or walk. The dementia manifests as memory impairment, inattentiveness, slowness, paucity of thought, and word-finding difficulties without aphasia. The sphincteric incontinence was described as "cerebral type," in which patients are unaware of the contents of the bowel or bladder. Lumbar puncture on these patients documented normal CSF pressure (less than 180 mm of water). Despite this, patients improved significantly following ventricular shunt therapy.[10]

The etiology of normal pressure hydrocephalus is multifactorial. Arachnoiditis, meningitis, ependymitis, encephalitis, subarachnoid hemorrhage, trauma, tumors and cysts within or adjacent to the ventricle, and stenosis of the aqueduct have been implicated. Perhaps more commonly, causes are idiopathic.

Planar imaging of these patients most frequently reveals ventriculomegaly and enlargement of CSF spaces in a pattern consistent with that of communicating hydrocephalus. Patients with normal pressure hydrocephalus have prominent CSF flow void within the cerebral aqueduct. This is thought in part to be due to increased ventricular volume as well as decreased ventricular compliance and actually greater flow through the aqueduct during the cardiac cycle. Patients with normal pressure hydrocephalus and prominent flow void have been proven to respond more favorably to CSF shunting.[11] Despite this, there does not appear to have been any change in the postoperative appearance of the magnitude of the flow void. Clinical recovery after shunting has been correlated to increased cerebral blood flow.[12]

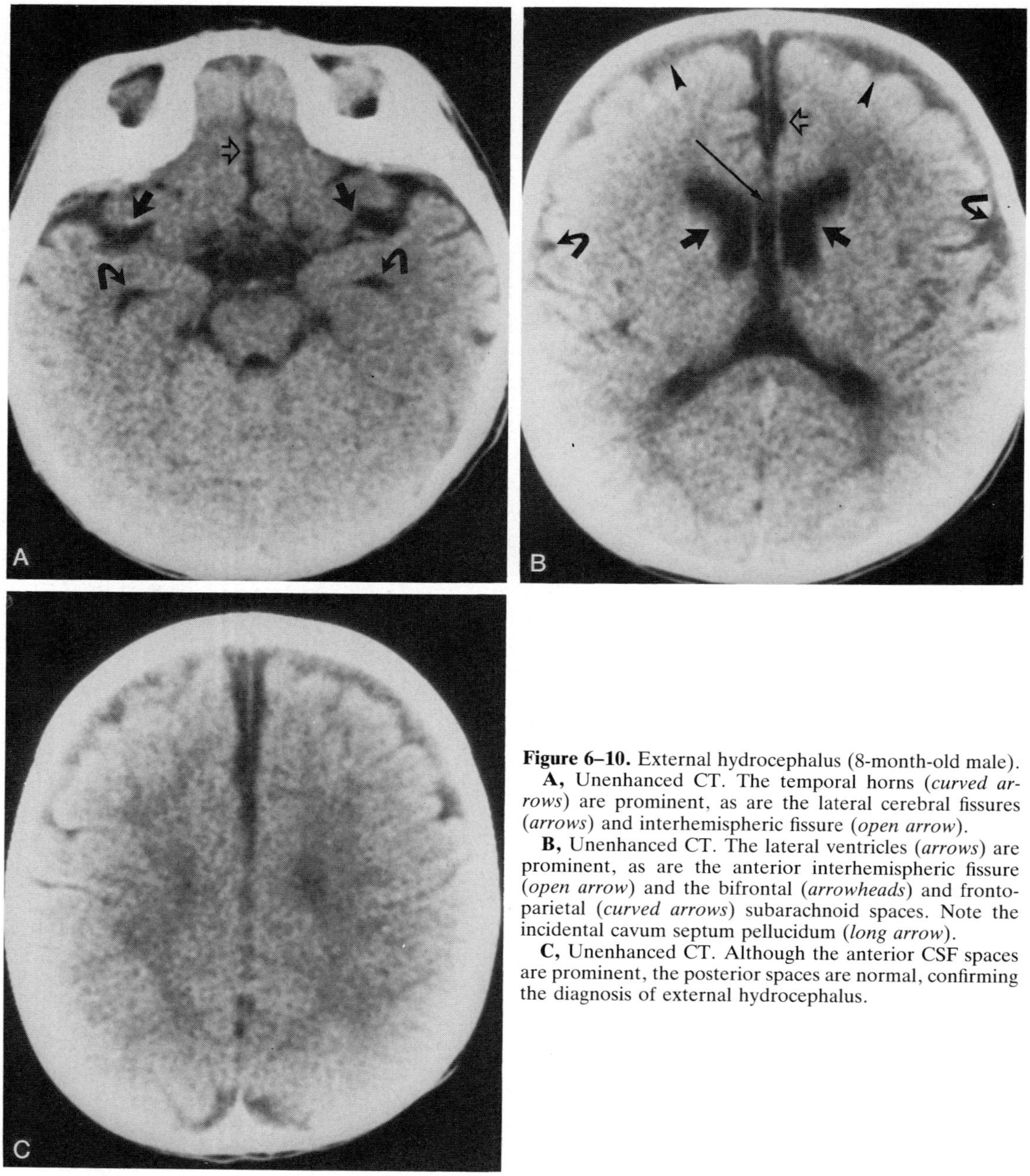

Figure 6–10. External hydrocephalus (8-month-old male).

A, Unenhanced CT. The temporal horns (*curved arrows*) are prominent, as are the lateral cerebral fissures (*arrows*) and interhemispheric fissure (*open arrow*).

B, Unenhanced CT. The lateral ventricles (*arrows*) are prominent, as are the anterior interhemispheric fissure (*open arrow*) and the bifrontal (*arrowheads*) and frontoparietal (*curved arrows*) subarachnoid spaces. Note the incidental cavum septum pellucidum (*long arrow*).

C, Unenhanced CT. Although the anterior CSF spaces are prominent, the posterior spaces are normal, confirming the diagnosis of external hydrocephalus.

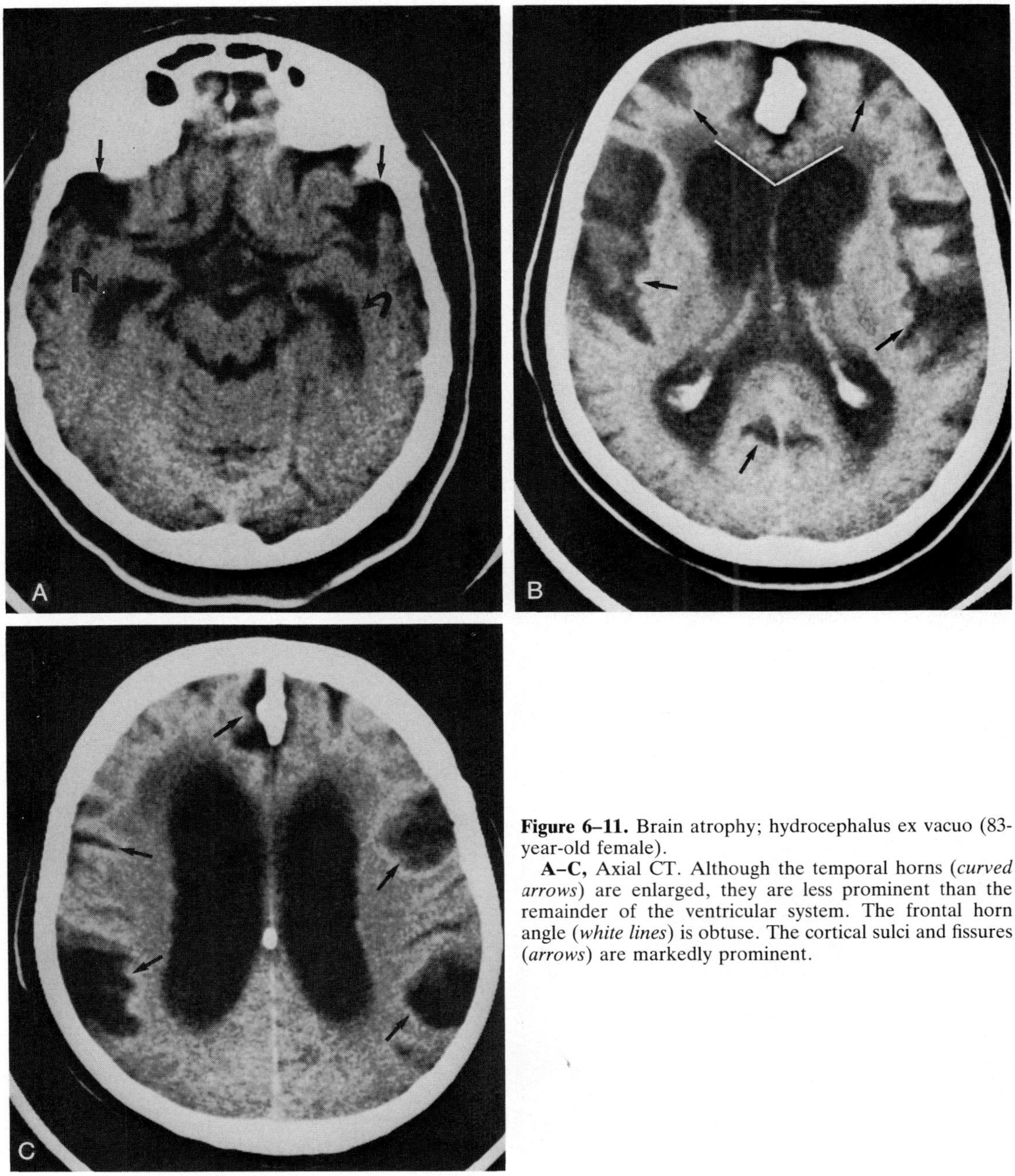

Figure 6–11. Brain atrophy; hydrocephalus ex vacuo (83-year-old female).

A–C, Axial CT. Although the temporal horns (*curved arrows*) are enlarged, they are less prominent than the remainder of the ventricular system. The frontal horn angle (*white lines*) is obtuse. The cortical sulci and fissures (*arrows*) are markedly prominent.

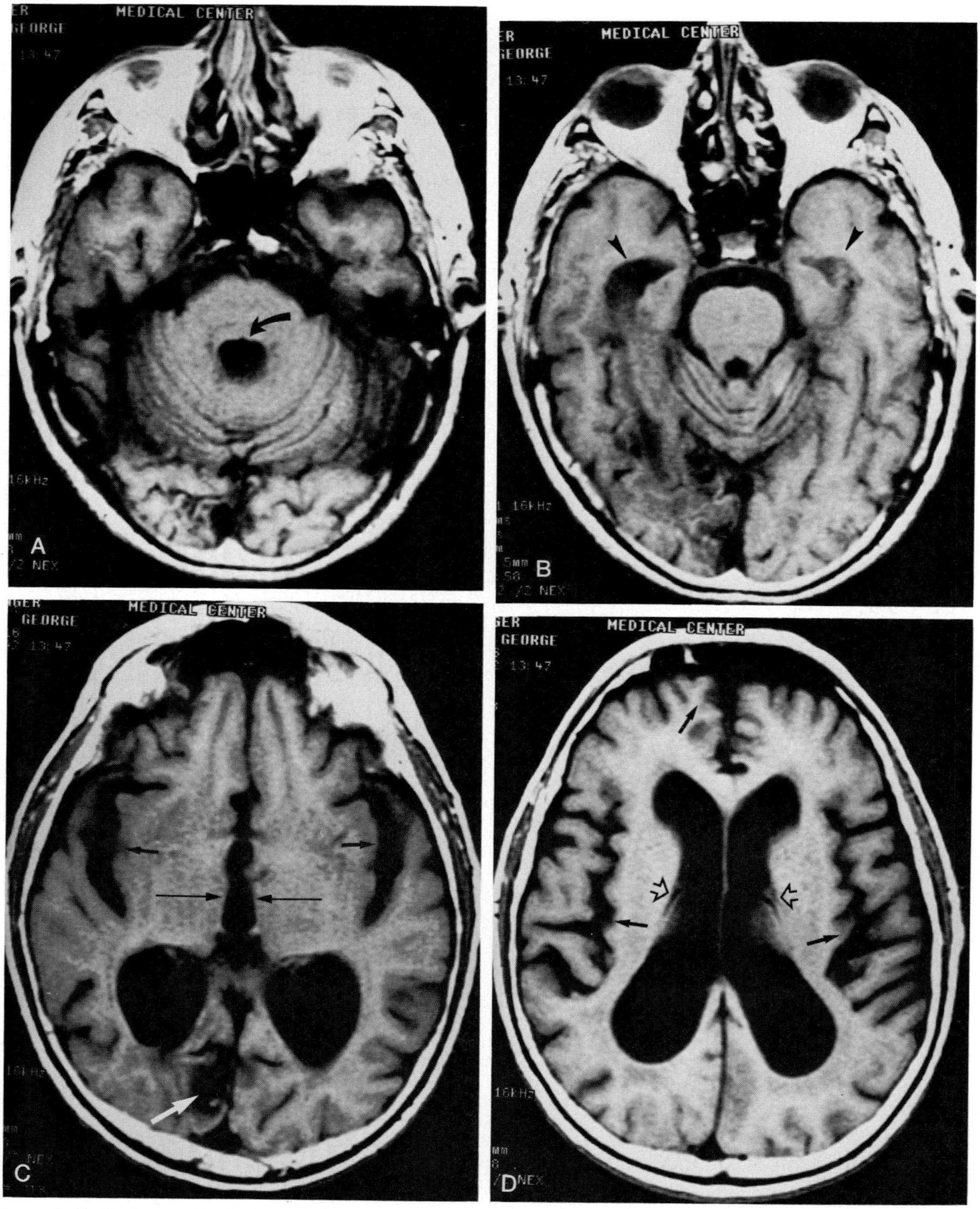

Figure 6–12. Brain atrophy; hydrocephalus ex vacuo (79-year-old male).

A–D, Axial T1. The CSF spaces are diffusely enlarged, indicative of generalized atrophy. The fourth ventricle (*curved arrow*) and bodies of the lateral ventricles (*open arrows*) are large. The temporal horns (*arrowheads*), though distended, are less prominent than the ventricular bodies. The lateral walls of the third ventricle (*long arrows*) are parallel. The superficial CSF spaces (*arrows*) are markedly prominent. Note the chronic right visual cortex infarction (*white arrow*).

External Hydrocephalus

This is a self-limiting condition that occurs in young patients before the closure of the sutures. The pathophysiology is speculative, but it is thought to be related to transient defect of CSF resorption at the level of the arachnoid villi. The patients exhibit a rapidly enlarging head as the sutures separate. The condition usually resolves in 2 to 3 years without need for intervention.

Planar imaging depicts mild ventricular enlargement and focal prominence of the bifrontal, frontal parietal, and interhemispheric fissure CSF spaces[13] (Fig. 6–10). External hydrocephalus can be distinguished radiographically from atrophy via the focality of the CSF space enlargement. Atrophy is usually holohemispheric with involvement of all cortical sulci. Clinical distinction between atrophy and external hydrocephalus is based on an enlarging head circumference or the presence of megalocephaly.

ATROPHY—HYDROCEPHALUS EX VACUO

Brain atrophy may also result in ventriculomegaly. Brain atrophy is usually most commonly related to decreased global perfusion seen with senescence. Brain atrophy results in loss of cerebral parenchyma with commensurate enlargement of the adjacent CSF spaces. Generally, atrophy tends to be diffuse and symmetric, although some neurodegenerative disorders have a predilection for specific regions of the brain.

The distinction between atrophy and communicating hydrocephalus may be problematic. In both conditions the ventricles and subarachnoid spaces may be enlarged. The distinguishing feature relates to the pattern of ventricular enlargement. Brain atrophy tends to spare the temporal lobes with relative preservation of the temporal horns. Although the temporal horns may be larger than normal, they are often disproportionately small when compared with the remainder of the lateral ventricle (Fig. 6–11). In addition, the frontal horns enlarge symmetrically owing to the parenchymal loss. The frontal horn angle at the level of the superior third ventricle is usually obtuse, greater than 95 degrees.[5] The third ventricle may be diffusely generous, yet the walls of the third ventricle remain parallel or only mildly convexed. The cortical sulci are generally more capacious with atrophy (Fig. 6–12) than with communicating hydrocephalus. White matter ischemic changes frequently accompany global atrophic processes.

References

1. Carpenter MB, Sutin J: *Human Neuroanatomy*, 8th ed. 1983, Williams & Wilkins, Baltimore.
2. Citrin CM, Sherman JL, Gangarosa RE, et al: Physiology of the CSF flow-void sign: Modification by cardiac gating. AJNR 1986; 7:1021–1024.
3. Atlas SW, Mark AS, Fram EK: Aqueductal stenosis: Evaluation with gradient-echo rapid MR imaging. Radiology 1988; 169:449–453.
4. Enzmann DR, Pek NJ: Normal flow patterns of intracranial and spinal cerebrospinal fluid defined with phase-contrast Cine MR imaging. Radiology 1991; 178:467–474.
5. Heinz ER, Ward A, Drayer BP, et al: Distinction between obstructive and atrophic dilatation of ventricles in children. J Comput Assist Tomogr 1980; 4:320–325.
6. Sjaastad O, Skalpe IO, Engeset A: The width of the temporal horn in the differential diagnosis between pressure hydrocephalus and hydrocephalus ex vacuo. Neurology 1987; 19:1087–1093.
7. Jinkins JR: Clinical manifestations of hydrocephalus caused by impingement of the corpus callosum on the falx: An MR study in 40 patients. AJNR 1991; 12:331–340.
8. El Gammal T, Allen MB, Brooks BS, et al: MR evaluation of hydrocephalus. AJNR 1987; 8:591–597.
9. Hakim S, Adams RD: The special clinical problem of symptomatic hydrocephalus with normal cerebrospinal fluid pressure, observations on cerebrospinal fluid dynamics. J Neurol Sci 1965; 2:307–327.
10. Adams RD, Fisher CM, Hakim S, et al: Symptomatic occult hydrocephalus with "normal" cerebrospinal fluid pressure: A treatable syndrome. N Engl J Med 1965; 273:117–126.
11. Bradley WG, Whittemore AR, Kortman KE, et al: Marked cerebrospinal fluid void: Indicator of successful shunt in patients with suspected normal-pressure hydrocephalus. Radiology 1991; 178:459–466.
12. Meyer JS, Kitagawa Y, Tanahaski N, et al: Evaluation of treatment of normal-pressure hydrocephalus. J Neurosurg 1985; 62:513–521.
13. Maytal J, Alvarez LA, Elkin CM, et al: External hydrocephalus: Radiologic spectrum and differentiation from cerebral atrophy. AJNR 87; 8:271–278.

7

CEREBROVASCULAR DISEASE

By comparison to other organ systems, the brain is a metabolically active organ that receives 15% of the resting cardiac output, accounts for 20% of oxygen consumption, and yet comprises only 2% of the adult total body weight.[1] The brain requires a constant supply of oxygen and glucose. Cerebrovascular disease indicates disruption of the oxygen and glucose supplied to the brain and may be the result of multiple causes, atherosclerosis being the most common. Cerebrovascular disease is the most common etiology of acute neurology hospital admissions in the United States.

Stroke denotes a focal, nonconvulsive neurologic deficit that may be abrupt in onset or may peak in minutes to days.[2] Focal neurologic deficits that resolve within 24 hours are called transient ischemic attacks (TIAs). Those that resolve beyond 24 hours are called reversible ischemic neurologic deficits (RINDs). Stroke affects approximately 400,000 Americans annually. After myocardial infarction and cancer, stroke is the leading cause of death,[3] accounting for 10% of deaths annually. Most strokes (80%) occur secondary to ischemia. Stroke is less commonly (20%) a result of intracranial hemorrhage, most often due to hypertension. This chapter will present the ischemic disease processes of the brain; the intracranial hemorrhages have been discussed in Chapter 4.

PATHOPHYSIOLOGY

Cellular Response

The multiple complex cellular functions of the brain depend on a continuous supply of oxygen and glucose. In the presence of oxygen, glucose undergoes oxidation (Krebs cycle) to form adenosine triphosphate (ATP) molecules. These high-energy phosphate mitochondrial products fuel cellular maintenance and cellular function. The brain is unable to store sufficient quantities of oxygen or glucose; therefore, the supply of these substrates must be uninterrupted. Absence of oxygen leads to anaerobic glycolysis resulting in less efficient energy production as well as the rapid formation and accumulation of lactic acid, an unwanted byproduct.

Vascular patency and systolic blood pressure have the dominant effect on flow. Blood flow to the resting gray matter is approximately 55 ml/100g per minute. This flow is maintained over a wide variation in systolic blood pressure (45 to 160 mm Hg).[4] Autoregulation of flow is achieved through a myogenic response of the arteriolar wall. As the systolic pressure increases, the vessels constrict, increasing vascular resistance and thereby diminishing blood flow. Alternatively, as the blood pressure decreases, the blood vessels dilate, decreasing the vascular resistance and increasing flow.

Local regulation of cerebral blood flow is also mediated by tissue carbon dioxide (CO_2) and hydrogen ion concentration. Accumulation of these products results in vasodilatation and increased flow to effectively reduce or remove these substrates. Conversely, a decrease in the tissue CO_2 and hydrogen concentration results in vasoconstriction and accumulation of these substrates to a homeostatic level.

Deprived of required substrates, a predictable cascade of cellular and subcellular events takes place. The sodium-potassium pump, which is responsible for maintenance of the electrical gradient across the cell membrane, fails. Ions are released from intracellular binding sites, and there is an efflux of intracellular potassium and an influx of extracellular sodium.[2] Water accumulates within the cell owing to the osmotic gradients produced by intracellular lactate and sodium. Initially, the intracellular water represents a redistribution from the capillary and extracellular compartments with only a minimal net increase in the amount of local water. Increasing tissue acidosis and osmolality lead to mitochondrial destruction, which may occur within the first 30 minutes following significant flow reduction. The cell rapidly loses its electrical activity, and unless flow is reinstituted, cell death is imminent. Net increase in local water (extracellular edema) occurs with reperfusion. As edema accumulates, local tissue pressure and mass effect increase, further compromising microcirculatory effectiveness. The blood-brain barrier (BBB) may be irreversibly disrupted after 4 to 6 hours of ischemia. To reiterate, ischemic edema is initially intracellular and subsequently becomes both intracellular and extracellular.[5]

Pathologic examination of the brain yields two distinct patterns of ischemic brain damage. One pattern consists of a global or widespread injury resulting from reduction or cessation of flow to all or most of the brain. This type of injury is usually from extracranial causes such as systemic hypotension, cardiac arrhythmia, or cardiac arrest. The other pattern is one in which ischemic changes are focal in nature, corresponding to a known arterial or venous distribution. This focal pattern may be associated with thrombotic or embolic events. Thrombosis most commonly results from atherosclerotic disease of the carotid arteries and less commonly from fibromuscular dysplasia (FMD), trauma, carotid dissection, vasculitis, or radiation.[6] Emboli are most commonly cardiac or carotid in origin.

Regardless of the pattern of ischemic injury, the gross and microscopic appearances are similar. On gross examination, the affected area is pale and swollen, the gray white junction may be indistinct, and the brain is softened[1] (Fig. 7–1). The adjacent cerebrospinal fluid (CSF) spaces are effaced. Resolution of the acute event is associated with progressive tissue liquefaction and cyst formation.

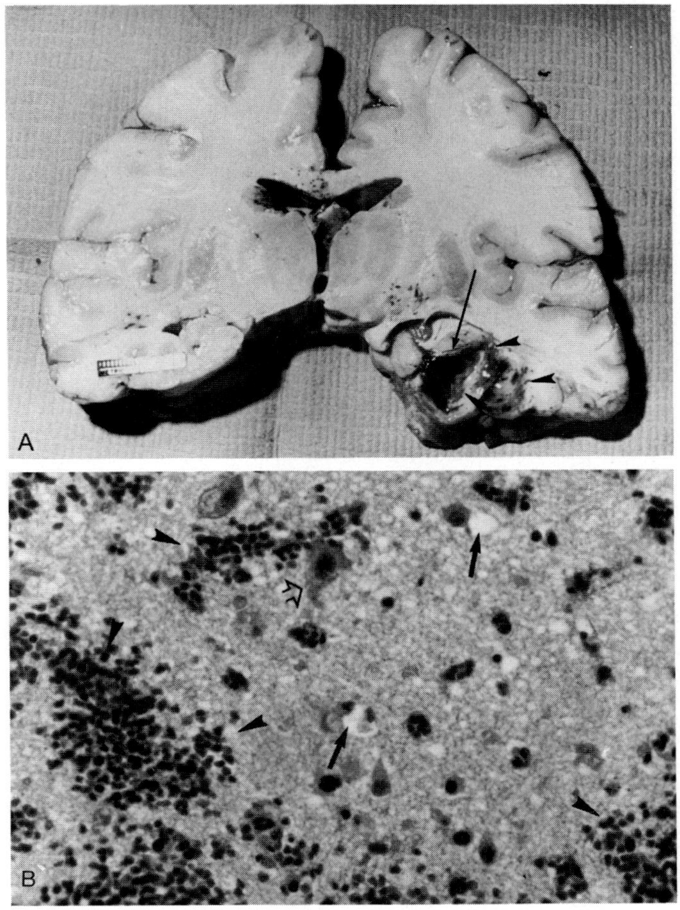

Figure 7–1. Acute infarction (pathology).

A, Gross coronal section. The left temporal lobe is soft and diffusely swollen. The infarcted center (*arrow*) fragmented during brain fixation. Acute petechial hemorrhage (*arrowheads*) surrounds the infarct.

B, Microscopic (Hematoxylin and eosin [H/E] original × 310). Pallor, glial cell vacuolization and swelling (*arrows*), parenchymal red cell extravasation (*arrowheads*), and neuronal eosinophilic necrosis (*open arrow*) corroborate acute cerebral infarction. (Courtesy of P. J. Cera, M. D., Department of Pathology, Geisinger Medical Center.)

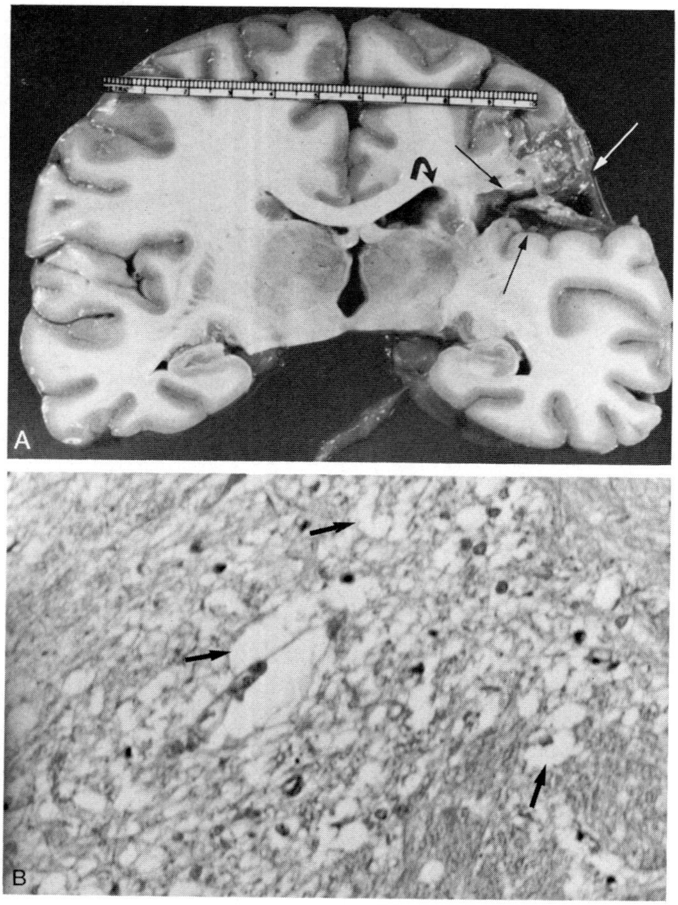

Figure 7–2. Chronic infarction (pathology).

A, Gross coronal section. Focal volume loss (*arrows*) with cystic changes are present in the left parietal lobe. The ipsilateral lateral ventricle (*curved arrow*) is commensurately enlarged, reflecting the focal volume loss.

B, Microscopic (H/E, original × 310). Microcystic change (*arrows*) and glial cell dropout are noted in this chronic cerebral infarction. (Courtesy of P. J. Cera, M. D., Department of Pathology, Geisinger Medical Center.)

The microscopic appearance is heralded by eosinophilic necrosis of neurons in which the cytoplasm becomes intensely eosinophilic and the nucleus pyknotic. Reactive changes include transient inflammatory cell infiltration, vascular and astrocytic proliferation, and phagocytic mobilization.[2] The necrotic tissue is phagocytized, and endothelial proliferation repairs damaged vessels.

The end-stage result of ischemic disease is a well-demarcated focus of soft, cavitated tissue. The surrounding CSF spaces are enlarged to compensate for the parenchymal volume loss (Fig. 7–2). The parenchyma does not scar, as collagen is not elaborated by astrocytes. Fibroblasts are distributed perivascularly, are not present in significant concentrations within the brain, and do not play a significant role in resolution of cerebral infarcts. Microscopically, fibrillary astrocytes replace the infarcted parenchyma.

It is estimated that 20% of infarctions may be associated with parenchymal hemorrhage. In truth, petechial hemorrhage may be detected microscopically in most infarcts. Gross hemorrhagic infarctions commonly result from embolic or venous occlusive disease. In the former, the embolus is lodged within a vessel of similar size. In the absence of well-defined collaterals, the endothelium and parenchyma distal to the embolus undergo ischemic changes. The embolus is lysed within 2 to 3 days, and when flow is reinstituted, arterial pressure will exceed the ability of the damaged endothelium to contain the blood within the vessel, resulting in parenchymal hemorrhage. Venous occlusive disease results in congestion, stasis, and vascular disruption as the continued egress of blood from the arterial side accumulates within the parenchyma.

Finally, two points warrant mention in this discussion. The first is the concept of selective vulnerability. Clearly, some neurons or cell populations are more sensitive to ischemia than are others. The areas most vulnerable to ischemia include the neurons within the third and fifth cortical layers of the cerebral cortex along the sulcal valleys and arterial border zones, pyramidal cells within Sommer's sector of the hippocampus, and the cerebellar Purkinje's cells. The concept of selective vulnerability is not new, yet the responsible pathophysiologic mechanism(s) remains controversial. Factors that may be responsible in part or in concert include the following: (1) Regions vary with respect to metabolism; (2) regions in the distal-most arterial supply and border zones are last to receive flow and hence are most susceptible to hypoperfusion[2]; and (3) neurotransmitters or exicotoxins (specifically glutamate and aspartate) may be released, exacerbating the local effects of ischemia.[1]

A final concept to mention is that of the ischemic penumbra. In the acute stage of infarction, the central necrotic tissue is often surrounded by a zone of nonfunctional but viable tissue. Current therapeutic regimens are directed toward the salvage of this precariously situated zone of viable tissue. The flow threshold for failure of normal electrical activity is higher than that for failure of energy metabolism.[7] Electrical function may be absent even though the neurons may be viable.

Imaging

Planar imaging provides a means to distinguish arterial vascular zones. The anterior, middle, and posterior cerebral arteries and the border zones between these vessels are presented in Figure 7–3. Knowledge of these vascular territories is extremely practical in evaluating patients with cerebral infarction and in predicting the etiology of the infarction.

In general, the anterior cerebral artery supplies the majority of the frontal lobes. The posterior cerebral artery supplies the majority of the occipital lobes as well as the base of the temporal lobes. The anterior two thirds of the parenchyma along the interhemispheric fissure is supplied by the anterior cerebral artery; the posterior third is supplied by the posterior cerebral artery. The middle cerebral artery supplies the majority of the supratentorial parenchyma, including most of the parietal and temporal lobes and portions of the frontal and occipital lobes. The basal ganglia and deep white matter are supplied by perforating lenticulostriate arteries from the anterior and middle cerebral arteries and the thalmoperforators and thalmogeniculate arteries from the posterior communicating and posterior cerebral arteries, respectively.

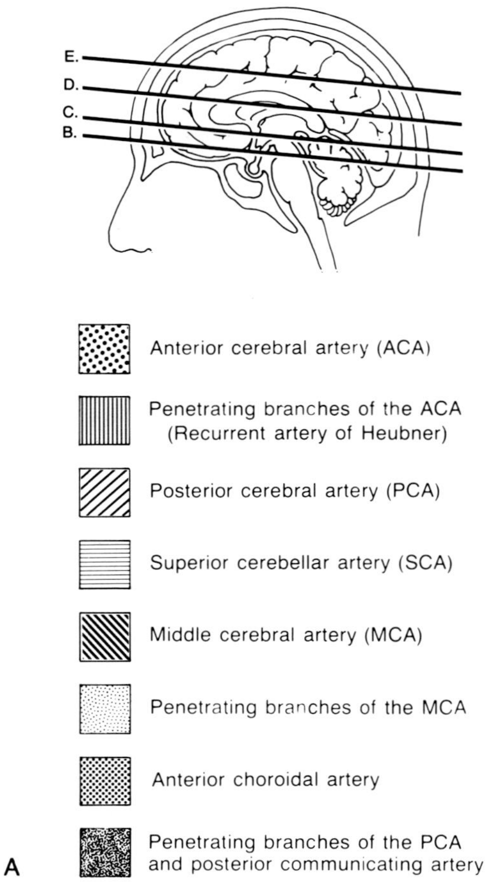

Figure 7–3. Vascular territories; axial planar imaging.

Computed Tomography

One of the initial applications of computed tomography (CT) was in the evaluation of patients with suspected cerebral infarction. As recently as 1988, 20% of all cranial CT examinations were performed to confirm stroke, and 80% of clinically diagnosed strokes were corroborated by CT.[8] The major role of CT in these patients is to exclude inflammatory or neoplastic processes that clinically may masquerade as cerebral infarction.

The initial CT findings of cerebral infarction include a vague, poorly circumscribed hypodensity. The gray-white junction may be obscured and minimal local mass effect may be evident as sulcal or ventricular compression or displacement.[8–10] It is important to note that the CT findings may lag behind the clinical findings by up to 48 hours. As the intracellular and extracellular water accumulates, the edema and mass effect become better delineated. The infarct becomes more hypodense and may assume a wedge shape, conforming to a known vascular distribution (Figs. 7–4, 7–5, 7–6). The degree of mass effect will peak by 3 days.

Evaluation of subtle gray-white matter junction changes in the periphery is hampered by beam-hardening artifact from the overlying calvarium. The basal ganglia and insular cortex are deep to the inner table, where beam-hardening artifacts are diminished. Accordingly, ischemic changes in these deep gray matter structures have been reported as early as 6 hours postictus. Partial or complete obscuration of the lentiform nucleus[11] and insular ribbon[12] may be the first indicator of a perforating or middle cerebral artery (MCA) infarction (Fig. 7–7). This sign is frequently detected earlier than similar changes in the peripheral gray-white junction.

A frequently reported secondary sign of cerebral infarction is the dense MCA sign[13–16] (Fig. 7–8). This sign may be present in thrombotic or embolic infarcts and may precede the

Text continued on page 213

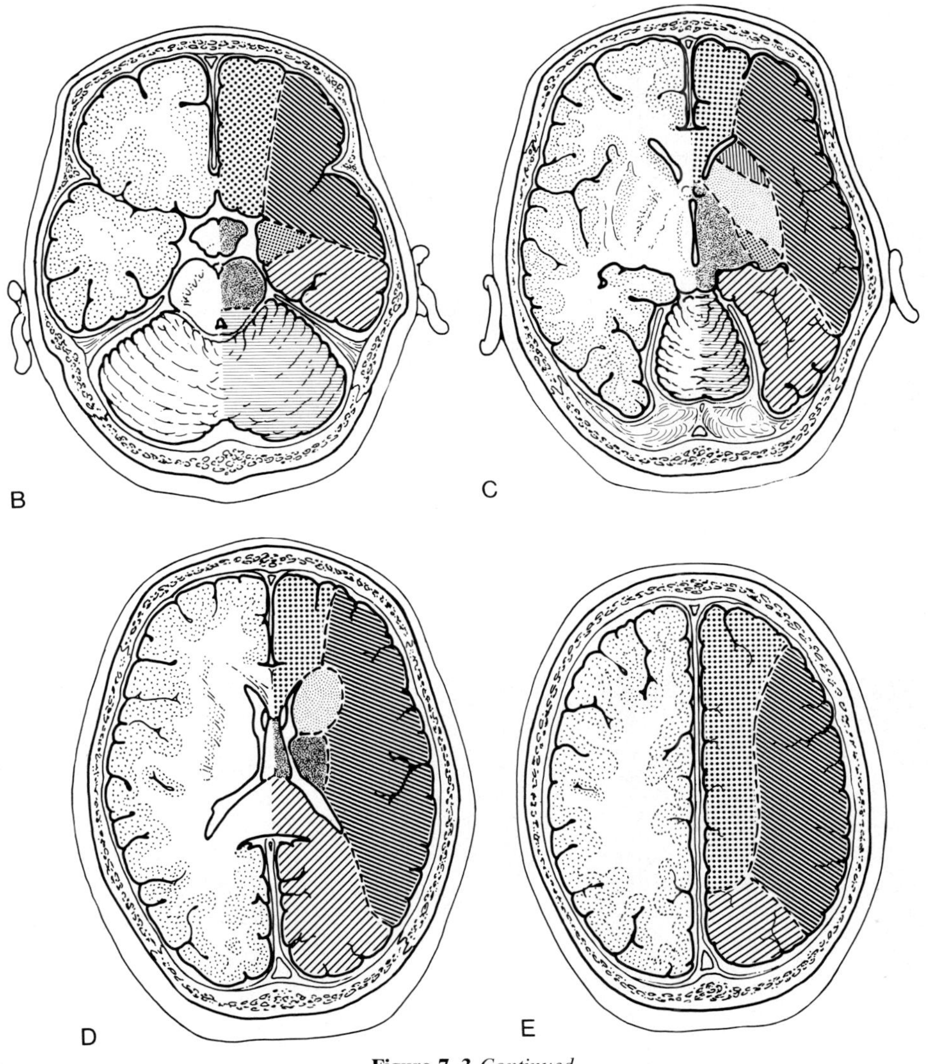

Figure 7–3 *Continued*

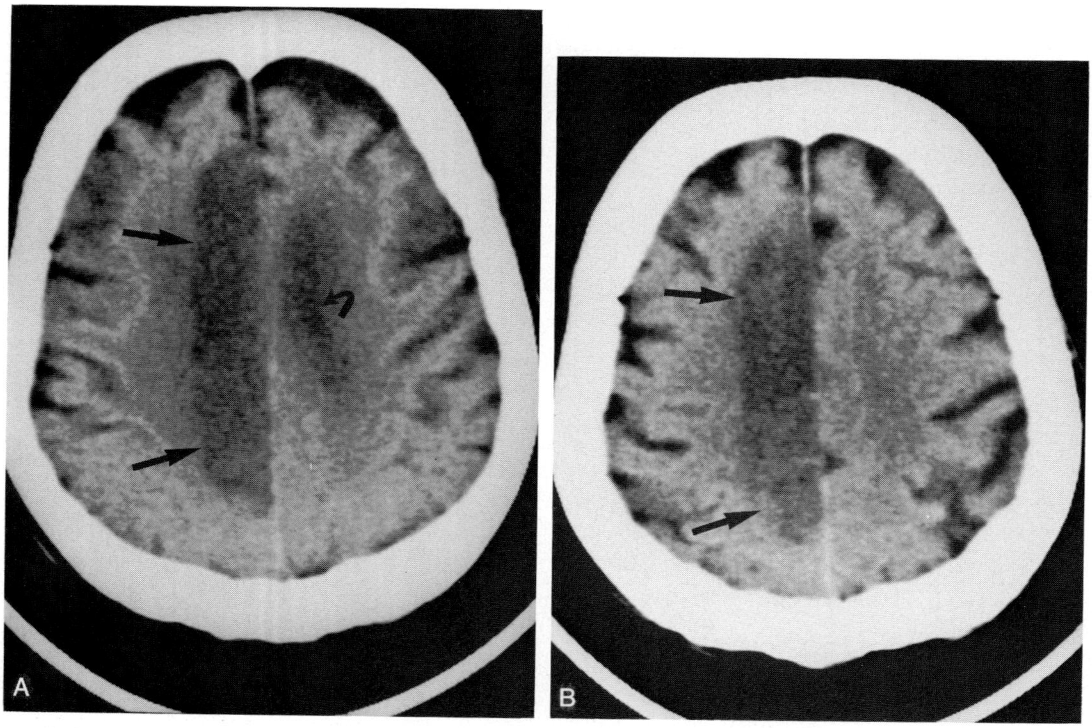

Figure 7–4. Subacute right anterior cerebral artery (ACA) infarction (65-year-old female).

A, B, Unenhanced computed tomography (CT). A hypodensity (*arrows*) involving the white matter and cortex of the interhemispheric surface of the right parietal lobe is noted, corresponding to the right ACA distribution. The adjacent sulci are compressed, indicating the subacute nature of this lesion. The hypodensity in the left cerebral hemisphere (*curved arrow*) represents the cephalad-most portion of the left lateral ventricle.

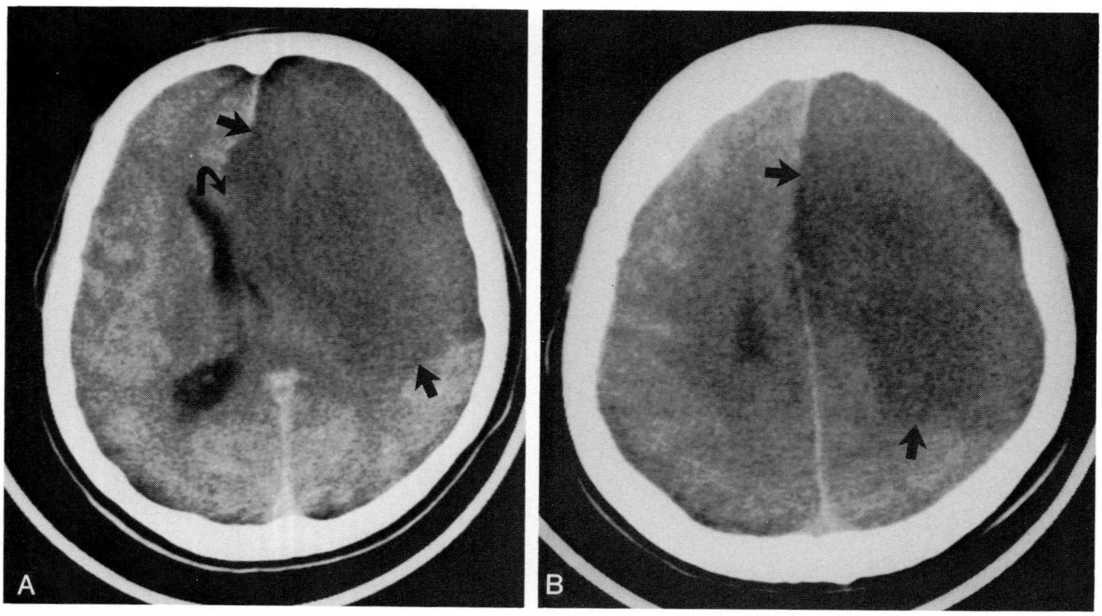

Figure 7–5. Subacute left ACA and middle cerebral artery (MCA) infarct (60-year-old male).

A, B, Unenhanced CT. A large, wedge-shaped hypodensity (*arrows*) involving both gray and white matter is present in the left frontal and parietal lobes. Left-to-right subfalcial herniation (*curved arrow*) is noted. The posterior cerebral artery (PCA) and distal portions of the MCA are spared from this ischemic edema.

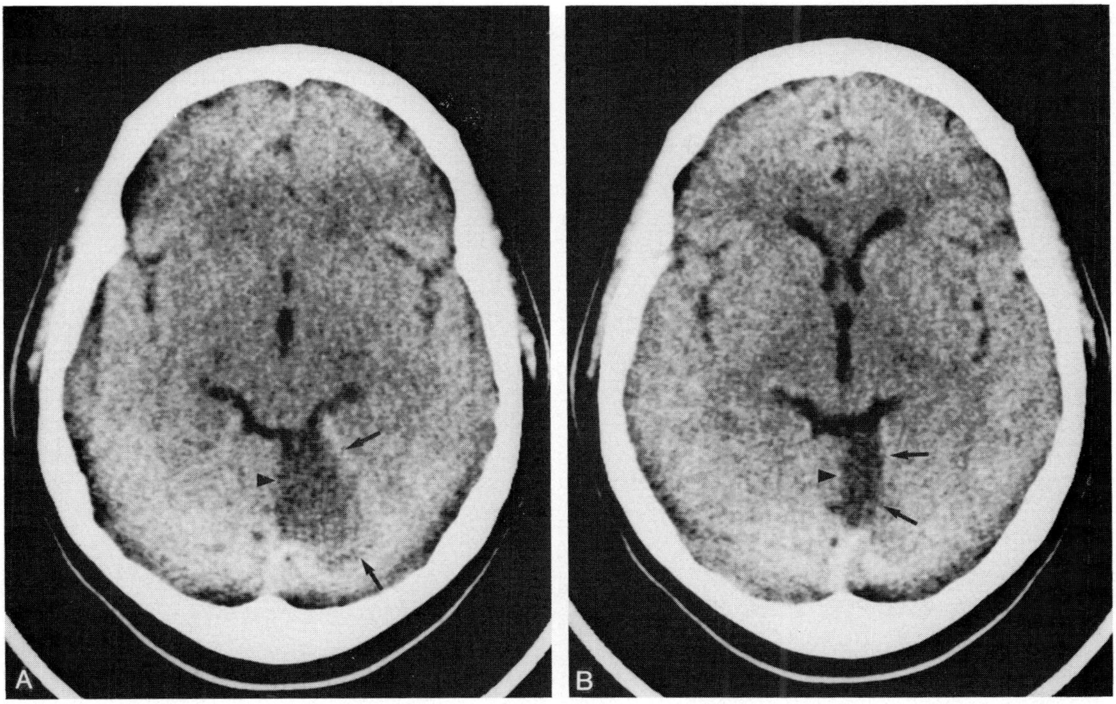

Figure 7–6. Subacute superior cerebellar artery infarction (44-year-old female).
A, B, Unenhanced CT. A hypodensity is present in the left paramedian superior cerebellar hemisphere. The ischemic edema respects the midline (*arrowhead*) and the tentorium (*arrows*).

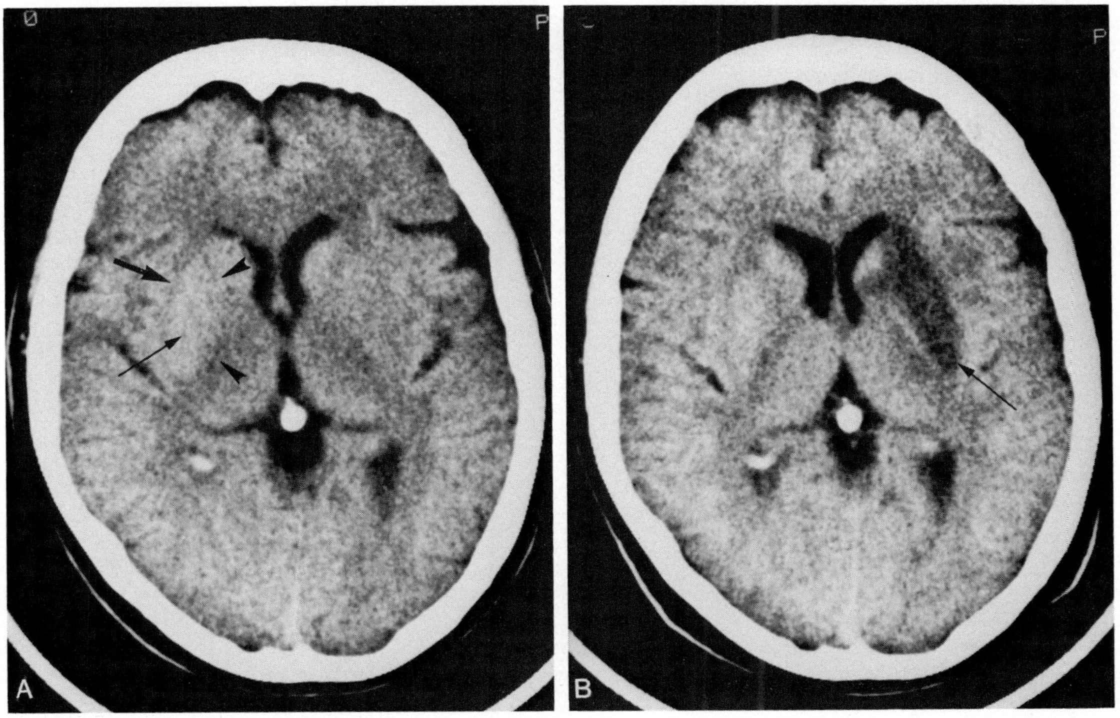

Figure 7–7. Acute left MCA infarction (65-year-old female).
A, Unenhanced CT (2 hours postictal). The density of the left lentiform nucleus is diminished and nearly indistinguishable from the adjacent white matter tracks. Note the normal right lentiform nucleus (*long arrow*) and the internal capsule (*arrowheads*) medially and the external/extreme capsule (*short arrow*) laterally.
B, Unenhanced CT (48 hours postictal). Ischemic edema is present in the left lentiform nucleus (*arrow*) signifying the presence of a subacute lateral lenticulostriate artery infarction.

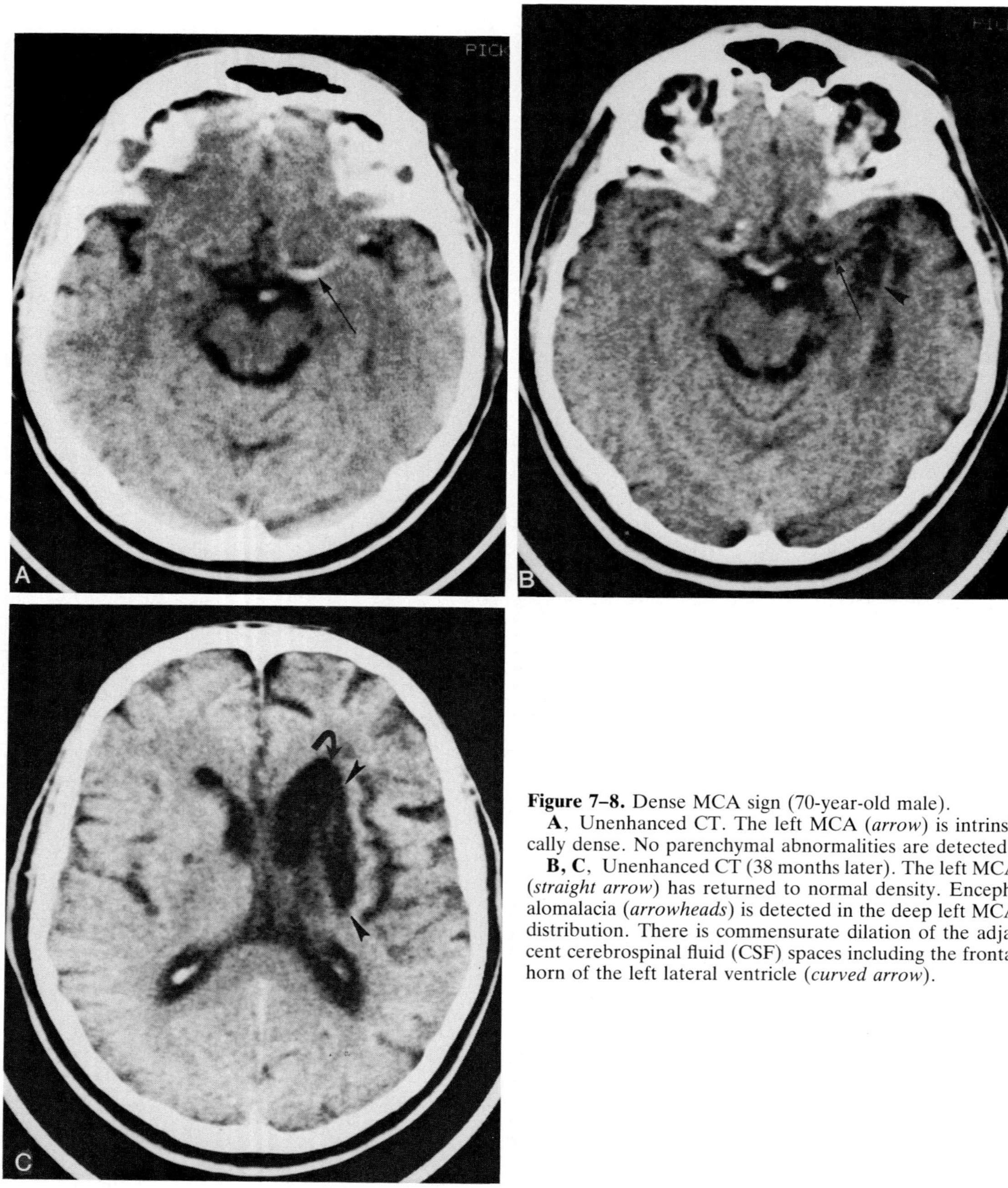

Figure 7–8. Dense MCA sign (70-year-old male).

A, Unenhanced CT. The left MCA (*arrow*) is intrinsically dense. No parenchymal abnormalities are detected.

B, C, Unenhanced CT (38 months later). The left MCA (*straight arrow*) has returned to normal density. Encephalomalacia (*arrowheads*) is detected in the deep left MCA distribution. There is commensurate dilation of the adjacent cerebrospinal fluid (CSF) spaces including the frontal horn of the left lateral ventricle (*curved arrow*).

eminent parenchymal changes. Anecdotal reports suggest this sign is a poor prognostic indicator as it implies major vessel occlusion.[16] This sign has a relatively low sensitivity and specificity and should be used with caution as MCA density may be due to atherosclerotic calcification and partial volume averaging of the contralateral MCA[14] (Fig. 7–9).

The edema begins to diminish after 4 to 5 days. Within a week to 10 days following an infarction, the edema continues to resolve to the point that the infarct, initially hypodense, may become isodense to adjacent normal parenchyma. Commensurate diminution in mass effect occurs, potentially rendering the infarct inconspicuous.

The CT properties of hemorrhage have been discussed in Chapter 4. Hemorrhage typically occurs 2 to 4 days postictus and is most commonly seen in patients receiving anticoagulant therapy (Fig. 7–10) or in patients in whom reperfusion of a damaged endothelial bed is observed. Reperfusion may be secondary to embolus lysis or collateral circulation (Fig. 7–11). The hemorrhage is often poorly marginated, interspersed among hypodense, infarcted, edematous parenchyma. The blood may be deposited heterogeneously within the cortex or subcortical region rather than forming a focal hematoma.

Chronic infarctions are manifest by volume loss (encephalomalacia). Generally, a well-circumscribed hypodensity is present with expansion of the adjacent CSF spaces including the sulci and the ventricle (Figs. 7–12, 7–8*C*). Rarely calcifications of varying size and number have been reported in chronic infarcts.[17]

Another finding associated with large chronic infarction is wallerian degeneration. When the nerves of the motor cortex undergo cell death, the axons that extend from the cortex through the brainstem undergo lysis by 1 week. The surrounding axon sheath is absorbed by 6 months.[18] Loss of these axons and surrounding myelin sheath results in volume loss, with a decreased size of the ipsilateral midbrain and pons.

Although our routine evaluation of patients with suspected stroke is performed without contrast, iodinated intravenous (IV) contrast may play an important role in the detection of cerebral infarction. In an early report,[19] 11%

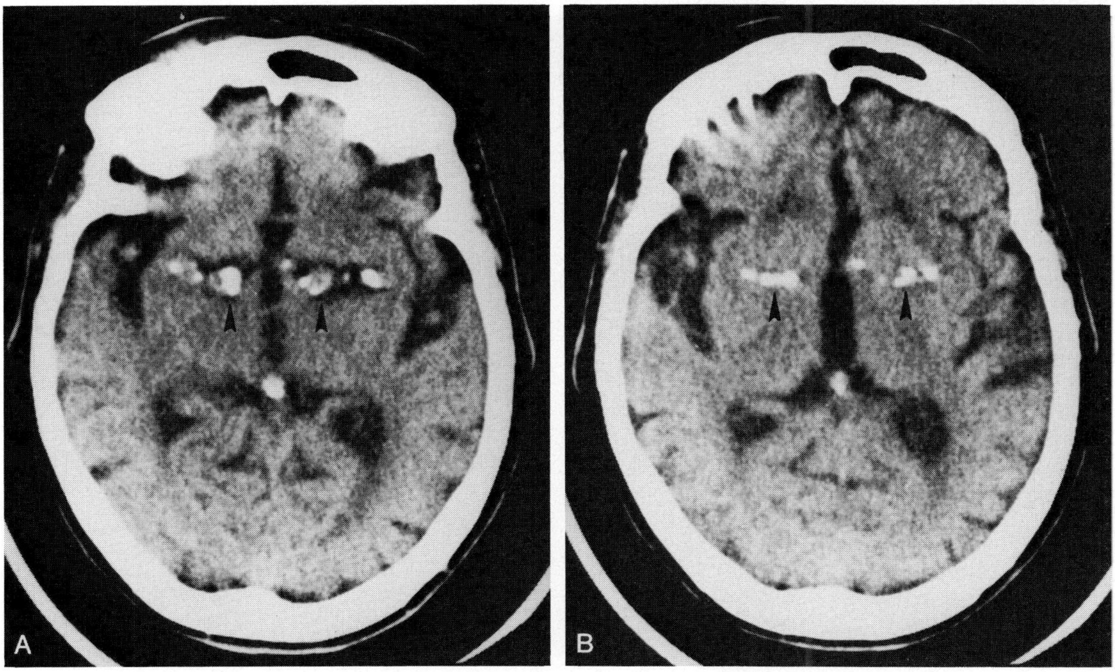

Figure 7–9. Diffuse atherosclerotic calcification of the MCAs (76-year-old male).

A, B, Unenhanced CT. Marked calcification of the MCAs (*arrowheads*) is present bilaterally. This is one of many conceivable pitfalls in the diagnosis of the dense MCA sign.

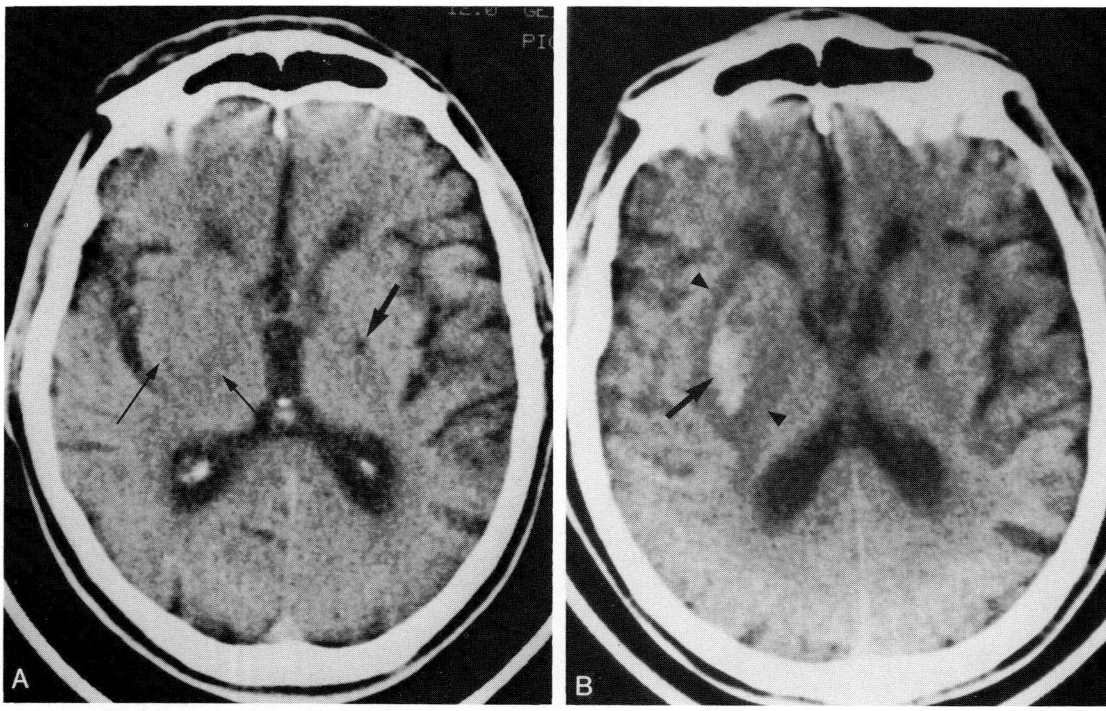

Figure 7–10. Hemorrhagic infarction (64-year-old male).

A, Unenhanced CT. Initially interpreted as normal, scan shows a vague hypodensity (*long arrows*) in the right lentiform nucleus. Incidentally, a chronic lacunar infarct (*short arrow*) is present in the posterior limb of the left internal capsule.

B, Unenhanced CT. Four days following therapeutic anticoagulation, a parenchymal hemorrhage (*arrow*) is evident with surrounded edema (*arrowheads*).

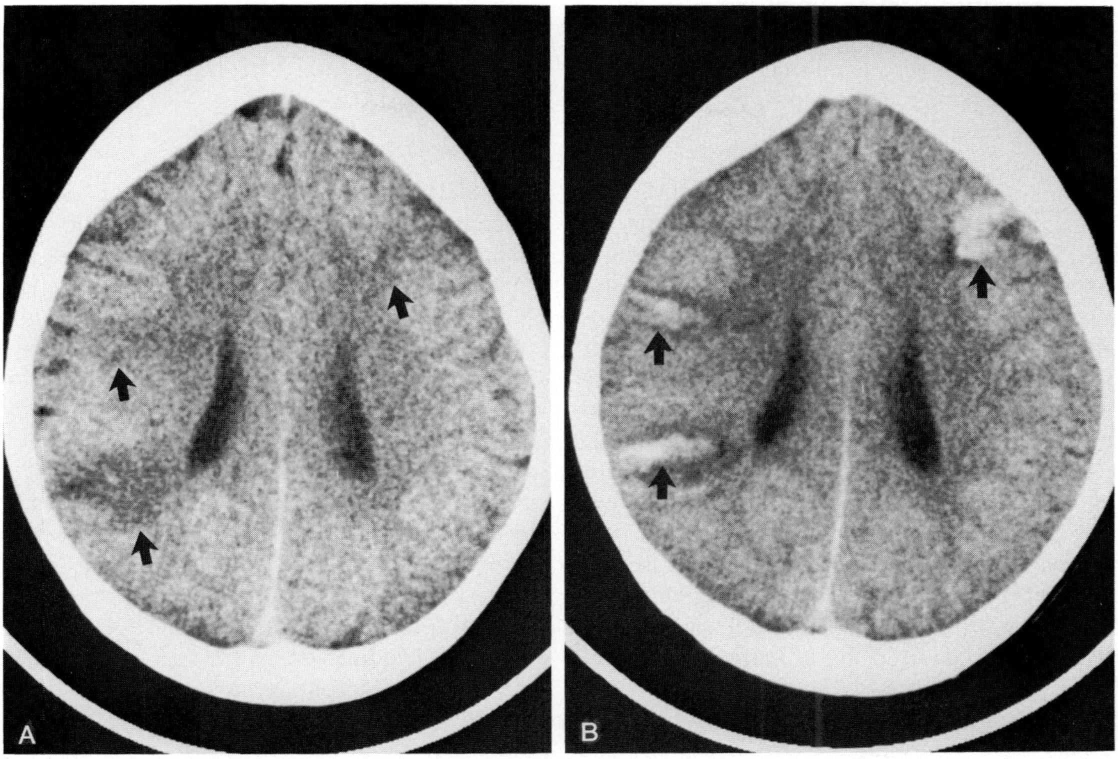

Figure 7–11. Hemorrhagic infarction (9-year-old male with sickle cell disease and cardiac thrombus).

A, Unenhanced CT (24 hours postictal). Ill-defined hypodensities (*arrows*) are present in the right and left MCA distribution. Multivessel disease suggests an embolic source.

B, Unenhanced CT (72 hours postictal). Parenchymal hemorrhage (*arrows*) has occurred in the interval with evidence of mild local mass effect and surrounding edema.

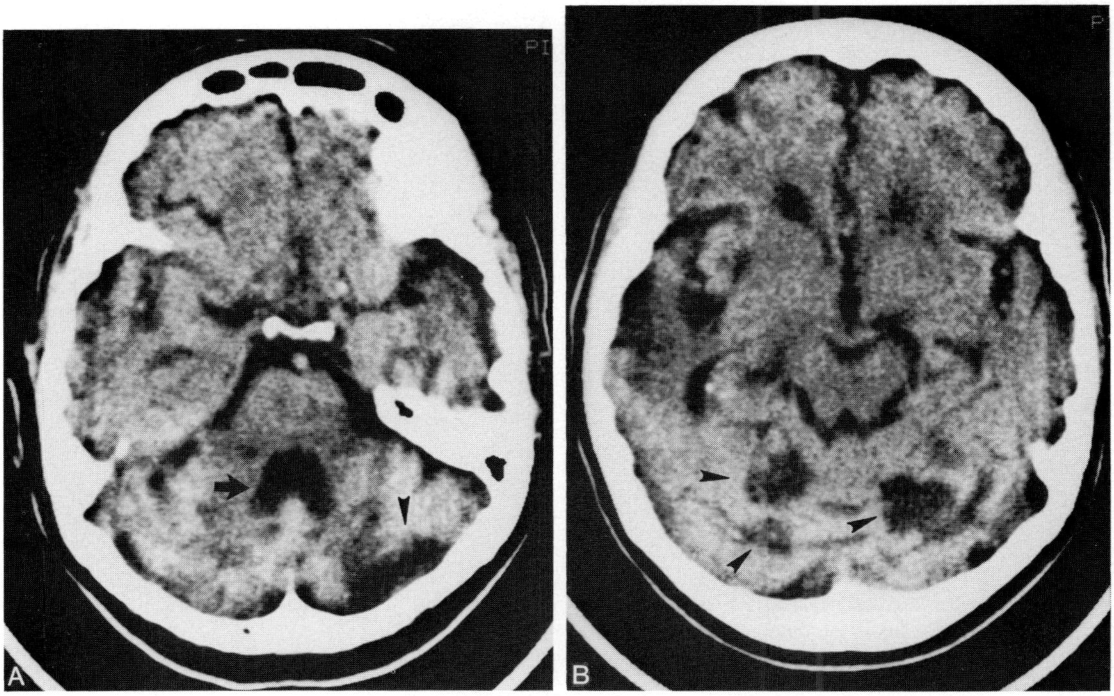

Figure 7–12. Chronic cerebellar infarction (81-year-old female).

A, B, Unenhanced CT. Multiple foci of encephalomalacia (*arrowheads*) are present in the cerebellar hemispheres bilaterally. The fourth ventricle (*arrow*) is commensurately enlarged, reflecting the parenchymal volume loss.

of patients with recent infarcts could be diagnosed only on the postcontrast scan. The patterns of enhancement vary. Although enhancement is predominantly peripheral or serpentine, the infarct may enhance centrally homogeneously, or heterogeneously[20] (Fig. 7–13). The timing of enhancement is also quite variable, appearing as early as 1 day and persisting as long as 9 months.[20] Several mechanisms are responsible for the enhancement that occurs after cerebral infarction. Luxury perfusion[21] refers to a hyperemic state from the vasodilatation that follows a period of vascular arrest. This may be partly related to loss of autoregulation of the cerebral blood flow triggered by tissue acidosis. Luxury perfusion may be seen immediately after reperfusion and is responsible for the early enhancement seen with infarction. Disruption of the BBB occurs 4 to 6 hours after prolonged ischemia and may also lead to parenchymal enhancement. In the reparative stage, new vessels form in attempts to reperfuse the parenchyma. These vessels frequently lack normal BBB and may be partially responsible for enhancement that occurs later than 1 week after ictus.

Magnetic Resonance Imaging

Initial experimental[22] and clinical[23] studies document the improved clinical utility that magnetic resonance imaging (MRI) provides in the detection of acute cerebral infarction. Not surprisingly, MRI is particularly sensitive to the water that accumulates within an acute infarct and surpasses CT in the early detection of infarct.[24–26] Signal changes on spin density and T2 images have proved to be relatively sensitive at documentation of infarction,[22, 23, 26] occurring as early as 2 to 4 hours after infarct in animal embolization models[22] and as early as 8 hours after infarct in clinical studies[27] (Fig. 7–14). Initially the increased signal is subtle, becoming more apparent as the edema accumulates. The high-signal changes often involve the cortex and usually respect arterial distributions. Spin density images have been reported to be more effective than T2-weighted images in defining the regional anatomy of an infarction.[26]

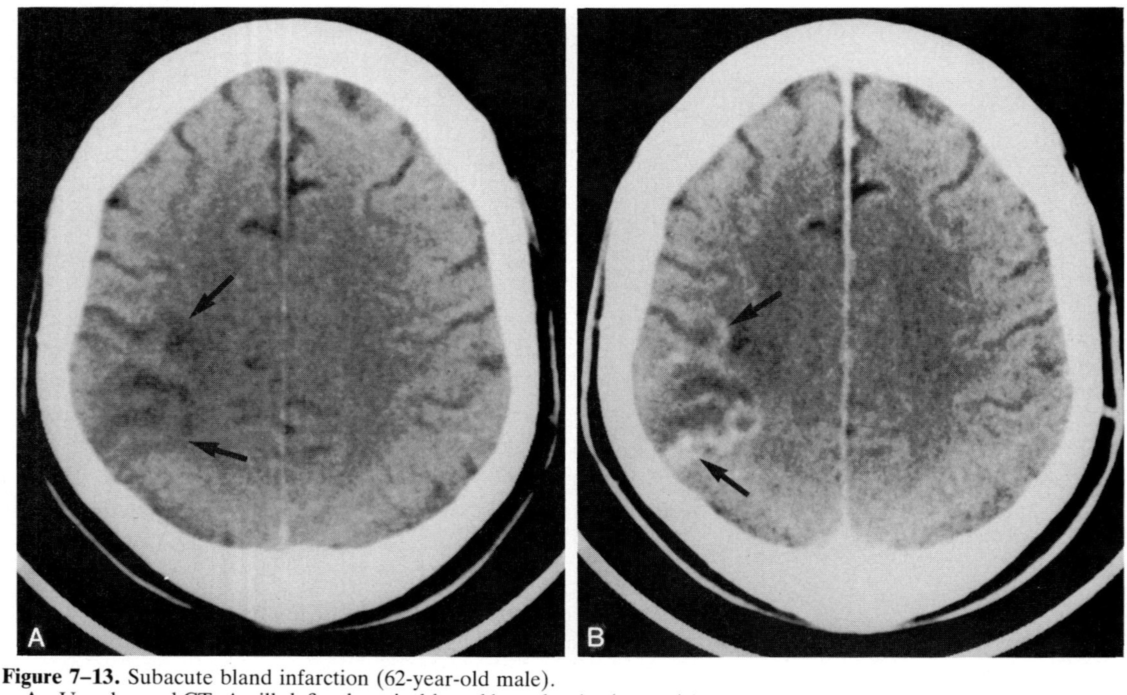

Figure 7–13. Subacute bland infarction (62-year-old male).

A, Unenhanced CT. An ill-defined cortical-based hypodensity (*arrows*) is present with local sulcal effacement indicating mass effect.

B, Enhanced CT. Serpentine cortical/subcortical enhancement (*arrows*) is the most common pattern of enhancement with a cerebral infarction.

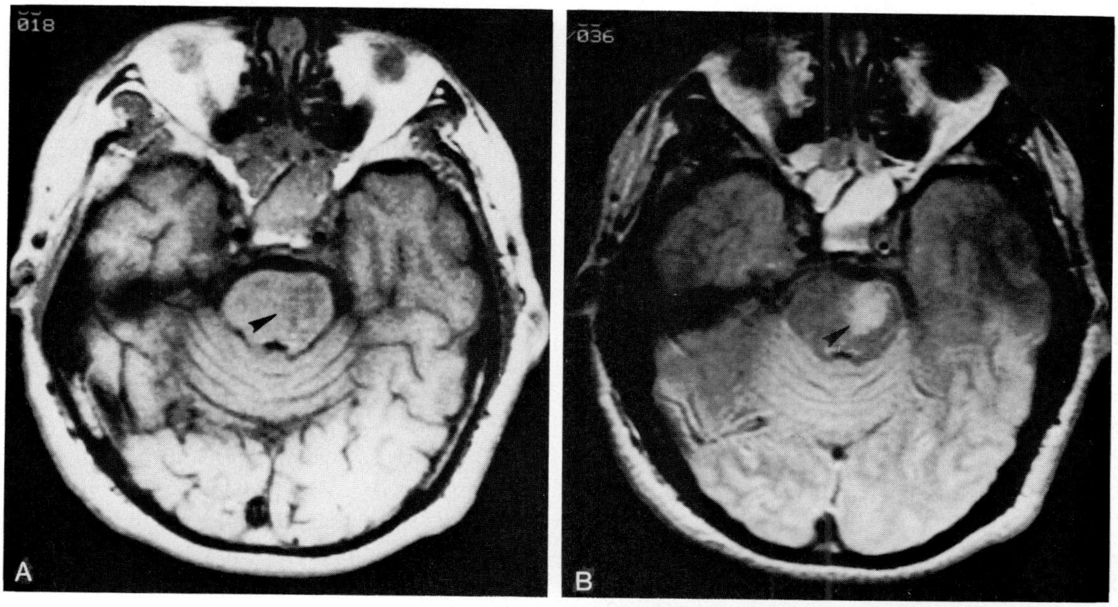

Figure 7–14. Subacute left pontine infarction (66-year-old male).

A, Axial T1. Subtle hypodensity (*arrowhead*) is evident in the left upper pons. There is mild enlargement of the pons on the left.

B, C, Axial spin density (SD) and T2. Corresponding high-signal foci (*arrowhead*) indicate the presence of an acute infarction of the deep perforating paramedian arteries, which arise from the basilar artery.

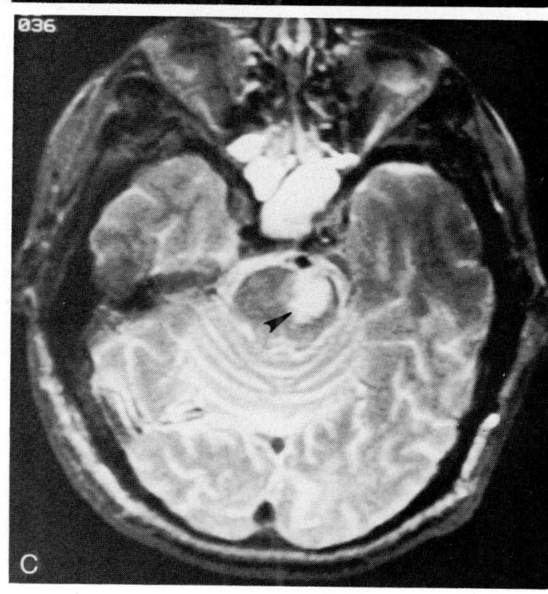

According to one author[27] the sensitivity of the T1 image in detecting infarction has been underestimated. Although actual signal changes may not occur until 16 to 24 hours postictus on the T1 images, the presence of brain swelling may be detected as early as 2 to 4 hours postictus—much sooner than the T2 signal changes just described. Brain swelling is manifest as enlargement of structures or, more commonly, distortion of normal adjacent structures. The mechanism of brain swelling in the absence of T2 signal changes is not understood. It is postulated that the water is bound to macromolecules and may not permit significant prolongation of T2 relaxation time.

Gadolinium has proven a useful adjunct in the evaluation of acute infarction. Although the initial focus of gadolinium was evaluation of parenchymal enhancement,[25, 28–30] more recent work[27, 31–33] has concentrated on vascular and meningeal enhancement. Interestingly, the presence of vascular enhancement proximal or distal to the infarct may precede other findings of acute infarction.[27, 33] This vascular enhancement is more common with cortical infarction[33] and may be accompanied by loss of arterial flow void within the adjacent arteries (Fig. 7–15). Arterial enhancement is usually transient, lasting less than 3 days.[31] Transient meningeal enhancement has been reported adjacent to larger infarctions between 2 to 6 days postictus.[31] Early parenchymal enhancement occurs by the third postictal day, unless associated with a border zone infarction, and is usually associated with minimal or reversible neurologic changes[33] (Fig. 7–16). Delayed parenchymal enhancement occurs after 7 days and is associated with more severe neurologic deficit.

The earliest reported sign of cerebral infarction is related to the blood vessel. Loss of flow void within the supplying artery or arteries may be detected as early as minutes following ictus.[33]

Chronic infarction has a variable appearance on MRI. Encephalomalacia with enlargement of surrounding CSF spaces corroborates chronicity (Fig. 7–17). The encephalomalacic cavity is isointense to CSF on T1 images. Adjacent CSF spaces are enlarged. The infarcted tissue may remain high signal on spin density and T2 images. Alternatively, if the infarct undergoes cystic necrosis, the central portion of the lesion may become isointense to CSF. A rim of gliosis may surround the lesion. The gliosis is most apparent on the spin density images as an irregular, often incomplete border of high signal.

Some investigators have demonstrated a tendency for MRI to underestimate the extent of ischemic neuronal damage. Histopathologic examination of infarcts in the rabbit model demonstrated normal spin density and T2 signal in areas of early neuronal injury. This was particularly true in the peripheral penumbra of the infarct.[34] Significant neuronal injury may occur in the face of normal MRI. This point was also corroborated in clinical series of acute infarcts in which two thirds of the patients receiving follow-up MRI demonstrated interval increase in size of the infarct. Bryan and coworkers[26] attributed this to the inability to reliably identify surrounding areas at risk for infarction.

Approximately 20% of cerebral infarctions are considered grossly hemorrhagic. The MRI signal characteristics of hemorrhage have been reviewed in Chapter 4. Unlike focal parenchymal hematomas, the hemorrhage associated with infarction is generally distributed heterogeneously throughout the infarction, often distributed in a serpentine fashion adjacent to or within the gray matter. MRI is quite sensitive in evaluating the paramagnetic moieties of subacute and chronic hematoma (Fig. 7–18). The MRI signal changes may be markedly abnormal in the face of a "normal" CT examination.

Petechial hemorrhage may be seen in most infarctions, and recently high-signal changes have been reported within infarctions on T1 images.[26, 35] These have been reported within the first 24 hours but occur more commonly in the subacute stage. There are no associated T2 signal changes detected with these lesions. These are thought to represent petechial hemorrhage from diapedesis of red blood cells from the damaged endothelium into the surrounding parenchyma.[26]

In addition to the encephalomalacic changes, excess iron deposition and wallerian degeneration may be detected in patients with chronic infarction. Excessive central iron deposition has been reported in five children who suffered from a severe ischemic event.[36] It is

Text continued on page 223

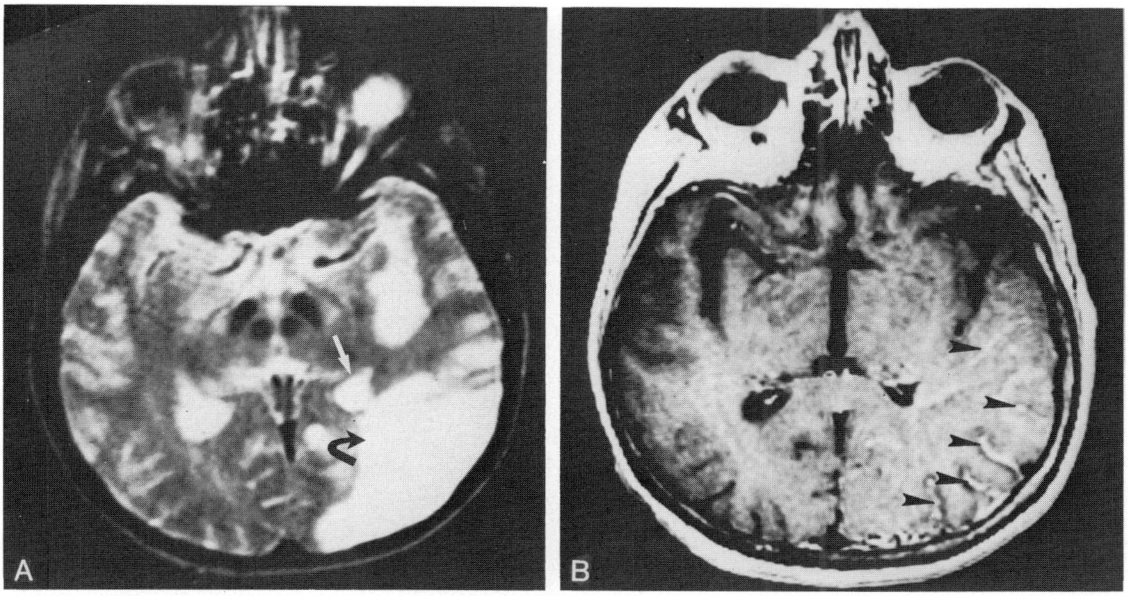

Figure 7–15. Acute left MCA infarction (62-year-old male).

A, Axial T2. High-signal ischemic edema (*curved arrow*) extends in a wedge-shaped distribution from the left atrium (*white arrow*) to the cortical surface. Moderate local mass effect is present.

B, Enhanced Axial T1. Linear foci of enhancement (*arrowheads*) are noted corresponding to pial vessels within cortical sulci. Sulcal effacement and mild compression of the left atrium corroborate the presence of local mass effect.

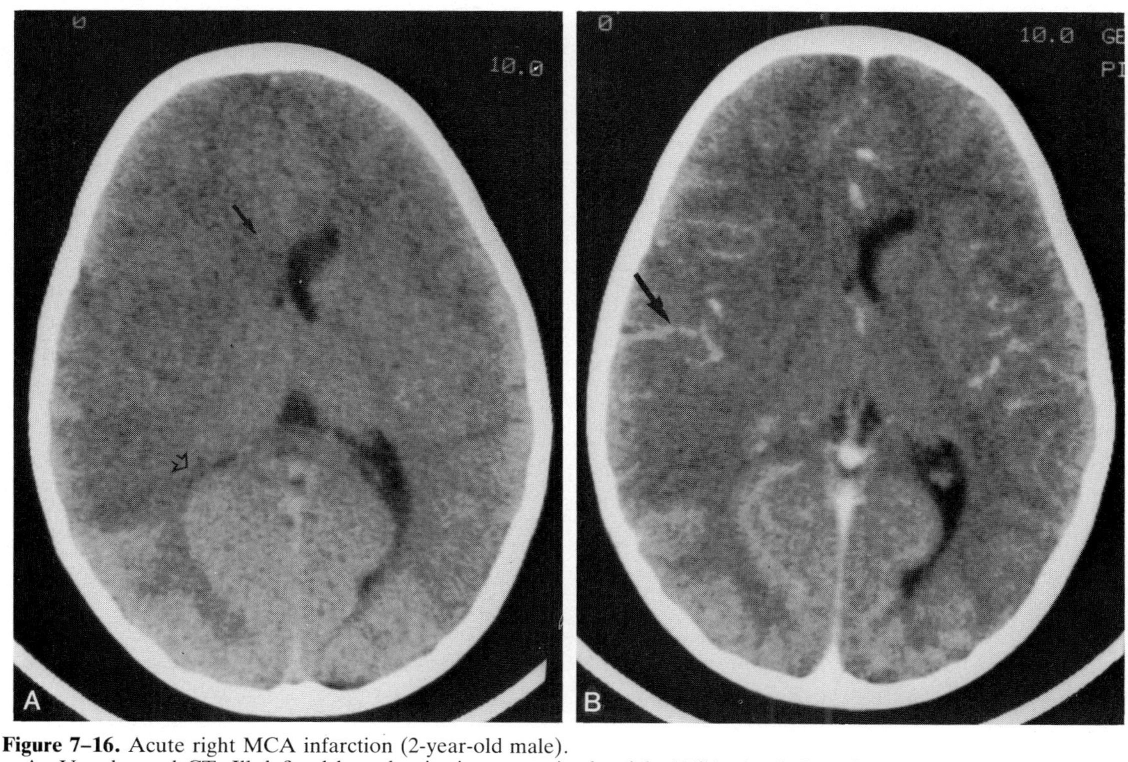

Figure 7–16. Acute right MCA infarction (2-year-old male).

A, Unenhanced CT. Ill-defined hypodensity is present in the right MCA circulation. Compression of the ipsilateral frontal horn (*closed arrow*) and atrium (*open arrow*) indicate mass effect.

B, Enhanced CT. MCA vessels (*arrow*) are prominent, yet no parenchymal enhancement is noted.

Illustration continued on following page

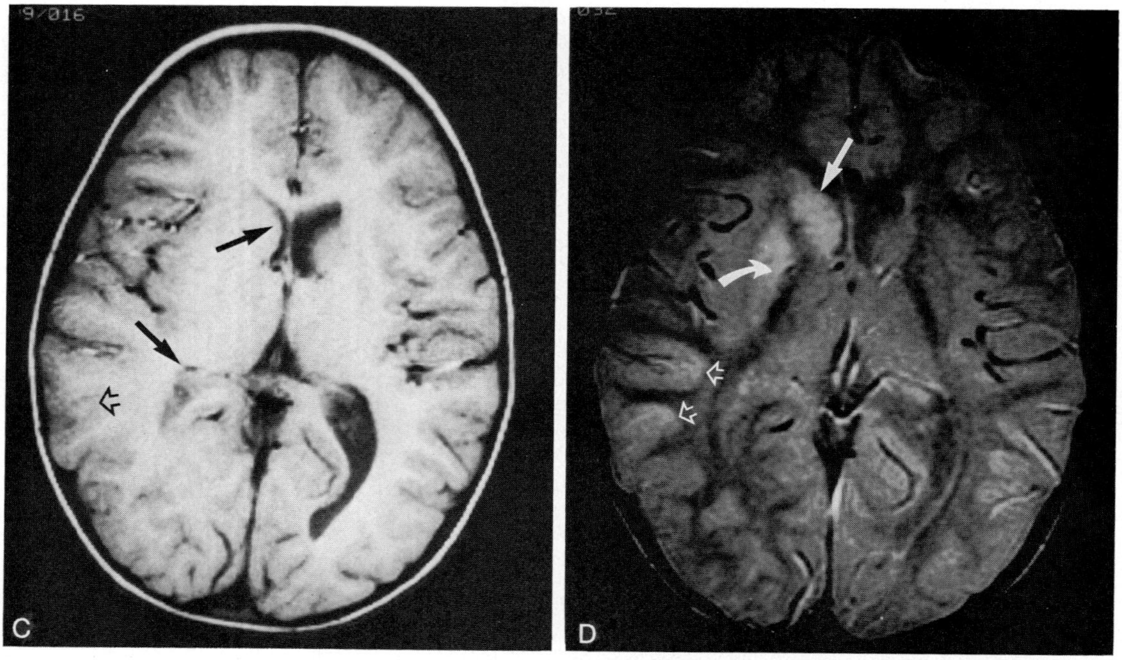

Figure 7–16 *Continued*

C, Axial T1. Mass effect is noted with compression of the ventricle (*solid arrows*) and effacement of adjacent sulci (*open arrow*).

D, Axial SD. Ischemic edema is present in the caudate head (*straight arrow*), lentiform nucleus (*curved arrow*), and over the parietal cortex (*open arrows*) on the right.

E, Enhanced axial T1. Enhancement is noted in the caudate head (*straight arrow*), lentiform nucleus (*curved arrow*), and within the affected cortical sulci (*open arrows*).

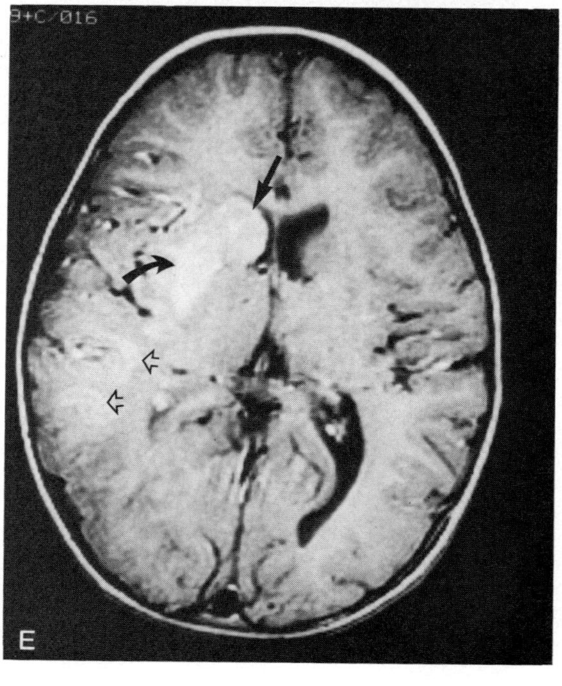

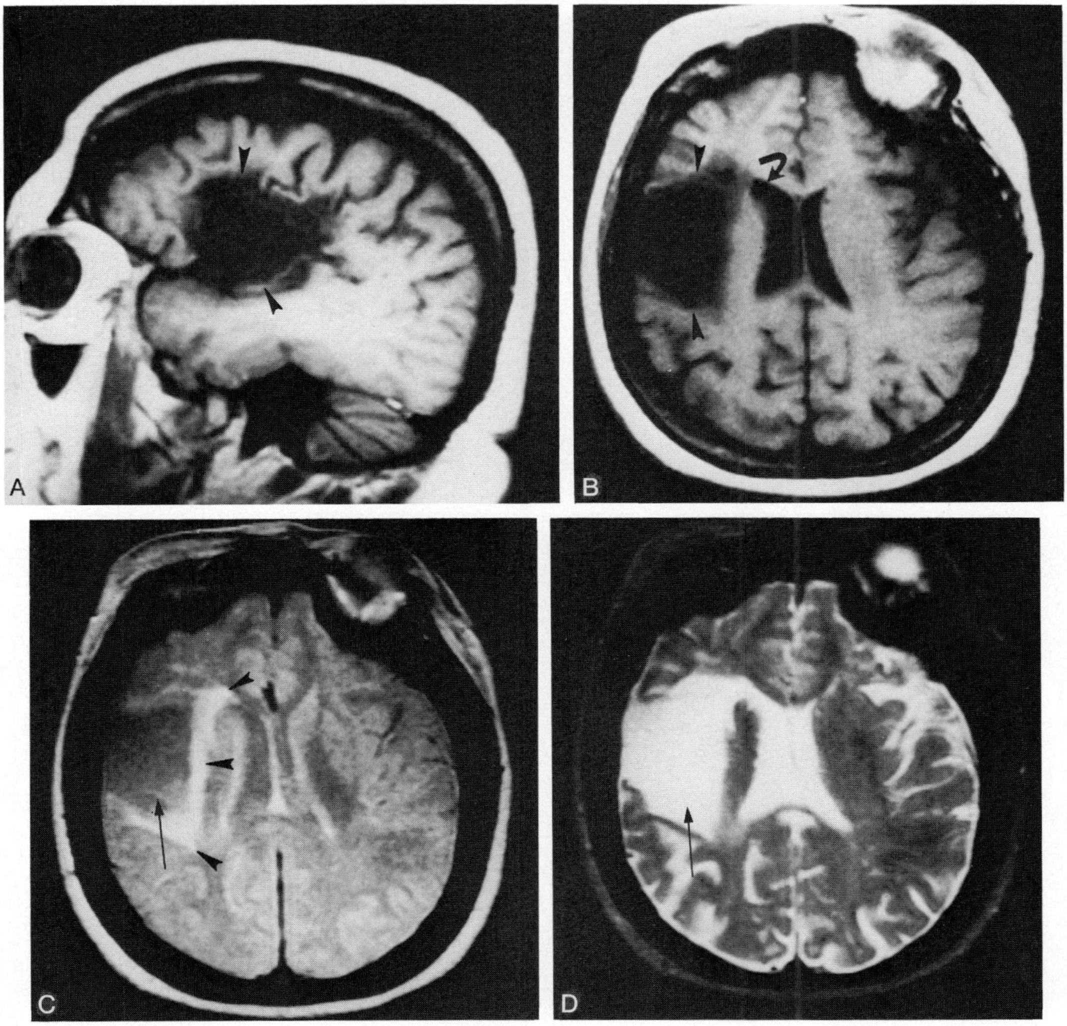

Figure 7–17. Chronic right MCA infarction (54-year-old female).

A, Parasagittal T1. An isointense-to-CSF encephalomalacic cavity (*arrowheads*) arises in place of the insular cortex.

B, Axial T1. The relationship of the cavity (*arrowheads*) to the commensurately enlarged right lateral ventricle (*curved arrow*) is noted.

C, D, Axial SD and T2. The cavity (*arrow*) remains isointense to CSF on both sequences. A halo of high signal (*arrowheads*) surrounds the parenchymal margin of the cavity. This is most conspicuous on SD image and presumably represents gliosis.

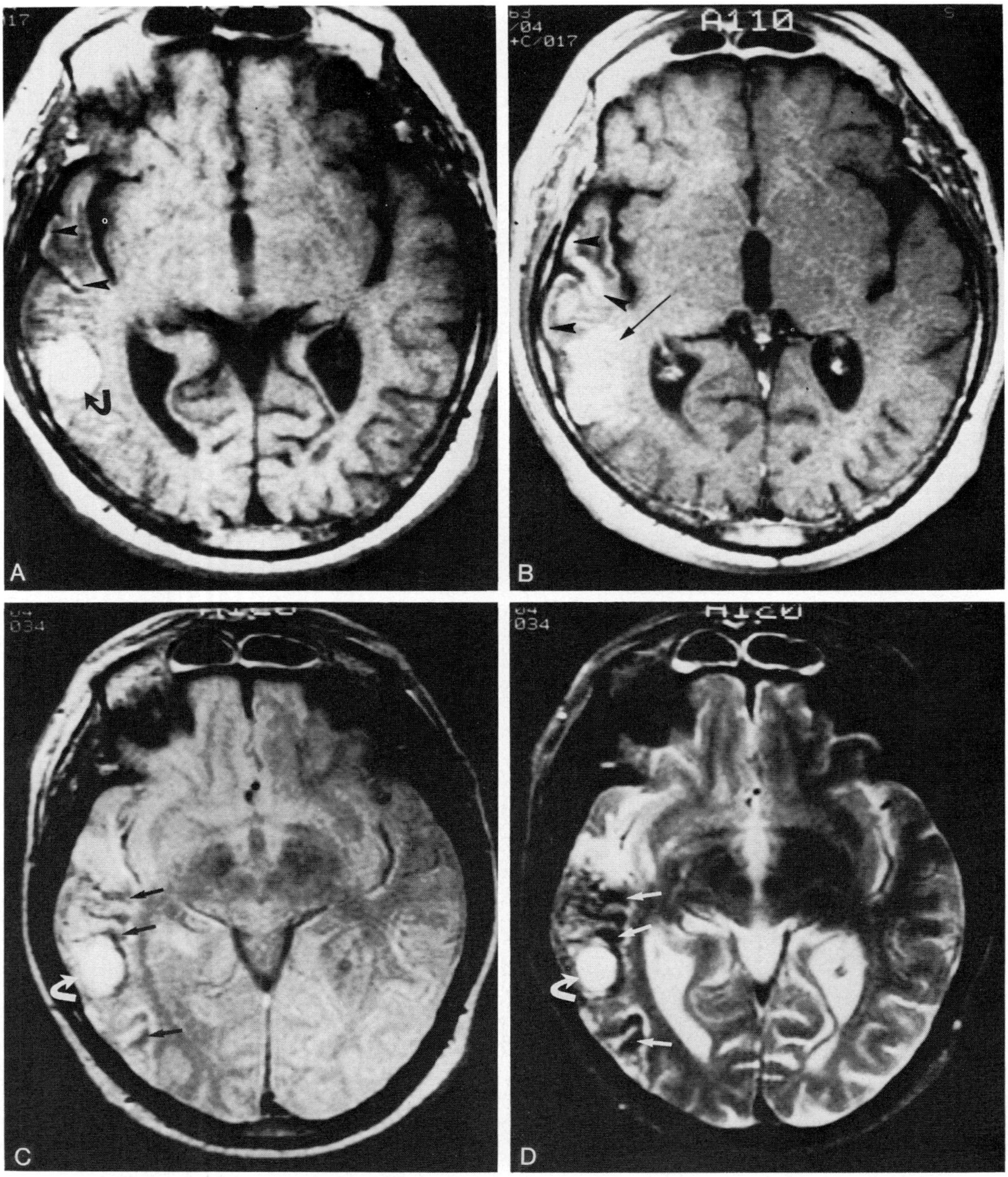

Figure 7–18. Hemorrhagic infarction (58-year-old male).

A, Axial T1. A 1.5-cm focus of increased signal intensity (*curved arrow*) indicative of methemoglobin is present in the left posterior temporal lobe. Subtle cortical foci of high signal (*arrowheads*) are also present over the anterior temporal cortex.

B, Enhanced axial T1. Serpentine enhancement over the temporal gyri (*arrowheads*) is noted, as is enhancement within the parenchyma (*arrow*).

C, D, Axial SD and T2. In addition to the extracellular methemoglobin (*curved arrow*) within the parenchyma, intracellular methemoglobin, or more likely hemosiderin/ferritin (*straight arrows*), is noted over the temporal parietal cortical mantle.

postulated that normal central to cortical axonal transport of iron ceases and iron accumulates within the basal ganglia, thalamus, and central white matter. Iron will diminish the T2 signal intensity in the corresponding regions.

Wallerian degeneration has been described in part in the preceding section. As the bulk of axonal degeneration takes place in the ipsilateral compact white matter tracts, mesencephalon and pons, and contralateral medulla along the cortical spinal tracts, MRI is ideally suited to evaluate the extent of disease, particularly within the posterior fossa.[37–40] The end-stage MRI manifestations of wallerian degeneration include atrophy (most apparent on T1 images) and high T2 signal intensity (owing to increased local water and to gliosis). Of note, a transient period (4 to 14 weeks) exists after infarction during which wallerian degeneration is manifest as low signal on T2 images. This is postulated to be secondary to myelin protein breakdown with preservation of the myelin lipids and creation of a hydrophobic tissue environment.[37]

Angiography

Despite rapid advances in magnetic resonance angiography (MRA), conventional angiography remains, at present, the procedure of choice in evaluating cerebrovascular occlusive disease in most institutions.[41] In many centers MRA has augmented carotid ultrasound for noninvasive carotid screening. In some centers, MRA findings guide surgical decisions (Fig. 7–19). Further refinement of MRA techniques, more experience with MRA, greater availability of MRA, and adjunctive use of carotid ultrasound may be necessary before conventional angiography is eliminated from the routine workup of patients with cerebrovascular disease.

The role of conventional angiography is to diagnose, localize, and quantify cerebrovascular occlusive disease.[41] The angiogram should be tailored to evaluate specific areas of suspected disease in each patient. The extracranial and intracranial course of the suspected pathologic vessels should be opacified to detect lumen narrowing (Fig. 7–20).

The chief angiographic findings of cerebral infarction include stenosis or occlusion of the arterial supply and/or alteration in circulation time, collateral circulation, and mass effect. The most common locations of atherosclerotic disease, in decreasing order, are the carotid bifurcation, carotid siphon, and circle of Willis. Quantification of arterial stenosis is imprecise, although best methods take into account a

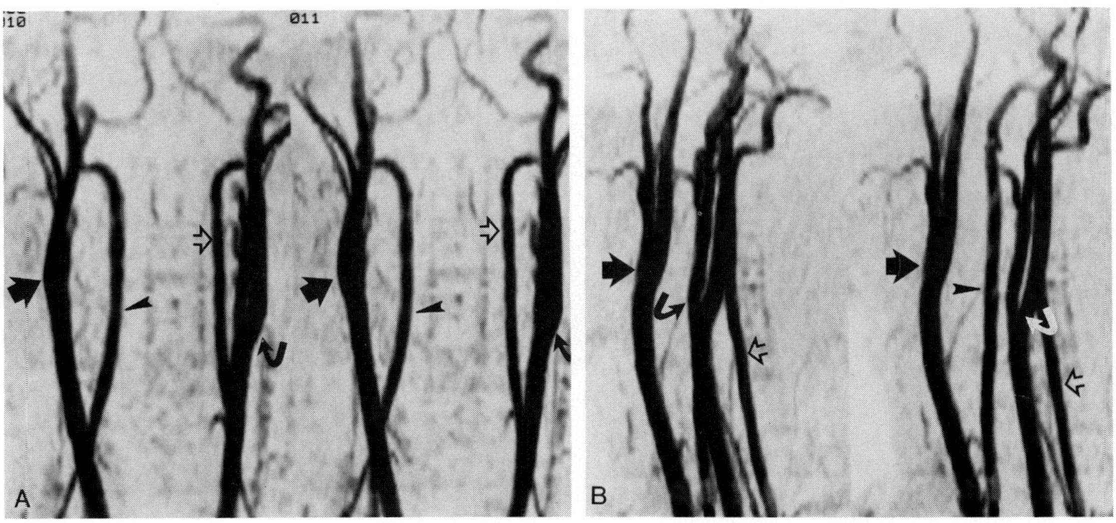

Figure 7–19. Normal magnetic resonance angiography (MRA). Two-dimensional (2D) time of flight. Neck (19-year-old-male).

A, B, In four projections, the right carotid (*arrow*) and left carotid (*curved arrow*) bifurcations are seen. Right (*arrowhead*) and left (*open arrow*) vertebral arteries are depicted.

Illustration continued on following page

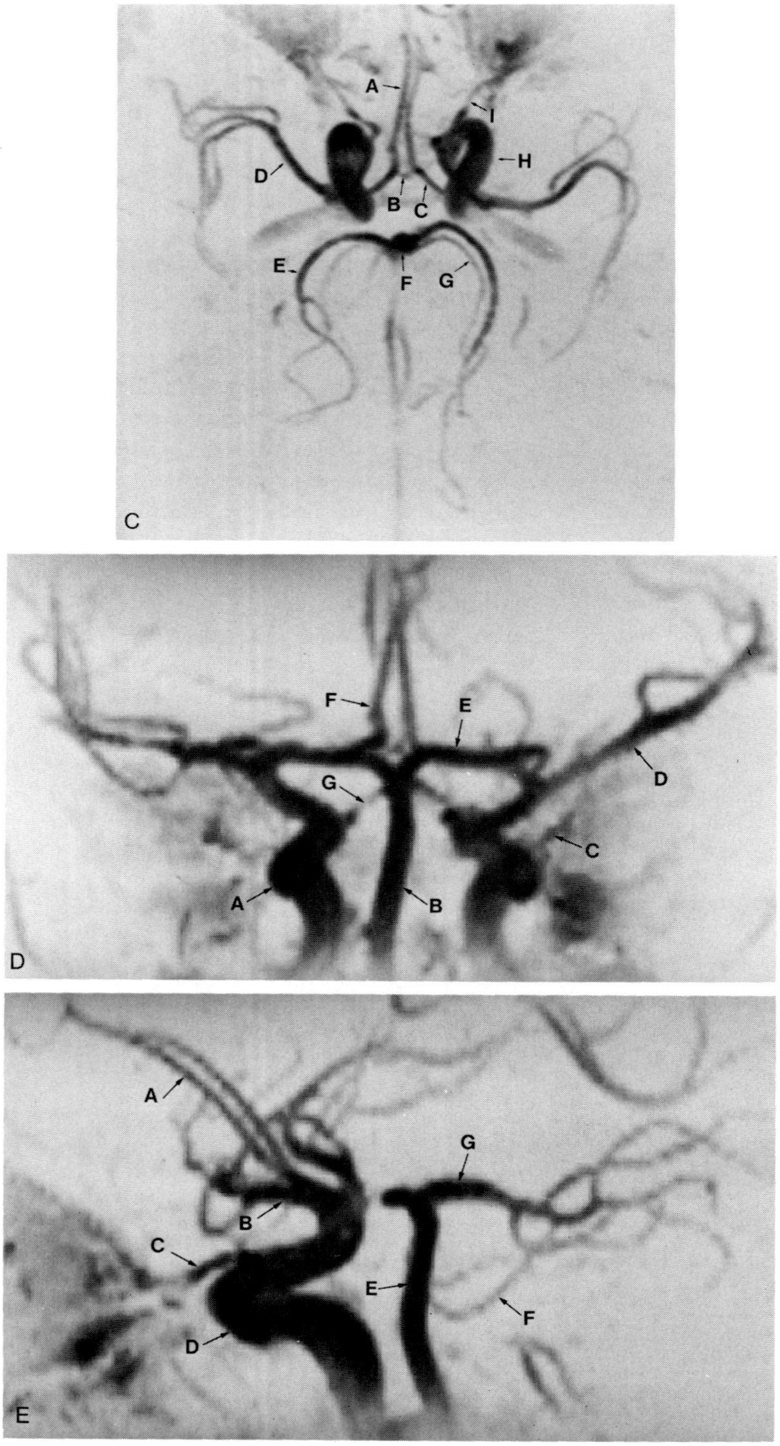

Figure 7–19 *Continued*
Three-dimensional (3D) phase contrast; circle of Willis.

C, Collapsed base view. (*A*) right A2 (ACA), (*B*) anterior communicating artery, (*C*) left A1 (ACA), (*D*) right MCA, (*E*) right PCA, (*F*) basilar, (*G*) left superior cerebellar, (*H*) left carotid siphon, (*I*) left ophthalmic artery.

D, Frontal projection view. (*A*) carotid siphon; (*B*) basilar artery; (*C*) left ophthalmic artery; (*D*) left MCA; (*E*) composite, left A1 (ACA) and left PCA; (*F*) right A2 (ACA); (*G*) right superior cerebellar.

E, Lateral projection view. (*A*) A2 (ACA), (*B*) MCA, (*C*) ophthalmic artery, (*D*) carotid siphon, (*E*) basilar artery, (*F*) superior cerebellar, (*G*) PCA.

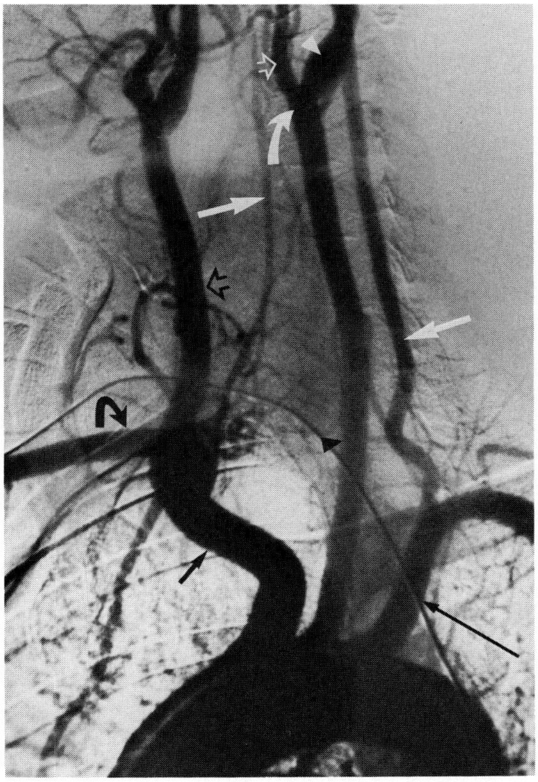

Figure 7–20. Right posterior oblique (RPO) arch aortogram (54-year-old female). The arch and takeoff of the great vessels are normal. The innominate artery (*short arrow*) and its branches, the right subclavian (*curved arrow*), and right common carotid artery (*open arrow*) are normal. The left common carotid artery (*arrowhead*) and left subclavian artery (*long arrow*) are also normal. The vertebral arteries (*white arrows*) are normal; the left is dominant. The left carotid bifurcation (*curved white arrow*) and the internal (*white arrowhead*) and external carotid arteries (*open white arrow*) are normal.

cross-sectional area referable to the normal vessel area (Fig. 7–21). The total vascular resistance depends on peripheral vascular resistance. Thus, moderate degrees of large vessel stenosis may be tolerated with a disproportionately small impact on the total resistance.[42] Although subclinical stenosis of 50 to 70% may not diminish flow or pressure, it may disrupt laminar flow, create turbulence, and predispose patients to endothelial cell injury and thrombus formation. In vivo and in vitro studies have determined that flow and pressure will be decreased in the face of a 70 to 90% stenosis of cross-sectional area.[6, 43–45] The larger the parent vessel, the greater the degree of stenosis required for flow and pressure drops.[44] When the cross-sectional area is less than 2 mm^2, blood flow will be reduced.[42, 43]

Arterial ulceration is a manifestation of atherosclerotic disease and may accompany arterial stenoses. Ulceration is secondary to endothelial or intimal loss and may result in platelet aggregation and fibrin thrombus formation. The aggregate may dislodge, resulting in distal embolization. Angiographic findings of arterial ulceration include irregularity of the arterial wall and, if advanced, a niche or outpouching of the vessel contour and delayed washout of contrast. Arterial ulceration is a gross or histologic diagnosis explaining in some cases the relatively poor correlation between the angiographic findings and the surgical findings. Only approximately 60% of surgical specimens showing ulceration are detected on angiography.[46] The overall accuracy of angiography at predicting ulceration is about 50%.

Cerebral emboli may be carotid or cardiac in origin. Angiographic findings of emboli include multiple branch occlusions within one or separate arterial vascular distributions.

Circulation time is often affected as a result of cerebral infarction.[47] Luxury perfusion[21] refers to the cerebral hyperemia that results from cerebral infarction. This concept has been described earlier in reference to the mechanism of contrast enhancement in stroke. This hyperemic state may persist for 2 weeks following infarction. The angiographic finding is local vasodilatation and early-draining vein(s) (Fig. 7–22). In addition, the circulation time to the ipsilateral or contralateral hemisphere may be prolonged, even in the absence of mass effect. Circulation to a specific region may be prolonged secondary to relative blockage at the arteriolar-capillary level.

Collateral circulation refers to the alternative pathways available for delivery of blood and substrates to a target region when the primary arterial channel is occluded. Collateral pathways develop with need. In the presence of a slowly progressive stenosis (atherosclerotic disease with thrombosis), collateral pathways may develop sufficiently over time to prevent ischemia in a region distal to an occlusion.[43] Alternatively, emboli are usually acute events. If sufficient collateral pathways are not already present, the distal parenchyma is at risk for infarction. The four major types of collateral channels include external carotid–internal carotid (EC-IC), leptomeningeal, intraparenchymal, and transdural (Fig. 7–23).

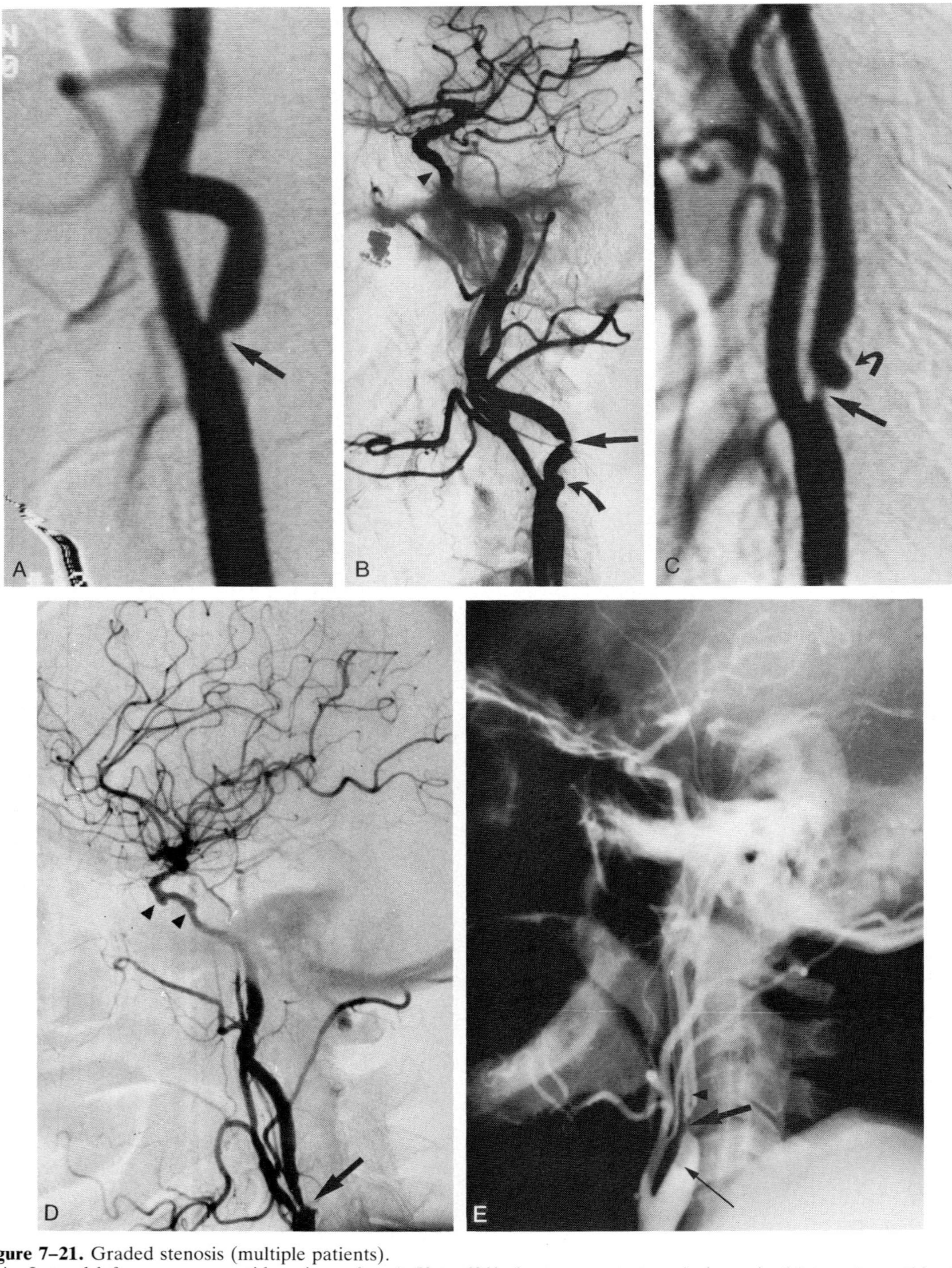

Figure 7–21. Graded stenosis (multiple patients).

A, Lateral left common carotid angiography. A 50 to 60% short-segment stenosis (*arrow*) of internal carotid artery (ICA) origin is present.

B, Lateral left common carotid angiography. Long-segment atherosclerotic disease of the left distal common and proximal ICA is present with foci of stenosis (*straight arrow*) and possible ulceration (*curved arrow*). Mild atherosclerotic irregularity of the carotid siphon (*arrowhead*) is noted.

C, Lateral left common carotid angiography. Eighty percent short-segment stenosis (*straight arrow*) of the ICA origin is present with possible distal ulceration (*curved arrow*).

D, Lateral left common carotid angiography. Moderate stenosis (*arrow*) of the ICA origin is present with concomitant atherosclerotic disease involving the carotid siphon (*arrowheads*).

E, Lateral left common carotid angiography. A short-segment, high-grade stenosis (*thick arrow*) of the left ICA is present, 2 to 3 cm cephalad to the vessel origin. Filling defects proximal (*long arrow*) and distal (*arrowhead*) to the stenosis represent intraluminal thrombus.

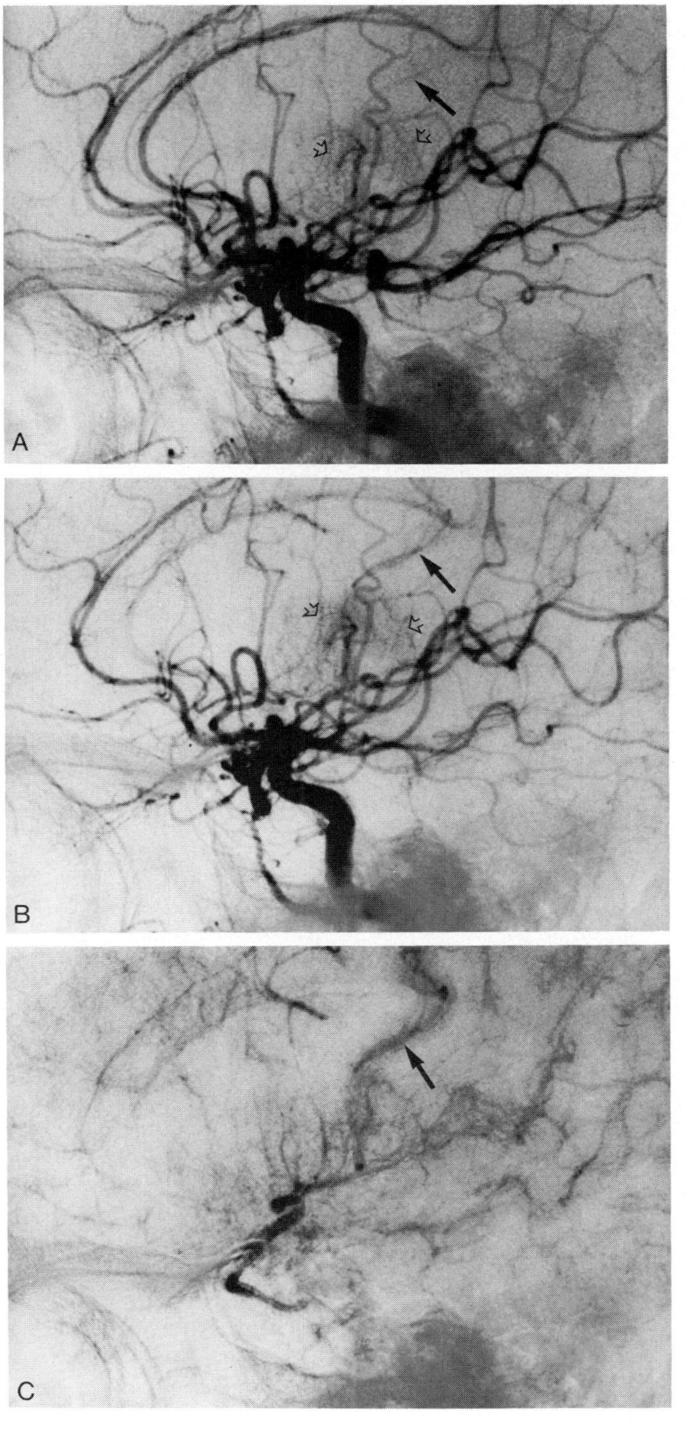

Figure 7–22. Luxury perfusion; lateral left common carotid angiography (54-year-old female 5 days postictal).

A, Early arterial phase. A faint parenchymal blush (*open arrows*) is present, and the branches of the sylvian fissure are diminished in number. An early draining vein (*closed arrow*) is present.

B, Late arterial phase. Parenchymal blush (*open arrows*) and early draining vein (*closed arrow*) are more apparent.

C, Venous phase. The early draining vein (*arrow*) indicating a hyperemic state remains quite prominent well into the venous phase.

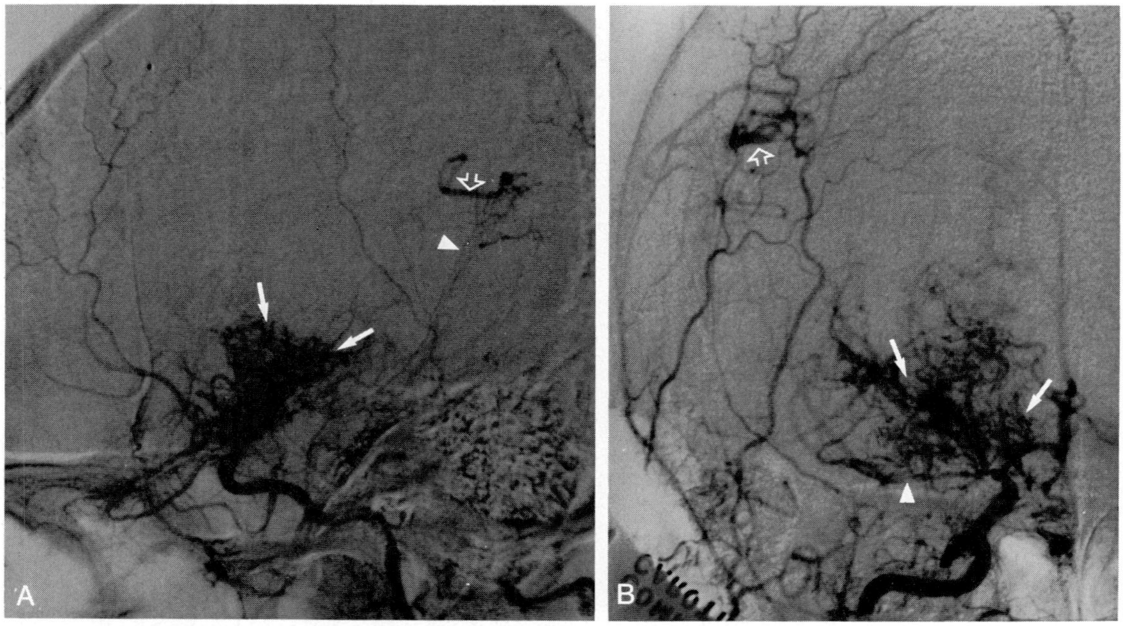

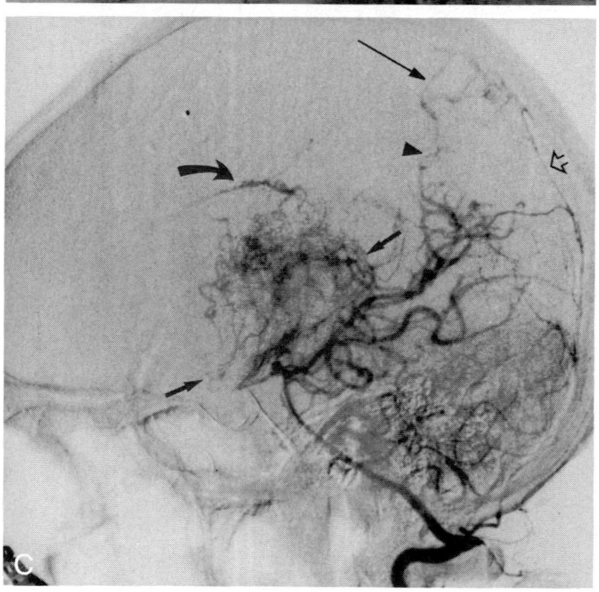

Figure 7–23. Collaterals; moyamoya disease–sickle cell disease (12-year-old male).

A, Lateral right carotid angiography. The ICA terminates in a racemose bundle of parenchymal collaterals (*closed arrows*), creating the "puff of smoke," which arise from the ICA and proximal A1 and M1 segments. The distal angular artery (*open arrow*) fills from the posterior middle meningeal (*arrowhead*) (transdural collaterals).

B, Anteroposterior (AP) right carotid angiography. The M1 segment (*arrowhead*) is markedly stenotic, providing no significant native flow to the parenchyma. The parenchymal collaterals (*arrows*) are well depicted. The angular artery (*open arrow*) fills via transdural collaterals.

C, Lateral left vertebral angiography. Parenchymal collaterals from the circle of Willis and choroidal vessels (*short arrows*) reconstitute the dorsal pericallosal artery (*curved arrow*). Transdural (*open arrow*) collaterals and leptomeningeal collaterals from the parietal occipital artery (*arrowhead*) supply the distal ACA (*long arrow*).

ETIOLOGY

Arterial Infarcts

These are supply-side infarcts, most frequently the result of thromboembolism causing infarctions that respect the arterial vascular territories. Hypotensive infarcts most commonly affect the border zone between arterial territories.

Extracranial Stenosis

The workup of these patients includes planar imaging to evaluate the intracranial sequelae of the flow-restrictive lesion, as well as angiography to document the etiology and extent of arterial disease.

Atherosclerosis. Atherosclerosis is the most common cause of extracranial and intracranial stenoses. This is an omnipresent disease, affecting multiple organ systems. It begins early in life and continues to, and often precipitates, death. The basic pathophysiology is the deposition of lipidlike material and plaques along the vessel wall. This is a systemic disease with a predilection for involvement of the great vessels from the arch, the renal arteries, and the coronary arteries. There is a predilection for extracranial sites of involvement in whites and in men. Intracranial involvement is more commonly seen in women and in blacks.[49]

The plaques increase in size at the expense of the cross-sectional area of the arterial lumen. The plaque may progress to cause a flow-restrictive lesion or to completely occlude the lumen. Even in the absence of flow-restrictive lesion, turbulence and stress may precipitate endothelial ulceration. The platelets are, thus, exposed to the collagen, which thereby induces platelet aggregation and thrombus formation. Thrombus may propagate, causing significant stenosis or occlusion of the parent artery. Alternatively, the thrombus may fragment and embolize into the downstream circulation, often resulting in a hemorrhagic infarction.

Planar imaging of cerebral infarction has been described. Angiographically, stenosis is frequently encountered. The carotid bifurcation is the most common site, followed by the siphon and the proximal MCA.

Fibromuscular Dysplasia (FMD). Hyperplasia of the media of the arterial wall is the hallmark of FMD. The mechanism remains unclear but is not related to an atherosclerotic or an inflammatory process. Patients may present with stroke, TIA, or subarachnoid hemorrhage, or may be asymptomatic. Women are affected more often than men. The lesions are usually located in the upper portions of the carotid or vertebral arteries from the C1 to the C3 level, rarely extending into the skull base. The lesions are bilateral in 65 to 86% of cases.[48, 50] Concurrent cerebral aneurysms may be detected in approximately one third of patients. Arterial stenosis may predispose to vascular insufficiency with carotid dissection or occlusion.

The diagnosis is established with angiography. The vessel contour appears as a "string of beads" consisting of concentric stenoses with multiple intervening arterial dilatations (Fig. 7–24). Less commonly, segmental fusiform dilatation of the artery may be present or a small intraluminal septum detected.[50] Progression of stenosis may be documented on follow-up angiography.

Trauma. Blunt or penetrating injury may lead to arterial stenosis. Subintimal hemorrhage (dissection) or vascular disruption may occur.[51]

The angiographic findings of trauma include vascular occlusion, extravasation of contrast material into the surrounding soft tissue, or pseudoaneurysm formation.

Arterial Dissection. Disruption of the intima and subintimal dissection of hemorrhage may be spontaneous or post-traumatic. This is frequently seen in patients following chiropractic manipulation of the neck. Patients may present with acute stroke or transient ischemic attack (TIA). The carotid or vertebral vessels may be involved. The dissection is often self-limiting and may clear without treatment. Alternatively, the dissected vessel may undergo complete occlusion.[52] Turbulent or slow flow through the true lumen may lead to thrombus formation and downstream embolization. A pseudoaneurysm may develop anywhere along the course of the dissection.

The angiographic findings of arterial dissection include irregular narrowing or tapering to occlusion of the involved vessel. The abnormality may be focal or diffuse, usually beginning in the neck and extending a variable distance to or rarely through the skull base

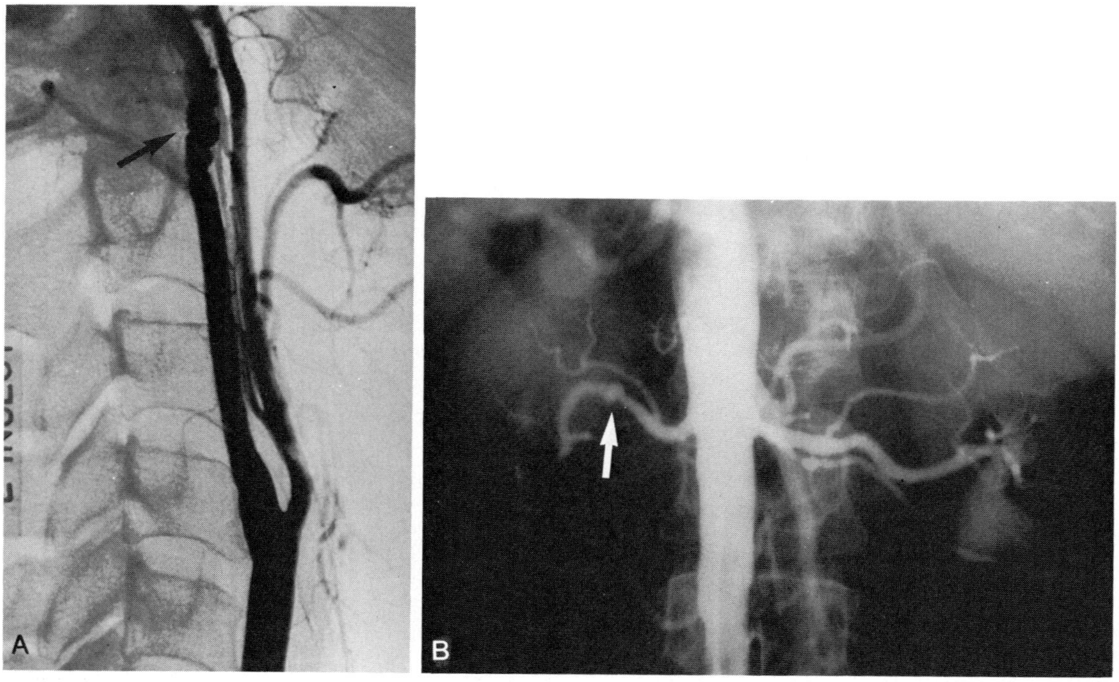

Figure 7–24. Fibromuscular dysplasia (44-year-old female).
A, Lateral left internal carotid angiography. A focal "string-of-beads" (*arrow*) appearance of the cephalad-most extracranial ICA is present.
B, AP aortogram. Similar segmental stenosis (*arrow*) is present involving the distal-most portion of the right renal artery.

(Fig. 7–25). Pseudoaneurysm appears as a focally contained collection of contrast material beyond the normal confines of the arterial wall.[53] These are usually less than a centimeter in greatest dimension, yet rarely may be larger (Fig. 7–26). It may be possible to detect the intimal flap, silhouetted between the patent true lumen and the false lumen. Delayed distal filling may be detected with intraluminal thrombus or distal vessel occlusion from emboli.[54]

Arteritis. Takayasu's arteritis is nonspecific, most likely autoimmune in origin, affecting young women. The aorta and its major branches are usually affected by this biphasic disease process.[55] In the first phase, the preocclusive stage, patients may have systemic signs and symptoms such as fever, night sweats, weakness, and chest or abdominal pain. In this phase of the disease, the histologic findings consist of diffuse granulation tissue and inflammatory infiltrative plasma cells and lymphocytes that invade and destroy the functioning arterial wall. The second phase is the occlusive stage, in which fibrosis predominates. Fibrous retraction and intimal thickening lead to significant reduction in the cross-sectional area of the lumen.

Angiographic findings consist of arterial stenoses of varying degrees of severity, fusiform or saccular aneurysms, or a combination of stenosis and aneurysm.[48, 55, 56] The arch and branch vessels, particularly the subclavian and the carotid arteries, are most commonly involved (Fig. 7–27). The left branch vessels of the arch tend to be more frequently involved and more severely affected than those on the right. In up to 80% of patients more than one branch vessel is involved.

Radiation. Patients who have received radiation for head and neck tumors may subsequently develop radiation-induced carotid or vertebral disease. Patients may have arterial changes indistinguishable from atherosclerosis and may present with signs and symptoms of cerebrovascular insufficiency.[57] The arterial changes are progressive and may be due to a periarterial fibrosis, direct damage to the arterial wall, occlusion of the vasa vasorum, and acceleration of atherosclerosis.[58] Three major

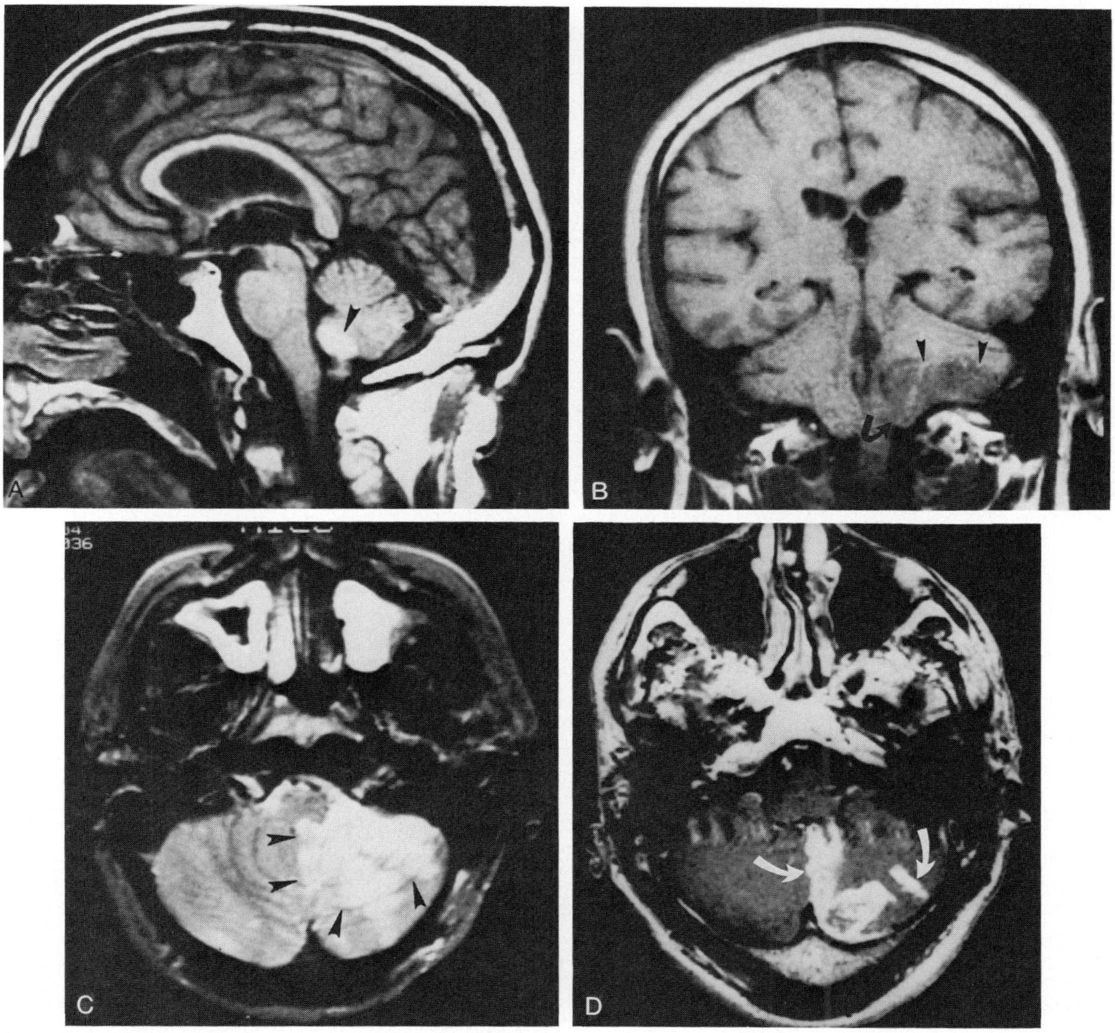

Figure 7–25. Left vertebral dissection (44-year-old male).

A, Parasagittal T1. A 1.5-cm focus of methemoglobin (*arrowhead*) is present in the anterior inferior vermis.

B, Coronal T1. Subtle decrease signal is present in the anterior left cerebellar hemisphere (*arrowheads*), extending into the tonsil (*curved arrow*).

C, Axial T2. High-signal foci (*arrowheads*) indicate ischemic edema in the cerebellar hemisphere. The infarct extends to but not beyond the midline.

D, Enhanced axial T1. Irregular parenchymal enhancement (*curved arrows*) is identified in the subacute stage.

Illustration continued on following page

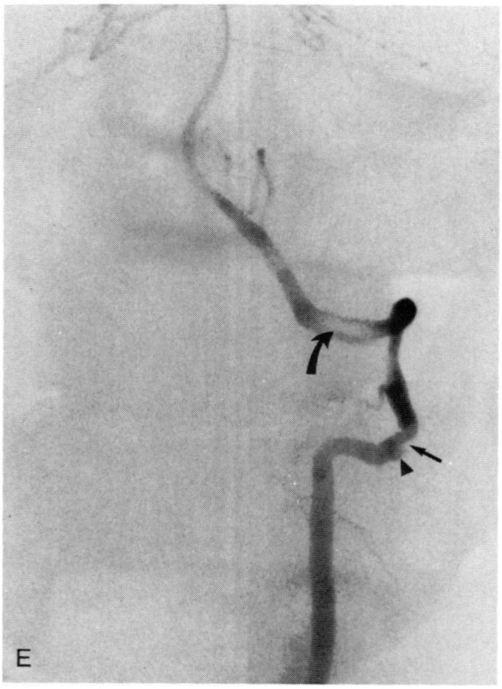

Figure 7–25 *Continued*

E, Transfacial left vertebral angiography. Irregular stenosis (*straight arrow*) and pseudoaneurysm (*arrowhead*) are present in the cephalad left vertebral artery. Distal thrombus (*curved arrow*) is also noted within the intradural segment of the left vertebral artery.

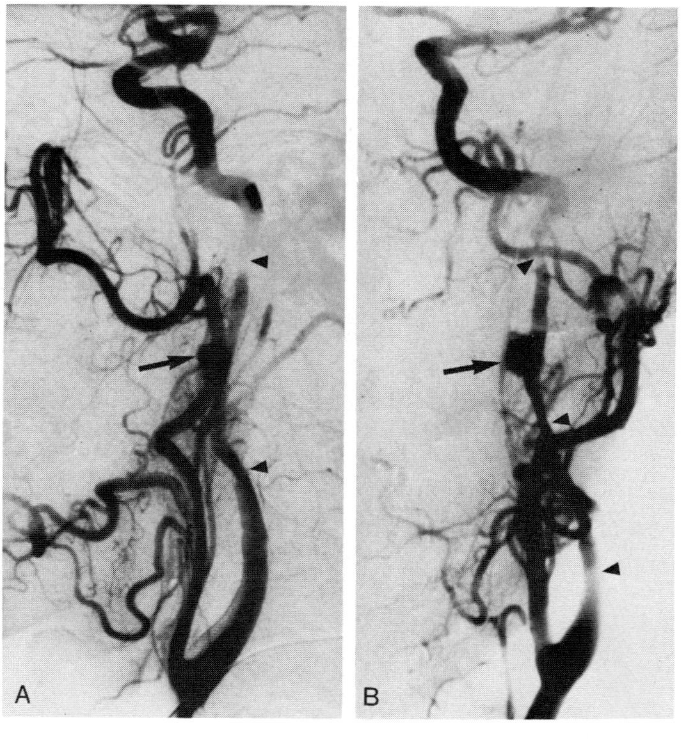

Figure 7–26. Left ICA dissection (55-year-old male).

A, B, Lateral and oblique left common carotid angiography. The ICA (*arrowheads*) tapers shortly beyond its origin throughout its course to the carotid canal. A pseudoaneurysm (*arrow*) is present at the C1–2 level within the midportion of the dissection.

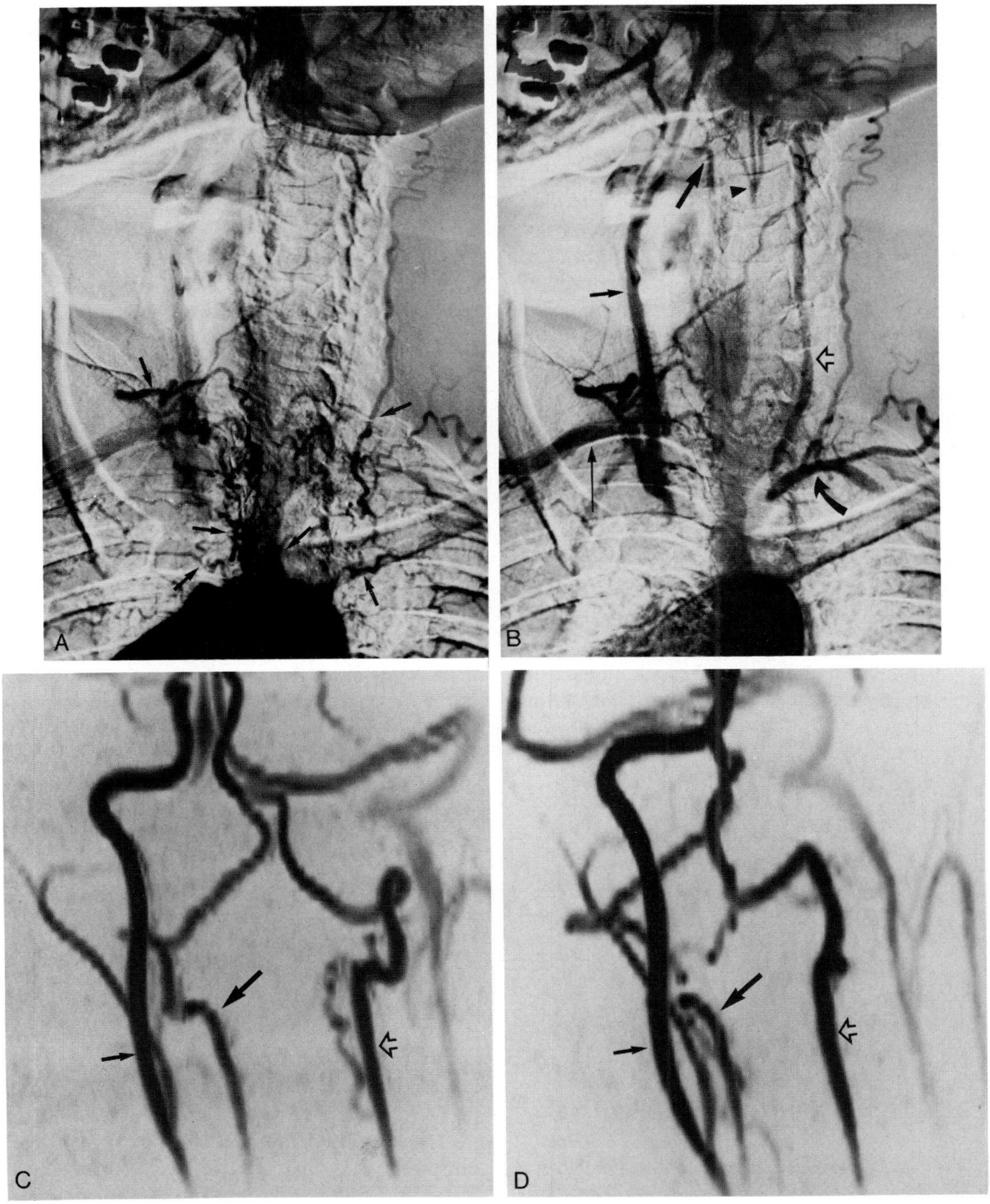

Figure 7–27. Takayasu's disease (55-year-old female).

A, RPO arch, early arterial phase. This demonstrates multiple collaterals (*arrows*) that arise from the arch without evidence of proximal great vessel opacification.

B, RPO arch, late arterial phase. The right subclavian (*long arrow*) and right common carotid (*short arrow*) arteries fill via collaterals. The left subclavian (*curved arrow*) and left vertebral (*open arrow*) fill via collaterals. The left external carotid artery (*arrowhead*) is present with occlusion of the left ICA and the left common carotid artery. The cephalad-most right vertebral (*large arrow*) is opacified.

C, D, Two-dimensional time of flight MRA-(projection images); AP and right anterior oblique (RAO) views. The left (*open arrow*) and right (*large arrow*) vertebral arteries are patent. The right carotid system (*small arrow*) is also patent. The left carotid system is not visualized with certainty. There is no indication of the severity of the occlusive disease affecting the origin of the great vessels on this sequence.

patterns of arterial injury have been documented: (1) intimal damage with mural fibrosis within 5 years of therapy, (2) fibrotic occlusion within 10 years of therapy, and (3) development of atheroma and periarterial fibrosis after 20 or more years of radiation.[59]

The angiographic findings are similar to those of atherosclerosis. Arterial narrowing, which may be smooth or irregular in contour, may be present. The lesions are usually focal, within the therapy port. Ulceration may be detected. These findings may occur in locations less commonly seen with atherosclerosis, such as distal to the carotid bifurcation.[60]

Intracranial Stenosis

The most common cause of stenosis of the intracranial arterial system is atherosclerosis. This most commonly involves the ICA at the siphon or branch point to the proximal portion of the MCA, anterior cerebral artery (ACA), and posterior cerebral artery (PCA), and basilar artery. Nonatheromatous causes of intracranial stenosis are relatively uncommon.[61]

Mechanical Compression. Mechanical compression results from various processes that may displace the vessel from its normal location and compress it against a relatively rigid structure. Supratentorial lesions that lead to descending transtentorial herniation compress the PCA against the tentorium as the brain is displaced caudally through the tentorial incisura and results in PCA infarction (Fig. 7–28). Also, parasellar neoplasms may compress the cavernous or supraclinoid ICA against the body of the sphenoid bone. More malignant, invasive lesions of the skull base (chordoma, metastasis, squamous cell carcinoma, rhabdomyosarcoma) may rarely directly invade the ICA and compromise the arterial lumen.

Inflammatory Disease. ***Primary Arteritis.*** Giant cell arteritis may primarily affect the arteries of the central nervous system in a focal or generalized pattern (Fig. 7–29). Systemic lupus erythematosus and polyarteritis nodosa may also affect the cerebral vessels.

Secondary Arteritis. This results from inflammatory changes within the subarachnoid space and pial surface, often causing a purulent meningitis with secondary inflammation of the adjacent vessels. These occur most commonly in superficial vessels, often within the Virchow-Robin spaces. The responsible organisms are usually bacterial (pneumococcus, *Haemophilus influenzae*, meningococcus, and staphylococcus). Less commonly they are fungal (mucormycosis, coccidioidomycosis, actinomycosis, and aspergillosis) or due to tuberculosis, sarcoidosis, or syphilis.

Angiographic findings of arteritis are nonspecific and include irregular narrowing and beading of cerebral vasculature. Rarely, these processes result in complete occlusion of the vessel. Primary infection of the vessel may lead to mycotic aneurysm formation.

Small Vessel Occlusive Disease

Lacunar Infarctions. Lacunar infarctions are small infarcts that result from occlusion of the minute arteries that penetrate the brain parenchyma. It is estimated that 16 to 19% of all infarctions are lacunar.[62–64] Multiple risk factors have been identified in this population and include, in decreasing frequency, hypertension, diabetes mellitus, and heart disease.[4, 63, 65]

Lacunar infarction is most often diagnosed based on clinical grounds due to the distinct clinical syndromes that result from the size and unique location of this type of infarct.[66] The most common clinical symptoms include pure motor hemiparesis, pure hemisensory stroke, sensorimotor deficit, ataxic hemiparesis, and dysarthria–"clumsy hand."[64, 66, 67]

The pathophysiology of lacunar infarction is multifactorial. Perhaps the most common etiology accounting for 80 to 90% of lacunar infarction is lipohyalinosis.[66–68] Lipohyalinosis is a hypertensive cerebral vasculopathy affecting vessels less than 200 μ in diameter, resulting in stenosis and ultimate arteriolar occlusion. Lipoid material is deposited within the arteriolar wall, and the vascular media thickens at the expense of the lumen.

This condition has been compared with the atheromatous changes that occur in larger vessels.[66] Fibrinoid necrosis, microatheromata, or large vessel atheromatous changes with occlusion of the penetrating arteries may be responsible for the remaining 10 to 20% of lacunar infarctions.[66]

The vessels most at risk for occlusion are the perforating vessels that arise from the circle of Willis and basilar artery. These include the lenticulostriate arteries from the anterior and

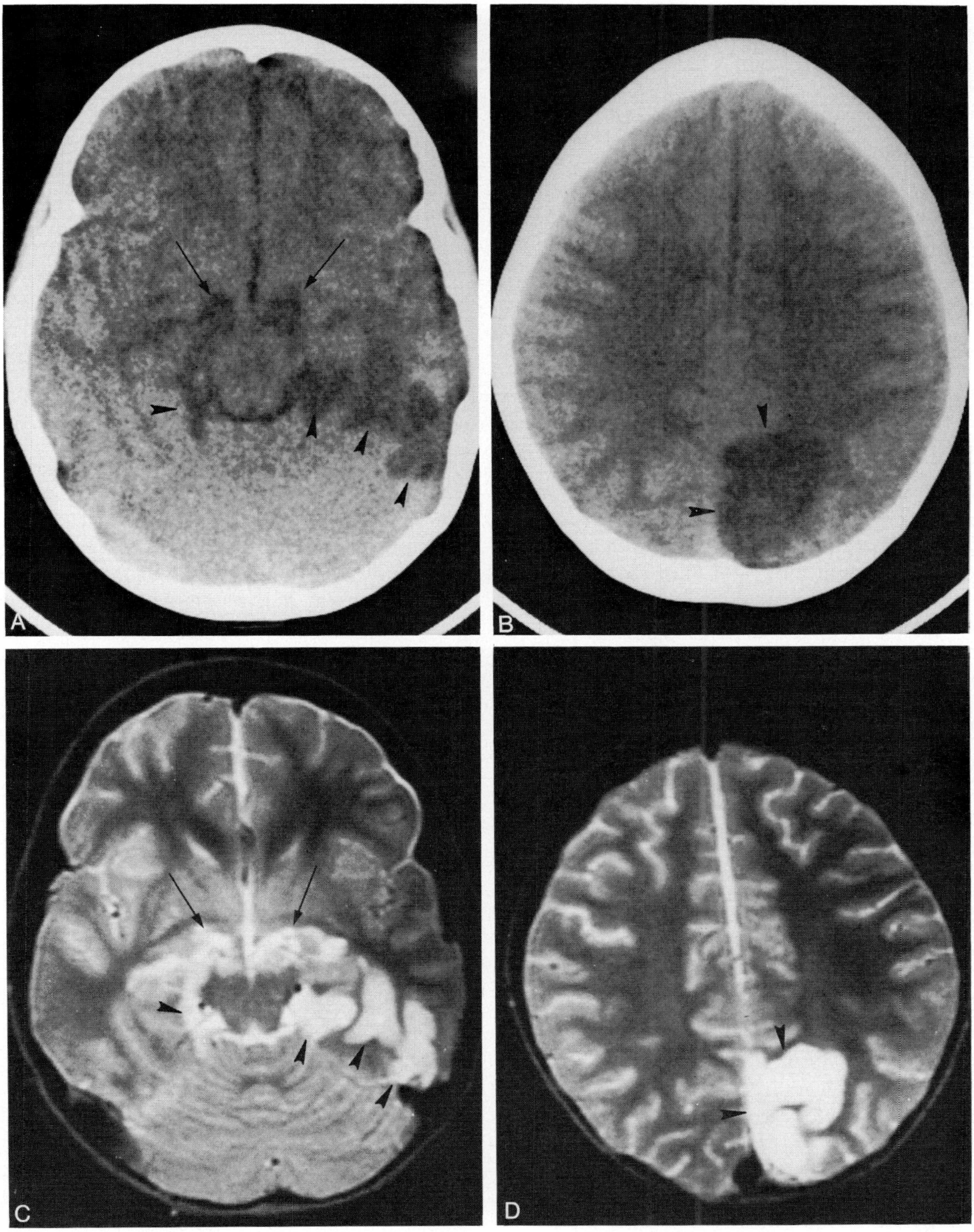

Figure 7–28. Bilateral PCA infarctions (the result of transient descending transtentorial herniation in an 8-year-old diabetic male).

A, Unenhanced CT. Ill-defined hypodensities are identified in the left PCA distribution bilaterally involving the posterior temporal lobes (*arrowheads*) and base of the posterior perforating substance (*arrows*).

B, Unenhanced CT. Infarct is present in the medial left occipital lobe (*arrowheads*).

C, Axial T2. The ischemic changes in the bilateral PCA distribution are again noted in the posterior temporal lobe (*arrowheads*) and the perforating substance (*arrows*).

D, Axial T2. The ischemic edema of the medial occipital lobe infarct (*arrowheads*) is noted.

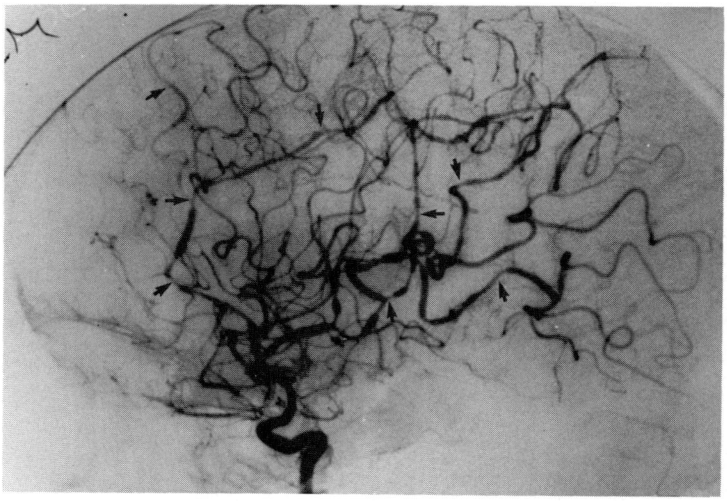

Figure 7–29. Giant cell arteritis (42-year-old female); lateral left ICA angiography. Florid changes of vasculitis are present involving multiple vessels. Luminal abnormalities with irregular beading and narrowing of multiple vessels (*arrows*) are noted. The arteries do not taper in the normal pattern.

middle cerebral arteries that enter the anterior perforating substance; the thalamoperforating and thalamogeniculate arteries from the posterior communicator and posterior cerebral arteries that enter the posterior perforating substance; and the paramedian branches that arise from the basilar artery and penetrate the pons. Accordingly, the most common location for lacunar infarcts, in decreasing order, are the putamen, caudate, thalamus, pons, internal capsule, and convolutional white matter.[67]

Multiple studies[64, 69] have demonstrated superiority of MRI in detecting lacunar infarction, particularly in the acute stage. In the acute state, MRI purportedly detected 92% of lacunar infarcts, none of which were apparent on CT.[69] Overall, MRI detected 74 to 78%, whereas CT detected 15 to 44% of clinically apparent lacunar infarctions. MRI manifestations include slitlike or ovoid foci, less than 1 cm in greatest linear dimension, which are high signal on T2 and spin density images. T1 sequences are useful to detect chronic infarct that manifest as foci of diminished signal.[64, 65, 69] CT is sensitive mainly to chronic lacunar infarcts that are depicted as foci of diminished attenuation (see Fig. 7–10).

Ischemic White Matter Disease. Like in small vessel lacunar disease and large vessel atherosclerotic disease, a collage of white matter changes is seen with increased frequency in patients with advanced age, hypertension, diabetes mellitus, and coronary artery disease.[70, 71] These abnormalities often do not represent actual infarction with necrosis but rather ischemic changes. Pathologic examination may detect arteriolar sclerosis, dilated perivascular spaces, vascular ectasia, gliosis, and demyelination.[72–74] Many of these entities may be present in patients with documented large and small vessel infarcts. It is most likely that these findings represent a spectrum of chronic cerebrovascular insufficiency.

Dilated perivascular (Virchow-Robin) spaces or état criblé are associated with hypertension and are seen at the base of the brain within the perforating substance and along the course of the deep medullary arteries. The vessels become ectatic and the surrounding brain shrinks, forming a space that subsequently fills with fluid. These isointense-to-CSF foci are noted immediately above the bifurcation of the ICA into the anterior and middle cerebral arteries on MRI.

Virchow-Robin spaces may be differentiated from lacunar infarcts based on size, shape, location, and signal intensity on spin density images. Virchow-Robin spaces are usually smaller than lacunar infarctions and are round or linear.[75] Virchow-Robin spaces remain isointense to CSF on spin density images, whereas lacunar infarcts most often are of high-signal intensity. Dilated perivascular spaces may also occur within the deep white matter. The MRI appearance of these deep lesions is similar to those at the base of the brain.[73]

Gliosis and perivascular demyelination may be induced by vascular insufficiency. These may be confluent or nonconfluent foci of increased signal on intermediate and T2 images in the periventricular or deep white matter (Fig. 7–30).

In summary, white matter changes are nonspecific on MRI and are seen with increased frequency in patients with cardiovascular risk factors and a history of completed stroke. In certain studies,[75] there is poor correlation between the clinical state and the extent of white matter lesions depicted on MRI. It is speculated that a majority of hyperintense punctate white matter lesions on MRI in the elderly are related to ischemia or infarction.[72]

Subcortical Atherosclerotic Encephalopathy (SAE), or Binswanger's Disease. In his original 1894 publication,[76] Binswanger described eight patients with a stepwise deterioration in mentation and motor function, all with white matter atrophy and hydrocephalus. Gross pathology was available in only one patient (who incidentally had syphilis). The histologic findings were not addressed. Subsequently, great controversy exists regarding the etiology, clinical presentation, and pathologic findings in these patients. Is Binswanger's disease a separate entity or merely an extreme expression

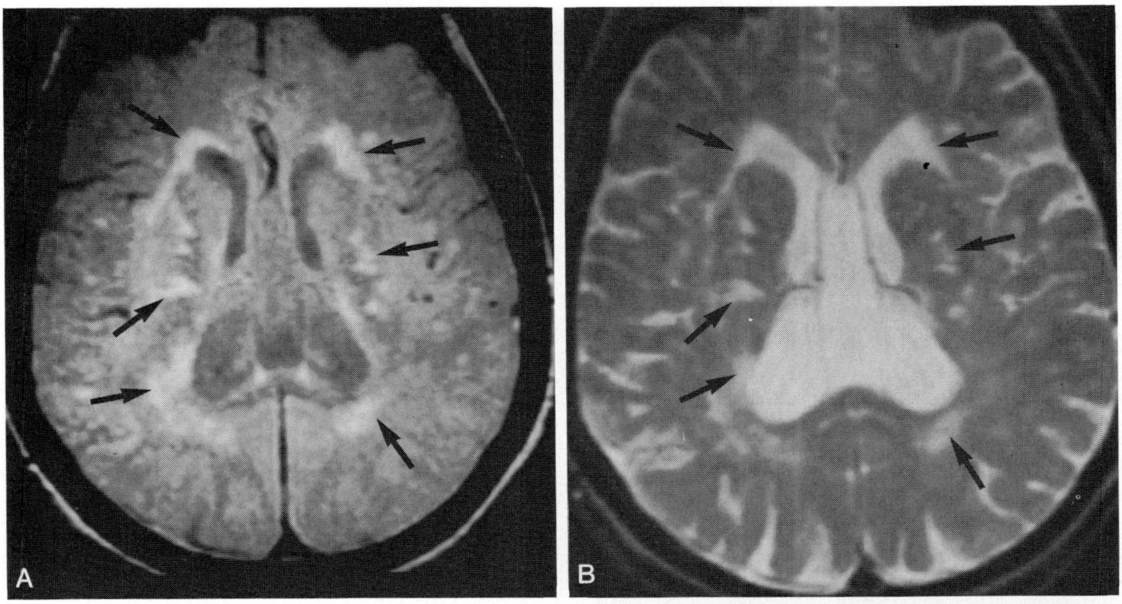

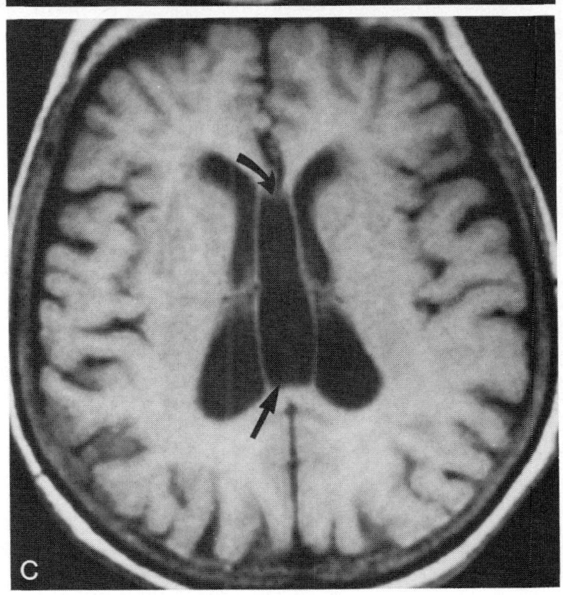

Figure 7–30. Ischemic white matter changes (69-year-old female).

A, B, Axial SD and T2. Confluent and discrete foci of high signal (*arrows*) are identified in the periventricular and deep white matter. Distinction between the ischemic change and the ventricle is more apparent on SD images.

C, Axial T1. The ischemic changes are largely inapparent on the T1-weighted sequence. Note the incidental cavum septum pellucidum (*curved arrow*) and cavum septum vergae (*straight arrow*).

of white matter ischemic disease? Is the diagnosis of Binswanger's disease based primarily on clinical or on histologic findings?

Classically, patients with SAE present with the gradual onset of neurologic deficits, which may plateau or actually improve.[77] Mental changes are present and variable, with periods of mania and defective judgment that may be followed by abulia, aphasia, and amnesic episodes. Patients display asymmetric weakness with pyramidal signs and pseudobulbar palsy. Ventriculomegaly secondary to white matter volume loss, without a significant degree of cortical atrophy, may be present. Patients often have hypertension or other vascular risk factors and may also present with acute stoke. The disease may be lengthy, with an average duration in one series[77] of approximately 6.5 years.

The classic gross morphologic finding of SAE is regional loss of white matter with gliosis. Infarcts may be discrete and/or confluent and involve the deep white matter, basal ganglia, and thalamus. There is relative sparing of the arcuate subcortical U fibers. Atrophic changes are central with relatively normal cortex. Ex vacuo hydrocephalus is present. Histologic examination reveals advanced arteriosclerotic changes in the perforating vessels to the subcortical gray and deep white matter.

The role of planar imaging is to exclude other treatable causes of disease. CT findings include varying degrees of periventricular hypodensity and ventriculomegaly.[78-80] Concurrent lacunar infarcts are common. MRI is more sensitive to these white matter and basal ganglionic changes with confluent and discrete foci of high signal on long repetition time (TR) images (Fig. 7–31). Similar high-signal changes occur in the central mid to upper pons.[68]

Hypotension

Hypotensive cerebrovascular disease results from an extracranial event, most often cardiac arrest. The central nervous system effects may be global, depending on the degree and duration of hypotension. Pre-existing significant vascular stenosis exacerbates the effects of hypotension. The distal-most parenchyma in an arterial territory will be the first to manifest the sequelae of hypoperfusion. These end arteries are located in the border zones between the anterior, middle, and posterior cerebral arteries. In addition to these cortical and subcortical locations, the penetrating deep medullary arteries are also end arteries that supply the periventricular white matter, head of caudate, putamen, and internal capsule. Accordingly, these structures are relatively sensitive to hypoperfusion.

Planar imaging findings of global hypoperfusion include diffuse mass effect with effacement of CSF-containing spaces and loss of gray-white junction, as well as focal ischemic changes in the basal ganglia and arterial border zones.[81] As edema accumulates in the basal ganglia and arterial border zones, the parenchyma becomes hypodense on CT and of increased signal intensity on T2 (Fig. 7–32). If the patient survives, focal encephalomalacic changes may occur in the basal ganglia and arterial border zones, or global supratentorial atrophy may be manifest. Hypoperfusion may cause laminar necrosis, which can be detected on enhanced CT as diffuse cortical enhancement.[82]

Venous Infarcts

Venous infarctions are usually the result of sinus thrombosis. The supply side is normal and continues to deliver blood to the parenchyma despite inability to drain this blood adequately into the sinuses or through collateral pathways. The volume of blood increases within the affected venous drainage territory. Ultimately, the ability of the endothelium to contain the blood within the vascular system is exceeded, resulting in intraparenchymal hemorrhage. The growing parenchymal hemorrhage further increases local tissue pressure, adversely affecting the perfusion pressure. The result is cerebral infarction and further parenchymal hemorrhage. These hemorrhagic infarcts are often superficial and may be multiple; they do not respect arterial border zones.

Signs of dural sinus occlusion, as described in Chapter 4, may be present; these include the "delta sign" on enhanced CT and loss of flow void on MRI (Fig. 7–33). Secondary collateral pathways may be dilated in an attempt to divert venous blood from the affected sinus. The CT and MRI appearances of hemorrhagic infarct are described in Chapter 4.

Text continued on page 243

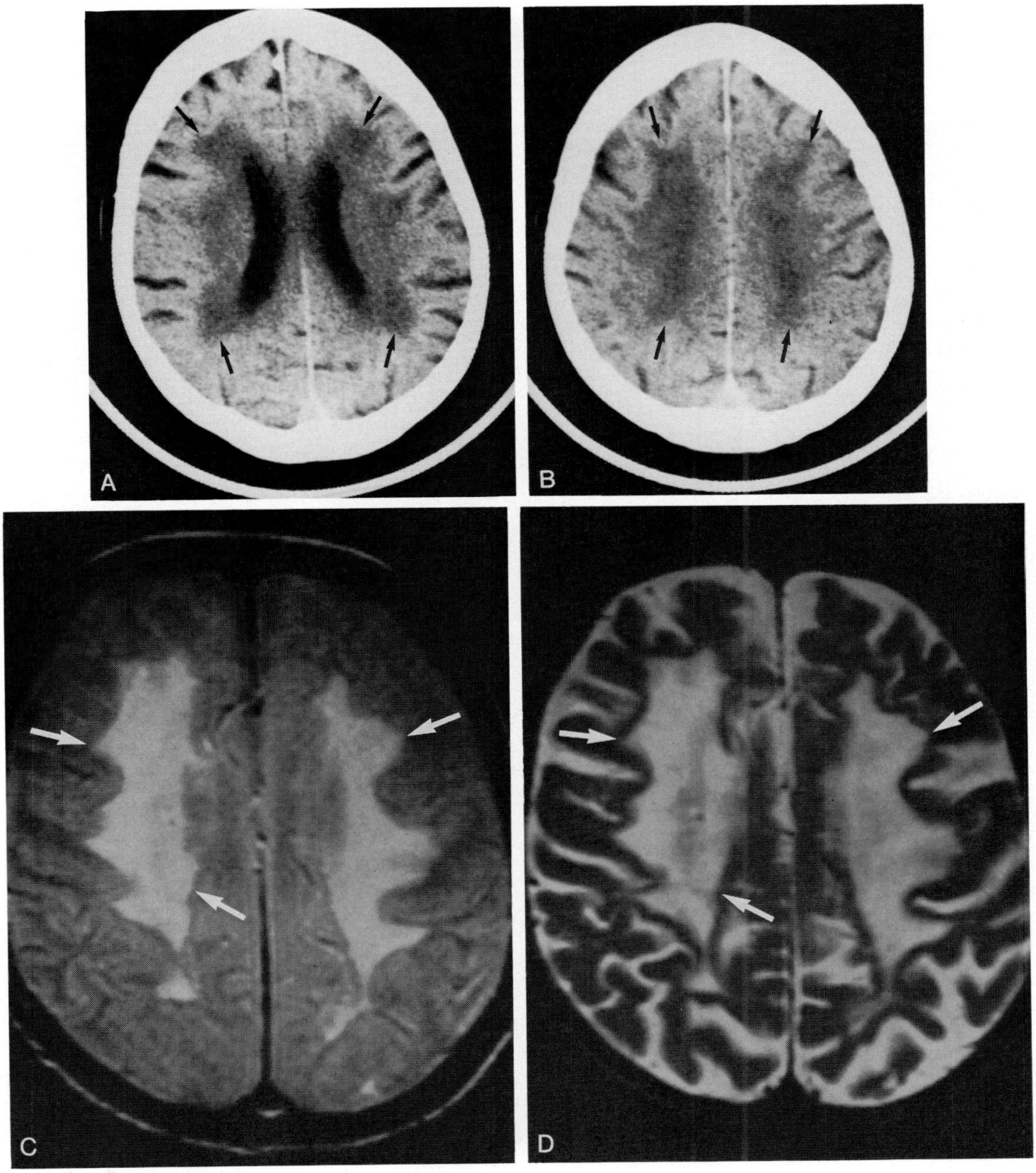

Figure 7–31. Subcortical arteriosclerotic encephalopathy (65-year-old male).

A, B, Unenhanced CT. Marked confluent hypodensity (*arrows*) is present throughout the white matter of both cerebral hemispheres.

C, D, SD and T2. Confluent high signal (*arrows*) is present in the cerebral white matter.

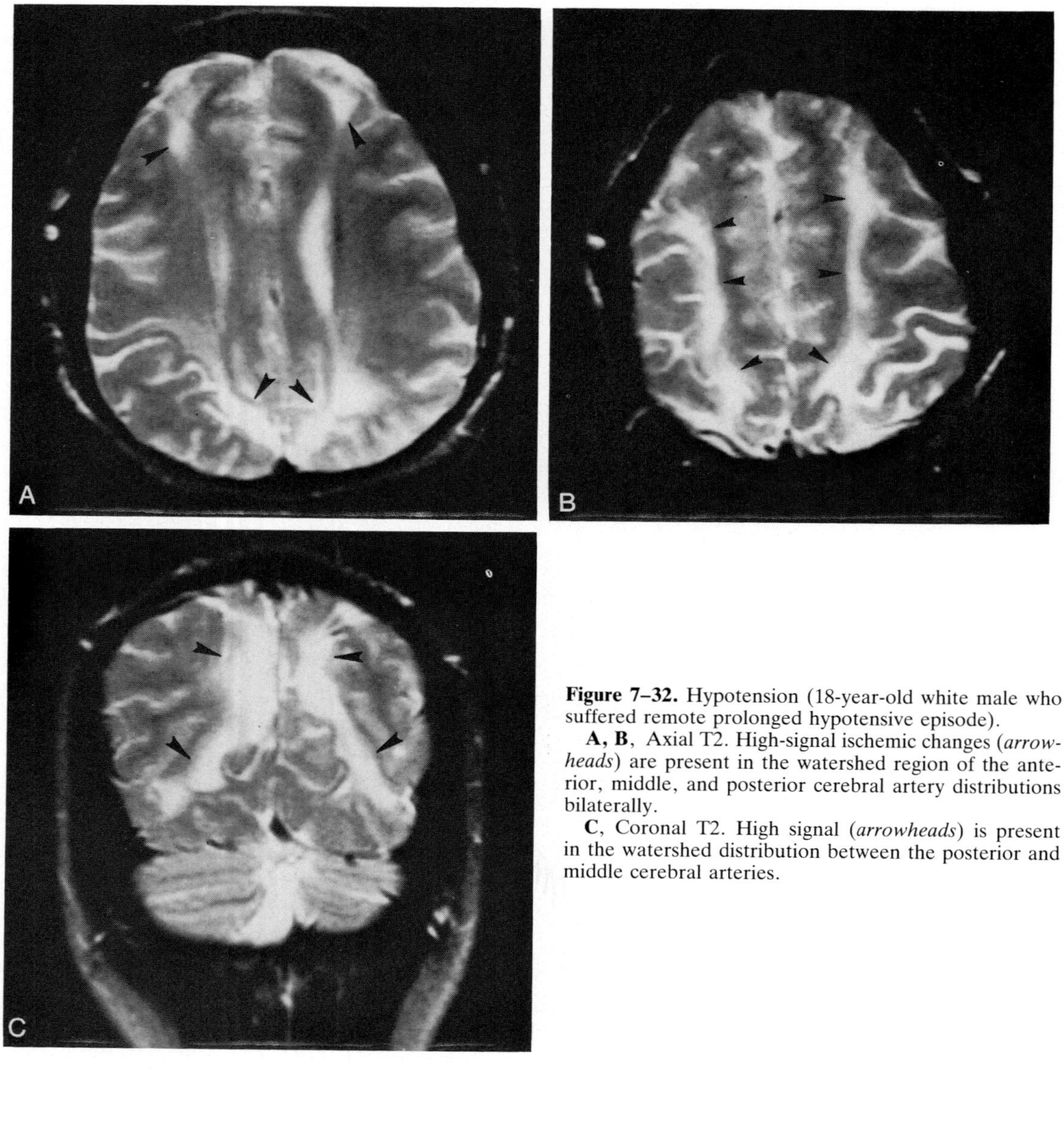

Figure 7–32. Hypotension (18-year-old white male who suffered remote prolonged hypotensive episode).

A, B, Axial T2. High-signal ischemic changes (*arrowheads*) are present in the watershed region of the anterior, middle, and posterior cerebral artery distributions bilaterally.

C, Coronal T2. High signal (*arrowheads*) is present in the watershed distribution between the posterior and middle cerebral arteries.

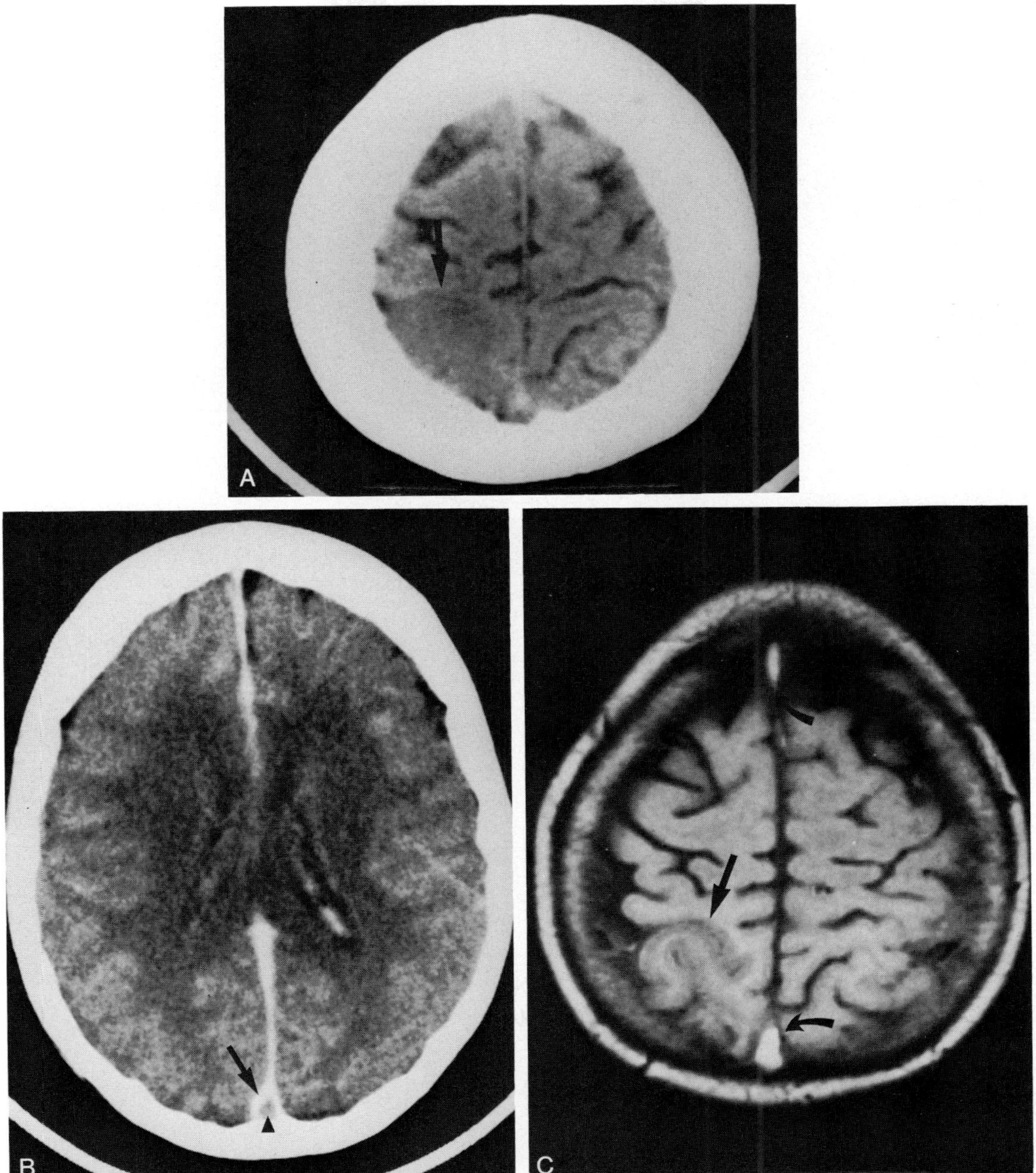

Figure 7–33. Venous infarction (26-year-old female with Crohn's disease and dehydration).

A, Unenhanced CT. A wedge-shaped hypodensity (*arrow*) is present in the right parietal vertex. The subacute infarct crosses the anterior and middle cerebral artery vascular territory, suggesting a venous etiology.

B, Enhanced CT. The superior sagittal sinus enhances peripherally (*arrow*) with inability to opacify the central thrombus (*arrowhead*). This has been termed the "delta" sign.

C, Axial T1. The parenchymal lesion is detected as local mass effect (*arrow*). The superior sagittal sinus contains high signal (*curved arrows*), which may represent slow flow or methemoglobin from recent occlusion.

Illustration continued on following page

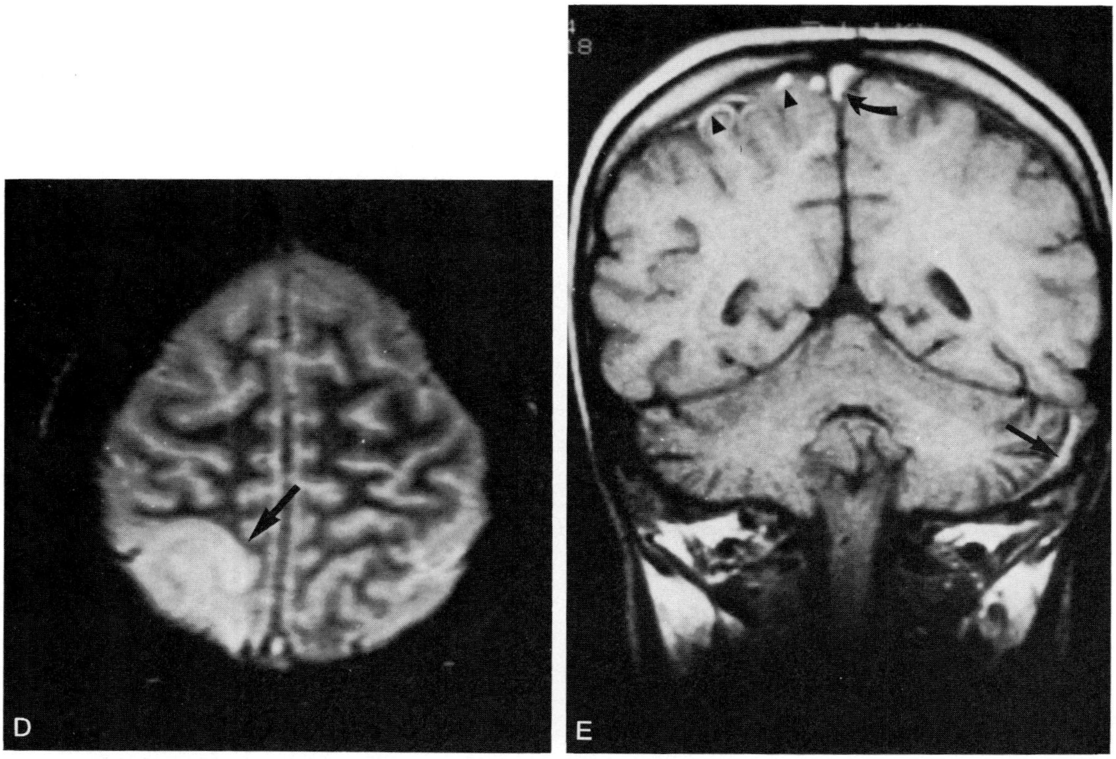

Figure 7–33 *Continued*
D, Axial T2. The parenchymal lesion (*arrow*) is confirmed.
E, Coronal T1. High signal is present in the superior sagittal sinus (*curved arrow*) and left sigmoid sinus (*straight arrow*). In conjunction with the images shown on CT and axial MRI, this suggests thrombosis. Linear high signal (*arrowheads*) is also present over the infarcted cortex, which may represent slow flow within or thrombosis of cortical veins.

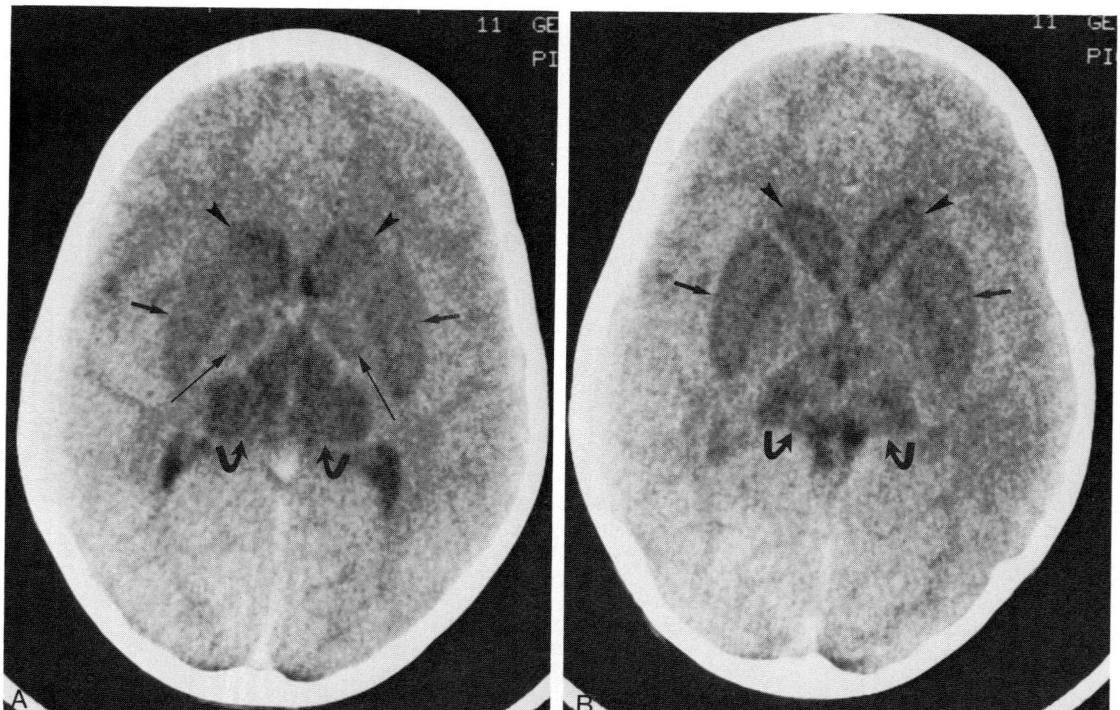

Figure 7–34. Near drowning (2-year-old female).
A, B, Unenhanced CT. Symmetric hypodensity is noted in the head of the caudate nucleus (*arrowheads*), lentiform nuclei (*short arrows*), subthalamic nuclei (*long arrows*), and thalami (*curved arrows*).

Miscellaneous Conditions

Near-Drowning

Alveolar oxygen exchange is interrupted in the near-drowning victim; this leads to cerebral hypoxia-anoxia, which rapidly precipitates cardiac arrest and diminished cerebral perfusion.

Planar imaging is often performed in these patients to assess the extent of cerebral damage. Although the initial examination may be normal,[83] parenchymal changes develop rapidly. Most commonly, ischemic edema in the basal ganglia and hippocampus may be detected as bilateral low-density changes on CT[84] and high-signal changes on T2 MRI within the basal ganglia and medial temporal lobes (Fig. 7–34). The thalami and cortical layers 3 and 5 (laminar necrosis) may be affected.[85] Diffuse cerebral edema may be seen, with loss of the gray-white junction.

Follow-up studies document progressive volume loss, which may be focal within the cortex and basal ganglia or global in distribution.

Carbon Monoxide

Carbon monoxide binds to the same site on the hemoglobin molecule as oxygen, forming carboxyhemoglobin. Carbon monoxide binds the carrier molecule hemoglobin with more than 200 times the affinity of oxygen. Displacing the oxygen, carboxyhemoglobin induces hypoxia; the oxygen dissociation curve is then shifted to the left, further decreasing the amount of oxygen released to tissues. Characteristic foci of cellular vulnerability can be detected within the globus pallidus, white matter, layers of the cerebral cortex, and hippocampus.

CT depicts regions of diminished density within the globus pallidus, hippocampus, and centrum semiovale. These are more frequently bilateral but may be unilateral.[86, 87] Rarely the lesions are isodense and may not be identified until iodinated contrast has been administered.[88] T2 MRI depicts high-signal lesions in all of the aforementioned areas. Laminar necrosis has also been detected as high-signal cortical foci.[89] Bilateral thalamic lesions have also been reported with MRI.[90]

Periventricular Leukomalacia (PVL)

This is a white matter destructive process resulting from ischemic injury to the periventricular arterial border zones and occurring in premature infants. Immature autoregulation and hypotension may play an important role in the development of PVL. The periatrial white matter and the white matter adjacent to the foramen of Monro are particularly susceptible. Clinically, patients with periatrial lesions affect the geniculocalcarine tracts with development of cortical blindness. White matter lesions adjacent to the foramen of Monro result in diplegia or paraplegia.

Ultrasound is particularly well suited to evaluate the periventricular changes in the neonate. The ischemic changes manifest initially as periventricular foci of increased echogenicity. Subsequently, multiple cystic encephalomalacia cavities of varying size may develop as the ventricles enlarge in an ex vacuo pattern.

The CT characteristics of PVL include ventriculomegaly; scalloped, irregular contours to the bodies of the lateral ventricles; decreased periventricular white matter volume (most marked at the trigone); and deep prominent sulci that may extend to the lateral ventricle.[91, 92]

MRI findings more accurately demonstrate the atrophic changes as well as the adjacent white matter lesions. Small periventricular cysts may be detected that may communicate with the ventricular body. Also, high-signal T2 and spin density changes in the immediate periventricular white matter are frequently noted, probably indicating gliosis related to the ischemic event[93, 94] (Fig. 7–35).

Radiation White Matter Disease

The pathophysiology of injury to the brain that results from therapeutic radiation remains controversial; however, most investigators attribute this to an underlying vascular injury. The endothelial cells and glial cells (most notably the oligodendroglial cells) are radiation sensitive.[95, 96] The damaged endothelium undergoes a reparative response that ultimately results in hyalinization, fibrosis, and mineralization of the vessel walls.[97, 98] This leads to relative tissue ischemia, demyelination, and, in severe cases, necrosis of the brain parenchyma.

The patterns of brain injury are varied and may be temporally divided into three stages: acute, early delayed, and late delayed (radiation necrosis).[97] Acute injury usually occurs within days to weeks of therapy and is the

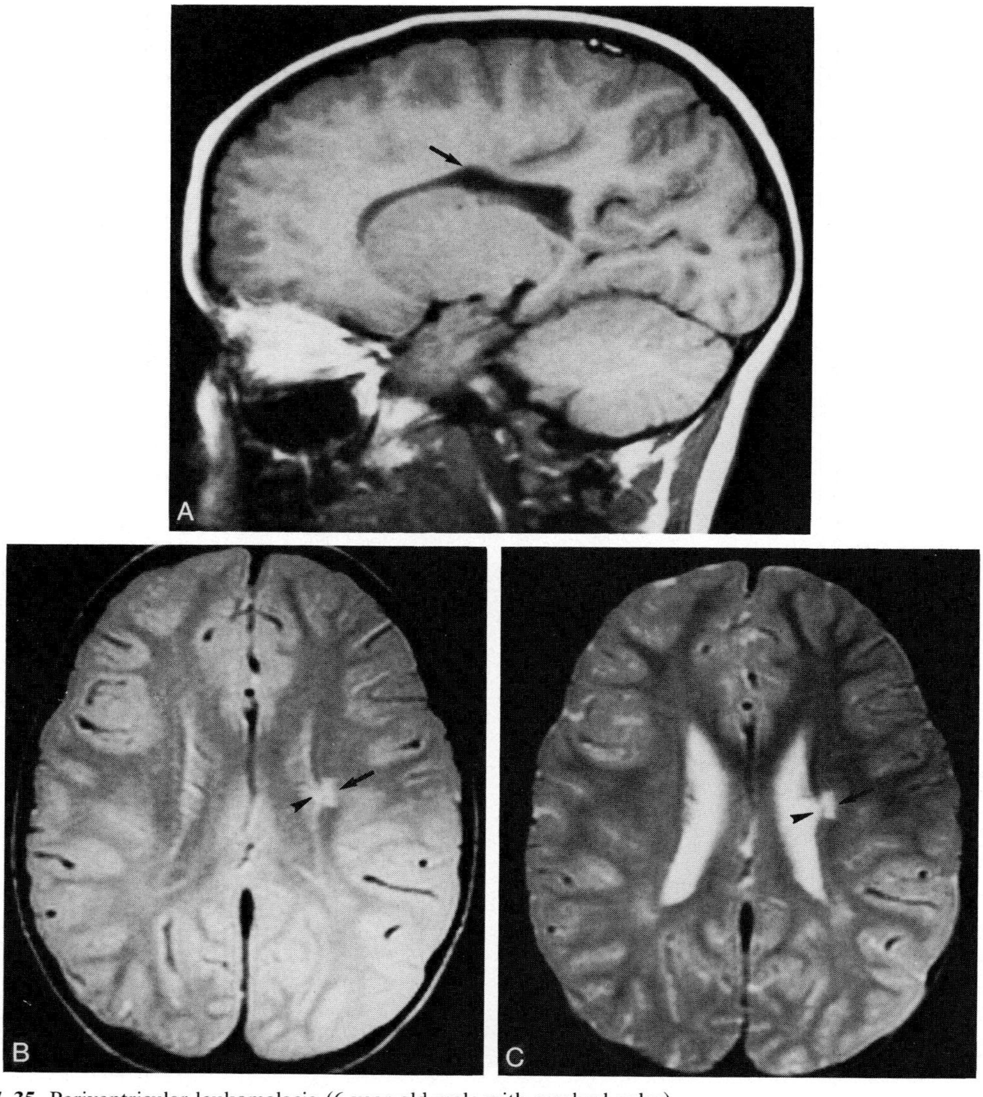

Figure 7–35. Periventricular leukomalacia (6-year-old male with cerebral palsy).

A, Parasagittal T1. Focal dilatation (*arrow*) of the body of the left lateral ventricle is noted.

B, C, Axial SD and T2. A focus of high signal (*arrow*) is noted in the left periventricular white matter, representing the sequelae of prior periventricular ischemia. Focal dilatation of the ventricle (*arrowhead*) is present.

result of capillary damage and disruption of the BBB. Vasogenic edema and transient enhancement are detected on planar imaging.

Early delayed effects occur weeks to months following therapy, resulting in axon demyelination. Microscopically discrete regions of demyelination are detected with pronounced microglial and astrocytic proliferation. Perivascular lymphocytic and plasma cell infiltrates are present in absence of degenerative vascular changes. Not surprisingly, MRI is markedly more sensitive than CT at detecting these predominantly white matter alterations.[96, 99–101] CT may document focal or diffuse hypodensity throughout the white matter. The ventricles and sulci may enlarge secondary to progressive loss of brain parenchyma. High signal changes on long TR images are noted focally or diffusely, symmetrically or asymmetrically throughout the white matter, generally sparing the basal ganglia, corpus callosum, and internal capsule. The gray matter may be involved in extreme cases. There is generally no evidence of mass effect. The white matter changes may be most marked remote from the tumor bed[101] and in the periventricular region where end artery blood flow is the most tenuous.[100]

Delayed effects of therapeutic radiation may occur months to years following therapy, occurring in 5% of patients at a median of 14 months following the radiation in one study.[102] One group[103] noted a twofold increase in the incidence of radiation necrosis (8.7% to 3.4%) in patients receiving standard regimens versus hyperfractionated doses. In addition, patients receiving conventional treatment regimens developed radiation necrosis sooner than did patients who received hyperfractionated doses (8.5 vs 21 months). Microscopically, progressive vascular alterations are noted, including heterogeneous endothelial hyperplasia, fibrinoid necrosis of penetrating arterioles, vascular occlusions, and morphologic changes suggestive of those seen with large vessel atherosclerosis. The BBB is disrupted, and vasogenic edema and mass effect are noted.[102] Cerebral necrosis is present and may contain foci of hemorrhage. CT depicts low attenuation, vasogenic edema, and patchy or irregular enhancement that may be accompanied by mass effect.[104] MRI more accurately depicts the mass effect, contrast enhancement, and edema.

There are no reliable clinical or radiographically detectable morphologic criteria to differentiate recurrent or residual tumor from radiation necrosis. This distinction is best based on evaluating the metabolism of the lesion utilizing positron emission tomography (PET).[105, 106] ^{18}F-deoxyglucose (FDG) is a marker of cellular metabolism. FDG will concentrate in regions of tumor (hypermetabolic) and not areas of radiation necrosis (hypometabolic).

References

1. Morris JH: The nervous system. *Robbins Pathologic Basis of Disease*. Cotran RS, Kumar V, Robbins SL (eds): 4th ed, 1989, WB Saunders, Philadelphia.
2. Nelson JS: Pathology of the nervous system. *Anderson's Pathology*. Kissane JM (ed): 9th ed, 1990, CV Mosby, St Louis.
3. Kricheff II: Arteriosclerotic ischemic cerebrovascular disease. Radiology 1987; 162:101–109.
4. Garcia JH: Ischemic injuries of the brain. Arch Pathol Lab Med 1983; 107:157–161.
5. O'Brien MD: Ischemic cerebral edema. A review. Stroke 1979; 10:623–628.
6. Grady PA: Pathophysiology of extracranial cerebral arterial stenosis—a critical review. Stroke 1984; 15:224–236.
7. Astrup J, Siesjö K, Symon L: Thresholds in cerebral ischemia—the ischemic penumbra. Stroke 1981; 12:723–725.
8. Wang AM, Lin JC, Rumbaugh CL: What is expected of CT in the evaluation of stroke? Neuroradiology 1988; 30:54–58.
9. Wall SD, Brant-Zawadzki M, Jeffrey RB, et al: High frequency CT findings within 24 hours after cerebral infarction. AJR 1982; 138:307–311.
10. Yock DH, Marshall WH: Recent ischemic brain infarcts at computed tomography: Appearance pre- and post-contrast infusion. Radiology 1975; 117:599–608.
11. Tomura N, Vemura K, Inugami A, et al: Early CT findings in cerebral infarction: Obscuration of the lentiform nucleus. Radiology 1988; 168:463–467.
12. Truwit CL, Barkovich AJ, Gean-Marton A, et al: Loss of the insular ribbon: Another early CT sign of acute middle cerebral artery infarction. Radiology 1990; 176:801–806.
13. Pressman BD, Tourje EJ, Thompson JR: An early CT sign of ischemic infarction: Increased density in a cerebral artery. AJNR 1987; 8:645–648.
14. Tomsick TA, Brott TG, Chambers AA: Hyperdense middle cerebral artery sign on CT: Efficacy in detecting middle cerebral artery thrombosis. AJNR 1990; 11:473–477.
15. Granström P: CT visualization of thrombus in cerebral artery. J Comput Assist Tomogr 1986; 10:541–542.
16. Schuierer G, Huk W: The unilateral hyperdense middle cerebral artery: An early CT-sign of embolism or thrombosis. Neuroradiology 1988; 30:120–122.
17. Kuzuhara S, Naito Y, Namura Y, et al: CT demonstration of calcification within old cerebral infarcts. J Comput Assist Tomogr 1985; 9:268–271.
18. Stovring J, Fernando LT: Wallerian degeneration of

the corticospinal tract region of the brain stem: Demonstration by computed tomography. Radiology 1983; 149:717–720.
19. Wing SD, Norman D, Pollock JA, et al: Contrast enhancement of cerebral infarcts in computed tomography. Radiology 1976; 121:89–92.
20. Norton GA, Kishore PRS, Lin J: CT contrast enhancement in cerebral infarction. AJR 1978; 131:881–885.
21. Lassen NA: The luxury-perfusion syndrome and its possible relation to acute metabolic acidosis localized within the brain. Lancet 1966; 2:1113–1115.
22. Unger EC, Gado MH, Fulling KF, et al: Acute cerebral infarction in monkeys: An experimental study using MR imaging. Radiology 1987; 162:789–795.
23. Bryan RN, Willcott MR, Schneiders NJ, et al: Nuclear magnetic resonance evaluation of stroke. Radiology 1983; 149:189–192.
24. Kertesz A, Black SE, Nicholson L, et al: The sensitivity and specificity of MRI in stroke. Neurology 1987; 37:1580–1585.
25. McNamara MT, Brant-Zawadzk M, Berry I, et al: Acute experimental cerebral ischemia: MR enhancement using Gd-DTPA. Radiology 1986; 158:701–705.
26. Bryan RN, Levy LM, Whitlow WD, et al: Diagnosis of acute cerebral infarction: Comparison of CT and MR imaging. AJNR 1991; 12:611–620.
27. Yuh WTC, Crain MR, Loes DJ, et al: MR imaging of cerebral ischemia: Findings in the first 24 hours. AJNR 1991; 12:621–629.
28. Imakita S, Nishimura T, Yamoda N, et al: Magnetic resonance imaging of cerebral infarction: Time course of Gd-DTPA enhancement and CT comparison. Neuroradiology 1988; 30:372–378.
29. Virapongse C, Mancuso A, Quisling R: Human brain infarcts: Gd-DTPA-enhanced MR imaging. Radiology 1986; 161:785–794.
30. Imakita S, Nishimura T, Naito H, et al: Magnetic resonance imaging of human cerebral infarction: Enhancement with Gd-DTPA. Neuroradiology 1987; 29:422–429.
31. Elster AD, Moody DM: Early cerebral infarction: Gadopentetate dimeglumine enhancement. Radiology 1990; 177:627–632.
32. Sato A, Takahashi S, Soma Y, et al: Cerebral infarction: Early detection by means of contrast-enhanced cerebral arteries at MR imaging. Radiology 1991; 178:433–439.
33. Crain MR, Yuh WTC, Greene GM, et al: Cerebral ischemia: Evaluation with contrast-enhanced MR imaging. AJNR 1991; 12:631–639.
34. DeLaPaz RL, Shibata D, Steinberg GK, et al: Acute cerebral ischemia in rabbits: Correlation between MR and histopathology. AJNR 1991; 12:89–95.
35. Nabatame H, Fujimoto N, Nakamura K, et al: High intensity areas on noncontrast T1-weighted MR images in cerebral infarction. J Comput Assist Tomogr 1990; 14:521–526.
36. Dietrich RB, Bradley WG: Iron accumulation in the basal ganglia following severe ischemic-anoxic insults in children. Radiology 1988; 168:203–206.
37. Kuhn MJ, Mikulis DJ, Ayoub DM, et al: Wallerian degeneration after cerebral infarction: Evaluation with sequential MR imaging. Radiology 1989; 172:179–182.
38. Inove Y, Matsumura Y, Fukuda T, et al: MR imaging of Wallerian degeneration in the brain stem: Temporal relationships. AJNR 1990; 11:897–902.
39. Titelbaum DS, Frazier JL, Grossman RI, et al: Wallerian degeneration and inflammation in rat peripheral nerve detected by in vivo MR imaging. AJNR 1989; 10:741–746.
40. Kuhn MJ, Johnson, KA, Davis KR: Wallerian degeneration: Evaluation with MR imaging. Radiology 1988; 168:199–202.
41. Caplan LR, Wolpert SM: Angiography in patients with occlusive cerebrovascular disease: Views of a stroke neurologist and neuroradiologist. AJNR 1991; 12:593–601.
42. Brice JG, Dowsett DJ, Lowe RD: Haemodynamic effects of carotid artery stenosis. Br Med 1964; 28:1363–1366.
43. Brice JG, Dowsett DJ, Lowe RD: The effects of constriction on carotid blood-flow and pressure gradients. Lancet 1964; 1:84–85.
44. Tindall GT, Odom GL, Cupp HB, et al: Studies on carotid artery flow and pressure. J Neurosurg 1962; 19:917–923.
45. May AG, DeWeese JA, Rob CG: Hemodynamic effects of arterial stenosis. Surgery 1963; 53:513–524.
46. Edwards JH, Kricheff II, Riles T, et al: Angiographically undetected ulceration of the carotid bifurcation as a cause of embolic stroke. Radiology 1979; 132:369–373.
47. Taveras JM, Gilson JM, Davis DO, et al: Angiography in cerebral infarction. Radiology 1969; 93:549–558.
48. Osborne AG: *Introduction to Cerebral Angiography*. 1980. Harper & Row, Hagerstown, MD.
49. Caplan LR, Gorelick PB, Hier DB: Race, sex, and occlusive cerebrovascular disease: A review. Stroke 1986; 17:648–655.
50. So EL, Toole JF, Dalal P, et al: Cephalic fibromuscular dysplasia in 32 patients. Arch Neurol 1981; 38:619–622.
51. Hughes JT, Brownell B: Traumatic thrombosis of the internal carotid artery in the neck. J Neurol Neurosurg Psychiatry 1968; 31:307–314.
52. Ehrenfeld WK, Wylie EJ: Spontaneous dissection of the internal carotid artery. Arch Surg 1976; 111:1294–1301.
53. Bradac GB, Kaernbach A, Bolk-Weischedel D, et al: Spontaneous dissecting aneurysm of cervical cerebral arteries. Neuroradiology 1981; 21:149–154.
54. Traflet RF, Babaria AR, Bell RD, et al: Vertebral artery dissection after rapid head turning. AJNR 1989; 10:650–651.
55. Lande A, Rossi P: The value of total aortography in the diagnosis of Takayasu's arteritis. Radiology 1975; 114:287–297.
56. Deutsch V, Wexler L, Deutsch H: Takayasu's arteritis. AJR 1974; 122:13–28.
57. McCready RA, Hyde GL, Bivins BA, et al: Radiation-induced arterial injuries. Surgery 1983; 93:306–312.
58. Kalman PG, Lipton IH, Provan JL, et al: Radiation damage to large arteries. Can J Surg 1983; 26:88–91.
59. Butter MJ, Lane HS, Webster JHH: Radiation injury to large vessels. Br J Surg 1980; 67:341–343.
60. Silverberg GD, Britt RH, Goffinet DR: Radiation-induced carotid artery disease. Cancer 1978; 41:130–137.

61. Momose KJ, New PFJ: Non-atheromatous stenosis and occlusion of the internal carotid artery and its main branches. AJR 1973; 118:550–566.
62. Olsen TS, Skriver EB, Herning M: Cause of cerebral infarction in the carotid territory. Its relation to the size and location of the infarct and to the underlying vascular lesion. Stroke 1985; 16:459–466.
63. Mohr JP, Caplan LR, Melski JW, et al: The Harvard Cooperative Stroke Registry: A prospective registry. Neurology 1978; 28:754–762.
64. Arboix A, Marti-Vilalta JL, Garcia JH: Clinical study of 227 patients with lacunar infarcts. Stroke 1990; 21:842–847.
65. Braffman BH, Zimmerman RA, Trojanowski JQ, et al: Brain MR: Pathologic correlation with gross and histopathology. 1. Lacunar infarction and Virchow-Robin spaces. AJNR 1988; 9:621–628.
66. Mohr JP: Lacunes. Stroke 1982; 13:3–11.
67. Fisher CM: Lacunar strokes and infarcts: A review. Neurology 1982; 32:871–876.
68. Solomon A, Yeates AE, Burger PC, et al: Subcortical arteriosclerotic encephalopathy: Brain stem findings with MR imaging. Radiology 1987; 165:625–629.
69. Rothrock JF, Lyden PD, Hesselink JR, et al: Brain magnetic resonance imaging in the evaluation of lacunar stroke. Stroke 1987; 18:781–786.
70. Fazekas F, Niederkorn K, Schmidt R, et al: White matter signal abnormalities in normal individuals: Correlation with carotid ultrasonography, cerebral blood flow measurements, and cerebrovascular risk factors. Stroke 1988; 19:1285–1288.
71. Awad IA, Spetzler RF, Hodak JA, et al: Incidental subcortical lesions identified on MRI in the elderly. I. Correlation with age and cerebrovascular risk factors. Stroke 1986; 17:1084–1089.
72. Braffman BH, Zimmerman RA, Trojanowski JQ, et al: Brain MR: Pathologic correlation with gross and histopathology. 2. Hyperintense white matter foci in the elderly. AJNR 1988; 9:629–636.
73. Awad IA, Johnson PC, Spetzler RF, et al: Incidental subcortical lesions identified on MRI in the elderly. II. Postmortem pathological correlations. Stroke 1986; 17:1090–1097.
74. Fazekas F, Kleinert R, Offenbacher H, et al: The morphological correlate of incidental punctate white matter hyperintensities on MR. AJNR 1991; 12:915–921.
75. Kobari M, Meyer JS, Ichijo M, et al: Leukoaraiosis: Correlation of MR and CT findings with blood flow, atrophy, and cognition. AJNR 1990; 11:273–281.
76. Binswanger O: Die Abrenzung der allgemeinen progressiven Paralyse. Berl Klin Wochenschr 1894; 31:1103–1105, 1137–1139, 1180–1186.
77. Caplan LR, Schoene WC: Clinical features of subcortical arteriosclerotic encephalopathy (Binswanger disease). Neurology 1978; 28:1206–1215.
78. Lotz PR, Ballinger WE, Quisling RG: Subcortical arteriosclerotic encephalopathy: CT spectrum and pathologic correlation. AJNR 1986; 7:817–822.
79. Kinkel WR, Jacobs L, Polachini I, et al: Subcortical arteriosclerotic encephalopathy (Binswanger's disease). Arch Neurol 1985; 42:951–959.
80. Loizou LA, Kendall BE, Marshal J: Subcortical arteriosclerotic encephalopathy: A clinical and radiological investigation. J Neurol Neurosurg Psychiatr 1981; 44:294–304.
81. Kjos BO, Brant-Zawadzki M, Young RG: Early CT findings of global central nervous system hypoperfusion. AJNR 1983; 4:1043–1048.
82. Liwnicz BH, Mouradian MD, Ball JB: Intense brain cortical enhancement on CT in laminar necrosis verified by biopsy. AJNR 1987; 8:157–159.
83. Taylor SB, Quencer RM, Holzman BH, et al: Central nervous system anoxic-ischemic insult in children due to near-drowning. Radiology 1985; 156:641–646.
84. Murray RR, Kapila A, Blanco E, et al: Cerebral computed tomography in drowning victims. AJNR 1984; 5:177–179.
85. Fitch ST, Gerald B, Magill HL, et al: Central nervous system hypoxia in children due to near drowning. Radiology 1985; 156:647–650.
86. Miura T, Mitomo M, Kawai R, et al: CT of the brain in acute carbon monoxide intoxication: Characteristic features and prognosis. AJNR 1985; 6:739–742.
87. Taylor R, Holgate RC: Carbon monoxide poisoning: Asymmetric and unilateral changes on CT. AJNR 1988; 9:975–977.
88. Zeiss J, Brinker R: Role of contrast enhancement in cerebral CT of carbon monoxide poisoning. J Comput Assist Tomogr 1988; 12:341–343.
89. Horowitz AL, Kaplan R, Sarpel G: Carbon monoxide toxicity: MR imaging in the brain. Radiology 1987; 162:787–788.
90. Tuchman RF, Moser FG, Moshé SL: Carbon monoxide poisoning: Bilateral lesions in the thalamus on MR imaging of the brain. Pediatr Radiol 1990; 20:478–479.
91. Schouman-Claeys E, Picard A, Lalande G, et al: Contribution of computed tomography in the etiology and prognosis of cerebral palsy in children. Br J Radiol 1989; 62:248–252.
92. Flodmark O, Roland EH, Hill A, et al: Periventricular leukomalacia: Radiologic diagnosis. Radiology 1987; 162:119–124.
93. Flodmark O, Lupton B, Li B, et al: MR imaging of periventricular leukomalacia in childhood. AJNR 1989; 10:111–118.
94. Barkovich AJ, Truwit CL: Brain damage from perinatal asphyxia: Correlation of MR findings with gestational age. AJNR 1990; 11:1087–1096.
95. Constine LS, Konski A, Ekholm S, et al: Adverse effects of brain radiation correlated with MR and CT imaging. Int J Radiat Oncol Biol Phys 1988; 15:319–330.
96. Curran WJ, Hecht-Leavitt C, Schut L, et al: Magnetic resonance imaging of cranial radiation lesions. Int J Radiat Oncol Biol Phys 1987; 13:1093–1098.
97. Lampert PW, Davis RL: Delayed effects of radiation on the human central nervous system, "early" and "late" delayed reaction. Neurology 1964; 14:912–917.
98. Hecht-Leavitt C, Grossman RI, Curran WJ, et al: MR of brain radiation injury: Experimental studies in cats. AJNR 1987; 8:427–430.
99. Dooms GC, Hecht S, Brant-Zawadzki M, et al: Brain radiation lesions: MR imaging. Radiology 1986; 158:149–155.
100. Curnes JT, Laster DW, Ball MR, et al: Magnetic resonance imaging of radiation injury to the brain. AJNR 1986; 7:389–394.
101. Tsuruda JS, Kortman KE, Bradley WG, et al: Radiation effects on cerebral white matter: MR evaluation. AJNR 1987; 8:431–437.
102. Marks JE, Baglan RJ, Prassad SC, et al: Cerebro-

radionecrosis: Incidence and risks in relation to dose, time, fractionation and volume. Int J Radiat Oncol Biol Phys 1981; 7:243–252.
103. Safdari GH, Fuentes JM, Dubois JB, et al: Radiation necrosis of the brain: Time of onset and incidence related to total dose and fractionation of the radiation. Neuroradiology 1985; 27:44–47.
104. Kingsley DPE, Kendall BE: CT of the adverse effects of therapeutic radiation of the central nervous system. AJNR 1981; 2:453–460.
105. Di Chiro G, Oldfield E, Wright DC, et al: Cerebral necrosis after radiotherapy and/or intra-arterial chemotherapy for brain tumors: PET and neuropathologic studies. AJNR 1987; 8:1083–1091.
106. Doyle WK, Budinger TF, Valk PE, et al: Differentiation of cerebral radiation necrosis from tumor recurrence by [^{18}F]-FDG and ^{82}Rb positron emission tomography. J Comput Assist Tomogr 1987; 11:563–570.

8

CENTRAL NERVOUS SYSTEM INFECTION AND INFLAMMATION

INFECTION

The brain is encased by bone, enveloped in dura, and protected from the systemic circulation by the blood-brain barrier (BBB). Unique to the brain is the absence of draining lymphatic channels. A wide variety of organisms, including bacteria, viruses, fungi, and parasites, may infect the central nervous system (CNS). The organism may arrive at the site of infection by a hematogenous route, by direct extension of a sinus or mastoid infection, or by penetrating injury.

Multiple compartments of the CNS may serve as sites for an infection. The parenchyma, the extra-axial spaces, or the meninges may be involved, either alone or in any combination. If appropriate treatment is delayed or inadequate, infectious processes frequently extend from one to adjacent compartments.

Histologic and Radiographic Findings

Cerebritis and Abscess

Once an organism gains access to the cerebral parenchyma, a predictable series of histologic events occurs. The brain mounts a cellular and vascular response to confine and destroy the inoculum. The rapidity and effectiveness of this response are a function of the patient's immunocompetence and the virulence of the organism.[1]

The parenchymal response may be divided into two major stages: cerebritis and capsule formation. Cerebritis is the earliest stage of a pyogenic infection, lasting 7 to 10 days following inoculation. Initially a central area of coagulative necrosis develops with surrounding areas of inflammatory infiltrate including polymorphonuclear lymphocytes and plasma cells. These changes are most marked in the cerebral white matter (Fig. 8–1). Perivascular infiltrates appear that ultimately lead to thrombosis of large and small arteries and veins in the surrounding region. Fibroblasts elaborate reticulum in the perivascular spaces, which forms the template for the subsequent deposition of collagen that occurs late in the cerebritis stage. The core of the inflammatory reaction undergoes liquefaction necrosis as vasogenic edema accumulates at the periphery.

The computed tomographic (CT) appearance of cerebritis in animal models[2, 3] and in clinical experience[4–6] has been reported. In early cerebritis, ill-defined regions of hypodensity appear with mild mass effect. Heterogeneous or ring enhancement may occur following contrast administration. In the late cerebritis stage, collagen deposition is significantly advanced to render the early capsule isodense or hyperdense to surrounding brain on the precontrast examination. Vasogenic edema and mass effect increase and there is evidence of ring enhancement surrounding a necrotic center. With time, the contrast may diffuse into the necrotic center.

Magnetic resonance imaging (MRI) depicts the changes of cerebritis more accurately and earlier than does CT.[6, 7] The edema will be apparent as regions of increased signal intensity on spin density and T2 images. The early mass effect will be best demonstrated on T1 images. Heterogeneous contrast enhancement is present in the early stages of cerebritis, becoming ringlike in the later stage.

The second stage of the parenchymal response is capsule formation. This generally occurs 10 to 14 days after inoculation. As the infection matures, necrotic debris and pus accumulate within the central abscess cavity (Fig. 8–2). The granulation tissue and fibrocollagenous capsule thicken. Reactive astrocytosis, neovascularity, and vasogenic edema may be found in the parenchyma adjacent to the capsule.[1] Blood supply to the gray matter is approximately four to five times greater than that to the white matter. This results in increased local delivery of inflammatory cells, allowing the abscess capsule closest to the gray matter to be thicker than that located along the ventricular surface. The capsule may actually appear to point to the ventricular surface in an attempt to capture the spreading organism.[3]

Otogenic abscesses appear in the temporal lobe or cerebellum. Rhinogenic abscesses are located in the frontal lobe. Hematogenous abscesses most often involve the gray-white junction of the middle cerebral artery (MCA) distribution, although they may occur anywhere. Hematogenous abscesses may be multiple or solitary. Otogenic or rhinogenic abscesses are usually solitary.[1]

On CT, the dense capsule is identified silhouetted between the hypodense necrotic center and the peripheral edema (Fig. 8–3). In general, the size of the capsule and the degree of surrounding edema may decrease compared with the late stage of cerebritis. After contrast administration, ring enhancement occurs, demonstrating a thin regular capsule. The central zone of necrosis does not enhance on delayed images.

MRI depicts the necrotic core as intermediate signal intensity between white matter and cerebrospinal fluid (CSF) on T1 images (Fig. 8–4). On T2 the signal intensity of the core is greater than that of gray matter.[8] The abscess capsule is isointense to hyperintense to brain on T1 images, and isointense to hypointense to white matter on T2. Although the etiology of the diminished signal of the abscess ring on T2 images is speculative, there is evidence to support the presence of paramagnetic free radical, released from macrophages during phagocytosis as the precipitating cause.[6, 8]

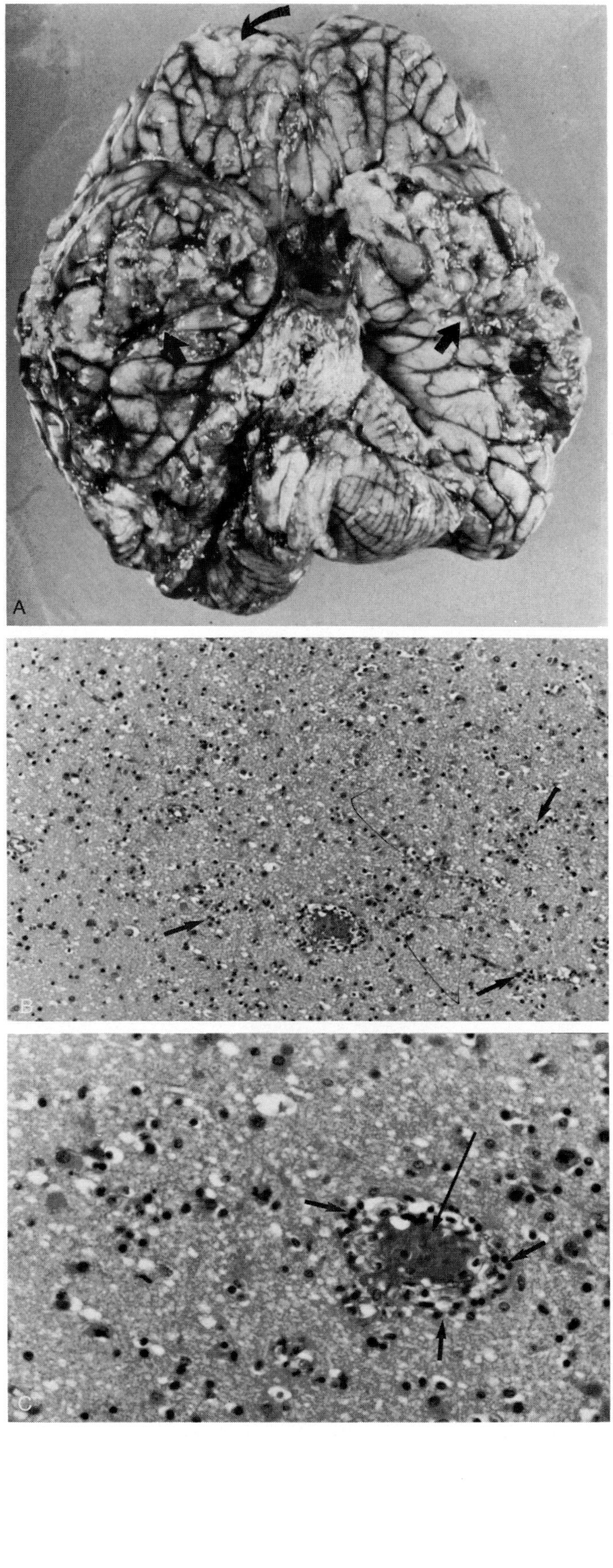

Figure 8–1. Cerebritis (pathology).

A, Gross. Diffuse marked edema is present with flattening of gyri and brain destruction in the bilateral temporal *(arrows)* and right frontal *(curved arrow)* lobes.

B, Microscopy (hematoxylin and eosin [H/E], original ×125). There is diffuse infiltration of inflammatory cells *(arrows)* including mononuclear and polymorphonuclear leukocytes into the cerebral parenchyma.

C, Microscopy (H/E, original ×310). Perivascular inflammatory cells *(arrows)* are responsible for the arterial thrombosis *(long arrow)*. (Courtesy of P. J. Cera, M.D., Department of Pathology, Geisinger Medical Center.)

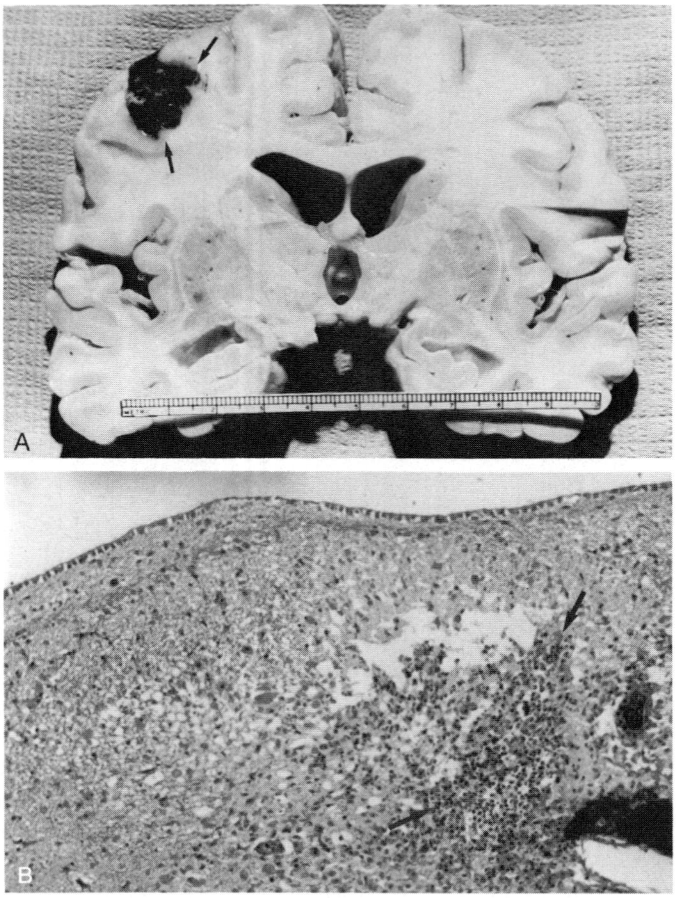

Figure 8–2. Abscess (pathology).

A, Gross (coronal section). A peripheral, well-organized abscess cavity *(arrows)* has erupted into the subarachnoid space. The abscess cavity has filled with hemopurulent material.

B, Microscopic (H/E, original ×125). Foci of neutrophils and necrosis *(arrows)* are present, indicating maturation of the inflammatory process. (Courtesy of P. J. Cera, M.D., Department of Pathology, Geisinger Medical Center.)

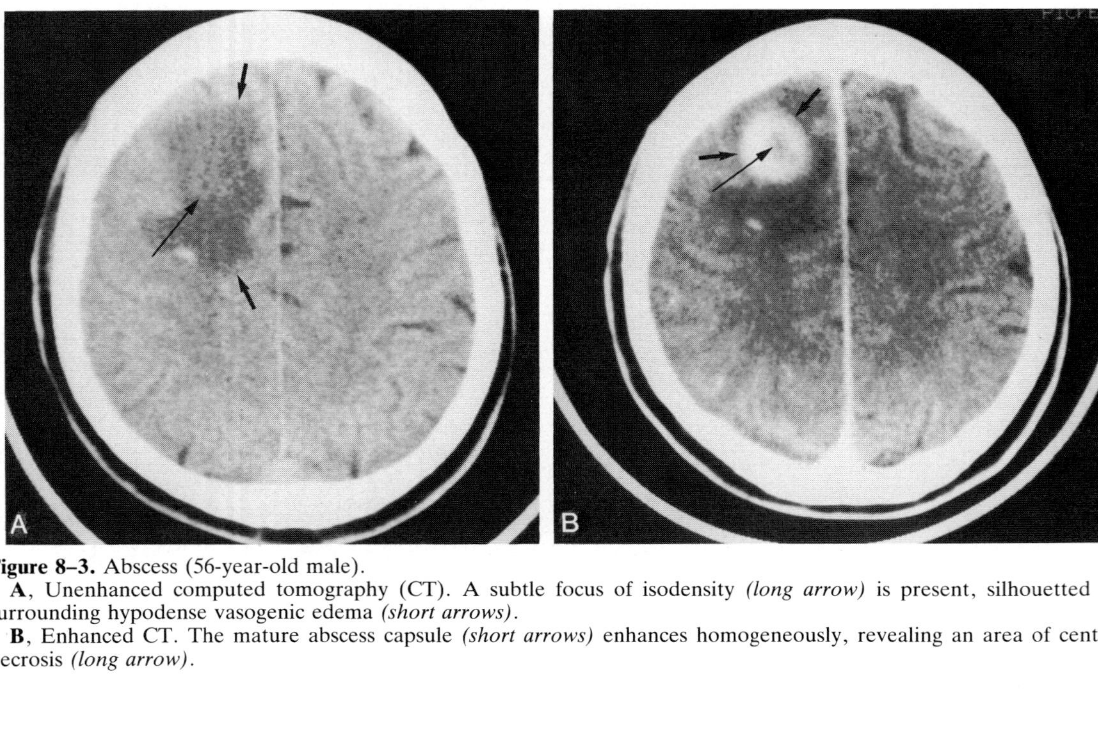

Figure 8–3. Abscess (56-year-old male).

A, Unenhanced computed tomography (CT). A subtle focus of isodensity *(long arrow)* is present, silhouetted by surrounding hypodense vasogenic edema *(short arrows)*.

B, Enhanced CT. The mature abscess capsule *(short arrows)* enhances homogeneously, revealing an area of central necrosis *(long arrow)*.

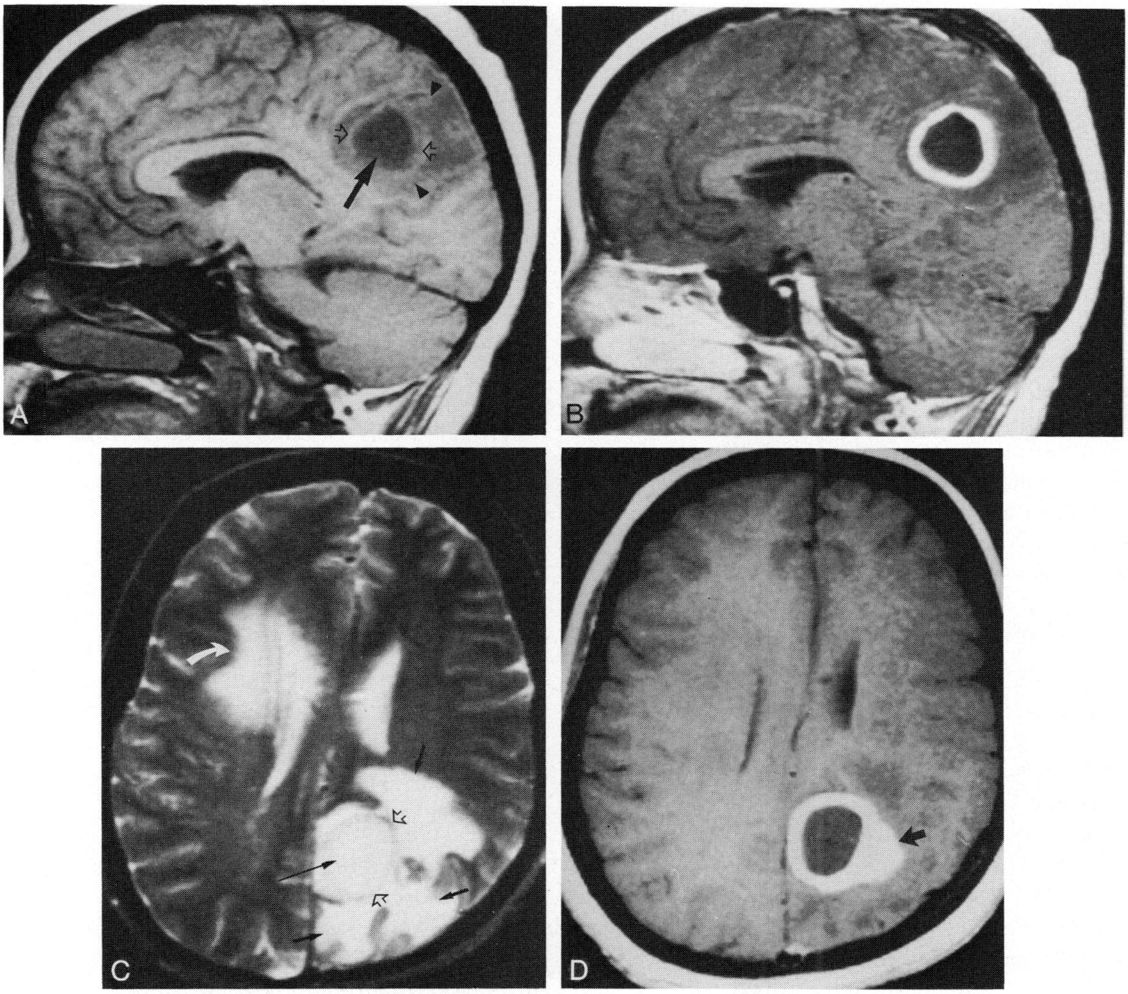

Figure 8–4. Abscess; *Staphylococcus aureus* (47-year-old male).

A, Parasagittal T1. A hypointense mass *(arrow)* is present in the parietal lobe. The mass is surrounded by a thin, isointense ring *(open arrows)*, which is marginated by ill-defined vasogenic edema *(arrowheads)*.

B, Enhanced parasagittal T1. The thin capsule of the abscess enhances homogeneously.

C, Axial T2. The necrotic center of the abscess cavity *(long arrow)*, like the surrounding vasogenic edema *(short arrows)*, is high signal intensity. The abscess capsule *(open arrows)* is isointense to parenchyma. A second focus of vasogenic edema *(curved arrow)* signifies a second lesion in the right parietal lobe.

D, Enhanced axial T1. A portion of the enhancing capsule *(arrow)* extends into the deep white matter.

In addition to establishing the diagnosis of an abscess, CT and MRI are useful in optimizing the timing of surgical intervention, determining effect of surgical and/or medical therapy, and detecting postoperative complications.[9] Intraventricular rupture with subsequent ependymitis may be detected as periventricular enhancement on contrast-enhanced CT. MRI depicts intraventricular and/or subarachnoid spread as increased signal intensity referable to CSF on T1 and T2. Contrast enhancement will more accurately localize the ependymal or pial surface involvement. In a small study, the mortality from brain abscesses in the pre-CT era was approximately 44%, compared with 0% in the post-CT era.[9] Interestingly, CT did not improve the 33% morbidity rate in intracerebral abscesses.

Steroids tighten the zona occludens of the endothelial cells, effectively decreasing the permeability of the BBB. Steroid therapy will decrease the pattern and magnitude of enhancement in the cerebritis stage.[4, 10] However, neovascularity is present by the time the capsule matures. These neovascular channels lack a normal BBB. Thus, administration of steroids will not have a significant effect on the enhancement in the capsule stage.[10]

Encephalitis

Encephalitis is generally the result of a viral infection that may induce an acute, subacute, or chronic inflammation of the brain parenchyma. The virus usually gains access to the CNS through a hematogenous route. The severity and location of the inflammatory process may be specific for each virus.[1]

Although the brain may appear normal on gross examination, diffuse or focal inflammatory infiltrates may be present in the gray and white matter and in Virchow-Robin spaces.[1] Monocytes, lymphocytes, and plasma cells may be present in the early infiltrate with varying degrees of neuronal necrosis and neovascularity. Definitive diagnosis depends on isolation of the virus, usually from biopsy.

In the United States, common viral agents responsible for acute encephalitis are the picornaviruses, togaviruses, herpesviruses, paramyxoviruses, and arenaviruses.[1]

The planar imaging appearance of encephalitis resembles that of cerebritis. The inflammatory process is poorly contained; vasogenic edema, mass effect, and heterogeneous enhancement are present to varying degrees.

Meningitis

This acute or chronic inflammation of predominantly the pia and arachnoid membranes may be caused by multiple organisms. Patients may present with stiff neck, fever, headache, and evidence of increased intracranial pressure.

Acute meningitis is usually purulent with an exudate identified in the subarachnoid space over the convexities shortly after inoculation. The subarachnoid vessels are congested and the brain is swollen. Polymorphonuclear leukocytes and fibrin accumulate early, followed by mononuclear and plasma cells. Acute meningitis is usually bacterial.[1]

Chronic meningitis is most often the result of tuberculosis or cryptococcus. Both acute and chronic inflammatory cells may be detected. The organisms are usually identified within the exudate.

The proximity of this inflammatory reaction to the dural veins and subarachnoid spaces leads to frequent complications. Interruption of the CSF pathway by inflammatory debris over the vertex may lead to communicating hydrocephalus. Reflux of inflammatory material into the ventricular system may create a noncommunicating hydrocephalus, as well as ventriculitis.

Dural veins may become thrombosed, resulting in subsequent cerebral infarctions. These infarctions are usually venous and superficial, and may be hemorrhagic in nature (Fig. 8–5). Some organisms have predilection for the basilar meninges. In these cases, the lenticulostriate arteries that enter the anterior perforating substance may be thrombosed, resulting in arterial infarctions of the basal ganglia and internal capsule.

The Virchow-Robin spaces that surround the penetrating arteries and invest the perforating substance may serve as conduits, permitting a primary meningeal infection entrance to the parenchyma with resultant cerebritis or abscess. Finally, subdural effusions may occur as a complication of meningitis (Fig. 8–6). These occur most frequently in children with *Haemophilus influenzae* meningitis[7] and are most often sterile.[6]

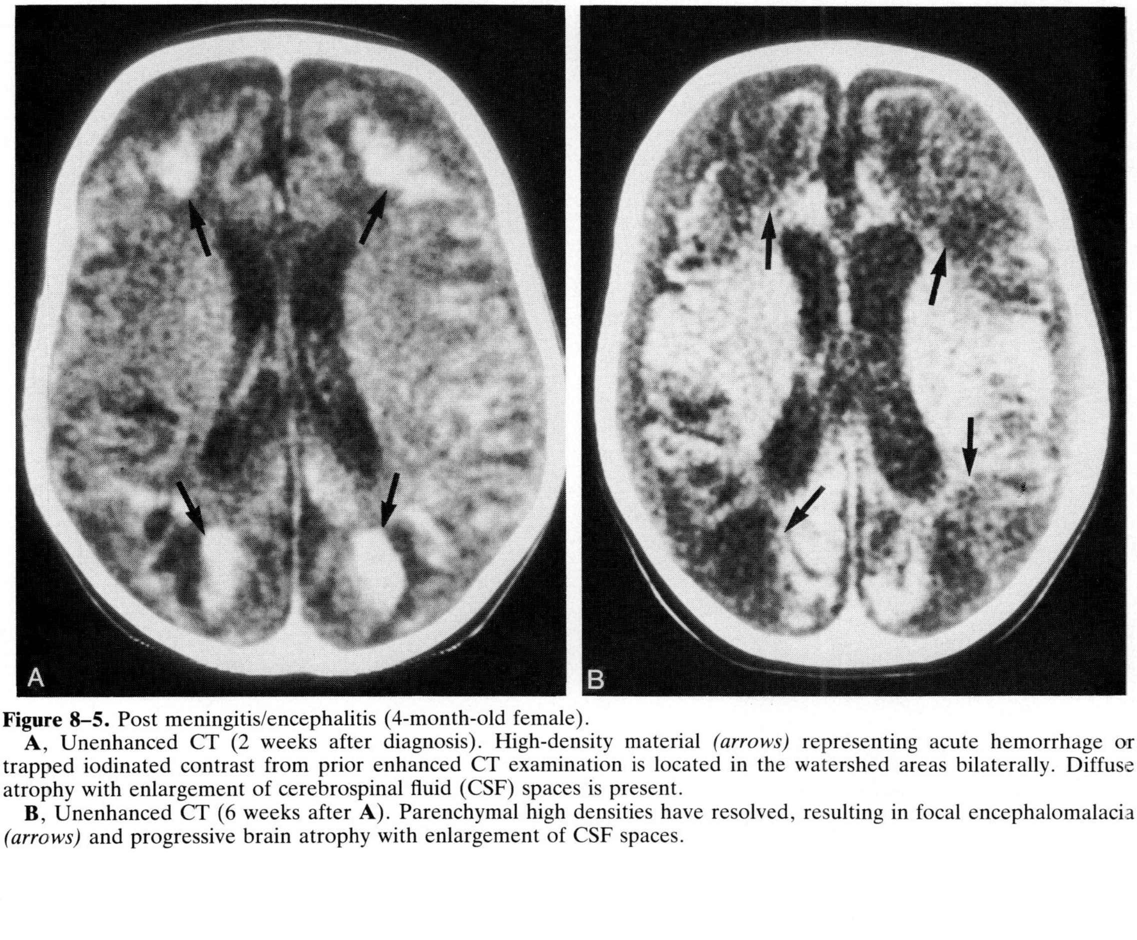

Figure 8–5. Post meningitis/encephalitis (4-month-old female).

A, Unenhanced CT (2 weeks after diagnosis). High-density material *(arrows)* representing acute hemorrhage or trapped iodinated contrast from prior enhanced CT examination is located in the watershed areas bilaterally. Diffuse atrophy with enlargement of cerebrospinal fluid (CSF) spaces is present.

B, Unenhanced CT (6 weeks after **A**). Parenchymal high densities have resolved, resulting in focal encephalomalacia *(arrows)* and progressive brain atrophy with enlargement of CSF spaces.

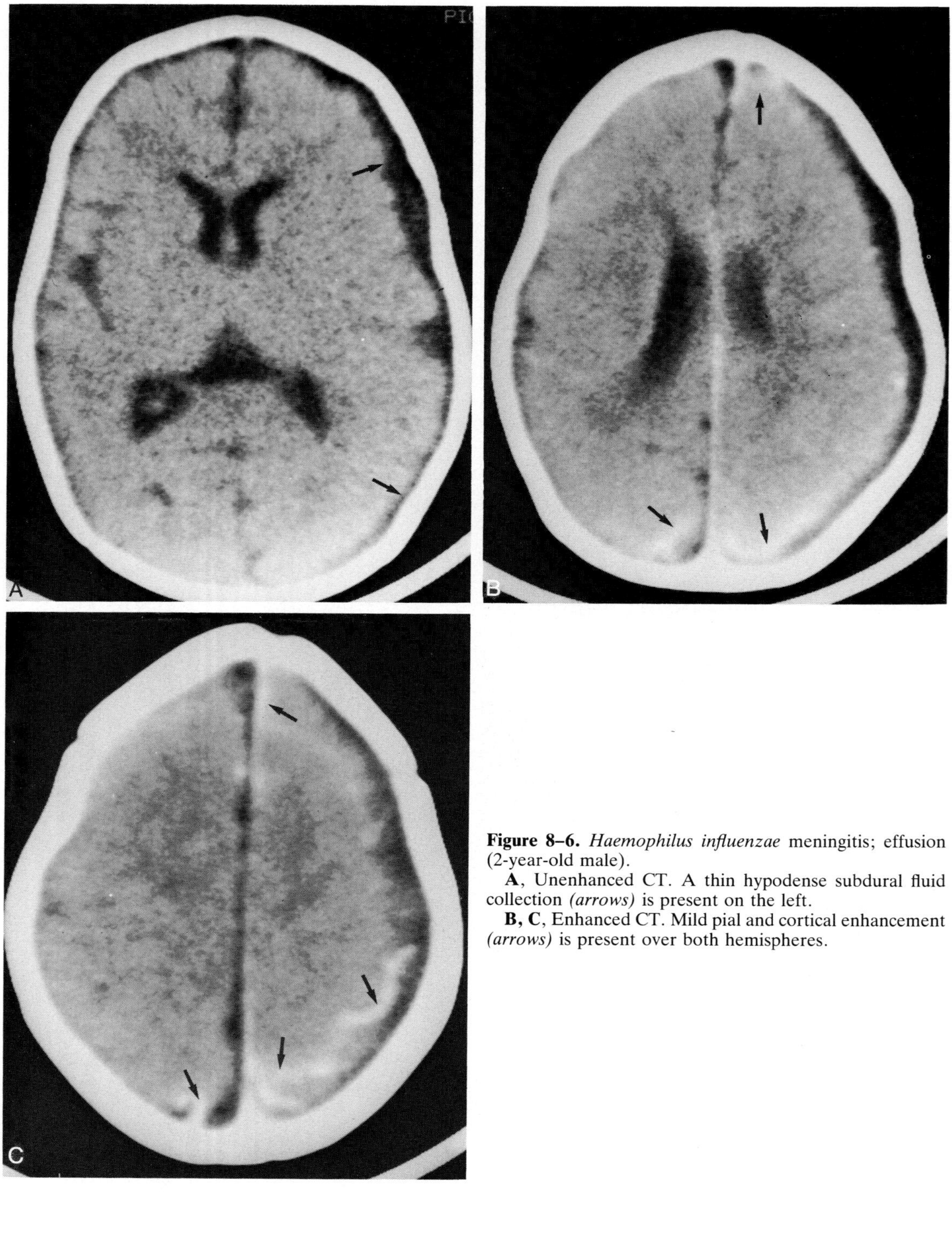

Figure 8–6. *Haemophilus influenzae* meningitis; effusion (2-year-old male).

A, Unenhanced CT. A thin hypodense subdural fluid collection *(arrows)* is present on the left.

B, C, Enhanced CT. Mild pial and cortical enhancement *(arrows)* is present over both hemispheres.

The CT examination in patients with meningitis may be normal.[7] Subtle regions of increased density in the basilar cisterns or sylvian fissures may be present secondary to inflammatory debris. Administration of contrast material is extremely useful in patients with suspected meningitis because the involved meninges may enhance vividly.[11] The normal symmetric architecture of the circle of Willis may be obscured by the enhancement (Fig. 8–7). The tentorium may enhance excessively. The normal discrete "dot-dash" pattern of the middle cerebral branches that course perpendicular and parallel to the plane of imaging in the sylvian fissure may be obscured by heterogeneous enhancement.

Ventricular dilatation secondary to hydrocephalus may be the only abnormal finding in patients with meningitis. If venous thrombosis extends to the dural sinus, a "delta sign" may be identified on CT, secondary to inability to opacify the thrombosed sinus.[12] Ischemic edema in the cortical and subcortical white matter crossing arterial vascular territories suggests venous infarction. Focal areas of increased density within the infarction are secondary to hemorrhage. The infarctions that occur in the anterior perforating substance are usually bland arterial infarcts in the lenticulostriate artery distribution of the anterior and/or middle cerebral arteries.

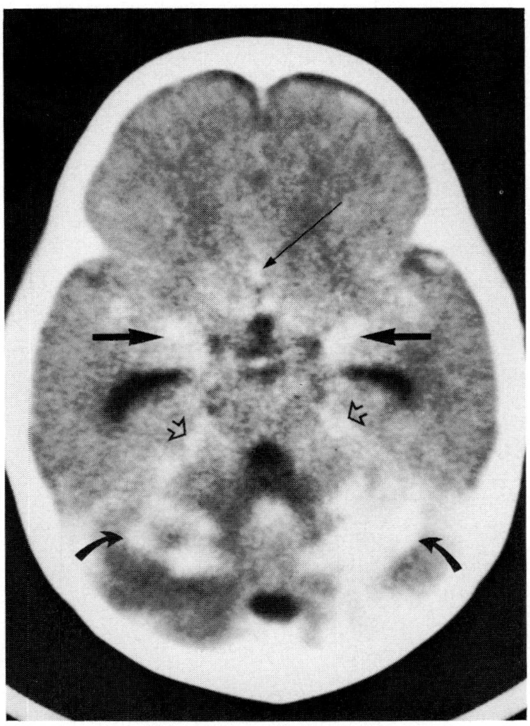

Figure 8–7. Pneumococcal meningitis-cerebritis (6-month-old female). Enhanced CT; diffuse irregular enhancement is present in the lateral cerebral fissure bilaterally *(solid arrows)*, in the interhemispheric fissure *(long arrow)*, and along the tentorium *(open arrows)*. Enhancement *(curved arrows)* in the superior aspect of the cerebellum confirms parenchymal involvement.

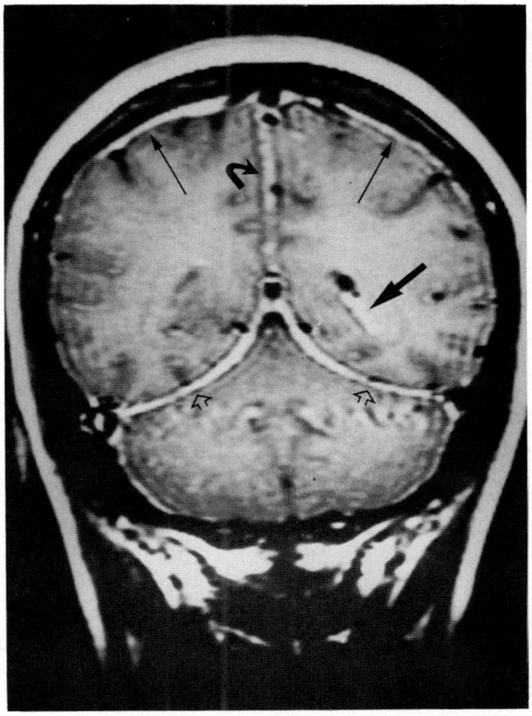

Figure 8–8. Meningitis; viral (42-year-old female). Enhanced coronal T1; there is diffuse meningeal enhancement over the convexities *(long arrows)*, falx cerebri *(curved arrow)*, and tentorium *(open arrows)*. Excessive enhancement in the left atrium *(solid arrow)* signifies ependymitis.

MRI is superior to CT in evaluating patients with meningitis and the resultant complications.[13] T2 images are sensitive at delineating infarct, abscess, and edema. Unenhanced T1 images detect mass effect and hemorrhage. Gadolinium-enhanced T1 images are sensitive at identifying areas of active inflammation and focal parenchymal lesions (Fig. 8–8). Dural venous thrombosis may be diagnosed if flow void is consistently absent and there is increased signal intensity within the dural channels on T1 images.[14]

MRI depicts ventriculitis as abnormal high signal of the ependyma and CSF on spin density and T2 images. Contrast enhancement of the ependymal surface will corroborate ventriculitis.[15]

Empyema

The accumulation of inflammatory debris may occur in the subdural and, less frequently, in the epidural compartment. Patients with empyemas may present with two distinctly different clinical scenarios, contingent on the etiology of the infection.[6, 16, 17] The patients with otorhinologic infections and subsequent retrograde thrombophlebitis and infection in the subdural compartment present with fever, lethargy, meningismus, headache, altered levels of consciousness, seizures, focal neurologic deficits, and rapid deterioration to coma and death. The dura is relatively resistant to the penetration of antibiotics. Consequently, this is a surgical emergency and should be addressed before secondary extension into the brain occurs with potential venous thrombosis, infarction, and abscess.

Patients with empyema may also present with a more indolent course. This occurs in patients months to years after craniotomy or drainage of a traumatic extra-axial hemorrhage. Patients present with slowly increasing mass effect and may exhibit insidious onset of seizures without evidence of systemic illness. In these patients, a well-formed inner subdural membrane is present from the prior hemorrhage or surgery and protects the underlying parenchyma and cortical vessels from the noxious, inflammatory debris.[16, 17]

The mortality rate for patients with subdural empyemas is 10 to 15%,[18] a twofold to fourfold decrease from the pre-CT era. On CT, the small extra-axial collection is isodense to CSF and may be crescentic or lentiform in shape (Fig. 8–9). The degree of mass effect is often greater than expected for the size of the inflammatory collection. The empyema is often more obvious when it occurs in the interhemispheric fissure, along the falx where it is not obscured by artifact from the adjacent bone. A well-defined medial border of enhancement[19, 20] is present that may extend into the subjacent parenchyma. Parenchymal involvement may occur secondary to retrograde venous thrombophlebitis with resultant abscess or infarction. The MRI examination accurately depicts the mass effect on the T1 sequence. The extra-axial collection is usually intermediate signal intensity between brain and CSF on T1. The collection is hyperintense to brain on T2.[6] High signal may occur in the subjacent cortex indicating ischemia or inflammation, both of which may be reversible.

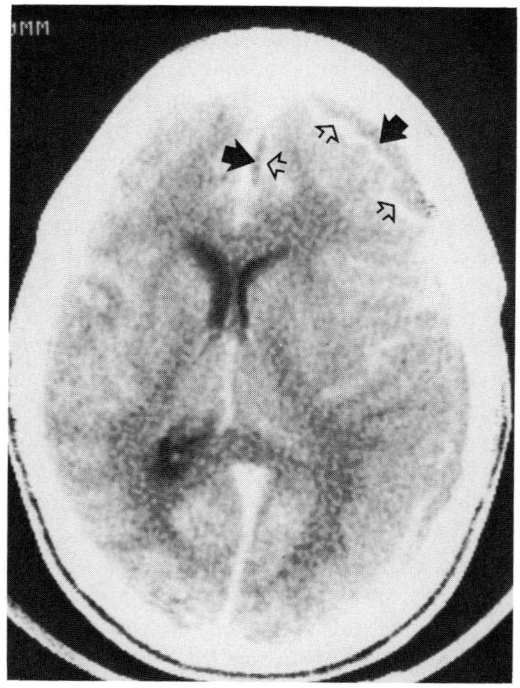

Figure 8–9. Subdural empyema (32-year-old female). Enhanced CT; a thin, low-density fluid collection *(solid arrows)* is present in the subdural space of the left frontal region. Leptomeningeal enhancement *(open arrows)* is present. The degree of mass effect (subfalcial herniation) is out of proportion to the small extracerebral empyema.

Common Causative Organisms

Bacterial

Aerobic or anaerobic streptococci are the most common bacterial organisms isolated in cerebral abscesses.[1] Eighty per cent of nontraumatic abscesses are due to anaerobic organisms.

Staphylococcus aureus is an aerobic gram-positive coccus that is often responsible for CNS abscesses. The organism commonly gains access to the CNS hematogenously, usually from an upper respiratory tract infection that may or may not be symptomatic. In experimental studies,[2] *S. aureus* brain abscesses may differ from typical pyogenic abscesses in some respects. The organism is more virulent than most and thus has a tendency to form larger abscesses and have a delayed course of healing. Inflammation frequently escapes the collagen capsule, and early ependymitis may be detected.

Listeria monocytogenes is a facultative anaerobic gram-positive rod. Spontaneous infections may occur in humans[21] and have been associated with immunocompromised patients or individuals with lymphoma. The mode of infection is unknown.[22] The organism is phagocytized but not killed by neutrophils and other phagocytic cells. Remaining viable, this organism is transported throughout the host. The organism may incite a meningoencephalitis in the presence or absence of bacteremia. In addition to cerebral parenchymal involvement,[23] the rhombencephalon[24] may be affected, resulting in rhombencephalitis (Fig. 8–10).

Bacteria are the most common cause of purulent meningitis. In neonates and newborns, *Escherichia coli* and other gram-negative enteric organisms, group B streptococci, and *L. monocytogenes* are isolated. *H. influenzae* may be isolated in infants and children. *Streptococcus pneumoniae* and *Neisseria meningitidis* may be responsible for meningitis in infants, children, and adults.[1]

Viral

Viral infections of the CNS usually incite encephalitis. Unlike pyogenic infections, which are contained by the host capsule, encephalitis is a diffuse parenchymal lesion that may spread rapidly throughout the cerebral parenchyma.[6] Viral infections may result from an acute infection or from reactivation of a latent virus.

Herpes Encephalitis

Herpes encephalitis is the most common nonepidemic fatal encephalitis in North America. Herpes simplex virus type I (HSV-I) causes this disease, and patients may present with global confusion, clouded sensorium, disorientation, and incoherent thought processes. Mental status deteriorates rapidly to coma.[25]

The infection may result from a primary infection or reactivation of a latent infection

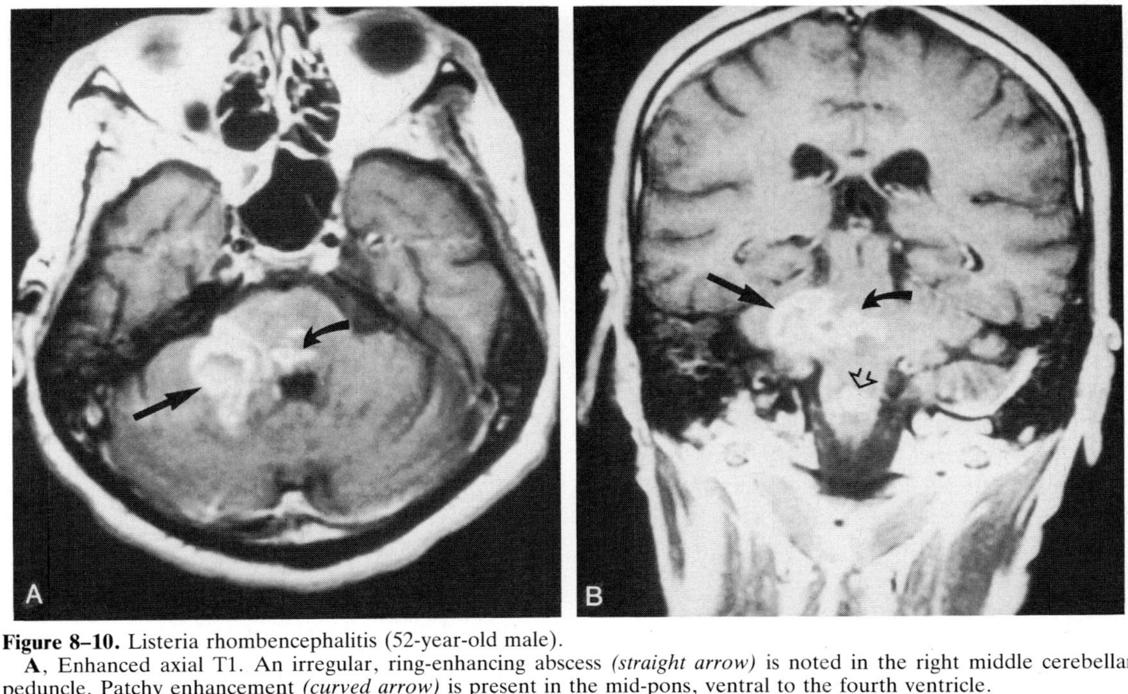

Figure 8–10. Listeria rhombencephalitis (52-year-old male).

A, Enhanced axial T1. An irregular, ring-enhancing abscess *(straight arrow)* is noted in the right middle cerebellar peduncle. Patchy enhancement *(curved arrow)* is present in the mid-pons, ventral to the fourth ventricle.

B, Enhanced coronal T1. The ring lesion *(straight arrow)* in the cerebellar peduncle and mid-pons *(curved arrow)* is present. A separate focus of inflammation *(open arrow)* in the mid-medulla is noted.

of the trigeminal ganglion.[26] Herpes encephalitis usually involves the temporal lobes, the insular cortex (sparing the lentiform nucleus), and orbital surface of the frontal lobe. Bilateral disease occurs in more than 50% of patients if not appropriately treated. Histologically, a diffuse meningoencephalitis is present with lymphocytic infiltrate of meninges, Virchow-Robin spaces, and subjacent brain. Hemorrhagic neuronal necrosis is a prominent feature, and microglial nodules and eosinophilic intranuclear inclusion bodies may be identified.[26]

Cross-sectional imaging reveals ill-defined areas of edema, mild mass effect, and heterogeneous linear enhancement (Fig. 8–11).[26, 27] Conspicuous sparing of the lentiform nucleus is highly suggestive of this disease.[27] MRI detects the encephalitis more accurately and earlier than CT[6] and may be used to monitor the response to therapy.[28] Parenchymal destructive changes may be widespread and result in significant morbidity.

The role of planar imaging in these patient is merely a corroborative one. In order for patients to avoid irreversible neuronal damage, empiric medical treatment (acyclovir administration) must commence before abnormalities are apparent on imaging studies. Left untreated, the mortality rate for HSV-I encephalitis is 70%.[1]

Fungal

Fungi are ubiquitous organisms that may be encountered in the household, soil, food, and air. Certain fungi are known to infect the normal host, including *Coccidioides*, histoplasmosis, and blastomycosis. These and other fungi *(Cryptococcus, Aspergillus, Mucor*, and *Candida)* may infect the immunocompromised host.[6]

Most fungal infections present as self-limiting pulmonary, sinus, or cutaneous syndromes; the CNS is only rarely involved. The organism is inhaled and phagocytized but is not killed by neutrophils or macrophages. It uses the reticuloendothelial system as a vehicle to reach any target organ.

The radiographic manifestations of CNS fungal infections are multifold and nonspecific. In most cases, it is impossible to be organism specific based on radiographic findings. In general, fungi may induce a meningitis, meningoencephalitis, formation of granulomata, abscess, vasculitis, aneurysm formation, infarction, or intracranial hemorrhage.

Coccidioidomycosis

Coccidioides immitis is a soil fungus endemic to the arid southwestern United States and Latin America. The dust-borne arthrospores are inhaled, most often leading to an asymptomatic respiratory infection that is self-limiting. Less frequently, an influenzalike illness may occur with fever, night sweats, malaise, cough, generalized aches, and anorexia.[21, 22] Dissemination occurs in a small percentage of cases. The intracranial structures serve as the target organ in less than 0.2% of patients. The most common radiographic findings are communicating hydrocephalus; enhancing, soft tissue density material in the basilar cisterns; and periventricular or focal white matter lesions.[29]

Histoplasmosis

Histoplasma capsulatum is a dimorphic soil fungus that is inhaled by the host. The organism is phagocytized by the alveolar macrophages and most frequently remains an acute or chronic pulmonary disease. Rapid dissemination throughout the body may occur, with most patients remaining asymptomatic.[21] Less than 25% of patients with disseminated disease will have CNS involvement. Miliary granulomas, basal leptomeningitis, and solitary granulomas may occur.[30]

Blastomycosis (North American)

Blastomyces dermatitidis is a dimorphic soil fungus that may cause a self-limiting disease like histoplasmosis. In addition, cutaneous lesions may develop on the face and trunk.[21] Once disseminated by the reticuloendothelial system, there is a propensity for blastomycosis to involve the male genital tract.[22] Intracranial disease is rare, with formation of meningitis or abscess (Fig. 8–12).

Cryptococcosis

See under Immunocompromised Host.

Aspergillosis

Aspergillus fumigatus is a ubiquitous fungus found on decaying vegetables. This opportu-

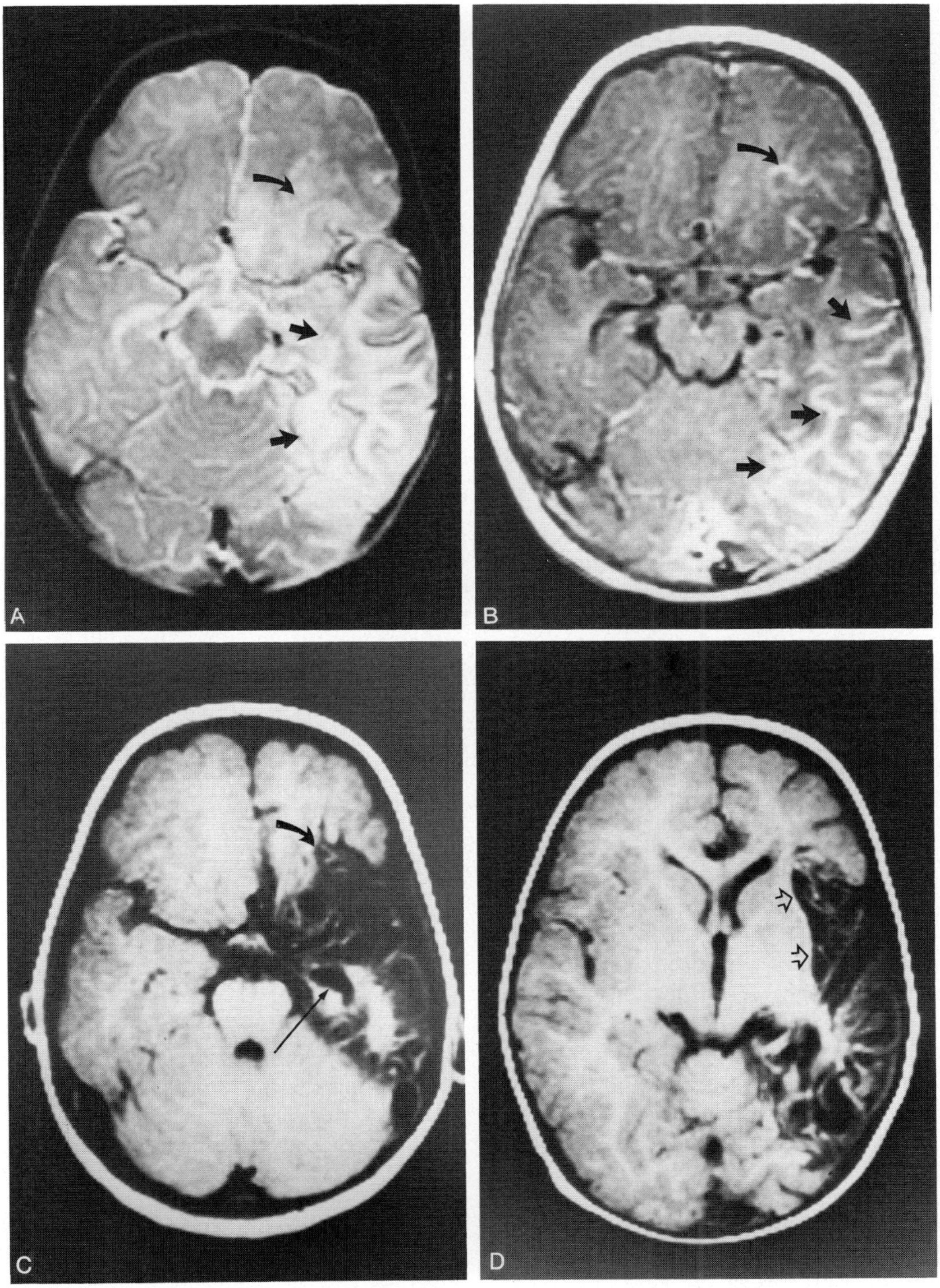

Figure 8–11. Herpes encephalitis HSV-I (1-year-old male).

A, Axial T2. Diffuse high signal in the left frontal *(curved arrow)* and left temporal lobes *(straight arrows)*, representing edema and inflammation, is noted 7 days following presentation.

B, Enhanced axial T1. Serpentine enhancement in the left frontal *(curved arrow)* and left temporal lobe *(straight arrows)* corroborates disruption of the blood-brain barrier (BBB) owing to active inflammation.

C, Axial T1 (3 weeks later). Marked encephalomalacic changes in the left frontal lobe *(curved arrow)* and left temporal lobe are present. Commensurate enlargement of the left temporal horn *(straight arrow)* is noted.

D, Axial T1. Sparing of the left lentiform nucleus *(open arrows)*, a finding that corroborates herpes simplex virus I (HSV-I), is demonstrated. There is marked volume loss of the left temporal lobe, insular cortex, and parietal lobe.

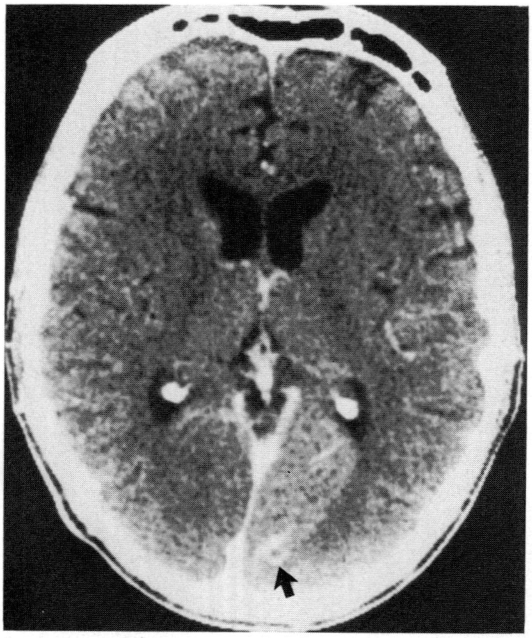

Figure 8–12. Blastomycosis (49-year-old male). Enhanced CT; a 1-cm ring-enhancing abscess *(arrow)* is noted in the left occipital lobe.

nistic invader of the immunocompromised host most frequently involves the lung, where at least three distinct forms of the disease may be identified.[21] Aspergillosis may also extend into the CNS by contiguous involvement from the sinuses.[6] Aspergillosis has a proclivity to invade the endothelium, with resultant thrombosis, infarct, and/or abscess formation. Infarctions may be hemorrhagic.[31] Vasculitis and aneurysm formation have been reported.[32] Diffuse leptomeningitis is uncommon.[11]

Mucormycosis

Mucorales fungi is an opportunistic organism that, like *Aspergillus*, invades and proliferates in the walls of blood vessels. It is found in patients with diabetes, extensive burns, lymphoma or leukemia, and immunosuppression.[21] The intracranial disease is most commonly a result of extension from the necrotizing vasculitis of the nose and sinuses that has extended into the orbital apex and cavernous sinus.[33–35] A rare blood-borne form of the disease exists with intracranial involvement without concomitant sinus disease.[35] Abscesses and bland, and/or hemorrhagic infarcts characterize this infection (Fig. 8–13).

Candidiasis

Candida albicans is an opportunistic organism that may invade any organ system in the debilitated or immunocompromised host.[21, 22]

Basilar CSF spaces are the most common site of granulomata and leptomeningeal thickening. Vascular occlusion may occur. High-density material, present in the CSF space, may enhance vividly. Infarcts and, less frequently, abscesses may occur in the distribution of the MCA.[36]

Parasitic

The frequency of parasitic infections in the United States is relatively rare compared with that of Third World countries. Cysticercosis is the most common parasite to involve the CNS. Cysticercosis is caused by the pork tapeworm *Taenia solium*. The larval stage enters humans, the intermediate hosts, through poorly prepared infected pork. Once attached to the small bowel mucosa, an adult tapeworm develops in 1 to 3 months. The adult liberates its oncospheres, which may be absorbed by the bowel wall, gaining access to the mesenteric circulation. The oncospheres may lodge in any tissue, voluntary muscle being the most common, followed by the CNS. CNS infection has been reported in more than 70% of patients with cysticercosis.[37]

Cysticercosis may involve the cerebral parenchyma or the CSF spaces (cisterns and ventricles). Although the reported frequency of parenchymal involvement varies,[38–40] the intraventricular form is by far the least common.

Owing to the varied patterns of CNS involvements, patients may present with multiple symptoms, most commonly seizures related to a focal mass lesion. In addition, patients may present with symptoms of increased intracranial pressure, vertigo, paresthesias, paraparesis, visual disturbances, or mental status deterioration.[37, 40]

As the larvae initially invade the CNS parenchyma, they may incite a mild inflammatory process with attendant local edema and mass effect. There is usually no evidence of enhancement on CT. MRI is more sensitive than CT at detecting the early active stage of the disease.[38, 39] The larvae subsequently form a cyst or bladder up to 2 to 3 cm in diameter. The scolex projects inward, attaching along

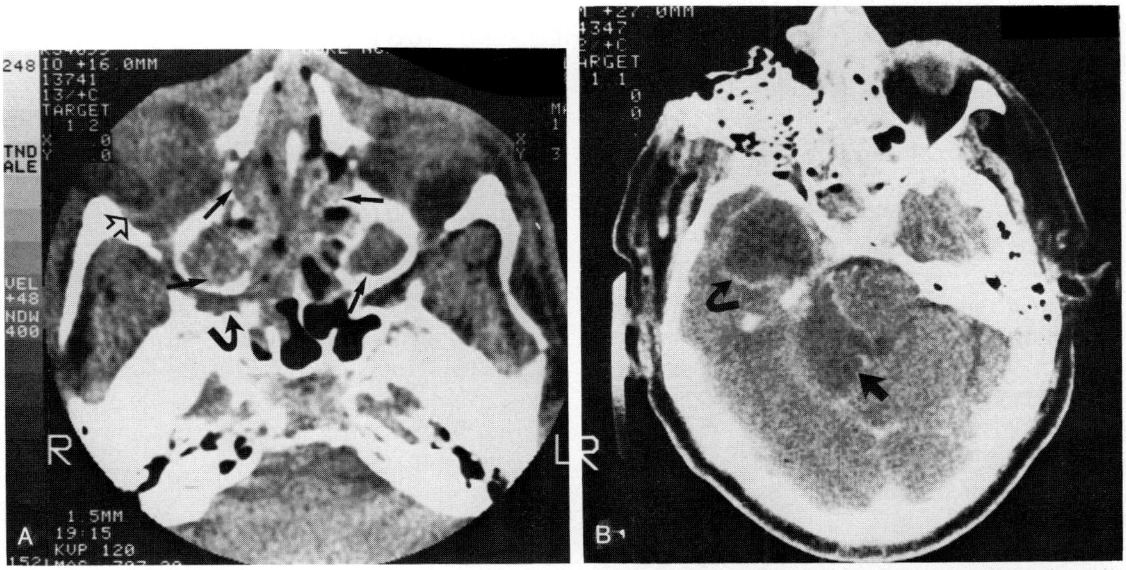

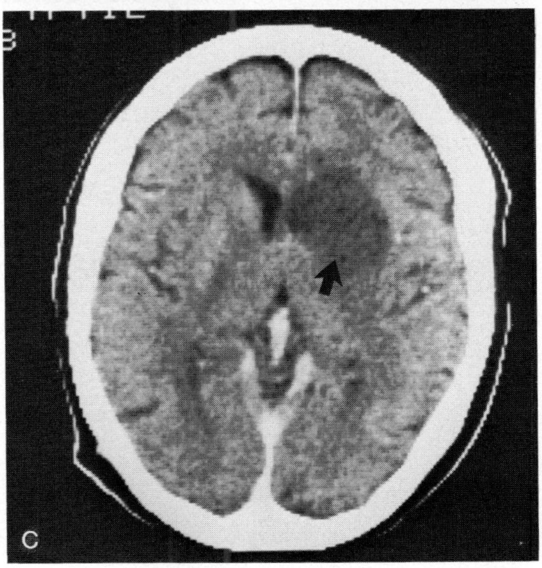

Figure 8–13. Mucormycosis (diabetic).

A, Enhanced CT (58-year-old male). Soft tissue density fills the paranasal sinuses *(straight arrows)*, the right retrobulbar region *(open arrow)*, and the right pterygopalatine fossa *(curved arrow)*.

B, Enhanced CT (61-year-old male). A thin rim of enhancement corroborates the presence of right temporal *(curved arrow)* and right superior cerebellar hemispheric *(straight arrow)* abscesses. Note the infected right globe has been removed.

C, Enhanced CT (32-year-old male). A bland infarct *(arrow)* is present in the left basal ganglia indicative of thrombosis of the anterior perforating vessels from leptomeningeal inflammation. (From Gamba JL, Woodruff WW, Djang WT, et al: Craniofacial mucormycosis: Assessment with CT. Radiology, 1986; 160:207–212, with permission.)

the wall of the cyst. Little surrounding tissue edema is noted at this stage. CT depicts spheric CSF-density cysts. The scolex may be visualized as a small focal nodule of increased density.[41] MRI depicts the viable cyst as isointense to CSF on all spin echo sequences (Fig. 8–14). The scolex may be visualized as a high-intensity nodule within the cyst on T1 images.[38, 39, 42]

As the cyst degenerates and the organism begins to die, the ability to mask its antigenic surface is lost and a discrete inflammatory reaction can be detected. Granulomatous changes and a chronic lymphocytic infiltrate accumulate. The lesion will begin to ring enhance, and edema will appear. The accumulation of protein within the cyst will shorten the T1 relaxation time, increasing the signal intensity of the cyst on T1 images.[6, 38, 39, 42] The degenerative cyst and edema may completely resolve or may later reappear as a punctate focus of calcification.[6, 37] CT is more effective than MRI in evaluating this stage of the disease process (Fig. 8–15).[38, 42] The calcification may appear as an inconspicuous focus of signal void on MRI.

Cysticercosis may occur primarily within the subarachnoid spaces of the basal cisterns. The racemose cysts that occur are nonviable, multilobular, and substantially larger than their intraparenchymal counterparts. The cysts are sterile and lack a scolex.[6] They may attain sufficient size within the basal cisterns to obstruct CSF spaces, resulting in hydrocephalus. The cysts are isointense to CSF on spin echo MRI (Fig. 8–16). In some instances, as the cysts degenerate, there is a leptomeningeal inflammatory and fibrotic reaction, which will appear as high signal around the periphery of the cyst on T2 sequences.

If the larval stage gains access to the ventricular system, an intraventricular cyst may occur. The cysts are isointense to CSF and, as with their parenchymal counterparts, a high-signal-intensity mural nodule representing the scolex may be seen on T1. The cysts may be position dependent and cause a noncommunicating hydrocephalus involving all or part of the ventricular system.

Degeneration of these intraventricular cysts may cause adjacent high signal on T2, repre-

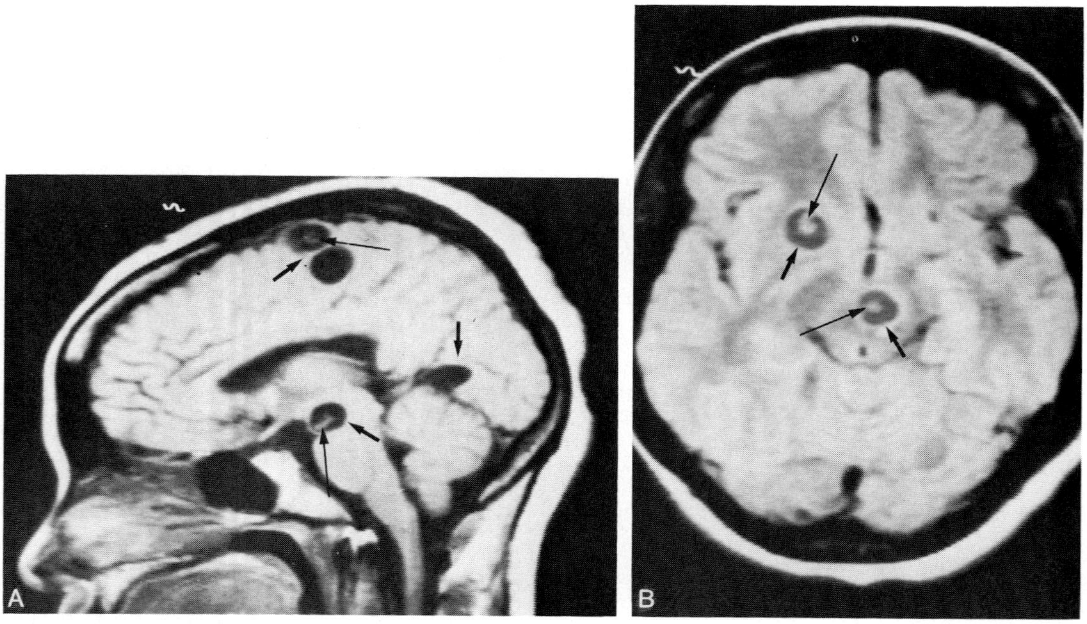

Figure 8–14. Parenchymal cysticercosis (age unknown).
A, B, Parasagittal and axial T1. Multiple isointense-to-CSF parenchymal cysts *(short arrows)* are present. The scolex *(long arrows)* of the organism is detected as foci of increased signal within multiple cysts. (From Lotz J, Hewlett R, Alheit B, et al: Neurocysticercosis: Correlative pathomorphology and MR imaging. Neuroradiology 1988; 30:35–41, with permission.)

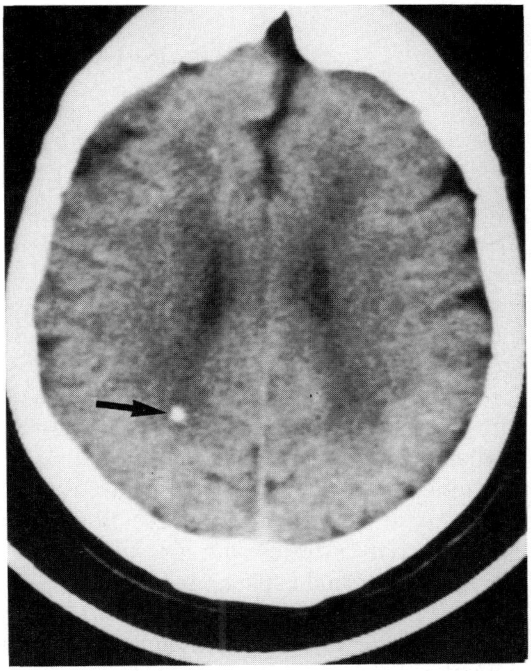

Figure 8–15. Cysticercosis; inactive (47-year-old male). Unenhanced CT; a punctate calcification *(arrow)* is noted in the right periatrial white matter.

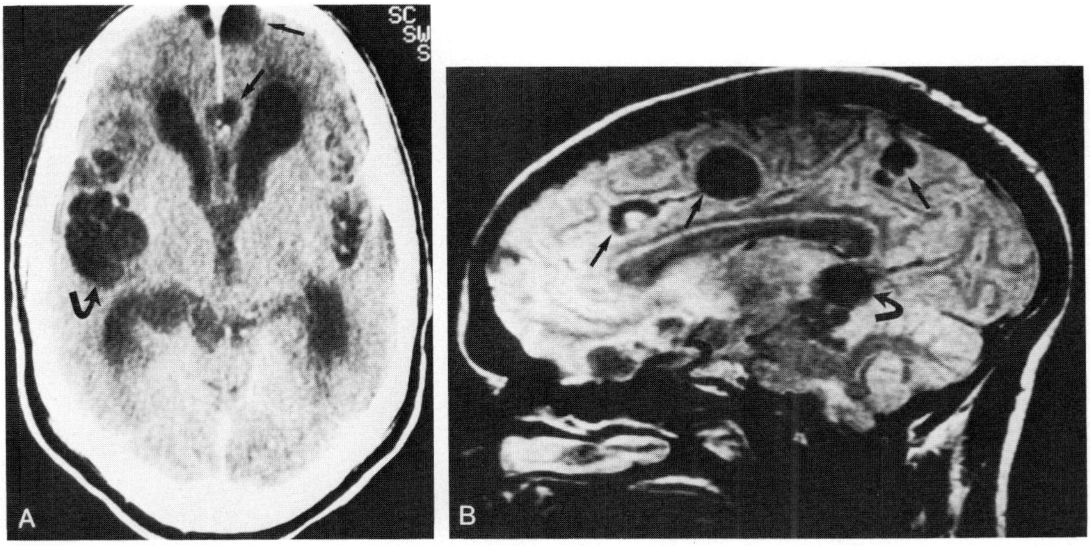

Figure 8–16. Racemose cysticercosis (age unknown).

A, Enhanced CT. Multiple large CSF-density cysts are present in the right sylvian fissure *(curved arrow)* and interhemispheric fissure *(short arrows)*.

B, Parasagittal T1. Large isointense-to-CSF cysts are present in the quadrigeminal cistern *(curved arrow)* and interhemispheric fissure *(straight arrows)*. (From Lotz J, Hewlett R, Alheit B, et al: Neurocysticercosis: Correlative pathomorphology and MR imaging. Neuroradiology 1988; 30:35–41, with permission.)

senting edema, gliosis, or inflammation.[39] MRI is more sensitive than CT in detecting and characterizing these intraventricular cysts.[39, 43]

Granulomatous

Tuberculosis

Tuberculosis (TB) enters the CNS by hematogenous dissemination. The three forms of TB infection[44, 45] are meningitis, tuberculoma, and encephalitis. Tuberculous meningitis, the most common form to involve the CNS, tends to involve the leptomeninges of the base of the brain, filling the subarachnoid space with a purulent exudate.[26] These patients present with signs and symptoms of meningitis with cranial nerve involvement. In addition to spreading throughout the subarachnoid spaces, the exudate may induce a vasculitis of the lenticulostriate arteries with a resultant infarction in the internal capsule or basal ganglia or both.

The second most common form of TB involvement of the CNS is parenchymal tuberculoma. These may occur separately or concurrently with leptomeningeal disease. The tuberculoma may be located anywhere in the supratentorial or infratentorial parenchyma and is characterized by a slowly expansile caseous mass surrounded by a rim of firm granulation tissue. These patients may present with signs and symptoms of intracranial mass including headache, papilledema, seizures, or focal neurologic deficits. The patient may be afebrile.[26]

TB encephalitis is rare, being the least common expression of CNS tuberculosis.[44, 45] These patients present with a rapidly progressive, edematous or hemorrhagic encephalopathy. TB encephalitis is often accompanied by meningitis and almost uniformly leads to coma.

Tuberculous exudates increase the density of the subarachnoid space on CT, most notably in the suprasellar cistern. Vivid enhancement of the meninges occurs following contrast administration (Fig. 8–17).[13, 45] Communicating hydrocephalus and/or infarctions in the basal ganglia are common findings (Fig. 8–18). The exudate increases the signal intensity of the suprasellar cistern on T1, and the postgadolinium examination demonstrates marked enhancement of the exudate and leptomeninges (Fig. 8–19). The T2 images are sensitive at

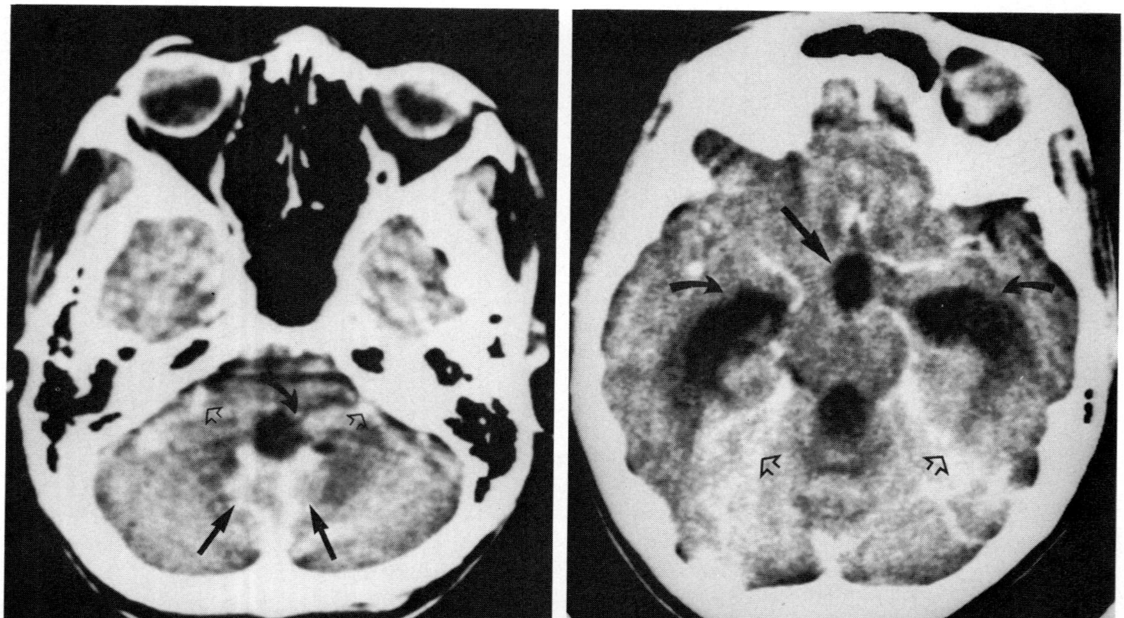

Figure 8–17. Tuberculosis (TB) (30-year-old female).

A, Enhanced CT. The fourth ventricle *(curved arrow)* is enlarged and irregular enhancement is present along the vermis *(straight arrows)* and cerebellopontine angle (CPA) *(open arrows)*.

B, Enhanced CT. Prominent enhancement over the tentorium *(open arrows)* is noted with enlargement of the third ventricle *(straight arrow)* and temporal horns *(curved arrows)*, indicating acute obstructive hydrocephalus.

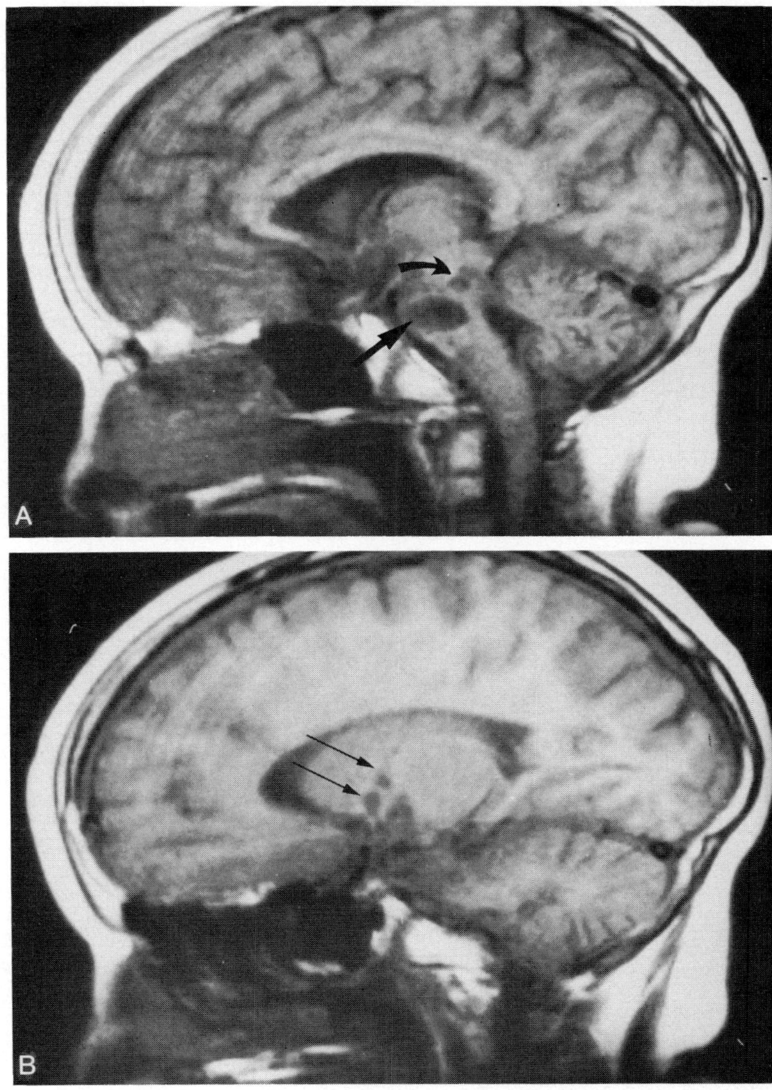

Figure 8–18. Tuberculosis (5-year-old male).

A, Parasagittal T1. Infarcts of varying size are located in the pons *(straight arrow)* and mesencephalon *(curved arrow)* as a result of remote TB meningitis.

B, Parasagittal T1. Similar encephalomalacic changes are present in the right basal ganglia *(arrows)* secondary to inflammatory exudate, which resulted in thrombosis of the lenticulostriate arteries.

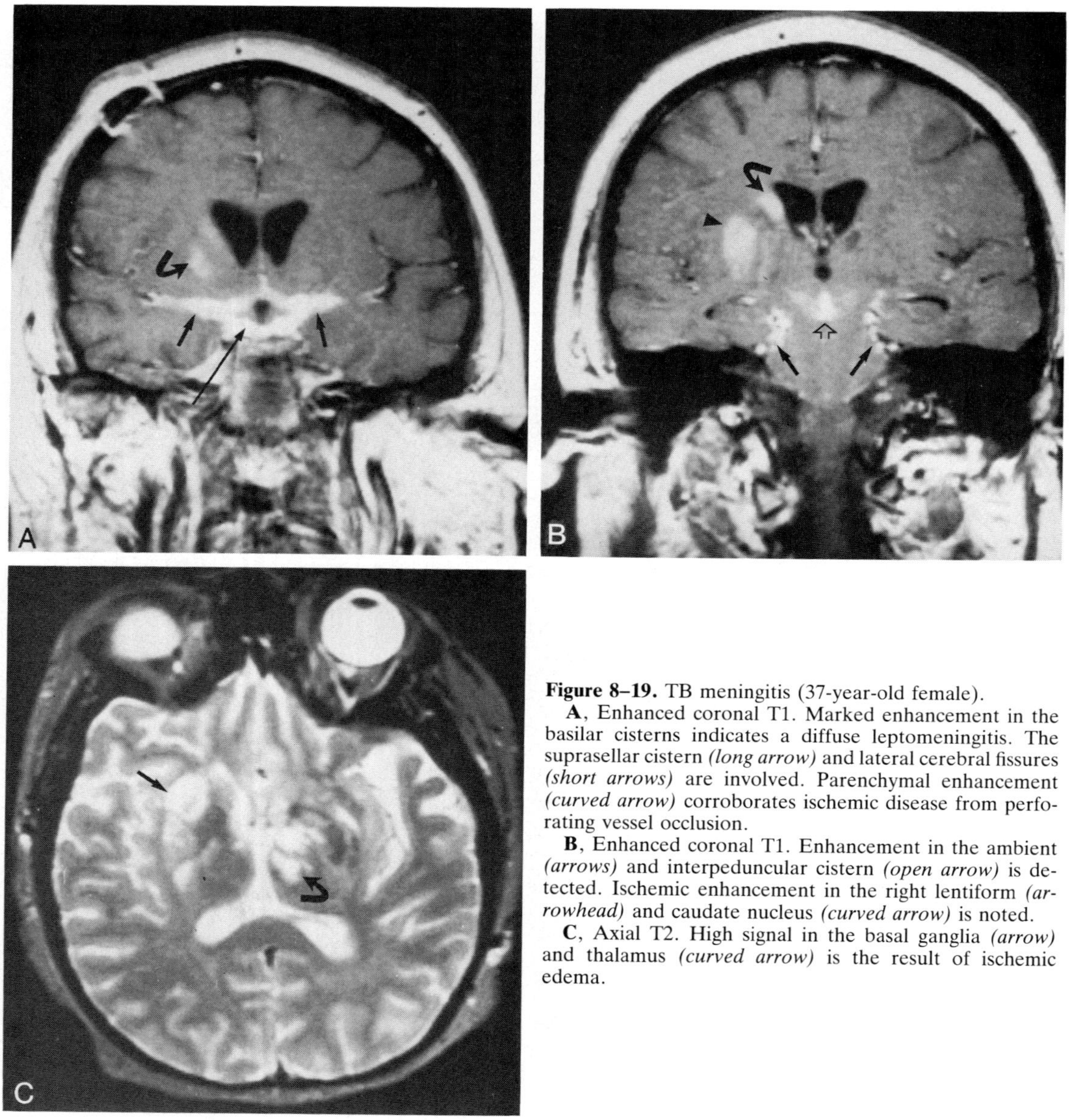

Figure 8–19. TB meningitis (37-year-old female).

A, Enhanced coronal T1. Marked enhancement in the basilar cisterns indicates a diffuse leptomeningitis. The suprasellar cistern *(long arrow)* and lateral cerebral fissures *(short arrows)* are involved. Parenchymal enhancement *(curved arrow)* corroborates ischemic disease from perforating vessel occlusion.

B, Enhanced coronal T1. Enhancement in the ambient *(arrows)* and interpeduncular cistern *(open arrow)* is detected. Ischemic enhancement in the right lentiform *(arrowhead)* and caudate nucleus *(curved arrow)* is noted.

C, Axial T2. High signal in the basal ganglia *(arrow)* and thalamus *(curved arrow)* is the result of ischemic edema.

detecting adjacent inflammatory or ischemic reactions in the parenchyma. Communicating hydrocephalus and infarcts in the basal ganglia can be adroitly displayed.[13]

Tuberculomas are most frequently solitary but may be multiple and clustered in a single group. They rarely calcify or exceed 2 cm in greatest linear dimension. Perilesional edema and mass effect are minimal. Smaller lesions enhance homogeneously and larger lesions enhance peripherally. The lesions are isointense to brain on T1 images (Fig. 8–20). Larger lesions are of low signal intensity and smaller lesions are of high signal intensity on T2.[46] The lesions ring enhance. TB encephalitis produces a diminished density in an irregular distribution on CT. Early and progressive edema and mass effect are apparent.[45]

Sarcoidosis

This granulomatous inflammatory disease clinically involves the CNS in 1 to 5% of patients with systemic sarcoidosis.[6, 47] Asymptomatic CNS involvement discovered at autopsy may exceed 60%.[47] The meninges are the most common focus of involvement, with a predilection for the base of the brain. The meninges may be thickened and/or discrete masses may be present.[26] Patients may present with visual disturbance, uveitis, gate ataxia, incoordination, diabetes insipidus, seizures, and cranial (especially facial nerve) neuropathies.[47] Communicating or noncommunicating hydrocephalus due to interruption of CSF pathways may occur. Deposition of noncaseous granuloma in the adventitia and media of small arteries and veins may lead to vessel occlusion with subsequent infarction.

Focal granulomatous masses may occur in the parenchyma. These lesions frequently occur subjacent to CSF spaces in the periventricular or subcortical white matter. Subcortical disease is most likely secondary to extension into the Virchow-Robin spaces that surround the arteries investing the parenchyma.[48]

The most common finding of CNS sarcoidosis on unenhanced CT is hydrocephalus.[49] Contrast enhancement delineates areas of leptomeningeal disease and granulomatous parenchymal masses.

The most common MRI finding in CNS sarcoidosis is enhancing meningeal disease.[50, 51] Enhancing intra-axial and extra-axial masses

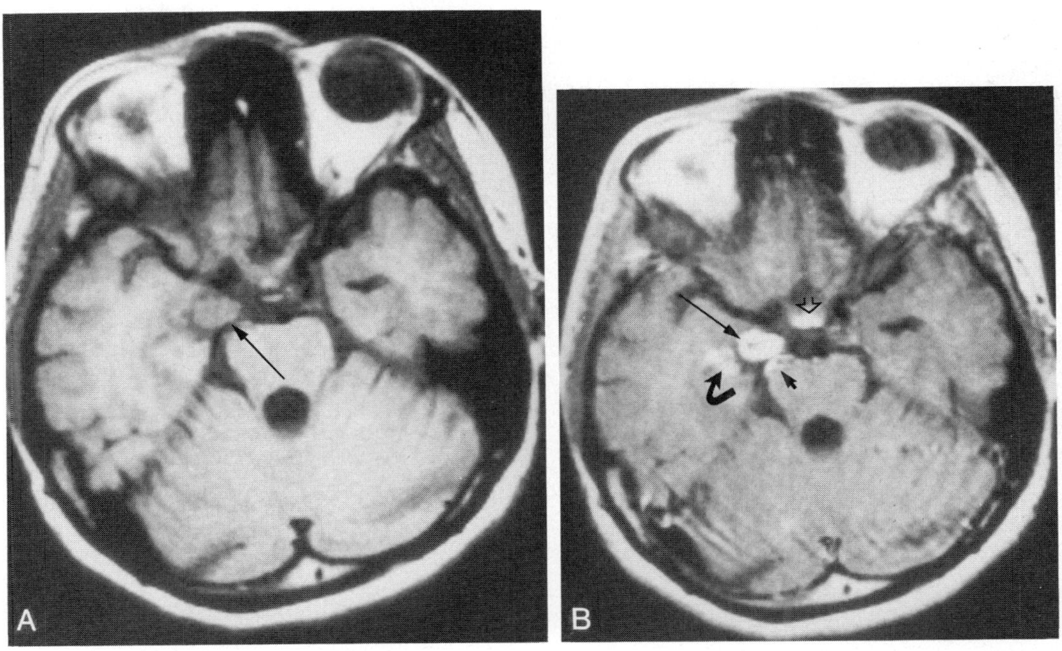

Figure 8–20. Tuberculoma (38-year-old female).

A, Axial T1. An isointense-to-gray matter mass *(arrow)* is present in the medial right temporal lobe, slightly deforming the suprasellar cistern.

B, Enhanced axial T1. The mass ring enhances *(long arrow)* with evidence of enhancement in the adjacent temporal parenchyma *(curved arrow)*, mesencephalon *(short arrow)*, and suprasellar cistern *(open arrow)*.

often involve the hypothalamus, optic chiasm, infundibulum, pituitary gland, and ventricular ependyma (Fig. 8–21). Additionally, discrete high-signal-intensity lesions on T2 images, indistinguishable from multiple sclerosis, have been reported.[47] Gadolinium enhancement is required in all patients undergoing planar evaluation of CNS sarcoidosis because the unenhanced examination may be normal.[50, 51]

Immunocompromised Host

With the advent of the acquired immunodeficiency syndrome (AIDS) epidemic, the "immunocompromised host" has taken on new meaning. In addition to patients receiving immunosuppressants for transplants or those being treated for primary neoplasms, individuals infected with the AIDS virus (human immunodeficiency virus [HIV]) make up a significant share of immunocompromised patients. This disease will serve as a model for the immunocompromised patient.

In general, immunosuppressed patients lack the ability to mount a normal host response. The host response may be incomplete or delayed, permitting extension of normal pathogens or opportunistic infections into adjacent brain parenchymal or CSF spaces before the infection can be effectively contained.

More than one third of patients with AIDS will develop signs and symptoms of CNS in-

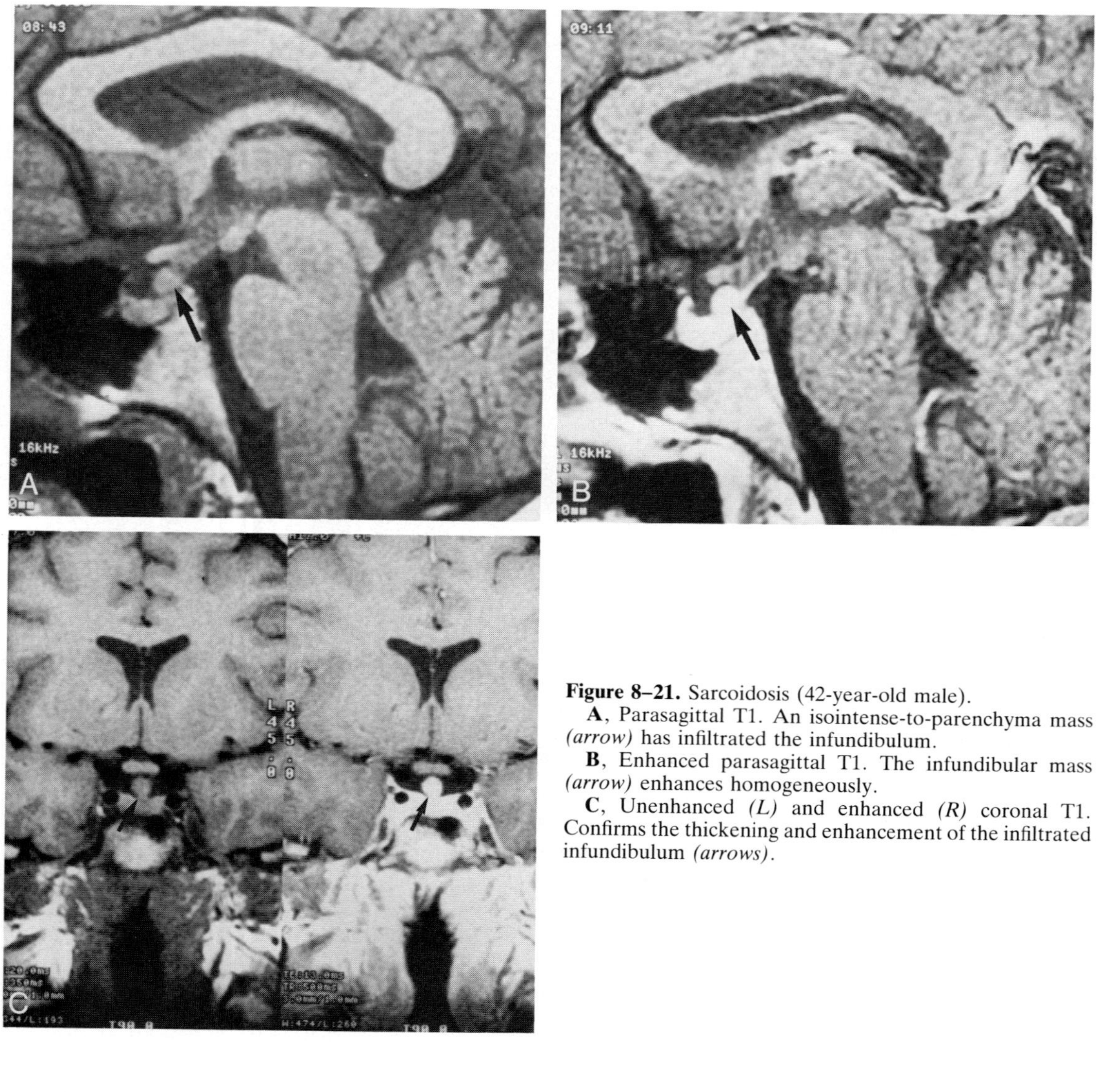

Figure 8–21. Sarcoidosis (42-year-old male).

A, Parasagittal T1. An isointense-to-parenchyma mass *(arrow)* has infiltrated the infundibulum.

B, Enhanced parasagittal T1. The infundibular mass *(arrow)* enhances homogeneously.

C, Unenhanced *(L)* and enhanced *(R)* coronal T1. Confirms the thickening and enhancement of the infiltrated infundibulum *(arrows)*.

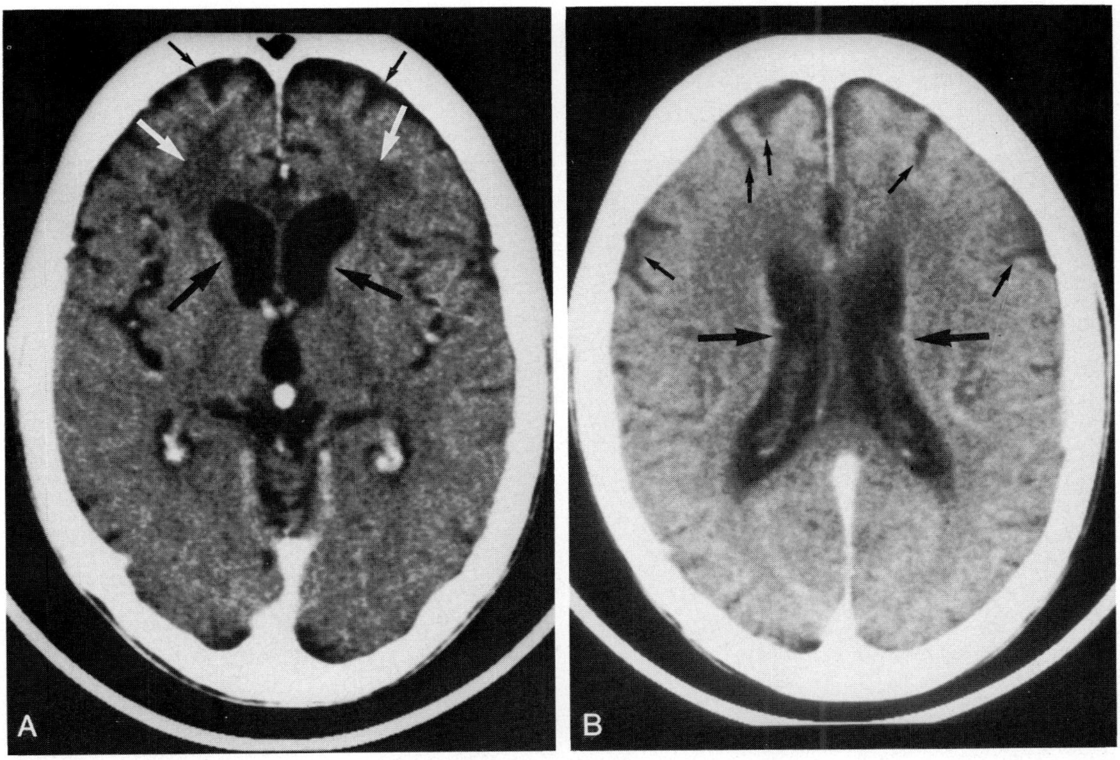

Figure 8–22. Human immunodeficiency virus (HIV) (32-year-old male).

A, B, Enhanced CT. No focal areas of enhancement are noted. The CSF spaces, including the ventricles *(bold black arrows)* and sulci *(thin black arrows)*, are enlarged, indicating a degree of atrophy far advanced for the patient's age. There are ill-defined white matter hypodensities *(white arrows)* in the frontal lobes.

volvement over the course of their disease. Radiographic findings in the CNS may be related to the presence of multiple organisms. In general, four patterns of involvement of the CNS are common, including atrophy, mass lesion, white matter disease, and/or leptomeningeal or ependymal disease.[52] The more common CNS infections associated with AIDS are presented here.

Human Immunodeficiency Virus (HIV)

HIV, the virus responsible for AIDS, is neurotropic. Patients present with progressive encephalopathy, somnolence, slow speech, word-finding difficulty, flat affect, and diminished attention.[18] The organism may be isolated in the brain within multinucleated giant cells and microglial cells. There is a predilection for the deep white and gray matter structures, with relative sparing of the subcortical white and cortical gray matter.[18]

The radiographic correlate of this involvement is central atrophy out of proportion to the patient's age. The ventricles are enlarged in an ex vacuo pattern.[18, 53] CT may also depict low-density parenchymal lesions without mass effect (Fig. 8–22). MRI is much more sensitive than CT at detecting the findings of HIV encephalitis.[18, 53] High-signal foci may be focally or diffusely present throughout the white matter on T2 (Fig. 8–23). The subinsular and periatrial white matter may be disproportionately involved.[54] Diffuse atrophy involving the cerebellum, cerebrum, or brainstem is common. Enhanced cross-sectional imaging is necessary to detect aseptic meningitis, which may occur secondary to HIV infection.

In general, there is a poor correlation between the extent of atrophy and the severity of the dementia that these patients may exhibit.[18] However, symptomatic HIV-positive patients are more likely (46%) than are asymptomatic HIV-positive patients (13%) to have

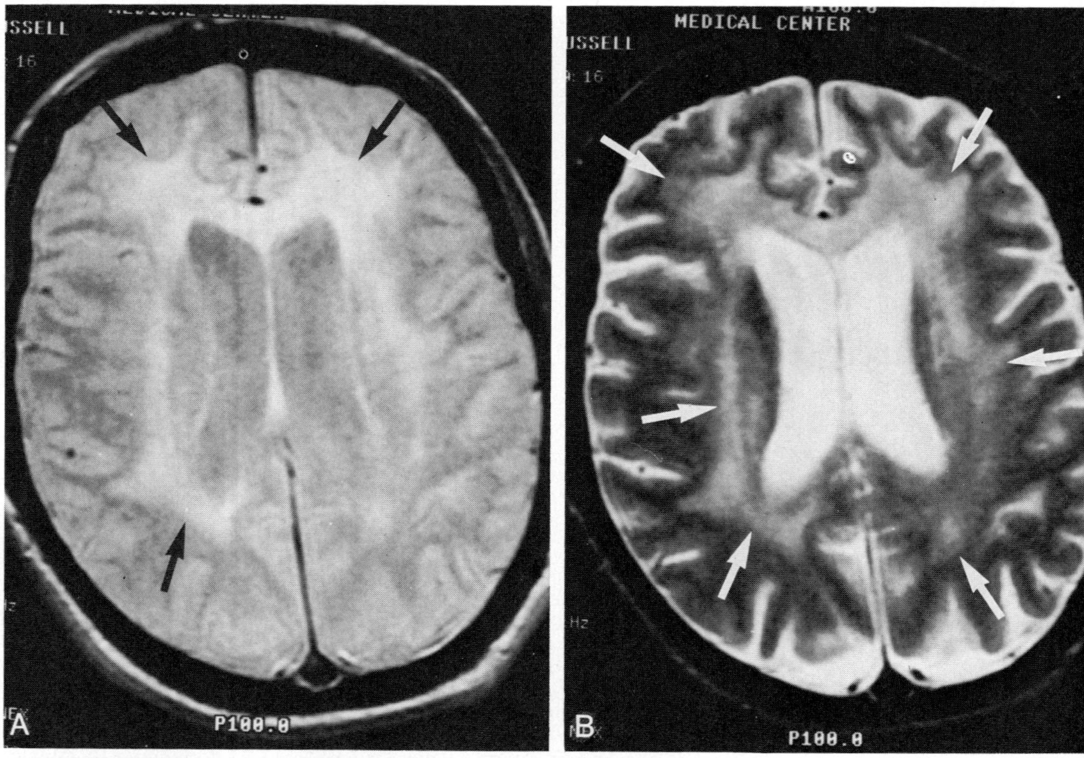

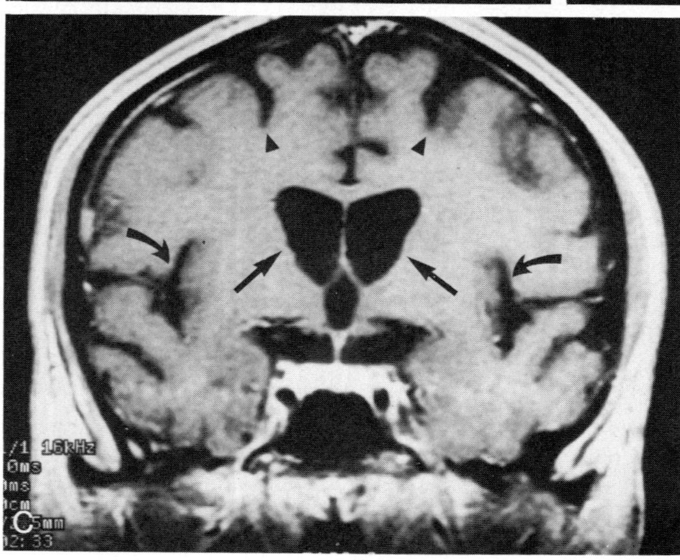

Figure 8–23. HIV (37-year-old male).

A, B, Axial SD and T2. Asymmetric high-signal white matter abnormalities *(arrows)* are detected bilaterally in the cerebral parenchyma.

C, Enhanced coronal T1. Marked parenchymal atrophy is present with enlargement of the ventricles *(arrows)*, sulci *(arrowheads)*, and sylvian fissures *(curved arrows)*. There is no evidence of pathologic enhancement.

abnormal MRI examinations.[55] CNS-screening MRI of neurologically asymptomatic patients is not cost effective.

Cytomegalovirus (CMV)

This opportunistic virus is second only in prevalence to the HIV organism in patients with AIDS in affecting the central nervous system. This organism typically occurs in the periventricular distribution, may coexist with HIV, and may be partly responsible for the acute encephalitis of these patients. Pathologically, intranuclear inclusions can be isolated.

MRI remains the cross-sectional imaging procedure of choice when evaluating patients with CMV; CT is somewhat insensitive to the periventricular hypoattenuation. However, it is nevertheless impossible to separate the white matter changes of CMV from those caused by HIV. But, ependymitis is more common with CMV and may be detected following administration of contrast material.

Toxoplasmosis

Toxoplasma gondii is a ubiquitous obligate intracellular protozoan infecting a large majority of the adult population. Patients usually harbor this organism in a dormant state for life, without sequelae. Reactivation may occur in immunocompromised patients, leading to a necrotizing encephalitis. Toxoplasmosis incites a vasculitis with perivascular infiltrates, peripheral astrocytosis, and edema. Toxoplasmosis is the most common cause of a focal parenchymal mass lesion in patients with AIDS.[6, 52, 56]

Patients may present with signs and symptoms of a focal mass effect, including seizures, focal neurologic deficits, and declining mental status. Patients can be treated successfully with sulfadiazine and pyrimethamine, although symptoms will return if treatment is discontinued.

Cross-sectional imaging demonstrates solitary or multiple masses that may occur anywhere in the supratentorial or infratentorial parenchyma (Fig. 8–24). These lesions have a predilection for the basal ganglia and deep gray matter[6, 56] and are associated with a moderate amount of edema and mass effect. The lesion is usually isodense to brain on the unenhanced CT examination and will enhance in

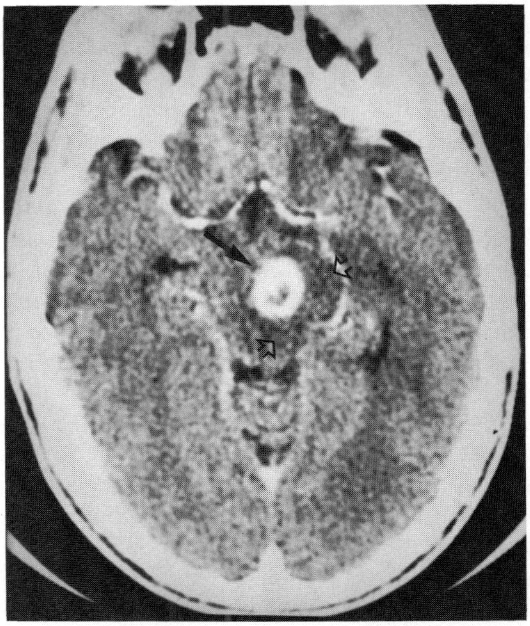

Figure 8–24. Toxoplasmosis (32-year-old male). Enhanced CT; a 1.3-cm ring-enhancing lesion *(solid arrow)* is present in the left mesencephalon, surrounded by vasogenic edema *(open arrows)*.

a ring or nodular pattern following contrast administration. MRI depicts the lesion, vasogenic edema, and pattern of enhancement more accurately than CT. The lesion and edema are hypointense on T1 and hyperintense on T2 images. After administration of contrast material, ring or nodular enhancement is readily detected.[52]

Lymphoma

CNS lymphoma is discussed in Chapter 3. CNS lymphoma is the second most common enhancing parenchymal lesion encountered in AIDS patients. As previously stated, the lymphoma associated with AIDS tends to be multiple and larger and to occur more frequently in the basal ganglia and temporal lobe than does non-AIDS lymphoma.

Distinguishing lymphoma from toxoplasmosis may not always be possible. Patients with enhancing parenchymal mass lesions therefore are given a trial course of medication. If the lesion does not respond after 2 weeks, biopsy is often performed as lymphoma is the next most likely cause of the mass. Planar imaging features that favor lymphoma over toxoplasmosis are increased density on unenhanced CT and a focal enhancing mass with subependymal spread on CT or MRI (Fig. 8–25).[57]

Progressive Multifocal Leukoencephalopathy (PML)

Two related papovaviruses (JC and SV40-PML) have been isolated in PML lesions.[26] This is a universal childhood infection that is reactived in the immunosuppressed patient.[6] There is a predilection to begin as multiple, small, subcortical white matter lesions and to progress to larger confluent areas of involvement in the white matter. The multiple subcortical sites of involvement account for the varied clinical presentations of these patients, including seizures, blindness, hemiparesis, intellectual dysfunction, and cerebellar or brainstem dysfunction. Patients with PML exhibit a progressive downhill course usually resulting in death in 6 months.

The virus attacks the oligodendroglial cells. Eosinophilic inclusion bodies may be identified in the distorted oligodendroglial cells. Death of these cells accounts for the large areas of demyelination encountered in PML.[58] There is a conspicuous lack of perivenous inflammation[59]; therefore, the BBB is normal.

CT reveals asymmetric hypodense abnormalities that may be solitary or multiple, located predominantly in the superficial white matter. PML is hypointense on T1 and hyperintense on spin density and T2. The intact BBB in these patients explains the absence of edema, mass effect, and contrast enhancement—the most common radiographic manifestations of this disease (Figs. 8–26, 8–27).

Cryptococcosis

Cryptococcus neoformans is an opportunistic fungus found in the soil that enters the host through the respiratory system. This is the

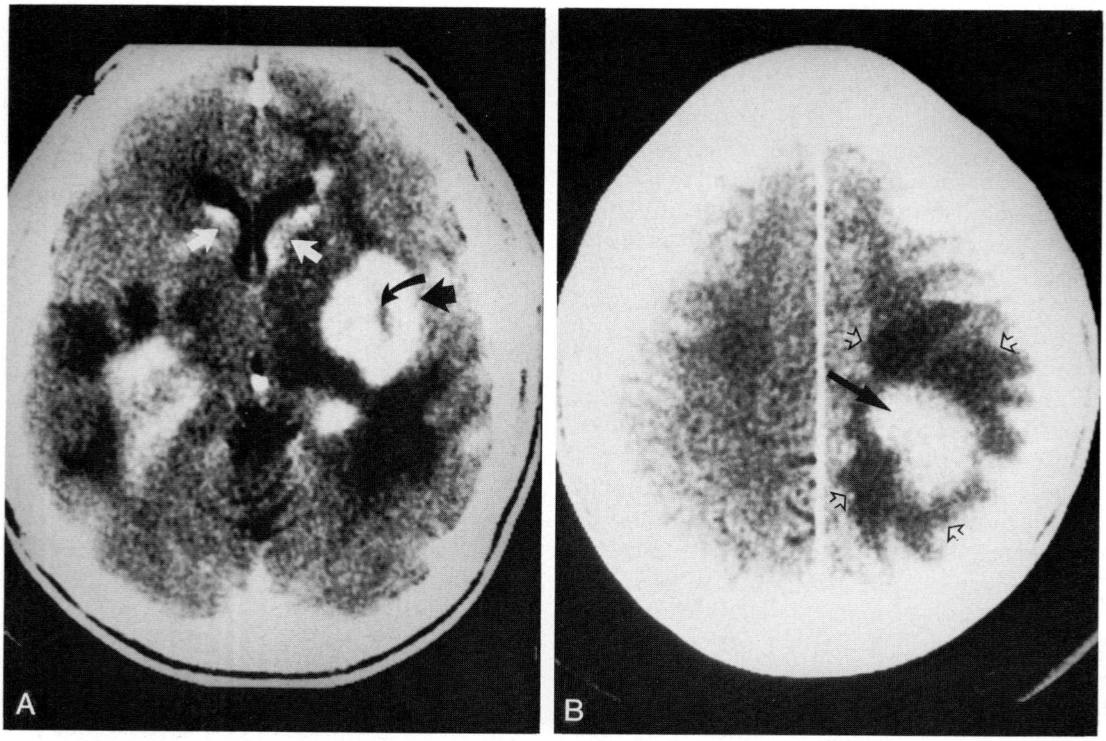

Figure 8–25. Lymphoma (immunoblastic, 28-year-old male).

A, Enhanced CT. Multiple enhancing lesions are present. The left basal ganglia lesion *(black arrow)* contains a region of central necrosis *(curved arrow)*. Enhancement of the head of the caudate nuclei bilaterally *(white arrows)* corroborates subependymal spread of immunoblastic lymphoma.

B, Enhanced CT. A homogeneously enhancing vertex lesion *(arrow)* is present. Vasogenic edema *(open arrows)* surrounds the lesion.

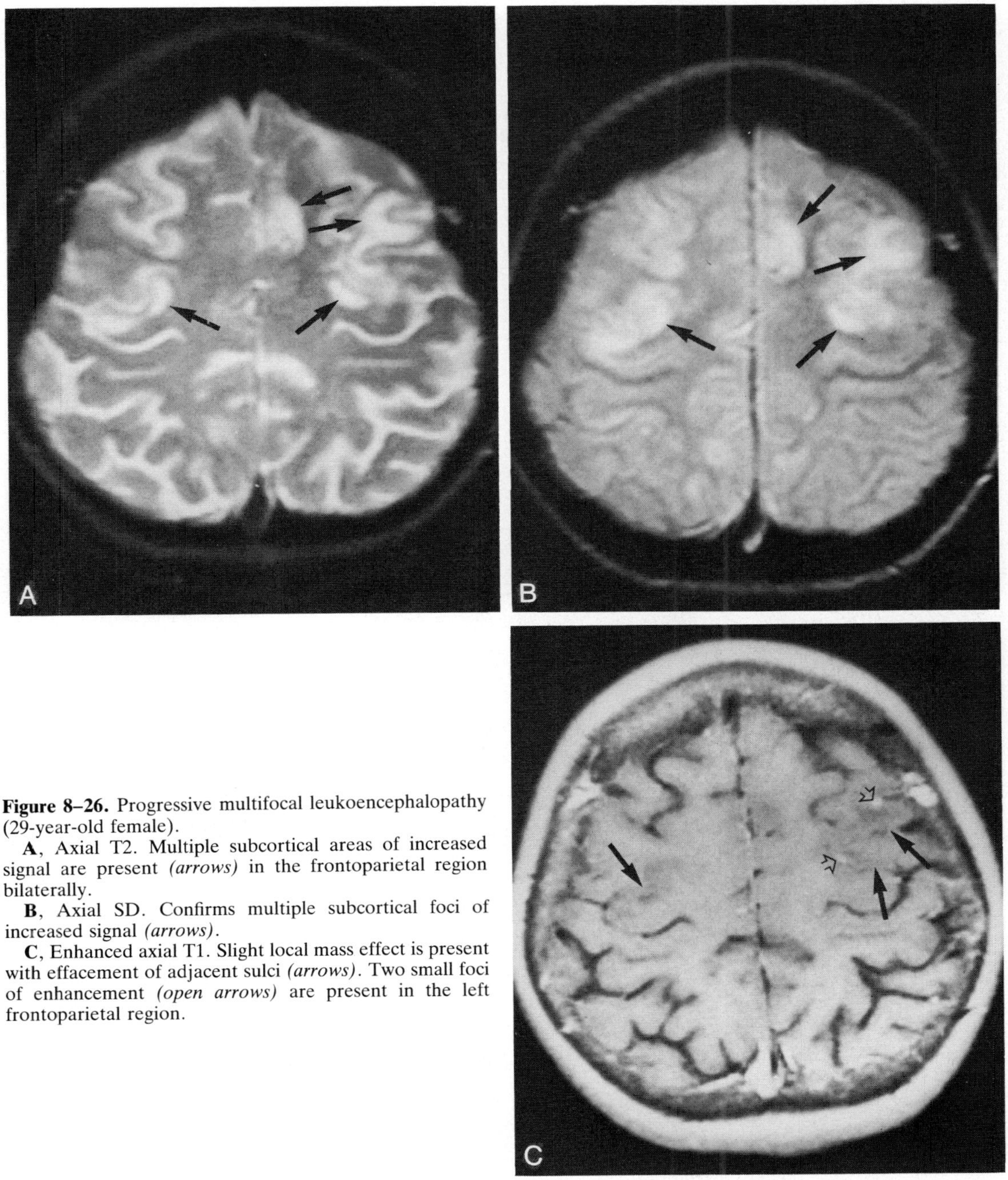

Figure 8–26. Progressive multifocal leukoencephalopathy (29-year-old female).

A, Axial T2. Multiple subcortical areas of increased signal are present *(arrows)* in the frontoparietal region bilaterally.

B, Axial SD. Confirms multiple subcortical foci of increased signal *(arrows)*.

C, Enhanced axial T1. Slight local mass effect is present with effacement of adjacent sulci *(arrows)*. Two small foci of enhancement *(open arrows)* are present in the left frontoparietal region.

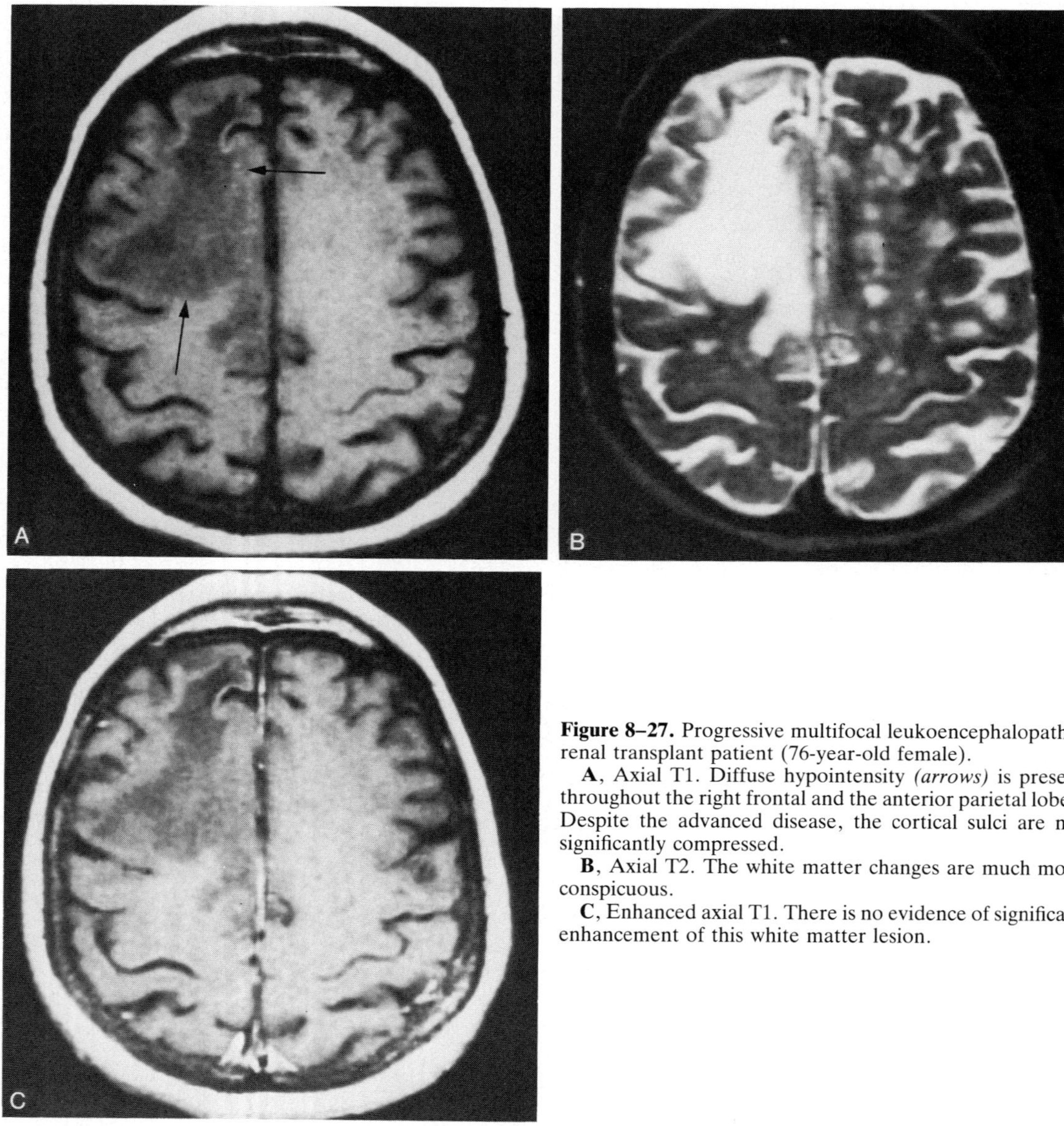

Figure 8–27. Progressive multifocal leukoencephalopathy; renal transplant patient (76-year-old female).

A, Axial T1. Diffuse hypointensity *(arrows)* is present throughout the right frontal and the anterior parietal lobes. Despite the advanced disease, the cortical sulci are not significantly compressed.

B, Axial T2. The white matter changes are much more conspicuous.

C, Enhanced axial T1. There is no evidence of significant enhancement of this white matter lesion.

most common fungal infection of the CNS[60] and is also the most common nonviral cause of meningitis in AIDS patients. Cryptococcosis incites a granulomatous meningitis,[6] resulting in meningeal thickening and hyperemia. The choroid is frequently involved, but the brain usually escapes direct infection. In about 10% of patients, however, the infection enters the Virchow-Robin spaces and forms cryptococcoma.[61] Patients may present with headache, altered mental status, and fever. Focal parenchymal lesions may lead to seizures. Communicating or noncommunicating hydrocephalus may develop. It is postulated that cryptococcus may involve the optic nerve and sheath primarily, accounting for the high frequency of patients with papilledema who do not exhibit radiographic evidence of hydrocephalus.

The CT findings are often normal in 40 to 50% of patients with cryptococcus meningitis.[61, 62] Common planar imaging findings include atrophy, hydrocephalus, gyral enhancement, and focal parenchymal nodules (Fig. 8–28). Decreased white matter attenuation on CT and corresponding increased T2 MRI signal are present.[61–63] The focal or diffuse enhancement in the meninges may be the only indication of a meningeal process in these patients.

Intrauterine Neonatal Infections

The fetus is immunologically inactive, incapable of antibody production for the first 30 weeks of gestation. Passive fetal immunity depends on transplacental transfer of maternal antibodies. Maternal antibodies do not reach detectable levels in the fetal circulation until 16 to 17 weeks of gestation.

"TORCH" is used to denote a common group of pathogens that induce fetal or neonatal infections: *t*oxoplasma, *r*ubella, *c*ytomegalovirus, *h*erpes simplex type II (HSV-II), and *o*ther infections, most commonly *Listeria* and *Treponema*.

Infectious entities may enter the fetus through the maternal bloodstream and placenta, from an ascending route through the

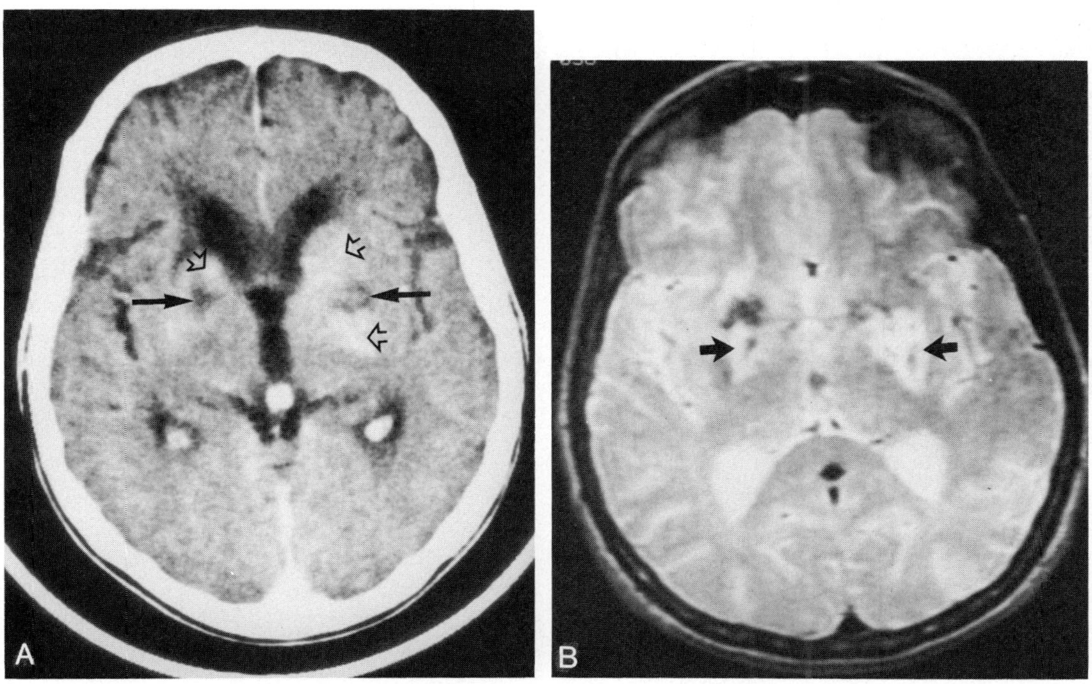

Figure 8–28. Cryptococcal meningitis (42-year-old male).

A, Enhanced CT. Focal infarcts *(arrows)* in the basal ganglia with adjacent irregular enhancement *(open arrows)* signify both chronic and acute changes in the parenchyma secondary to ischemic changes in the lenticulostriate artery distribution.

B, Axial T2. Heterogeneous signal *(arrows)* emanates from the basal ganglia bilaterally, secondary to postinflammatory infarct.

cervix and across fetal membranes, or as the fetus passes through an infected birth canal. The TORCH infections occur during gestation via a transplacental route (except for HSV-II, which most commonly occurs during birth[65, 66]). The earlier in gestation that an organism enters the fetus, the more pronounced the chromosomal or teratogenic effects. Finally, some organisms possess an affinity for specific organ systems.[64]

Neonatal Toxoplasmosis

This protozoan infection may be transmitted in macrophages via a transplacental route, resulting in multiple organ system involvement. Patients usually present by 4 months of age with hepatosplenomegaly, pneumonia, anemia, thrombocytopenia, and skin rash. Microcephaly, hydrocephalus, chorioretinitis, meningoencephalitis, and seizures have been reported.[67] Parenchymal calcifications may occur in a periventricular pattern[68] or more diffusely throughout the parenchyma.[67] MRI depicts multiple destructive lesions in the periventricular white matter (Fig. 8–29). Extensive porencephaly may result from widespread parenchymal destruction.

Rubella

This virus enters the fetus at any time during gestation through a transplacental route. The earlier the infection occurs, the more extensive the ramifications, with stillbirth and abortion the most common sequelae of first-trimester infection. Multisystem involvement is common, including hepatosplenomegaly, low birth weight, congenital heart disease, deafness, cataracts, and micro-ophthalmia.[67] The organism incites a vasculopathy with mural deposition of mucopolysaccharide and calcium.[1] The most common CNS lesions are chronic leptomeningitis, encephalitis, myelin retardation, and microcephaly.[64] Hydrocephalus and deep and superficial gray matter calcifications are common.

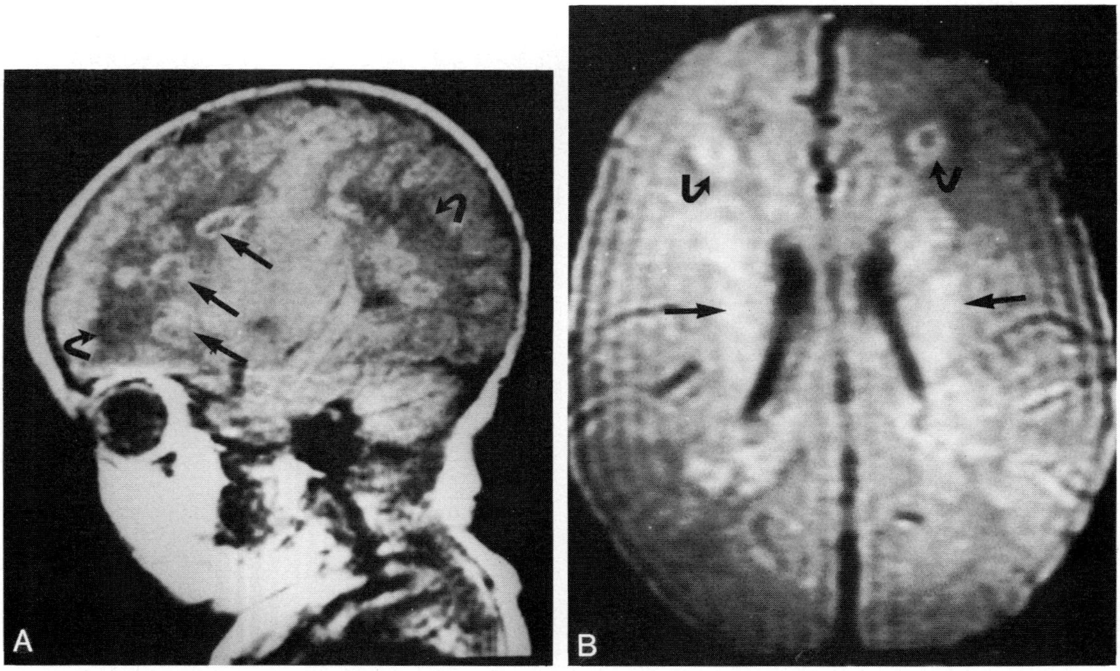

Figure 8–29. Toxoplasmosis (1-year-old female).

A, Parasagittal T1. High-signal rings *(straight arrows)* are present in the periventricular frontal white matter. The high signal may be secondary to methemoglobin. Diffuse decreased signal intensity *(curved arrows)* is present in the periventricular white matter anteriorly and posteriorly.

B, Axial SD. Diffuse periventricular increased signal *(solid arrows)* with rings of increased signal *(curved arrows)* is noted.

Cytomegalic Inclusion Disease

This omnipresent virus enters the fetus through a transplacental or ascending route. Most patients with congenital CMV infections do not exhibit signs or symptoms. If these infants do become symptomatic, however, hepatosplenomegaly, thrombocytopenia, pneumonia, chorioretinitis, and anemia occur.

Multinucleated giant cells with intranuclear inclusions are found in areas of inflammation and cytolysis.[64] Microcephaly is a common finding, although it may not be apparent until the first year of life. The virus has an affinity for the ependymal lining of the ventricles, resulting in cerebral calcifications that occur in a periventricular location.[67] Calcifications may also be found in the basal ganglia and cortical and subcortical regions. These calcifications are readily detected on CT, as are brain atrophy and various degrees of cerebellar hypoplasia (Fig. 8–30).

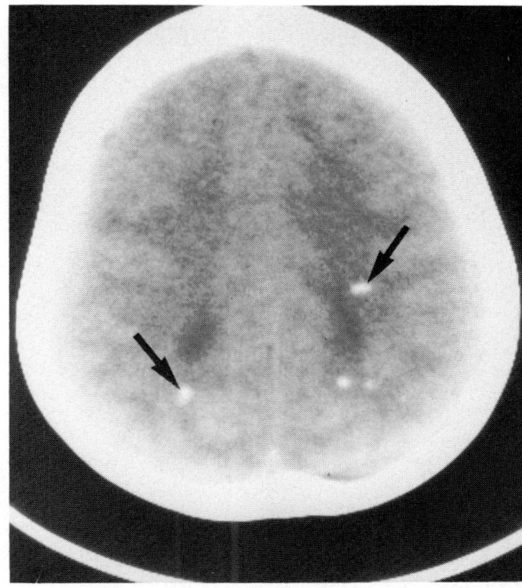

Figure 8–30. Cytomegalovirus (CMV) (3-year-old male). Unenhanced CT; multiple punctate periventricular calcifications *(arrows)* are present.

MRI demonstrates atrophy, disruption of normal gyri formation, and delayed myelination (Fig. 8–31).[69] The cortical sulci and lateral ventricles are enlarged, reflecting volume loss. Pachygyria may be detected, as well as persistent abnormally high signal in the periventricular white matter resulting

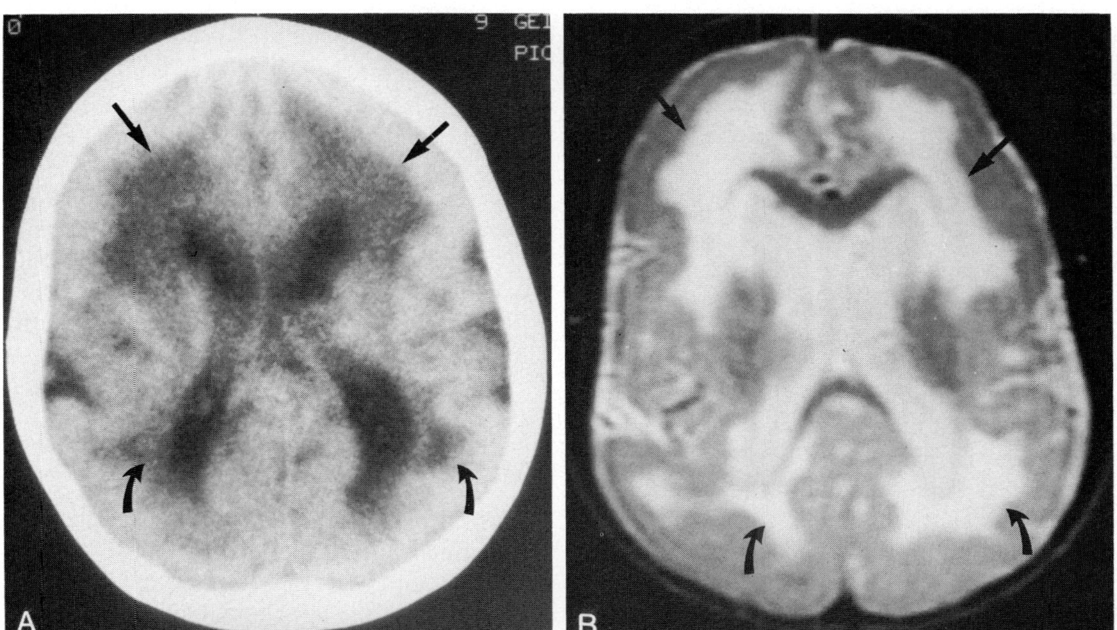

Figure 8–31. CMV (3-month-old female).

A, Unenhanced CT. There is diffuse hypodensity in the frontal *(straight arrow)* and periatrial *(curved arrow)* white matter bilaterally. The lateral ventricles are enlarged.

B, Axial T2. White matter changes become more apparent with involvement of all the frontal *(straight arrows)* white matter and left-greater-than-right periatrial white matter *(curved arrows)*. Pachygyria is noted in the frontal and occipital lobes.

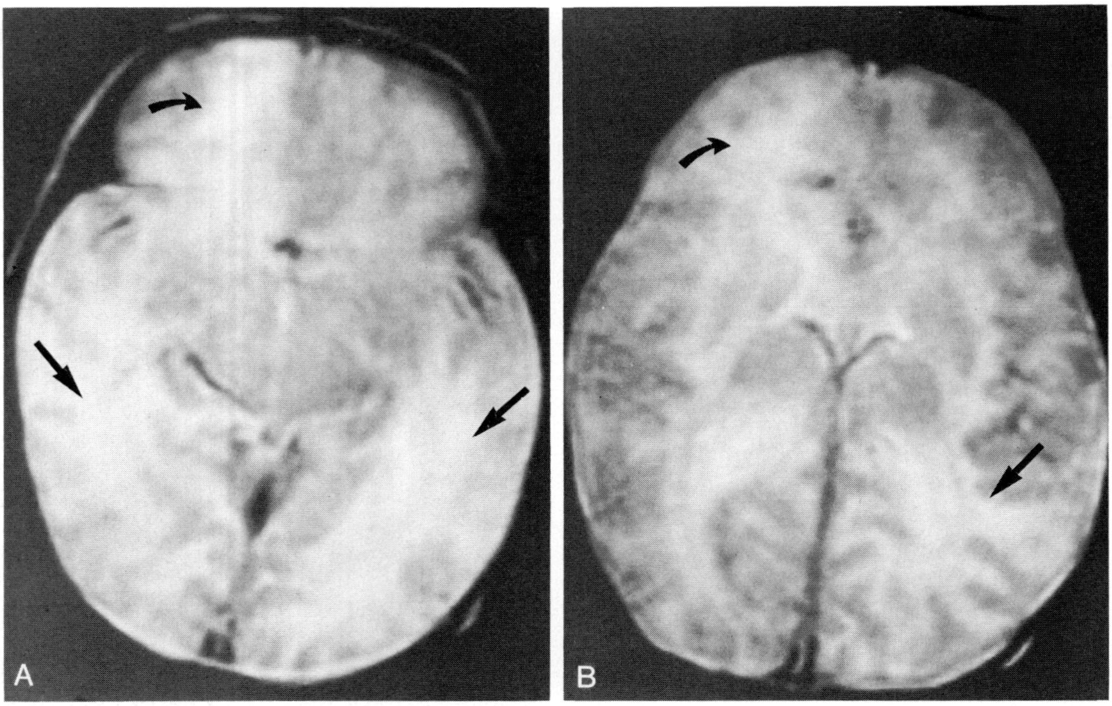

Figure 8–32. Neonatal herpes; HSV-II (2-month-old female).

A, Axial SD. Asymmetric, diffuse high-signal intensity is noted in the right frontal *(curved arrow)* and right-greater-than-left temporoparietal region *(straight arrows)*.

B, Axial SD. Right frontal white matter *(curved arrow)* and left-greater-than-right periatrial white matter *(straight arrow)* changes are present.

from delayed or pathologic myelination. Paraventricular cystic lesions adjacent to the occipital horns have been reported.[69]

Herpes Simplex Virus Type II

HSV-II is most commonly contracted in the neonatal period, during passage through an infected birth canal. In 30% of patients with HSV-II, the CNS may be involved, either alone or together with other organ systems. Patients may present with lethargy, irritability, and seizures at 2 to 4 weeks of age.[65] This rapidly progressive disease begins in the white matter and extends to involve adjacent parenchyma. Periventricular and cortical mononuclear cell infiltration can be demonstrated.

CT demonstrates areas of decreased attenuation in the cerebral white matter with fingerlike regions of increased attenuation in the cortex.[65, 66] The high-density material in the cortex may be secondary to hemorrhage, gyral calcification, sequestered contrast material, or a combination thereof. A meningeal pattern of enhancement occurs. MRI depicts widespread white matter signal abnormalities (Fig. 8–32). The white matter changes progress rapidly, causing extensive parenchymal destruction and resulting in multicystic encephalomalacia (Fig. 8–33).

An in utero congenital form of HSV-II also exists. These patients display microcephaly, periventricular calcifications, micro-ophthalmia, and chorioretinitis.[64]

INFLAMMATION

Multiple Sclerosis (MS)

MS is an inflammatory process of the brain and spinal cord that affects primarily the white matter. Although the etiology of this disease remains elusive, it is most likely autoimmune related. The disease is 1.4 to 1.9 times more common in women,[70] affects patients between 10 and 50 years of age, and is seen most frequently in northern parts of Europe and the United States.

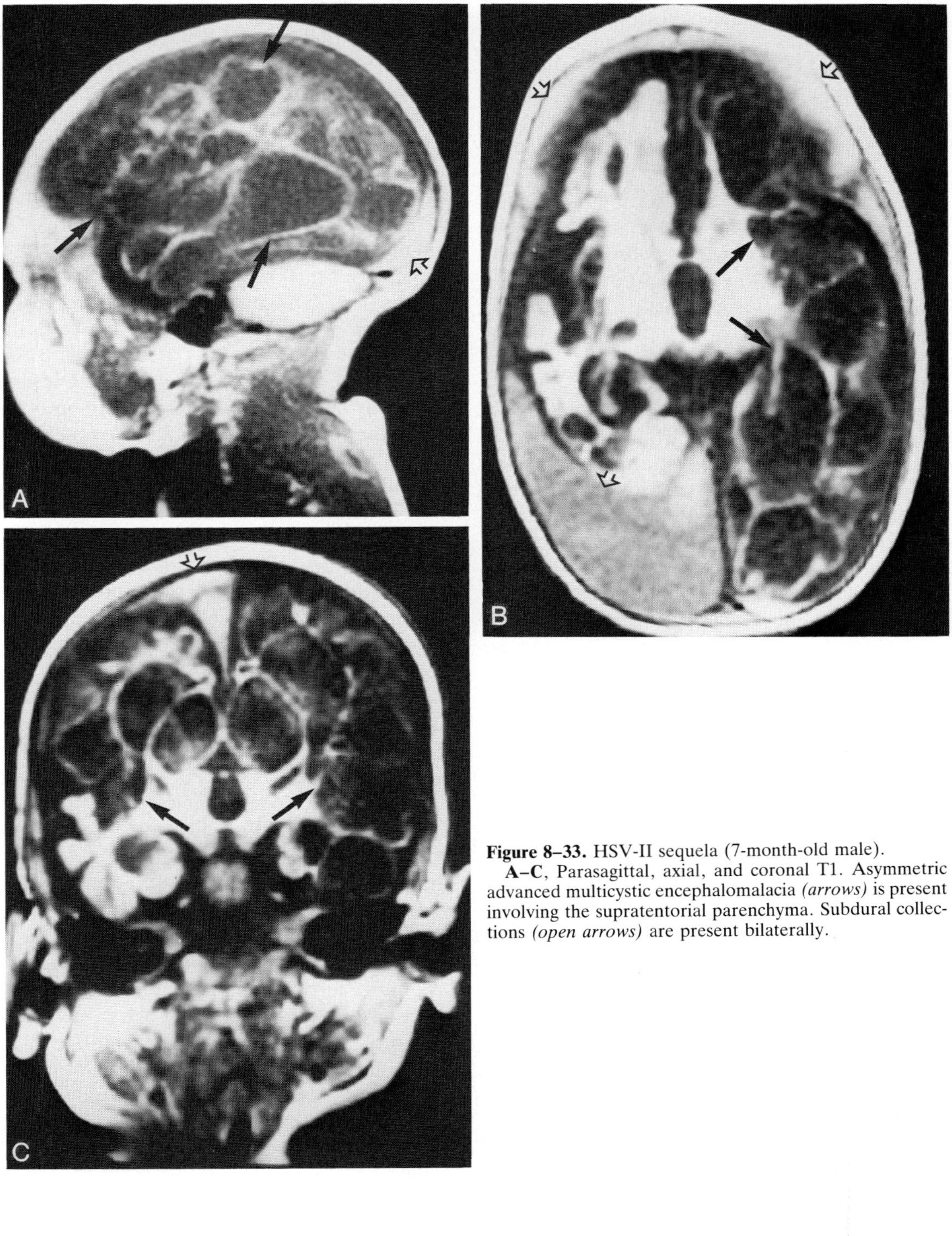

Figure 8–33. HSV-II sequela (7-month-old male).
A–C, Parasagittal, axial, and coronal T1. Asymmetric advanced multicystic encephalomalacia *(arrows)* is present involving the supratentorial parenchyma. Subdural collections *(open arrows)* are present bilaterally.

The clinical hallmark of this disease is lesions that are separate with respect to time and space.[1] Patients may present with weakness or paresthesias in one or more extremities, visual disturbances, and/or incoordination. The natural history of MS is variable, although it most commonly assumes a relapsing, remitting course with progressive disability over time. Alternatively, patients may present with an acute attack that is followed by a rapidly progressive downhill course.

The diagnosis of MS may be established clinically. In light of the varied manifestations of this disease, it may be considered a diagnosis of exclusion. Visual evoked response may be abnormal. Patients may present with elevated immunoglobulin G synthesis in the form of oligoclonal bands within the CSF.

The earliest pathologic changes are marked by mononuclear cell and lymphocytic accumulation in the perivenular white matter, most commonly adjacent to the anterior and posterior horns of the lateral ventricles.[71] Less commonly, there may be involvement at the cortical white matter junction, pons, cerebellar peduncles, central white matter, optic nerves, and spinal cord.[1] Initially, the myelin membrane is the point of destruction, with relative sparing of the oligodendroglial cells.[1] Lipid-laden macrophages containing myelin debris begin to accumulate as myelin loss progresses. There is relative sparing of the axons with evidence of astrocytic proliferation. Chronic lesions are characterized by profound myelin loss, absence of oligodendroglia, and scattered fibrillary astrocytes. The perivenous infiltrates and macrophages are absent in the chronic stage.

Cross-sectional imaging has contributed a wealth of knowledge toward the diagnosis of MS and to documentation of its response to therapy. Hypodensities in the central white matter may be detected on unenhanced CT. BBB is disrupted in the presence of acute lesions; consequently, intravenously enhanced CT is more sensitive than unenhanced cranial CT at diagnosing the active lesions. Double-dose delay techniques offer increased sensitivity at lesion detection.[72] Atrophy, focal or diffuse, may be detected in patients with chronic disease.

Multiple clinical studies have established MRI sensitivity up to 96%[73] and specificity 95 to 99%[74] in evaluating patients with MS. In the acute stage of perivenous inflammation, discrete high signal intensity lesions will be present on T2 images (Fig. 8–34). These lesions may diminish somewhat in size during the stage of demyelination, but will maintain an ovoid appearance with their long axis perpendicular to the ventricular surface (Dawson's fingers).[75] T1 images will remain normal until a significant amount of myelin loss has occurred. Enhancement may be detected in this early stage following administration of gadolinium (Fig. 8–35).[76] The active lesions are of high signal intensity on spin density and T2 images. Confluent and/or focal lesions of the inferior surface of the corpus callosum were reported in 93% of patients with MS versus 2.4% of control patients.[77] The lesions radiate from the ventricular surface into the overlaying corpus callosum and are most conspicuous on the spin density images in the sagittal plane (Fig. 8–36).

Distinction between active and chronic lesions is not possible on spin density and T2 images, as both lesions will appear as high signal intensity. Active lesions are generally inapparent on T1 images, are enhanced following gadolinium administration, are generally nonconfluent, and may be associated with minimal mass effect. Chronic lesions, on the other hand, are identified as well-defined hypodensities on T1 images, do not enhance following gadolinium administration,[78] tend to be confluent, and are more frequently associated with focal parenchymal loss (Fig. 8–37).

Diminished T2 signal has been reported[79] in the thalamus and putamen in patients with chronic MS (Fig. 8–38). The presence of this decreased signal correlated with the advanced degree of white matter involvement. The deposition of ferric iron within the putamen and thalamus may be responsible for this signal change.

It is important to realize that foci of inflammation need not necessarily progress to foci of demyelination.[80] This may account for transient areas of increased signal intensity on long repetition time (TR) images that resolve to normal appearance on subsequent examinations.[73, 76] It is also estimated that 75% of MRI-detectable lesions are clinically asympto-

Text continued on page 287

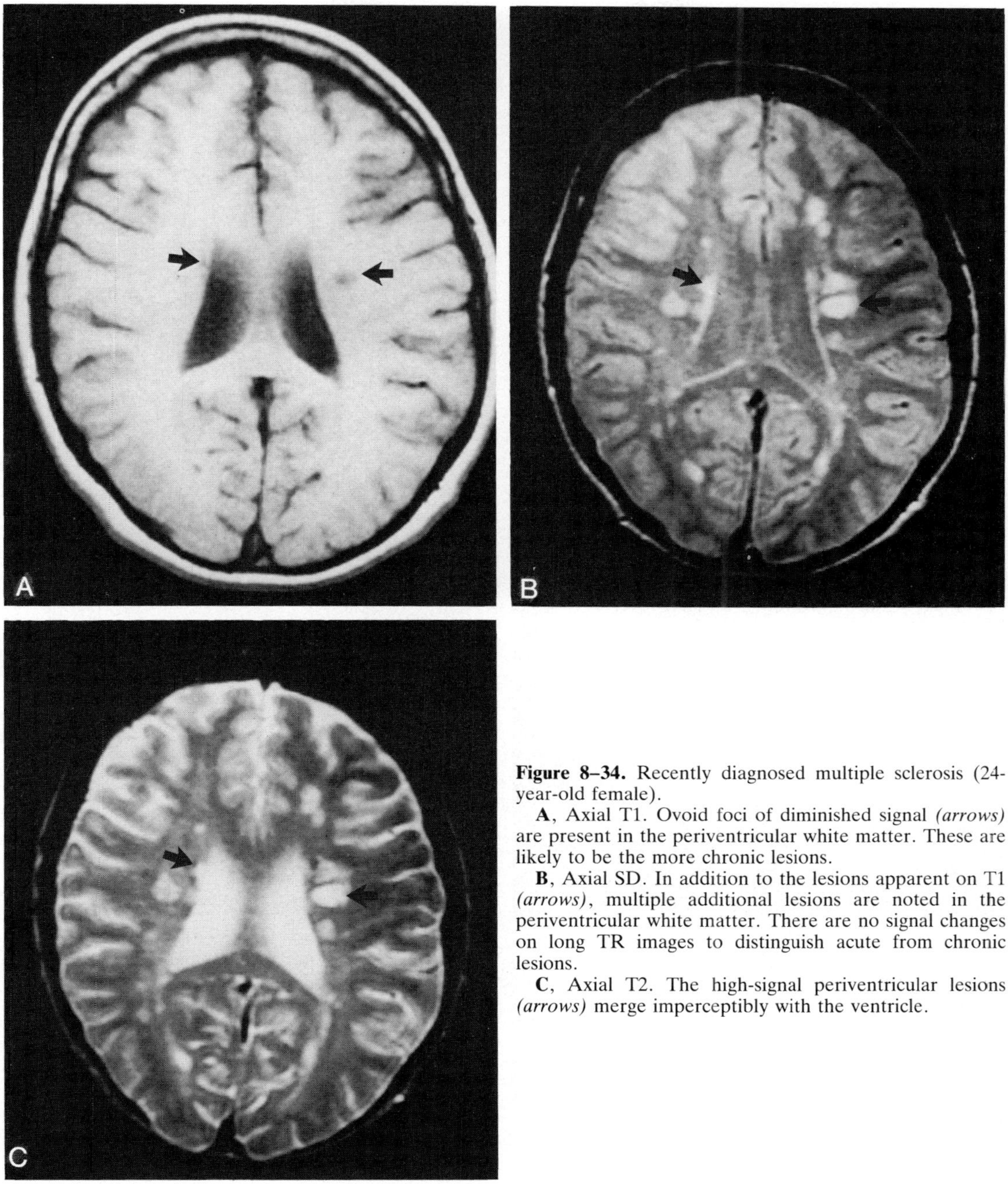

Figure 8–34. Recently diagnosed multiple sclerosis (24-year-old female).

A, Axial T1. Ovoid foci of diminished signal *(arrows)* are present in the periventricular white matter. These are likely to be the more chronic lesions.

B, Axial SD. In addition to the lesions apparent on T1 *(arrows)*, multiple additional lesions are noted in the periventricular white matter. There are no signal changes on long TR images to distinguish acute from chronic lesions.

C, Axial T2. The high-signal periventricular lesions *(arrows)* merge imperceptibly with the ventricle.

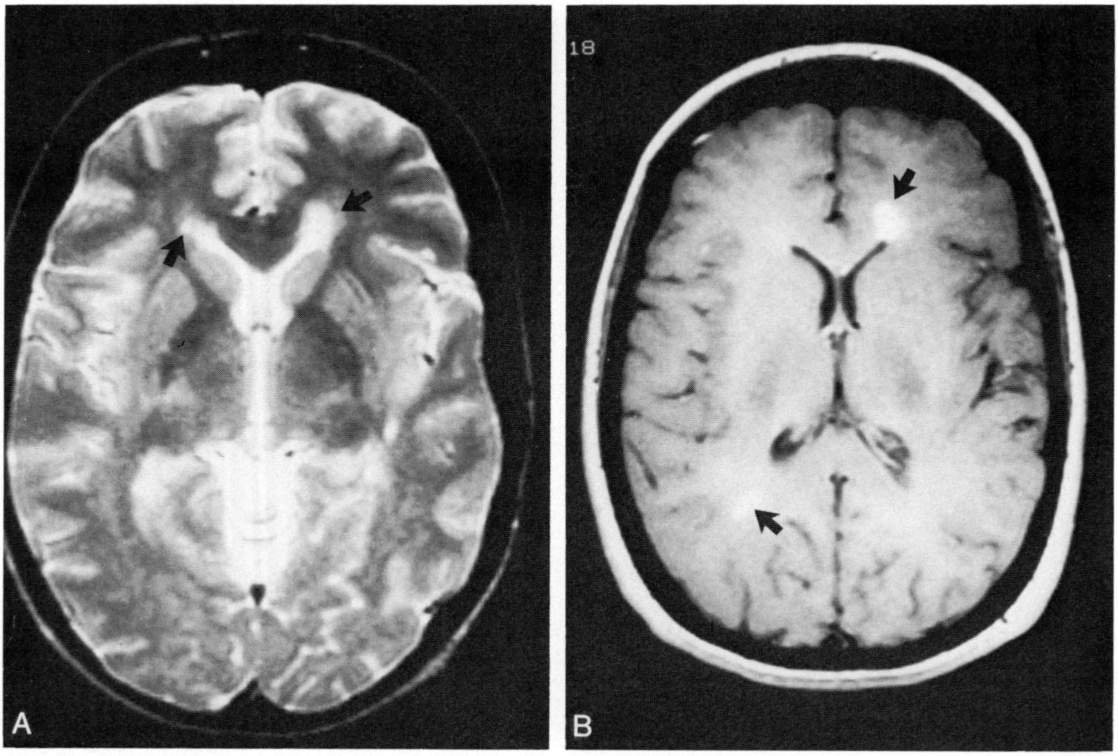

Figure 8–35. Multiple sclerosis (23-year-old female).

A, Axial T2. Periventricular foci of demyelination *(arrows)* are manifest as regions of high signal.

B, Enhanced axial T1. The foci of acute demyelination *(arrows)* enhance, indicating an acute process associated with disruption of the BBB.

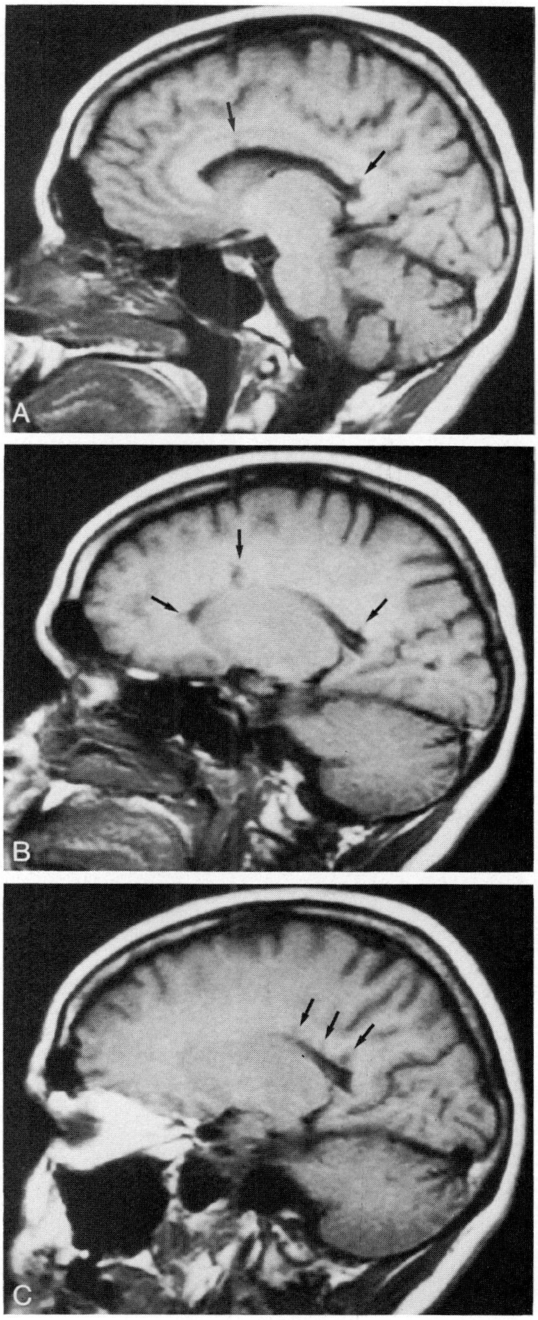

Figure 8–36. Multiple sclerosis (27-year-old female).
A–C, Parasagittal T1. Multiple regions of diminished signal *(arrows)* radiate from the ventricular surface into the corpus callosum and periventricular white matter.

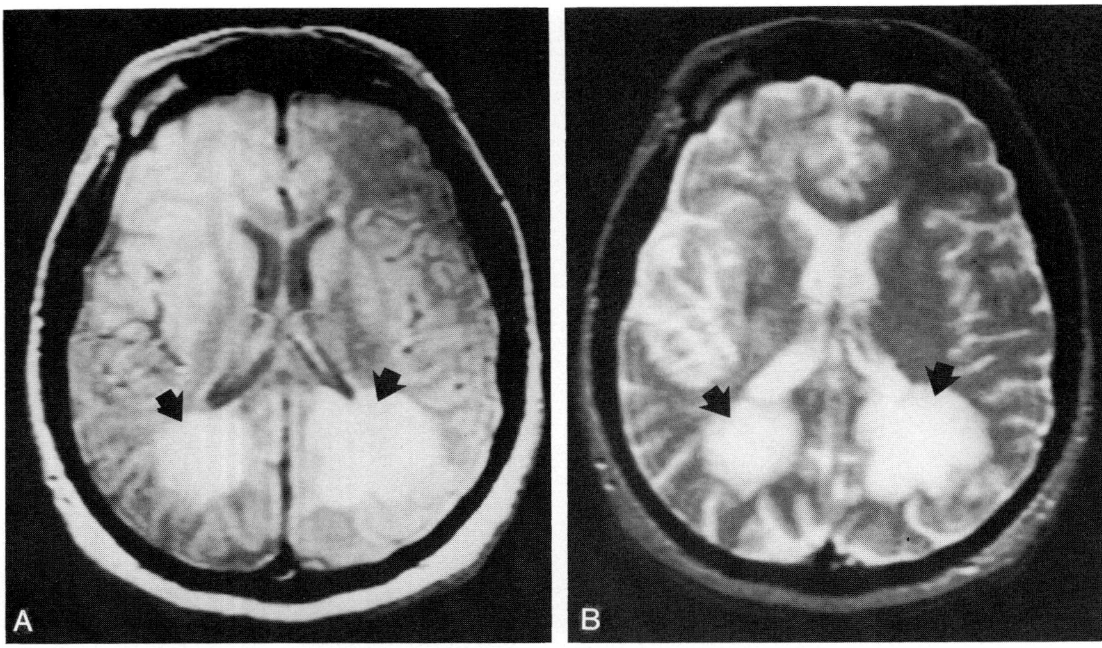

Figure 8–37. Multiple sclerosis (34-year-old female with a 10-year history of the disease).

A, Axial SD. Large plaques *(arrows)* are present in the periatrial white matter. There is a tendency for smaller plaques to coalesce into larger lesions with chronicity.

B, Axial T2. Similar foci *(arrows)* of high signal are noted in the periatrial white matter.

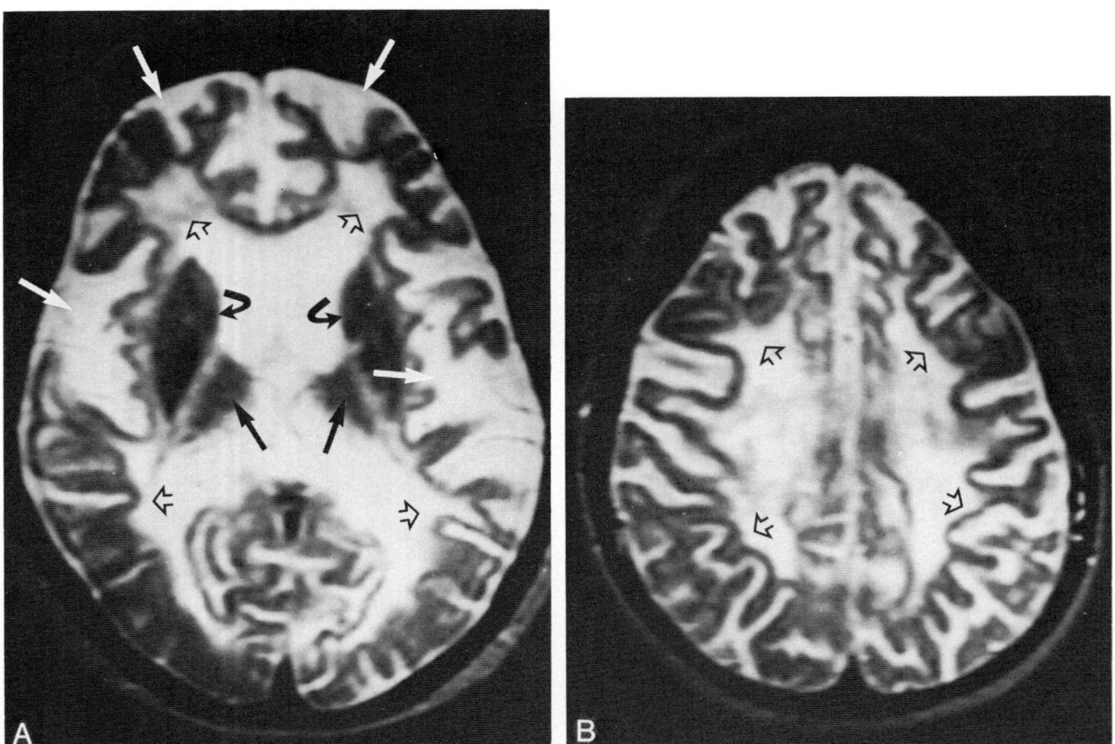

Figure 8–38. Multiple sclerosis (25-year-old female with chronic, end-stage disease).

A, Axial T2. Advanced white matter changes *(open arrows)*, diffuse enlargement of the CSF-containing spaces *(white arrows)*, and markedly diminished signal of the thalamus *(solid arrows)* and lentiform nuclei *(curved arrows)* corroborate the presence of advanced multiple sclerosis.

B, Axial T2. Advanced white matter changes *(open arrows)* extend to the subcortical white matter.

matic.[81] Also, thorough microscopic review at autopsy commonly reveals multiple small gyral lesions that are below the resolution of current imaging instruments.[70] This accounts for MRI evidence of progressive disease in patients undergoing clinical remission.[73] The parenchymal lesions of the posterior fossa tend to be more frequently associated with symptoms.[81] The total number of lesions detected are no indication of the duration or severity of the disease.[70]

References

1. Nelson JS: *Anderson's Pathology*. Kissane JM, ed. 9th ed, 1990. CV Mosby, St Louis.
2. Enzmann DR, Britt RR, Obana WG, et al: Experimental staphylococcus aureus brain abscess. AJNR 1986; 7:395–402.
3. Britt RH, Enzmann DR, Placone RC, et al: Experimental anaerobic brain abscess—computerized tomographic and neuropathologic correlations. J Neurosurg 1984; 60:1148–1159.
4. Enzmann DR, Britt RH, Placone RC: Staging of human brain abscess by computed tomography. Radiology 1983; 146:703–708.
5. Whelan MA, Hilal SK: Computed tomography as a guide in the diagnosis and follow-up of brain abscesses. Radiology 1980; 135:663–671.
6. Sze G, Zimmerman RD: The magnetic resonance imaging of infections and inflammatory diseases. Radiol Clin North Am 1988; 26:839–859.
7. Cockrill HH, Dreisbach J, Lowe B, Yamauchi T: Computed tomography in leptomeningeal infections. AJR 1978; 130:511–515.
8. Haimes AB, Zimmerman RD, Morgello S, et al: MR imaging of brain abscesses. AJNR 1989; 10:279–291.
9. Rosenblum ML, Hoff JT, Norman D, et al: Decreased mortality from brain abscesses since the advent of computerized tomography. J Neurosurg 1978; 49:658–668.
10. Enzmann DR, Britt RH, Placone RC, et al: The effects of short-term corticosteroid treatment on the CT appearance of experimental brain abscesses. Radiology 1982; 145:79–84.
11. Enzmann DR, Norman D, Mani J, Newton TH: Computed tomography of granulomatous basal arachnoiditis. Radiology 1976; 120:341–344.
12. Goldberg AL, Rosenbaum AE, Wang H, et al: Computed tomography of dural sinus thrombosis. J Comput Assist Tomogr 1986; 10:16–20.
13. Chang KH, Han MH, Roh JK, et al: Gd-DTPA-enhanced MR imaging of the brain in patients with meningitis: Comparison with CT. AJNR 1990; 11:69–76.
14. Macchi PJ, Grossman RI, Gomori JM, et al: High field MR imaging of cerebral venous thrombosis. J Comput Assist Tomogr 1986; 10:10–15.
15. Barloon TJ, Yuh WTC, Knepper LE, et al: Cerebral vasculitis: MR findings. J Comput Assist Tomogr 1990; 14:272–275.
16. Weingarten K, Zimmerman RD, Becker RD, et al: Subdural and epidural empyemas: MR imaging. AJNR 1989; 10:81–87.
17. Post EM, Modesti LM: "Subacute" postoperative subdural empyema. J Neurosurg 1981; 55:761–765.
18. Chrysikopoulos HS, Press GA, Grafe MR, et al: Encephalitis caused by human immunodeficiency virus: CT and MR imaging manifestations with clinical and pathologic correlation. Radiology 1990; 175:185–191.
19. Zimmerman RD, Leeds NE, Danziger A: Subdural empyemas: CT findings. Radiology 1984; 150:417–422.
20. Sadhu VK, Handel SF, Pinto RS, Glass TF: Neuroradiologic diagnosis of subdural empyema and CT limitations. AJNR 1980; 1:39–44.
21. Jawetz E, Melnick JL, Adelberg EA: *Review of Medical Microbiology*, 13th ed. 1978. Lange Medical Publications, Los Altos, CA.
22. Youmans GP, Paterson PY, Sommers HM: *The Biological and Clinical Basis of Infectious Disease*. 1975. WB Saunders, Philadelphia.
23. Haykal H, Zamani A, Wang AM, et al: CT features of early *Listeria monocytogenes* cerebritis. AJNR 1987; 8:279–282.
24. Just M, Krämer G, Higer HP, et al: MRI of Listeria rhombencephalitis. Neuroradiology 1987; 24:401–402.
25. Davis JM, Davis KR, Kleinman GM, et al: Computed tomography of herpes simplex encephalitis, with clinicopathological correlation. Radiology 1978; 129:409–417.
26. Berger PC, Vogel FS: *Surgical Pathology of the Nervous System and Its Coverings*, 2nd ed. 1982. John Wiley & Sons, New York.
27. Zimmerman RD, Russell EJ, Leeds NE, Kaufman D: CT in the diagnosis of herpes simplex encephalitis. AJR 1980; 134:61–66.
28. Lester JW, Carter MP, Reynolds TL: Herpes encephalitis: MR monitoring of response to acyclovir therapy. J Comput Assist Tomogr 1988; 12:941–943.
29. Dublin AB, Phillips HE: Computed tomography of disseminated cerebral coccidioidomycosis. Radiology 1980; 135:361–368.
30. Dion FM, Venger BH, Landon G, Handel SF: Thalamic histoplasmoma: CT and MR imaging. J Comput Assist Tomogr 1987; 11:193–195.
31. Enzmann DR, Brant-Zawadski M, Britt RH: CT of central nervous system infections in immunocompromised patients. AJNR 1980; 1:239–243.
32. Jinkins JR, Siqueira E, Al-Kawi MZ: Cranial manifestations of aspergillosis. Neuroradiology 1987; 29:181–185.
33. Press GA, Weindling SM, Hesselink JR, et al: Rhinocerebral mucormyocosis: MR manifestations. J Comput Assist Tomogr 1988; 12:744–749.
34. Gamba JL, Woodruff WW, Djang WT, Yeates AE: Craniofacial mucormycosis: Assessment with CT. Radiology 1986; 160:207–212.
35. Ginsberg F, Peyster RG, Hoover ED, Kinkelstein SD: Isolated cerebral mucormycosis: Case report with CT and pathologic correlation. AJNR 1987; 8:558–560.
36. Whelan MA, Stern J, deNapoli RA: The computed tomographic spectrum of intracranial mycosis: Correlation with histopathology. Radiology 1981; 141:703–707.
37. Kramer LD, Locke GE, Byrd SE, Daryabagi J: Cerebral cysticercosis: Documentation of natural history with CT. Radiology 1989; 171:459–462.
38. Martinez HR, Rangel-Guerra R, Elizondo G, et al: MR imaging in neurocysticercosis: A study of 56 cases. AJNR 1989; 10:1011–1019.

39. Teitelbaum GP, Otto RJ, Lin M, et al: MR imaging of neurocysticercosis. AJNR 1989; 10:709–718.
40. Carbajal JR, Palacios E, Azar-Kia B, Churchill R: Radiology of cysticercosis of the central nervous system including tomography. Radiology 1977; 125:127–131.
41. Lotz J, Hewlett R, Alheit B, Bowen R: Neurocysticercosis: Correlative pathomorphology and MR imaging. Neuroradiology 1988; 30:35–41.
42. Suss RA, Maravilla KR, Thompson J: MR imaging of intracranial cysticercosis: Comparison with CT and anatomopathologic features. AJNR 1986; 7:235–242.
43. Rhee RS, Kumasaki DY, Sarwar M, et al: MR imaging of intraventricular cysticercosis. J Comput Assist Tomogr 1987; 11:598–601.
44. Draouat S, Abdenabi B, Ghanem M, Bourjat P: Computed tomography of cerebral tuberculoma. J Comput Assist Tomogr 1987; 11:594–597.
45. Suss RA, Resta S, Diehl JT: Persistent cortical enhancement in tuberculous meningitis. AJNR 1987; 8:716–720.
46. Gupta RK, Jena A, Sharma A, et al: MR imaging of intracranial tuberculomas. J Comput Assist Tomogr 1988; 12:280–285.
47. Smith AS, Meisler DM, Weinstein MA, et al: High-signal periventricular lesions in patients with sarcoidosis: Neurosarcoidosis or multiple sclerosis? AJNR 1989; 10:485–490.
48. Mirfakhraee M, Crofford MJ, Guinto FC, et al: Virchow-Robin space: A path of spread in neurosarcoidosis. Radiology 1986; 158:715–720.
49. Hayes WS, Sherman JL, Stern BJ, et al: MR and CT evaluation of intracranial sarcoidosis. AJNR 1987; 8:841–847.
50. Sherman JL, Stern BJ: Sarcoidosis of the CNS: Comparison of unenhanced and enhanced MR images. AJNR 1990; 11:915–923.
51. Seltzer S, Mark AS, Atlas SW: CNS sarcoidosis: Evaluation with contrast-enhanced MR imaging. AJNR 1991; 12:1227–1233.
52. Federle MP: A radiologist looks at AIDS: Imaging evaluation based on symptom complexes. Radiology 1988; 166:553–562.
53. Donovan Post MJ, Tate LG, Quencer RM, et al: CT, MR, and pathology in HIV encephalitis and meningitis. AJNR 1988; 9:469–476.
54. Flowers CH, Mafee MF, Crowell R, et al: Encephalopathy in AIDS patients: Evaluation with MR imaging. AJNR 1990; 11:1235–1245.
55. Donovan Post MJ, Berger JR, Quencer RM: Asymptomatic and neurologically symptomatic HIV-seropositive individuals: Prospective evaluation with cranial MR imaging. Radiology 1991; 178:131–139.
56. Levy RM, Rosenbloom S, Perrett LV: Neuroradiologic findings in AIDS: A review of 200 cases. AJR 1986; 147:977–983.
57. Dina TS: Primary central nervous system lymphoma versus toxoplasmosis in AIDS. Radiology 1991; 179:823–828.
58. Carroll BA, Lane B, Norman D, Enzmann D: Diagnosis of progressive multifocal leukoencephalopathy by computed tomography. Radiology 1977; 122:137–141.
59. Mark AS, Atlas SW: Progressive multifocal leukoencephalopathy in patients with AIDS: Appearance on the MR images. Radiology 1989; 173:517–520.
60. Levy RM, Bredesen DE, Rosenblum ML: Neurological manifestations of the acquired immunodeficiency syndrome (AIDS): Experience at UCSF and review of the literature. J Neurosurg 1985; 62:475–495.
61. Popovich MJ, Arthur RH, Helmer E: CT of intracranial cryptococcosis. AJNR 1990; 11:139–142.
62. Tan CT, Kuan BB: Cryptococcus meningitis, clinical-CT scan considerations. Neuroradiology 1987; 29:43–46.
63. Tien RD, Chu PK, Hesselink JR: Intracranial cryptococcosis in immunocompromised patients: CT and MR findings in 29 cases. AJNR 1991; 12:283–289.
64. Krasinski K: Fetal infections. In *Disorders of the Developing Nervous System: Diagnosis and Treatment.* Hoffman HJ, Epstein F, eds. 1986. Blackwell Scientific Publications, Boston.
65. Herman TE, Cleveland RH, Kushner DC, Taveras JM: CT of neonatal herpes encephalitis. AJNR 1985; 6:773–775.
66. Noorbehesht B, Enzmann DR, Sullender W, et al: Neonatal herpes simplex encephalitis: Correlation of clinical and CT findings. Radiology 1987; 162:813–819.
67. Overall JC, Glasgow LA: Virus infections of the fetus and newborn infant. J Pediatr 1970; 7:315–333.
68. Collins AT, Cromwell LD: Computed tomography in the evaluation of congenital cerebral toxoplasmosis. J Comput Assist Tomogr 1980; 4:326–329.
69. Boesch C, Issakainen J, Kewitz G, et al: Magnetic resonance imaging of the brain in congenital cytomegalovirus infection. Pediatr Radiol 1989; 19:91–93.
70. Uhlenbrock D, Seidel D, Gehlen W, et al: MR imaging in multiple sclerosis: Comparison with clinical, CSF and visual evoked potential findings. AJNR 1988; 9:59–67.
71. Morris JH: The nervous system. In *Robbins Pathologic Basis of Disease*. Cotran RS, Kumar V, Robbins SL, eds. 4th ed, 1989, WB Saunders, Philadelphia.
72. Sears ES, McCammon A, Bigelow R, Hayman LA: Maximizing the harvest of contrast enhancing lesions in multiple sclerosis. Neurology 1982; 32:815–820.
73. Uhlenbrock D, Herbe E, Seidel D, Gehlen W: One-year MR imaging follow-up of patients with multiple sclerosis under cortisone therapy. Neuroradiology 1989; 31:3–7.
74. Yetkin FZ, Haughton VM, Papke RA, et al: Multiple sclerosis: Specificity of MR for diagnosis. Radiology 1991; 178:447–451.
75. Horowitz AL, Kaplan RD, Grewe G, et al: The ovoid lesion: A new MR observation in patients with multiple sclerosis. AJNR 1989; 10:303–305.
76. Grossman RI, Braffman BH, Brorson JR, et al: Multiple sclerosis: Serial study of gadolinium-enhanced MR imaging. Radiology 1988; 169:117–122.
77. Gear-Marton AD, Vezina LG, Marton KJ, et al: Abnormal corpus callosum: A sensitive and specific indicator of multiple sclerosis. Radiology 1991; 180:215–221.
78. Nesbit GM, Forbes GS, Scheithauer BW, et al: Multiple sclerosis: Histopathologic and MR and/or CT correlation in 37 cases at biopsy and three cases at autopsy. Radiology 1991; 180:467–474.
79. Drayer B, Berger P, Horwitz B, et al: Reduced signal intensity on MR images of thalamus and putamen in multiple sclerosis: Increased iron content? AJNR 1987; 8:413–419.
80. Poser CM, Kleefield J, O'Reilly GV, Jelesz F: Neuroimaging and the lesion of multiple sclerosis. AJNR 1987; 8:549–552.
81. Jacobs L, Kinkel WR, Polachini I, Kinkel RP: Correlations of nuclear magnetic resonance imaging, computerized tomography, and clinical profiles in multiple sclerosis. Neurology 1986; 36:27–34.

9

THE ORBIT AND VISUAL APPARATUS

ANATOMY

Orbit

The orbit is the bony cavity that contains and protects the anterior visual system. The orbit is composed of seven separate bones and is roughly conical[1]; the apex is directed posterior superomedial, toward the suprasellar cistern (Fig. 9–1). The majority of the orbital roof is composed of the broad, convexed-upward orbital surface of the frontal bone. The posterior one fifth of the orbital roof is composed of the lesser wing of the sphenoid bone. The lateral wall of the orbit contains the

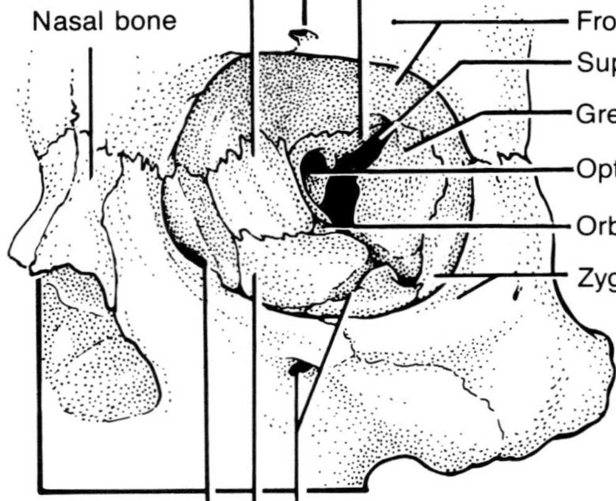

Figure 9–1. Frontal drawing of bony orbit.

greater wing of the sphenoid bone posteriorly and the thick zygomatic bone anteriorly. The zygomatic bone continues medially to form the lateral one third of the floor and rim of the orbit. The maxilla forms the medial two thirds of the orbital floor and orbital rim. The orbital process of the palatine bone forms the small posterior-most segment of the floor. The ethmoid bone forms the posterior four fifths of the medial wall of the orbit. The lacrimal bone forms the anterior one fifth of the medial orbital wall.

Optic Canal and Superior and Inferior Orbital Fissures

The optic canal resides in the cephalad medial apex of the orbit. The canal is 8 to 10 mm long and is surrounded superiorly and laterally by the lesser wing of the sphenoid bone. The body of the sphenoid bone forms the medial aspect of the optic canal. The optic nerve and the ophthalmic artery enter the orbit through the optic canal.

The superior and inferior orbital fissure together form a "V," the apex of which is directed medially. The superior orbital fissure is marginated by the lesser wing of the sphenoid bone above and the greater wing of the sphenoid bone below. The optic strut separates the optic canal from the superior orbital fissure. The oculomotor (III), trochlear (IV), ophthalmic (V_1), and abducens (VI) nerves exit the cavernous sinus and enter the orbital apex through the superior orbital fissure. The superior ophthalmic vein exits the orbit through the superior orbital fissure to enter the cavernous sinus.

The inferior orbital fissure lies at the junction of the lateral wall and floor of the orbit and is marginated by the greater wing of the sphenoid bone posterolaterally and the maxilla and orbital process of the palatine bone anteromedially. The maxillary branch of the trigeminal nerve (V_2) enters the orbit through the inferior orbital fissure before exiting into the inferior orbital canal. The infraorbital artery enters and the inferior ophthalmic vein variably exits the orbit through the inferior orbital fissure.

Septum

The periorbita is the periosteum of the orbit. The fibrous sheet is loosely applied along the surface of the orbit, except at suture lines where the periosteum is rigidly adherent to the edge of the bone. The septum is a fibrous extension of the periorbita that extends from the anterior orbital margin centripetally to the tarsal plates of the upper and lower lids (Fig. 9–2). The septum offers a relative barrier to

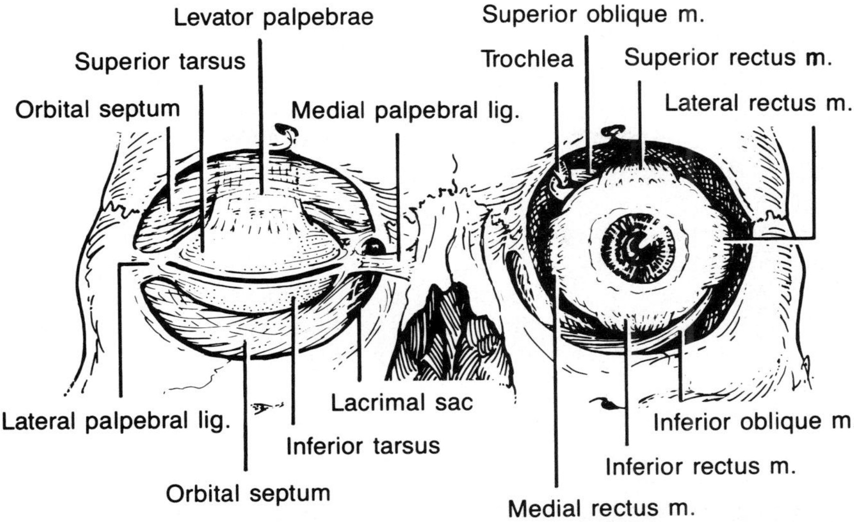

Figure 9–2. Frontal drawing of soft tissue anatomy (tarsal plates and orbital septum removed on patient's left).

the spread of infection and tumor between the subcutaneous soft tissues anterior to the septum (preseptal) and those located posterior to the septum (postseptal).

Globe

The globe is a three-layered sphere composed (from superficial to deep) of the cornea-sclera, the choroid, and the retina (Fig. 9–3). The sclera covers the posterior 80% of the globe, providing a rigid matrix of support. The cornea is contiguous with the sclera and covers the anterior 20% of the globe, providing a transparent medium through which to transmit light. The sclera is enveloped by Tenon's capsule, a thick fibrous sheath that serves as secondary support and an insertion for the extraocular muscles. The choroid comprises a layer of blood vessels and nerve fibers that supports the metabolic needs of the retina. The retina is the photoreceptive layer composed of rods and cones upon which the light is focused. A point-to-point relationship exists between the retina and the visual cortex of the occipital lobes.

The globe is positioned in the anterior orbit. The globe should not normally extend more than 21 mm anterior to the interzygomatic line (the line that connects the zygoma at the level of the orbital equator in the axial plane).[2]

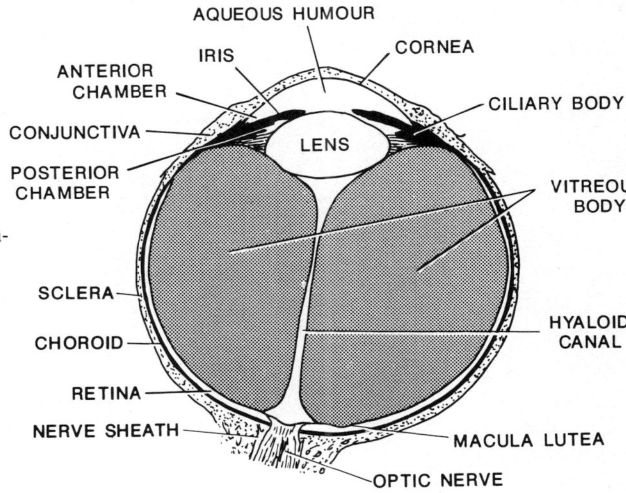

Figure 9–3. Axial drawing of globe (medical illustration by Diane Blue).

Anterior extension beyond this point constitutes proptosis.

The lens is a biconvexed 4.5 × 10 mm structure composed of densely packed hexagonal fibers surrounded by an elastic capsule. The lens is suspended by the ciliary body, a triangular structure that separates the aqueous humor anteriorly from the vitreous humor posteriorly. The more anterior aqueous humor is further subdivided by the pigmented iris into the anterior and posterior chambers. The vitreous humor fills the globe posterior to the lens.

Current planar imaging lacks the resolution to distinguish among the three layers of the globe and to differentiate the anterior and posterior chambers of the aqueous humor. The lens is intrinsically dense on computed tomography (CT) (Fig. 9–4), becoming more dense with age. The fibroelastic composition of the lens renders it intermediate signal on T1-weighted and low signal on T2-weighted magnetic resonance imaging (MRI)[3] (Fig. 9–5). The fluid-filled globe has a prolonged T1 and T2 relaxation time.

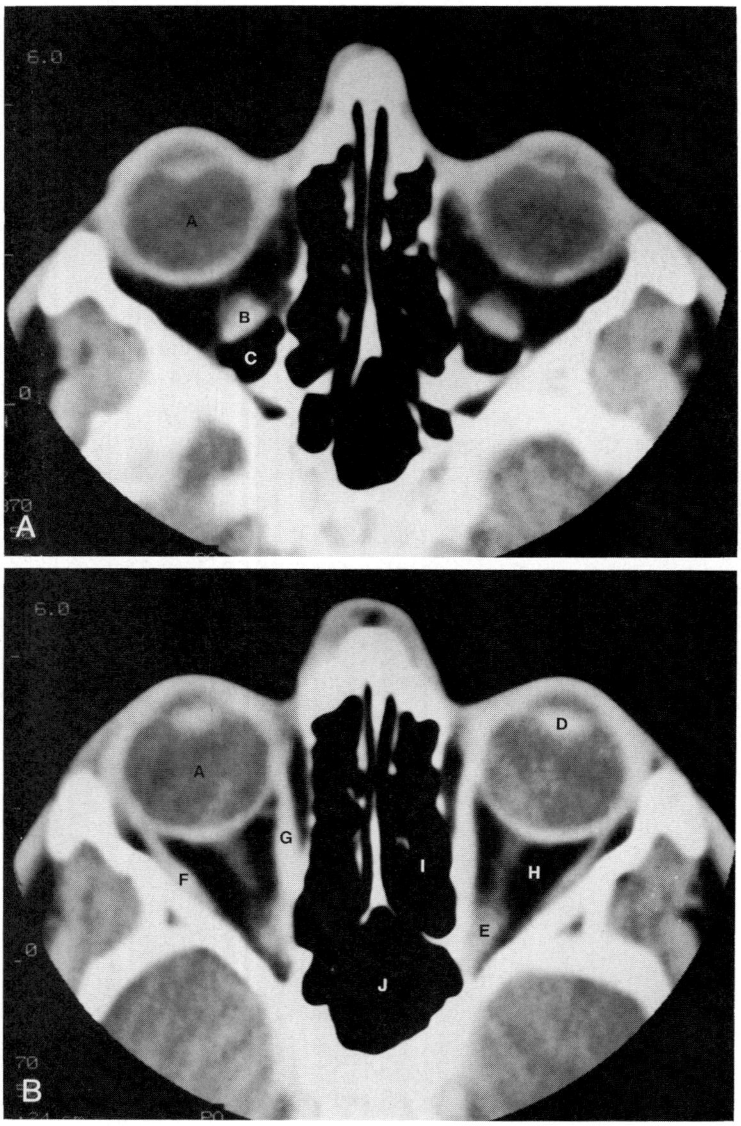

Figure 9–4. Computed tomographic (CT) anatomy.

A–D, Enhanced axial CT (inferior to superior). *(A)* globe, *(B)* inferior rectus muscle, *(C)* maxillary sinus, *(D)* lens, *(E)* optic nerve, *(F)* lateral rectus muscle, *(G)* medial rectus muscle, *(H)* retrobulbar fat, *(I)* ethmoid sinus, *(J)* sphenoid sinus, *(K)* lacrimal gland, *(L)* frontal sinus, *(M)* trochlea for superior oblique muscle, *(N)* superior ophthalmic vein, *(O)* superior rectus–levator muscle complex, *(P)* anterior clinoid.

Optic Nerve and Sheath

The optic nerve is a centrifugal extension of the central nervous system (CNS) into the orbit. The nerve extends from the optic chiasm through the optic canal and annulus of Zinn to the posterior globe forming the ophthalmoscopically apparent optic disc. The dural membranes surround the nerve such that the subarachnoid space investing the nerve is contiguous with the remainder of the cerebrospinal fluid (CSF), providing a potential pathway of tumor dissemination.[4] The nerve measures approximately 4 to 6 mm in diameter and not infrequently has a tortuous intraconal course to the globe.

Extraocular Muscles

Seven radiographically distinguishable muscles are present in the orbit, one of which elevates the upper lid (superior levator palpebrae) (Fig. 9–6). In addition, four rectus and two oblique muscles are responsible for positioning the globe. The rectus muscles arise from a small fibrous ring at the apex of the orbit, called the annulus of Zinn.[5] These mus-

Text continued on page 299

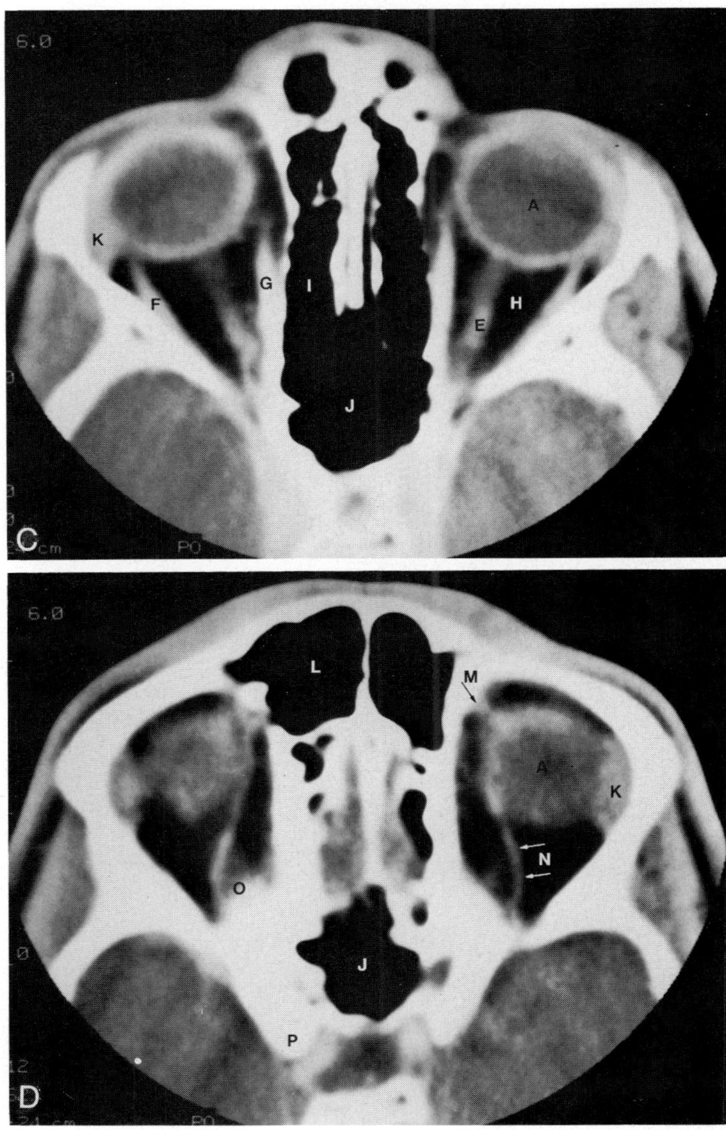

Figure 9–4 *Continued*

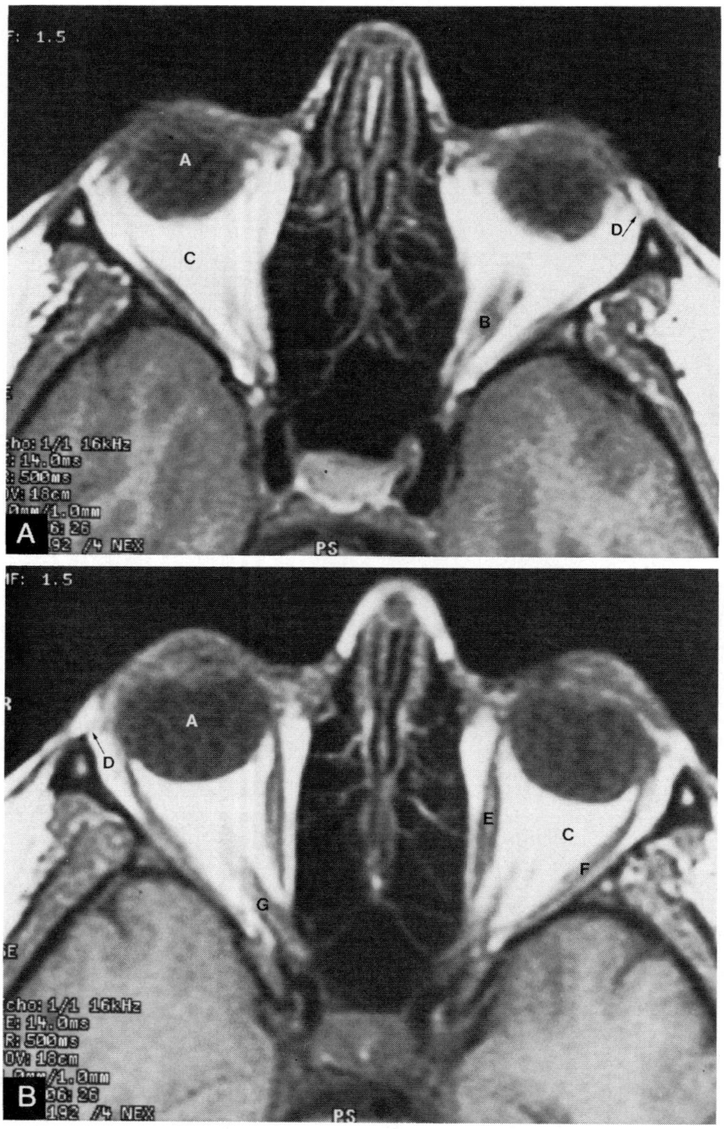

Figure 9–5. Magnetic resonance imaging (MRI) anatomy.

A–E, Axial T1 (inferior to superior).

F–I, Coronal T1 (anterior to posterior). *(A)* globe, *(B)* inferior rectus muscle, *(C)* retrobulbar fat, *(D)* orbital septum, *(E)* medial rectus muscle, *(F)* lateral rectus muscle, *(G)* optic nerve, *(H)* ophthalmic artery, *(I)* infundibulum, *(J)* superior oblique muscle, *(K)* lacrimal gland, *(L)* superior rectus–levator muscle complex, *(M)* lens, *(N)* superior ophthalmic vein, *(O)* optic chiasm.

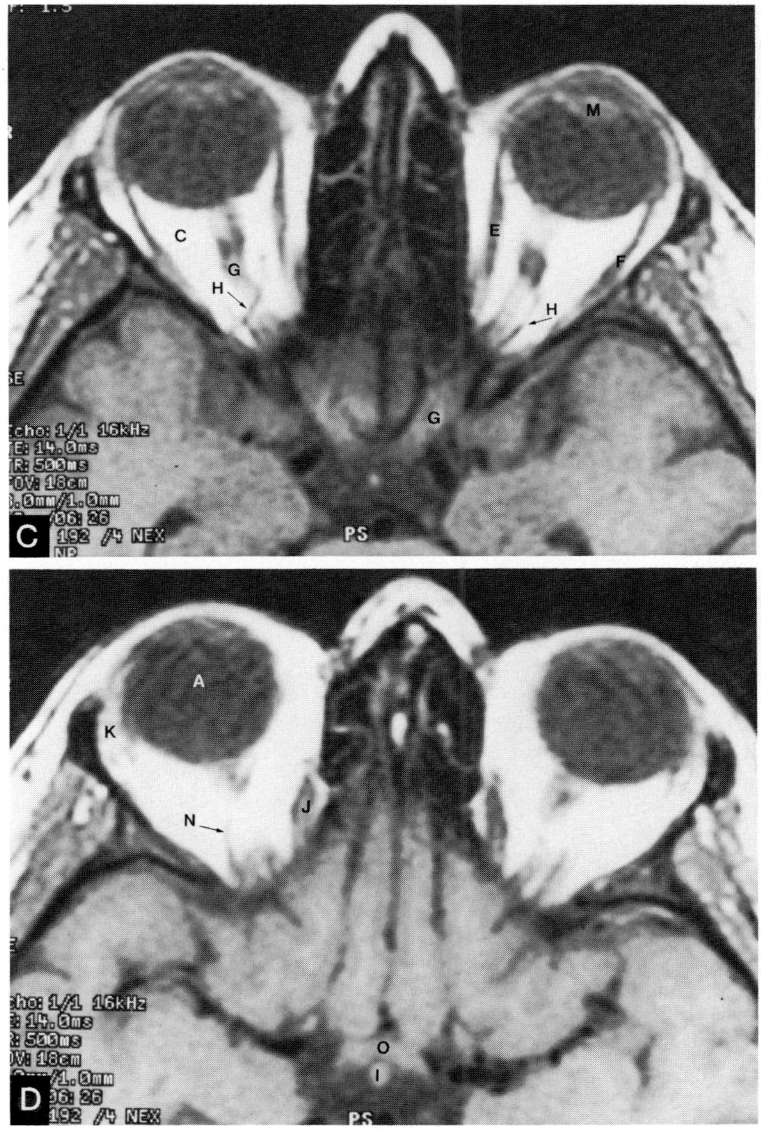

Figure 9–5 *Continued*

Illustration continued on following page

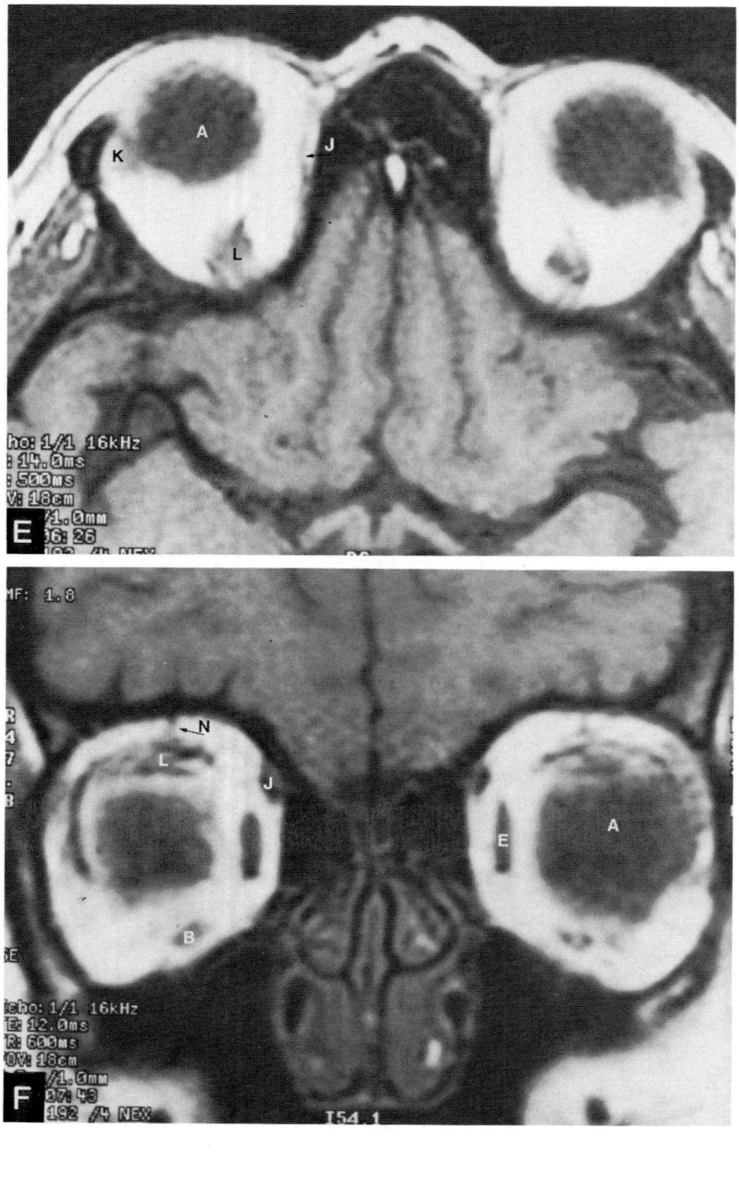

Figure 9–5 *Continued*

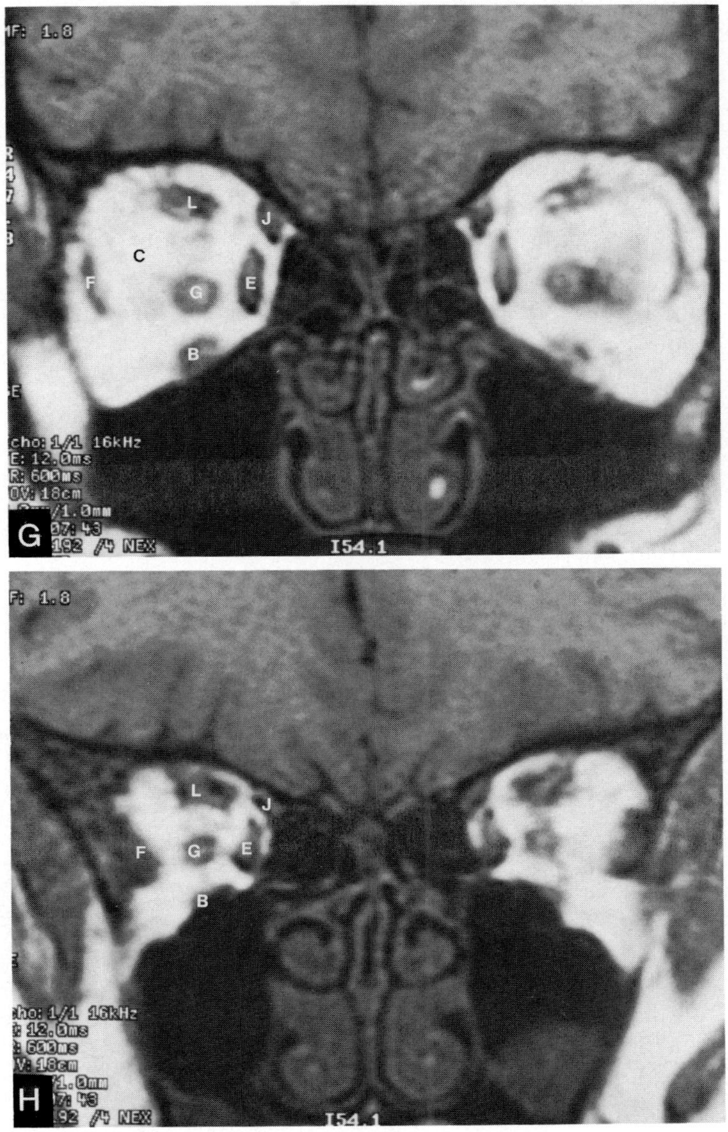

Figure 9–5 *Continued*
Illustration continued on following page

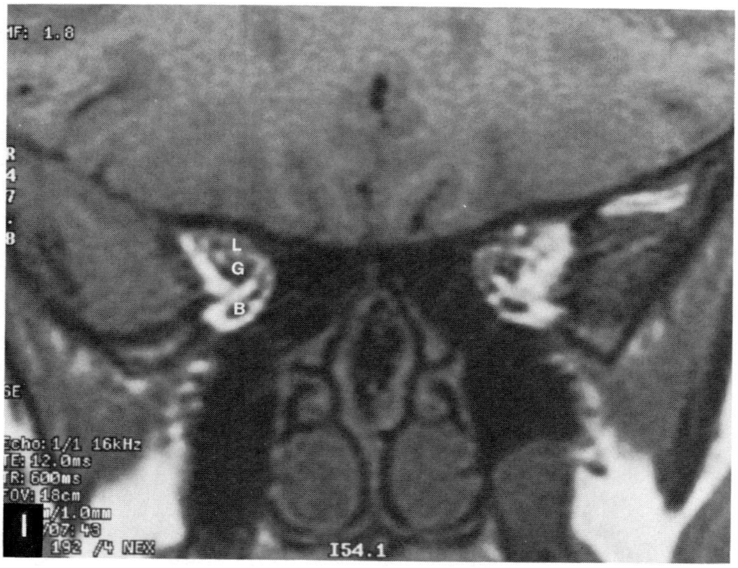

Figure 9–5 *Continued*

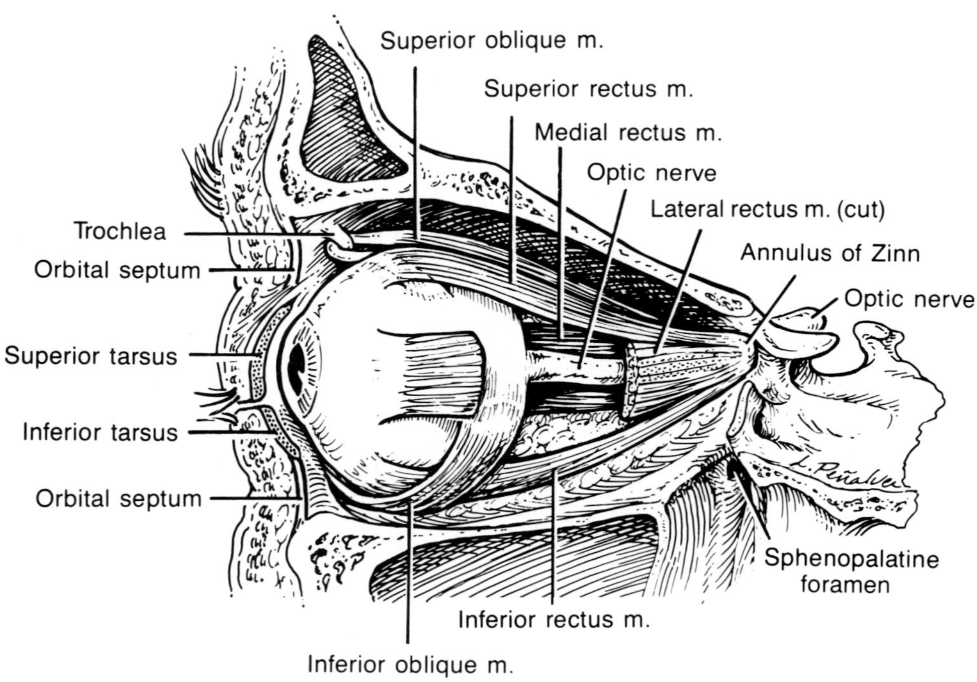

Figure 9–6. Lateral drawing of orbit.

cles converge on the four quadrants of the globe from the medial, lateral, superior, and inferior positions. Two oblique muscles, the inferior and superior oblique, attach to the globe. The inferior oblique muscle arises from the medial anterior aspect of the orbit along the lacrimal bone. This is the shortest of the extraocular muscles and the only one that does not arise within the orbital apex. The superior oblique muscle arises from the superior medial apex periorbita and courses along the medial aspect of the orbit to reach the fibrous trochlea before continuing posterolaterally to insert on the globe. A fascial sheath surrounds each extraocular muscle and extends between muscle sheaths to form the intermuscular septum. The extraocular muscles enhance more vividly than do other skeletal muscles,[6] secondary to increased vascularity necessary to permit the high-speed movement and nonfatiguing tonus.

Vascular Structures

Two consistently identifiable vascular structures may be identified within the orbit. The ophthalmic artery enters the orbit inferior to the optic nerve through the optic canal. The proximity of this structure to the optic nerve aids in its identification. The ophthalmic artery represents the major vascular supply to the orbital contents as it arborizes into the central retinal artery, which pierces the dura and lies within the center of the optic nerve. The lacrimal, muscular, ciliary, ethmoid, and supraorbital arteries arise from the ophthalmic artery.

The superior ophthalmic vein has a tortuous course extending from anteromedial to posterolateral. Anteriorly, the vessel is extraconal. Midway along its course, it pierces the intramuscular septum to become intraconal. The superior ophthalmic vein drains a portion of the face and the orbital contents through the superior orbital fissure into the cavernous sinus.

The inferior ophthalmic vein is not readily identifiable on planar images unless a high flow state exists. The inferior ophthalmic vein also drains into the cavernous sinus through either the inferior or the superior orbital fissure.

Lacrimal Apparatus

The lacrimal gland is a postseptal, almond-shaped structure that resides in the lacrimal fossa along the medial surface of the zygomatic process of the frontal bone. The gland is 10 × 5 mm in size and is separated from the globe by the lateral rectus muscle.

The gland secretes tears that are conveyed to the surface of the eyeball by 10 to 12 small ducts. The tears travel medially to exit the orbit into the nasal cavity. The tears enter a small orifice (punctum) located on the medial aspect of the upper and lower lid. These puncta communicate with the lacrimal sac (a preseptal structure) via the superior and inferior canaliculi. The fluid then enters the nasolacrimal duct and descends to exit Hasner's valve, below the inferior turbinate into the nasal cavity.[7]

Optic Chiasm and Visual Pathways

The optic nerves converge at the optic chiasm, which is located in the suprasellar cistern, a variable distance anterior to the pituitary infundibulum. The medial retinal (nasal) fibers decussate at the chiasm (Fig. 9–7). The lateral retinal (temporal) fibers remain ipsilateral to their origin. The optic tracts extend from the optic chiasm to the ipsilateral lateral geniculate body. The optic radiations travel from the lateral geniculate body to the posterior portion of the internal capsule along the lateral aspect of the occipital horn of the lateral ventricle until they terminate on the visual cortex of the medial occipital lobe.[8] The fibers are initially compactly arranged at the internal capsule and become progressively more divergent as they fan out toward the visual cortex. Point-to-point localization is maintained from the retina to the visual cortex.

IMAGING STRATEGY

The retrobulbar structures are surrounded by extraocular fat. This provides natural CT and MRI contrast differentiation among fat, muscle, and nerve. CT is most useful for calcified lesions, still an area of relative insensitivity for MRI. Unenhanced CT examinations may be conducted with thin (1- to 2-mm) increments in an axial plane, if the suspected pathology is medial or lateral. The coronal plane is most sensitive at characterizing pathology in the superior and inferior portions of the orbit. A limited contrast-enhanced ex-

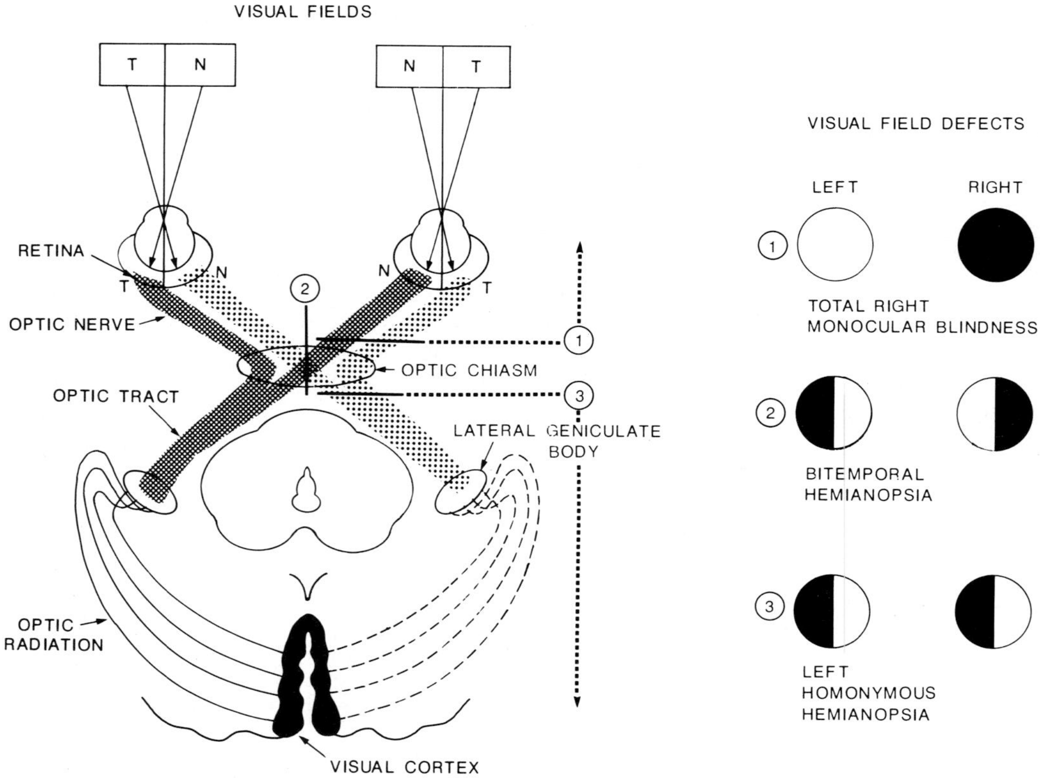

Figure 9–7. Drawing of visual pathways (medical illustration by Diane Blue; modified from Langer BG, Charletta DA, Mafee MF, et al: MRI of the normal optic pathway. Seminars in Ultrasound, CT and MRI 1988; 9:401–412.)

amination in one plane may be useful to characterize the enhancing pattern of a given lesion detected on the unenhanced study.

MRI may be performed with a small annular surface coil if the globe is the area of suspected pathology and with a head coil if retrobulbar or intracranial disease is suspected. MRI is more sensitive than CT in characterizing the anatomy and pathology in the orbital apex, superior orbital fissure, and optic canal. MRI may be useful in characterizing hemorrhagic lesions, detecting flow, determining with greater sensitivity the intracranial extent of optic neoplasms, and distinguishing pseudotumor from neoplasm.[9–11] MRI should be performed with high-resolution T1 images in at least two planes. If gadolinium is used, fat suppression technique will distinguish enhancement from intrisically high-signal retrobulbar fat. The T2 sequence can be performed in one plane, although it is less useful than the gadolinium-enhanced sequence in most patients.

PATHOLOGY

A location approach to orbital pathology is presented here. The major anatomic divisions are the globe, the intraconal space (which will include the extraocular muscles), and the extraconal space (Fig. 9–8). In some instances, disease may extend through the muscular cone or globe, or both, to involve more than one space.

Globe

Neoplastic

Retinoblastoma

Retinoblastoma is a neuroectodermal tumor of childhood that arises from the retina. Retinoblastoma is the most common intraocular malignant tumor of childhood, occurring at a rate of 1 to 15 per 30,000 people.[12] The average age at the time of diagnosis is 13 months, with 90% detected before 5 years of age. The lesion

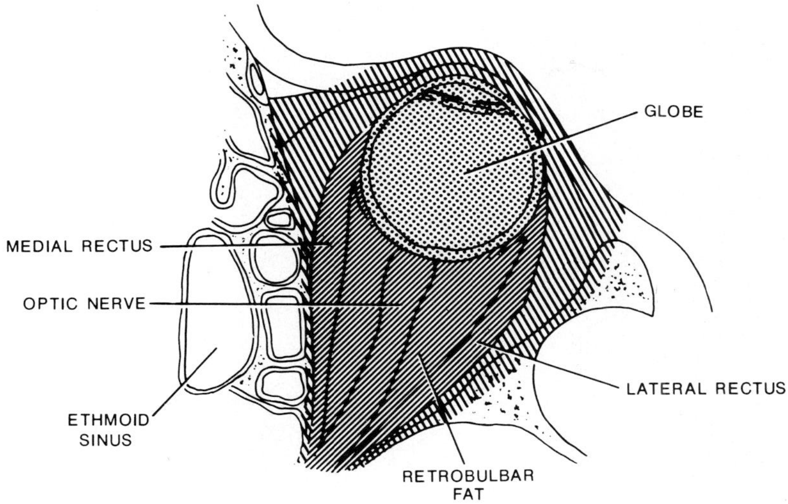

COMMON ORBITAL MASS LESIONS

LOCATION

AGE	GLOBE	INTRACONAL *	EXTRACONAL
CHILDREN	RETINOBLASTOMA	OPTIC NERVE GLIOMA RHABDOMYOSARCOMA	LYMPHANGIOMA RHABDOMYOSARCOMA METASTASIS
ADULTS	MELANOMA METASTASIS ENDOPHTHALMITIS	MENINGOMA HEMANGIOMA GRAVE'S ORBITOPATHY PSEUDOTUMOR	LYMPHOMA LACRIMAL GLAND TUMOR METASTASIS DERMOID
*	INCLUDES MUSCLE CONE		

Figure 9–8. Differential diagnosis of common orbital mass lesions (medical illustration by Diane Blue).

occurs with equal frequency in males and females. In 10 to 15% the lesions are familial, and in 25 to 33% they are multifocal, either within one globe or bilateral. A rare trilateral form exists in which a histologically similar neuroectodermal tumor develops within the pineal region. Patients present with leukocoria (white reflex) on fundoscopic examination. Early diagnosis is imperative in children afflicted with retinoblastoma, as disease confined to the globe is curable in 80 to 95% of cases[13] with 5-year survival of 92%.[12] Violation of the globe with spread to contiguous or noncontiguous structures results in nearly 100% mortality.[14] Retinoblastoma can extend through the choroid or along the subarachnoid space surrounding the optic nerve and may result in diffuse meningeal dissemination.[14, 15] Distant spread to the lung, bone, brain, and liver may occur.[13]

On CT evaluation a homogeneous mass slightly hyperdense to vitreous is present (Fig. 9–9). The mass is peripherally located, indicating its retinal origin. Release of DNA from the necrotic tumor results in calcification, which can be detected in 80 to 90% of cases. The tumor enhances homogeneously, but only to a slight degree. On CT, it is difficult to differentiate retinoblastoma from retinal detachment, which frequently accompanies retinoblastoma.

The MRI appearance of retinoblastoma is

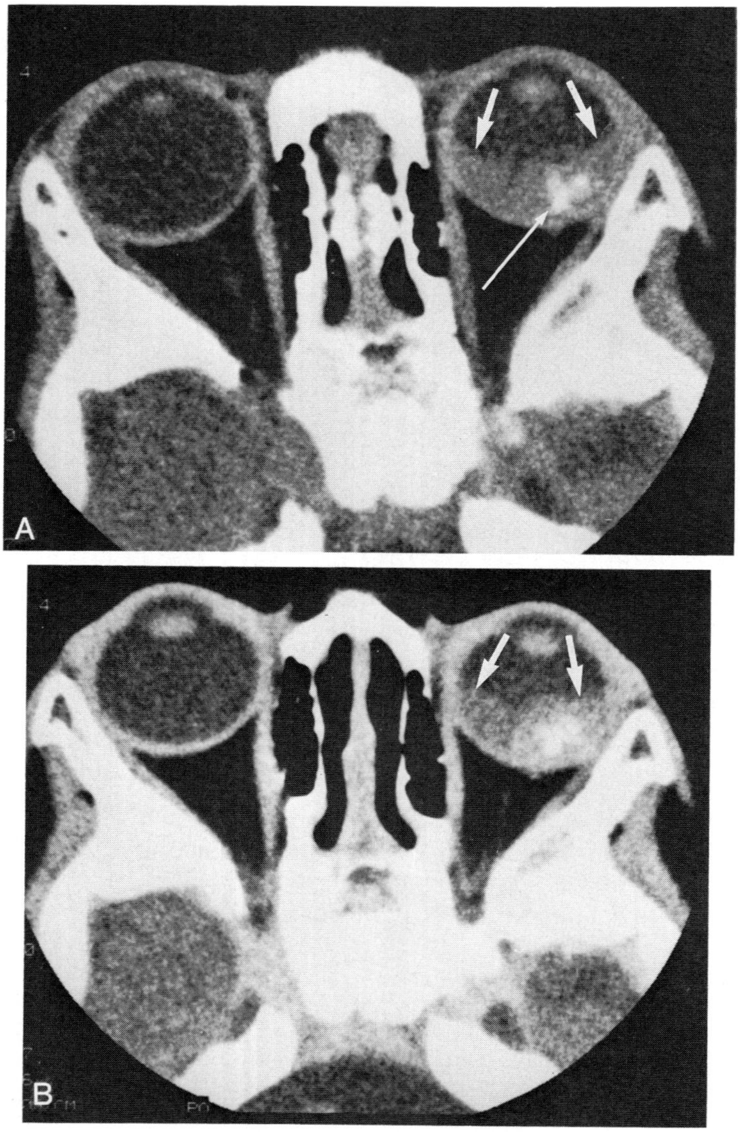

Figure 9–9. Retinoblastoma (1-year-old male).

A, Unenhanced CT. An exophytic intravitreal mass *(short arrows)* is present on the left. Amorphic calcification *(long arrow)* is present within the matrix of the tumor.

B, Enhanced CT. The mass *(arrows)* enhances homogeneously, more accurately delineating tumor margin from the vitrous.

that of a peripheral, exophytic mass of variable size (Fig. 9–10). The mass is isointense to hyperintense to vitreous on T1 and hypointense to vitreous on T2.[12, 16, 17] Dense calcification may decrease to some degree both T1 and T2 relaxation times. The subretinal proteinaceous effusion or hemorrhage that may occur with retinal detachment is usually easily distinguishable from tumor, appearing as a homogeneous collection of material that is high signal on T1- and T2-weighted images. Contrast may also help, as tumor will enhance and an effusion will not.

Melanoma

Melanoma is the most common primary orbital malignancy of the globe, usually affecting patients in their seventh decade. Melanoma arises from the pigmented choroid of the uvea. This condition occurs 15 times more frequently in whites than in blacks. Melanoma of the choroid may arise from a pre-existing nevus.[18] Patients are often asymptomatic but may experience decreased vision and glaucoma secondary to associated retinal detachment. The single most important prognostic factor is tu-

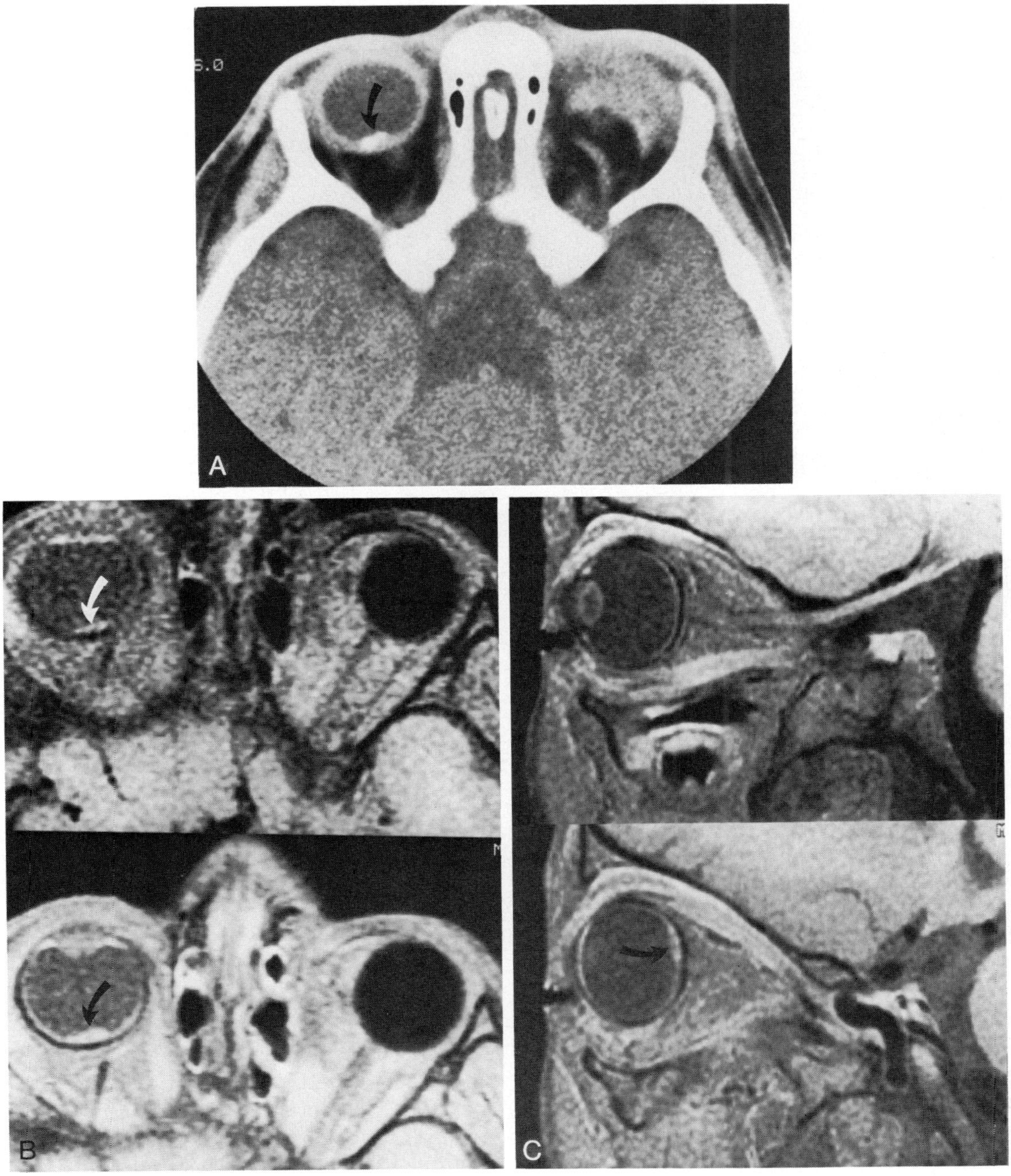

Figure 9–10. Retinoblastoma (4-year-old female).

A, Axial CT. A small exophytic calcification *(arrow)* is present in the right globe.

B, Axial fat-saturated T1. *Top*, Unenhanced; a thin crescentic focus of increased signal *(arrow)* is present along the posterior right globe. The high signal may be due in part to subretinal effusion or blood. The left globe has been resected and replaced by a prosthesis. *Bottom*, Enhanced; the thin tumor mass *(arrow)* is more readily apparent on the enhanced examination.

C, Parasagittal fat-saturated T1. The thin enhancing tumor mass *(arrow)* is confined to the globe without extension into contiguous structures.

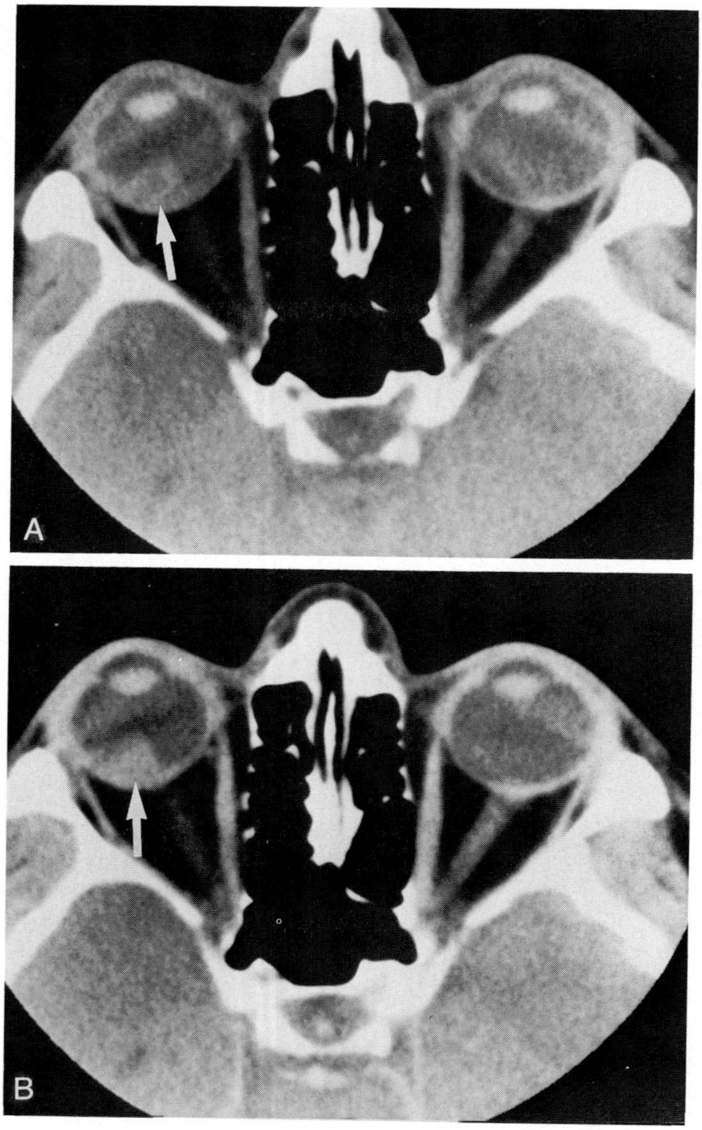

Figure 9–11. Melanoma (44-year-old female).

A, Unenhanced CT. An intrinsically dense exophytic intraocular mass *(arrow)* is present on the right. The posterior margin of the globe remains smooth and well marginated.

B, Enhanced CT. The mass *(arrow)* enhances homogeneously.

mor size, underscoring the importance of early detection.[19] These are unifocal lesions. Extraocular extension at the time of diagnosis occurs in less than 15%.

CT imaging reveals an elevated hyperdense, noncalcified, sharply marginated mass (Fig. 9–11). The lesion may enhance to a moderate degree. The mass may appear as a focal thickening of the posterior ocular wall or extend a variable distance into the vitreous. Associated retinal detachment with exudative subretinal effusion may be indistinguishable from tumor on unenhanced CT. Intravenous (IV) contrast may be useful to distinguish this relationship.

The MRI appearance of uveal melanoma is variable, depending on the chemical makeup of the tumor and presence of associated hemorrhage. Melanotic melanomas have shortened T1 and T2 relaxation times, so that, relative to vitreous, these lesions are high signal on T1- and low signal on T2-weighted images.[11, 18–20] Amelanotic melanomas may exhibit a signal intensity slightly higher than that of vitreous on T1-weighted images and may be rendered inapparent on T2-weighted images. One group[19] found that the postgadolinium T1-weighted sequence was the most sensitive at detecting uveal melanoma and at distinguishing it from subretinal collections, the latter of which did not enhance.

Metastasis

Metastasis to the globe most commonly arises secondary to invasion from tumor rising in contiguous regions. The globe is, however, the most common orbital structure to be involved by hematogenous metastatic dissemination. Ocular metastases are more common in adults than in children and arise from the heart, lung, and gastrointestinal and genitourinary systems.[21, 22] Bilateral metastases are rare.

Most lesions are microscopic, beyond the resolution of CT and MRI instruments. The CT appearance of macroscopic metastasis is variable, ranging from a focal thickening of the globe to an infiltrative, poorly marginated hyperdense mass (Fig. 9–12). The mass enhances moderately and is rarely calcified. MRI depicts a mass of slightly greater signal intensity than that of vitreous on T1 and diminished signal relative to vitreous on T2. MRI excels at differentiating bright T1 subretinal fluid from tumor.

Inflammatory

Endophthalmitis

This inflammatory condition of the globe usually results from intraocular surgery or penetrating trauma. Endophthalmitis may also result from seeding of a systemic source of infection or extension from a contiguous structure. Common bacterial pathogens include staphylococci, streptococci, meningococci, and gram-negative organisms.

Planar imaging findings include thickening and enhancement of the uveal-scleral junction (Fig. 9–13). The density of the vitreous may increase and the density of the lens may decrease.[15, 23]

Developmental

Coloboma

Incomplete fusion of the embryonic fissure or primitive choroidal fissure results in a gap or diverticulum in the posterior globe. This may occur at the optic nerve or elsewhere along the retinochoroidal junction, often inferior nasal to the optic nerve.[24–27] The resulting cyst is surrounded by sclera lined by a dysmorphic neuroectodermal layer. Visual acuity is variable, ranging from normal to loss of light perception. Colobomas may be bilateral and result in microphthalmos.[25] Colobomas account for 11.5% of patients with leukocoria from causes other than retinoblastoma.[28]

Planar imaging reveals a diverticulum of varying size extending into the retrobulbar region from the posterior globe (Fig. 9–14). The contents of the diverticulum resemble the vitreous regarding CT density and MRI signal.

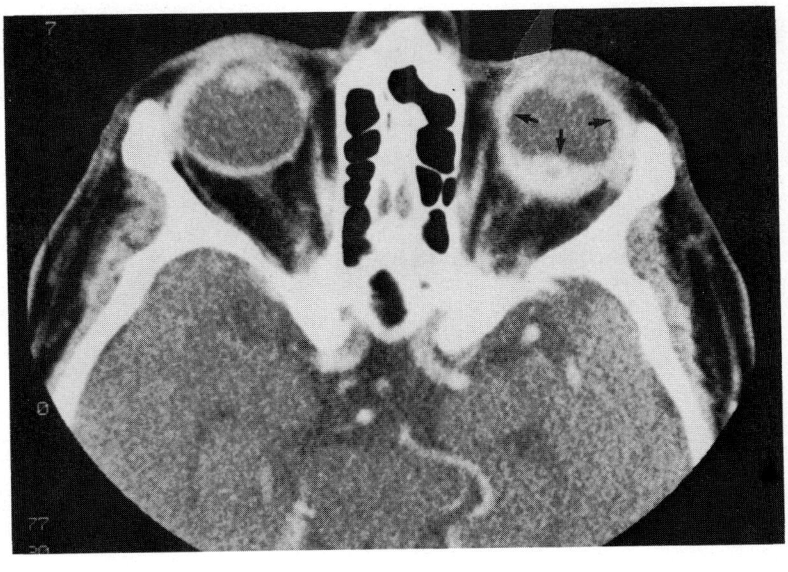

Figure 9–12. Metastasis; breast (70-year-old female). Enhanced CT; diffuse thickening of the globe *(arrows)* is present with more focal enhancement and soft tissue mass noted posteriorly.

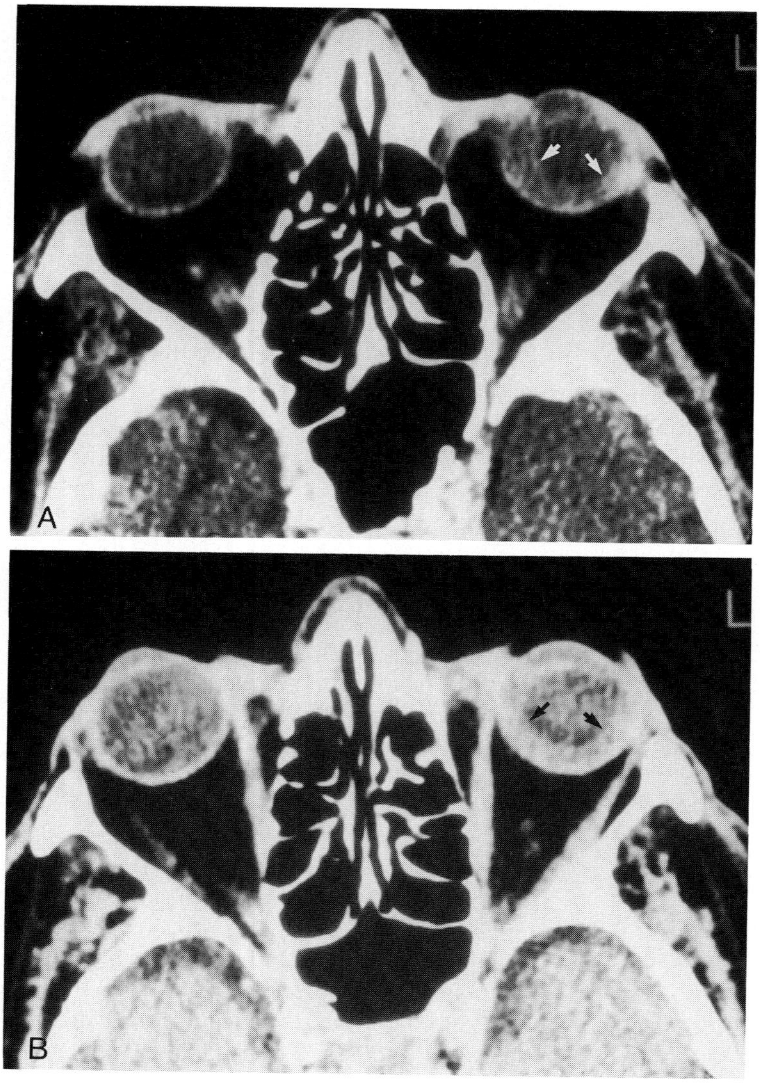

Figure 9–13. Viral endophthalmitis (42-year-old female).

A, Unenhanced CT. A subtle collar of high density *(arrows)* lines the vitreous body of the left globe.

B, Enhanced CT. The collar of inflammatory tissue *(arrows)* becomes more apparent following contrast administration.

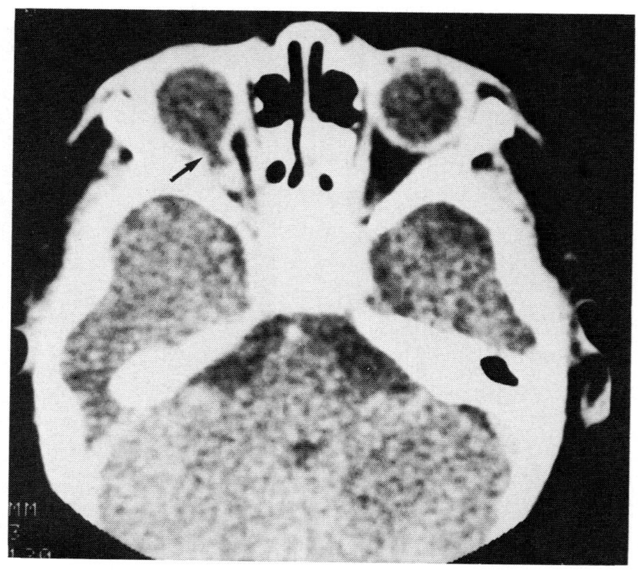

Figure 9–14. Coloboma (4-month-old male). Enhanced CT; a prominent diverticulum *(arrow)* extends posteriorly from the globe. The diverticulum is contiguous with the vitreous and is lined by radiographically similar material to the posterior globe.

Persistent Hyperplastic Primary Vitreous (PHPV)

The hyaloid vascular system is the embryonic intraocular mechanism that supplies nutrients to the developing lens, vitreous, and optic nerve. These vessels normally regress before 8 months of gestation as the vascular system matures. Failure of regression of the hyaloid vascular system results in PHPV. The primary vitreous is an extremely vascular mesenchymal tissue that proliferates, resulting in a retrolental mass of varying size.[15, 24, 29–31] The mass may be funnel-shaped, with the apex directed toward the lens, outlining Cloquet's canal, the embryonic course of the hyaloid artery. PHPV may result in blindness and leukocoria. PHPV is the second most common cause (19%) of leukocoria not attributed to retinoblastoma.[28] The friability of the hyperplastic vascular system may result in intraocular hemorrhage. The average age at time of diagnosis is 4 months. PHPV is bilateral in 4% of affected patients.

CT depicts an enhancing, irregular, noncalcified soft tissue intravitreal mass (Figs. 9–15, 9–16). Microphthalmos, a small lens, and a normal to small optic nerve are present. PHPV results in high signal on T1- and T2-weighted images.[20]

Features that distinguish PHPV from retinoblastoma are microphthalmos, a shallow anterior chamber, prominent retinal vessels, unilaterality, lack of calcification, funnel-shaped intravitreal mass, increased density of the vitreous on CT, and high T2 signal intensity (Table 9–1).

Coats' Disease

Coats' disease is a primary vascular anomaly of the retina characterized by telangiectasias that are unusually permeable, resulting in the accumulation of lipoproteinaceous exudate in the retina and subretinal space. Males are affected more commonly than females. Patients are usually asymptomatic until the retina detaches, which explains the fact that children

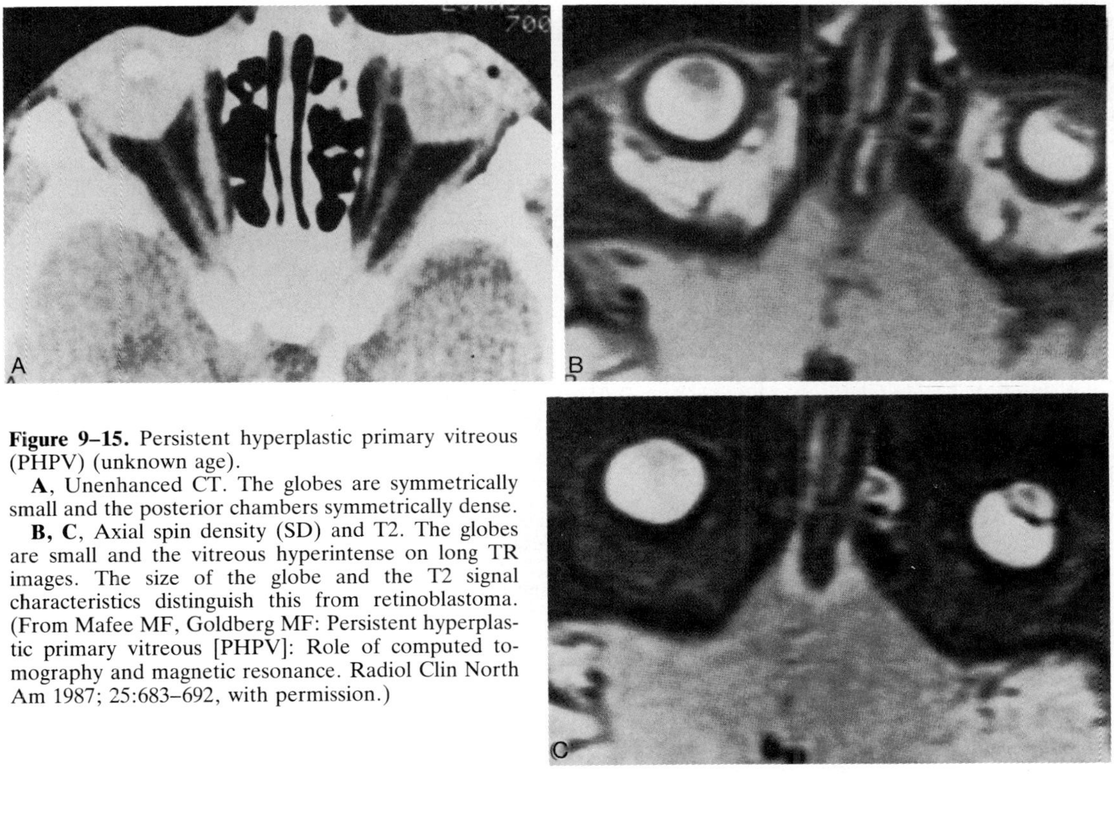

Figure 9–15. Persistent hyperplastic primary vitreous (PHPV) (unknown age).
A, Unenhanced CT. The globes are symmetrically small and the posterior chambers symmetrically dense.
B, C, Axial spin density (SD) and T2. The globes are small and the vitreous hyperintense on long TR images. The size of the globe and the T2 signal characteristics distinguish this from retinoblastoma. (From Mafee MF, Goldberg MF: Persistent hyperplastic primary vitreous [PHPV]: Role of computed tomography and magnetic resonance. Radiol Clin North Am 1987; 25:683–692, with permission.)

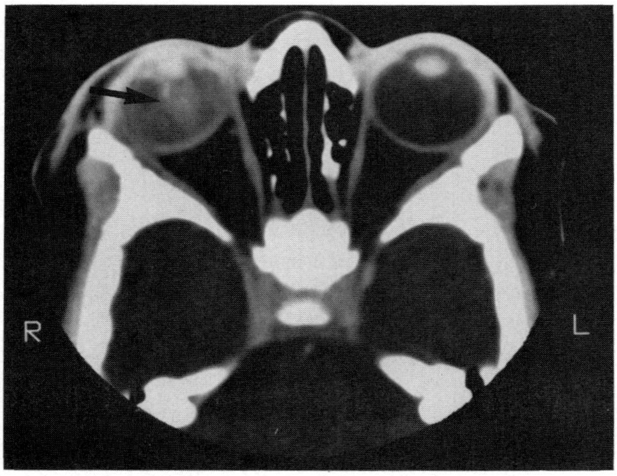

Figure 9–16. PHPV (6-week-old male). Enhanced axial CT; the band of increased attenuation *(arrow)* in the small right globe represents the embryonic hyaloid vascular system remnant. (From Wells RG, Miro P, Brummond R: Color-flow doppler sonography of persistent hyperplastic primary vitreous. J Ultrasound Med 1991; 10:405–407, with permission.)

with this disease come to medical attention slightly later (at age 4 to 8 years) than do those with retinoblastoma. Patients present with leukocoria, strabismus, decreased vision, and glaucoma.[29] Coats' disease is a relatively uncommon cause (4%) of leukocoria.[28]

CT demonstrates a noncalcified increased density of the vitreous without a focal mass[24] (Fig. 9–17). The MRI signal characteristics include hyperintensity on T1- and T2-weighted images. Although the CT appearance of Coats' disease may be similar to that of noncalcified retinoblastoma, T2 signal characteristics will differentiate these lesions.

Trauma

Orbital trauma may be blunt or penetrating and result in a broad spectrum of abnormalities involving the globe, retrobulbar soft tissues, or bony perimeter of the orbit.

Ocular trauma may lead to globe disruption, lens dislocation, intraocular foreign body, or hemorrhage (Figs. 9–18 to 9–20). End-stage ocular trauma, termed phthisis bulbi, results in a nonfunctioning shrunken calcified globe (Fig. 9–21).

Trauma may result in orbital fractures, involving the orbital rim, floor, or walls of the orbit, depending on the location and magnitude of the vector of force. Blunt trauma directed toward the globe may increase the orbital pressure, resulting in a blow-out fracture. Orbital floor blow-out fractures were found to be nearly twice as common as medial wall blow-out fractures in one series.[32] Floor and medial wall fractures frequently occur in the same patient (Fig. 9–22).

Although conventional wisdom supports the premise that CT is more sensitive at detecting orbital fractures, surface coil MRI has been demonstrated to be superior to CT in fracture

Table 9–1. LEUKOCORIA: DISTINGUISHING CHARACTERISTICS OF COMMON CAUSES

	Retinoblastoma	PHPV*	Coloboma	Coats' Disease
Relative frequency	23.5	5.1	3.6	1
Age	1 yr (90% by 5 yr)	4 mo	< 1 yr	4–8 yr
Sex	Male = female	Male:female, 2:3	Male = female	Male:female, 3:2
Imaging	Globe normal size Exophytic peripheral mass Bilateral 30% Calcification 80–90% T1: isointense-hyperintense T2: hypointense	Microphthalmos Unilateral Funnel-shaped vitreal mass T2: hyperintense	Globe normal → small Retrobulbar diverticulum	Globe normal → small Vitreous increased density T2: hyperintense

*PHPV = persistent hyperplastic primary vitreous.

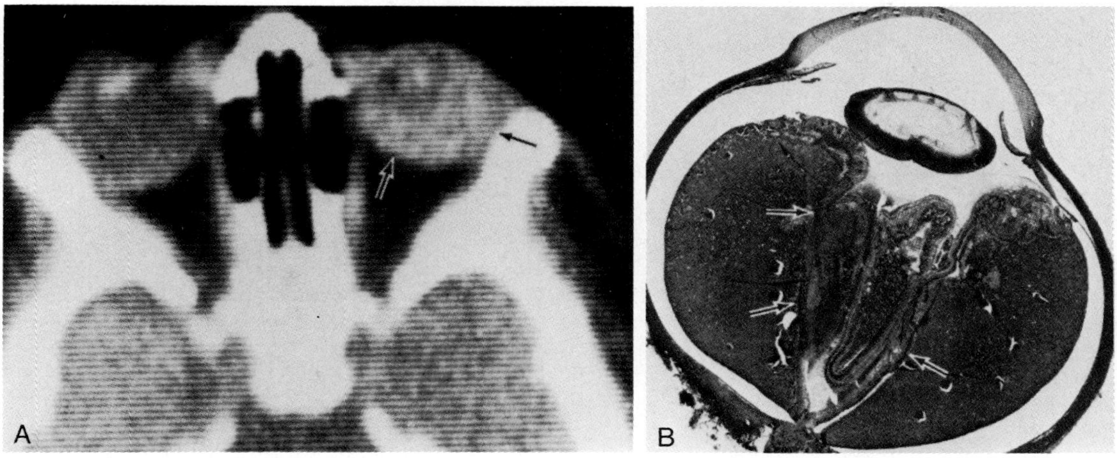

Figure 9–17. Coats' disease (7-month-old male).

A, Unenhanced CT. The vitreous body of the left globe is partially filled with a hyperdense mass *(arrows)*.

B, Photomicrograph demonstrates an exudative detachment of the retina *(arrows)*. (From Sherman JL, McLean IW, Brallier DR: Coats' disease: CT pathologic correlation in two cases. Radiology 1983; 146:77–78, with permission.)

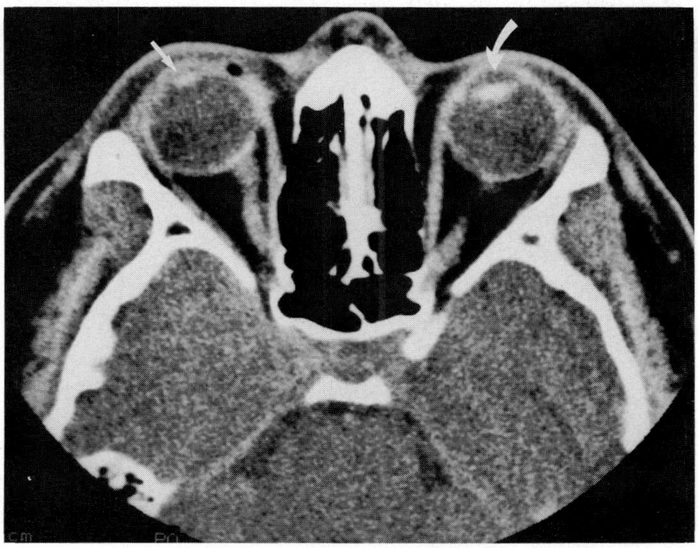

Figure 9–18. Trauma (18-year-old male). Unenhanced CT; a puncture wound to the cornea has deflated the aqueous humor *(arrow)*. The size of the normal aqueous is demonstrated anterior to the lens on the left *(curved arrow)*.

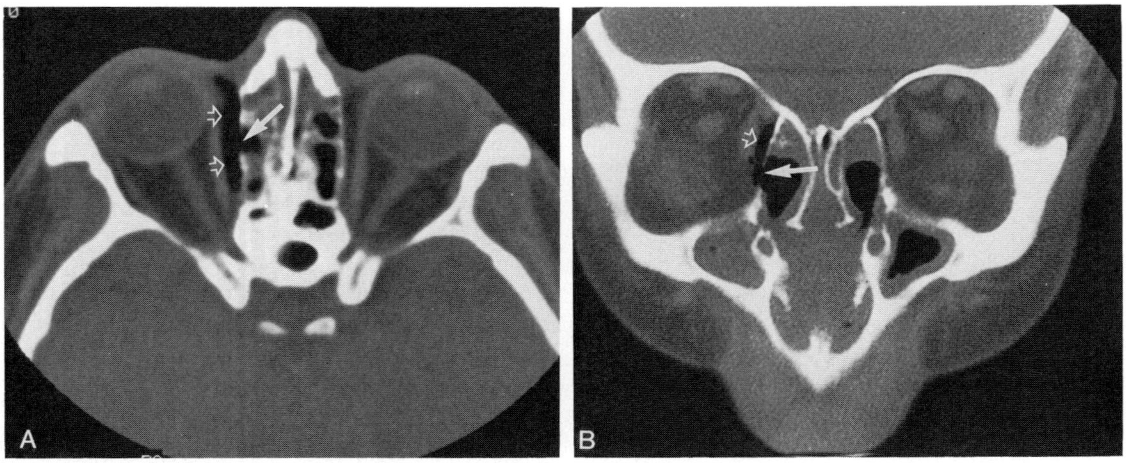

Figure 9–19. Iatrogenic trauma following functional endoscopic sinus surgery (23-year-old male).
A, Axial CT. A defect in the medial orbital wall *(arrow)* and extraconal orbital gas *(open arrows)* are noted.
B, Coronal CT. The rent in the lamina papyracea *(arrow)* is visualized. Note the medial extraconal gas *(open arrow)*.

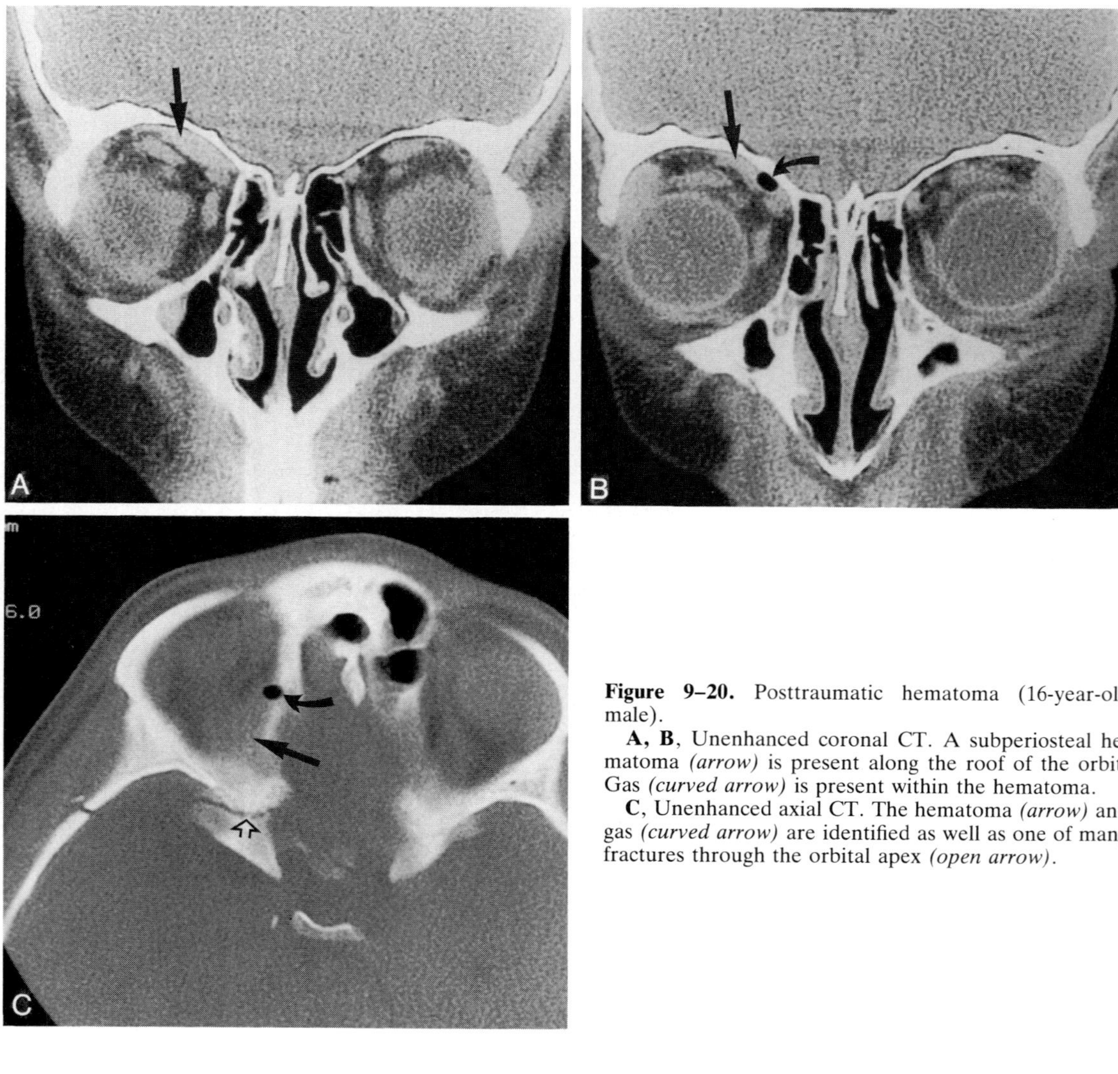

Figure 9–20. Posttraumatic hematoma (16-year-old male).

A, B, Unenhanced coronal CT. A subperiosteal hematoma *(arrow)* is present along the roof of the orbit. Gas *(curved arrow)* is present within the hematoma.

C, Unenhanced axial CT. The hematoma *(arrow)* and gas *(curved arrow)* are identified as well as one of many fractures through the orbital apex *(open arrow)*.

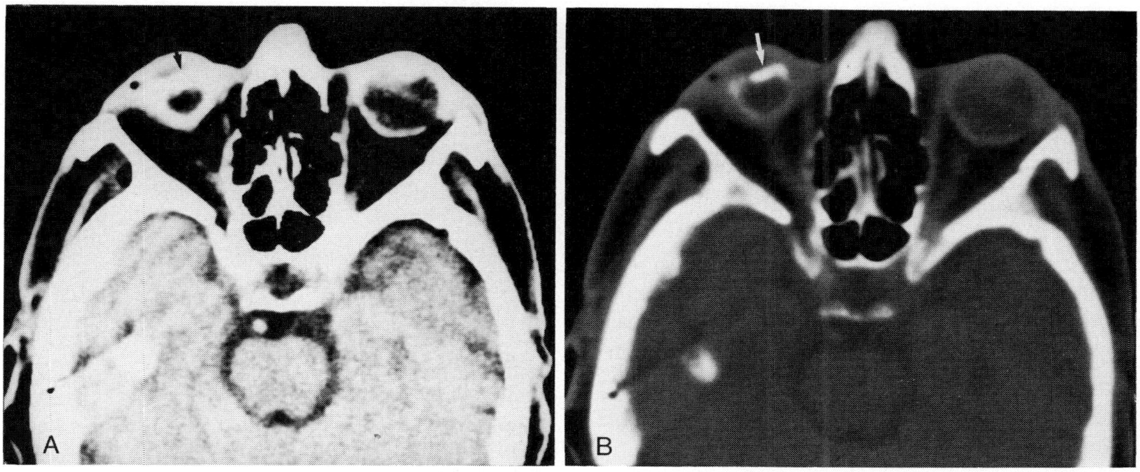

Figure 9–21. Phthisis bulbi (71-year-old female, veteran of barroom brawl 30 years earlier).
A, B, Enhanced CT. The right globe is atretic and partially calcified *(arrow)*.

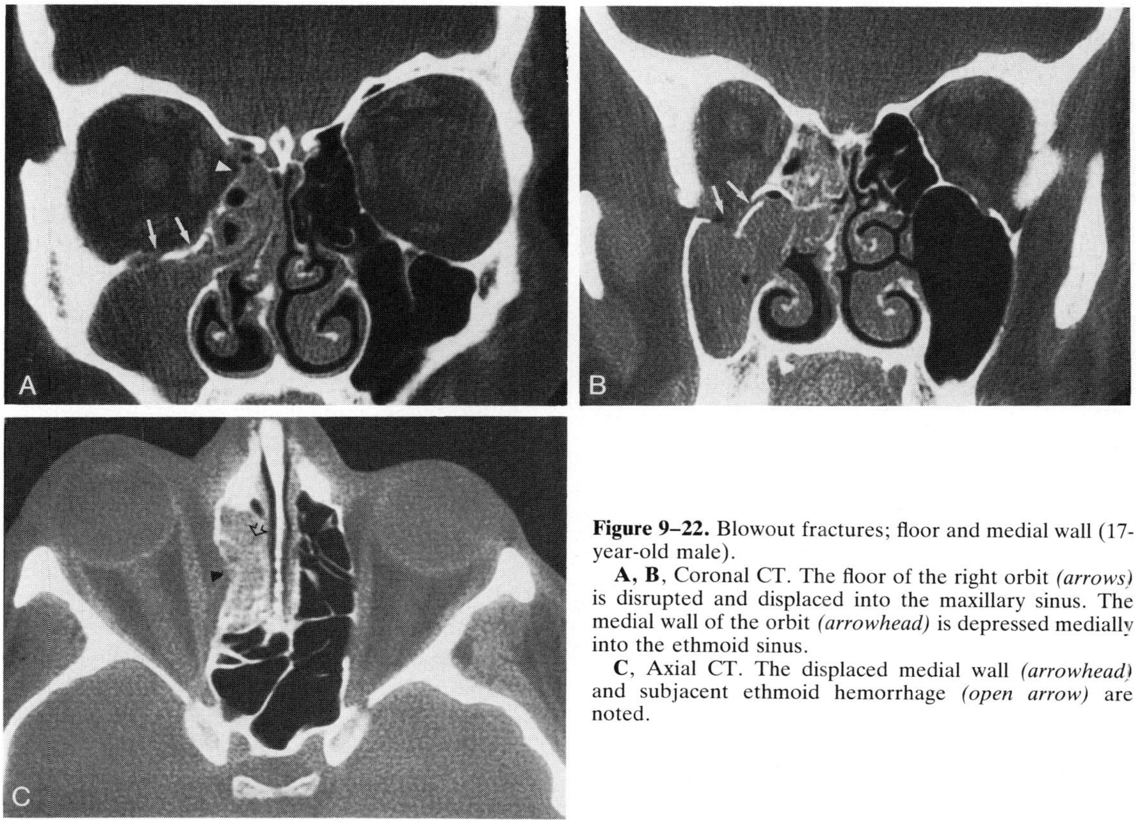

Figure 9–22. Blowout fractures; floor and medial wall (17-year-old male).

A, B, Coronal CT. The floor of the right orbit *(arrows)* is disrupted and displaced into the maxillary sinus. The medial wall of the orbit *(arrowhead)* is depressed medially into the ethmoid sinus.

C, Axial CT. The displaced medial wall *(arrowhead)* and subjacent ethmoid hemorrhage *(open arrow)* are noted.

detection.[33] MRI is also very helpful in detecting fat and muscle that have prolapsed through a blow-out fracture, possibly causing entrapment[33, 34] and decreased ocular motility. MRI is also superior for detection of optic nerve injury and orbital hematoma.[11]

Hematic cysts are the result of incompletely resorbed subperiosteal hematomas. Although not always secondary to trauma, this is the most common etiology. The orbital roof is the most common location for a hematic cyst as the roof is concaved and the periorbita is not as firmly adherent to the bone.[35, 36] With time, the chronic granulomatous reaction is surrounded by fibrous tissue, and benign bony resorption and remodeling of the orbit may occur.[37]

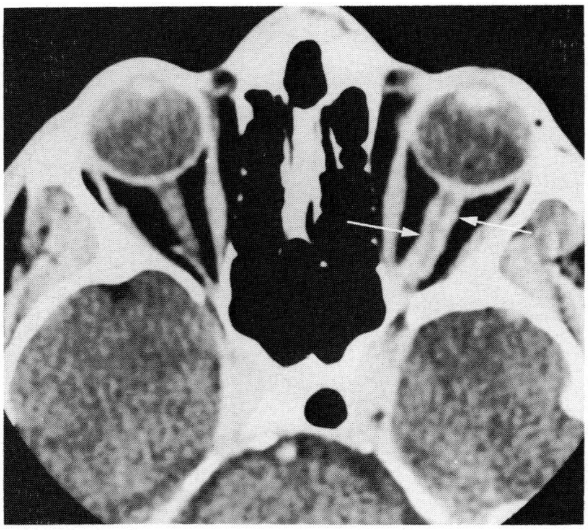

Figure 9–23. Meningioma (45-year-old female). Enhanced CT; the left optic nerve sheath complex is thickened and enhances in a tram-track pattern *(arrows)*. Although not pathognomonic for meningioma, this is characteristic of this entity.

Intraconal

Neoplastic

Meningioma

Orbital meningiomas arise from meningothelial cells found beneath the dural sheath that surrounds the optic nerve. Less commonly, meningiomas may arise from ectopic rests, located anywhere within the orbit. Orbital meningiomas may also result from direct extension of an intracranial meningioma through the optic canal or superior orbital fissure. Orbital meningiomas present most often in the fourth to fifth decade, occurring twice as commonly in females. Bilaterality implicates neurofibromatosis. Patients present with insidious onset of decreased visual acuity, proptosis, and limitation of ocular movement, papilledema, or optic atrophy.[38] Rarely, optic nerve meningiomas present in childhood. These lesions tend to be clinically and radiographically more aggressive.

Optic nerve meningiomas most commonly result in well-defined tubular thickening of the nerve (64%) or fusiform enlargement (23 to 30%) on CT[4, 39] (Fig. 9–23). The tram-track pattern of increased density and enhancement encasing the hypodense nerve is common for meningioma but is nonspecific, as optic neuritis and pseudotumor may present similarly. Optic nerve meningiomas may be partially or completely calcified. The intrinsic high density resulting from calcification may obscure any detectable contrast enhancement. Meningiomas that occur near the bony apex or extend through the optic canal or superior orbital fissure may induce adjacent bony sclerosis or erosion.[40] The MRI appearance of orbital meningiomas is variable, depending largely on the size of the lesion and the amount of calcification. The tumors are generally hypointense to fat on T1-weighted images and isointense to hyperintense to fat on T2-weighted images[20, 21, 41] (Fig. 9–24). Small, densely calcified lesions may be more apparent on CT than on MRI.[16] Gadolinium-enhanced MRI,[4] particularly that employing fat saturation techniques, is very sensitive at detecting these lesions.

Optic Nerve Glioma

Optic nerve gliomas are generally well-differentiated, slow-growing tumors of childhood. They have a benign juvenile pilocytic histology. From 80 to 90% of patients present by the first decade with low-grade proptosis, visual field obscuration with eye movement,[40] optic atrophy, and decreased vision.[39] Bilaterality confirms neurofibromatosis. At diagnosis, 30 to 40% of tumors are confined to the orbit.[15] Alternatively, the tumor may extend through the optic canal into the optic chiasm, along the optic tracks to the lateral geniculate body and onward along the optic radiations.[42] A rare malignant form of optic nerve glioma exists in adults, which results in early intracranial extension and death within 1 year.

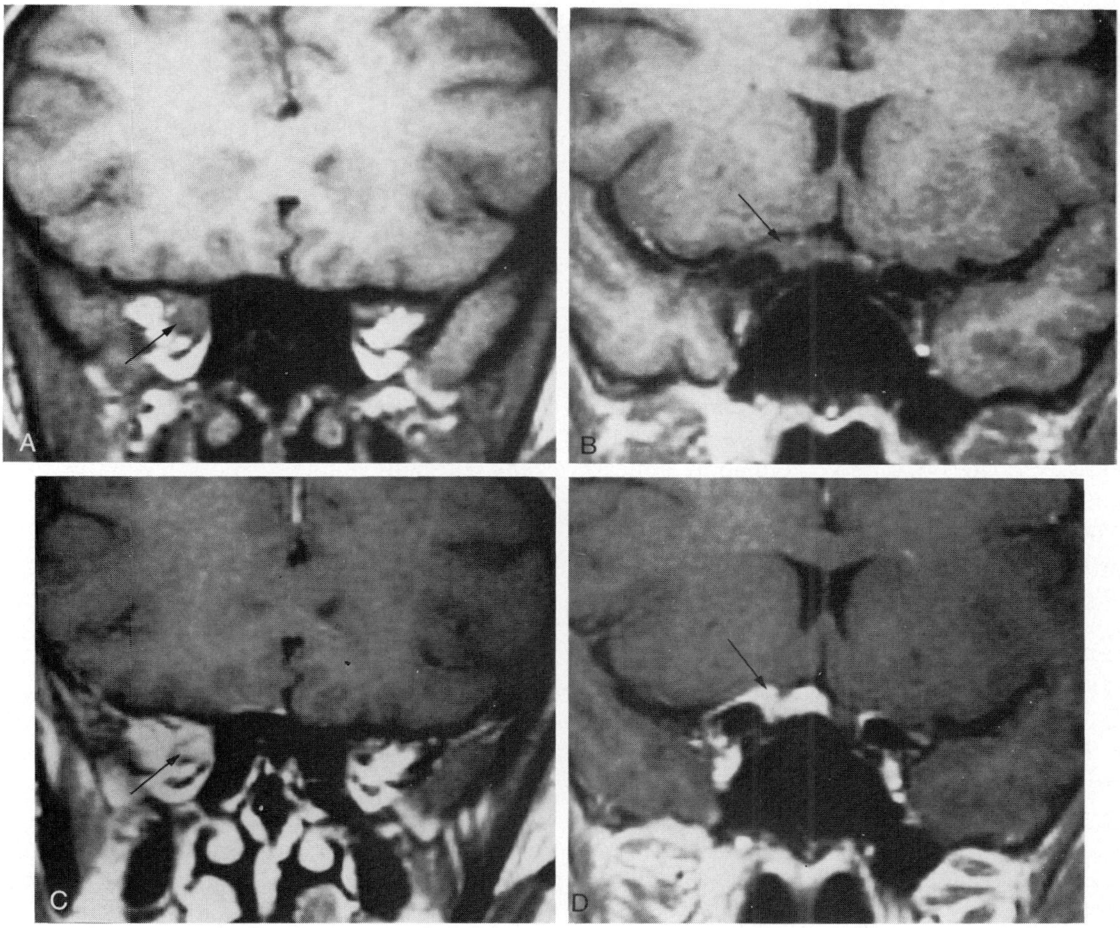

Figure 9–24. Meningioma (37-year-old female).

A, B, Coronal T1. Asymmetric soft tissue *(arrow)* is present in the right orbital apex, extending intracranially along the planum.

C, D, Enhanced coronal T1. The intraorbital component of the mass *(arrow)* enhances heterogeneously, whereas the intracranial component enhances homogeneously.

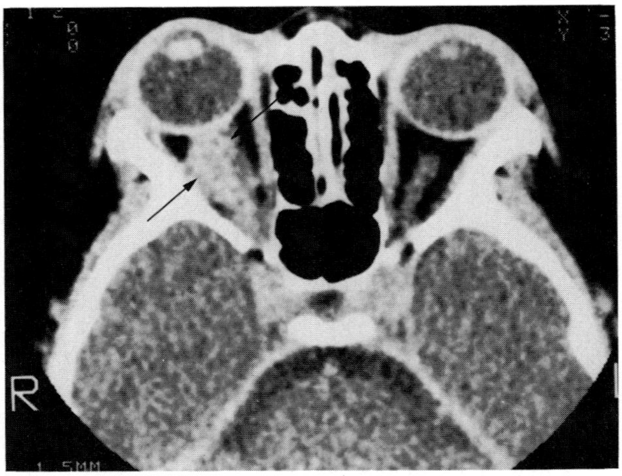

Figure 9–25. Optic nerve glioma (6-year-old female). Enhanced CT; fusiform enlargement of the right optic nerve complex *(arrows)* is present with mild proptosis. The mass enhances heterogeneously.

Tumor growth results in diffuse tortuous enlargement of the nerve.[35, 43] The actual intraorbital tumor mass may be much smaller than suspected by planar imaging as meningeal hyperplasia, mucin production, and reactive gliosis may contribute to the dimension of the mass.[39, 44] The optic nerve commonly appears kinked or buckled, secondary to the pliant nature of the mucin-rich tumor. CT may detect lucent regions within the tumor mass secondary to tumor necrosis and/or high mucin content (Figs. 9–25, 9–26). Calcium is rarely detected and enhancement is absent to mild (Table 9–2).

Table 9–2. MENINGIOMA–OPTIC NERVE GLIOMA: DISTINGUISHING CHARACTERISTICS

	Meningioma	Optic Nerve Glioma
Age	30–50 yr	First decade of life
Sex	Female:male, 2–4:1	Female ≥ male
Clinical presentation	Decreased visual acuity Proptosis Decreased ocular motility	Decreased visual acuity Low-grade proptosis
Imaging	Segmental or diffuse Hyperdense Calcification Hyperostosis Moderate homogeneous enhancement Tram-track pattern T1: isointense-hyperintense	Fusiform enlargement Tortuous hypodense nerve No calcification Canal erosion Mild enhancement T1: hypointense

The MRI appearance of intraorbital optic nerve glioma is isointense to slightly hyperintense to white matter on T1- and T2-weighted images. The intracranial component of the tumor is, however, markedly hyperintense on T2-weighted images.[4, 11, 39] Enhancement varies and is usually minimal.

Hemangioma

Cavernous hemangiomas are the most common benign orbital neoplasms. These lesions usually occur in patients between the second and fourth decades of life and are slightly more common in females. These tumors grow very slowly, resulting in unilateral proptosis, diplopia, and decreased visual acuity.[21, 35] The tumors are composed of large dilated vascular channels, lined by thin attenuated endothelial cells and covered by a fibrous pseudocapsule. Rarely, hemangiomas may become isolated from the systemic circulation resulting in thrombus, phlebolith formation, fibrosis, and hemosiderin deposition.

The lesion appears well demarcated, smoothly marginated, homogeneous, and round, ovoid, or lobulated on planar imaging (Fig. 9–27). The mass is intrinsically highly dense on CT with a variable degree of enhancement. The lesion is intraconal and displaces but does not invade the optic nerve or extraocular muscles.[2, 24] MRI demonstrates a low-signal, isointense-to-muscle mass on T1 that is markedly hyperintense on T2.[11, 16, 20, 41, 45]

Capillary hemangiomas are uncommon le-

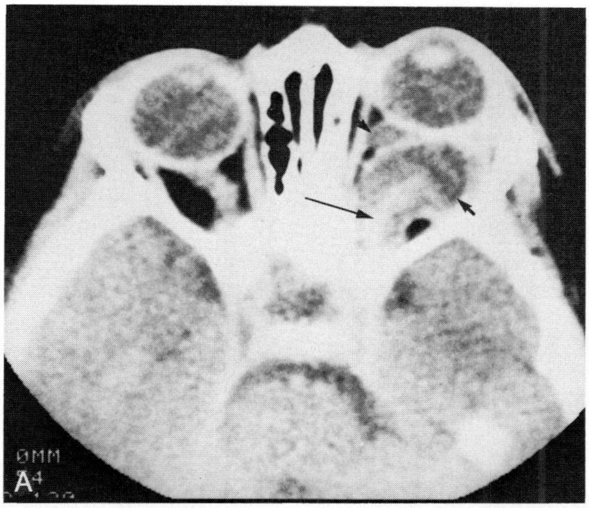

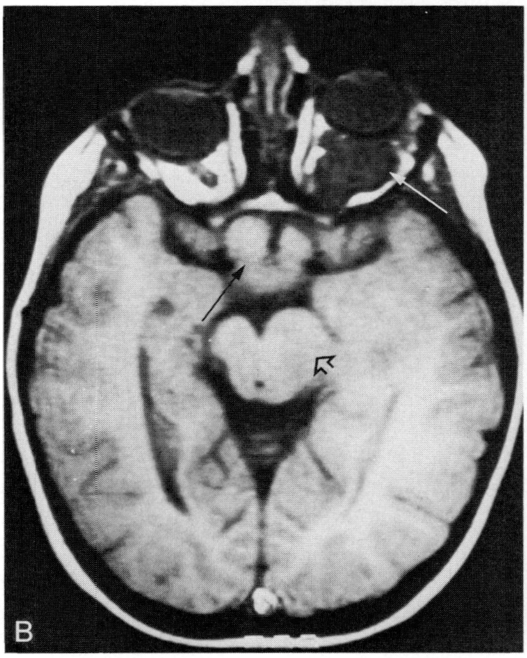

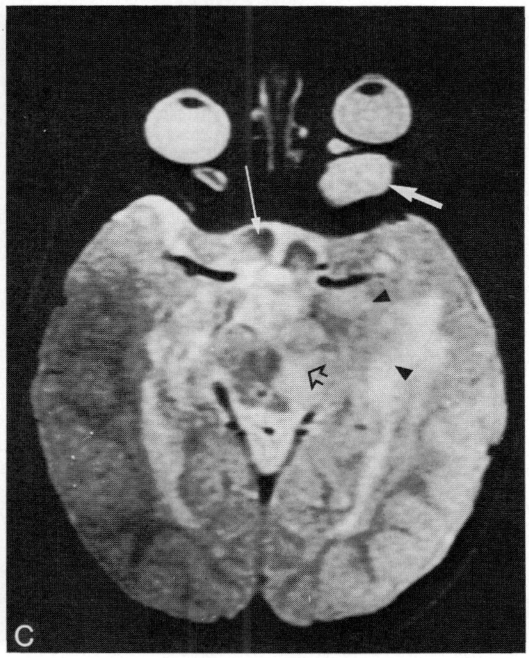

Figure 9–26. Optic nerve glioma (2-year-old male).

A, Enhanced CT. The optic nerve *(long arrow)* is silhouetted by a fusiform hypodense mass *(short arrows)*, which surrounds the nerve.

B, Axial T1. The intraorbital mass *(long white arrow)* is nearly isointense to vitreous. The intracranial extension of the mass is apparent with marked enlargement of the optic chiasm *(long black arrow)* and left mesencephalon *(open arrow)*.

C, Axial T2. The intraorbital component of the mass *(short white arrow)* remains isointense to vitreous. High-signal changes are identified in the left temporal lobe *(arrowheads)*, indicating tumor extension toward the lateral geniculate body. The left mesencephalon *(open arrow)* is enlarged secondary to extension from the geniculate body. The optic chiasm *(long white arrow)* is enlarged.

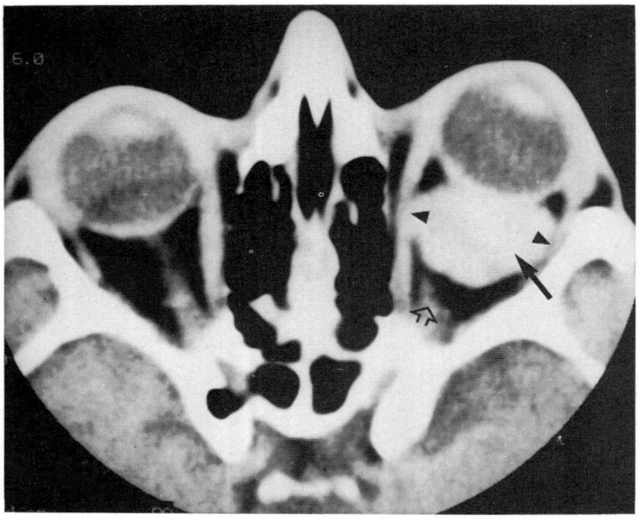

Figure 9–27. Cavernous hemangioma (37-year-old male). Enhanced CT; a well-circumscribed homogeneously enhancing intraconal mass *(arrow)* displaces the optic nerve *(open arrow)* and rectus muscles *(arrowheads)*.

sions that occur in the neonate. These lesions are usually confined to the superficial orbital structures and are associated with diffusely dilated capillaries and chemosis. These poorly encapsulated lesions may appear aggressive. Endothelial and capillary proliferation surround small capillary-sized vascular channels. The lesions may increase in size for 6 to 10 months before beginning to regress. They may involute completely in 1 to 3 years.[2, 15, 35]

Planar imaging demonstrates an irregular mass, which may be well to poorly marginated (Fig. 9–28). The mass is usually extraconal and enhances homogeneously and early on dynamic CT scanning.[46]

Peripheral Nerve Sheath Tumors

Peripheral nerve sheath tumors may have a varied histology and include neurilemomas (schwannomas), neurofibromas, or plexiform neurofibromas. The optic nerve, which contains no Schwann cells, is primarily unaffected by these peripheral nerve sheath tumors.

Neurilemomas or schwannomas are well-encapsulated neoplasms composed of Schwann cells and surrounded by a compressed perineural tissue capsule.[35] These lesions occur anywhere within the orbit but most commonly are intraconal. Neurofibromas are nonencapsulated, poorly defined tumors that may merge imperceptibly with adjacent tissues. These tumors tend to be less cellular than schwannomas and tend to occur anywhere within the orbit but are usually extraconal and in the superior quadrants. Plexiform neurofibromas differ from simple neurofibromas in that a cellular perineural sheath separates these tumors into discrete neuromatous units. Plexiform neurofibromas are diffusely infiltrative overgrowths of all elements of the peripheral nerve, resulting in enlargement of the orbit and a thickening of the lids, periorbita, and extraocular muscles.[47] Plexiform neurofibroma is pathognomonic for neurofibromatosis (von Recklinghausen's disease).

Despite histologic differences, the planar images of neurilemomas and neurofibromas may be similar. A fusiform, retrobulbar mass, elongated in the long axis of the orbit, with variable enhancement and benign orbital enlargement may be either neurilemoma or neurofibroma. Neurilemomas tend to be intraconal, however, and larger than neurofibromas. Neurofibromas more often involve the bony apex and the upper orbit and are more commonly extraconal.[48]

Orbital plexiform neurofibromas involve any portion of the orbit, are poorly marginated and infiltrative, extend centripetally, and enhance moderately. These lesions may be associated with various degrees of orbital dysplasia, pulsatile exophthalmos, congenital glaucoma (buphthalmos), and other orbital neoplasms including optic nerve glioma and meningioma.[49, 50]

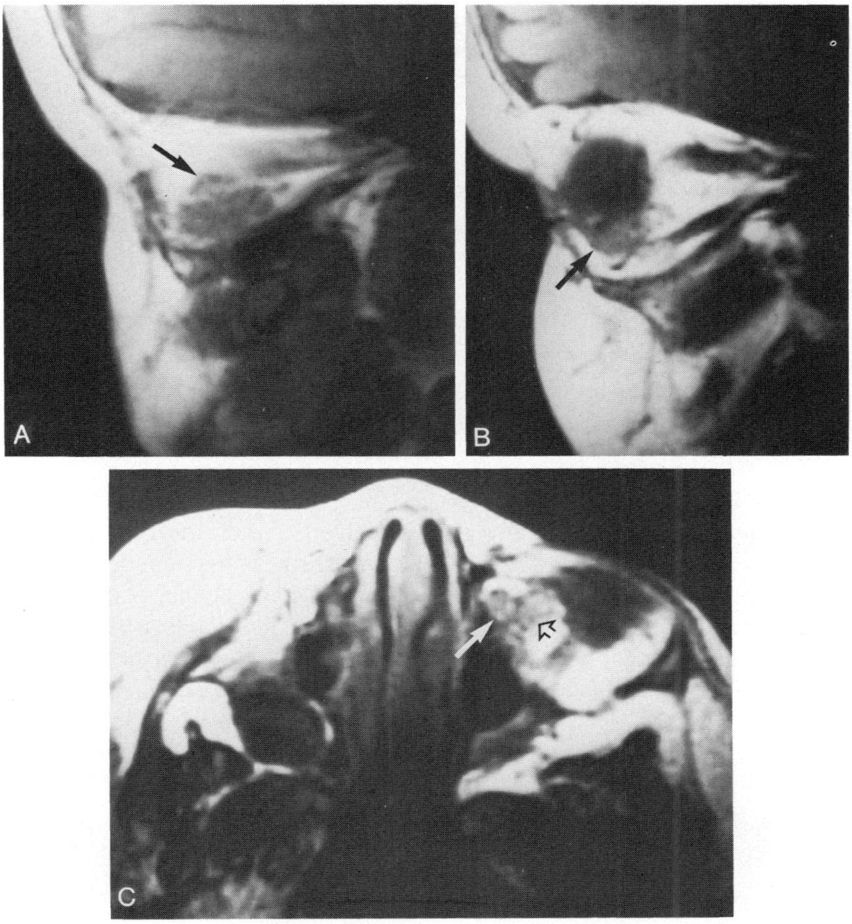

Figure 9–28. Capillary hemangioma (8-month-old female).

A, B, Parasagittal T1. An infiltrative isointense-to-muscle mass *(arrow)* is present in the inferior medial portion of the orbit.

C, Axial T1. The mass *(open arrow)* is predominantly intraconal, although there is some medial extraconal extension *(closed arrow)*.

Inflammatory

Pseudotumor

Orbital pseudotumor is the most common cause of intraorbital mass lesion in the adult population and results from an idiopathic inflammatory reaction that may involve any or all orbital structures. Although likely to be autoimmune, this process may be associated with several systemic diseases including sarcoidosis, Wegener's granulomatosis, lymphoma, fibrosing mediastinitis, thyroiditis, cholangitis, and vasculitis.[21, 24] Although patients with pseudotumor may present at any age, most do so between 20 and 40 years of age. Males and females are affected equally. Patients present with acute onset of painful proptosis, chemosis, and decreased motility of the extraocular muscles.[11, 51] Pseudotumor is unilateral in 85% of cases. In the acute stage, patients are markedly sensitive to steroids, a distinguishing clinical feature of this disease.

Histologically, the acute phase is characterized by a hypocellular pleomorphic infiltrate. Although lymphocytes predominate, eosinophils, polymorphonuclear lymphocytes, and plasma cells are present. Subacute and chronic phases are characterized by the presence of fibrosis.[52]

From the imaging perspective, orbital pseudotumor is the chameleon of orbital disease. The orbital contents may be affected alone or in any combination.[52–54] Enhancing soft tissue thickening of the sclera, optic nerve, extraocu-

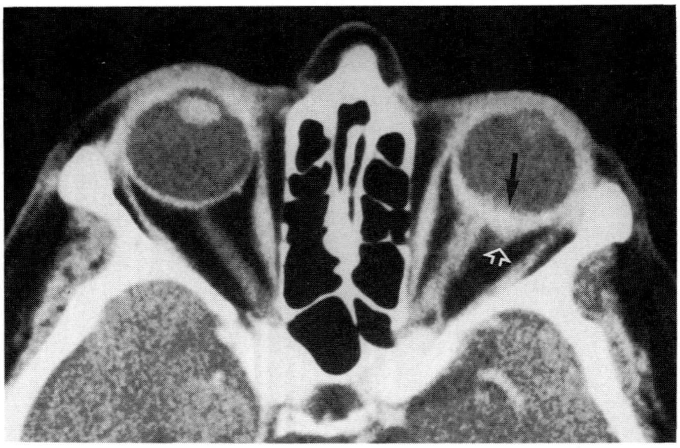

Figure 9–29. Pseudotumor; scleritis (47-year-old female). Enhanced axial CT; scleral thickening *(arrow)* is present on the left. There is extension of the inflammatory process *(open arrow)* into the retrobulbar soft tissues.

lar muscle(s), and lacrimal gland may be present (Figs. 9–29 to 9–31). A discrete soft tissue mass may be detected within the retrobulbar fat. The density of the retrobulbar fat may be increased. When the extraocular muscles are involved, the entire muscle, including the tendon sheath, is thickened. There is no predilection for involvement of a specific muscle. Destructive bony lesions and intracranial extension from the orbit have been reported.[55]

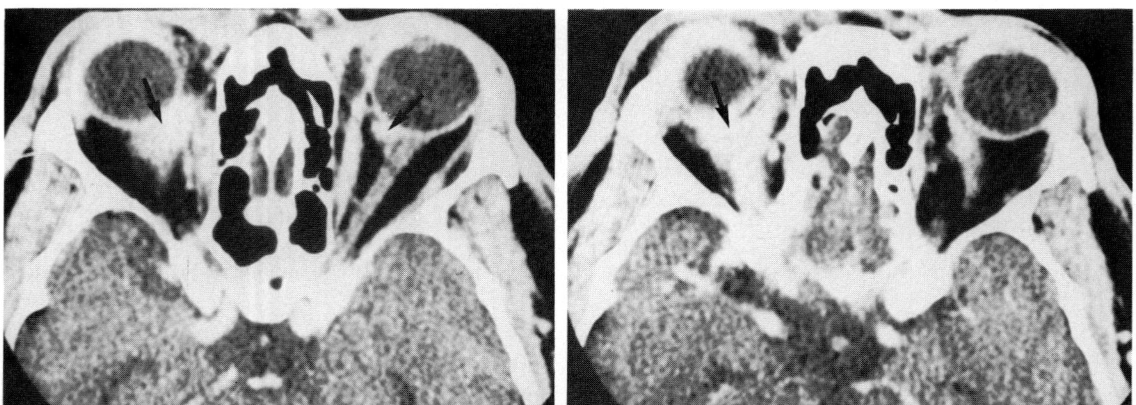

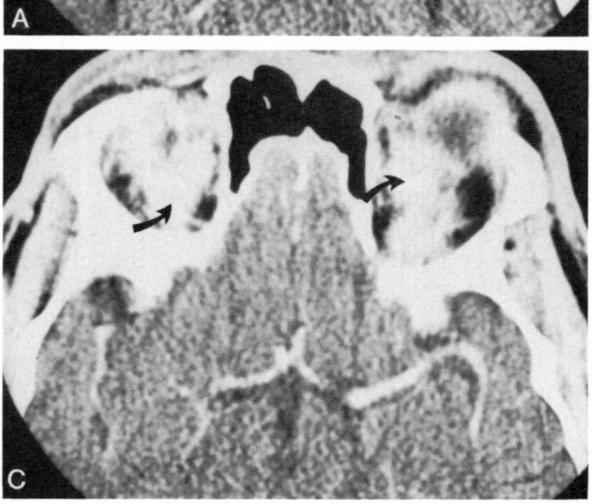

Figure 9–30. Pseudotumor (62-year-old male).

A–C, Enhanced axial CT. Bilateral asymmetric involvement is noted, with heterogeneous soft tissue masses *(arrows)* in both intraconal compartments. The superior rectus–levator complex *(curved arrows)* is markedly thickened bilaterally.

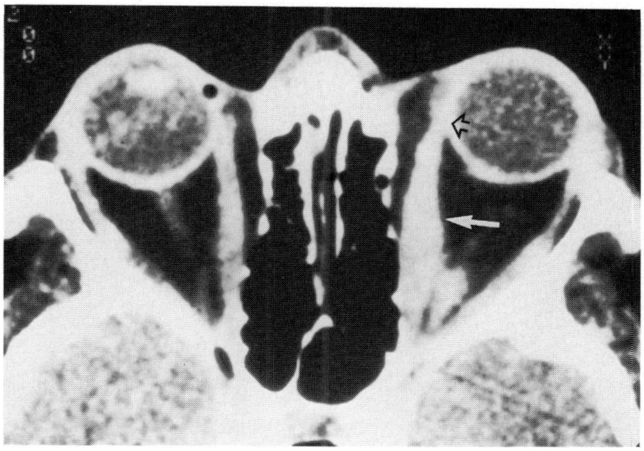

Figure 9–31. Pseudotumor (28-year-old male). Enhanced axial CT; the left medial rectus muscle *(arrow)* is enlarged. The tendinous insertion of the muscle *(open arrow)* is also markedly thickened.

The MRI demonstrates an isointense-to-muscle mass on T1 that becomes isointense to fat on T2.[10, 11, 20, 21, 56]

Optic Neuritis

Optic neuritis is an acute, nonspecific inflammatory process of the optic nerve. In childhood, optic neuritis is often related to a neurologic or systemic illness such as meningitis, encephalitis, or multiple sclerosis (MS). Optic neuritis in adults is a nonspecific phenomenon resulting from ischemia, systemic lupus erythematosus, radiation, sarcoidosis, syphilis, or, most commonly, MS.[57] Patients present with impaired visual acuity, pain, abnormal color vision, and/or afferent pupillary defects.

Planar imaging may demonstrate an enlarged optic nerve.[4, 39, 58, 59] The nerve may enhance on CT in a tram-track or heterogeneous pattern. Enhanced T1 MRI has demonstrated small linear foci of enhancement within the optic nerve and optic chiasm.[59, 60] Enhancement of the optic nerve may be inapparent on conventional T1 spin echo sequences; however, on enhanced fat-suppressed T1 images, the abnormal nerve may enhance to the same degree as the extraocular muscles[61] (Fig. 9–32). Patients with this disease require a screening T2-weighted sequence of the brain to evaluate for the white matter changes of MS.

Developmental

Septo-optic Dysplasia (SOD)

SOD is considered by some to be the mildest form of holoprosencephaly. This midline developmental defect involves the septum pellucidum, optic nerves, chiasm, and infundibulum. Patients with SOD may be blind and exhibit hypothalamic pituitary axis dysfunction.[24]

Absence of the septum pellucidum is readily demonstrated on planar imaging (Fig. 9–33). Additional findings include hypoplasia of the optic nerves and prominence of the suprasellar cistern.

Varix

Vascular malformations of the orbit are rare and may be associated with high-flow intracranial vascular malformations. Orbital varix may be congenital or acquired. Patients may exhibit exophthalmos that is intermittent, associated with activities that increase venous pressure such as the Valsalva maneuver or coughing.

Planar imaging demonstrates enlarged dilated tortuous intraconal vascular channels that are distensible with a Valsalva maneuver. These densely enhance on CT and may display flow effects on MRI contingent on flow velocity. Diagnostic angiography may be performed by cannulating a superficial facial vein and performing orbital venography (Fig. 9–34).

Metabolic

Graves' disease

Graves' disease, or thyroid ophthalmopathy, is the most common cause of bilateral or unilateral proptosis in the adult population. Bilateral disease occurs in 85% of cases. Patients may present either in a euthyroid state

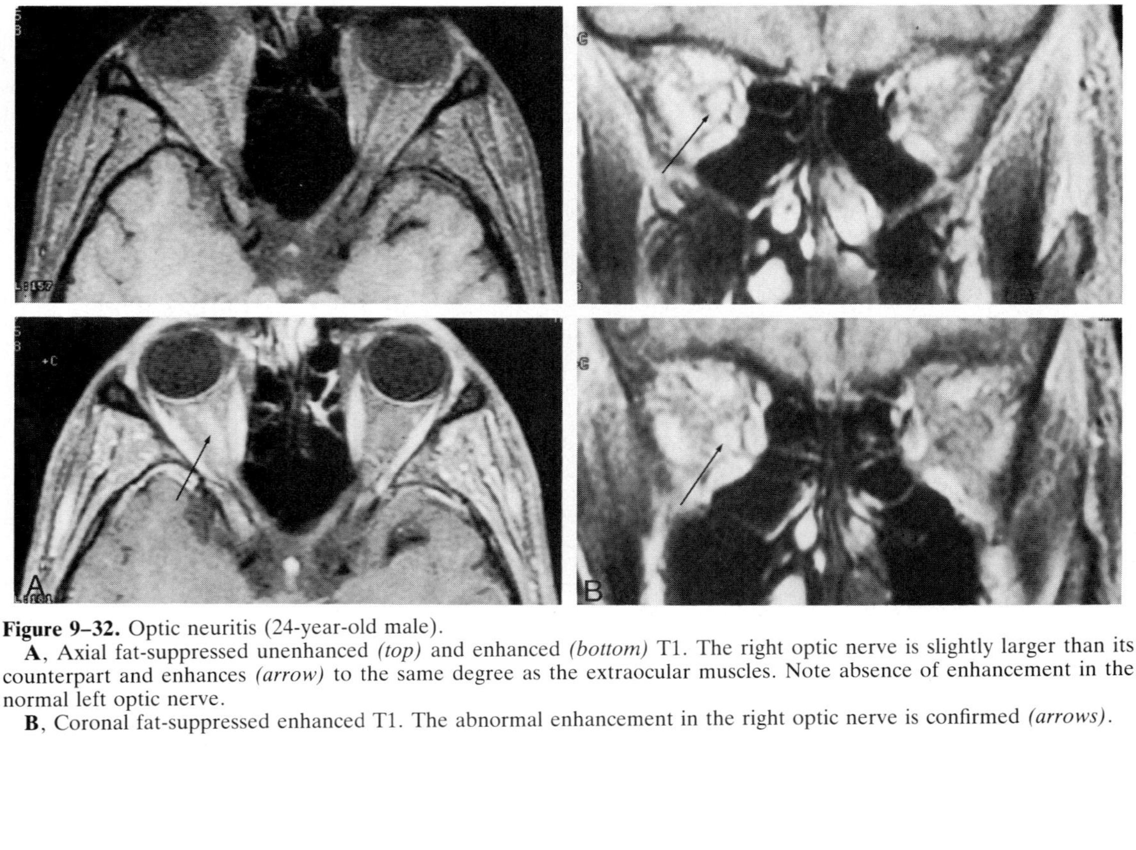

Figure 9–32. Optic neuritis (24-year-old male).

A, Axial fat-suppressed unenhanced *(top)* and enhanced *(bottom)* T1. The right optic nerve is slightly larger than its counterpart and enhances *(arrow)* to the same degree as the extraocular muscles. Note absence of enhancement in the normal left optic nerve.

B, Coronal fat-suppressed enhanced T1. The abnormal enhancement in the right optic nerve is confirmed *(arrows)*.

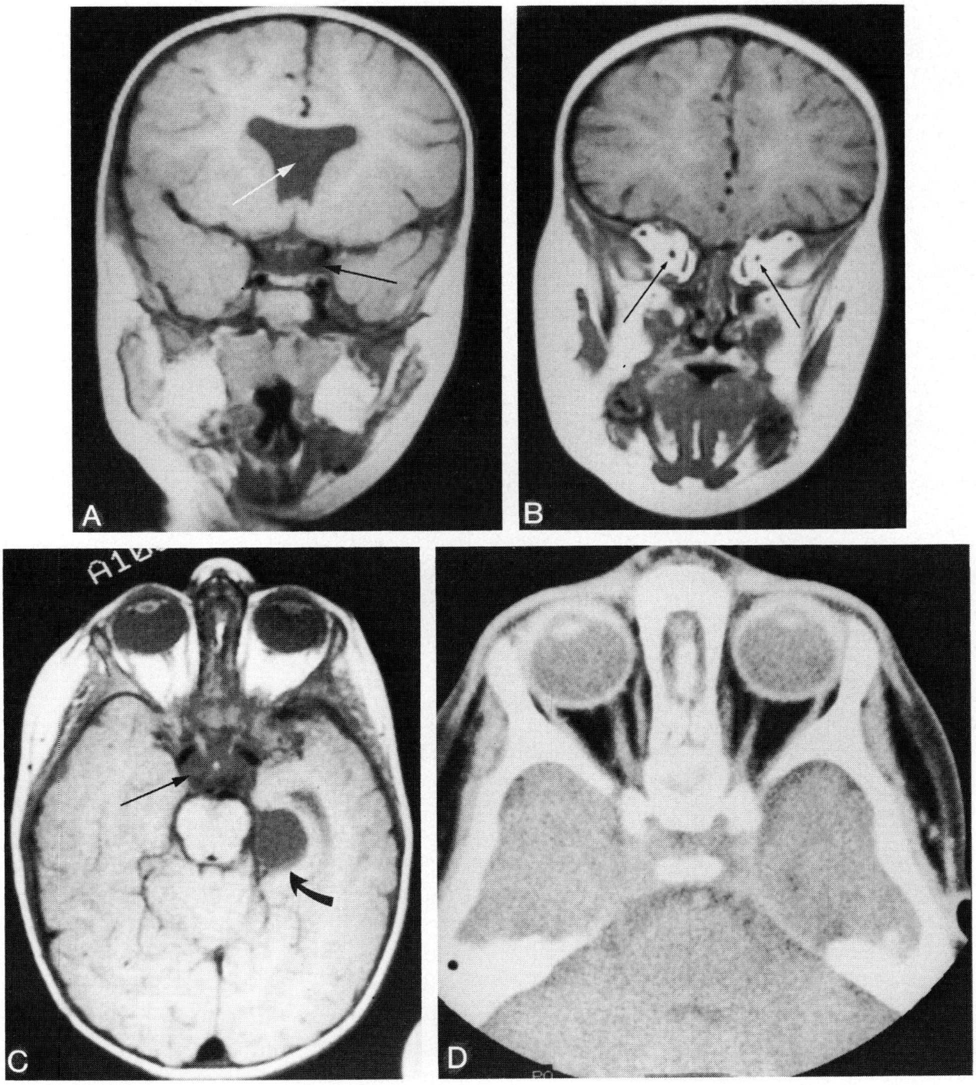

Figure 9–33. Septo-optic dysplasia (1-year-old male).

A, Coronal T1. The septum pellucidum *(white arrow)*, which normally separates the anterior portion of the lateral ventricles, is absent. The suprasellar cistern *(black arrow)* is prominent.

B, Coronal T1. The optic nerves *(arrows)* are hypoplastic bilaterally.

C, Axial T1. The suprasellar cistern *(straight arrow)* is prominent. An incidental arachnoid cyst *(curved arrow)* is present in the left middle fossa.

D, Unenhanced CT. Hypoplasia of the optic nerves is more difficult to detect on the axial image due to partial volume averaging.

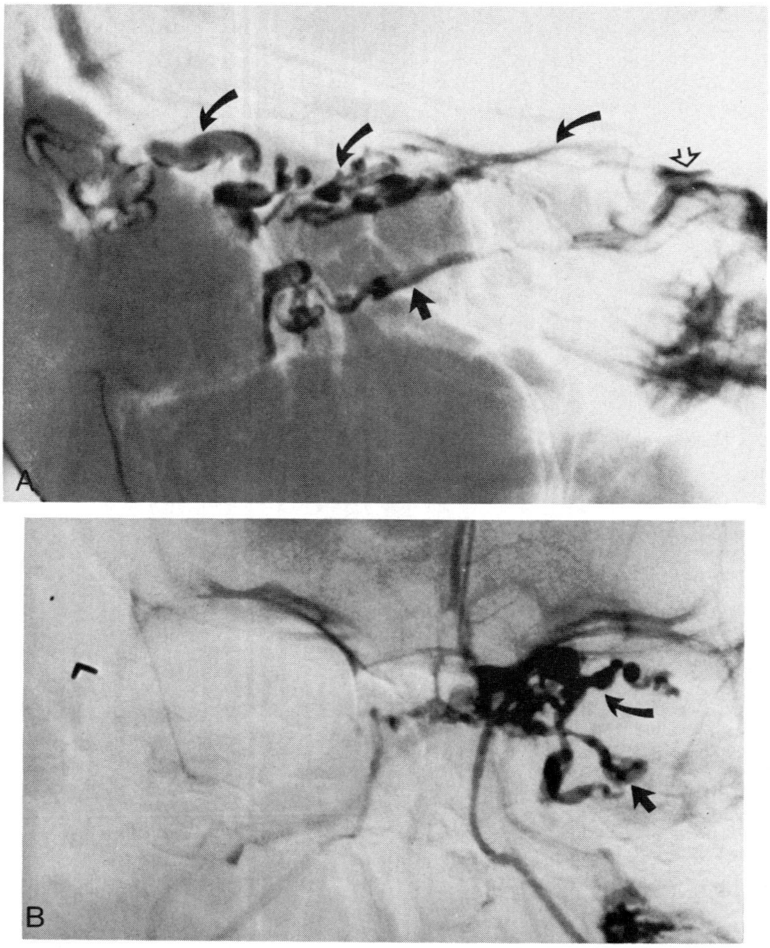

Figure 9–34. Varix (22-year-old female).

A, B, Lateral and anteroposterior (AP) orbital venography. Markedly ectatic, tortuous, superior ophthalmic *(curved arrows)* and inferior ophthalmic *(straight arrow)* veins drain into the cavernous sinus *(open arrow)*.

or with clinical signs of hyperthyroidism including weight loss, smooth skin, lid retraction, and increased heart rate.[21] Graves' disease occurs four times more frequently in women. Symptoms of Graves' ophthalmopathy include proptosis, decreased range of motion, and diplopia. Rarely, patients present with pain.[52] Symptoms usually develop within 1 year following onset of hyperthyroidism and usually resolve in 3 to 36 months.[62]

The orbital target structures include the extraocular muscles and retrobulbar fat. The extraocular muscles may be diffusely enlarged and the volume of the retrobulbar fat may be markedly increased. An optic neuropathy may be manifest, most probably secondary to muscle hypertrophy and compression of the optic nerve.[63, 64] The optic nerve may actually enlarge in late-stage Graves' disease secondary to distention of the optic nerve sheath by trapped CSF.[4, 39] Optic neuropathy requires prompt treatment with steroids, radiation, and/or decompression.[65] The lacrimal gland may less commonly be enlarged.

Pathologic examination reveals various degrees of thickening of the extraocular muscles. Lymphocytic and plasmocytic infiltration and edema within the endomysium lead to fibroblast activation and production of mucopolysaccharides, collagen, and glycoproteins that increase the bulk of the extraocular muscles. Progressive fibrosis may occur later in the disease, as may focal fatty infiltration of the muscles.[62, 66] The volume of the retrobulbar fat also increases.

Planar imaging clearly demonstrates fusiform enlargement of the extraocular muscles. The muscles are smoothly marginated, taper-

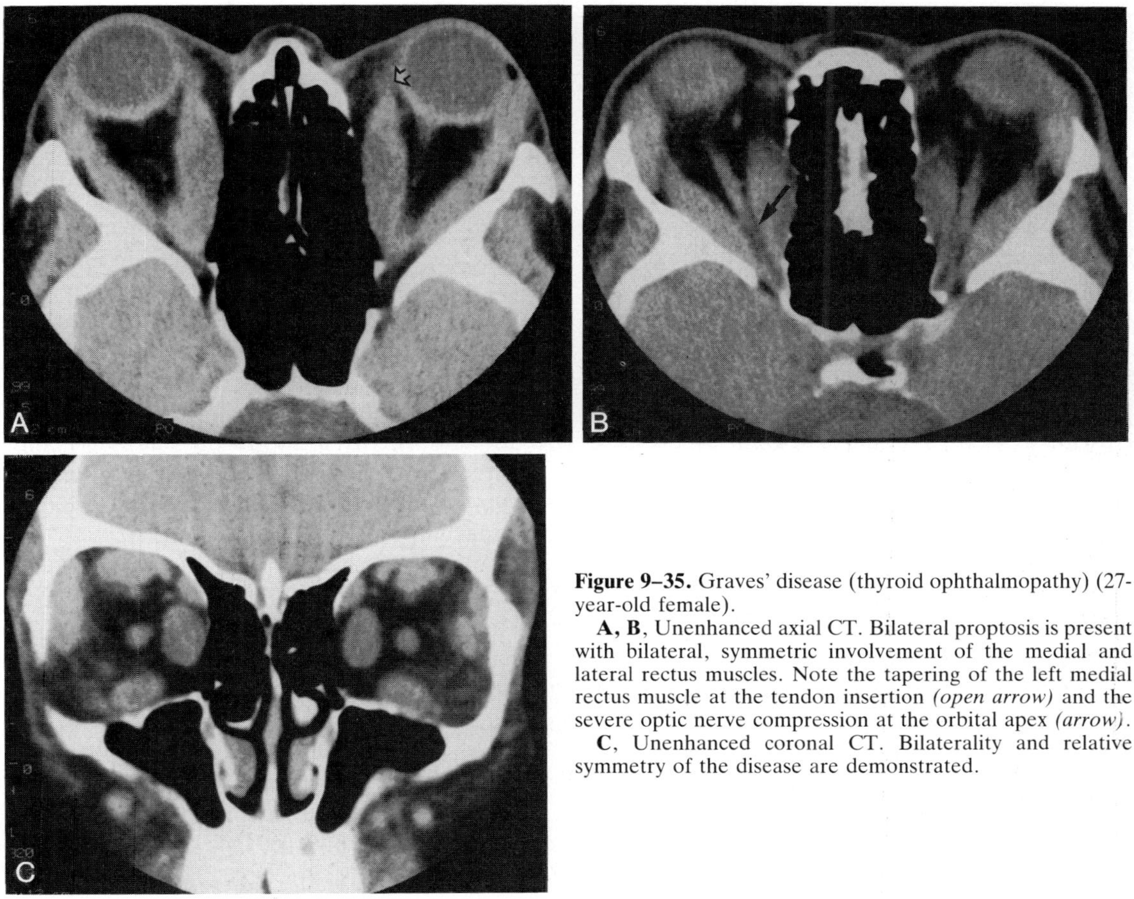

Figure 9–35. Graves' disease (thyroid ophthalmopathy) (27-year-old female).

A, B, Unenhanced axial CT. Bilateral proptosis is present with bilateral, symmetric involvement of the medial and lateral rectus muscles. Note the tapering of the left medial rectus muscle at the tendon insertion *(open arrow)* and the severe optic nerve compression at the orbital apex *(arrow)*.

C, Unenhanced coronal CT. Bilaterality and relative symmetry of the disease are demonstrated.

ing normally to their insertion at Tenon's capsule (Fig. 9–35). By conventional wisdom the incidence and severity of muscle enlargement have followed a predictable sequence: the *i*nferior rectus, *m*edial rectus, *s*uperior rectus, *l*ateral rectus, and *oblique* muscles (mnemonic IM SLO) are most commonly and severely involved.[21] However, a more recent study[64] demonstrated the most common pattern was enlargement of all muscles. The superior muscle group was more commonly involved than any other, and when only one muscle was involved, it was the superior rectus.

The MRI appearance of Graves' disease is that of fusiform enlargement of the muscle. The affected muscles are isointense to normal muscle on T1-weighted images. Focal fatty inclusions of muscle may be detected in chronic cases. On T2-weighted images the enlarged muscles are isointense or minimally hyperintense to fat.[16, 20, 67] Features that distinguish Graves' disease from pseudotumor are listed in Table 9–3.

Table 9–3. GRAVES' DISEASE AND PSEUDOTUMOR: DISTINGUISHING CHARACTERISTICS

	Graves' Disease	Pseudotumor
Age	20–40 yr	20–40 yr
Sex	Female:male, 4:1	Female = male
Clinical presentation	± Hyperthyroidism Proptosis Decreased ocular motility Diplopia	Painful proptosis Decreased ocular motility Steroid responsive
Bilaterality	85–90%	10–15%
Imaging	Fusiform enlargement, extraocular muscles (IM-SLO) Tapers to tendon Increased density and volume of retrobulbar fat	Multiple forms: Myositic (involves tendon) Scleral Lacrimal gland Retrobulbar mass

Extraconal

Neoplastic

Lacrimal Gland Tumor

The lacrimal gland may give rise to epithelial or lymphoid origin neoplasms.[24, 68, 69] Epithelial origin tumors account for 50% of lacrimal gland masses. Half of the epithelial tumors are pleomorphic (benign mixed) adenomas. The remaining epithelial tumors are malignant, the most common of which is adenoid cystic carcinoma. Other malignant epithelial neoplasms include mucoepidermoid, adenocarcinoma, squamous cell carcinoma, and anaplastic cancer. Fifty per cent of lacrimal gland masses are lymphoid or inflammatory. The histology of these masses varies, ranging from reactive lymphoid hyperplasia to malignant lymphoma. Bilateral lacrimal gland masses should suggest pseudotumor, sarcoidosis, or lymphoma.[22]

No reliable radiographic criteria exist to distinguish lacrimal gland masses. Although a benign mixed tumor is generally homogeneous and well marginated and may cause bony erosion, a highly aggressive anaplastic carcinoma may present in the same fashion. Aggressive bone destruction corroborates malignancy. Otherwise, size, margination, and enhancement are nonspecific at differentiating lacrimal gland tumors (Fig. 9–36).

Lymphoma

Lymphoma represents 10 to 15% of orbital masses[22, 70] and is a leading cause of proptosis in the adult.[21] Lymphoma may have primary involvement in the orbit or may involve the orbit secondarily in approximately 3% of patients with systemic lymphoma. Lymphoma is a disease of older patients in the sixth to seventh decades, causing subacute, painless swelling; proptosis; and diplopia. Lymphoid tissue is normally found in the lacrimal gland, soft tissue of the eyelid, and conjunctiva. Accordingly, these are the most common sites of orbital lymphoma.

As mentioned with lacrimal gland tumors, a spectrum of lymphoproliferative disease exists. Histologically, it may be difficult to distinguish reactive disease from malignancy.[71] Accordingly, no planar imaging characteristics reliably differentiate these lesions. The tumors are usually homogeneous, high-density masses with sharp margins exhibiting mild mass effect (Figs. 9–37, 9–38). The tumors are soft and pliable, conforming to the contour of sur-

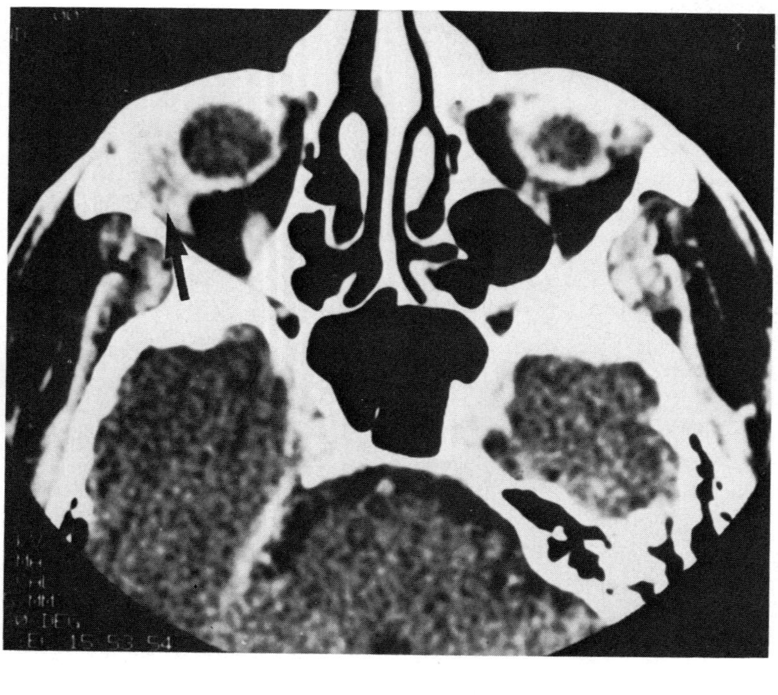

Figure 9–36. Benign mixed tumor of the lacrimal gland (46-year-old male). Enhanced CT; the right lacrimal gland *(arrow)* is markedly enlarged and enhances heterogeneously. A discrete mass is not identified.

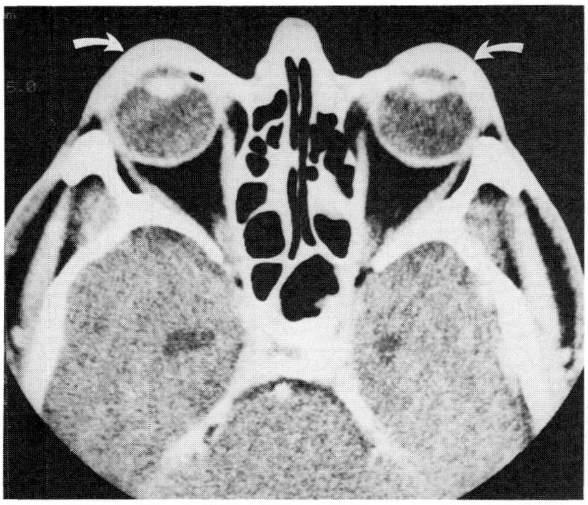

Figure 9–37. Conjunctival lymphoma (50-year-old female). Enhanced CT; conjunctival, preseptal soft tissue thickening *(curved arrows)* is present bilaterally.

rounding structures.[72] The lesions are generally extraconal but may be intraconal as well.[24] The signal characteristics are variable and may be indistinguishable from pseudotumor.[21] MRI depicts an isointense-to-muscle lesion on T1-weighted images that become hyperintense on T2-weighted images.[16, 20, 21, 41]

Lymphangioma

Lymphangiomas are lesions of children and young adults, consisting of dysplastic, epithelial-lined, lymph-filled channels and smooth muscle bundles. The lesions are poorly marginated and result in irregular growth into the surrounding connective tissue stroma.[35, 73] The tumor may occur in the conjunctiva, eyelid, or retrobulbar region. Patients present with slowly progressive unilateral proptosis, diplopia, decreased visual acuity, and lid swelling.[21] The lymphoid component of the tumor may undergo hyperplasia in response to a systemic infection resulting in increased proptosis. In addition, intratumoral hemorrhage may result from rupture of friable dysplastic vessels, causing acute onset of proptosis.

The mass is heterogeneous and poorly marginated, and it infiltrates soft tissue planes on CT (Fig. 9–39). Contrast enhancement is minimal and in most cases is present only if there is history of prior hemorrhage. Enhancement tends to be peripheral, often outlining the small hemorrhagic cystic cavities.

Bony changes and intratumoral calcification are rare.[35] MRI depicts a heterogeneous mass that is increased signal relative to muscle on T1 and relative to fat on T2.[15, 35, 56]

Rhabdomyosarcoma

Rhabdomyosarcoma is the most common orbital malignancy in children.[24] The patients average 7 years of age at diagnosis, with 90% of cases diagnosed by the age of 16 years.[15, 74] The tumor may arise primarily within the orbit or by secondary extension from contiguous structures. Children present with rapidly progressive unilateral proptosis, ptosis, palpable mass, and ophthalmoplegia.

Planar imaging demonstrates a highly aggressive soft tissue mass (Fig. 9–40). The mass may be extraconal or intraconal, or both, with possible extension into the paranasal sinuses or cranium, accompanied by marked bone destruction. The mass is isodense to muscle on CT and may enhance moderately. The neoplasm is isointense to muscle on T1 MRI and isointense to hyperintense to muscle on T2.

Metastasis

Metastases in adults are often ocular. In children, however, metastases are frequently orbital, involving the bone through spread from contiguous structures. Systemic hematopoietic malignancies such as leukemia and multiple myeloma may also involve the orbit.

In children, neuroblastoma, Ewing's sarcoma, and histiocytosis may involve the orbit.[24]

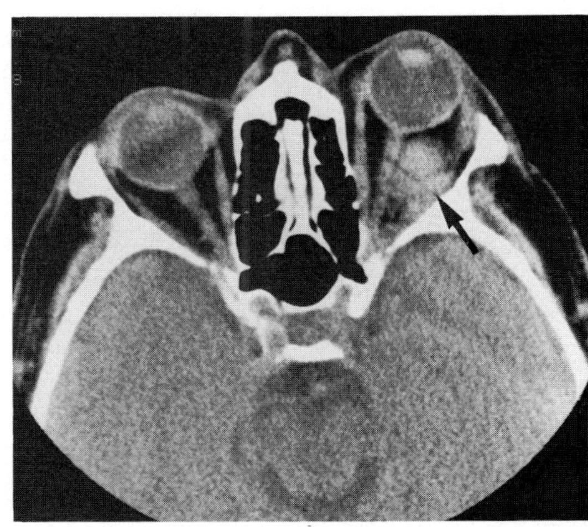

Figure 9–38. Lymphoma (78-year-old male). Unenhanced CT; a homogeneous, predominantly intraconal mass *(arrow)* is present in the left orbit, with resultant proptosis.

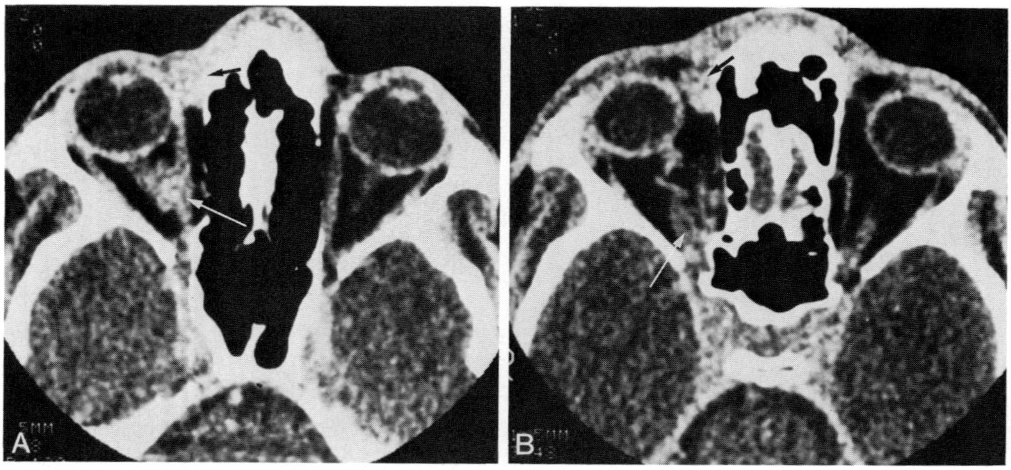

Figure 9–39. Lymphangioma (44-year-old female).
A, B, Enhanced CT. A heterogeneous, infiltrative, intraconal and extraconal mass *(white arrow)* is present in the right orbit, extending into the medial preseptal space *(black arrow)*.

Neuroblastoma typically affects children at 2 years of age. In 20% of patients with neuroblastoma, orbital metastases will develop, resulting in a spiculated periosteal new bone reaction. Ewing's sarcoma may rarely metastasize to the orbit, causing a raised periosteal reaction. Histiocytosis affects the orbit in approximately 10% of patients. The lesions may have the benign appearance of epidermoid cyst or may appear lytic and more aggressive if the patient has Hand-Schüller-Christian disease.

In adults any primary tumor may hematogenously metastasize to the soft tissue or bone of the orbit. Cancers of the breast, lung, and prostate are common primary tumors to metastasize to this region. Patients often present with proptosis and a history of prior malignancy. Multiple myeloma may also involve the orbit and periorbital region.[22, 75] In addition to the hematogenously disseminated neoplasms, direct extension of tumor from the paranasal sinuses, nasal cavity, nasopharynx, or face may occur.

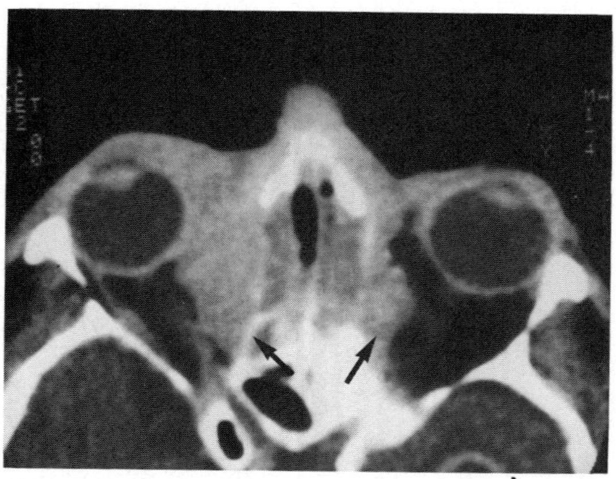

Figure 9–40. Rhabdomyosarcoma (1-year-old male). Enhanced axial CT; an infiltrative, aggressive soft tissue mass *(arrows)* invades both orbits and the ethmoid sinus. The right-sided disease is more advanced with invasion of the globe and proptosis.

Planar imaging demonstrates a mass of varying size, often with associated bone disruption (Figs. 9–41 to 9–43). The mass may be infiltrative or well defined, involving any portion of the orbit (Figs. 9–44, 9–45). The mass is usually noncalcified and enhances relatively homogeneously.

Inflammatory

Infectious processes of the orbit involve patients of all ages. The patients present with lid edema, painful proptosis, ophthalmoplegia, fever, and leukocytosis.[15] The majority (76%) of orbital infections are secondary to seeding from the paranasal sinuses.[23, 76] In children the ethmoid and maxillary sinuses are the most common source; the frontal sinuses are the most common source in adults.[77] A valveless venous plexus exists between the paranasal sinuses and the orbit, offering an effective conduit of transmission. Trauma[77] and spread from other contiguous structures account for a smaller percentage of orbital infection. *Staph-*

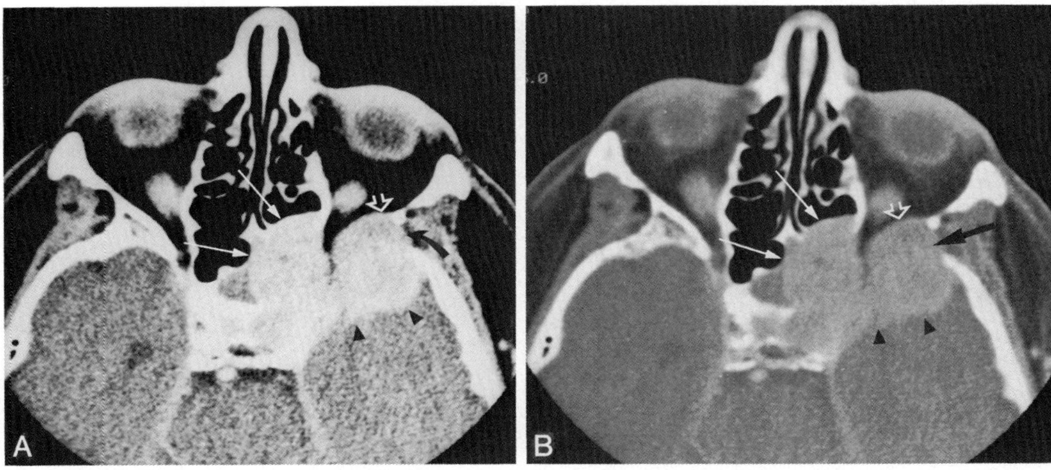

Figure 9–41. Plasmacytoma (65-year-old female).
A, B, Enhanced CT (soft tissue and bone windows). A homogeneously enhancing mass has destroyed the greater wing of the sphenoid bone *(straight black arrow)* and extends into the orbit *(open arrow)*, middle cranial fossa *(black arrowheads)*, temporal fossa *(curved black arrow)*, and paranasal sinuses *(straight white arrows)*.

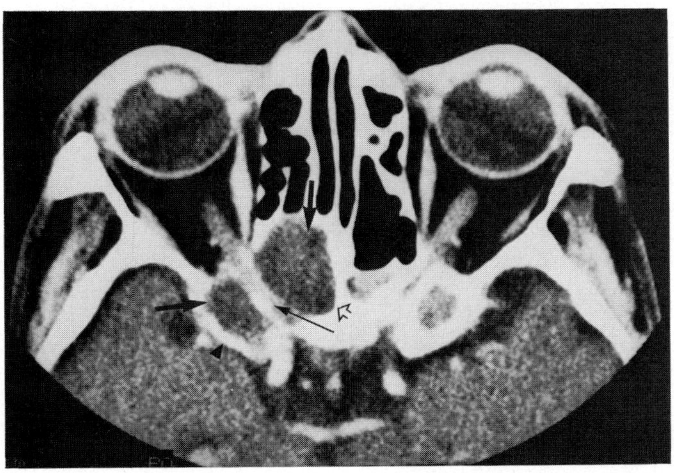

Figure 9–42. Sphenoid sinus carcinoma (76-year-old female). Enhanced CT; an infiltrative soft tissue mass *(short arrows)* has destroyed the anterior clinoid process *(arrowhead)* and planum *(open arrow)* as it surrounds the right optic nerve *(long arrow)*.

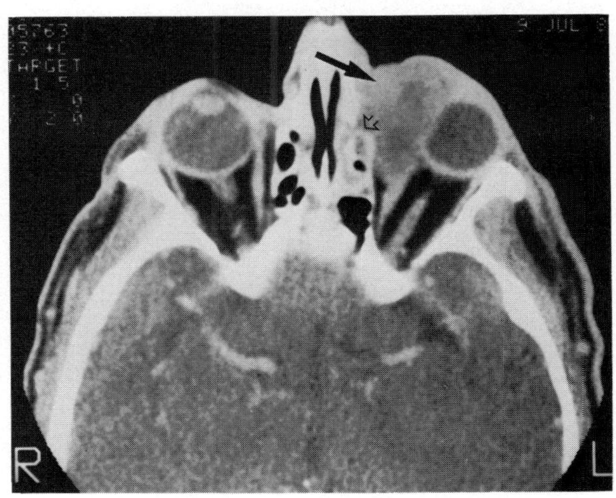

Figure 9–43. Undifferentiated carcinoma of the lacrimal sac (65-year-old male). Enhanced CT; heterogeneously enhancing mass *(arrow)* is present along the medial aspect of the left orbit. Bone destruction *(open arrow)* with extension into the left ethmoid sinus and compression of the globe with proptosis are present.

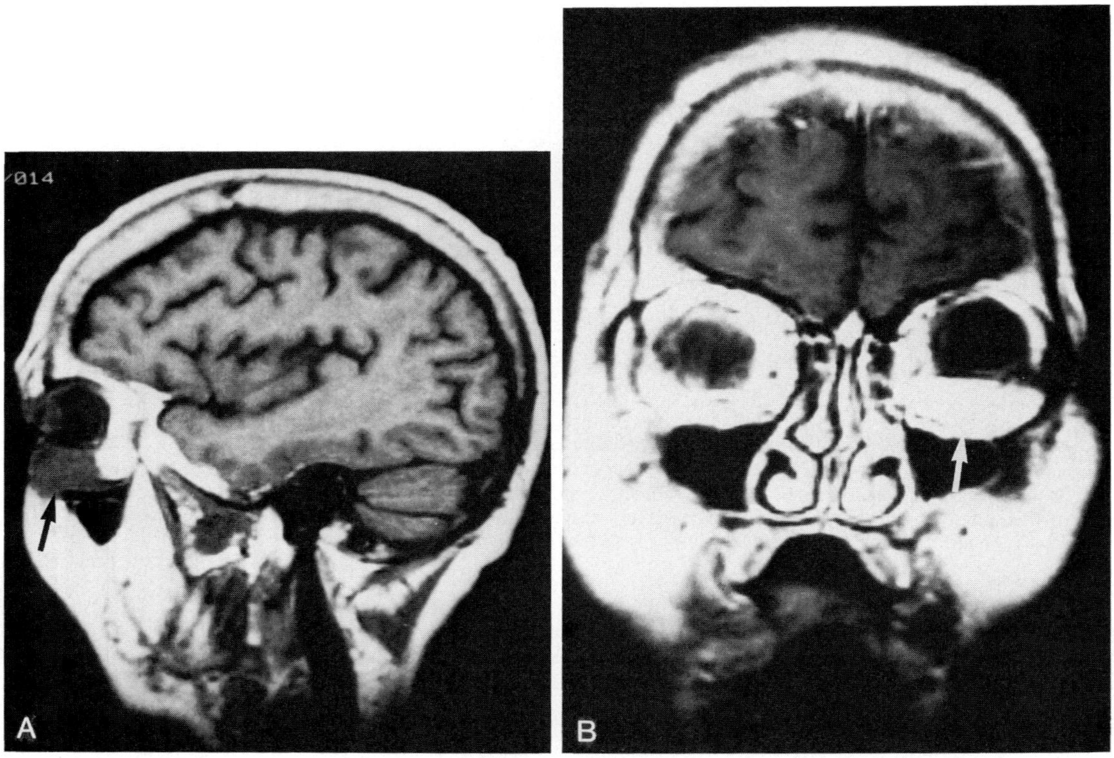

Figure 9–44. Metastatic breast cancer (65-year-old female).

A, Parasagittal T1. An extraconal intermediate signal intensity soft tissue mass *(arrow)* is present within the inferior anterior orbit. Commensurate displacement and compression of the globe are noted.

B, Enhanced coronal T1. The mass *(arrow)* enhances homogeneously.

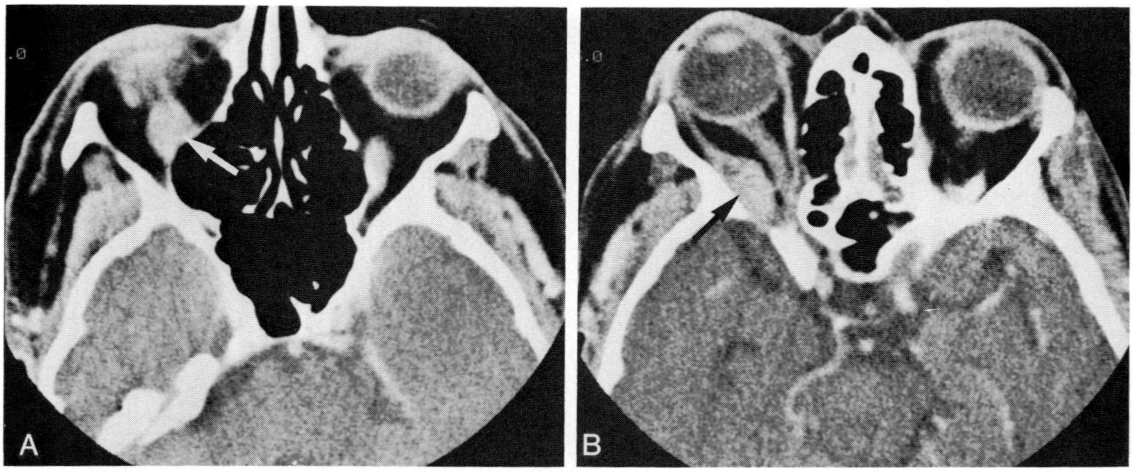

Figure 9–45. Metastatic breast cancer (65-year-old female).

A, B, Enhanced axial CT. There is evidence of homogeneously enhancing soft tissue metastases to the belly of the inferior rectus muscle *(white arrow)* and lateral rectus muscle *(black arrow)*. Commensurate displacement of the optic nerve is noted.

ylococcus and *Streptococcus* are common causes of orbital infection in children and adults; orbital infection in infants and toddlers is most commonly due to *Haemophilus influenzae*. Inadequate or delayed therapy may result in progression of an orbital cellulitis to an abscess with extension into the intracranial space or, rarely, may result in cavernous sinus thrombosis.

Although any component of the orbit may be involved, the infectious process usually starts peripherally and extends centripetally into the orbit. The periosteum and septum encase the orbital contents and offer the first line of defense against the spread of infection. This fibrous sheath often succeeds at protecting the orbital contents and confining the infection to either the preseptal or subperiosteal space. Preseptal disease involves the conjunctiva, lid, lacrimal sac, and other superficial periorbital soft tissues.[78, 79] Postseptal disease results in orbital cellulitis, which may involve any portion of the orbital contents. Subperiosteal disease is manifest by a collection of material that is contiguous with the paranasal sinuses and has a convex medial surface that displaces the medial rectus laterally.

Orbital cellulitis is often a diffuse process involving the periorbital soft tissues including the muscles and retrobulbar fat. The muscles may be thickened and the retrobulbar fat infiltrated with edema and inflammatory cells. Organization and encapsulation of the nidus lead to the formation of an abscess. The abscess is usually extraconal.

Cellulitis appears as an ill-defined region of increased density on CT (Fig. 9–46). The area may enhance heterogeneously, and local mass effect may be apparent. The inflammatory cells and edema elevate the density of the retrobulbar fat on CT and decrease the T1 and increase the T2 signal of the fat on MRI (Fig. 9–47).

Distinction between orbital cellulitis and abscess is important, as the former is effectively treated with antibiotics, whereas the latter may require surgical drainage. However, it may not be possible in every instance to make this distinction on planar imaging.[78] Abscesses usually appear as complex masses containing low-density central components and gas with a hyperdense, peripherally enhancing rim[20, 21, 78] (Fig. 9–48). Unfortunately, organizing cellulitis may have the same appearance if gas from the communicating paranasal sinus enters the cellulitis. MRI depicts a low-signal T1 mass with corresponding high T2 signal.

Abscess may occur anywhere within the orbit but most commonly occurs in the subperiosteal space.[15] The most common subperiosteal location is beneath the orbital roof.[79] Axial images have proven relatively insensitive at detecting and predicting the size of orbit roof abscesses. One investigator[79] demonstrated that more than one third of orbital roof abscesses detected on coronal CT were missed on axial imaging.

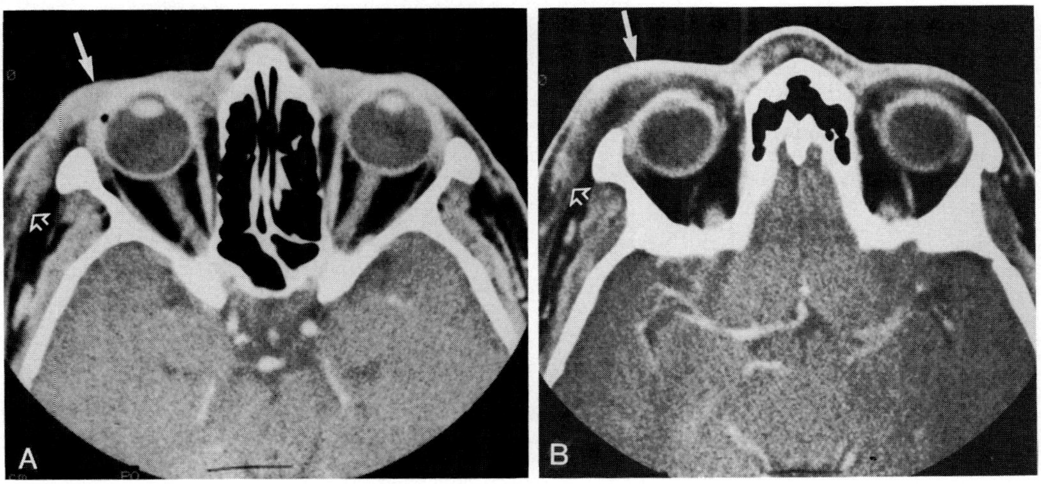

Figure 9–46. Preseptal cellulitis (32-year-old female).
A, B, Enhanced CT. Preseptal, subcutaneous soft tissue swelling *(arrow)* is present on the right. The soft tissue edema extends lateral to the zygoma into the temporal fossa *(open arrow)*.

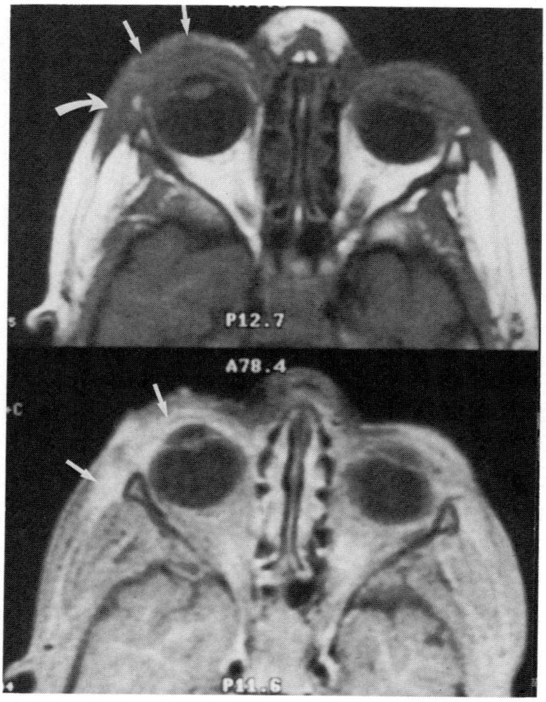

Figure 9–47. Preseptal cellulitis (3-year-old female).

Top, Axial T1. Soft tissue thickening *(arrows)* is present in the preseptal region of the right orbit. The soft tissue *(curved arrow)* extends toward the temporal fossa.

Bottom, Enhanced fat-saturated T1. The preseptal inflammatory tissue *(arrows)* enhances. There is no evidence of postseptal disease.

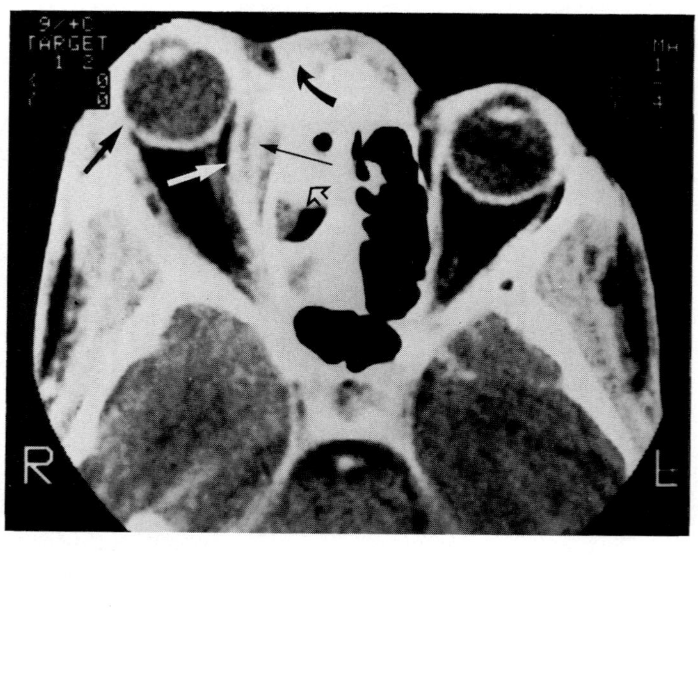

Figure 9–48. Subperiosteal abscess (67-year-old female). Enhanced CT; a peripherally enhancing subperiosteal abscess *(long thin arrow)* is present along the medial orbit, displacing the medial rectus muscle *(white arrow)* laterally. Ethmoid sinus opacification *(open arrow)*, preseptal extension *(curved arrow)*, and gross proptosis *(short black arrow)* are present.

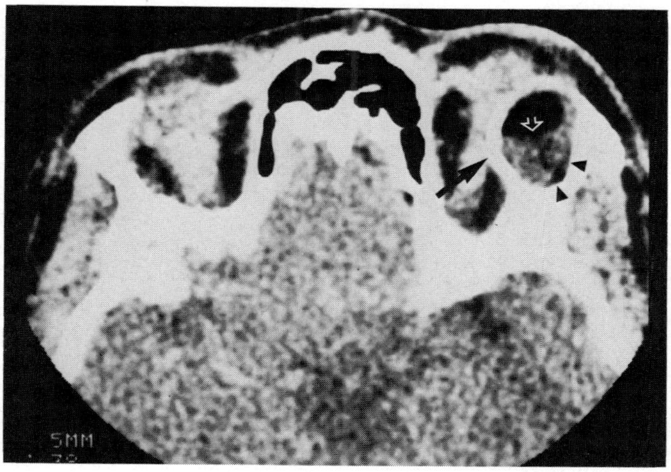

Figure 9–49. Dermoid (45-year-old female). Enhanced CT; a peripherally calcified upper outer quadrant mass *(arrow)* is present on the left. Benign bony erosion *(arrowheads)* and fat-matrix level *(open arrow)* confirmed the diagnosis.

Developmental

Dermoid Cyst

Dermoid cysts are the most common congenital lesions of the orbit, accounting for 1 to 2% of orbital masses.[80] They most commonly present as superficial periorbital lesions in children. Examination often detects painless subcutaneous nodules, often fixed to the periosteum. Rarely, these patients require diagnostic imaging.

Dermoid cysts may present also in adults, most commonly with symptoms of long-standing proptosis. In adults, the lesions are usually deep, located in the upper outer quadrant of the orbit, adjacent to the lacrimal fossa. These developmental lesions arise from germ cells trapped in the closing zygomaticofrontal suture.

The typical CT appearance of dermoid cyst is a well-defined, extraconal, centrally hypodense mass (Figs. 9–49, 9–50). The lesion may be peripherally calcified and benign bony erosion is common. A fat-fluid level may be present and is pathognomonic for dermoid cyst.[11, 80] On MRI the fat is high signal on T1 and floats on the gravity-dependent low-signal soft tissue or fluid moiety of the lesion.[15, 20, 35]

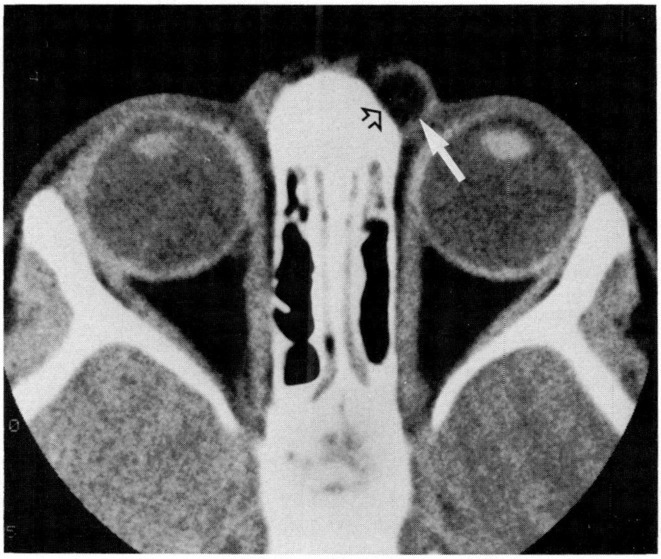

Figure 9–50. Superficial dermoid (3-year-old female). Unenhanced CT; a hypodense mass *(arrow)* is present in the subcutaneous tissues medial to the left globe. Subtle benign bony erosion *(open arrow)* is present.

References

1. Zonneveld FW, Koornneef L, Hillen B, et al: Normal direct multiplanar CT anatomy of the orbit with correlative anatomic cryosections. Radiol Clin North Am 1987; 25:381–407.
2. Hilal SK, Trokel SL: Computerized tomography of the orbit using thin sections. Semin Roentgenol 1977; 12:137–147.
3. Langer BG, Mafee MF, Pollock S, et al: MRI of the normal orbit and optic pathway. Radiol Clin North Am 1987; 25:429–446.
4. Azar-Kia B, Mafee MF, Horowitz SW, et al: CT and MRI of the optic nerve and sheath. Seminars in Ultrasound, CT, and MR 1988; 9:443–454.
5. Daniels DL, Yu S, Pech P, et al: Computed tomography and magnetic resonance imaging of the orbital apex. Radiol Clin North Am 1987; 25:803–817.
6. Kaissar G, Kim JH, Bravo S, et al: Histologic basis for increased extraocular muscle enhancement in gadolinium-enhanced MR imaging. Radiology 1991; 179:541–542.
7. Russell EJ, Czervionke L, Huckman M, et al: CT of the inferomedial orbit and the lacrimal drainage apparatus: Normal and pathologic anatomy. AJNR 1985; 6:759–766.
8. Langer BG, Charletta DA, Mafee MF, et al: MRI of the normal optic pathway. Seminars in Ultrasound, CT and MR 1988; 9:401–412.
9. Zimmerman RA, Bilaniuk LT: Ocular MR imaging. Radiology 1988; 168:875–876.
10. Atlas SW, Bilaniuk LT, Zimmerman RA, et al: Orbit: Initial experience with surface coil spin-echo MR imaging at 1.5 T. Radiology 1987; 164:501–509.
11. Atlas SW: MR of the orbit: Current imaging applications. Seminars in Ultrasound, CT, and MR 1988; 9:381–400.
12. Mafee MF, Goldberg MF, Greenwald MJ, et al: Retinoblastoma and simulating lesions: Role of CT and MR imaging. Radiol Clin North Am 1987; 25:667–681.
13. Atlas SW, Kemp SS, Rorke L, et al: Hemorrhagic intracranial retinoblastoma metastases: MR-pathology correlation. J Comput Assist Tomogr 1988; 12:286–289.
14. Meli FJ, Boccaleri CA, Manzitti J, et al: Meningeal dissemination of retinoblastoma: CT findings in eight patients. AJNR 1990; 11:983–986.
15. Wells RG, Sty JR, Gonnering RS: Imaging of the pediatric eye and orbit. Radiographics 1989; 9:1023–1044.
16. Sullivan JA, Harms SE: Surface coil MR imaging of orbital neoplasms. AJNR 1986; 7:29–34.
17. Haik BG, Louis LS, Smith ME, et al: Magnetic resonance imaging in the evaluation of leukocoria. Ophthalmology 1985; 92:1143–1152.
18. Peyman GA, Mafee MF: Uveal melanoma and similar lesions: The role of magnetic resonance imaging and computed tomography. Radiol Clin North Am 1987; 25:471–486.
19. Mihara F, Gupta KL, Murayama S, et al: MR imaging of malignant uveal melanoma: Role of pulse sequence and contrast agent. AJNR 1991; 12:991–996.
20. Sullivan JA, Harms SE: Characterization of orbital lesions by surface coil MR imaging. Radiographics 1987; 7:9–28.
21. Armington WG, Bilaniuk LT: The radiologic evaluation of the orbit: Conal and intraconal lesions. Seminars in Ultrasound, CT, and MR 1988; 9:455–473.
22. Peyster RG, Shapiro MD, Haik BG: Orbital metastasis: Role of magnetic resonance imaging and computed tomography. Radiol Clin North Am 1987; 25:647–662.
23. Weber AL, Mikulis DK: Inflammatory disorders of the paraorbital sinuses and their complications. Radiol Clin North Am 1987; 25:615–630.
24. Hopper KD, Haas DK, Sherman JL: The radiographic evaluation of congenital and pediatric lesions of the orbit. Seminars in Ultrasound, CT and MRI 1988; 9:413–427.
25. Wright DC, Yuh WTC, Thompson HS, et al: Bilateral microphthalmos with orbital cysts: MR findings. J Comput Assist Tomogr 1987; 11:727–729.
26. Mafee MF, Jampol LM, Langer BG, et al: Computed tomography of optic nerve colobomas, morning glory anomaly, and colobomatous cyst. Radiol Clin North Am 1987; 25:693–699.
27. Simmons JD, LaMasters D, Char D: Computed tomography of ocular colobomas. AJNR 1983; 4:1049–1052.
28. Howard GM, Ellsworth RM: Differential diagnosis of retinoblastoma. Am J Ophthalmol 1965; 60:610–618.
29. Sherman JL, McLean IW, Brallier DR: Coat's disease: CT pathologic correlation in two cases. Radiology 1983; 147:77–78.
30. Mafee MF, Goldberg MF, Valvassori GE, et al: Computed tomography in evaluation of patients with persistent hyperplastic primary vitreous (PHPV). Radiology 1982; 145:713–717.
31. Mafee MF, Goldberg MF: Persistent hyperplastic primary vitreous (PHPV): Role of computed tomography and magnetic resonance. Radiol Clin North Am 1987; 25:683–692.
32. Ball JB: Direct oblique sagittal CT of orbital wall fractures. ANJR 1987; 8:147–154.
33. Tonami H, Nakagawa T, Ohguchi M, et al: Surface coil MR imaging of orbital blowout fractures: A comparison with reformatted CT. AJNR 1987; 8:445–449.
34. Tonami H, Yamamoto I, Matsuda M, et al: Orbital fractures: Surface coil MR imaging. Radiology 1991; 179:789–794.
35. Mafee MF, Putterman A, Valvassori GE, et al: Orbital space-occupying lesions: Role of computed tomography and magnetic imaging. Radiol Clin North Am 1987; 25:529–559.
36. Wiot JG, Pleatman CW: Chronic hematic cysts of the orbit. AJNR 1989; 10:S37–S39.
37. Travis RC, Murray PI, Moseley IF, et al: Orbital intraconal haematic cysts in young people: Computed tomography and magnetic resonance imaging. Br J Radiol 1989; 62:521–525.
38. Jafar JJ, Crowell RM: Parasellar and optic nerve lesions: The neurosurgeon's prospective. Radiol Clin North Am 1987; 25:877–892.
39. Azar-Kia B, Naheedy MH, Elias DA, et al: Optic nerve tumors: Role of magnetic resonance imaging and computed tomography. Radiol Clin North Am 1987; 25:561–581.
40. Jakobiec FA, Depot MJ, Kennerdell JS, et al: Combined clinical and computed tomographic diagnosis of orbital glioma and meningioma. Ophthalmology 1984; 91:137–155.
41. Bilaniuk LT, Atlas SW, Zimmerman RA: Magnetic resonance imaging of the orbit. Radiol Clin North Am 1987; 25:509–528.
42. Lourie GL, Osborne DR, Kirks DR: Involvement of posterior visual pathways by optic nerve gliomas. Pediatr Radiol 1986; 16:271–274.

43. Hendrix LE, Kneeland JB, Haughton VM: MR imaging of optic nerve lesions: Value of Gadopentetate dimeglumine and fat-suppression technique. AJNR 1990; 11:749–754.
44. Daniels DL, Pech P, Kay MC, et al: Orbital apex: Correlative anatomic and CT study. AJNR 1985; 6:705–710.
45. Fries PD, Char DH, Norman D: MR imaging of orbital cavernous hemangioma. J Comput Assist Tomogr 1987; 11:418–421.
46. Mafee MF, Miller MT, Tan W, et al: Dynamic computed tomography and its application to ophthalmology. Radiol Clin North Am 1987; 25:715–731.
47. Reed D, Robertson WD, Rootman J, et al: Plexiform neurofibromatosis of the orbit: CT evaluation. AJNR 1986; 7:259–263.
48. Dervin JE, Beaconsfield M, Wright JE, et al: CT findings in orbital tumors of nerve sheath origin. Clin Radiol 1989; 40:475–479.
49. Linder B, Campos M, Schafer M: CT and MRI of orbital abnormalities in neurofibromatosis and selected craniofacial anomalies. Radiol Clin North Am 1987; 25:787–802.
50. Zimmerman RA, Bilaniuk LT, Metzger RA, et al: Computed tomography of orbital—facial neurofibromatosis. Radiology 1983; 146:113–116.
51. Bilaniuk LT, Schenck JF, Zimmerman RA, et al: Ocular and orbital lesions: Surface coil MR imaging. Radiology 1985; 156:669–674.
52. Curtin HD: Pseudotumor. Radiol Clin North Am 1987; 25:583–599.
53. Flanders AE, Mafee MF, Rao VM, et al: CT characteristics of orbital pseudotumor and other orbital inflammatory processes. J Comput Assist Tomogr 1989; 13:40–47.
54. Nugent RA, Rootman J, Robertson WD: Acute orbital pseudotumors: Classification and CT features. AJR 1981; 137:957–962.
55. Frohman LP, Kupersmith MJ, Lang J, et al: Intracranial extension and bone destruction in orbital pseudotumor. Arch Ophthalmol 1986; 104:380–384.
56. Sobel DF, Kelly W, Kjos BO, et al: MR imaging of orbital and ocular diseases. AJNR 1985; 6:259–264.
57. Merandi SF, Kudryk BT, Murtagh FR, et al: Contrast-enhanced MR imaging of optic nerve lesions in patients with acute optic neuritis. AJNR 1991; 12:923–926.
58. Howard CW, Osher RH, Tomsak RL: Computed tomographic features in optic neuritis. Am J Ophthalmol 1980; 89:699–702.
59. Miller DH, Newton MR, van der Poel JC, et al: Magnetic resonance imaging of the optic nerve in optic neuritis. Neurology 1988; 38:175–179.
60. Guy J, Mancuso A, Quisling RG, et al: Gadolinium-DTPA-enhanced magnetic resonance imaging in optic neuropathies. Ophthalmology 1990; 97:592–600.
61. Tien RD, Chu PK, Hesselink JR, et al: Intra- and paraorbital lesions: Value of fat-suppression MR imaging with paramagnetic contrast enhancement. AJNR 1991; 12:245–253.
62. Hosten N, Sander B, Cordes M, et al: Graves' ophthalmopathy: MR imaging of the orbits. Radiology 1989; 172:759–762.
63. Forbes G, Gorman CA, Breman MD, et al: Ophthalmopathy of Graves' disease: Computerized volume measurements of the orbital fat and muscle. AJNR 1986; 7:651–656.
64. Nugent RA, Belkin RI, Neigel JM, et al: Graves' orbitopathy: Correlation of CT and clinical findings. Radiology 1990; 177:675–682.
65. Barrett L, Glatt HJ, Burde RM, et al: Optic nerve dysfunction in thyroid eye disease: CT. Radiology 1988; 167:503–507.
66. Trokel SL, Jakobiec FA: Correlation of CT scanning and pathologic features of ophthalmic Graves' disease. Ophthalmology 1981; 88:553–564.
67. Atlas SW, Grossman RI, Savino PJ, et al: Surface-coil MR of orbital pseudotumor. AJNR 1987; 8:141–146.
68. Hesselink JR, Davis KR, Dallow RL, et al: Computed tomography of masses in the lacrimal gland region. Radiology 1979; 131:143–147.
69. Mafee MF, Haik BG: Lacrimal gland and fossa lesions: Role of computed tomography. Radiol Clin North Am 1987; 25:767–779.
70. Flanders AE, Espinosa GA, Markiewicz DA, et al: Orbital lymphoma: Role of CT and MRI. Radiol Clin North Am 1987; 25:601–613.
71. Mittal BB, Deutsch M, Kennerdell J, et al: Paraocular lymphoid tumors. Radiology 1986; 159:793–796.
72. Yeo JH, Jakobiec FA, Abbott GF, et al: Combined clinical and computed tomographic diagnosis of orbital lymphoid tumors. Am J Ophthalmol 1982; 94:235–245.
73. Graeb DA, Rootman J, Robertson WD, et al: Orbital lymphangiomas: Clinical, radiologic, and pathologic characteristics. Radiology 1990; 175:417–421.
74. Vade A, Armstrong D: Orbital rhabdomyosarcoma. Radiol Clin North Am 1987; 25:701–714.
75. Boyadjis TA, D'Altorio RA: Orbital involvement by multiple myeloma: case report. CT: The Journal of Computed Tomography 1986; 10:145–146.
76. Hirsch M, Lifshitz T: Computerized tomography in the diagnosis and treatment of orbital cellulitis. Pediatr Radiol 1988; 18:302–305.
77. Zimmerman RA, Bilaniuk LT: CT of orbital infection and its cerebral complications. AJR 1980; 134:45–50.
78. Towbin R, Han BK, Kaufman RA, et al: Postseptal cellulitis: CT in diagnosis and management. Radiology 1986; 158:735–737.
79. Langham-Brown JJ, Rhys-Williams S: Computed tomography of acute orbital infection: The importance of coronal sections. Clin Radiol 1989; 40:471–474.
80. Nugent RA, Lapointe JS, Rootman J, et al: Orbital dermoids: Features on CT. Radiology 1987; 165:475–478.

10

SELLAR AND JUXTASELLAR ANATOMY AND PATHOLOGY

ANATOMY

The pituitary gland resides in the sella turcica (Turkish saddle), a shallow depression along the cephalad dorsal-most aspect of the central ridge of the sphenoid bone, which bisects the middle cranial fossa, separating its respective halves.

Anterior to the sella, the planum sphenoidale extends posteriorly from the cribriform plate to the sphenoid bone limbus (Figs. 10–1 and 1–3). The chiasmatic sulcus and tuberculum sella are juxtaposed between the limbus and the anterior wall of the sella turcica. The middle clinoid processes are two small posterior projections from the tuberculum that lie medial to the internal carotid artery as it ascends from the cavernous sinus. Lateral to the tuberculum sella on each side are the dorsal-most extensions of the lesser wings of the sphenoid, the anterior clinoid processes. The optic canal lies between the anterior clinoid and the limbus. The optic canal is directed cephalad and medial from the orbital apex to the suprasellar cistern.

The sella is surrounded on three sides (anterior, inferior, and posterior) by bone, and on three sides (lateral walls and superior) by dura. The anterior wall, floor, and posterior wall form the bony saddle to contain the gland. The floor of the sella is of variable thickness, contingent on the degree of aeration of the underlying sphenoid sinus. The posterior wall of the sella extends from the floor to the dorsum sella. The dorsum sella terminates in two small lateral extensions, the posterior clinoid processes. The posterior clinoid processes extend anteriorly a variable distance from the dorsum and are more medial than are the larger anterior clinoid processes. The dorsal inferior-most extent of the body of the sphenoid is the clivus, which forms the midline anterior bony margin of the posterior fossa.

The sella is surrounded on three sides by dura. The lateral walls of the sella are com-

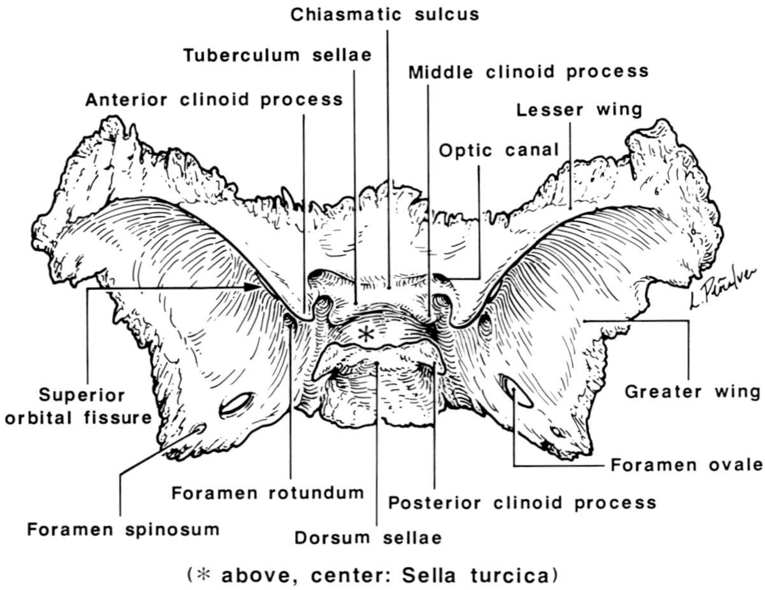

Figure 10–1. Bony anatomy; cephalad posterior view.

posed of a thin dural reflection that separates the contents of the sella from the cavernous sinus. Superiorly, the thin diaphragma sellae extends from the anterior to the posterior clinoid processes. A small orifice is present in the central diaphragma sellae, permitting the transmission of the pituitary infundibulum.

The sphenoid sinus first appears within the body of the sphenoid bone in the fourth intrauterine month; it is fully developed by young adulthood. The degree of sphenoid sinus aeration is variable. The sinus may extend superiorly to the anterior clinoid processes, the floor of the sella, and the dorsum. Alternatively, the sinus may be hypoplastic and not reach the anterior wall or floor of the sella. The sinus drains into the nasal cavity through the sphenoethmoidal recess above the superior turbinate.

From an embryologic, anatomic, and physiologic perspective, the anterior and posterior lobes of the pituitary gland are distinctive (Fig. 10–2). The anterior lobe (adenohypophysis) develops from the upward migration of an ectodermal lined diverticulum (Rathke's pouch) from the primitive mouth.[1] The cells within the adenohypophysis are arranged in cords and synthesize adrenocorticotropic hormone (ACTH), growth hormone (GH), prolactin, thyroid-stimulating hormone (TSH), follicle-stimulating hormone (FSH), and luteinizing hormone (LH). The hypothalamus mediates the synthesis and release of hormones from the adenohypophysis through chemical factors that travel via the bloodstream (hypothalamohypophyseal portal system) to the membrane receptors. With the exception of prolactin, the hypothalamus has a stimulatory effect on the production and release of the hormones of the adenohypophysis. The hypothalamohypophyseal portal system surrounds the infundibulum and lacks a blood-brain barrier (BBB).

The posterior lobe (neurohypophysis) is derived from neuroectoderm of the diencephalon at 3 to 4 weeks' gestational age. These cells migrate ventrally from the neurohypophyseal bud to form the supraoptic and paraventricular nuclei of the hypothalamus, the infundibulum, and the posterior lobe.[1] The pituicytes, which compose the neurohypophysis, are the terminal axonal projections of the cell bodies that make up these hypothalamic nuclei. Once produced by the organelles of the hypothalamic nuclei, antidiuretic hormone (ADH) and oxytocin are bound to neurophysin and, via axonal flow, are transported down the infundibulum to the neurohypophysis, which functions as a reservoir until hormonal release is dictated by the hypothalamus.[2]

Lateral to the sella turcica and medial to the temporal lobe lies the cavernous sinus. The sinus is a venous channel that extends from the clivus posteriorly to the greater and lesser

Text continued on page 341

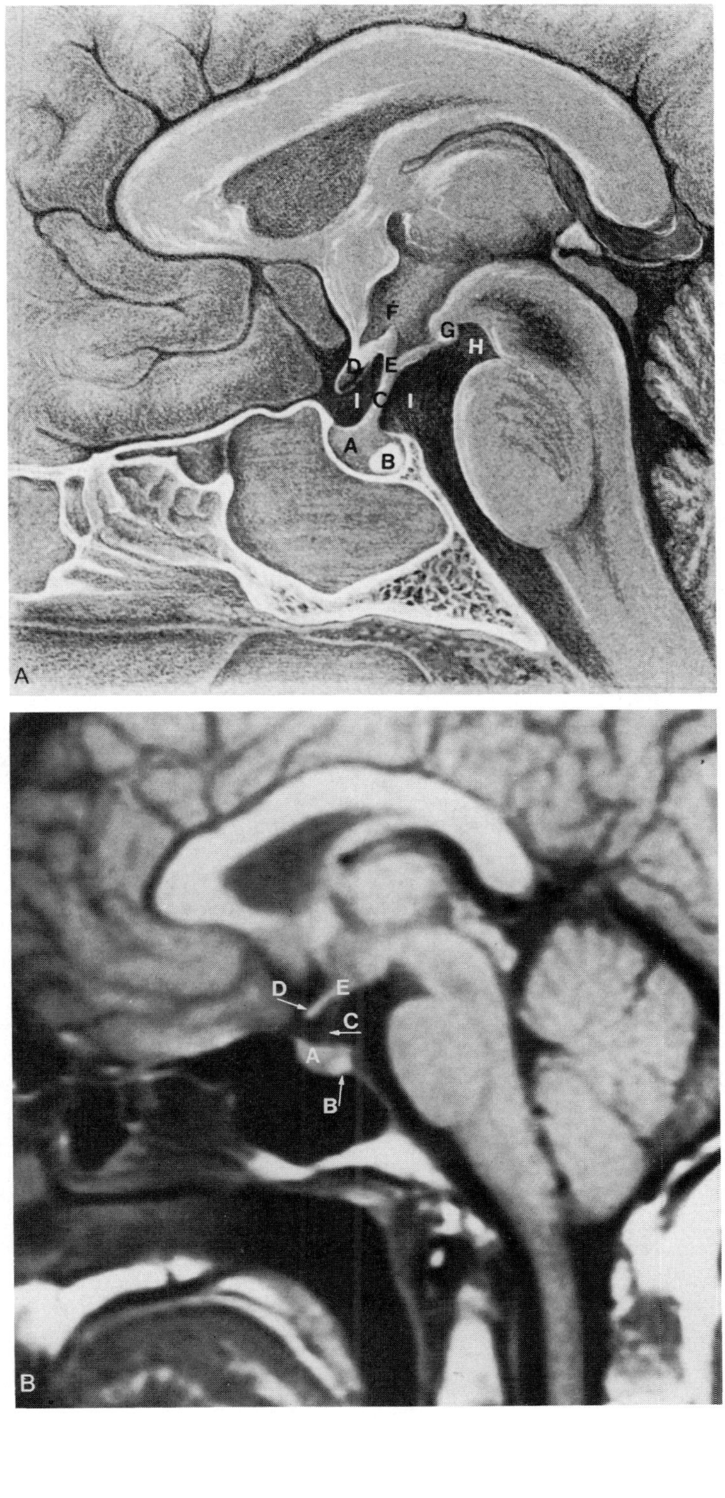

Figure 10–2. Anatomy; magnetic resonance imaging (MRI).

A, Sagittal drawing. *(A)* Adenohypophysis, *(B)* neurohypophysis, *(C)* infundibulum, *(D)* optic chiasm, *(E)* tuber cinereum, *(F)* anterior third ventricle, *(G)* mammillary bodies, *(H)* interpeduncular cistern, *(I)* suprasellar cistern.

B, Sagittal T1. *(A)* Adenohypophysis, *(B)* neurohypophysis, *(C)* infundibulum, *(D)* optic chiasm, *(E)* tuber cinereum.

Illustration continued on following page

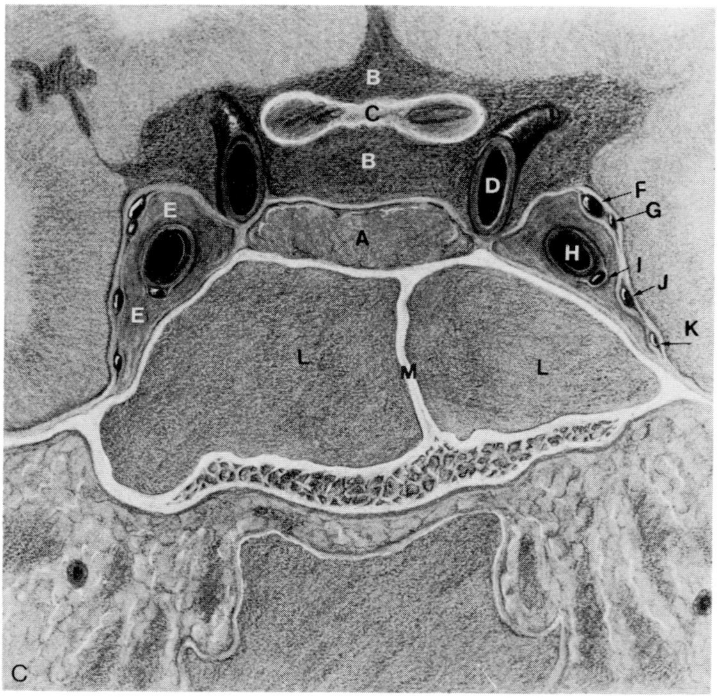

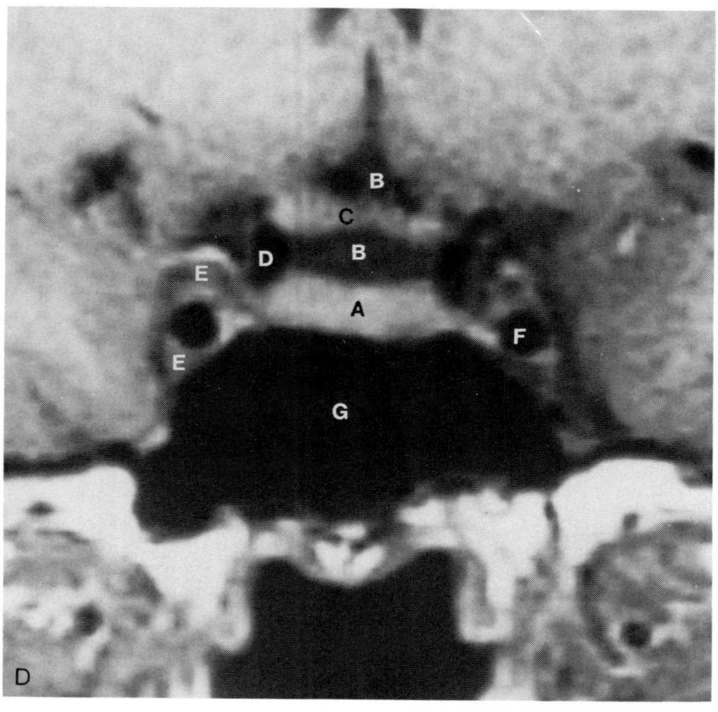

Figure 10–2 *Continued*

C, Coronal drawing (anterior sella). *(A)* Adenohypophysis, *(B)* suprasellar cistern, *(C)* optic chiasm, *(D)* supraclinoid internal carotid artery (ICA), *(E)* cavernous sinus, *(F)* oculomotor nerve, *(G)* trochlear nerve, *(H)* cavernous ICA, *(I)* abducens nerve, *(J)* ophthalmic nerve, *(K)* maxillary nerve, *(L)* sphenoid sinus, *(M)* sphenoid septum.

D, Coronal T1 (anterior sella). *(A)* Adenohypophysis, *(B)* suprasellar cistern, *(C)* optic chiasm, *(D)* supraclinoid ICA, *(E)* cavernous sinus, *(F)* cavernous ICA, *(G)* sphenoid sinus.

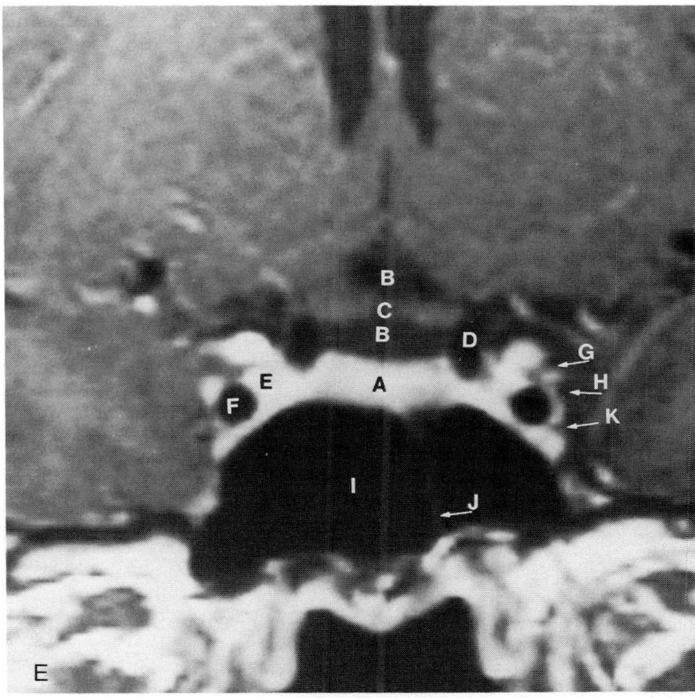

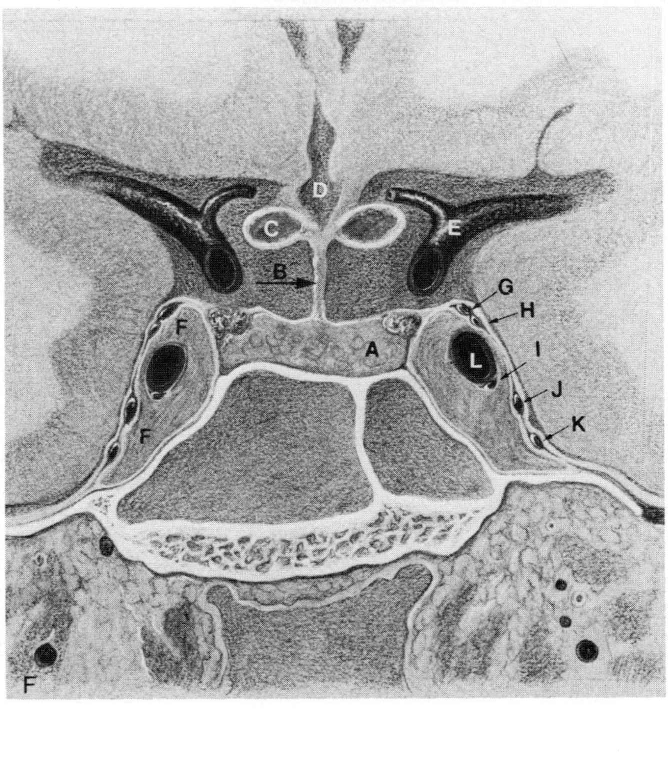

Figure 10–2 *Continued*

E, Enhanced coronal T1 (anterior sella). *(A)* Adenohypophysis, *(B)* suprasellar cistern, *(C)* optic chiasm, *(D)* supraclinoid ICA, *(E)* cavernous sinus, *(F)* cavernous ICA, *(G)* oculomotor-trochlear complex, *(H)* ophthalmic nerve, *(I)* sphenoid sinus, *(J)* sphenoid sinus septum, *(K)* maxillary nerve.

F, Coronal drawing (midsella). *(A)* Adenohypophysis, *(B)* infundibulum, *(C)* optic tract, *(D)* anterior third ventricle, *(E)* supraclinoid ICA bifurcation, *(F)* cavernous sinus, *(G)* oculomotor nerve, *(H)* trochlear nerve, *(I)* abducens nerve, *(J)* ophthalmic nerve, *(K)* maxillary nerve, *(L)* cavernous ICA.

Illustration continued on following page

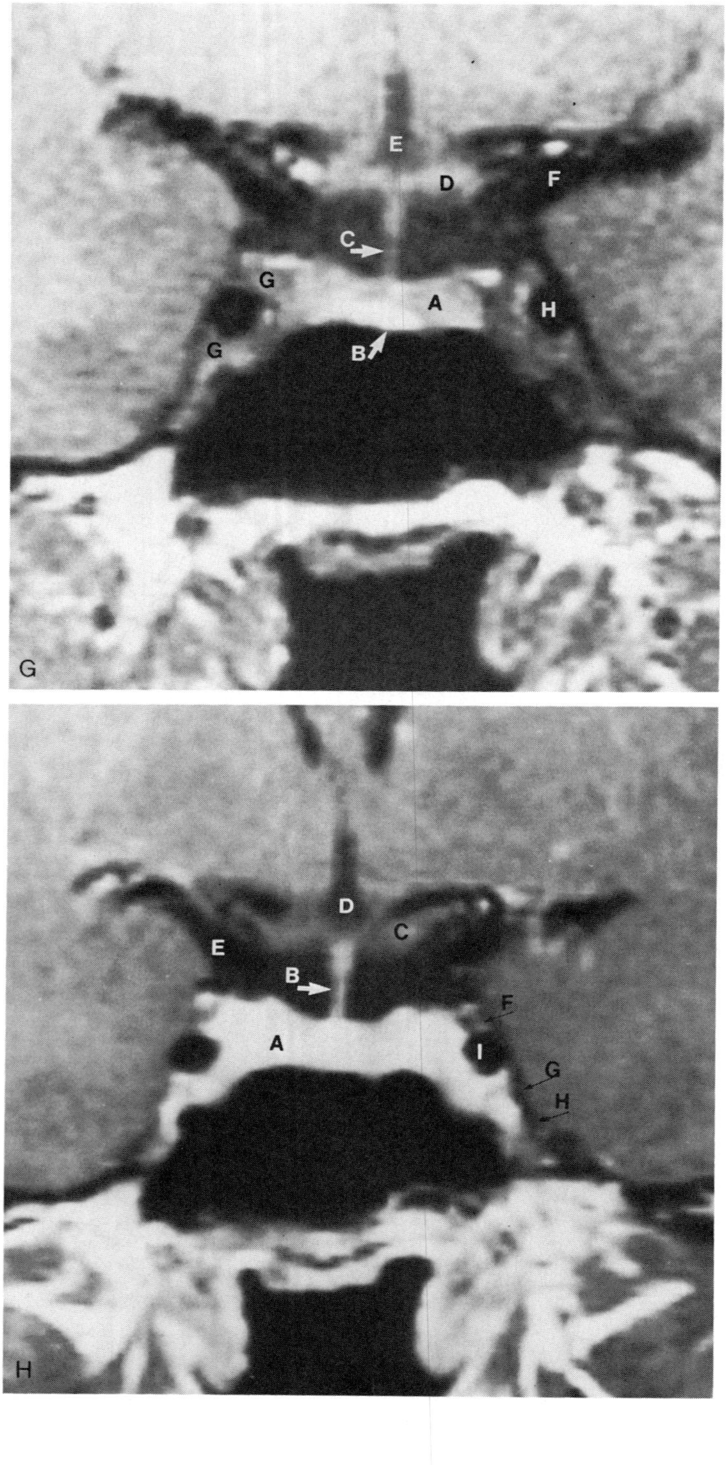

Figure 10–2 *Continued*

G, Coronal T1 (midsella). *(A)* Adenohypophysis, *(B)* neurohypophysis, *(C)* infundibulum, *(D)* optic tract, *(E)* anterior third ventricle, *(F)* supraclinoid ICA, *(G)* cavernous sinus, *(H)* cavernous ICA.

H, Enhanced coronal T1 (midsella). *(A)* Adenohypophysis, *(B)* infundibulum, *(C)* optic tract, *(D)* anterior third ventricle, *(E)* supraclinoid ICA, *(F)* oculomotor-trochlear complex, *(G)* ophthalmic nerve, *(H)* maxillary nerve, *(I)* cavernous ICA.

(From Johnsen DE, Woodruff WW, Allen IS, et al: MR imaging of the sellar and juxtasellar regions. Radiographics 1991, 11:727–758, with permission.)

wings anteriorly. Like other venous sinuses, the cavernous sinus is enclosed within a dural envelope. The medial wall is relatively thin and separates the sella from the cavernous sinus. The lateral wall is thicker and separates the cavernous sinus from the temporal lobe.

In addition to the venous channels that drain the orbit and portions of the face, the cavernous sinus contains the internal carotid artery as well as cranial nerves III, IV, first and second divisions of V (V_1, V_2), and VI. The cranial nerves enter the sinus lateral to the dorsum sella. With the exception of the second division of cranial nerve V, the remaining cranial nerves exit the cavernous sinus through the superior orbital fissure. Cranial nerve V_2 exits the midportion of the cavernous sinus through the foramen rotundum.

Posterior, lateral, and inferior to the cavernous sinus lies Meckel's cave. This cerebrospinal fluid (CSF) space contains the gasserian ganglion of the trigeminal nerve (V) and is enclosed superiorly and laterally by a band of dura. The CSF within Meckel's cave communicates freely with the subarachnoid space but not with the cavernous sinus.

Juxtaposed between the anterior perforating substance above and the diaphragma sellae below lies the suprasellar cistern. In the axial plane, it has been variably described as a five- or six-pointed star, contingent on the appearance of the posterior-most border of the cistern.[3] Anteriorly, the cistern is bounded by the posterior-most extent of the orbital surface of the frontal lobe, the rectus gyrus. The interhemispheric fissure demarcates the rectus gyrus medially, and the lateral cerebral fissure borders the rectus gyrus laterally. The uncus of the temporal lobe comprises the lateral borders of the suprasellar cistern. Axial images obtained at the level of the pons demonstrate a single posterior convexity that is demarcated by the crural fissures producing a five-pointed cistern. Alternatively, if the axial images are performed at the level of the mesencephalon, the star has a sixth point, the interpeduncular cistern.

The contents of the suprasellar cistern include, from anterior to posterior, the optic apparatus; the infundibulum, which is contiguous with the tuber cinereum; and the mammillary bodies of the hypothalamus. The optic nerves continue on a posterior medial course from the optic canals until they merge at the optic chiasm. The optic tracts extend posterolateral from the optic chiasm to surround the midbrain on their course to the lateral geniculate bodies.

Cephalad to the optic chiasm are the anterior inferior recesses of the third ventricle. The anterior wall of the third ventricle, or lamina terminalis, extends from the anterior commissure to the chiasmatic recess. The more dorsal infundibular recess is enclosed by a conical portion of the hypothalamus, the tuber cinereum. The tuber cinereum tapers as it extends inferiorly from the hypothalamus to terminate in the infundibulum. The infundibulum extends from the tuber cinereum, through the diaphragma sellae to the superior border of the pituitary gland.

The mammillary bodies are paired paramedian structures located dorsal to the tuber cinereum. They are approximately 5 mm long and extend into the dorsal-most aspect of the suprasellar cistern, just ventral to the cerebral peduncles.

IMAGING TECHNIQUES

Until recently, computed tomography (CT) has been regarded as the procedure of choice for evaluating the sellar and juxtasellar regions.[4, 5] However, magnetic resonance imaging (MRI) has rapidly become the standard of care in evaluating patients with suspected abnormalities of the sella or parasellar region.[6–9] In general, coronal images are the most sensitive at detecting intrasellar pathology as well as documenting the juxtasellar extent of lesions.

The CT examination should be conducted with the head in maximum extension and appropriate gantry angulation to permit coronal images through the sella. Frequently, the gantry will have to be angulated to avoid dental artifacts that may obscure the contents of the sella. Contiguous 1- to 2-mm collimated images from the clivus to the tuberculum should be performed immediately following intravenous (IV) administration of a bolus of contrast (Table 10–1).

When evaluating the sella with MRI, parasagittal and coronal T1-weighted high-resolu-

Table 10–1. IMAGING TECHNIQUE

A. **CT**
1. Bolus-drip—42 g iodine
2. Coronal 1–2 mm collimated contiguous images immediately following contrast administration

B. **MR**

Plane	TR/TE (ms)	Excitations	Matrix	FOV (cm)	Slice Thickness/ Gap*	Time	No. of Slices
Unenhanced:							
Sagittal	500/20	2	256^2	18	3/1	4:23	12
Coronal	500/20	4	256^2	18	3/1	8:35	12
Enhanced:							
Coronal	500/20	2	256^2	18	3/1	4:23	12

*Millimeters

tion (256^2 matrix, 18-cm field of view (FOV), four excitations, ≤3-mm thickness) techniques should be used. Following administration of gadolinium, a repeat coronal T1-weighted sequence should be performed. T2-weighted sequences are generally of limited use when evaluating sellar pathology and are not part of our routine imaging protocol. T2 sequences are helpful to evaluate for peritumoral edema and tumor extension into parenchyma before contrast administration.

RADIOGRAPHIC ANATOMY

CT will provide information regarding the bony anatomy of the sella (Fig. 10–3). The floor of the sella is generally well demonstrated against the soft tissue density of the gland above and the air within the sphenoid sinus below. The floor of the sella may normally be so thin its contiguity may be questioned. The anterior and posterior clinoid processes are well demonstrated. The anterior clinoid processes are larger and more laterally positioned than are the posterior clinoids.

On MRI, the sellar floor may not be well visualized because the signal void from the thin bone may merge imperceptibly with gas within the sphenoid sinus. Alternatively, if there is sinus disease or underpneumatization of the sinus, the floor can be demonstrated as a thin band of decreased signal. If marrow fills the dorsum sella or clinoid processes, or both, they may be depicted as areas of relatively high signal intensity on T1 images. Parasagittal T1 images offer an accurate depiction of the anteroposterior (AP) dimension of the sella.

The dural margins of the sella are not consistently identified on CT or MRI. The diaphragma sellae may be detected on coronal MRI images as a linear band of diminished signal intensity on long repetition time (TR)–short echo delay time (TE) spin echo sequences.[10] The decreased signal is derived from this thin dural membrane and possibly from the minute blood vessels that run above and below the roof of the sella. The thin lateral dural wall of the sella turcica is inconsistently identified on CT and MRI,[11] complicating our ability to detect cavernous sinus invasion by a primary intrasellar process.[12] However, one investigator has reported the ability to demonstrate the medial wall of the cavernous sinus in 90% of patients using a dynamic enhanced MRI technique.[13]

The CT appearance of the gland has been well described.[4] The gland is generally homogeneously dense and enhances homogeneously following IV administration of iodinated contrast material. The vertical dimension of the gland in the normal man should not exceed 7 mm. The height of the gland in premenopausal women should not exceed 10 mm. The gland becomes atretic in postmenopausal women, averaging approximately 5 mm in vertical dimension. The gland enlarges slightly during pregnancy to a peak height of 12 mm 1 week postpartum, and returns to normal size 3 weeks postpartum.[14]

MRI can distinguish the anterior and posterior lobes of the hypophysis.[6, 7, 15] The anterior lobe is isointense to gray matter on T1 images. A focal bright spot has been identified in the normal neurohypophysis on T1 images. This was originally thought to represent flow-related enhancement in the intercavernous sinus, a dorsal fat pad,[16] or lipoid material in the pituicytes.[17] However, lack of chemical

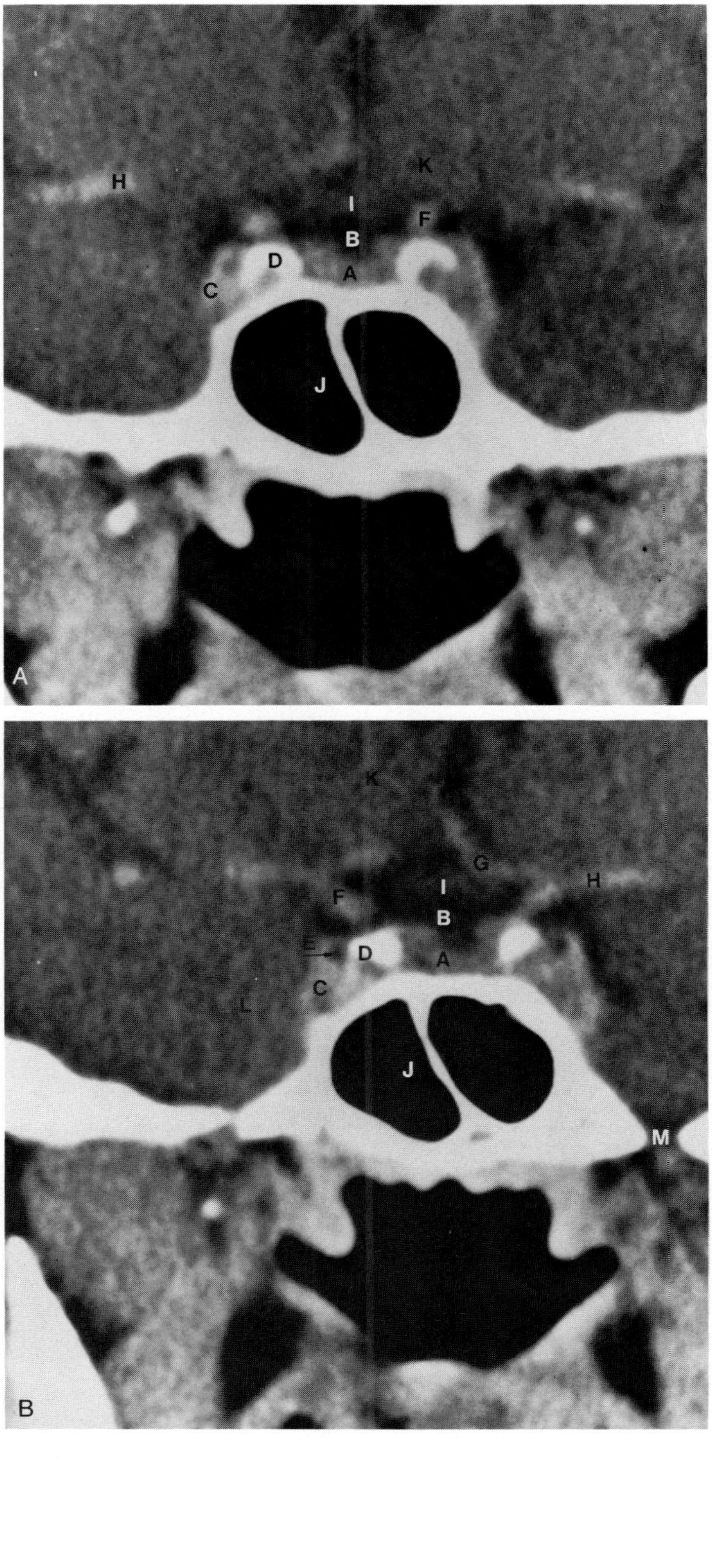

Figure 10–3. Anatomy; CT.

A, B. Coronal CT soft tissue and bone windows. *(A)* Pituitary gland, *(B)* suprasellar cistern, *(C)* cavernous sinus, *(D)* cavernous internal carotid artery (calcified), *(E)* III and IV nerve complex, *(F)* supraclinoid carotid artery, *(G)* anterior cerebral artery (ACA), *(H)* middle cerebral artery (MCA), *(I)* optic chiasm, *(J)* sphenoid sinus, *(K)* frontal lobe, *(L)* temporal lobe, *(M)* foramen ovale, *(N)* anterior clinoid process, *(O)* posterior clinoid process, *(P)* superior orbital fissure, *(Q)* inferior orbital fissure, *(R)* foramen rotundum, *(S)* vidian canal.

Illustration continued on following page

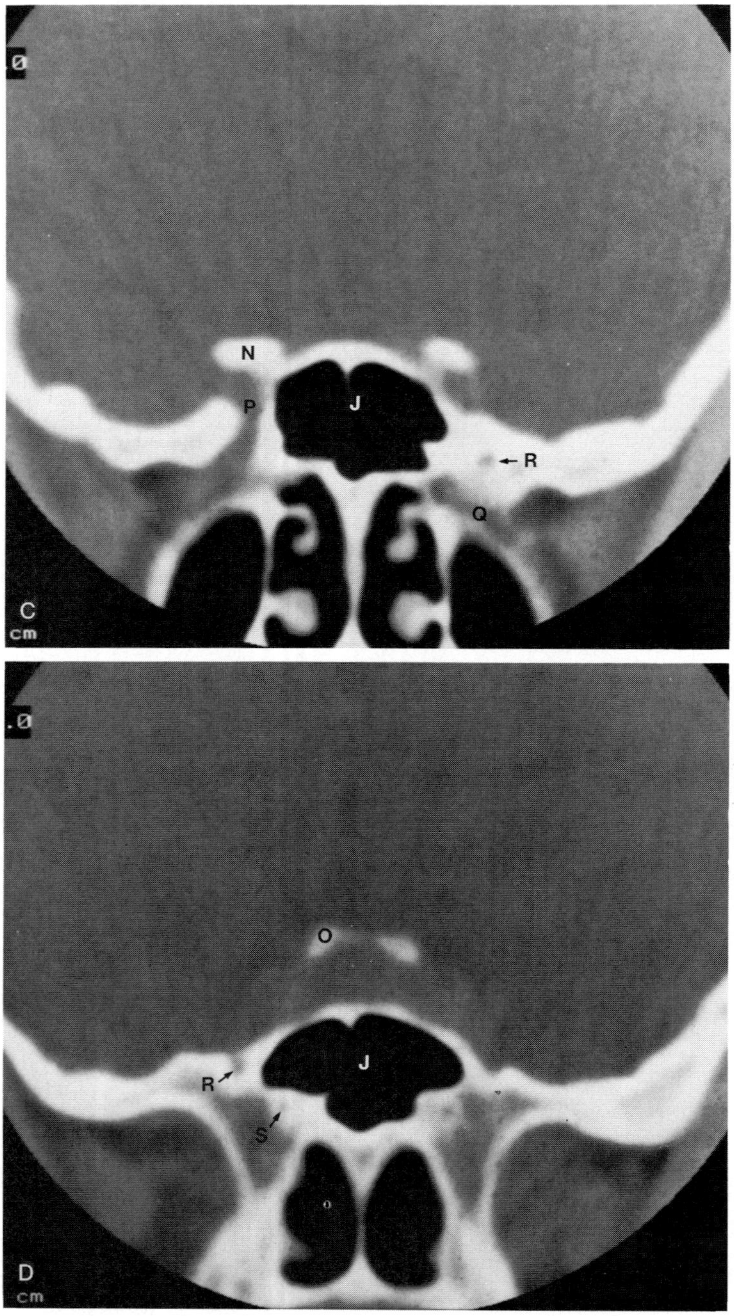

Figure 10–3 *Continued*
C, D. Coronal CT soft tissue and bone windows. *(A)* Pituitary gland, *(B)* suprasellar cistern, *(C)* cavernous sinus, *(D)* cavernous internal carotid artery (calcified), *(E)* III and IV nerve complex, *(F)* supraclinoid carotid artery, *(G)* anterior cerebral artery (ACA), *(H)* middle cerebral artery (MCA), *(I)* optic chiasm, *(J)* sphenoid sinus, *(K)* frontal lobe, *(L)* temporal lobe, *(M)* foramen ovale, *(N)* anterior clinoid process, *(O)* posterior clinoid process, *(P)* superior orbital fissure, *(Q)* inferior orbital fissure, *(R)* foramen rotundum, *(S)* vidian canal.

shift artifact in the frequency encoded direction[18] and conspicuous absence of this high signal in patients with diabetes insipidus[19] have led some investigators to conclude that this may be related to neurosecretory material within the hypothalamohypophyseal tract. More recently, fat- and water-suppression techniques have been applied to evaluate this high-signal material. No one technique was uniformly successful in suppressing this signal in all patients, leading the investigator to conclude the source of the high-intensity signal is variable.[20]

The pituitary gland, infundibulum, and cavernous sinus enhance relatively homogeneously following contrast administration.[21] Dynamic studies following gadopentetate dimeglumine bolus demonstrate regional variations in the uptake of contrast within the gland.[22] The posterior lobe enhances most rapidly followed by a centrifugal progression from the insertion of the infundibulum. The distinction between the gland and the cavernous sinus may be more apparent on the unenhanced images.

The cavernous sinus is best evaluated in the coronal plane. Cranial nerves III, IV, V_1, V_2, and VI may be detected as nonenhancing structures along the lateral wall of the cavernous sinus.[13, 23, 24] The cavernous internal carotid artery (ICA) may be hyperdense to the cavernous sinus on unenhanced CT. Atherosclerotic calcification may be of use in locating the cavernous carotid artery. IV contrast renders the ICA and cavernous sinus isodense on CT. MRI depicts the ICA as a well-circumscribed region of signal void within the cavernous sinus. Focal areas of fat may be identified within the cavernous sinus in 27% of normal patients.[25] The thick lateral dural membrane of the cavernous sinus is clearly identified on CT and MRI.

Meckel's cave and the gasserian ganglion are identified on CT as 1 cm in greatest dimension, hypodense elliptical structures posterior-inferior lateral to the cavernous sinus.[26] Administration of IV contrast material enhances the dural margin of Meckel's cave; intrathecal contrast material opacifies Meckel's cave. Meckel's cave is isointense to CSF on all spin echo sequences.

The parenchymal perimeter of the suprasellar cistern can be accurately identified on CT. Axial CT demonstrates an inverted V, representing the optic chiasm and proximal optic tracts. The infundibulum and third ventricle are well demonstrated. Conspicuity of the suprasellar contents can be increased following the administration of intrathecal water-soluble contrast.[27] Coronal CT demonstrates the horizontal orientation of the optic chiasm and the vertical orientation of the infundibulum.[3]

Parasagittal T1 images routinely demonstrate all major contents of the suprasellar cistern and are particularly useful when evaluating the lamina terminalis, the anterior inferior recesses of the third ventricle, the relationship of the optic chiasm to the infundibulum, and the size, shape, and contents of the sella.

Coronal T1 images accurately depict the uncus of the temporal lobes, anterior perforating substance, optic apparatus, infundibulum, and third ventricle.

COMMON PATHOLOGY

(Table 10–2)

Adenoma (Table 10–3)

Pituitary adenomas account for 10% of intracranial neoplasms and occur most frequently in patients between 20 and 50 years of age.[28] Pituitary adenomas are classified by size as microadenomas or macroadenomas. Microadenomas are 10 mm or less in greatest linear dimension. These tumors are generally active, producing a predictable constellation of clinical findings early, before the tumor attains significant size. The tumors most often secrete prolactin, GH, or ACTH. Prolactin-secreting adenomas are the most common microadenomas and induce amenorrhea and galactorrhea. Patients with ACTH tumors present with Cushing's disease. Tumors that produce GH cause acromegaly in adults and gigantism in adolescents.

The CT appearance of microadenoma has been described.[4] The most sensitive criterion for diagnosing a microadenoma is a focal region of hypodensity within the gland. This density difference may be accentuated immediately after contrast administration because the gland is more vascular than is the hypo-

Table 10–2. DISTINGUISHING THE COMMON SELLAR/JUXTASELLAR LESIONS

	Macroadenoma	Meningioma	Craniopharyngioma	Aneurysm
Incidence	10	3	2	1
Age	50	65	35	55
Sex (F:M)	1:1.3	3:1	1:1.6	3:2
MRI				
Location	Intrasellar Midline	Juxtasellar Eccentric	Juxtasellar/ intrasellar (4/1) Midline	Juxtasellar Eccentric
T1 signal	Homogeneous Isointense	Homogeneous Isointense	Heterogeneous ↑ & ↓	Flow void Thrombus
Enhancement	+ (Homogeneous/ heterogeneous)	+ (Homogeneous)	+ (Solid tumor)	± Periphery
CT				
Bone changes	Erosion	Hyperostosis	Rare	Rare
Ca^{2+}	Rare	Psammomatous	Concentric Mulberry	± Concentric
Enhancement	Homogeneous	Homogeneous	Heterogeneous	Lumen enhances

dense adenoma. The disparity in density of the gland and the adenoma is a transient phenomenon following contrast administration. After 2 to 3 minutes, the adenoma begins to trap sufficient amounts of iodine to render it isodense to the normal gland.

Secondary radiographic signs exist but offer a less sensitive means to detect pituitary microadenomas. A focal upward convexity of the superior border of the gland, deviation of the infundibulum away from the side of the lesion, an enlarged gland, and erosions of the bony perimeter of the sella may corroborate the presence of a microadenoma.[4] However, the smaller the lesion, the less obvious the secondary changes will appear. It is important to understand that a microadenoma may be present within the gland despite a normal high-resolution CT examination.

The MRI appearance of microadenomas has received a lot of attention.[11, 15, 21, 29–32] MRI has surpassed the sensitivity and specificity of CT to detect abnormalities of the sella.[31] The most sensitive sign of a microadenoma on unenhanced T1 images is a focal region of hypointensity within the gland (Fig. 10–4). This hypointensity will be more apparent if T1 images are obtained immediately after gadolinium administration.[21, 29] Enhanced T1 images better delineate microadenomas and may detect those that are isointense to gland and otherwise inapparent on the unenhanced examination.[33] The maximum contrast between enhancing gland and the hypovascular microadenoma occurs 3 minutes after bolus injection of gadolinium.[34] It is crucial to recognize that the microadenoma will at some point accumulate sufficient contrast material to render it isointense to the normal gland.[29] Some investigators have reported equal success at detecting microadenomas in examinations using half-dose gadopentetate dimeglumine (0.05 mmol/kg) compared with full-dose examinations.[35]

Table 10–3. DIFFERENTIATING ADENOMAS

	Micro	Macro
A. CT		
Size	≤1.0 cm	>1.0 cm
Density	↓	→
Enhancement	−	+, variable
B. MRI		
Signal: T1	↓	→
Enhancement	Initial −; late +	+, variable
C. Clinical		
Incidence	1	2.5
Signs/symptoms	Endocrinopathy	Chiasmal syndrome Endocrinopathy

The appearance of microadenomas on T2 is variable[11, 15, 30] and unpredictable. The microadenoma may be isointense to gland if solid or hyperintense to gland if semiliquid. The high signal of CSF and decreased signal to noise render the adenoma less conspicuous on the T2 images. It is unlikely that T2 images will offer additional information that cannot be obtained from the post–gadolinium-enhanced T1-weighted sequence in most instances.

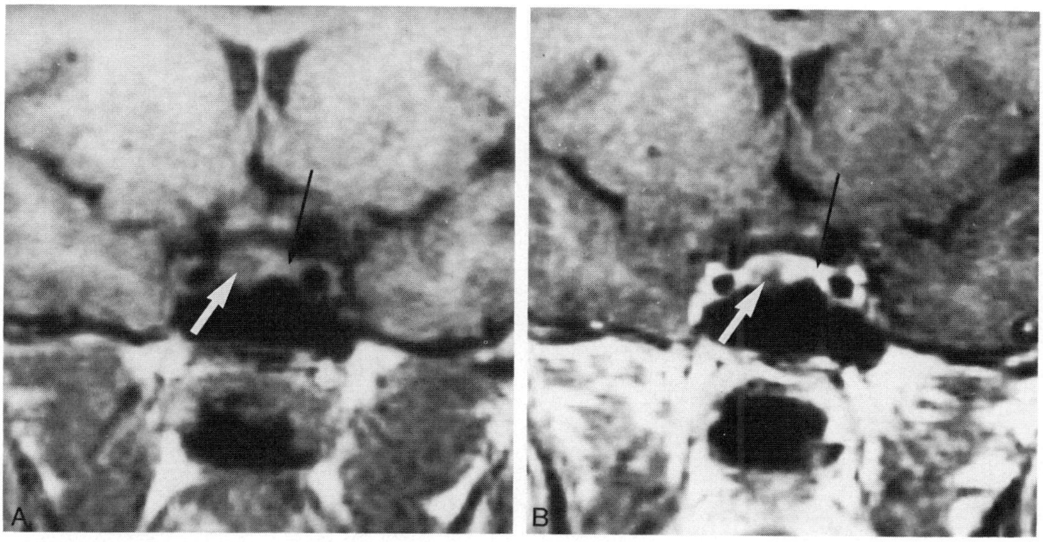

Figure 10–4. Microadenoma (28-year-old female).

A, Coronal T1. An ill-defined focus of diminished signal *(white arrow)* is noted to the right of midline within the gland *(black arrow)*.

B, Enhanced coronal T1. The lesion *(white arrow)* becomes more conspicuous as the gland *(black arrow)* enhances on the immediate postcontrast scan.

(From Johnsen DE, Woodruff WW, Allen IS, et al: MR imaging of the sellar and juxtasellar regions. Radiographics 1991; 11:727–758, with permission.)

The secondary signs of microadenoma described on CT have also been corroborated on MRI.[11] Asymmetric upward convexity of the gland, sloping of the sellar floor, and infundibular displacement may be evaluated. However, infundibular displacement or tilt also has been reported in 46% of normal patients.[36]

Macroadenomas (greater than 1 cm) are generally nonfunctioning adenomas that do not become evident until the tumor has attained sufficient size to compress the adjacent structures. The adenoma may attain enormous size and extend superiorly to compress the optic chiasm and infundibulum or laterally to invade the cavernous sinus. Benign bony erosive changes may be identified as the slowly growing mass exceeds the size of the bony sella.

Macroadenomas are isodense to brain parenchyma on CT (Fig. 10–5). By virtue of their slow growth and absence of hormonal production, they may attain dramatic size. Bony erosive changes are accurately depicted with CT. These lesions usually enhance homogeneously following contrast administration. Rarely do adenomas contain calcification.[4] The suprasellar and parasellar extensions of tumor can be effectively evaluated. Macroadenomas that exhibit suprasellar extension may have a dumbbell shape as they extend through the diaphragma sellae. Gross cavernous sinus invasion may be detected only if there is asymmetry of size or shape of the lateral wall of the sinus or a focal abnormal density within the sinus.[23]

On MRI, macroadenomas are isointense to hypointense to normal gland on T1 images[8, 11] (Fig. 10–6). The normal gland may be detected within the sella if it is not significantly compressed by the tumor. The neoplasm will generally enhance homogeneously. The tumor is variable in signal intensity on T2 images. With the exception of documenting the presence of the diaphragma sellae on spin density images, the long TR sequence is unlikely to offer additional significant diagnostic information. MRI is much more sensitive than CT at detecting the suprasellar extent of neoplasms.[6, 21, 31] MRI is also more sensitive than CT at detecting cavernous sinus invasion by macroadenomas[24] (Fig. 10–7). Inability to routinely visualize the medial dural wall of the cavernous sinus[11] and the variability in size and signal intensity of the normal cavernous sinus hinder our ability to detect cavernous sinus invasion. With the use of current MRI techniques, some authors[12] estimate our ability to accurately predict cavernous sinus invasion is 55%. The most specific

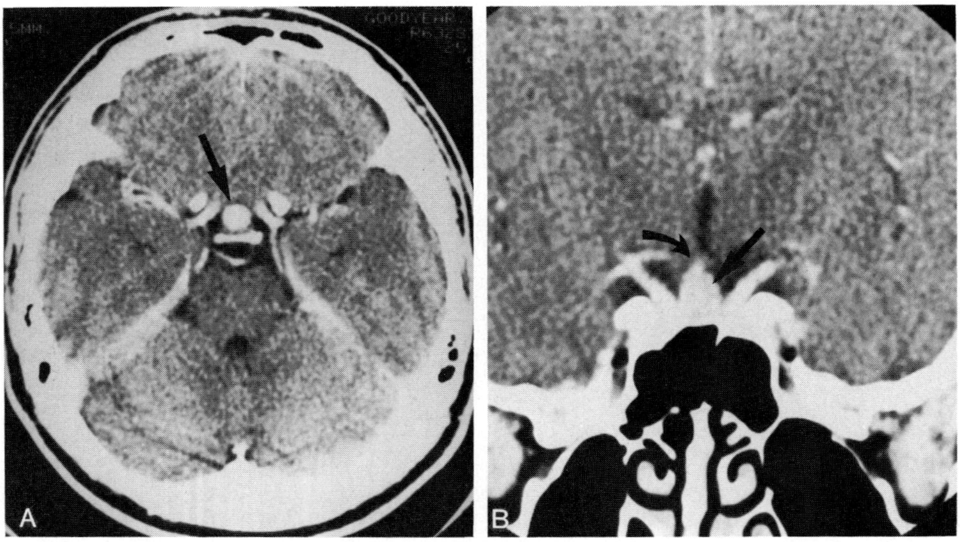

Figure 10–5. Macroadenoma (30-year-old male).
A, Enhanced axial CT. An 8-mm transverse dimension mass *(arrow)* fills the suprasellar cistern.
B, Enhanced coronal CT. The focal, convex, 12-mm homogeneously enhancing mass *(straight arrow)* extends to the hypothalamus *(curved arrow)*.

sign of cavernous sinus invasion is carotid artery encasement.[12] Contrast material may render the macroadenoma and cavernous sinus isointense, further hindering our ability to document invasion.[21] A clinically useful indicator of cavernous sinus invasion by prolactin-secreting tumors is elevation of the serum prolactin level above 2000 ng/ml.[37]

The ability to detect flow and hemoglobin degradation products on MRI has a major ramification in the workup of sellar and juxtasellar lesions. In nearly every incidence, MRI can accurately exclude an aneurysm, obviating the need for preoperative angiography.[31] The insensitivity of MRI to detect calcification may actually improve our ability to diagnose those rare adenomas that contain calcium.

The most common intracranial neoplasm to hemorrhage is pituitary adenoma. Intratumoral hemorrhage may occur in microadenomas or macroadenomas. In a series of 560 surgically proven cases, intratumoral hemorrhage occurred in nearly 17%.[38] Almost half of patients with histologic evidence of hemorrhage had no related symptoms. Smaller hemorrhages may be undetectable on CT. Acute hemorrhage within the gland will be hyperdense on CT. If CT is performed more than 2 weeks after the hemorrhagic event, the hemorrhage may be hypodense.[38] MRI is much more sensitive than CT at detecting small amounts of methemoglobin, which are hyperintense on T1 images (Fig. 10–8).

Pituitary apoplexy is a clinical syndrome of acute onset of headache, vomiting, visual impairment, diplopia, or a change in consciousness. Apoplexy is often a surgical emergency and results from infarct or more commonly hemorrhage into a pre-existing adenoma with a rapid accumulation of a mass. In a small series,[8] only 13% of patients with MRI-documented hemorrhage presented with apoplexy. CT demonstrates a sizable mass that may extend from the sella into the suprasellar cistern or cavernous sinus. If tumor necrosis and infarct are responsible for the mass, the lesion will be hypodense on CT and hypointense on T1 images (Figs. 10–9, 10–10). Alternatively, if tumoral hemorrhage is the precipitating factor, the CT will demonstrate increased density within the mass and the T1-weighted MRI will be high signal secondary to methemoglobin.[39]

Patients with prolactin-secreting tumors may respond to bromocriptine therapy. Although the mechanism of action of this dopamine agonist is not known, the proposed effect is selective inhibition of protein and hormonal synthesis in the prolactin-secreting cells.[40] Reduction of tumor size may be documented on

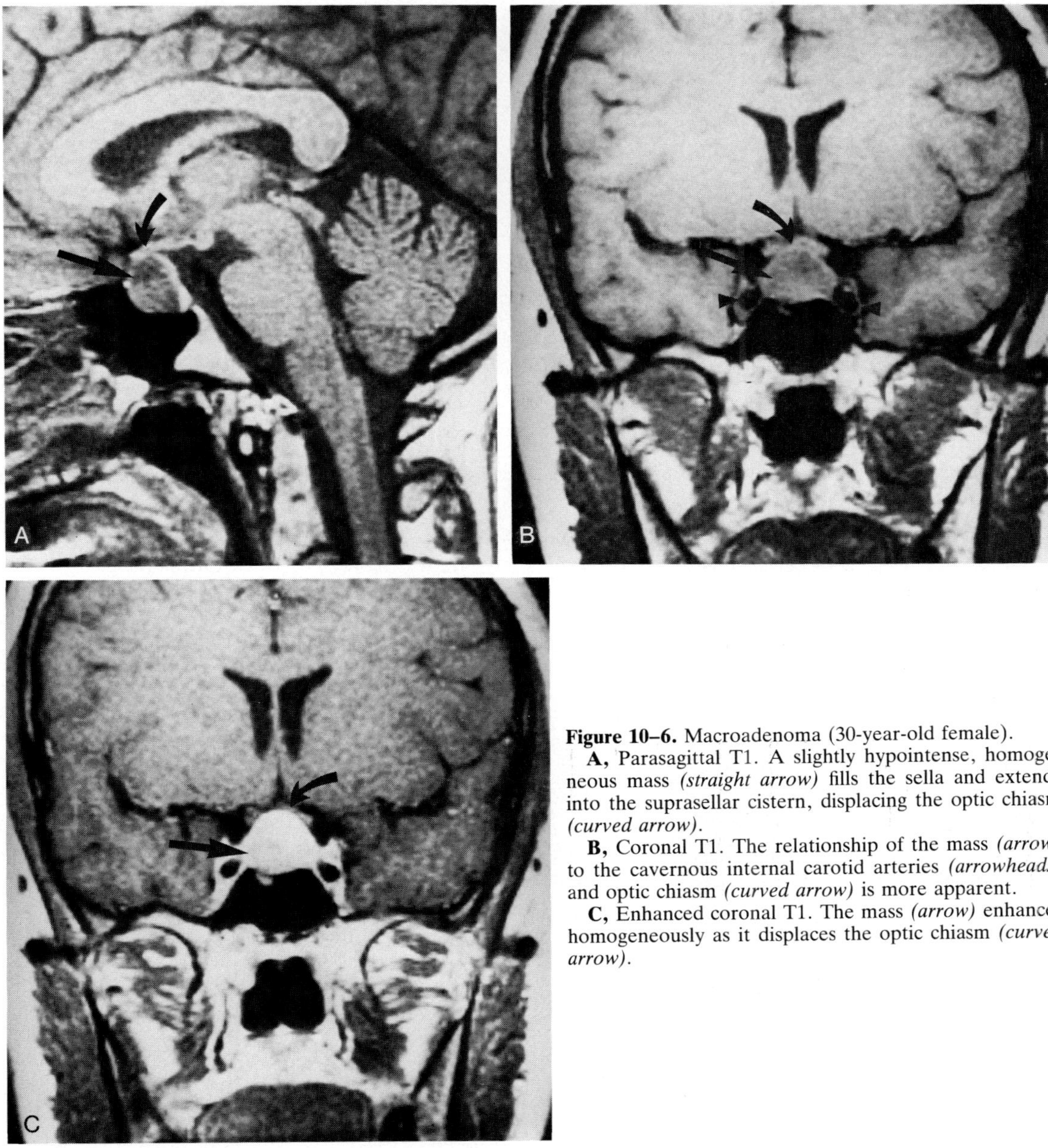

Figure 10–6. Macroadenoma (30-year-old female).

A, Parasagittal T1. A slightly hypointense, homogeneous mass *(straight arrow)* fills the sella and extends into the suprasellar cistern, displacing the optic chiasm *(curved arrow)*.

B, Coronal T1. The relationship of the mass *(arrow)* to the cavernous internal carotid arteries *(arrowheads)* and optic chiasm *(curved arrow)* is more apparent.

C, Enhanced coronal T1. The mass *(arrow)* enhances homogeneously as it displaces the optic chiasm *(curved arrow)*.

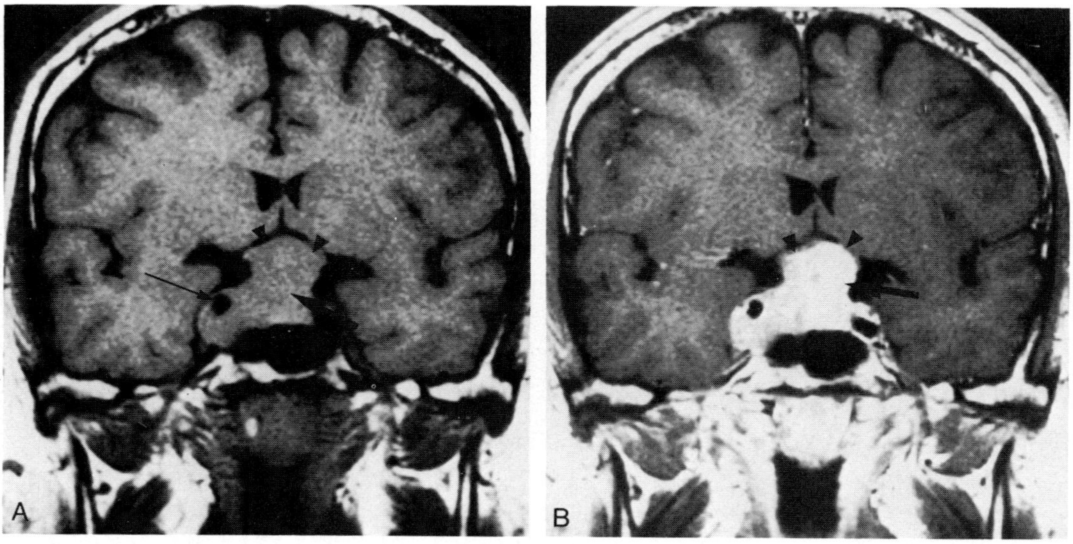

Figure 10–7. Macroadenoma with cavernous sinus extension (38-year-old female).

A, Coronal T1. An isointense–to–gray matter mass *(thick arrow)* fills the sella and extends cephalad to displace the optic chiasm *(arrowheads)* and laterally into the right cavernous sinus as it surrounds the cavernous internal carotid artery *(thin arrow)*.

B, Enhanced coronal T1. The mass *(arrow)* enhances homogeneously, revealing the displaced optic chiasm *(arrowheads)*.

(From Johnsen DE, Woodruff WW, Allen IS, et al: MR imaging of the sellar and juxtasellar regions. Radiographics 1991; 11:727–758, with permission.)

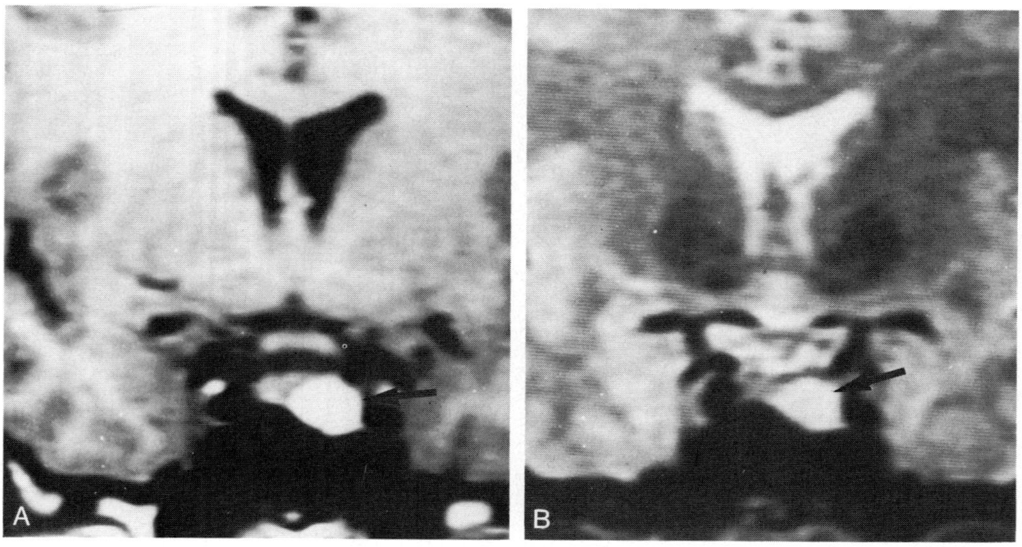

Figure 10–8. Hemorrhagic adenoma (30-year-old female).

A, Coronal T1. A focus of high signal *(arrow)* representing methemoglobin in a macroadenoma is noted. The floor of the sella is remodeled.

B, Coronal T2. The methemoglobin is extracellular, remaining high signal *(arrow)*. Unlike intraparenchymal hemorrhage, hemosiderin does not accumulate within the gland, as the lack of a blood-brain barrier permits the rapid removal of hemoglobin degradation products by macrophages.

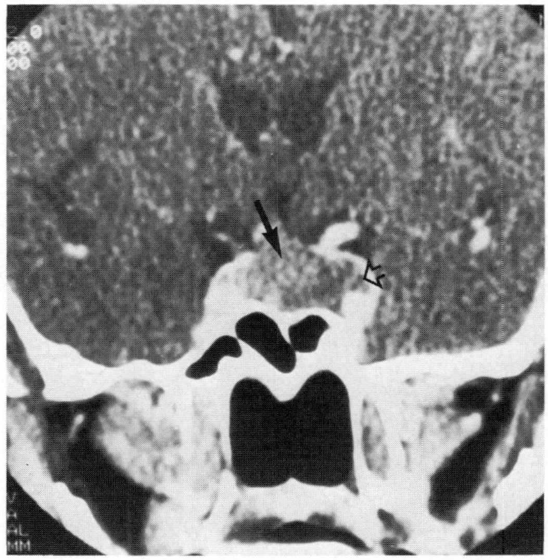

Figure 10–9. Pituitary apoplexy (30-year-old male). Enhanced coronal CT reveals a hypodense mass *(arrow)* extending into the left cavernous sinus *(open arrow);* the mass is responsible for acute ophthalmoplegia. The intrinsic hypodensity in this case indicates the ischemic rather than hemorrhagic nature of this process.

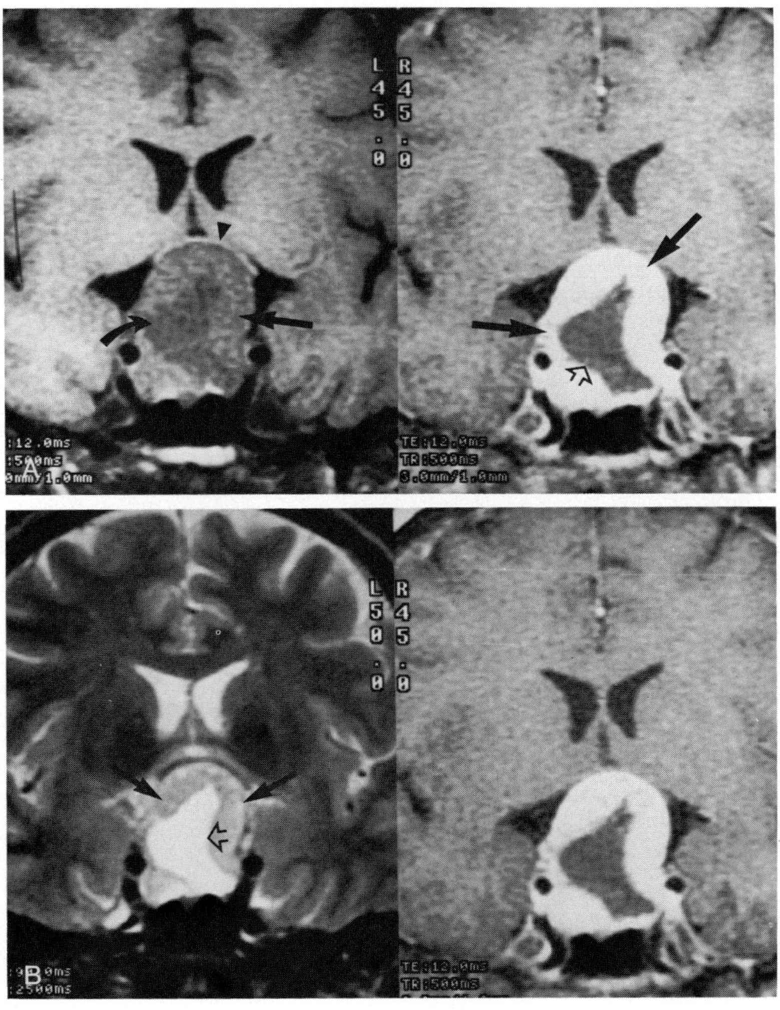

Figure 10–10. Pituitary infarct; necrosis (48-year-old male).

A, Coronal T1. *Left* (unenhanced), A large sellar mass *(arrow)* has extended into the suprasellar cistern, elevating the optic chiasm *(arrowhead)*. The central portion of the mass *(curved arrow)* is hypointense to the adenoma. *Right* (enhanced), The periphery of the adenoma enhances *(arrows)*, revealing a central infarcted region *(open arrow)*.

B, Coronal T2 *(left)* is the reverse of the gadolinium enhanced image *(right)*. The edematous necrotic tissue *(open arrow)* is higher signal than the adenoma *(arrows)*.

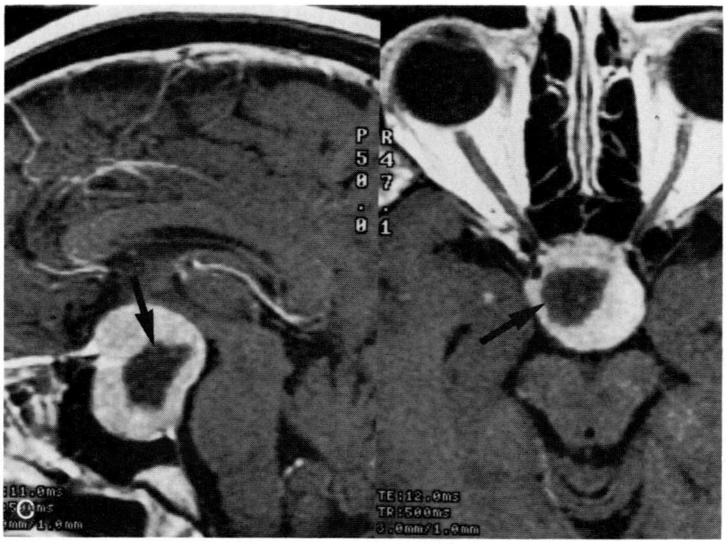

Figure 10–10 *Continued*
C, Enhanced parasagittal *(left)* and axial *(right)* T1. Absence of central enhancement *(arrow)* corroborates necrosis.

both CT and MRI[31, 40] following bromocriptine therapy (Fig. 10–11). The reduction of tumor size on MRI may also be accompanied by an increase in signal intensity of the tumor on T1 images and a variable increase or decrease of its signal intensity on T2 images. The etiology of the signal changes remain controversial. Cellular involutional changes, perhaps in concert with changes in the extracellular milieu, have been implicated by some.[41] Although bromocriptine is not tumoricidal and hemorrhage is not a prominent feature of the histology,[40] others speculate intratumoral hemorrhage may account for the signal changes.[31, 42]

Meningioma

Meningiomas represent 15 to 20% of intracranial neoplasms and may be suprasellar or parasellar in origin. Suprasellar meningiomas may arise locally from the diaphragma sellae or tuberculum sella. Larger meningiomas may extend into the suprasellar cistern from their origin in the base of the anterior cranial fossa or along the greater wing of the sphenoid bone. Tumors may extend into the middle fossa or posterior fossa, or both. They may be globoid or en placque in configuration. Meningiomas occur more commonly in women and after the third decade of life.[28]

The CT appearance of suprasellar meningiomas has been described.[3] These dural-based lesions are generally well circumscribed and isodense to hyperdense to cortex. The degree of hyperdensity correlates with the tumoral calcium content. Hyperostotic changes of the subjacent bone may occur in response to these lesions. Generally, dense homogeneous enhancement occurs after contrast administration. Vasogenic edema is an uncommon finding in patients with meningiomas of the suprasellar region.

MRI is superior to CT in evaluating the extent of suprasellar meningiomas[43] (Fig. 10–12). T1 images demonstrate a mass that is hypointense to isointense to cortex. On T2 images the mass is isointense to hyperintense to cortex.[44] The signal intensity of meningiomas may parallel that of the cortex, in which case smaller tumors may not be detected before the administration of contrast material. As on CT, the lesion generally enhances homogeneously on MRI (Fig. 10–13). Enhancement of the adjacent dura may corroborate the diagnosis of meningioma.[45, 46] The meningioma may extend into the cavernous sinus and encase the carotid artery. MRI is the method of choice to evaluate for encasement of the cavernous carotid artery[47] (Fig. 10–14).

Craniopharyngioma

Craniopharyngiomas are epithelial neoplasms that arise from squamous epithelial rests of Rathke's pouch and account for 2 to 3% of intracranial masses. Although these

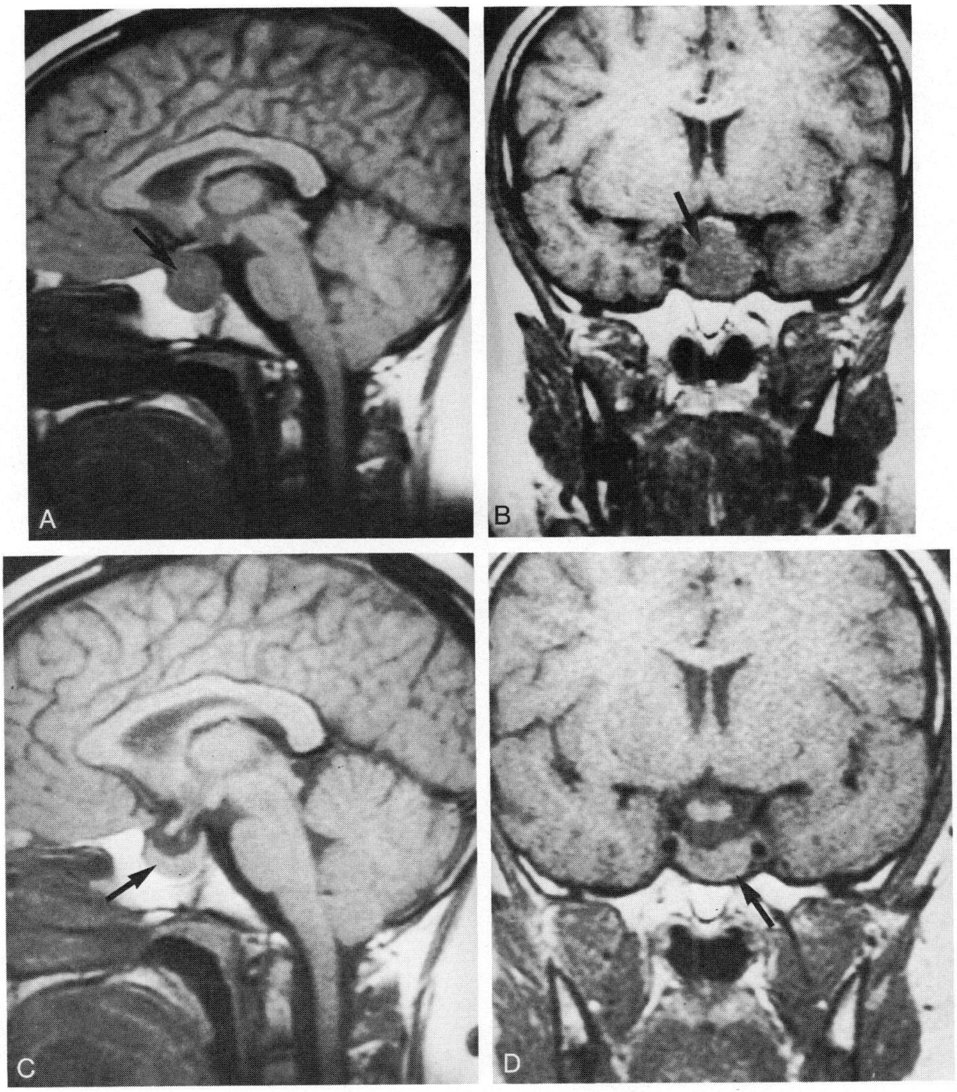

Figure 10–11. Macroadenoma; response to bromocriptine (15-year-old male).
A, Parasagittal T1. A homogeneous isointense mass *(arrow)* fills the sella and extends into the suprasellar cistern.
B, Coronal T1. Relationship of the mass *(arrow)* to the surrounding structures is more accurately depicted.
C, D, Parasagittal and coronal T1 2 months after bromocriptine therapy. Marked reduction in tumor size *(arrow)* is seen in response to treatment. There is no evidence of pituitary hemorrhage.

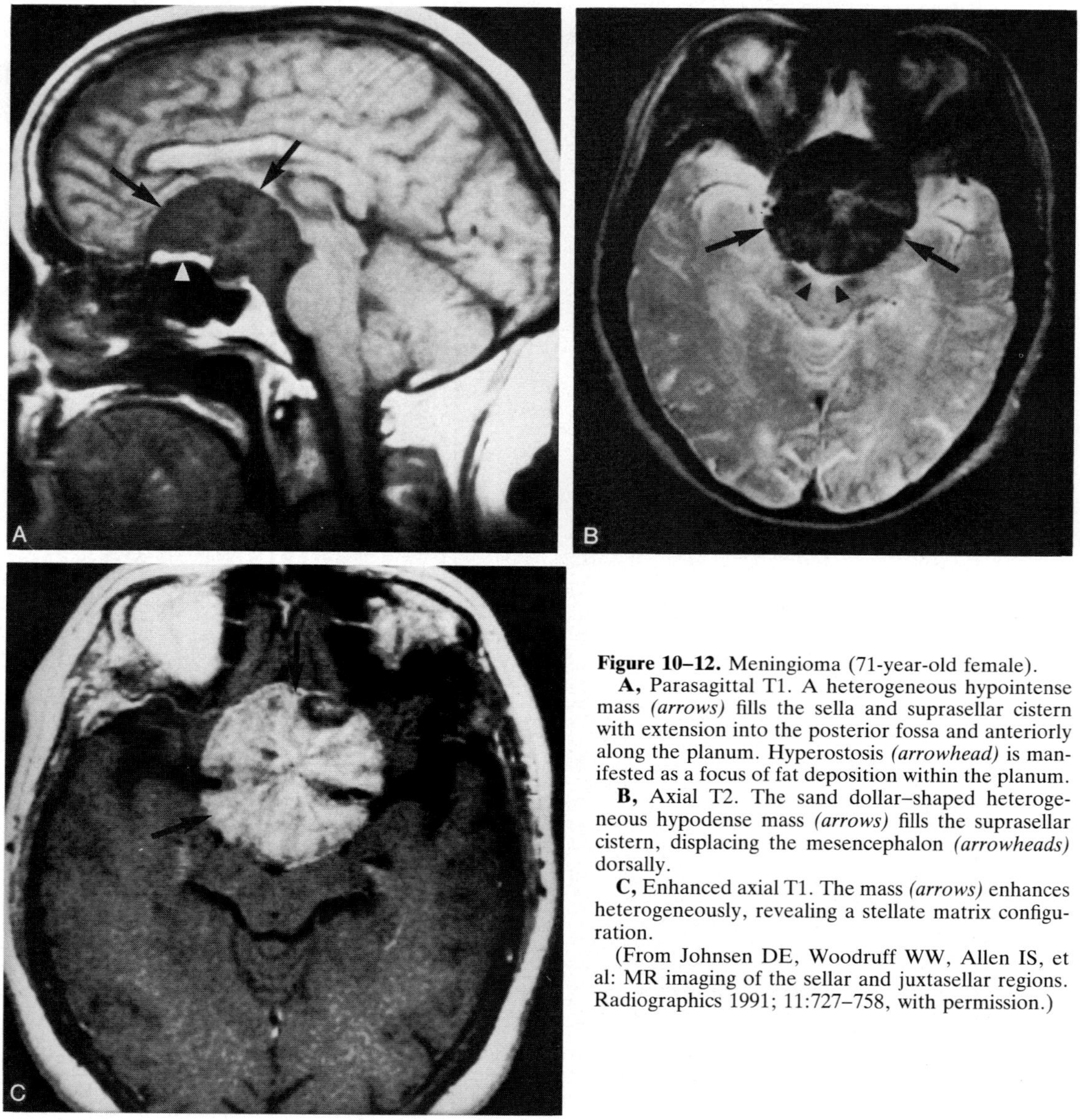

Figure 10–12. Meningioma (71-year-old female).

A, Parasagittal T1. A heterogeneous hypointense mass *(arrows)* fills the sella and suprasellar cistern with extension into the posterior fossa and anteriorly along the planum. Hyperostosis *(arrowhead)* is manifested as a focus of fat deposition within the planum.

B, Axial T2. The sand dollar–shaped heterogeneous hypodense mass *(arrows)* fills the suprasellar cistern, displacing the mesencephalon *(arrowheads)* dorsally.

C, Enhanced axial T1. The mass *(arrows)* enhances heterogeneously, revealing a stellate matrix configuration.

(From Johnsen DE, Woodruff WW, Allen IS, et al: MR imaging of the sellar and juxtasellar regions. Radiographics 1991; 11:727–758, with permission.)

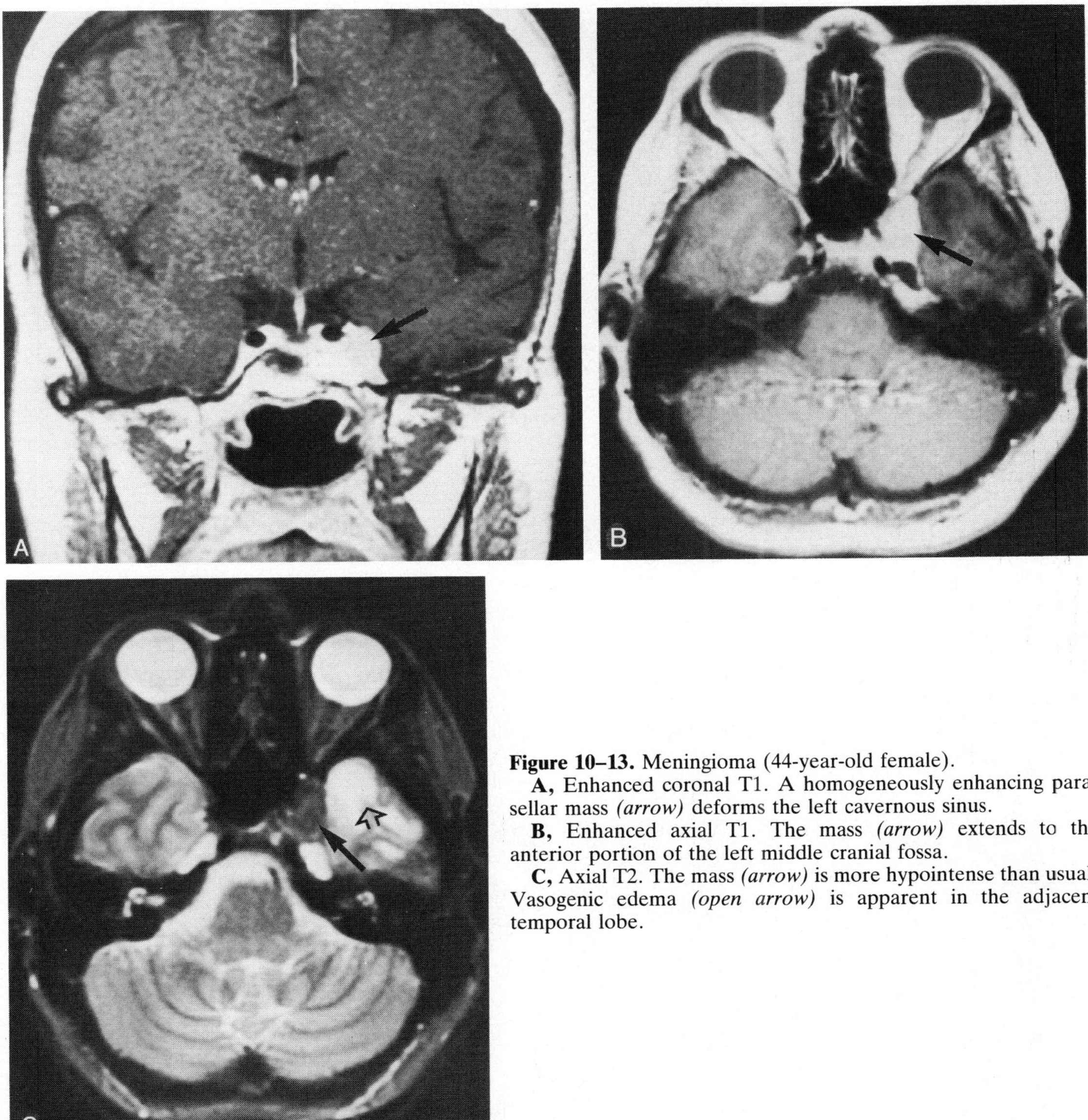

Figure 10–13. Meningioma (44-year-old female).

A, Enhanced coronal T1. A homogeneously enhancing parasellar mass *(arrow)* deforms the left cavernous sinus.

B, Enhanced axial T1. The mass *(arrow)* extends to the anterior portion of the left middle cranial fossa.

C, Axial T2. The mass *(arrow)* is more hypointense than usual. Vasogenic edema *(open arrow)* is apparent in the adjacent temporal lobe.

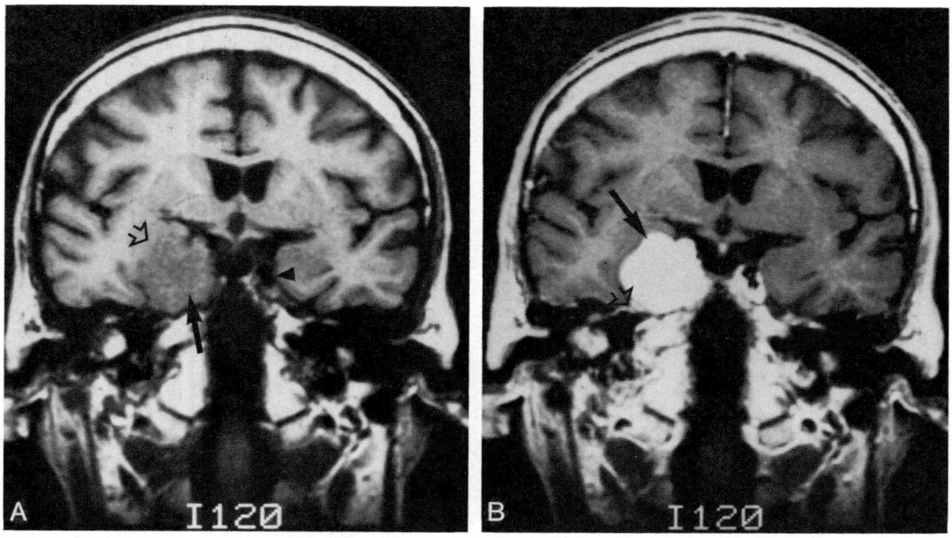

Figure 10–14. Meningioma (64-year-old female).

A, Coronal T1. An isointense–to–gray matter mass *(arrow)* fills the right cavernous sinus, displacing the uncus *(open arrow)* laterally. The flow void *(arrowhead)* identified in the contralateral carotid artery is absent on the right, secondary to invasion and occlusion.

B, Enhanced coronal T1. The mass *(arrow)* enhances homogeneously, revealing a small dural tail *(open arrow)*.

(From Johnsen DE, Woodruff WW, Allen IS, et al: MR imaging of the sellar and juxtasellar regions. Radiographics 1991; 11:727–758, with permission.)

lesions most frequently occur in patients under age 20, they may present in middle age.[28] These lesions are most commonly located between the brain and the pituitary gland and may cause visual disturbance, interruption of CSF flow, and/or hypothalamic-hypophyseal dysfunction.[28]

Plain films may demonstrate either a peripheral eggshell-type calcification or a more heterogeneous "mulberry" calcification. The sella may be enlarged secondary to direct tumor invasion or the effects of long-standing increased intracranial pressure.

Craniopharyngiomas are histologically and radiographically the most heterogeneous of all suprasellar lesions. On CT, areas of irregular calcification, hypodense cysts, and/or solid components of the mass may be identified.

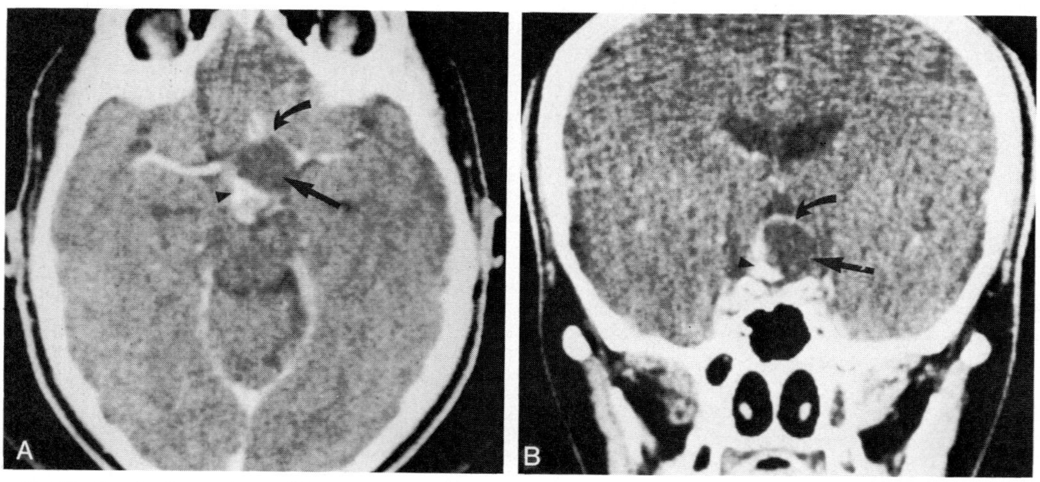

Figure 10–15. Craniopharyngioma (12-year-old male).

A, Enhanced axial CT. A heterogeneous, partially cystic *(arrow)*, partially calcified *(arrowhead)* suprasellar mass is present, with evidence of slight peripheral enhancement *(curved arrow)*.

B, Enhanced coronal CT. Calcified *(arrowhead)*, cystic *(arrow)*, and peripherally enhancing *(curved arrow)* moieties are present.

Incidence of tumoral calcification and cyst formation is twice as high (80%) when these lesions occur in childhood. The solid portion of the tumor commonly enhances after contrast administration[48] (Fig. 10–15). Twenty percent of these lesions may occur as a primary intrasellar process. Calcification and posterior superior extension of the lesion favor craniopharyngioma over adenoma[3] when this lesion involves the sella.

The MRI appearance of craniopharyngioma is variable. The T1 appearance of the lesion depends on the contents of the cysts (Figs. 10–16 to 10–18). Cholesterol or methemoglobin causes an increased signal intensity on T1 images[49]; alternatively, fluid or keratin diminishes the signal intensity on T1 images. T2 images most commonly demonstrate a lesion of high signal intensity. The presence of keratin or dense calcification will diminish the T2 signal.[49] Tumoral calcification may not be detected with MRI.

MRI has proved more efficacious than CT in evaluating the extension of the lesion into

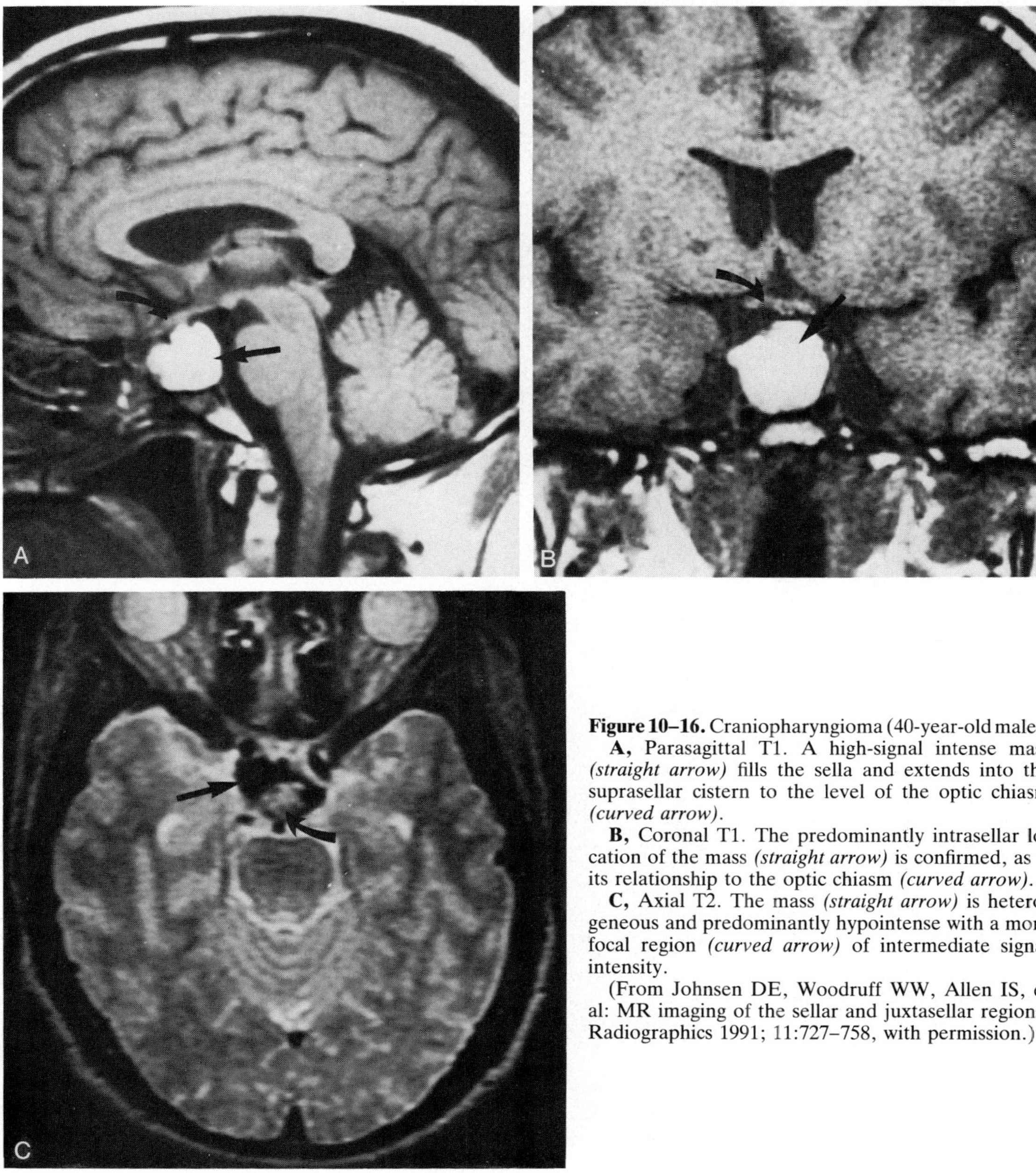

Figure 10–16. Craniopharyngioma (40-year-old male).

A, Parasagittal T1. A high-signal intense mass *(straight arrow)* fills the sella and extends into the suprasellar cistern to the level of the optic chiasm *(curved arrow)*.

B, Coronal T1. The predominantly intrasellar location of the mass *(straight arrow)* is confirmed, as is its relationship to the optic chiasm *(curved arrow)*.

C, Axial T2. The mass *(straight arrow)* is heterogeneous and predominantly hypointense with a more focal region *(curved arrow)* of intermediate signal intensity.

(From Johnsen DE, Woodruff WW, Allen IS, et al: MR imaging of the sellar and juxtasellar regions. Radiographics 1991; 11:727–758, with permission.)

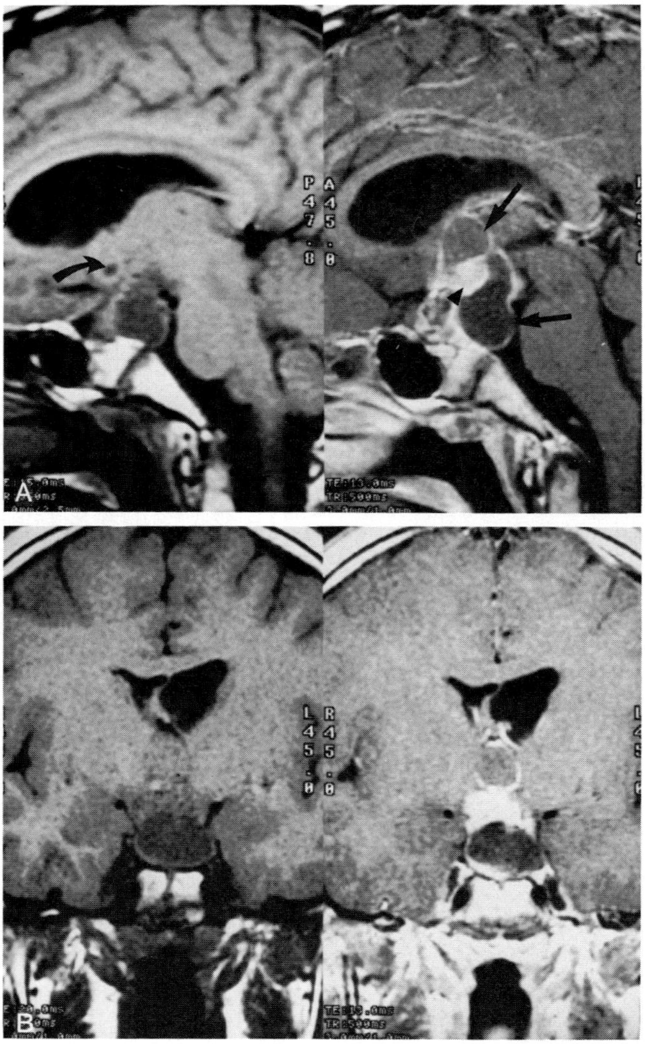

Figure 10–17. Craniopharyngioma (13-year-old female).

A, Parasagittal T1 (*left,* unenhanced; *right,* enhanced). A multicystic *(arrows),* peripherally and centrally enhancing *(arrowhead)* suprasellar mass is present. A focus of decreased signal may represent tumoral calcification *(curved arrow).* Notice the different signal intensities of the contents of the suprasellar cysts.

B, Coronal T1 (*left,* unenhanced; *right,* enhanced). The heterogeneity of the mass is corroborated.

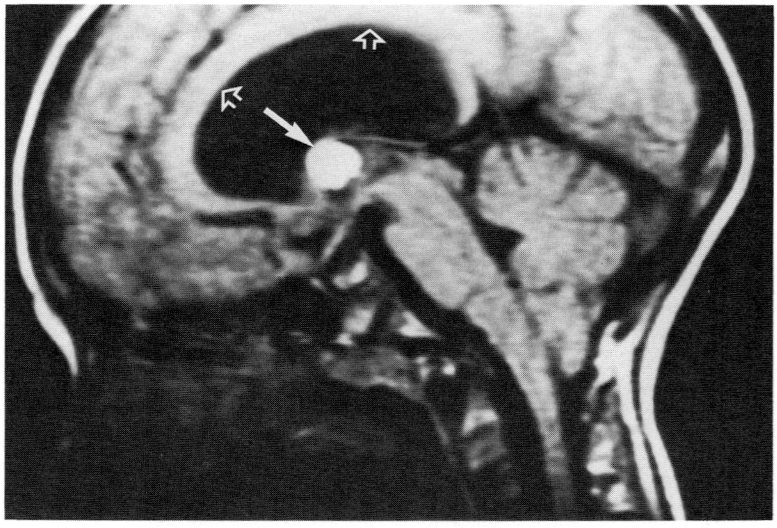

Figure 10–18. Craniopharyngioma; intraventricular (7-year-old male). Parasagittal T1; a homogeneously intense, midline periventricular mass *(solid arrow)* is present, with resultant obstructive hydrocephalus of the lateral ventricle and bowing of the corpus callosum *(open arrows).* The appearance of this lesion is more typical of a colloid cyst.

the cavernous sinus and retroclival area.[48–50] However, CT may provide a more specific diagnosis for craniopharyngioma owing to its ability to detect tumoral calcification.[48, 49]

Aneurysm

Aneurysms of the cavernous or supraclinoid ICA may present as juxtasellar masses. The aneurysms usually arise from the ICA and may be of variable size; this is the most common location for giant aneurysms (>2.5 cm). Patients may have symptoms of visual deficits or cranial nerve palsy.

CT depicts a paramedian, well-circumscribed hyperdense mass. Thrombus may form within the aneurysm, diminishing its lumen. Calcification may be detected in the wall of the aneurysm. After administration of contrast material, the patent lumen increases in density. In general, the thrombus remains hypodense. The enhancement pattern has the potential to mimic a necrotic pituitary adenoma.[4]

Marked sensitivity to flow and hemoglobin degradation products improves the specificity of MRI over CT (Figs. 10–19, 10–20). In virtually every case, MRI can obviate the need for angiography when evaluating sella or parasellar masses.[6, 50] The MRI appearance of a giant aneurysm has been described.[51] Flow void is present in cases of turbulent flow through the patent lumen. In regions of slow flow, even echo rephasing may occur in late echo images. Thrombus appears as alternating areas of medium to high signal intensity on T1 and low signal on T2 images, representing areas of methemoglobin and hemosiderin.

UNCOMMON PATHOLOGY

Optic Chiasm Glioma

Optic chiasm gliomas are generally low-grade astrocytic neoplasms occurring in childhood.[28] These tumors may extend through the optic canal to the optic chiasm and along the optic tracks. Bilaterality corroborates a diagnosis of neurofibromatosis (type I). The optic chiasm is also the site of a more malignant form of this lesion, which occurs in adults.[28] Patients usually present with decreasing visual acuity.

The optic chiasm may be enlarged. CT demonstrates hypodense to isodense lesions that generally enhance following contrast administration.[52] A minimally enhancing intraconal mass with concomitant proptosis may be detected in the orbit. MRI more accurately delineates optic chiasm enlargement and extension along the optic tracts as hypointense on T1 and hyperintense on T2 images (Fig. 10–21). The mass may enhance minimally.

Hypothalamic Glioma

Hypothalamic gliomas are tumors of childhood or adolescence. These patients usually present with hydrocephalus, diencephalic syndrome, or diabetes insipidus.

CT demonstrates an isodense-to-brain, noncalcified soft tissue mass with variable enhancement. MRI demonstrates a mass that is hypointense on T1 and hyperintense on T2 images[6] (Fig. 10–22). The mass may extend into the suprasellar cistern or the brain parenchyma, or both. The sella and hypophysis are usually normal despite the suprasellar mass. Enhancement is variable and may not be present (Fig. 10–23).

Chordoma

Chordomas are slowly growing neoplasms that arise from notochord remnants. Thirty-five percent arise along the clivus, the second most common site of chordoma origin after the sacrum.[28] Chordomas are twice as common in males and peak in the third to seventh decades.

CT demonstrates a mass of variable size, near the clivus, paramedian or midline in location. The mass is usually hyperdense to brain and locally aggressive with bone destruction. Calcification is present in 75% of patients, secondary to tumoral calcification formation or sequestered bone.[53] CT accurately depicts the bony changes. Contrast enhancement is present in nearly every case.

MRI demonstrates a mass that is nearly always high signal on T2 images (Fig. 10–24). On T1 images 75% of the lesions are isointense to brain; the remainder are hypointense.[54] MRI may help distinguish the typical physaliphorous subset (4-year survival) from the

Text continued on page 366

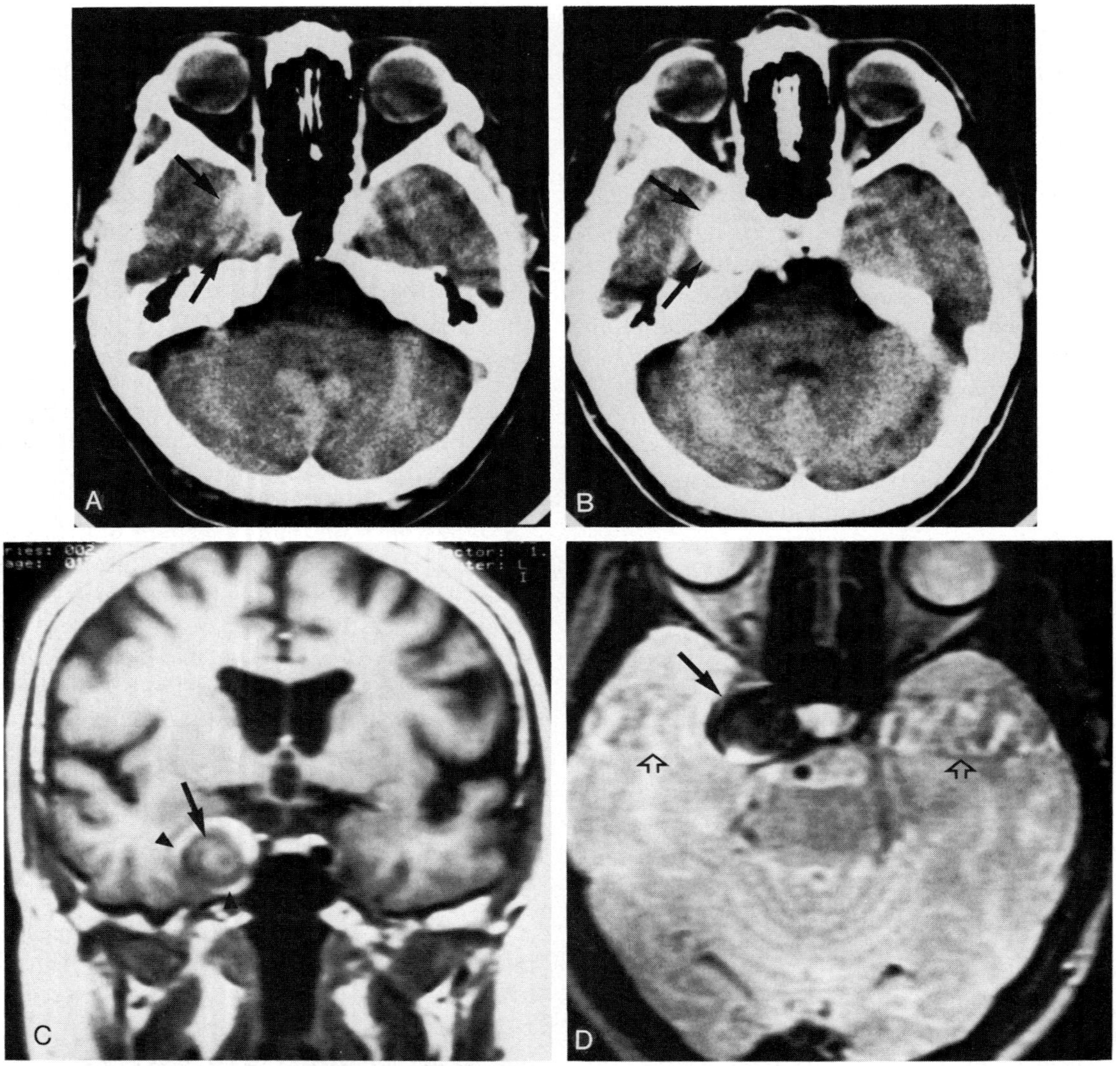

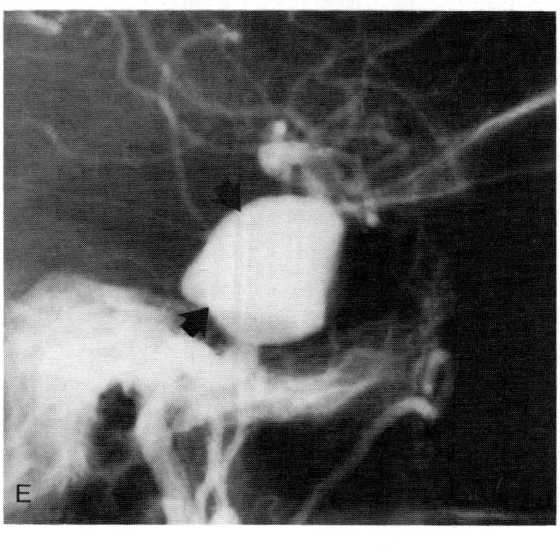

Figure 10–19. Aneurysm (73-year-old female).

A, Unenhanced CT. A poorly defined, intrinsically dense right cavernous sinus mass *(arrows)* is present.

B, Enhanced CT. The mass *(arrows)* enhances homogeneously, revealing a clearly defined lateral border.

C, Coronal T1. Heterogeneous signal *(arrow)* is secondary to turbulent flow. High-signal methemoglobin *(arrowheads)* is seen around the periphery of the aneurysm.

D, Axial T2. Flow void is noted within the aneurysm *(arrow),* as is flow artifact *(open arrows)* in the phase-encoded direction.

E, Right lateral common carotid angiogram reveals a large cavernous carotid aneurysm *(arrows).*

(From Johnsen DE, Woodruff WW, Allen IS, et al: MR imaging of the sellar and juxtasellar regions. Radiographics 1991; 11:727–758, with permission.)

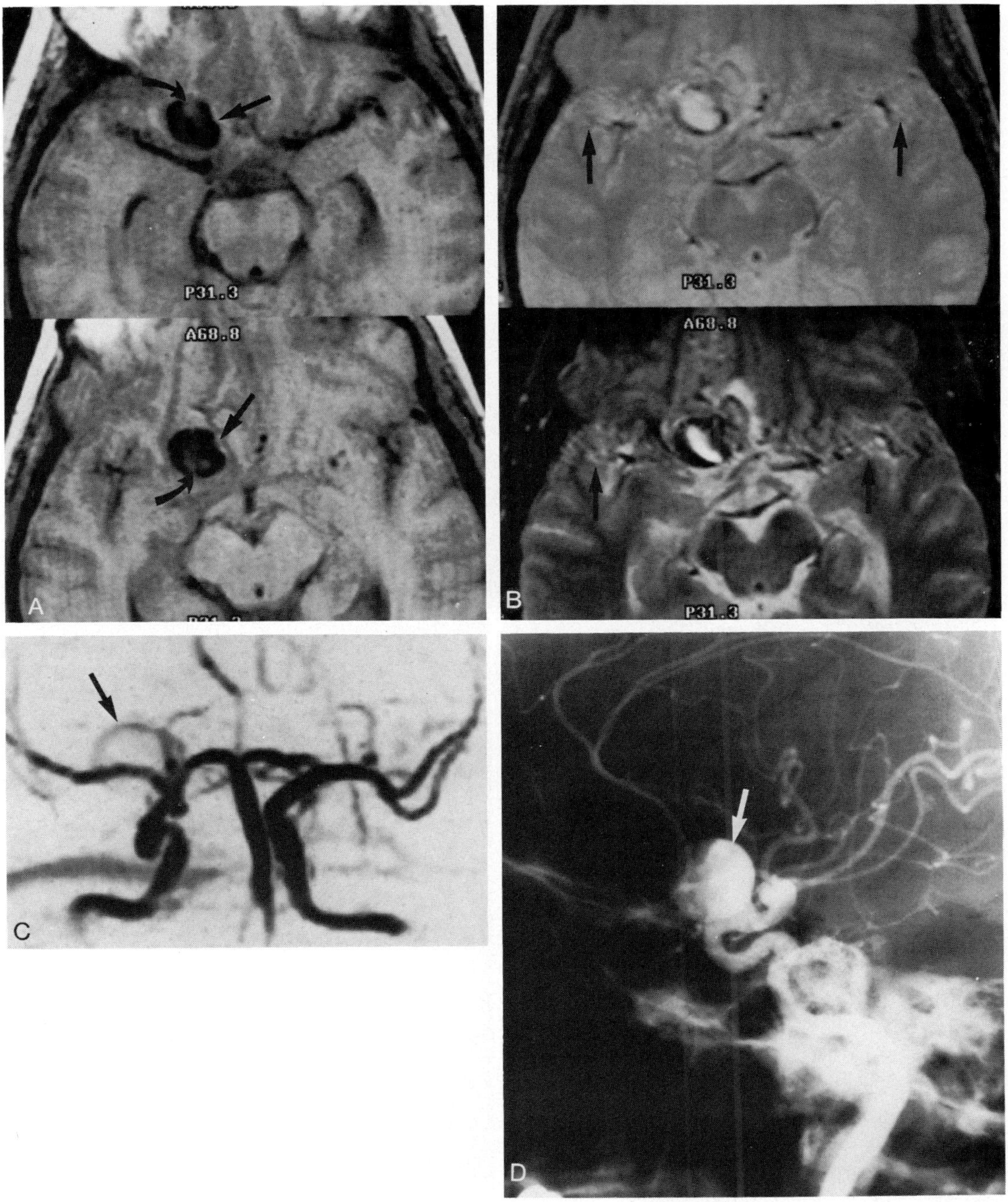

Figure 10–20. Aneurysm (45-year-old female).

A, Axial T1. A well-marginated focus *(arrow)* of flow void is present in the right parasellar region. Turbulence creates an intermediate signal *(curved arrow)* within the aneurysm.

B, Axial spin density (SD) *(top)* and T2 *(bottom)*. Flow artifact *(arrows)* is present in the phase-encoded direction. Flow and turbulence accounts for the signal changes within the aneurysm.

C, Frontal view 3-dimensional (3D) phase contrast magnetic resonance angiography (MRA). The rim of the aneurysm *(arrow)* can be detected.

D, Lateral right ICA arteriogram. A solitary supraclinoid artery aneurysm is opacified *(arrow)*.

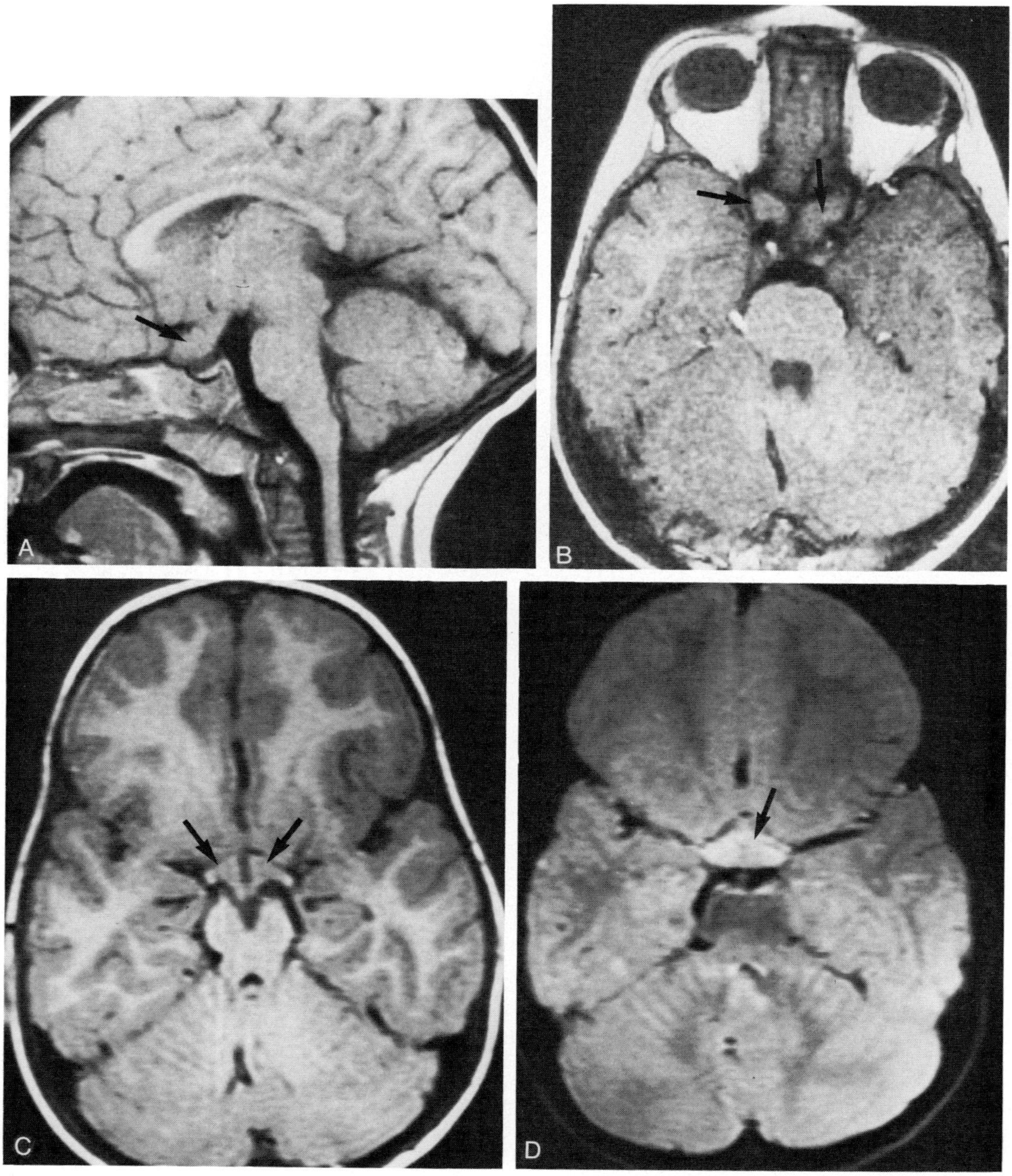

Figure 10–21. Optic chiasm glioma (18-month-old male).

A, Parasagittal T1. The optic chiasm *(arrow)* is enlarged three to four times its normal size.

B, Axial T1. The dorsal-most optic nerves *(arrows)* are enlarged bilaterally.

C, Axial T1. The proximal optic tracts *(arrows)* are also enlarged.

D, Axial SD. The signal intensity and the size of the optic chiasm *(arrow)* are abnormal, secondary to gliosis, tumor, or edema.

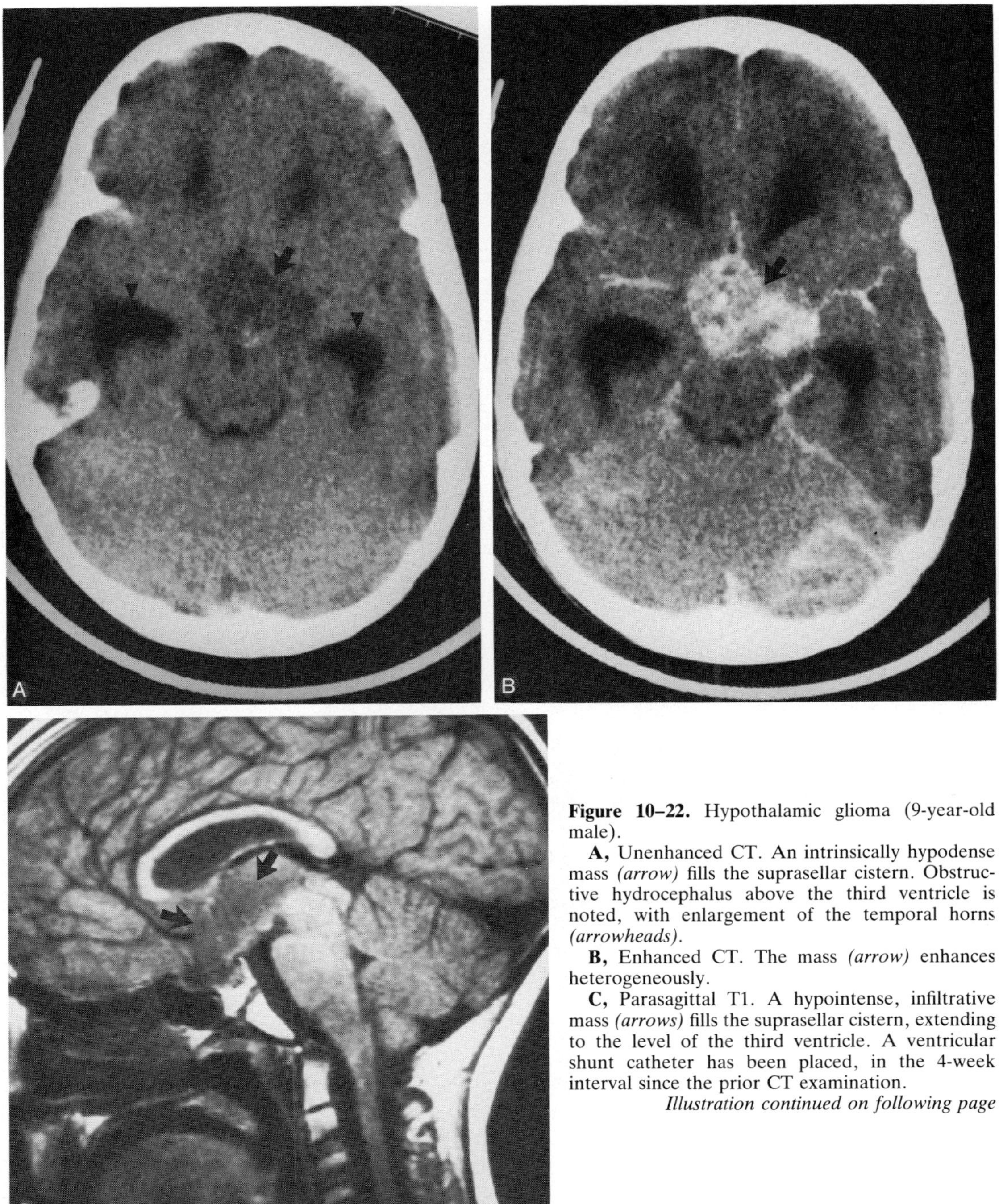

Figure 10–22. Hypothalamic glioma (9-year-old male).

A, Unenhanced CT. An intrinsically hypodense mass *(arrow)* fills the suprasellar cistern. Obstructive hydrocephalus above the third ventricle is noted, with enlargement of the temporal horns *(arrowheads)*.

B, Enhanced CT. The mass *(arrow)* enhances heterogeneously.

C, Parasagittal T1. A hypointense, infiltrative mass *(arrows)* fills the suprasellar cistern, extending to the level of the third ventricle. A ventricular shunt catheter has been placed, in the 4-week interval since the prior CT examination.

Illustration continued on following page

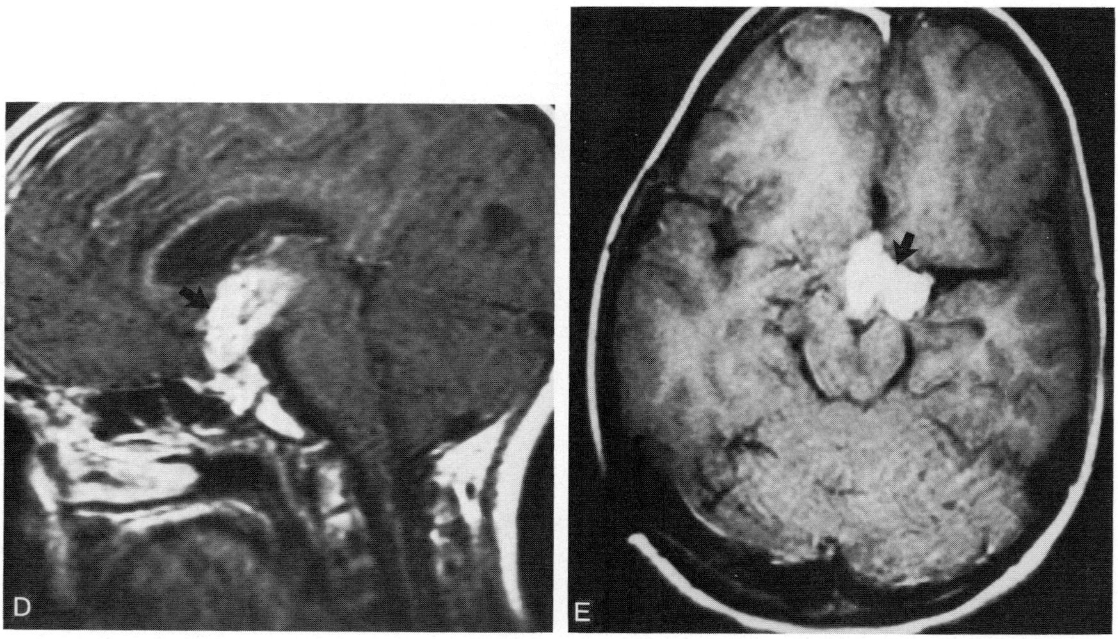

Figure 10–22 *Continued*

D, Enhanced parasagittal T1. Although degraded by motion, the boundaries of the tumor are more readily apparent (*arrow*).

E, Enhanced axial T1. The mass *(arrow)* has decreased in size over the 1-month treatment period and now enhances homogeneously.

(From Johnsen DE, Woodruff WW, Allen IS, et al: MR imaging of the sellar and juxtasellar regions. Radiographics 1991; 11:727–758, with permission.)

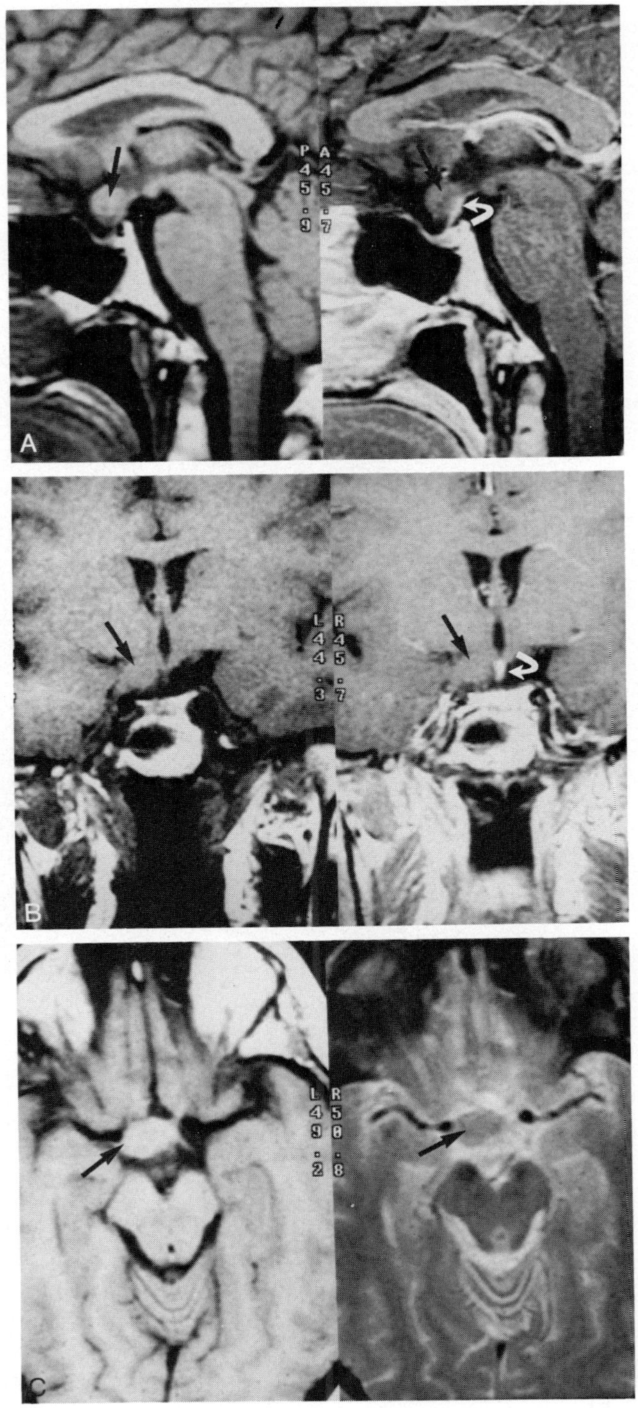

Figure 10–23. Hypothalamic glioma (20-year-old male).

A, Parasagittal T1 (*left,* unenhanced; *right,* enhanced). A 1-cm suprasellar mass *(arrows)* is present. The enhancing infundibulum *(curved arrow)* is located adjacent to the nonenhancing mass.

B, Coronal T1 (*left,* unenhanced; *right,* enhanced). The relationship of the eccentric tumor *(arrows)* and infundibulum *(curved arrow)* is more apparent.

C, Axial SD *(left)* and T2 *(right)*. The suprasellar mass *(arrows)* remains isointense to the adjacent parenchyma.

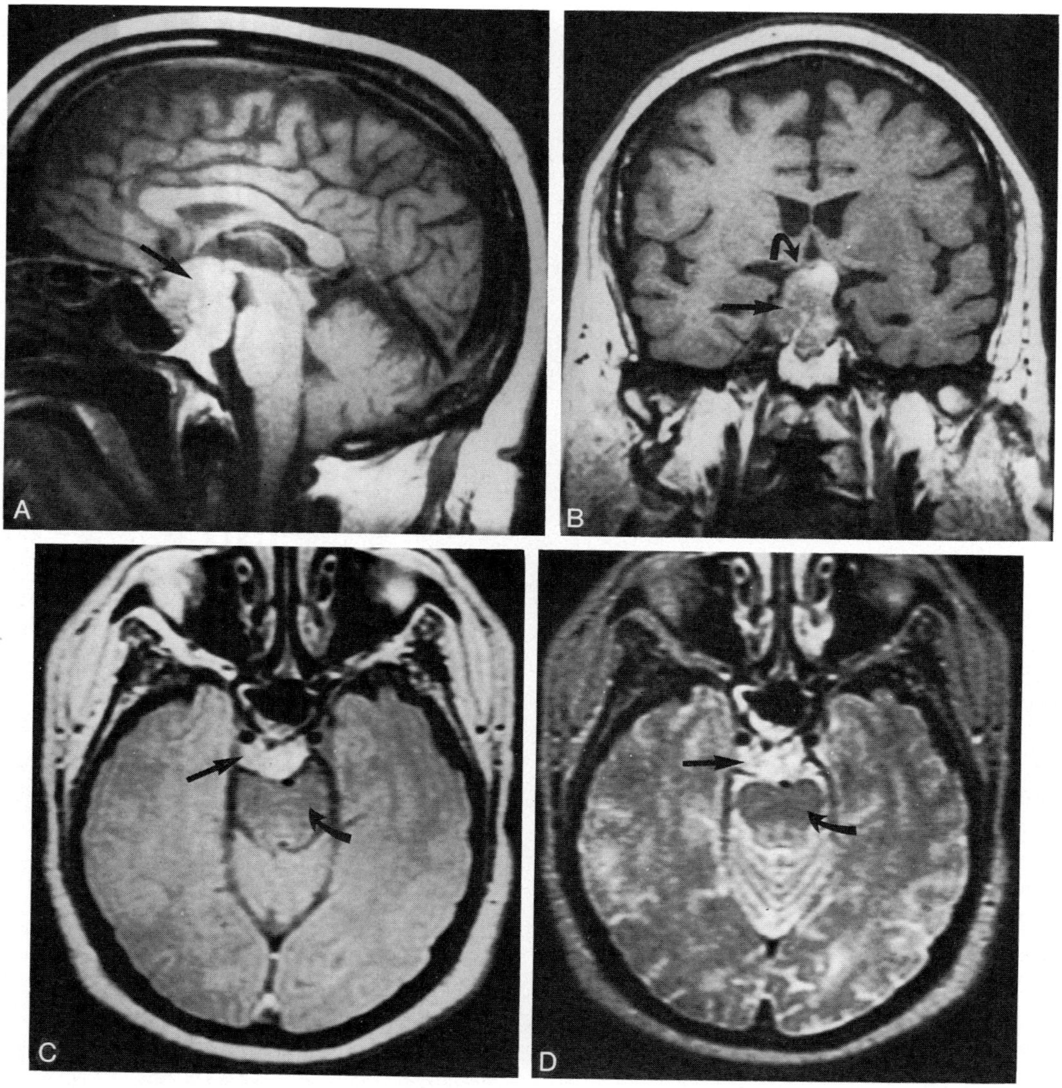

Figure 10–24. Chordoma (64-year-old male).

A, Parasagittal T1. A lobulated heterogeneous signal mass *(arrow)* arises from the clivus. The clivus is destroyed as the mass extends into the posterior fossa as well as the suprasellar cistern.

B, Coronal T1. The suprasellar extent of the mass *(straight arrow)* and displacement of the optic chiasm *(curved arrow)* are noted.

C, D, Axial SD and T2. The heterogeneous mass *(straight arrow)*, which is principally high signal, destroys the clivus and displaces the pons *(curved arrow)* dorsally.

chondroid chordoma (16-year survival). Chondroid chordomas contain cartilage that shortens the T1 and T2 relaxation times referable to the physaliphorous chordomas.

Hypothalamic Hamartoma

Hypothalamic hamartomas consist of congenital heterotopic gray matter that originates in the hypothalamus. These sessile or pedunculated masses may extend ventrally from the tuber cinereum.

Patients usually come to medical attention by age 10. Hamartomas are most often pedunculated and associated with precocious puberty. Patients with the less common sessile type may present with seizures.[55]

The typical CT appearance consists of an isodense-to-brain, nonenhancing soft tissue mass within the interpeduncular cistern.[56] The mass may be a few millimeters to a few centimeters in greatest dimension.

MRI provides better definition of the mass and its relationship to the tuber cinereum and mammillary bodies. The mass is usually isointense to gray matter on T1 and hyperintense to gray matter on T2 images[55–57] (Fig. 10–25). The mass does not enhance after administration of gadolinium.

Rathke's Cleft Cyst

As the invaginating Rathke's pouch ascends to the sella, it loses its communication with the primitive oral cavity. Upon reaching the sella, the anterior wall of the pouch proliferates to become the anterior lobe (adenohypophysis) and pars tuberalis. The posterior wall gives rise to the intermediate lobe of the gland. As the anterior wall of the pouch proliferates, the central lumen diminishes in size to become Rathke's cleft.[1] The cells of Rathke's cleft give rise to a spectrum of epithelial cysts from the single-walled Rathke's cleft cyst to the most complex of these epithelial neoplasms, the craniopharyngioma.[58]

Rathke's cleft cysts are rare lesions that most commonly are incidental postmortem findings. Infrequently, these cysts may grow large enough to compress the pituitary gland, optic chiasm, or hypothalamus.[28] Patients may present with hypopituitarism, diabetes insipidus, visual disturbances, or headache.[58]

The radiographic appearance of the lesion depends on the complexity of the wall of the cyst as well as the contents secreted by the cells lining the cyst. The cyst is usually located in the anterior portion of the sella and suprasellar cistern. CT most often demonstrates a homogeneous hypodense intrasellar cyst. The capsule of the cyst may enhance. Serous fluid–containing cysts are isointense to CSF on all spin echo MRI sequences (Fig. 10–26). Alternatively, the cysts may contain cholesterol, rendering the lesion hyperintense on T1 images (Fig. 10–27). The more complex the cyst wall, the more heterogeneous its contents. Complex cysts may perhaps represent a transition between Rathke's cleft cysts and craniopharyngiomas and will appear as peripherally enhancing masses that are isodense to slightly hyperdense to brain on CT. The MRI appearance of these lesions varies, with heterogeneous mixed intensities on T1 and T2 images.[58, 59]

Empty Sella

Although empty sella is not a true neoplasm, these patients may present with signs and

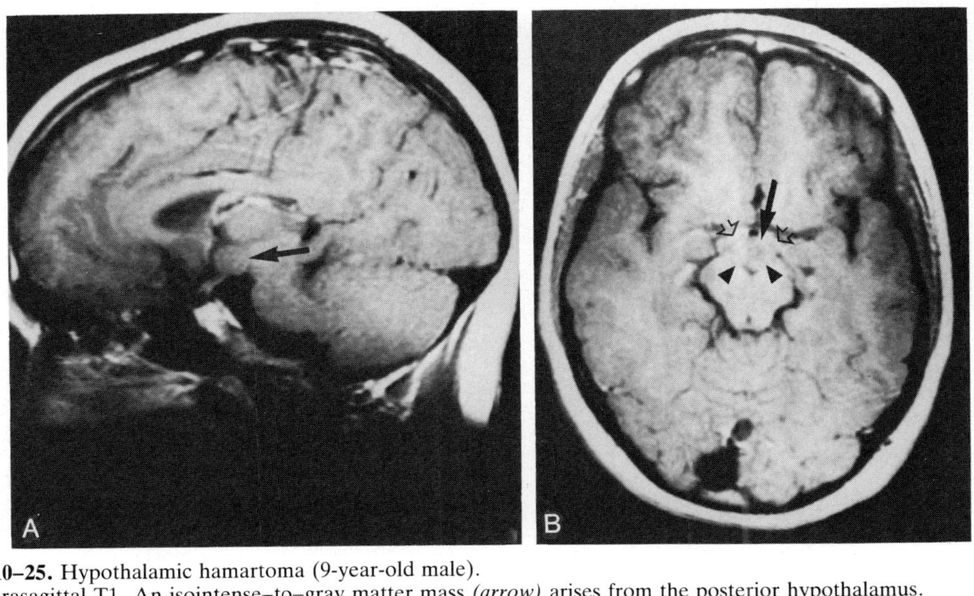

Figure 10–25. Hypothalamic hamartoma (9-year-old male).

A, Parasagittal T1. An isointense–to–gray matter mass *(arrow)* arises from the posterior hypothalamus.

B, Axial T1. The mass *(arrow)* fills the posterior suprasellar cistern and interpeduncular cistern. The proximal optic tract *(open arrows)* and cerebral peduncles *(arrowheads)* surround the mass.

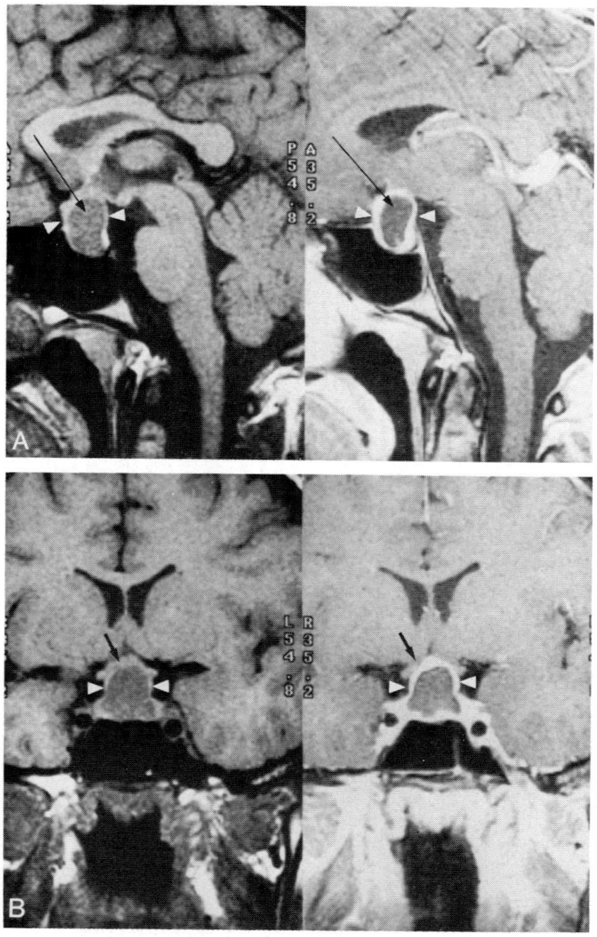

Figure 10–26. Rathke's cleft cyst (22-year-old female).

A, Parasagittal T1 (*left,* unenhanced; *right,* enhanced). An isointense-to-parenchyma intrasellar mass *(arrow)* has extended into the suprasellar cistern. The mass is surrounded by a thin capsule *(arrowheads)* that enhances.

B, Coronal T1 (*left,* unenhanced; *right,* enhanced). The relationship between the elevated optic chiasm *(arrow)* and the peripherally enhancing mass *(arrowheads)* is demonstrated.

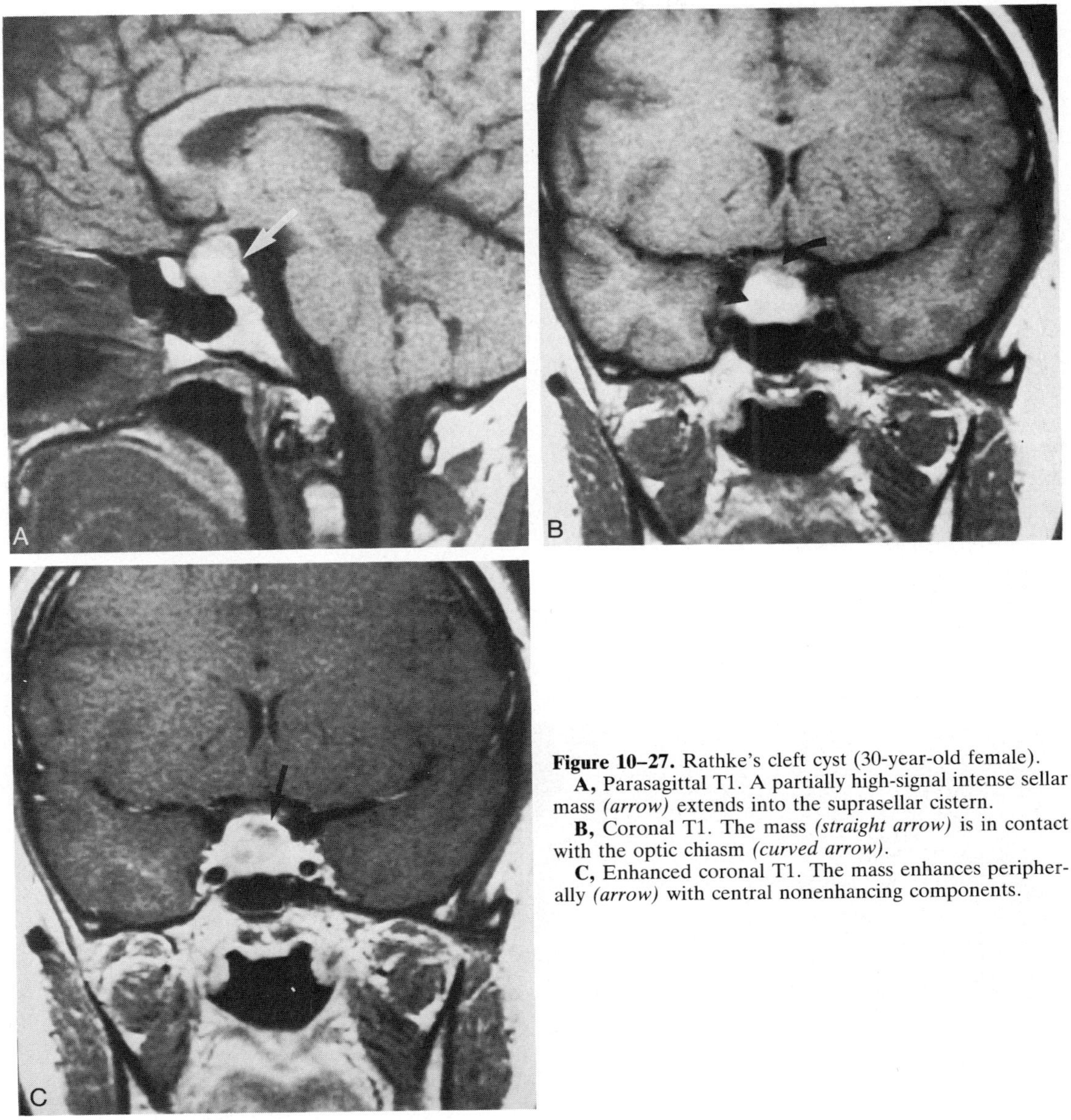

Figure 10–27. Rathke's cleft cyst (30-year-old female).

A, Parasagittal T1. A partially high-signal intense sellar mass *(arrow)* extends into the suprasellar cistern.

B, Coronal T1. The mass *(straight arrow)* is in contact with the optic chiasm *(curved arrow)*.

C, Enhanced coronal T1. The mass enhances peripherally *(arrow)* with central nonenhancing components.

symptoms of suprasellar mass. The empty sella may occur in patients as a primary or secondary phenomenon. Primary empty sella originates from a congenital defect in the diaphragma sellae, with resultant extension of CSF into the sella. Consequently, there may be enlargement of the sella turcica and compression of the normal gland into the posterior inferior aspect of the sellar floor. The optic chiasm and/or third ventricle rarely herniate into the sella in primary empty sella.

Secondary empty sella results from a specific cause. Most commonly, remote surgery, radiation, infarction of the gland, or infection may be implicated. CSF extends into the sella, the sella may be remodeled, and the gland is compressed. Optic chiasm herniation is more commonly associated with secondary empty sella, although the visual disturbances in these patients are not indicative of the presence or degree of herniation of the optic chiasm.[60]

Plain films and CT demonstrate sellar enlargement with remodeling of the floor and dorsum sella. With planar imaging, the gland may be identified along the posterior inferior sella, and the infundibulum may be identified extending into the sella.[4]

MRI more accurately depicts the repositioned gland, course of the infundibulum, and herniation of the optic chiasm into the sella (Figs. 10–28, 10–29).

Arachnoid Cyst

Arachnoid cysts are loculated collections of CSF within arachnoid membranes. These cysts most commonly occur in the middle cranial fossa and may extend secondarily into the suprasellar cistern. Alternatively, these cysts may occur primarily within the suprasellar cistern or the sella, displacing the adjacent sutures. Arachnoid cysts may be congenital or acquired and may attain sufficient size to cause symptoms related to the optic apparatus or hypothalamic hypophyseal axis.[61]

CT demonstrates a nonenhancing isodense-to-CSF mass and commensurate displacement of surrounding structures. Diagnosis may require intrathecal contrast administration.

MRI shows a smoothly marginated isointense-to-CSF mass[62] (Figs. 10–30, 10–31). The extra-axial origin and degree of mass effect are more accurately depicted with MRI. A primary intrasellar arachnoid cyst can be differentiated from an empty sella by the displacement of the gland and infundibulum out of the sella, a finding that occurs only in the former condition.

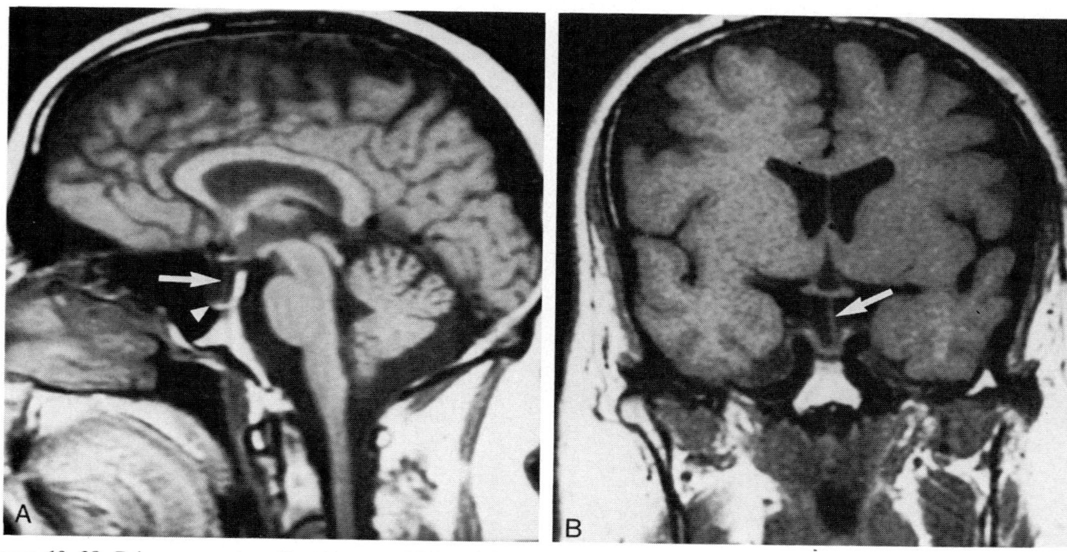

Figure 10–28. Primary empty sella (44-year-old female).

A, Parasagittal T1. The sella is enlarged, and the infundibulum *(arrow)* terminates in a small focus of glandular tissue *(arrowhead)*.

B, Coronal T1. The course of the infundibulum *(arrow)* and its termination in the sella are confirmed.

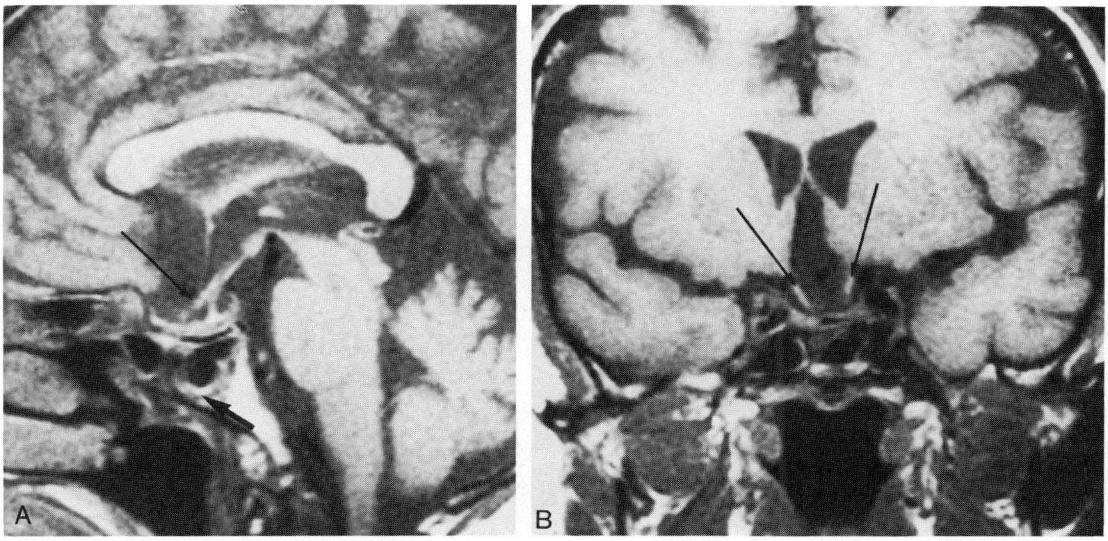

Figure 10–29. Secondary empty sella (37-year-old female).

A, Parasagittal T1. The sella is shallow and elongated, and postsurgical changes *(short arrow)* are noted in the sphenoid sinus. The optic chiasm *(long arrow)* has herniated into the sella.

B, Coronal T1. Herniation of the optic apparatus *(arrows)* into the sella is confirmed.

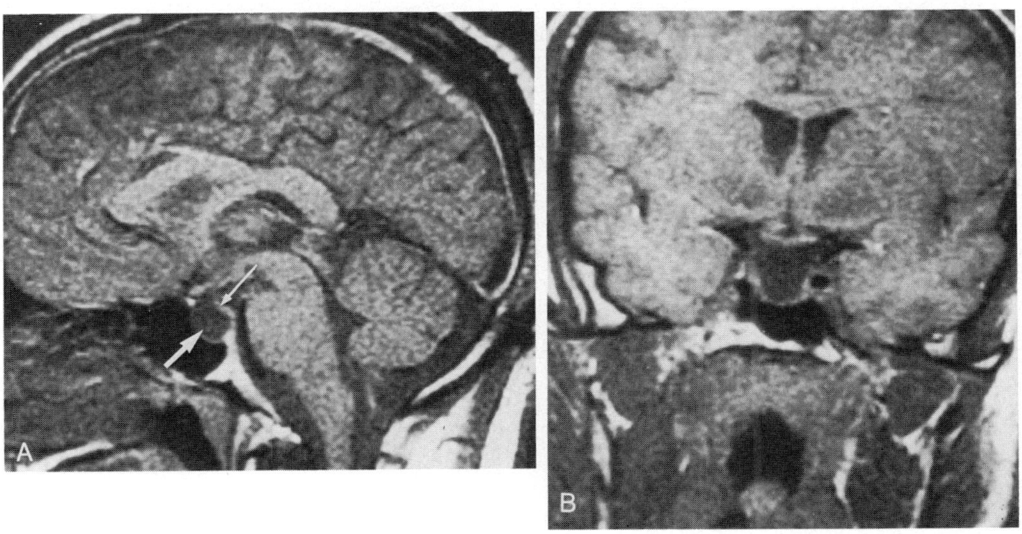

Figure 10–30. Intrasellar arachnoid cyst (45-year-old male).

A, Parasagittal T1. Cerebrospinal fluid (CSF)-signal-intensity material fills the slightly enlarged sella *(thick arrow)*. The local mass effect is corroborated by cephalad-dorsal displacement of the infundibulum and the atretic gland *(thin arrow)*.

B, Coronal T1. The infundibulum cannot be identified within the sella.

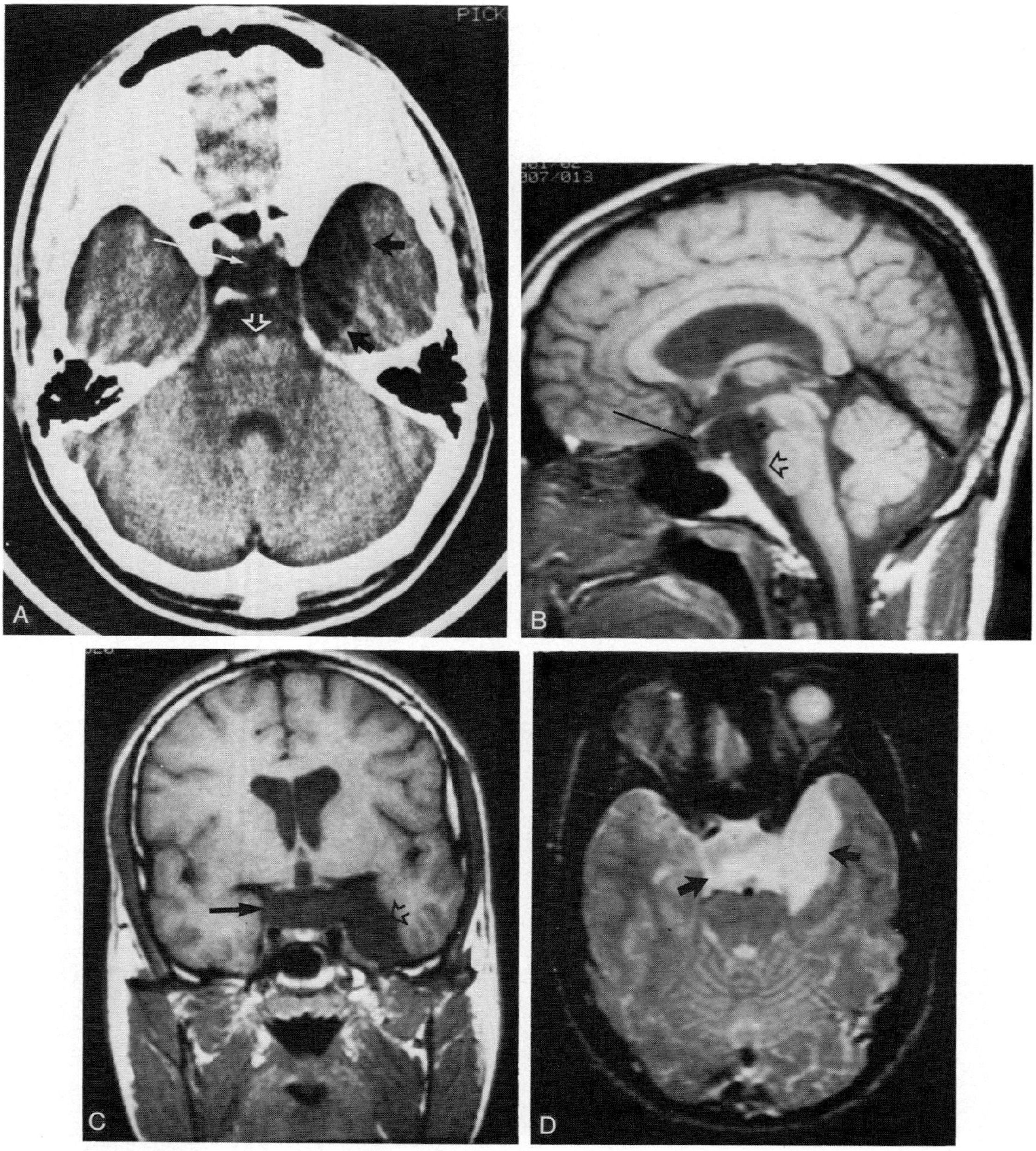

Figure 10–31. Arachnoid cyst (24-year-old male).

A, Enhanced CT. An isodense-to-CSF, well-circumscribed cyst *(black arrows)* fills the left middle cranial fossa and suprasellar cistern. The infundibulum *(long arrow)* is displaced ventrally, and the pons *(open arrow)* is displaced dorsally.

B, Parasagittal T1. The isointense-to-CSF mass displaces the infundibulum *(long arrow)* and pons *(open arrow)*.

C, Coronal T1. The suprasellar *(solid arrow)* and juxtasellar *(open arrow)* extent of the mass is apparent.

D, Axial T2. The mass (*arrows*) remains isointense to CSF.

Metastatic Disease

Metastatic disease may occur in the suprasellar cistern with primary involvement of the infundibulum. The patient may present with disruption of the hypothalamohypophyseal axis or visual symptoms or both. Corroborative history is helpful in securing the diagnosis. The infundibulum may be enlarged and a discrete enhancing mass may be identified. The degree of involvement is more effectively evaluated with MRI (Fig. 10–32).

Metastatic disease may also occur in the cavernous sinus, adjacent dura, and bone. The mode of transmission to the cavernous sinus varies. Hematogenous metastasis usually indicates advanced disease and heralds a poor prognosis.[63] A primary tumor from the sphenoid sinus or nasopharynx may also invade the cavernous sinus via direct extension. Metastatic disease may arrive in the cavernous sinus through the cranial nerves in the form of perineural tumor extension.[64] Pterygopalatine soft tissue involvement may corroborate the diagnosis. Planar imaging demonstrates a mass that may cause asymmetric convexity of the cavernous sinus (Fig. 10–33).

Granulomatous Disease

Tuberculosis or sarcoidosis may involve the suprasellar cistern and infundibulum. Corroborative history is useful in securing the diagnosis. The infundibulum may be selectively enlarged. The sarcoid patient presenting with diabetes insipidus and chiasmal dysfunction has a high likelihood of CNS involvement.[65]

The mass may be isodense to brain and may enhance vividly on CT.[66] MRI will more accurately depict the suprasellar cistern and involvement of its contents. The mass is generally isointense to brain on T1 and hyperintense on T2. Contrast enhancement is readily depicted on T1 (Fig. 10–34). Parenchymal granulomas or infarcts may support the diagnosis of basilar leptomeningeal disease.

Germ Cell Tumor

This is the most frequently occurring neoplasm of the pineal region, and when it occurs in the suprasellar cistern it is often called an ectopic pinealoma. The parasellar region is the most common location for intracranial germinoma in females. Lesions that occur primarily within the pineal gland may have secondary spread to the suprasellar region. This most commonly occurs in children who may present with diabetes insipidus and later visual loss and hypopituitarism.[28] The tumor is generally adherent to the optic chiasm and undersurface of the brain and may completely fill the suprasellar cistern.

Text continued on page 379

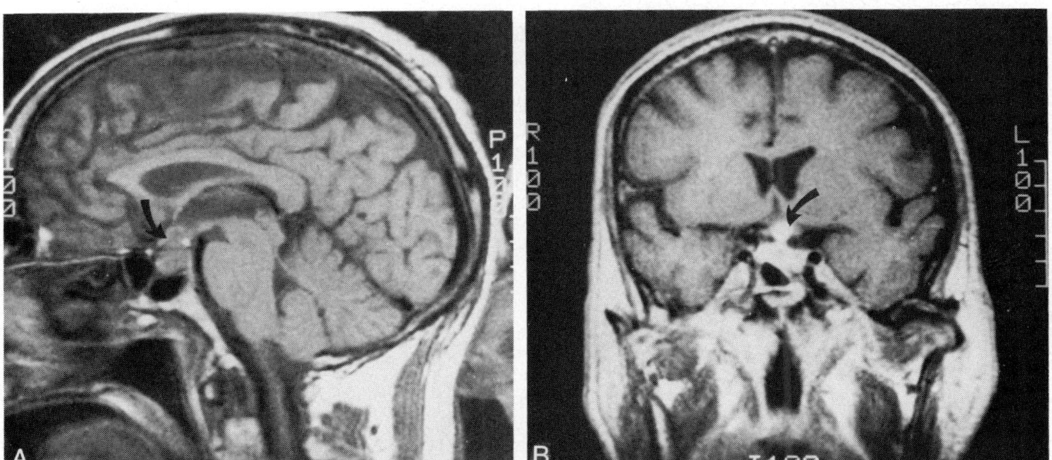

Figure 10–32. Metastatic small cell carcinoma from the lung (64-year-old male).

A, Parasagittal T1. An isointense-to-parenchyma mass *(arrow)* fills the suprasellar cistern, extending from the gland to the third ventricle.

B, Enhanced coronal T1. The infundibulum *(arrow)* is enlarged and enhances homogeneously.

(From Johnsen DE, Woodruff WW, Allen IS, et al: MR imaging of the sellar and juxtasellar regions. Radiographics 1991; 11:727–758, with permission.)

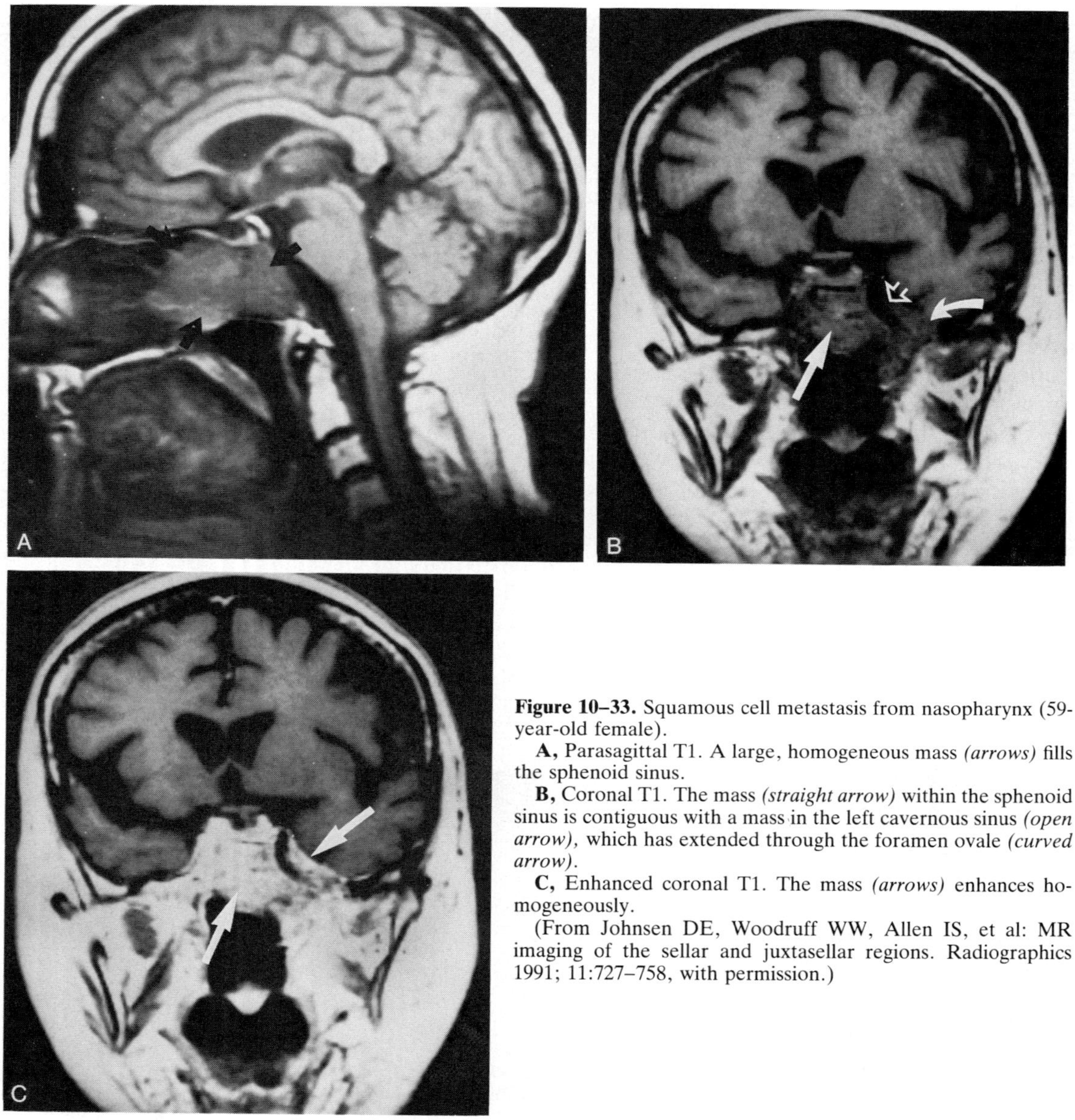

Figure 10–33. Squamous cell metastasis from nasopharynx (59-year-old female).

A, Parasagittal T1. A large, homogeneous mass *(arrows)* fills the sphenoid sinus.

B, Coronal T1. The mass *(straight arrow)* within the sphenoid sinus is contiguous with a mass in the left cavernous sinus *(open arrow),* which has extended through the foramen ovale *(curved arrow).*

C, Enhanced coronal T1. The mass *(arrows)* enhances homogeneously.

(From Johnsen DE, Woodruff WW, Allen IS, et al: MR imaging of the sellar and juxtasellar regions. Radiographics 1991; 11:727–758, with permission.)

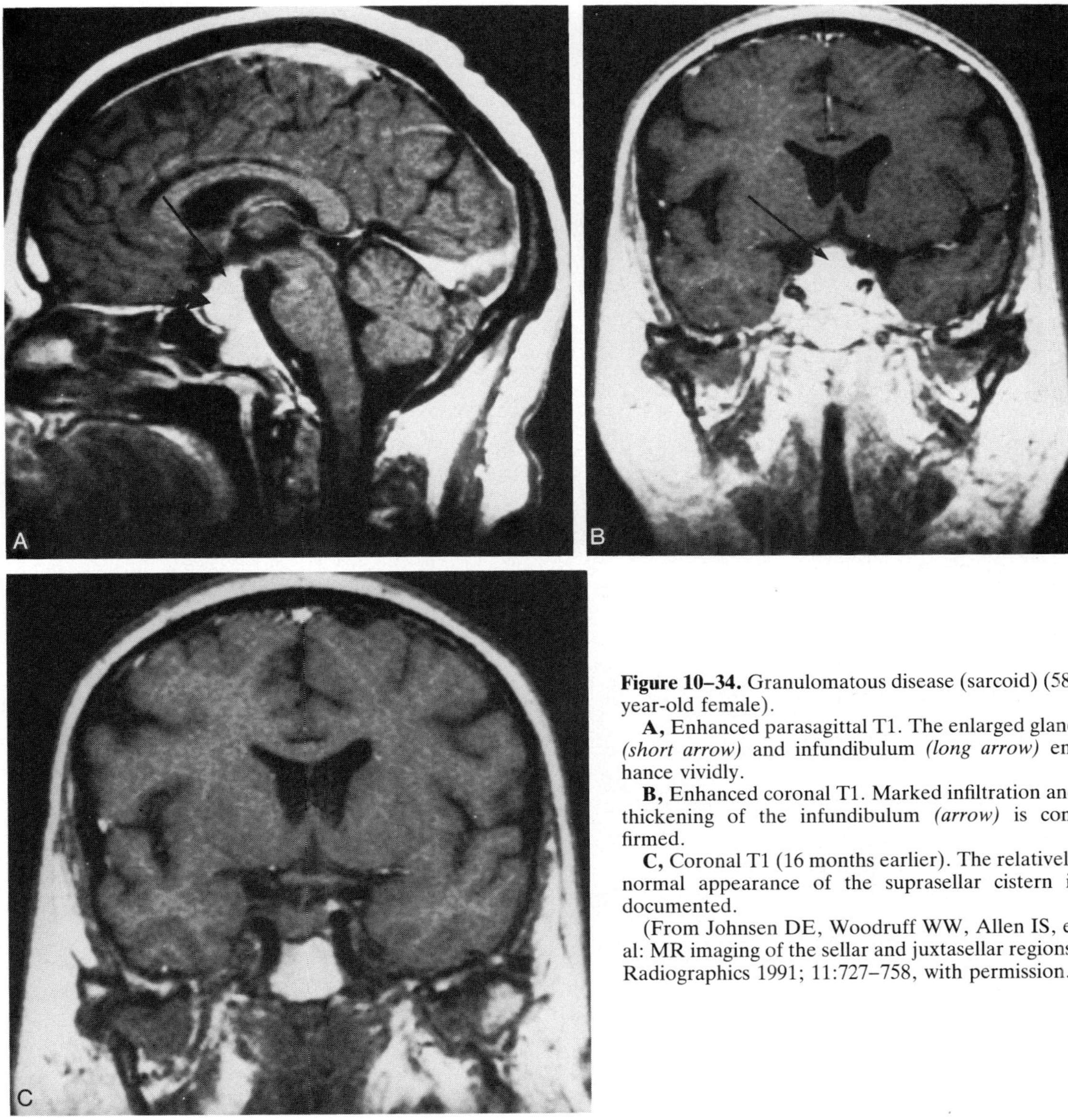

Figure 10–34. Granulomatous disease (sarcoid) (58-year-old female).

A, Enhanced parasagittal T1. The enlarged gland *(short arrow)* and infundibulum *(long arrow)* enhance vividly.

B, Enhanced coronal T1. Marked infiltration and thickening of the infundibulum *(arrow)* is confirmed.

C, Coronal T1 (16 months earlier). The relatively normal appearance of the suprasellar cistern is documented.

(From Johnsen DE, Woodruff WW, Allen IS, et al: MR imaging of the sellar and juxtasellar regions. Radiographics 1991; 11:727–758, with permission.)

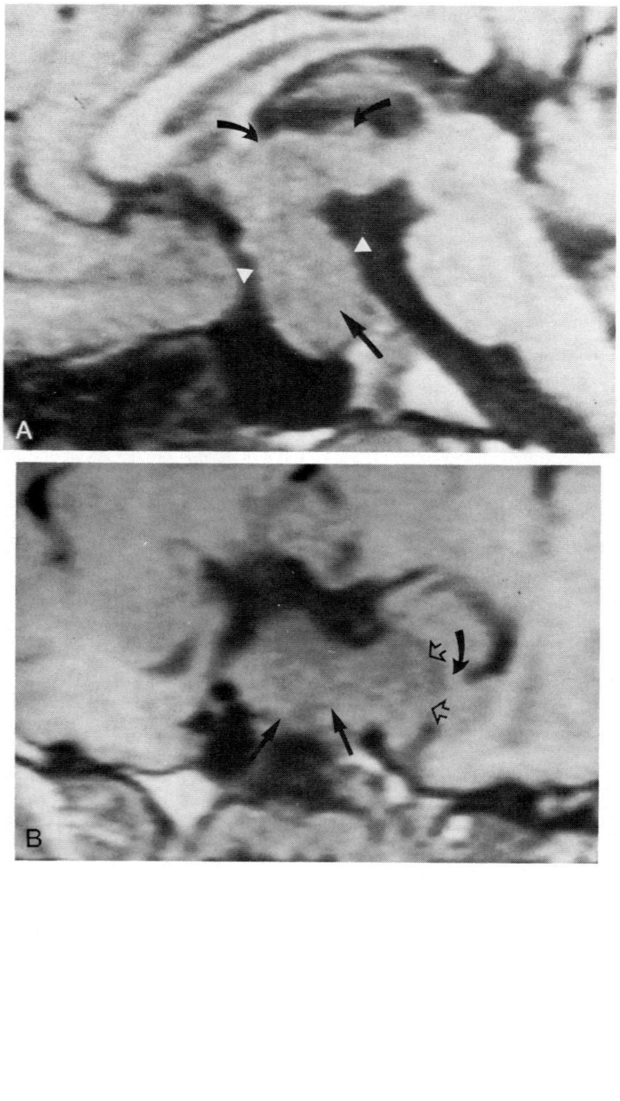

Figure 10–35. Germinoma (12-year-old male).

A, Parasagittal T1. A homogeneous lobulated isointense–to–gray matter mass extends from the sella *(straight arrow)* into the suprasellar cistern *(arrowheads)* and the third ventricle *(curved arrows).*

B, Coronal T1. The mass fills the sella *(straight arrows)* and extends into the left cavernous sinus *(open arrows),* displacing the uncus *(curved arrow)* laterally.

(From Johnsen DE, Woodruff WW, Allen IS, et al: MR imaging of the sellar and juxtasellar regions. Radiographics 1991; 11:727–758, with permission.)

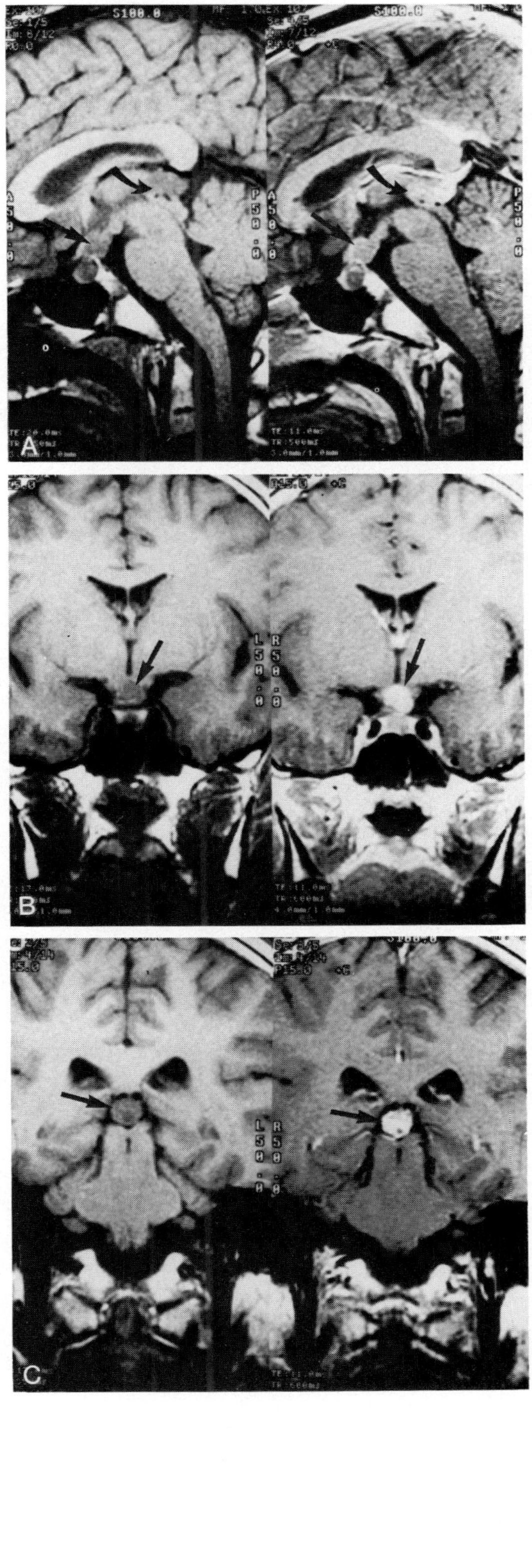

Figure 10–36. Germinoma (14-year-old male).

A, Parasagittal T1 (*left,* unenhanced; *right,* enhanced). Tandem, homogeneous, slightly hypointense masses are noted in the suprasellar *(straight arrow)* and pineal region *(curved arrow)*. The lesions enhance slightly after contrast administration.

B, Coronal T1 (*left,* unenhanced; *right,* enhanced). The suprasellar moiety *(arrow)* enhances homogeneously.

C, Coronal T1 (*left,* unenhanced; *right,* enhanced). The pineal primary *(arrow)* is slightly more heterogeneous than the suprasellar metastasis.

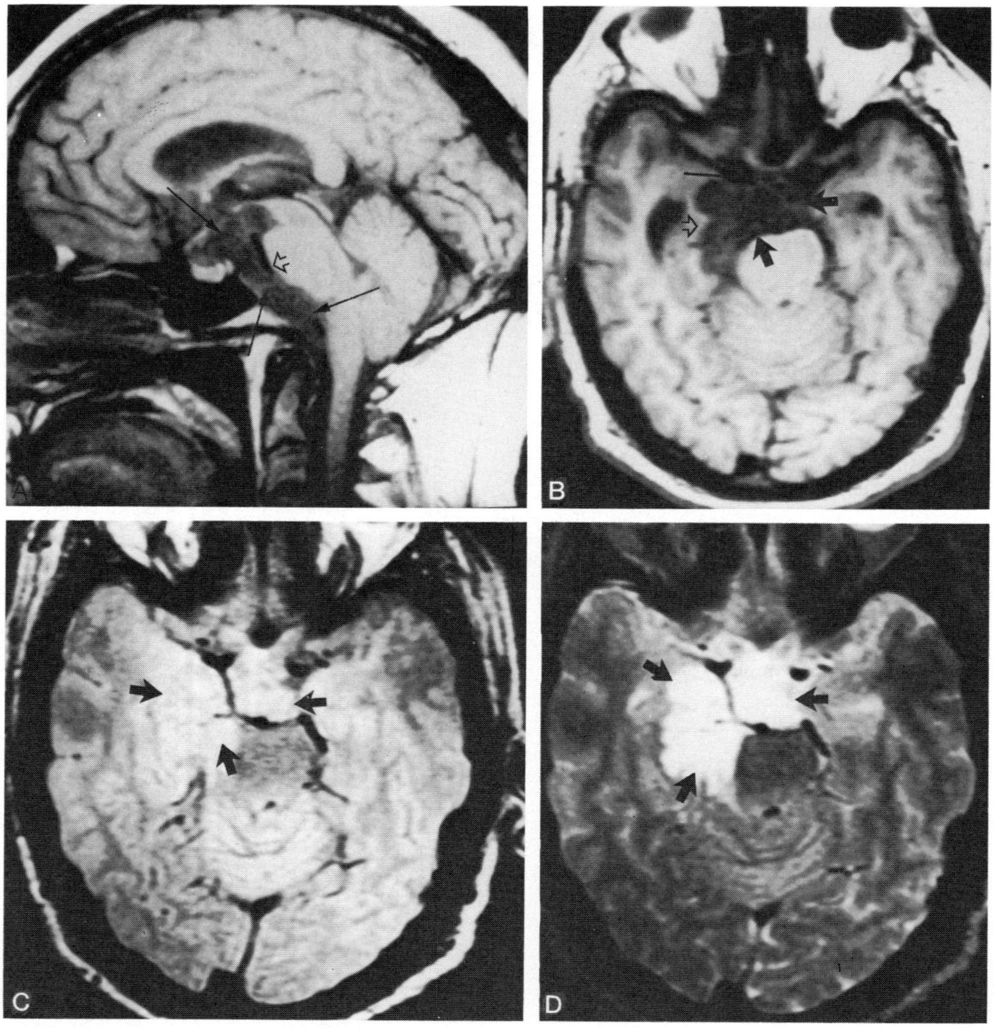

Figure 10–37. Epidermoid (50-year-old male).

A, Parasagittal T1. Isointense-to-CSF mass *(arrows)* displaces the pons *(open arrow)* and fills the dorsal suprasellar cistern.

B, Axial T1. The lobulated mass *(short arrows)* displaces the right temporal lobe *(open arrow)* laterally and the infundibulum *(thin arrow)* ventrally.

C, D, Axial spin density and T2. The mass *(arrows)* remains isointense to CSF.

(From Johnsen DE, Woodruff WW, Allen IS, et al: MR imaging of the sellar and juxtasellar regions. Radiographics 1991; 11:727–758, with permission.)

CT depicts a homogeneous soft tissue density mass that enhances uniformly. MRI depicts an isointense mass on T1 and slightly hyperintense mass to brain on T2. The tumor enhances homogeneously (Fig. 10–35). An enhancing pineal region mass may be detected in children (Fig. 10–36).

Epidermoid

Epidermoids are epithelial inclusion cysts that occur most commonly along the petrous apex, cerebellopontine angle, and juxtasellar region. The lesion is more common in men between 30 and 60 years of age. Epidermoid cysts are generally hypodense to brain on CT, approaching the density of CSF. Lesions that contain cholesterol may be hypodense to CSF.

MRI depicts well-defined lesions that may have irregular borders.[67] The signal intensity of the epidermoid cyst is contingent on the amount of cholesterol versus the amount of keratin within the lesion (Fig. 10–37). Increased concentration of cholesterol will commensurately shorten the T1 and T2 relaxation times. The T2 appearance of these lesions varies and may be hypointense to brain and CSF[67] or hyperintense to surrounding brain.[68] Epidermoid cysts do not enhance.

References

1. Moore KL: *The Developing Human,* 2nd ed, 1977. WB Saunders, Philadelphia.
2. Guyton AC: *Textbook of Medical Physiology,* 5th ed, 1976. WB Saunders, Philadelphia.
3. Naidich TP, Pinto RS, Kushner MJ, et al: Evaluation of sellar and parasellar masses by computed tomography. Radiology 1976; 120:91–99.
4. Taylor S: High resolution computed tomography of the sella. Radiol Clin North Am 1982; 20:207–236.
5. Swartz JD, Russell KB, Basile BA, et al: High resolution computed tomography of the intrasellar contents: Normal, near normal, and abnormal. Radiographics 1983; 3:228–247.
6. Lee BCP, Deck MDF: Sellar and juxtasellar lesion detection by MR. Radiology 1985; 157:143–147.
7. Hawkes RC, Holland GN, Moore WS, et al: The application of NMR imaging to the evaluation of pituitary and juxtasellar tumors. AJNR 1983; 4:221–222.
8. Johnsen DE, Woodruff WW, Allen IS, et al: MR imaging of the sellar and juxtasellar regions. Radiographics 1991; 11:727–758.
9. Zimmerman RA: Imaging of intrasellar, suprasellar, and parasellar tumors. Semin Roentgenol 1990; 25:174–197.
10. Daniels DL, Pojunas KW, Kilgore DP, et al: MR of the diaphragma sellae. AJNR 1986; 7:765–769.
11. Kucharczyk W, Davis DO, Kelly WM, et al: Pituitary adenomas: High resolution MR imaging at 1.5 T. Radiology 1986; 161:761–765.
12. Scotti G, Yu CY, Dillon WP, et al: MR imaging of cavernous sinus involvement by pituitary adenomas. AJNR 1988; 9:657–664.
13. Korogi Y, Takahashi M, Sakamoto Y, et al: Cavernous sinus: Correlation between anatomic and dynamic gadolinium-enhanced MR imaging findings. Radiology 1991; 180:235–237.
14. Elster AD, Sanders TG, Vines FS, et al: Size and shape of the pituitary gland during pregnancy and post partum: Measurement with MR imaging. Radiology 1991; 181:531–535.
15. Pojunas KW, Daniels DL, Williams AL, et al: MR imaging of prolactin-secreting microadenomas. AJNR 1986; 7:209–213.
16. Mark L, Pech P, Daniels D, et al: The pituitary fossa: A correlative anatomic and MR study. Radiology 1984; 153:453–457.
17. Colombo N, Berry I, Kucharczyk J, et al: Posterior pituitary gland: Appearance on MR images in normal and pathologic states. Radiology 1987; 165:481–485.
18. Nishimura K, Fujisawa I, Togashi K, et al: Posterior lobe of the pituitary: Identification by lack of chemical shift artifact in MR imaging. J Comput Assist Tomogr 1986; 10:899–902.
19. Fujisawa I, Nishimura K, Asato R, et al: Posterior lobe of the pituitary in diabetes insipidus: MR findings. J Comput Assist Tomogr 1987; 11:221–225.
20. Mark LP, Haughton VM, Hendrix LE, et al: High-intensity signals within the posterior pituitary fossa: A study with fat suppression. MR techniques. AJNR 1991; 12:529–532.
21. Davis PC, Hoffman JC, Malko JA, et al: Gadolinium—DTPA and MR imaging of pituitary adenoma: A preliminary report. AJNR 1987; 8:817–823.
22. Sakamoto Y, Takahashi M, Korogi Y, et al: Normal and abnormal pituitary glands: Gadopentetate dimeglumine–enhanced MR imaging. Radiology 1991; 178:441–445.
23. Kline LB, Acker JD, Donovan Post MJ, et al: The cavernous sinus: A computed tomographic study. AJNR 1981; 2:299–305.
24. Daniels DL, Pech P, Mark L, et al: Magnetic resonance imaging of the cavernous sinus. AJNR 1985; 6:187–192.
25. Stricof DD, Gabrielsen TD, Latack JT, et al: CT demonstration of cavernous sinus fat. AJNR 1989; 10:1199–1201.
26. Kapila A, Chakeres DW, Blanco E: The Meckel cave: Computed tomographic study. Radiology 1984; 152:425–433.
27. Drayer BP, Rosenbaum AE, Kennerdell JS, et al: Computed tomographic diagnosis of suprasellar masses by intrathecal enhancement. Radiology 1977; 123:339–344.
28. Burger PC, Vogel S: *Surgical Pathology of the Nervous System and Its Coverings.* 1982. John Wiley & Sons, New York.
29. Dwyer AJ, Frank JA, Doppman JL, et al: Pituitary adenomas in patients with Cushing's disease: Initial experience with Gd-DTPA–enhanced MR imaging. Radiology 1987; 163:421–426.
30. Doppman JL, Frank JA, Dwyer AJ, et al: Gadolinium DTPA–enhanced MR imaging of ACTH-secreting microadenomas of the pituitary gland. J Comput Assist Tomogr 1988; 12:728–735.

31. Mikhael MA, Ciric IS: MR imaging of pituitary tumors before and after surgical and/or medical treatment. J Comput Assist Tomogr 1988; 12:441–445.
32. Steiner E, Imhof H, Knosp E: Gd-DTPA enhanced high resolution MR imaging of pituitary adenomas. Radiographics 1989; 9:587–598.
33. Newton DR, Dillon WP, Norman D, et al: Gd-DTPA–enhanced MR imaging of pituitary adenomas. AJNR 1989; 10:949–954.
34. Miki Y, Matsuo M, Nishizawa S, et al: Pituitary adenomas and normal pituitary tissue: Enhancement patterns on gadopentetate-enhanced MR imaging. Radiology 1990; 177:35–38.
35. Davis PC, Gokhale KA, Joseph GJ, et al: Pituitary adenoma: Correlation of half-dose gadolinium-enhanced MR imaging with surgical findings in 26 patients. Radiology 1991; 180:779–784.
36. Ahmadi H, Larsson EM, Jinkins JR: Normal pituitary gland: Coronal MR imaging of infundibular tilt. Radiology 1990; 177:389–392.
37. Shucart WA: Implications of very high serum prolactin levels associated with pituitary tumors. J Neurosurg 1980; 52:226–228.
38. Wakai S, Fukushima T, Teramoto A, et al: Pituitary apoplexy: Its incidence and clinical significance. J Neurosurg 1981; 55:187–193.
39. Ostrov SG, Quencer RM, Hoffman JC, et al: Hemorrhage within pituitary adenomas: How often associated with pituitary apoplexy syndrome? AJNR 1989; 10:503–510.
40. Barrow DL, Tindall GT, Kovacs K, et al: Clinical and pathological effects of bromocriptine on prolactin-secreting and other pituitary tumors. J Neurosurg 1984; 60:1–7.
41. Weissbuch SS: Explanation and implications of MR signal changes within pituitary adenomas after bromocriptine therapy. AJNR 1986; 7:214–216.
42. Yousem DM, Arrington JA, Zinreich ST, et al: Pituitary adenomas: Possible role of bromocriptine in intratumoral hemorrhage. Radiology 1989; 170:239–243.
43. Yeakley JW, Kulkarni MV, McArdle CB, et al: High resolution MR imaging of juxtasellar meningiomas with CT and angiographic correlation. AJNR 1988; 9:279–285.
44. Spagnoli MV, Goldberg HI, Grossman RI, et al: Intracranial meningiomas: High-field MR imaging. Radiology 1986; 161:369–375.
45. Aoki S, Sasaki Y, Machida T, et al: Contrast-enhanced MR images in patients with meningiomas: Importance of enhancement of the dura adjacent to the tumor. AJNR 1990; 11:935–938.
46. Goldsher D, Litt AN, Pinto RS, et al: Dural "tail" associated with meningiomas on Gd-DTPA-enhanced MR images: Characteristics, differential diagnostic value and possible implications for treatment. Radiology 1990; 176:447–450.
47. Young SC, Grossman RI, Goldberg HI, et al: MR of vascular encasement in parasellar masses: Comparison with angiography and CT. AJNR 1988; 9:35–38.
48. Freeman MP, Kessler RM, Allen JH, et al: Craniopharyngioma: CT and MR imaging in nine cases. J Comput Assist Tomogr 1987; 11:810–814.
49. Pusey E, Kortman KE, Flannigan BD, et al: MR of craniopharyngiomas: Tumor delineation and characterization. AJNR 1987; 8:439–444.
50. Karnaze MG, Sartor K, Winthrop JD, et al: Suprasellar lesions: Evaluation with MR imaging. Radiology 1986; 161:77–82.
51. Olsen WL, Brant-Zawadski M, Hodes J, et al: Giant intracranial aneurysms: MR imaging. Radiology 1987; 163:431–435.
52. Azar-Kia B, Naheedy MH, Elias DA, et al: Optic nerve tumors: Role of magnetic resonance imaging and computed tomography. Radiol Clin North Am 1987; 25:561–581.
53. Oot RF, Melville GE, New PFJ, et al: The role of MR and CT in evaluating clival chordomas and chondrosarcomas. AJNR 1988; 9:715–723.
54. Sze G, Vichanco LS, Brant-Zawadski MN, et al: Chordomas: MR imaging. Radiology 1988; 166:187–191.
55. Boyko OB, Curnes JT, Oakes WJ, et al: Hamartomas of the tuber cinereum: CT, MR and pathologic findings. AJNR 1991; 12:309–314.
56. Burton EM, Ball WS, Crone K, et al: Hamartoma of the tuber cinereum: A comparison of MR and CT findings in four cases. AJNR 1989; 10:497–501.
57. Barral V, Brunelle F, Brauner R, et al: MR of hypothalamic hamartomas in children. Pediatr Radiol 1988; 18:449–452.
58. Kucharczyk W, Peck WW, Kelly WM, et al: Rathke cleft cysts: CT, MR imaging, and pathologic features. Radiology 1987; 165:491–495.
59. Mize W, Ball WS, Towbin RB, et al: Atypical CT and MR appearance of Rathke cleft cyst. AJNR 1989; 10:S83–S84.
60. Kaufman B, Tomsak RL, Kaufman BA, et al: Herniation of the suprasellar visual system and third ventricle into empty sellae: Morphologic and clinical considerations. AJNR 1989; 10:65–76.
61. Woodruff WW, Heinz ER, Djang WT, et al: Hyperprolactinemia: An unusual manifestation of suprasellar cystic lesions. AJNR 1987; 8:113–116.
62. Wiener SN, Pearlstein AE, Eiber A: MR imaging of intracranial arachnoid cysts. J Comput Assist Tomogr 1987; 11:236–241.
63. Donovan Post MJ, Mendez DR, Kline LB, et al: Metastatic disease to the cavernous sinus: Clinical syndrome and CT diagnosis. J Comput Assist Tomogr 1985; 9:115–120.
64. Woodruff WW, Yeates AE, McLendon RE: Perineural tumor extension to the cavernous sinus from superficial facial carcinoma: CT manifestations. Radiology 1986; 161:395–399.
65. Walker FO, McLean WT, Eister A, et al: Chiasmal sarcoidosis. AJNR 1990; 11:1205–1207.
66. Jinkins JR: Dynamic CT of tuberculous meningeal reaction. Neuroradiology 1987; 29:343–347.
67. Steffey DJ, DeFilipp GJ, Spera T, et al: MR imaging of primary epidermoid tumors. J Comput Assist Tomogr 1988; 12:438–440.
68. Vion-Dury J, Vincentelli F, Jiddane M, et al: MR imaging of epidermoid cysts. Neuroradiology 1987; 29:333–338.

11

TEMPORAL BONE

The temporal bone is a complex structure that houses the receptors for balance and hearing. Multiple vital vascular structures and nerves course within or adjacent to the temporal bone. The temporal bones form a portion of the skull base separating the middle and the posterior cranial fossae (Figs. 11–1 to 11–10).

ANATOMY

Temporal Bone Components

The temporal bone is a composite of four separate segments[1] (Figs. 11–1 to 11–4). The squamosal portion of the temporal bone is a broad, flat bone that delineates the lateral-most extent of the middle cranial fossa as it articulates with the greater wing of the sphenoid anteriorly and the parietal bone superiorly. The temporalis muscle inserts along the lateral surface of the bone. The zygomatic process is a thin anterior extension of bone that arises from the lateral surface of the squamosal temporal bone. The zygomatic process articulates anteriorly with the zygomatic bone. The middle meningeal artery enters the skull base through the foramen spinosum and courses along the medial surface of the temporal bone, beneath the periosteum (dura mater).

The petromastoid segment of the temporal bone is, by far, the most complex and houses the middle and inner ear structures. This temporal bone segment articulates anteriorly with the greater wing of the sphenoid, superiorly

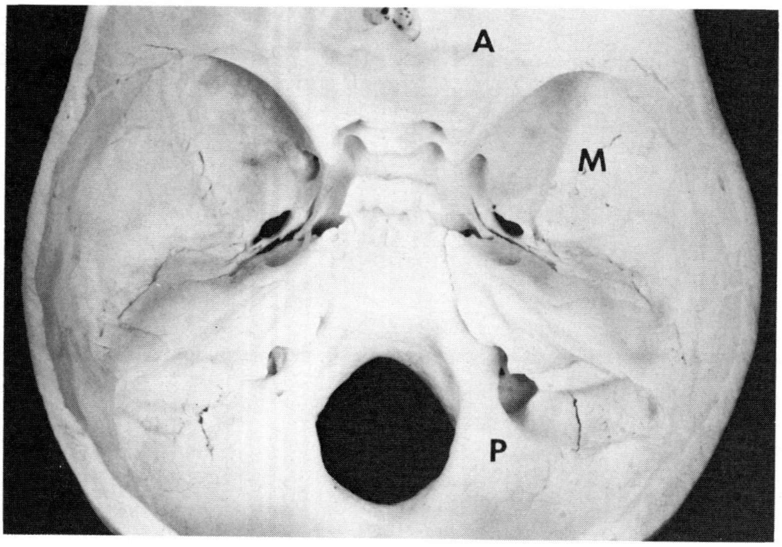

Figure 11–1. Intracranial anatomy. *(A)* Anterior cranial fossa, *(M)* middle cranial fossa, *(P)* posterior cranial fossa.

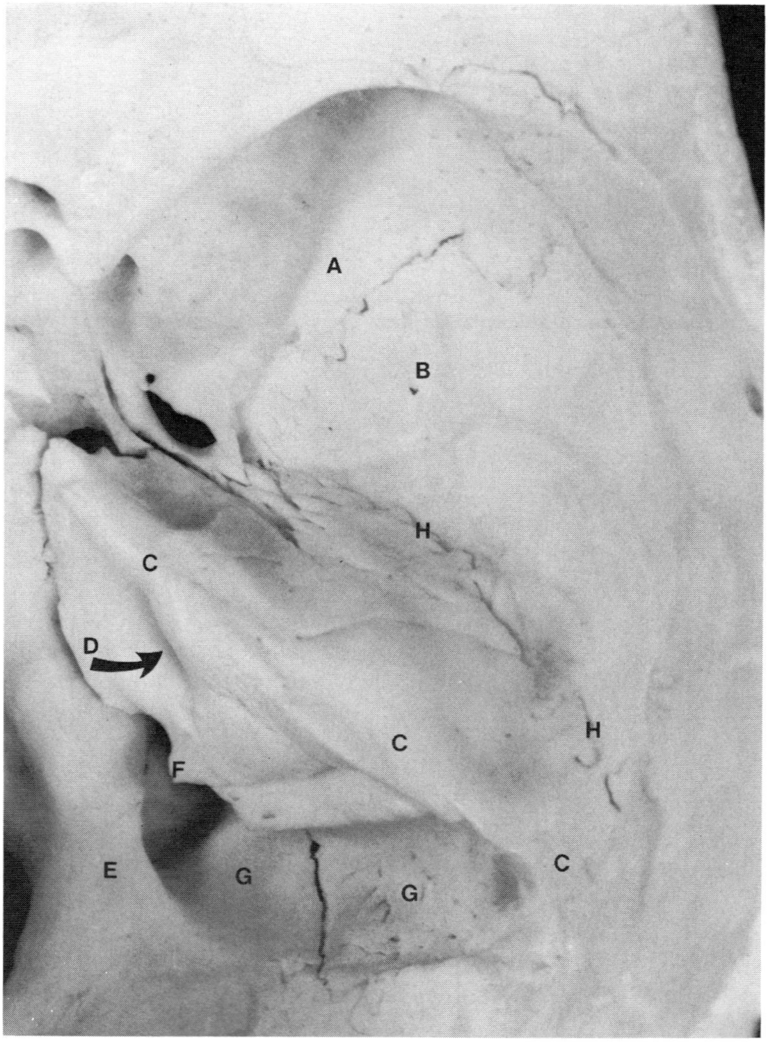

Figure 11–2. Blowup of left hemicalvarium. *(A)* Greater wing of sphenoid, *(B)* squamosal temporal bone, *(C)* petrous ridge, *(D)* internal auditory canal, *(E)* occipital bone, *(F)* jugular spine, *(G)* course of sigmoid sinus, *(H)* petrosquamosal suture.

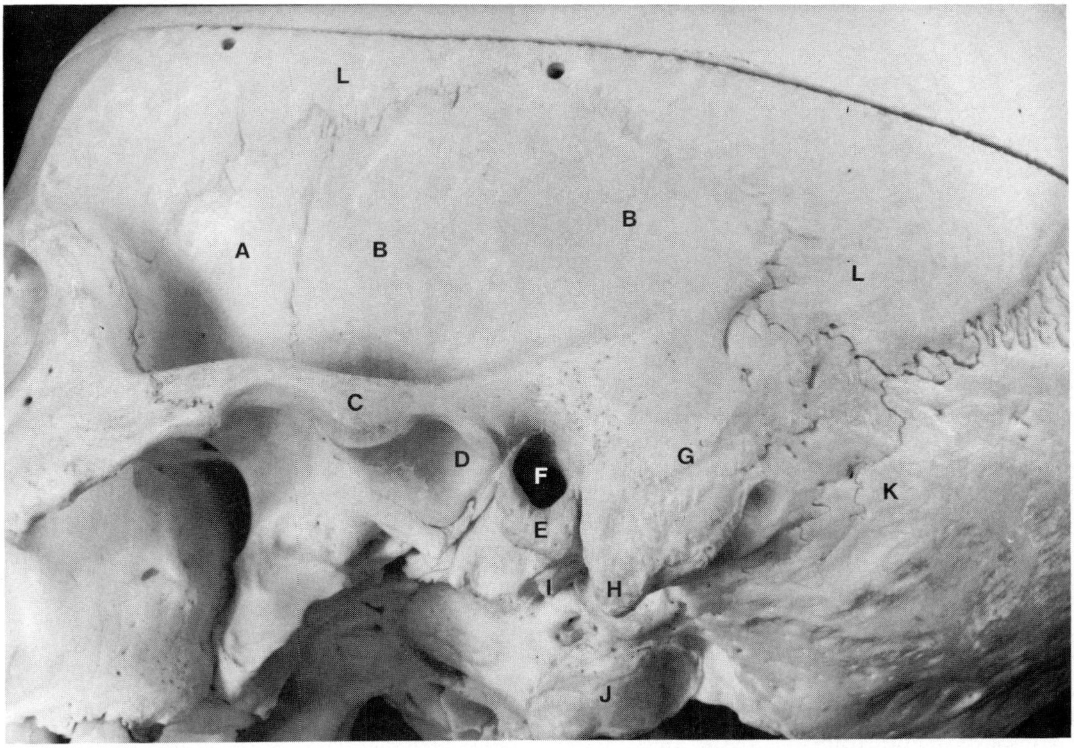

Figure 11–3. Lateral inferior oblique view of the temporal bone. *(A)* Greater wing of sphenoid, *(B)* squamosal temporal bone, *(C)* zygomatic process, *(D)* mandibular fossa, *(E)* tympanic temporal bone, *(F)* external auditory canal, *(G)* mastoid temporal bone, *(H)* mastoid process, *(I)* styloid process (fractured), *(J)* occipital condyle, *(K)* occipital bone, *(L)* parietal bone.

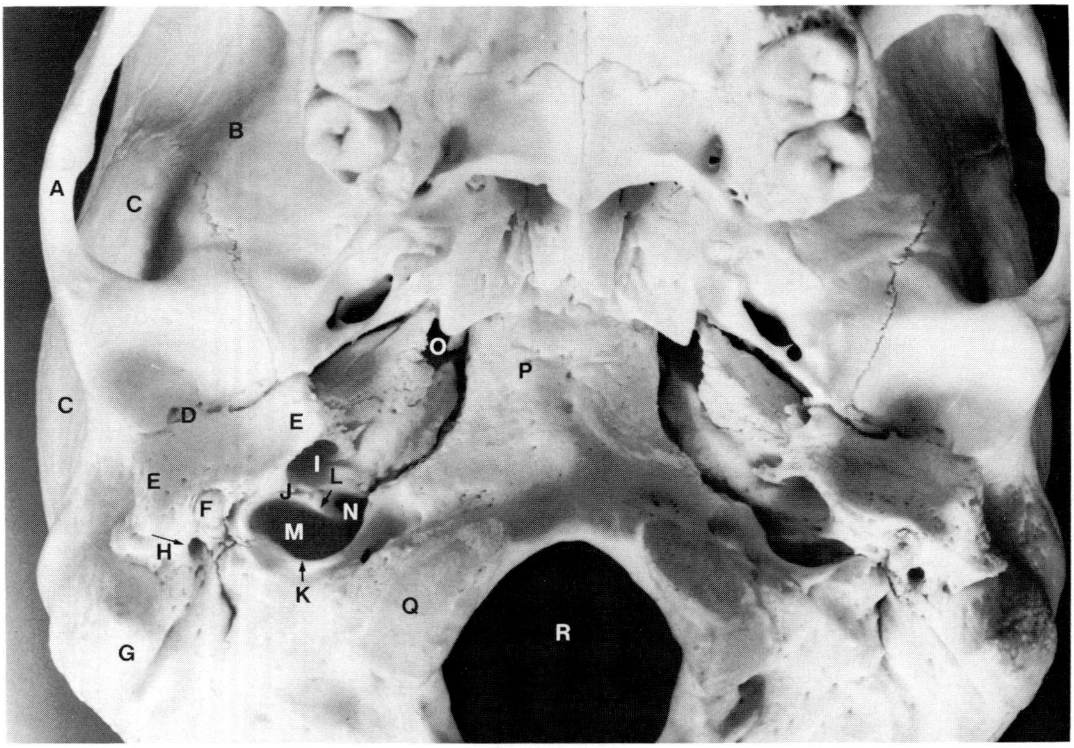

Figure 11–4. Base view of the petrous bone. *(A)* Zygomatic process, *(B)* greater wing of sphenoid, *(C)* squamosal temporal bone, *(D)* mandibular fossa, *(E)* tympanic temporal bone, *(F)* styloid process (fractured), *(G)* mastoid tip, *(H)* stylomastoid foramen, *(I)* carotid foramen, *(J)* caroticojugular spine, *(K)* jugular foramen, *(L)* jugular spine, *(M)* pars vascularis, *(N)* pars nervosa, *(O)* foramen lacerum, *(P)* base of clivus, *(Q)* occipital condyle, *(R)* foramen magnum.

with the parietal bone, and posteriorly and medially with the occipital bone. The mastoid process is an inferior extension of bone that houses the mastoid air cells. The powerful sternocleidomastoid muscle originates at the mastoid process.

The tympanic portion of the temporal bone is a small curved plate that resides inferior to the squamosal and anterior to the petromastoid portions of the temporal bone. The tympanic portion of the temporal bone forms the anterior wall, floor, and posterior portions of the external auditory canal. The posterior portion of the mandibular fossa is formed by the tympanic temporal bone.

The styloid process is a thin segment of bone directed anteriorly. The styloid averages 2.5 to 3 cm in length and is the site of attachment for the stylohyoid, styloglossus, and stylopharyngeus muscles. Juxtaposed between the styloid process and the mastoid process is the stylomastoid foramen. The styloid process is juxtaposed between the parotid gland located laterally and the vascular sheath located medially.

The bulk of the following discussion will be confined to the petromastoid segment of the temporal bone. Classically, the ear has been subdivided into the external, middle, and inner segments. The tympanic membrane demarcates the junction of the external and middle ear. The external and middle ear serve to collect and transmit sound waves. The oval window demarcates the middle and inner ear sections. The inner ear contains the cochlea and semicircular canals, the receptor organs for sound and balance, respectively.

External Ear

The external ear is composed of the fleshy, cartilaginous auricle and the external auditory canal. The medial two thirds of the external auditory canal is formed by the tympanic portion of the temporal bone. The lateral one third of the canal is cartilaginous, derived from the cartilage of the auricle. Small clefts are present in the floor of the cartilaginous external auditory canal known as the fissures of Santorini. These fissures provide for flexibility of the cartilage and secondarily serve as potential pathways for spread of tumor and infection.[2]

Middle Ear

The middle ear or tympanic cavity is juxtaposed between the tympanic membrane laterally and the oval window medially (Fig. 11–5). The tympanic cavity may be subdivided into the epitympanum (that portion of the tympanic cavity above the tympanic membrane), the mesotympanum (that portion of the tympanic cavity at the level of the tympanic membrane), and the hypotympanum (that portion of the tympanic cavity below the tympanic membrane).[3] The tympanic cavity is contiguous with the nasopharynx through the eustachian tube, which arises within the anteroinferior hypotympanum. The tympanic cavity is also in contact with the more posteriorly located mastoid air cells. The major contents of the tympanic cavity include the ossicles, the tensor tympani and stapedius muscles, the chordae tympani, the tympanic branch of the glossopharyngeal nerve (Jacobson's nerve), the auricular branch of the vagus nerve (Arnold's nerve), and the horizontal or tympanic portion of the facial nerve (Fig. 11–6). The salient bony landmarks and contents of the tympanic cavity are presented here in succession.

The anterior tympanic cavity contains the eustachian canal and the semicanal of the tensor tympani. The eustachian tube is more laterally located and parallels the course of the internal carotid artery (ICA) as it extends anteromedial to the nasopharynx. The semicanal is located medial to the eustachian canal and terminates in the cochleariform process, the origin of the tendon for the tensor tympani. The tensor tympani inserts on the neck of the malleus and functions to dampen or modulate sound transmission.

The otic capsule or bony labyrinth of the inner ear forms the medial wall of the tympanic cavity (Fig. 11–7). The cochlear promontory is a rounded elevation of thin bone that covers the lateral margin of the basal turn of the cochlea. The promontory is directed obliquely in a posterosuperior orientation. The oval window is a dehiscence in the bony vestibule located superior to the cochlear promontory. The footplate of the stapes covers the oval window. The round window is located inferior to the cochlear promontory. It is covered by the secondary tympanic membrane. The lateral semicircular canal forms the horizontal bulge

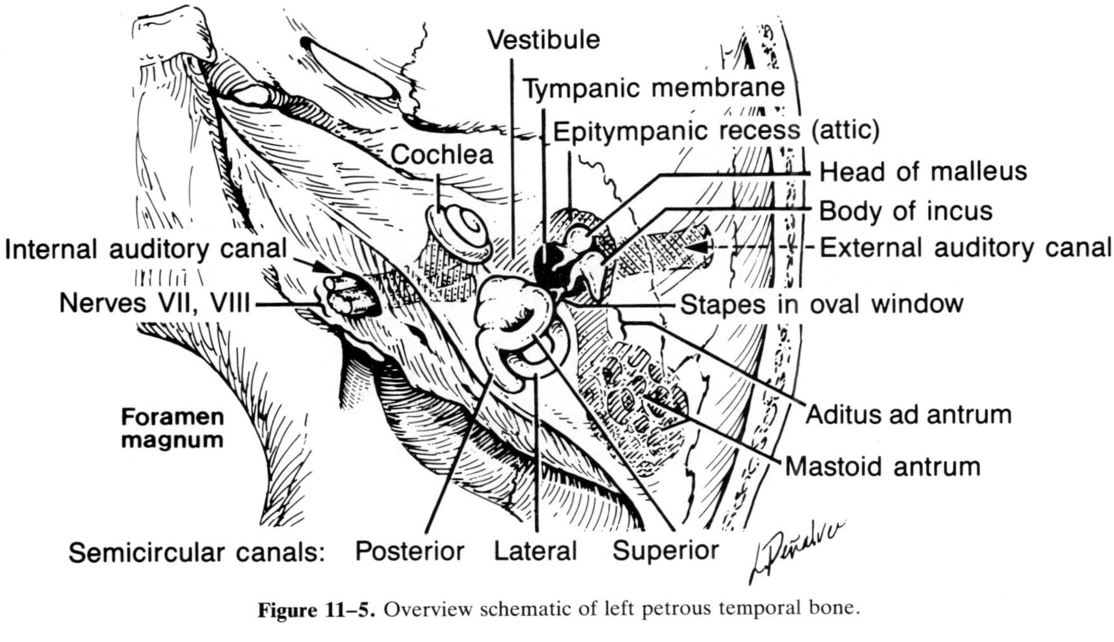

Figure 11–5. Overview schematic of left petrous temporal bone.

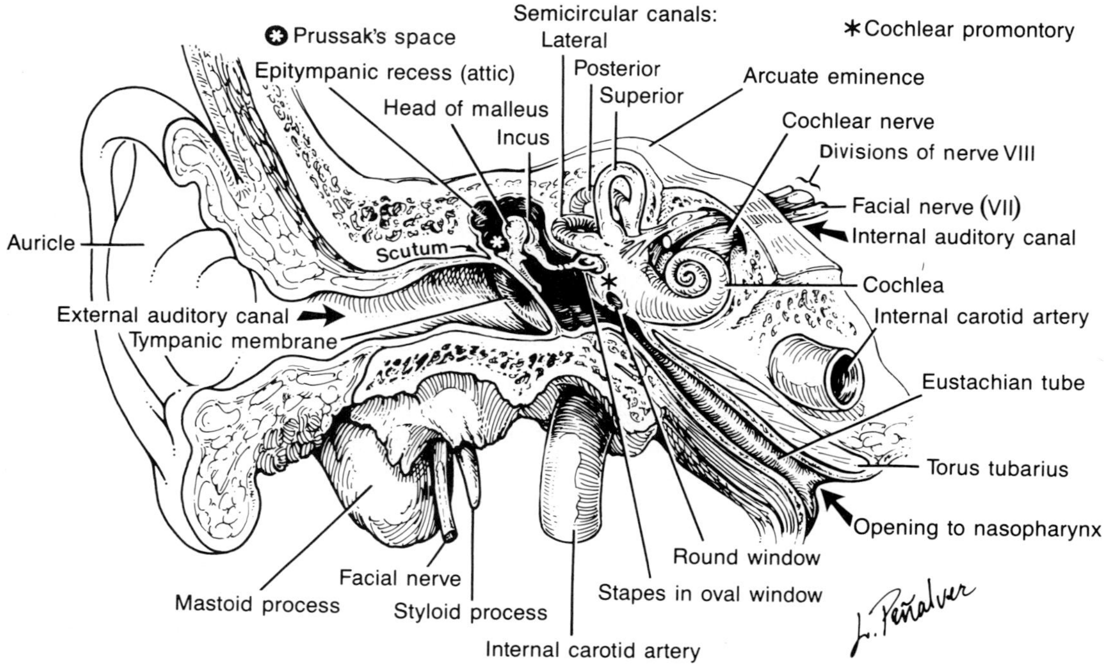

Figure 11–6. Coronal view of contents of right petrous temporal bone.

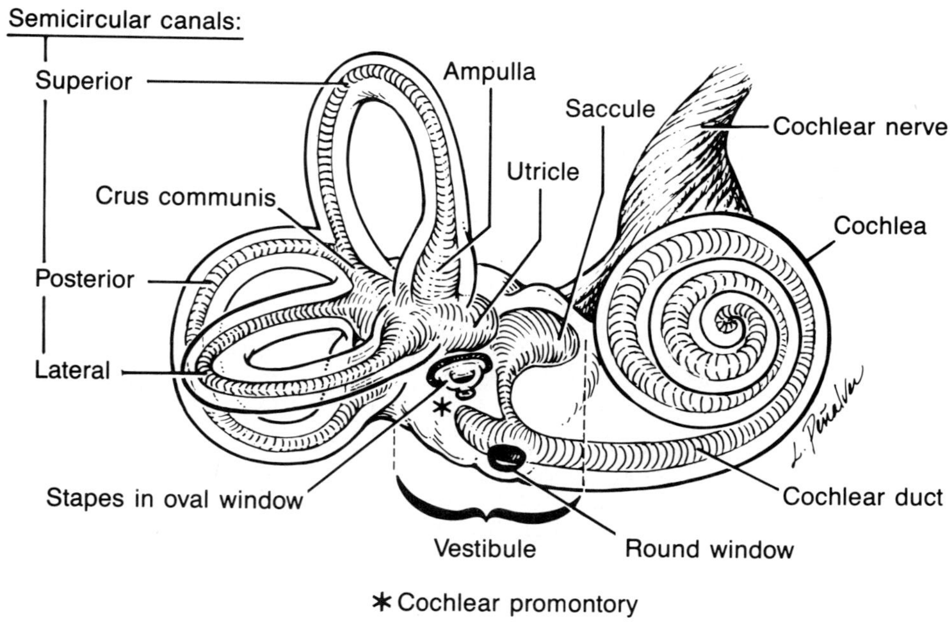

Figure 11–7. Lateral view of membranous and bony labyrinth.

located along the superior-most aspect of the medial wall of the epitympanum. A small, often partially dehiscent canal lies just inferior to the lateral semicircular canal and represents the canal for the tympanic portion of the facial nerve.

The posterior wall is composed of the pyramidal eminence, a bony ridge oriented in a vertical direction. The pyramidal eminence is anterior to the vertical facial nerve canal and serves as the site of origin of the stapedius muscle. The stapedius muscle inserts on the crus of the stapes. Like its counterpart, the tensor tympani, the stapedius modulates the mechanical transmission of sound. Medial to the pyramidal eminence is the sinus tympani. It is located posterior to the cochlear promontory and is contiguous with the oval window superiorly and the round window inferiorly. The facial recess is a shallow depression located lateral to the pyramidal eminence. The posterior wall of the tympanic cavity separates the middle ear from the mastoid air cells. The additus ad antrum is an irregular channel in the posterior wall of the tympanic cavity that permits communication of the epitympanic recess with the upper mastoid air cells.

The lateral wall of the tympanic cavity is formed, to a large part, by the conical tympanic membrane. The tympanic membrane is obliquely oriented in an inferomedial posterolateral location. The external surface of the tympanic membrane is covered with the stratified squamous epithelium found in the external ear. Respiratory epithelium, like that found in the middle ear, lines the inner surface of the tympanic membrane. A middle fibrous layer is present in the lower two thirds of the tympanic membrane (pars tensa). Fibers are arranged in a radial and circular pattern and are partly responsible for weaving the handle of the malleus into the medial aspect of the tympanic membrane. The pars flaccida is the upper third of the tympanic membrane that lacks the middle fibrous layer. As a result, the pars flaccida is a common site for acquired cholesteatomas. The scutum is a thin bony process that extends inferomedial from the roof of the external auditory canal (EAC) into the tympanic cavity and serves as the cephalad attachment site for the tympanic membrane. The limbus is a bony ridge in the floor of the EAC that serves as an attachment point for the inferior portion of the tympanic membrane. The oblique course of the tympanic membrane may be depicted on thin-cut computed tomography (CT) and coronal and axial planes. The scutum is best identified in the coronal plane and should terminate in a point (Fig. 11–8). Prussak's space is located between the scutum located laterally and the ossicles located medially.

The roof of the tympanic cavity is the tegmen tympani. This thin, bony plate separates the tympanic cavity below from the middle cranial fossa and temporal lobe above. The tegmen tympani is contiguous with the tegmen mastoideum (the roof of the mastoid antrum) via the additus ad antrum. Coronal images best depict the tegmen tympani and mastoideum. Often, they may be so thin that their competence is questioned. This represents a potential pathway of tumor and infection from the middle ear to the intracranial space.

The floor of the tympanic cavity is thin and featureless. The jugular foramen lies inferior to the hypotympanum. The jugular foramen may be divided into the small medial pars nervosa, which contains the glossopharyngeal nerve (IX) and the inferior petrosal sinus. The more lateral pars vascularis transmits the vagus nerve (X) and the spinal accessory (XI) nerve, the jugular bulb, and the meningeal branch of the ascending pharyngeal artery.[4] The jugular spine separates the pars nervosa from the pars vascularis. The caroticojugular spine separates the carotid canal from the jugular foramen. The relationship between the jugular bulb and the hypotympanum, as well as that between the carotid artery and cochlea, is demonstrated equally well on coronal and axial planar imaging. The carotid canal begins at the skull base anteromedial to the jugular foramen. The carotid courses anteromedial through the horizontal canal until it extends cephalad, above the foramen lacerum forming the precavernous segment.

The ossicles are composed of the malleus, incus, and stapes. The malleus contains a handle or manubrium that is vertically oriented in the mesotympanum. The manubrium is invested by fibrous tissue into the tympanic membrane. The head of the malleus articulates with the body of the incus in the epitympanic

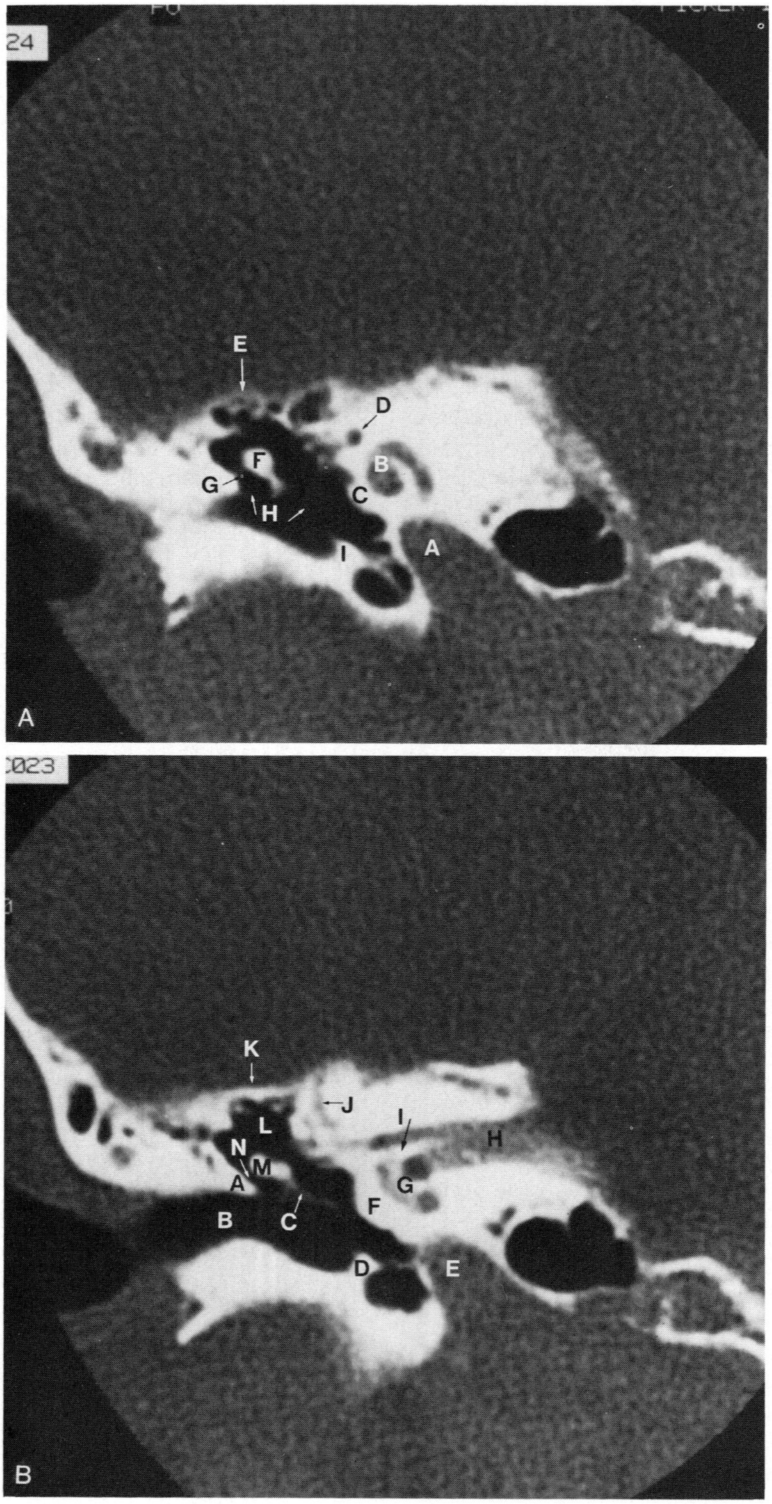

Figure 11–8. CT; coronal images (anterior to posterior).

A, *(A)* Internal carotid artery (ICA), *(B)* cochlea, *(C)* cochlear promontory, *(D)* geniculate ganglion, *(E)* tegmen tympani, *(F)* head of malleus, *(G)* Prussak's space, *(H)* tympanic membrane, *(I)* limbus.

B, *(A)* Scutum, *(B)* external auditory canal (EAC), *(C)* handle of malleus (applied to TM), *(D)* limbus, *(E)* ICA, *(F)* cochlear promontory, *(G)* cochlea, *(H)* internal auditory canal (IAC), *(I)* crista falciformis, *(J)* superior semicircular canal (anterior limb), *(K)* tegmen tympani, *(L)* epitympanic recess (attic), *(M)* malleus, *(N)* Prussak's space.

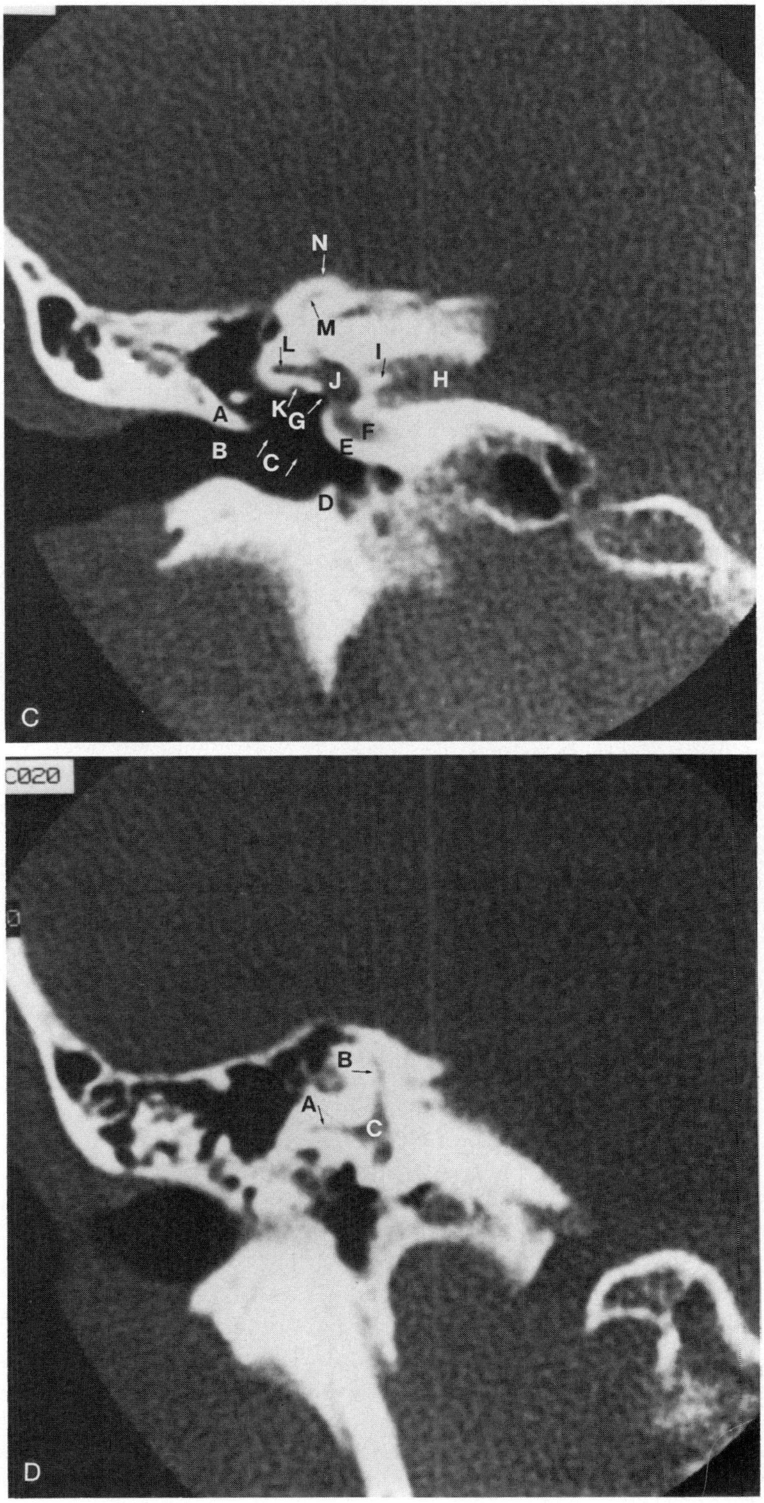

Figure 11–8 *Continued*

C, *(A)* Scutum, *(B)* EAC, *(C)* tympanic membrane, *(D)* limbus, *(E)* cochlear promontory, *(F)* basal turn of cochlea, *(G)* oval window, *(H)* IAC, *(I)* crista falciformis, *(J)* vestibule, *(K)* horizontal facial canal, *(L)* lateral semicircular canal, *(M)* superior semicircular canal, *(N)* arcuate eminence.

D, *(A)* Lateral semicircular canal, *(B)* crus communis, *(C)* vestibule.

Illustration continued on following page

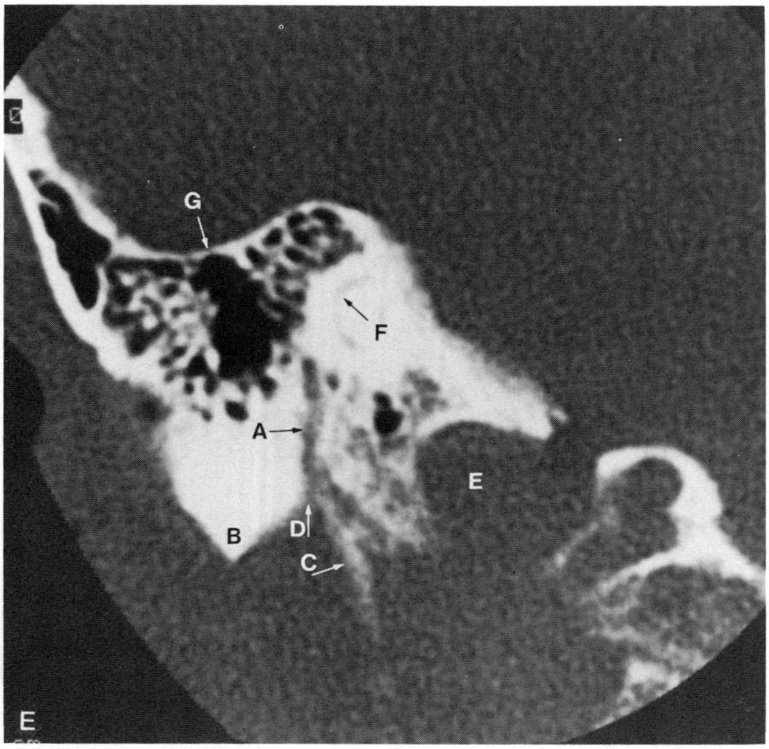

Figure 11–8 *Continued*
E, *(A)* Vertical facial canal, *(B)* mastoid tip, *(C)* styloid process, *(D)* stylomastoid foramen, *(E)* jugular foramen, *(F)* posterior semicircular canal, *(G)* tegmen mastoideum.

recess. The long process of the incus extends caudally, just posterior to the manubrium to articulate with the crus of the stapes. The stapes is shaped like a stirrup and its footplate articulates with the oval window. The head of the malleus and the body of the incus resemble an ice cream cone on axial CT: The incus constitutes the "cone" portion and is directed posterolaterally, and the head of the malleus represents the "ice cream" portion (Fig. 11–9). The axial images may depict the parallel course of the malleus and the long process of the incus, the latter of which is posterior and medial. The stapes is too small to be consistently visualized on planar imaging. The crus of the stapes may infrequently be identified as a Y-shaped structure on axial CT.

The nervous system invests the tympanic cavity. The chorda tympani is the final branch to arise from the seventh nerve before the latter exits the stylomastoid foramen. The chorda tympani enters the tympanic cavity from the posterior wall and courses medial to the tympanic membrane and the malleus to exit anterolaterally through the petrotympanic fissure. The chorda tympani supplies taste to the anterior two thirds of the tongue and parasympathetic stimulation to the sublingual and submandibular glands.

The tympanic branch of the glossopharyngeal nerve (Jacobson's nerve) and the auricular branch of the vagus nerve (Arnold's nerve) lie within the hypotympanum adjacent to the cochlear promontory. Both nerves may give origin to glomus tympanicum tumors.[5]

Inner Ear

The inner ear includes those structures between the oval window and the medial-most aspect of the internal auditory canal (IAC), which terminates in the cerebellopontine angle. The major components of the internal ear are the bony and membranous labyrinths. The bony labyrinth, also known as the otic capsule, is composed of thick, dense bone that predominantly supports and protects the membranous labyrinth (Fig. 11–7). The membranous labyrinth includes the organs of hearing (cochlea) and balance (vestibular system). The membranous labyrinth is bathed in perilymph, which communicates with the CSF via the cochlear

Text continued on page 395

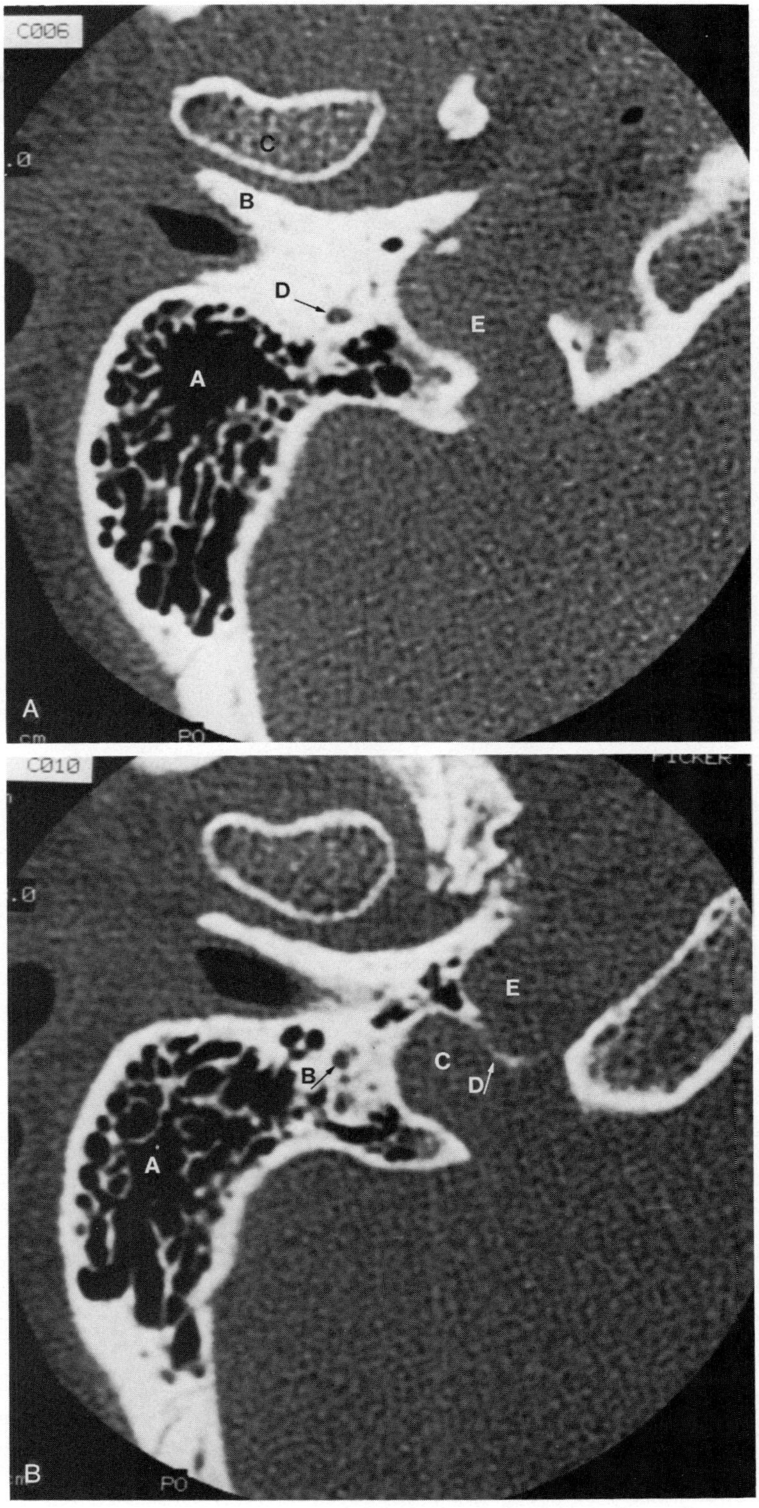

Figure 11–9. Computed tomography (CT); axial plane (inferior to superior).

A, *(A)* Mastoid air cells, *(B)* tympanic portion of the temporal bone (posterior border of mandibular fossa), *(C)* mandibular condyle, *(D)* vertical facial canal, *(E)* jugular foramen.

B, *(A)* Mastoid air cells, *(B)* vertical facial canal, *(C)* jugular foramen, *(D)* caroticojugular spine, *(E)* carotid foramen.

Illustration continued on following page

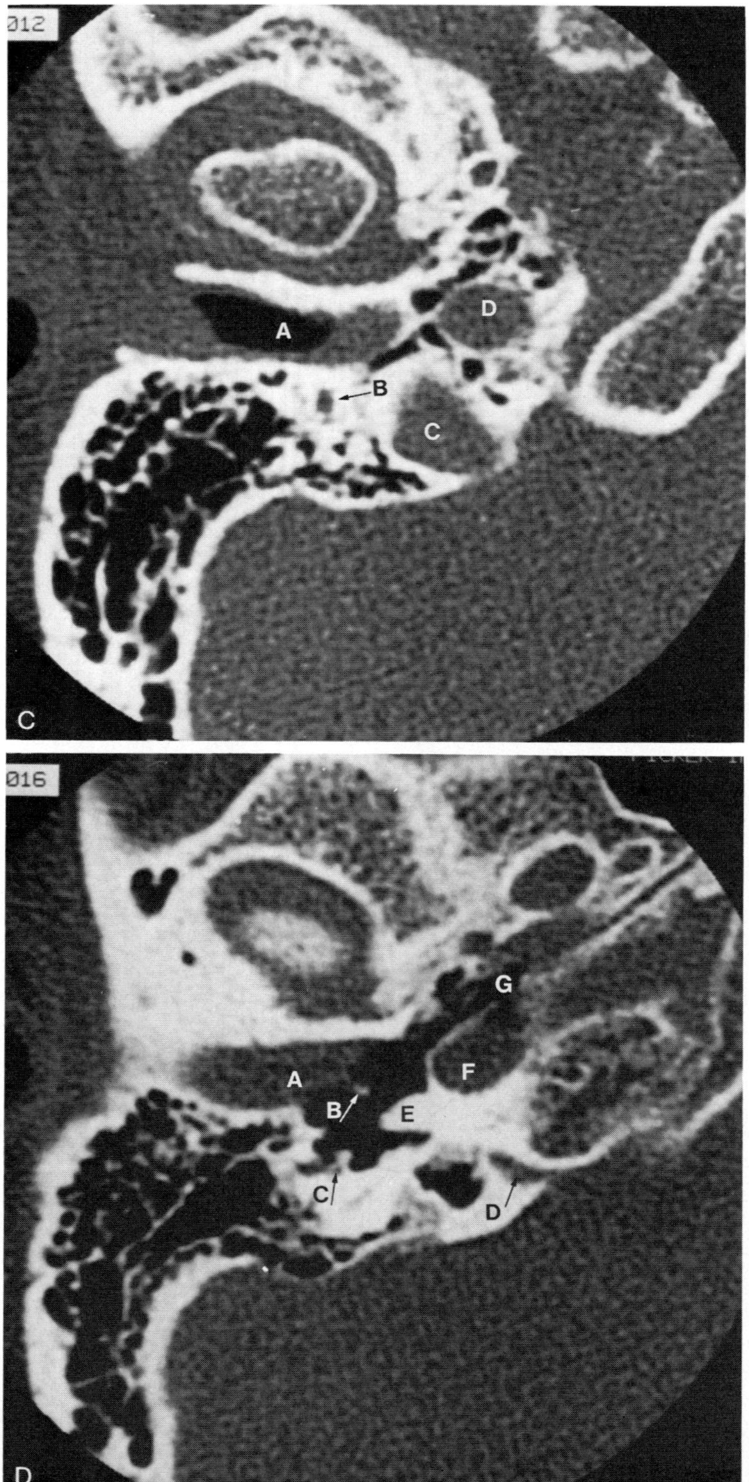

Figure 11–9 *Continued*

C, *(A)* External auditory canal, *(B)* vertical facial canal, *(C)* jugular foramen, *(D)* carotid canal.

D, *(A)* Soft tissue within the external auditory canal, *(B)* manubrium of malleus (applied to the tympanic membrane), *(C)* vertical facial canal, *(D)* cochlear aqueduct, *(E)* cochlear promontory, *(F)* carotid canal, *(G)* eustachian tube.

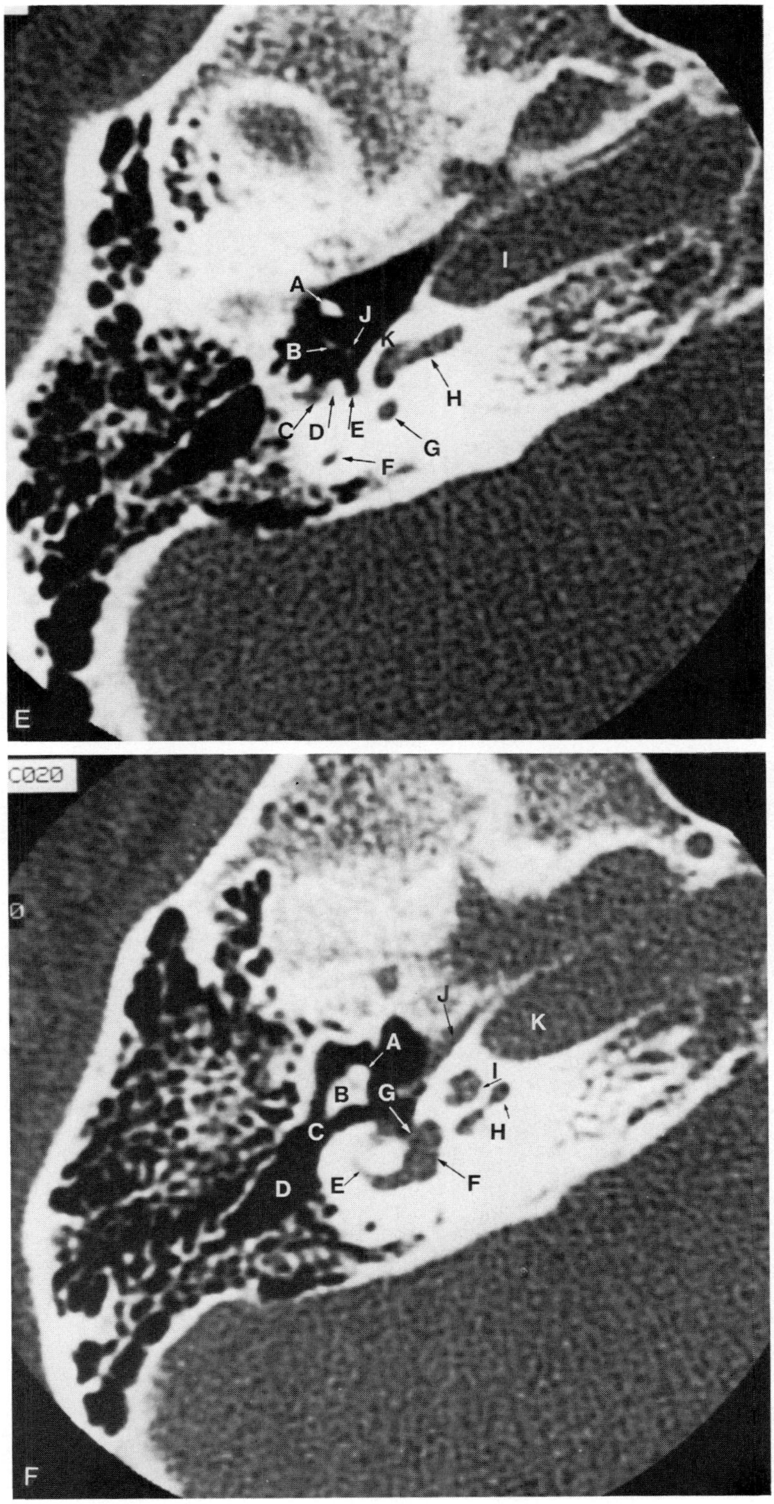

Figure 11–9 *Continued*

E, *(A)* Neck of malleus, *(B)* long process of incus, *(C)* vertical facial canal, *(D)* pyramidal eminence, *(E)* sinus tympany, *(F)* posterior semicircular canal, *(G)* ampulla of posterior semicircular canal, *(H)* basal turn of cochlea, *(I)* horizontal petrus carotid canal, *(J)* stapes, *(K)* cochlear promontory.

F, *(A)* Head of malleus, *(B)* body of incus, *(C)* additus ad antrum, *(D)* mastoid antrum, *(E)* lateral semicircular canal, *(F)* vestibule, *(G)* oval window, *(H)* basal turn of cochlea, *(I)* apical and second turns of cochlea, *(J)* stapedius muscle, *(K)* horizontal petrus carotid canal.

Illustration continued on following page

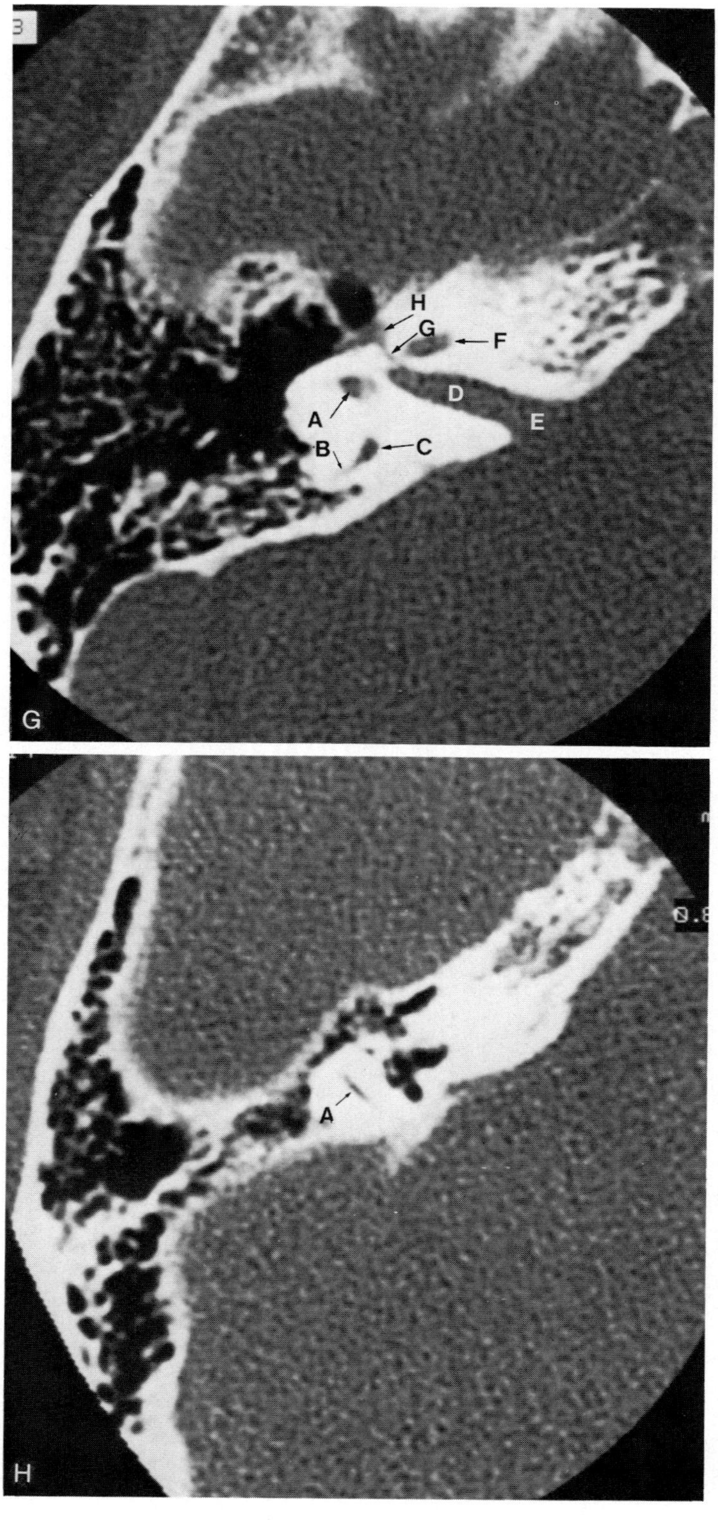

Figure 11–9 *Continued*

G, *(A)* Vestibule, *(B)* posterior semicircular canal, *(C)* crus communis, *(D)* internal auditory canal, *(E)* porus acusticus, *(F)* basal turn of cochlea, *(G)* facial canal, *(H)* geniculate ganglion.

H, *(A)* Superior semicircular canal.

aqueduct. Endolymph fills the membranous labyrinth.

Located anterior to the fundus of the IAC, the cochlea is a coiled, tubular structure shaped like a snail, with 2½ to 2¾ turns; the apex of the coiled tube is directed anterolateral. The cochlea contains three parallel fluid-filled ducts that are responsible for sound perception.

The basal turn of the cochlea and its bony covering form the most notable landmark in the medial aspect of the tympanic cavity, the cochlear promontory. The middle and apical turns are stacked on the basal turn and oriented anterolaterally.

The vestibular system, located posterolateral to the fundus of the IAC, includes the semicircular canals and the vestibule, which contains the saccule and utricle. The vestibule is the central portion of the osseous labyrinth and is juxtaposed between the cochlea located anteriorly and the semicircular canals located posteriorly. The vestibule communicates with the fundus of the IAC through the lamina cribrosa, a fenestrated plate through which the cochlear and vestibular nerves traverse. Laterally, two bony dehiscences are present in the vestibule that communicate with the tympanic cavity. The fenestra vestibuli, or oval window, is located anterosuperior to the cochlear promontory. The fenestra cochleae, or round window, is located posterior to the promontory and inferior to the oval window. The vestibule contains the saclike sense organs of acceleration—the saccule and utricle. The saccule is smaller and located anterior to the utricle.

The semicircular canals are arranged in orthogonal planes and include the lateral, superior, and posterior canals. These thin, arcuate structures originate and terminate in the utricle. The bulbous distal end of each canal contains the ampulla, the specialized organs responsible for the detection of angular acceleration. The posterior and superior canals share a common proximal limb, the crus communis. The cephalad-most arc of the superior canal forms a prominent bony landmark in the floor of the middle cranial fossa, which is called the arcuate eminence.

Because of the complex relationship of the semicircular canals, no single plane is accurate in detecting them in total. CT depicts small, round, or linear lucencies in the dense bony labyrinth. Magnetic resonance imaging (MRI) depicts punctate high-signal foci on T2 corresponding to endolymph and perilymph that are surrounded by areas of signal void representing the dense bony labyrinth (Fig. 11–10).

The porus acusticus is the opening of the IAC that permits the seventh and eighth cranial nerves to enter the canal from the cerebellopontine angle. The crista falciformis is a horizontally oriented thin bony septum that incompletely separates the fundus of the canal into the superior and inferior compartments.

The seventh cranial nerve arises in the pontomedullary junction and contains a small sensory and larger motor component. The course of the facial nerve through the petrous portion of the temporal bone is marked by three linear segments separated by two 90-degree turns. The facial nerve enters the anterosuperior quadrant of the porus acusticus from the cerebellopontine angle and extends horizontally to exit the fundus of the canal through the facial canal, a thin, arcuate lucency located above the cochlea and terminating in the geniculate ganglion. The nerve takes a 90-degree posterior turn to extend along the superior medial wall of the tympanic cavity, just beneath the lateral canal. The nerve may be housed within a thin, bony canal that may be dehiscent. Superolateral to the pyramidal eminence, the nerve makes a second 90-degree turn to extend inferiorly into the vertical portion of the facial nerve canal. The nerve exits the skull base at the stylomastoid foramen to enter the parotid gland before innervating the muscles of the face.

The greater petrosal nerve arises from the geniculate ganglion and innervates the lacrimal gland. The lesser petrosal nerve also arises from the geniculate ganglion and descends inferiorly to contribute to the tympanic plexus. The seventh cranial nerve gives off a small nerve to the stapedius muscle as well as the chorda tympani in the vertical facial canal.

The vestibulocochlear nerve lies within the lateral upper medulla. The cochlear division of the nerve enters the anteroinferior quadrant of the porus acusticus, beneath the facial nerve. The cochlear nerve returns sensory input from the spiral organ in the cochlea. The vestibular nerve occupies the posterior supe-

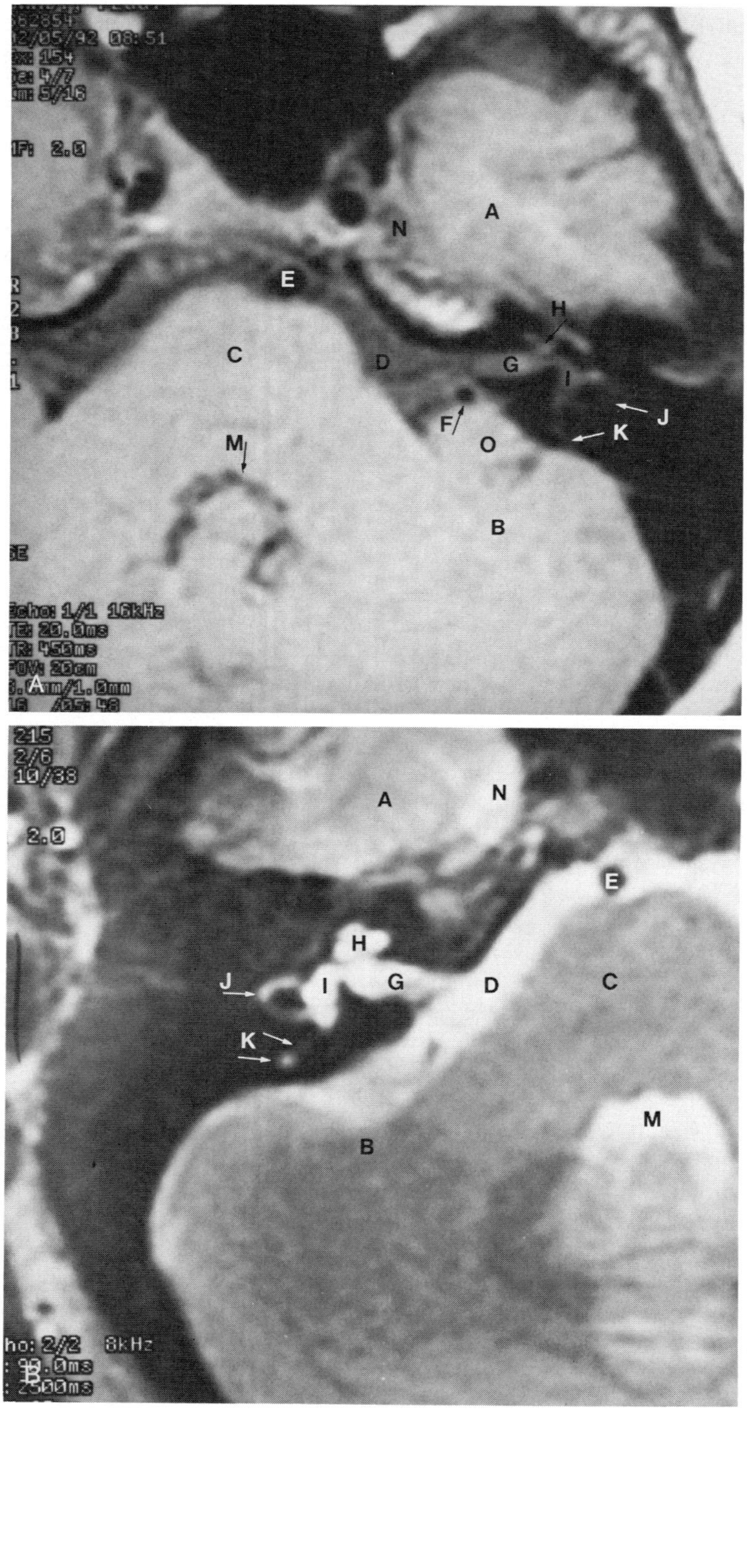

Figure 11–10. Magnetic resonance imaging (MRI) anatomy.

A, Axial T1. **B, C,** Axial T2. *(A)* Temporal lobe, *(B)* cerebellum, *(C)* pons, *(D)* cerebellopontine angle, *(E)* basilar artery, *(F)* anterior inferior cerebellar artery, *(G)* internal auditory canal, *(H)* cochlea, *(I)* vestibule, *(J)* lateral semicircular canal, *(K)* posterior semicircular canal, *(L)* superior semicircular canal, *(M)* fourth ventricle, *(N)* Meckel's cave, *(O)* flocculus.

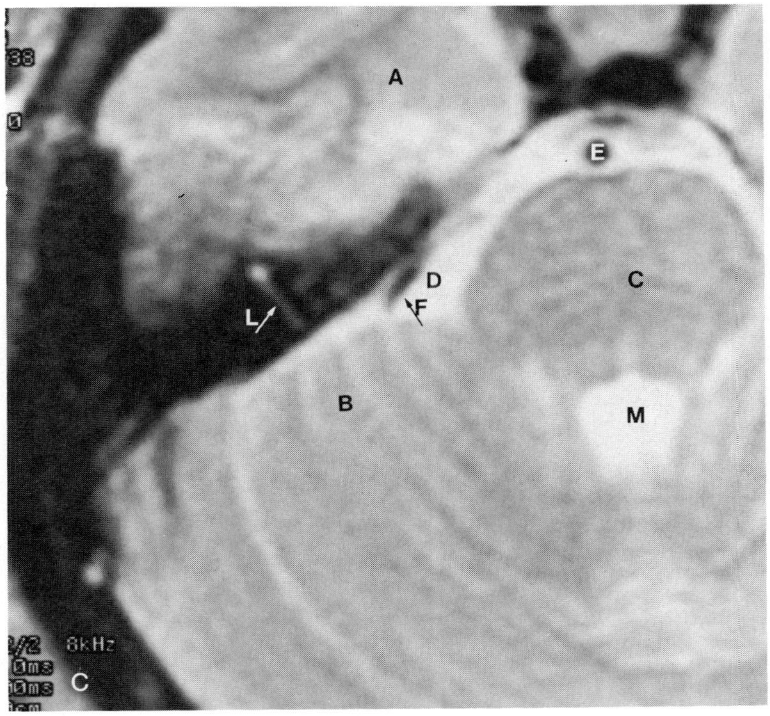

Figure 11–10 *Continued*

rior and inferior quadrants of the porus acusticus with separate superior and inferior branches. The saccule and posterior canal are innervated by the inferior branch. The superior branch innervates the utricle and the superior and lateral semicircular canals.

PATHOLOGY

Congenital

Mondini Malformation

Several anomalies may involve the petrous portion of the temporal bone. The best known is the Mondini malformation. This anomaly primarily affects the cochlea and may be due to multiple causes including in utero infection or vascular, toxic, metabolic, or chromosomal insults.[6] The insult may occur anytime during the sixth to 10th weeks of gestation, when the cochlea develops. Typically, the basal turn of the cochlea is normal, and the middle and apical turns are incomplete and fill an amorphic bony cavity in the otic capsule.[7] The degree of sensorineural hearing loss is variable, contingent on the degree to which the neuroepithelium develops. CT demonstrates lack of septation of middle and apical turns and an irregular bony cyst, often in the face of a normal basal turn (Fig. 11–11).

In addition to the Mondini malformation, an insult during the time of formation of the inner ear may lead to a variety of dysplastic conditions affecting any segment of the otic capsule (Fig. 11–12). The vestibule, vestibular aqueduct, and IAC may, in part or in combination, be affected.[6]

Vascular Anomalies

Internal Carotid Artery

The ICA enters the skull base through the vertical portion of the carotid canal. As the ICA ascends, it is separated from the tympanic cavity by the carotid plate, a thin bony covering often less than 0.5 mm thick. Rarely, the carotid artery may enter the tympanic cavity, appearing as a pulsatile reddish tympanic mass on otoscopic examination.[8] The carotid plate may be dehiscent and the carotid artery may be laterally herniated into the tympanic cavity. In such a case, the vertical canal of the carotid artery is present and appears normal.

Alternatively, the vertical portion of the carotid may have regressed during embryogenesis and the inferior tympanic branch of the

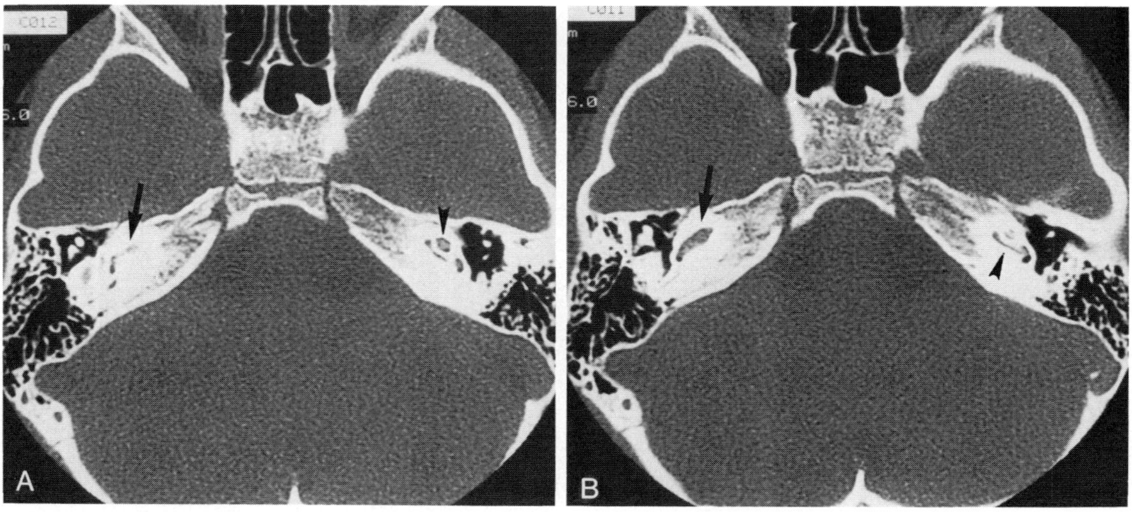

Figure 11–11. Mondini's syndrome (5-year-old male).
A, B, Axial CT. The normal cochlear turns are identified on the left *(arrowhead)*. The cochlea on the right is deformed. An ectatic basilar turn *(arrow)* is identified without evidence of the middle or apical turns.

ascending pharyngeal and caroticotympanic branch of the ICA (normally two small adjacent arteries that supply the middle ear) hypertrophy and anastomose to form an aberrant carotid artery.[9] In such a case, the vertical portion of the carotid canal is absent, the carotid plate is dehiscent, and the carotid takes an aberrant lateral course through the tympanic cavity.

Patients with an aberrant carotid artery are more commonly females (92%), the right side is more often affected (73%), and patients average 25 years of age at time of diagnosis.[10] Patients have tinnitus, hearing loss (most commonly conductive), and otalgia. An aberrant carotid artery was responsible for 8 of 107 patients presenting with pulsatile tinnitus in one series[8]; 7 were originally thought to have glomus tumors clinically.

The radiographic workup of patients with a

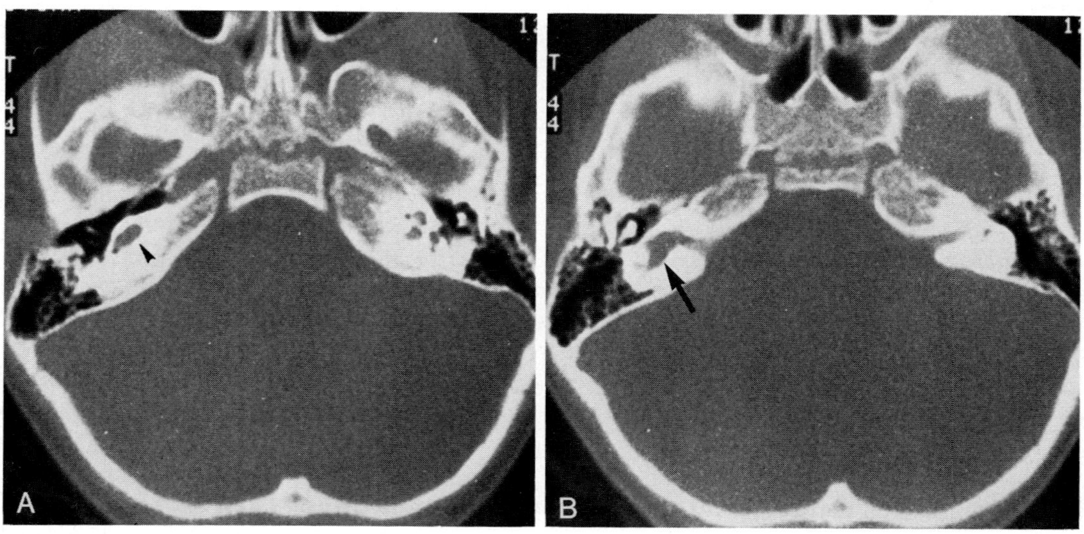

Figure 11–12. Mondini's variant (2-year-old male).
A, B, Axial CT. In addition to the solitary ectatic basilar turn of the cochlea *(arrowhead)*, the vestibule *(arrow)* is markedly enlarged and dysplastic.

vascular tympanic cavity mass must be precise to avoid biopsy of an aberrant carotid artery. CT demonstrates dehiscence of the carotid plate along the medial wall of the hypotympanum, herniation of the carotid artery into the hypotympanum, and the absence of the vertical carotid canal in cases of aberrant carotid artery (Fig. 11–13). Angiographically, lateral displacement of the genu of the vertical portion of the carotid artery may be demonstrated. The spin echo MRI sensitivity of detecting this disease has been expectedly disappointing because of the inability to consistently visualize bony landmarks.[8] However, MRI angiography has been employed to detect an aberrant ICA.[11]

Jugular Bulb

The jugular bulb normally lies below the tympanic cavity, separated from the tympanic cavity by the floor of the hypotympanum. In 6% of patients, the jugular bulb may extend above and elevate the floor of the hypotympanum.[12] Usually, the jugular bulb is covered by bone. Rarely, however, the bony floor of the hypotympanum may be dehiscent and the

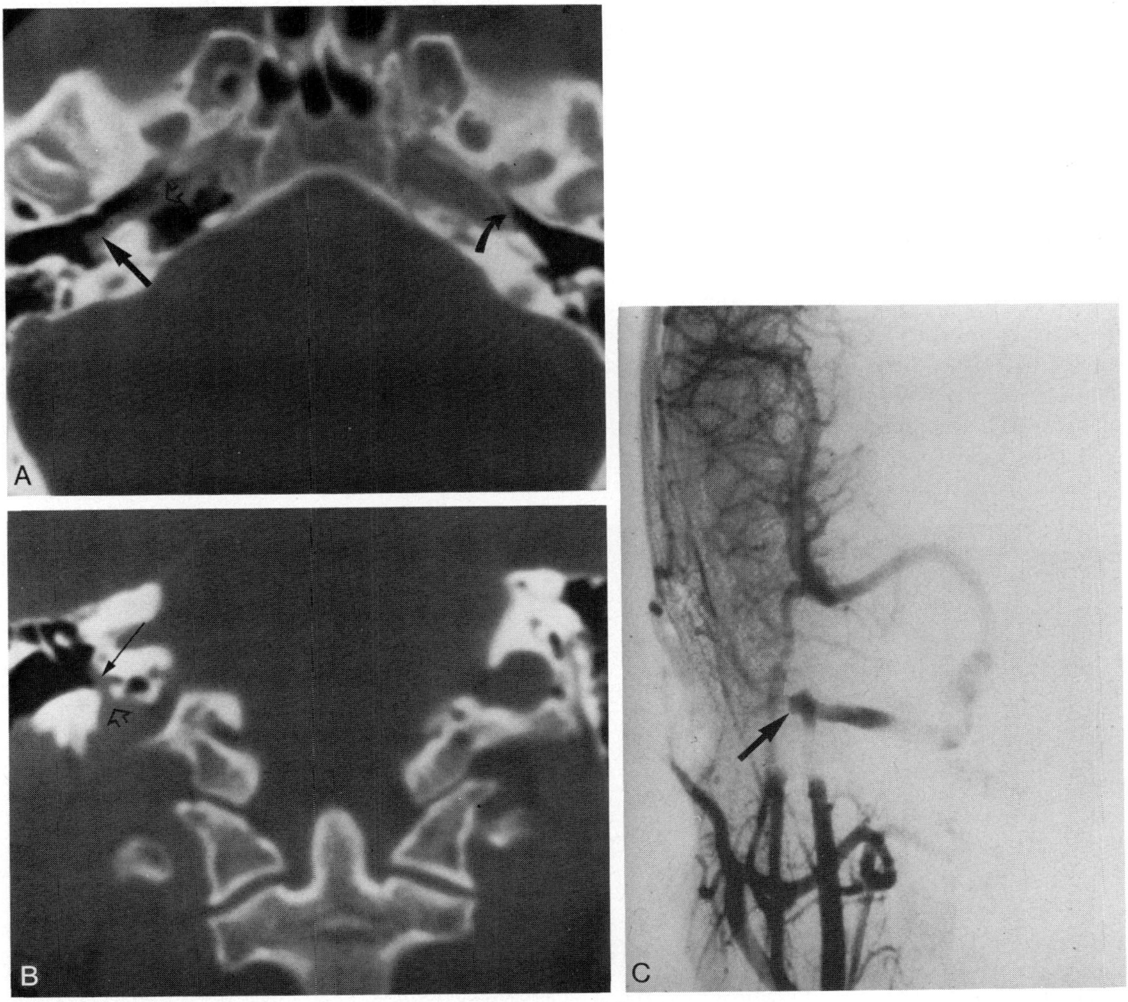

Figure 11–13. Laterally displaced carotid artery (38-year-old male).

A, Axial CT. A soft tissue mass *(arrow)* is present in the right hypotympanum. The mass is contiguous with the ICA *(open arrow)*. The carotid plate present on the left *(curved arrow)* is dehiscent on the right.

B, Coronal CT. The soft tissue mass *(arrow)* is contiguous with the carotid artery *(open arrow)*.

C, Anteroposterior (AP) right common carotid arteriography. A small knuckle of the genu of the ascending carotid *(arrow)* extends lateral from its normal location, revealing the etiology of this otoscopically identified pulsatile mass.

jugular bulb may protrude into the hypotympanum.[5, 13, 14]

CT is the most reliable way to establish a diagnosis of a high-riding or dehiscent jugular bulb. Contiguity of the hypotympanic mass with the jugular bulb and demonstration of bony dehiscence of the floor confirm the diagnosis (Fig. 11–14).

Inflammatory

Acute and Chronic Otitis Media

Acute otitis media is a common, clinically diagnosed infectious disorder of the middle ear that may secondarily involve the mastoid air cells (otomastoiditis). This condition is commonly caused by viral or bacterial organisms that ascend from the nasopharynx into the tympanic cavity through the eustachian tube. Once organisms have gained access to the tympanic cavity, an inflammatory reaction ensues with mucosal edema, leukocytic infiltration, hemorrhage, and accumulation of proteinaceous exudate. Mucosal edema may lead to eustachian tube obstruction, ultimately leading to decreased middle ear pressure and seepage of serous and mucous fluid from the mucosa. Typically, patients present with otalgia and a conductive hearing deficit. The diagnosis is established otoscopically, the patient is treated with an appropriate antibiotic, and the signs and symptoms resolve without sequelae.

Patients with uncomplicated acute otitis media do not require neuroimaging. If planar imaging is undertaken, however, mucosal thickening and gravity-dependent middle ear effusion may be detected. It would be abnormal to visualize mucosa on high-resolution CT because normal mucosa is too thin to visualize.[15] Dependent fluid should be distinguished from nondependent soft tissue, which may represent granulation tissue or cholesteatoma.[16] Dependent effusion is diagnosed by obtaining images with the patient in two separate positions or is suggested by detection of an air-fluid level. MRI demonstrates high-signal material on T2-weighted images (Fig. 11–15). The T1 signal characteristics of this material are variable, depending on the amount of glycoprotein within the effusion, which decreases T1 relaxation time.

Chronic otitis media may be seen in patients with allergy, altered immune states, eustachian tube dysfunction, and tympanic membrane perforation. Chronic mucosal irritation may result in soft tissue and bony response, which in some instances may cause irreversible damage to the middle ear structures. The periosteum of the tympanic cavity may be damaged from prolonged infection. In an attempt to repair the periosteum, the overlying mucosa

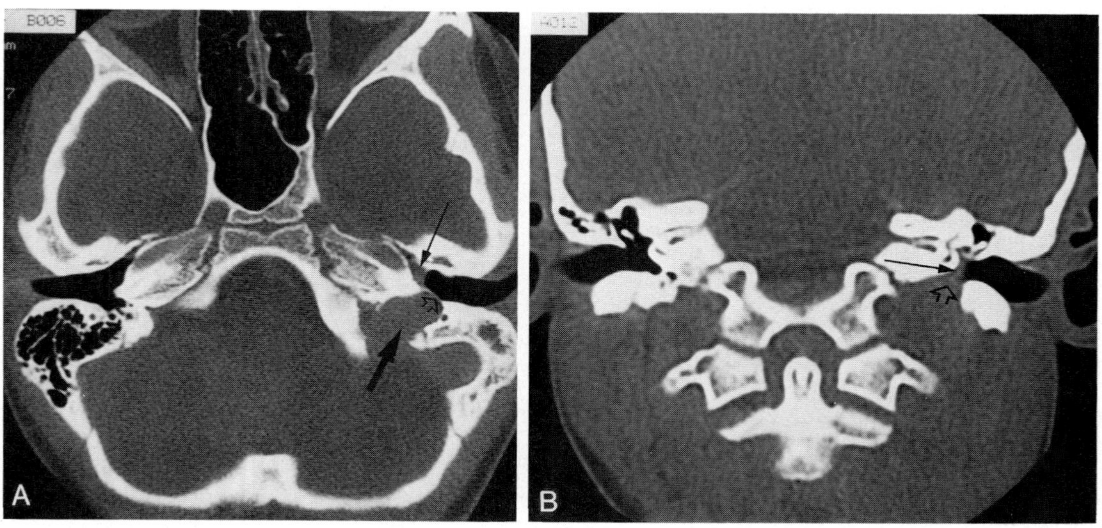

Figure 11–14. High-riding dehiscent jugular bulb (12-year-old male).

A, Axial CT. The left jugular bulb *(bold arrow)* is ectatic and high riding. The jugular plate *(open arrow)* separating the jugular fossa from the hypotympanum is significantly thinned. Soft tissue *(thin arrow)* is present in the hypotympanum.

B, Coronal CT. The contiguity of the soft tissue mass *(arrow)* and the jugular bulb *(open arrow)* is demonstrated.

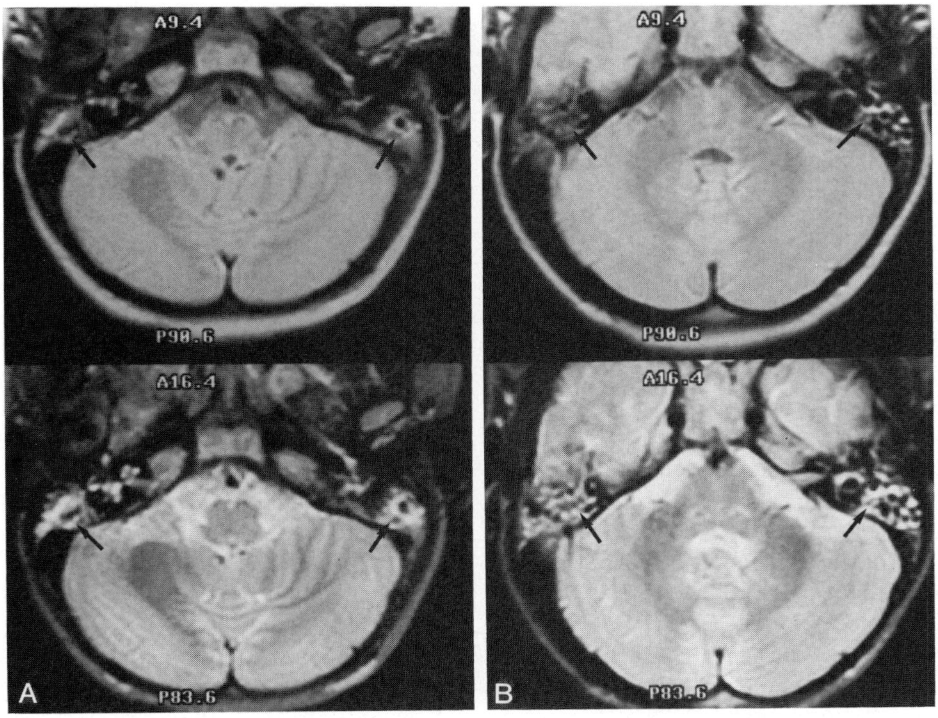

Figure 11–15. Otomastoiditis (4-year-old female).
A, B, *Top,* axial spin density (SD). *Bottom,* axial T2. High-signal inflammatory material *(arrows)* is noted bilaterally within the petromastoid temporal bones.

forms granulation tissue. Granulation tissue appears as nondependent soft tissue, usually without bone destruction on CT.[15] Granulation tissue consistently enhances on MRI, a distinguishing feature when considering cholesteatoma and cholesterol granuloma in the differential diagnosis.[17]

Chronic otitis media may result in ossicular fixation or dislocation. The repeatedly inflamed mucosa may form scar or fibrous tissue, which may reduce ossicular mobility. Alternatively, tympanosclerosis may result from submucosal fibroblast infiltration and subsequent deposition of calcium and phosphate. Tympanosclerosis may involve the tympanic membrane or the ligaments and tendons of the ossicular chain. Ossicular fixation is an irreversible, end-stage response to chronic otitis media.[15, 16] CT depicts a decrease in the number of aerated mastoid air cells with reactive sclerosis of the surrounding bone. Resorption of the otic capsule may be detected.

Chronic tympanic infection is frequently associated with cholesteatoma and cholesterol granuloma.

Cholesteatoma

"Cholesteatoma" is a misnomer. These soft tissue lesions are more accurately termed "keratomas." They consist of sacs of stratified squamous epithelium that contain keratinaceous debris and a fibrous stroma subepithelium.[15, 18, 19] Cholesterol is not present in cholesteatomas.

Cholesteatoma may be congenital or acquired. Only 2% of cholesteatomas are congenital.[20] Congenital cholesteatomas may result from either congenital inclusion of ectodermal debris that subsequently proliferates or from squamous metaplasia. By definition, the tympanic membrane is intact in patients with congenital cholesteatoma. Patients may present at any age, though this is usually discovered in childhood during a routine otoscopic examination or during middle ear exploration for a conductive hearing deficit.

Congenital cholesteatoma may affect any portion of the temporal bone including the petrous apex and the supralabyrinthine and parajugular regions. The most common place in which congenital cholesteatomas are detected, however, is the tympanic cavity—more specifically at the junction of the mesotympanum and epitympanum.[20] CT depicts a homogeneous, nonenhancing mass that is associated with ossicular dislocation in 75% of cases.

Ninety-eight percent of cholesteatomas are acquired.[6] The etiology of acquired cholesteatomas is still somewhat controversial. The end result is proliferation of stratified squamous cells within the tympanic cavity. Squamous cells reside within the external ear and are not normally found within the tympanic cavity. Accordingly, theories regarding the origin of these lesions are directed at explaining the cause of ectopic squamous cells within the tympanic cavity. Squamous cells may enter the tympanic cavity from the EAC through a tympanic perforation or encystment of retraction pockets of the tympanic membrane. Tympanic membrane retraction results when the pressure within the tympanic cavity falls below ambient pressure. This would naturally affect the weakest part of the tympanic membrane, the pars flaccida. Tympanic perforation more commonly occurs in the pars tensa and is associated with otitis media. Another potential explanation for the origin of squamous epithelium in the tympanic cavity is squamous metaplasia of the existing respiratory epithelium of the tympanic cavity. This may occur in response to recurrent or chronic infections.

Acquired cholesteatomas may be subclassified as primary or secondary. Primary acquired cholesteatomas occur in patients without prior history of otitis and involve the nonfibrous posterosuperior segment of the tympanic membrane, pars flaccida. Perhaps a result of tympanic retraction, these slowly enlarging soft tissue lesions are located medial and cephalad to the tympanic insertion, adjacent to the bony scutum.

As the lesions enlarge, they extend into Prussak's space, that region bordered by the tympanic membrane and scutum laterally, the malleus medially, and the epitympanic space superiorly. The lesion enlarges at the expense of the surrounding bone and often the adjacent scutum may be destroyed or ossicles dislocated. The bone destruction may result from direct pressure erosion and/or the reaction of the proteolytic enzyme, collagenase, which is produced by the subepithelial fibrous stroma.

Planar imaging depicts a nonenhancing homogeneous soft tissue mass in Prussak's space (Fig. 11–16). Coronal CT demonstrates resorption of the scutum or ossicles, or both. The mass is usually isointense to slightly hypointense to brain on T1 and isointense to hyperintense to brain on T2 MRI.

Secondary acquired cholesteatomas occur in patients with a history of prior otitis. The pars tensa of the tympanic membrane may be per-

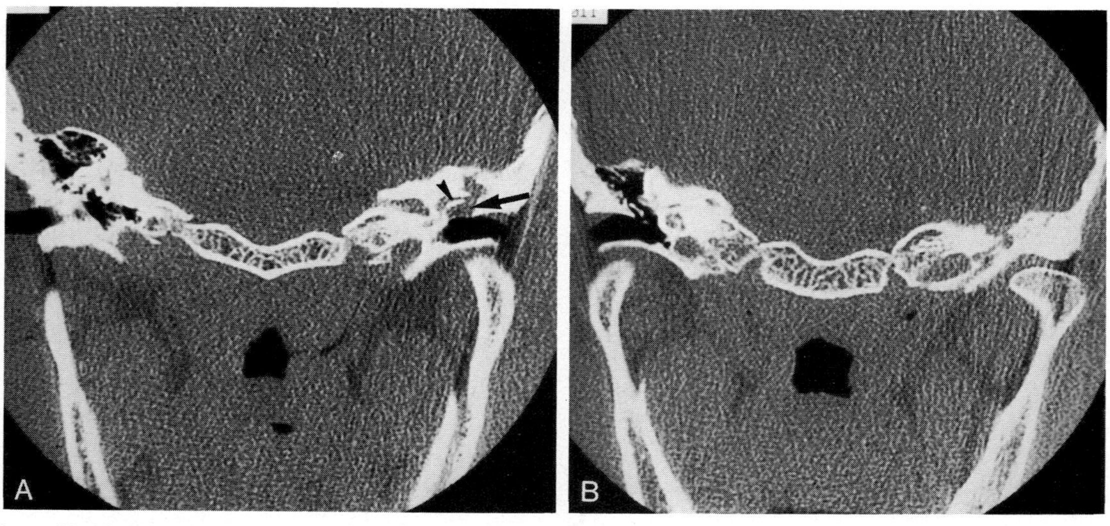

Figure 11–16. Cholesteatoma, primary acquired (49-year-old male).

A, Coronal CT. Soft tissue *(arrow)* fills Prussak's space and the epitympanic recess. The ossicles *(arrowhead)* are eroded and displaced mediosuperior.

B, Coronal CT. Demonstrates a normal-appearing right tympanic cavity.

forated with a soft tissue mass present in the mesotympanum. Prussak's space is usually normal.[16] The soft tissue mass may extend laterally through a bulging tympanic membrane, medially into the bony labyrinth, cephalad through the epitympanum and tegumen tympani, or anteriorly into the petrous apex[21] (Fig. 11–17). The ossicles may be dislocated or completely resorbed. Bone destruction is a hallmark of the lesion.

Complications of cholesteatoma include automastoidectomy, labyrinthine fistula, facial nerve palsy, meningitis, and dural sinus thrombosis.[21]

Grossly, congenital and acquired cholesteatomas differ significantly. Acquired cholesteatomas are usually foul-smelling, greasy, infected masses. Congenital cholesteatomas (epidermoidomas) are odorless, dry, and flaky with a nodular glistening surface.[22]

Cholesterol Granuloma

Cholesterol granulomas are the product of a nonspecific foreign body tissue reaction to cholesterol crystals. They result from inadequate drainage and ventilation of an aerated portion of the temporal bone, usually from mucosal edema and subsequent obstruction. The mucosa of the now-loculated, isolated air cells continue to resorb air, causing a chamber of negative pressure. This, in turn, results in local mucosal hypoxia and subsequent submucosal extravasation of blood and serum into the surrounding area. Local tissue necrosis ensues. The breakdown products from local

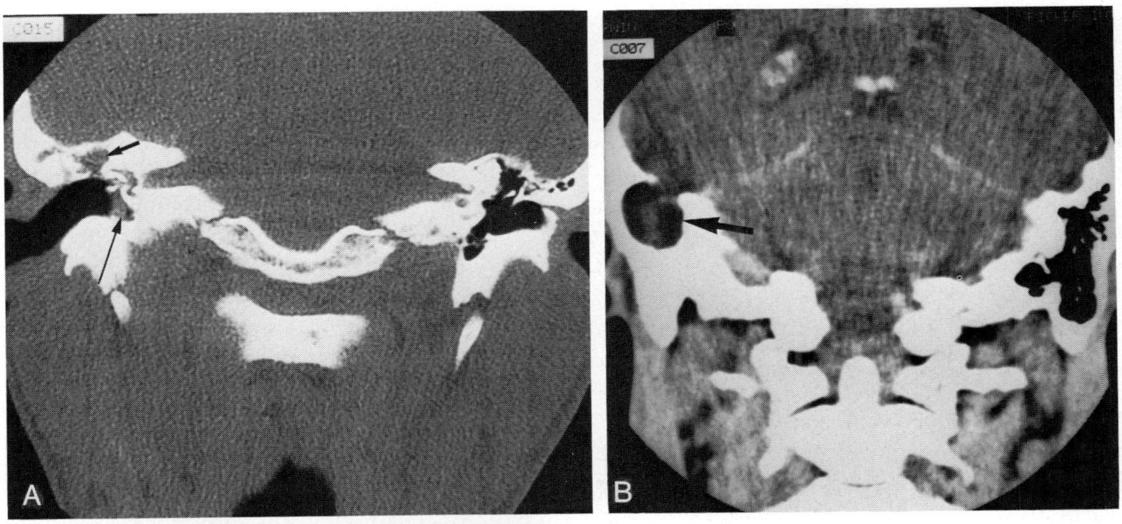

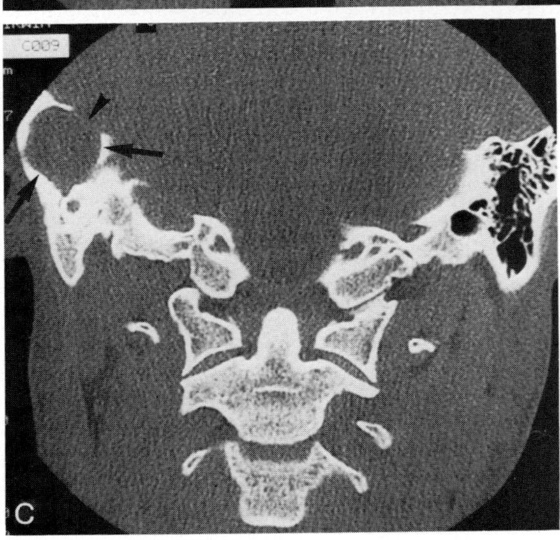

Figure 11–17. Cholesteatoma, secondary acquired (23-year-old male).

A, Coronal CT. Soft tissue fills the hypotympanum and mesotympanum *(long arrow)* and the epitympanic recess *(short arrow)*.

B, Coronal CT. The hypodense mass *(arrow)* extends posteriorly along the petrous ridge, eroding the surrounding bone.

C, Coronal CT. The benign bony erosive changes *(arrows)* are noted, with focal dehiscence of the inner table *(arrowhead)*.

tissues, blood vessels, and serum are the main source of cholesterol, which subsequently forms crystals and incites a sterile foreign body tissue reaction.[15, 23, 24] The cholesterol granuloma continues to enlarge as adjacent air cells are recruited. Macroscopically, these lesions consist of brownish-yellow semiliquid. Microscopically, cholesterol crystals are surrounded by foreign body giant cells and are embedded in fibrous connective tissue with hemosiderin-laden macrophages and chronic inflammatory cells and blood vessels.[18]

Cholesterol granulomas may occur anywhere within the aerated temporal bone, but do so most commonly in the middle ear cavity. Cholesterol granulomas of the tympanic cavity are frequently associated with acute and chronic otitis media, granulomatous mastoiditis, and cholesteatoma.[25] Accordingly, these lesions tend to be detected early and are usually confined to the middle ear or mastoid air cells. CT demonstrates a nonenhancing soft tissue mass with variable, but usually minimal, bony erosion. These lesions are usually indistinguishable on CT from cholesteatoma, paraganglioma, or herniation of brain through a dehiscent tegumen tympani. The MRI most commonly depicts a high-signal lesion on T1 and T2.[18]

Cholesterol granulomas of the petrous apex are less common than middle ear cholesterol granulomas. Nonetheless, this is the most common benign tumor of the petrous apex.[25] Because these lesions are usually not associated with other disease processes, they may reach enormous size before the patient seeks medical attention, with cerebellopontine angle (CPA) cranial nerve compression symptoms (hearing loss, tinnitus, vertigo, facial twitching).[23] The apex lesions tend to be significantly larger and associated with more bony erosive changes than their middle ear counterparts. The MRI signal intensity in this lesion is affected by the cholesterol content and the hemoglobin breakdown products. As mentioned previously, the lesions are usually bright on T1 and T2 sequences (Fig. 11–18). The hemosiderin tends to collect at the periphery of this lesion, often rendering the outer margin very low signal on T2 sequences. Postsurgically, the lesion is less bright on T1-weighted images, reflecting the successful drainage of cholesterol and the chronic hemorrhagic products.[25]

The nonpneumatized petrous apex normally contains marrow. This marrow is bright on T1, like the cholesterol granuloma. However, comparison of the "lesion" to fat on T2 sequence will distinguish apex marrow from the higher T2 signal cholesterol granuloma.[26]

Bell's Palsy

Bell's palsy is the most common cause of facial nerve paralysis, may occur at any age, usually has an acute onset, and typically resolves in 2 months. Resolution is usually complete. In most uncomplicated cases, patients with Bell's palsy do not require planar imaging. However, if symptoms are recurrent, prolonged, progressive, or associated with dysfunction of other cranial nerves, planar imaging is warranted.

Bell's palsy, although still considered idiopathic, and a diagnosis of exclusion, is usually viral. Herpes simplex virus type I and varicella zoster have been implicated.[27] The pathophysiology relates to neuronal edema, which causes a compressive neuropathy most often as the facial nerve traverses the facial canal from the IAC fundus to the geniculate ganglion.

The object of planar imaging is to exclude a mass lesion within or adjacent to the facial nerve from its brainstem origin to the parotid gland. Although initial reports[28] demonstrated no enhancement of the normal facial nerve, more recent data[28a] revealed enhancement of the facial canal seqment of the facial nerve in 76% of normal patients. Gadolinium-enhanced MRI has demonstrated abnormal enhancement in nearly 80% of patients with clinical Bell's palsy[27] (Fig. 11–19). The enhancement occurs most commonly in the labyrinthine segment and the descending facial nerve canal. Contrast enhancement may persist beyond the point of clinical improvement.

Malignant External Otitis

Malignant external otitis most commonly affects elderly diabetic patients.[29] *Pseudomonas aeruginosa* is the organism responsible for the entity that begins in the floor of the external ear cavity as an area of granulation tissue. As the infection progresses, the underlying bony and cartilaginous EAC becomes infected, with resultant osteomyelitis and chondritis. The infection spreads centrifugally through the fissures of Santorini,[15, 30] located

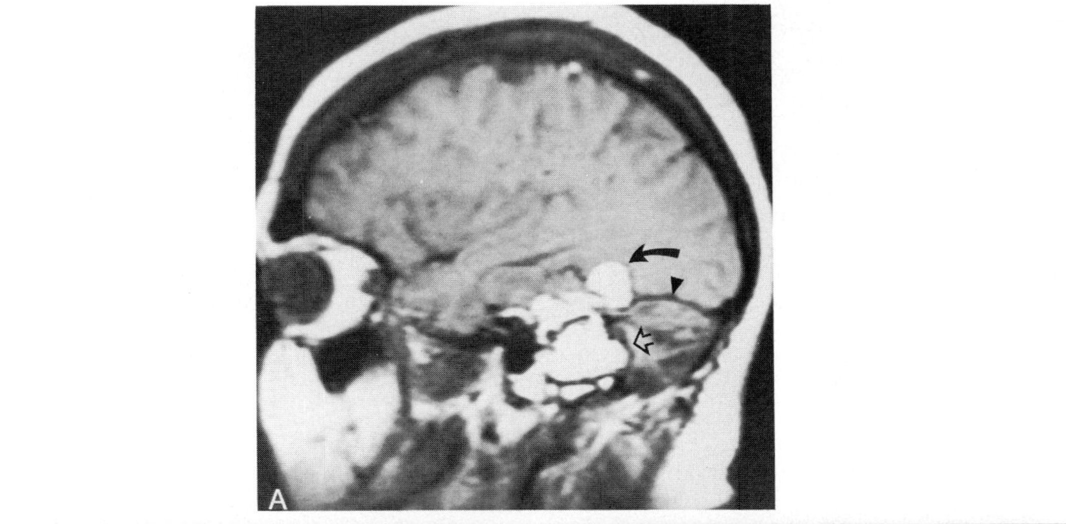

Figure 11–18. Cholesterol granuloma (34-year-old female).

A, Parasagittal T1. A complex high-signal mass is located within the petrous apex. The mass extends above *(curved arrow)* and below *(open arrow)* the tentorium *(arrowhead)*.

B, C, Axial T2. The multilocular mass is predominantly high signal, with scattered foci of diminished signal *(arrows)*, presumably representing hemosiderin.

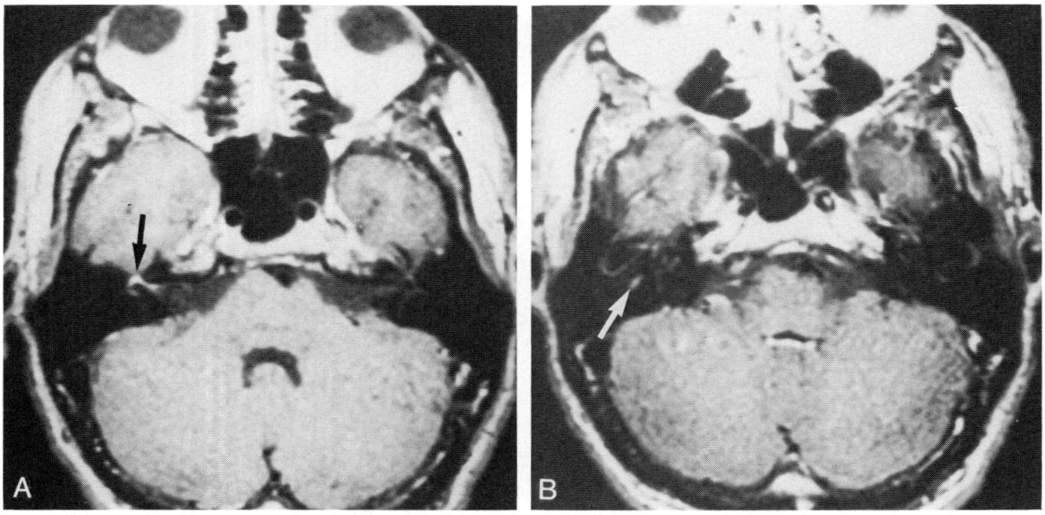

Figure 11–19. Bell's palsy (28-year-old male).

A, B, Enhanced axial T1. Abnormal enhancement of the labyrinthine *(black arrow)* and the proximal vertical portion of the right facial nerve *(white arrow)* is present. No mass lesion is identified.

in the cartilaginous floor of the EAC. The bacteria spread rapidly to the soft tissues at the base of the skull. The jugular bulb and sigmoid sinus may be involved, resulting in thrombosis. Patients may develop meningitis. Patients present with unrelenting otalgia, headache, purulent otorrhea that is unresponsive to topical antibiotics, and an increased erythrocyte sedimentation rate.[31] Local recurrence after administration of appropriate antibiotics occurs in 20% of patients.

Planar imaging demonstrates an infiltrative soft tissue reaction; loss of soft tissue fascial planes at the skull base; and soft tissue or fluid in the EAC, middle ear, and mastoid air cells, as well as adjacent to the eustachian tube. The infection is unilateral in 64% of patients.[31] Aggressive bone destruction may be present. MRI adroitly characterizes the enhancing infiltrative soft tissue abnormalities of this disease (Fig. 11–20).

Trauma

Temporal bone fractures may be classified into longitudinal or transverse. Longitudinal fractures account for 70 to 80% of all temporal bone fractures.[32–34] Longitudinal fractures run roughly parallel to the long axis of the petrous ridge and result from a direct blow to the temporal or parietal bones. The fracture usually begins in the posterior aspect of squamosal temporal bone extending to the posterosuperior roof of the EAC and extending medially through the roof of the middle ear cavity. The fracture passes anterolateral to the membranous vestibule, through the region of the geniculate ganglion, to end in the fibrous tissues of the foramen lacerum (Fig. 11–21). Depending on the magnitude of force, the fracture may extend a variable distance into the sphenoid bone.[35]

Approximately 20 to 30% of patients with longitudinal fractures present with facial paralysis that is usually delayed in onset. This is usually caused by a hematoma or edema and a compressive neuropathy, usually within the tympanic portion of the canal, distal to the geniculate ganglion. Complete recovery from paralysis occurs in 75% of patients. Conductive hearing loss may occur in up to 65% of patients,[34] but this is transient in nearly 80% of patients. However, 10 to 15% of cases of conductive hearing loss result from ossicular disruption and require surgical realignment.

Transverse fractures account for 10 to 20% of temporal bone fractures. These fractures result from a blow to the occipital or frontal bones and are more commonly associated with facial bone fractures. Transverse fractures course perpendicular to the axis of the petrous ridge, through the middle (lateral) or inner (medial) ear (Fig. 11–22). Lateral temporal bone fractures extend through the vestibule, resulting in complete, irreversible hearing loss or vertigo with spontaneous nystagmus, or

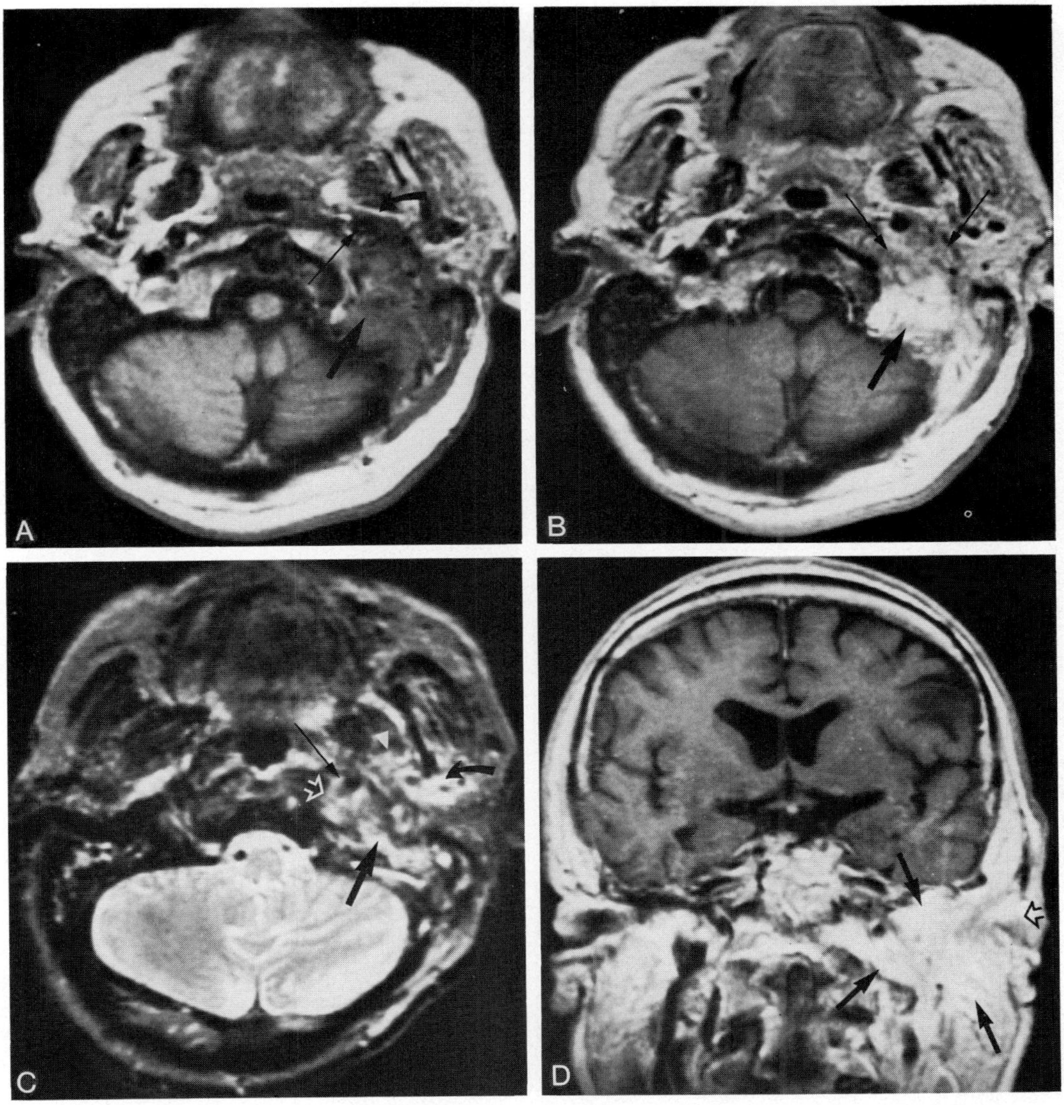

Figure 11–20. Malignant external otitis (74-year-old diabetic male).

A, Axial T1. An infiltrative isointense-to-muscle mass *(bold arrow)* is located in the soft tissues at the skull base on the left. The mass displaces the ICA *(long arrow)* anteriorly, obscures the internal jugular vein, and compresses the buccopharyngeal fascia *(curved arrow).*

B, Enhanced axial T1. The soft tissue mass *(bold arrow)* enhances homogeneously. The extracranial soft tissue *(thin arrows)* enhances heterogeneously.

C, Axial T2. Heterogeneous high signal *(bold arrow)* represents the soft tissue at the skull base. The inflammatory process has extended into the prevertebral fascia *(open arrow),* parotid gland *(curved arrow),* vascular sheath *(long arrow),* and lateral pterygoid muscle *(arrowhead).*

D, Enhanced coronal T1. The enhancing soft tissue *(arrows)* is contiguous with and extends from the skull base. The external auditory canal is filled with enhancing soft tissue *(open arrow).*

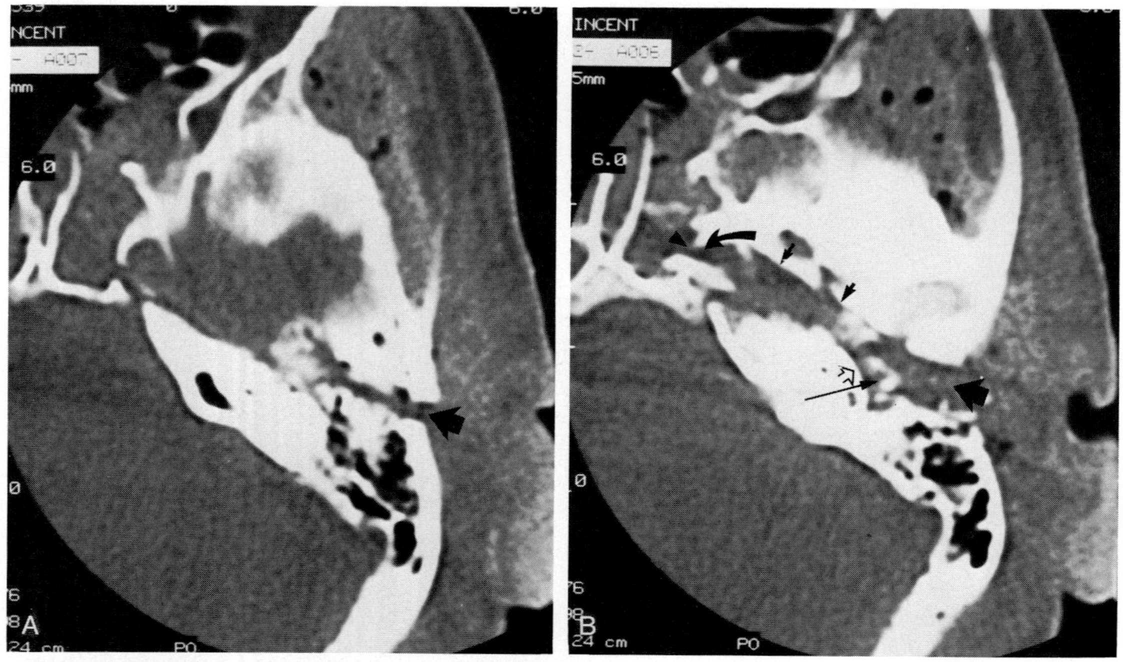

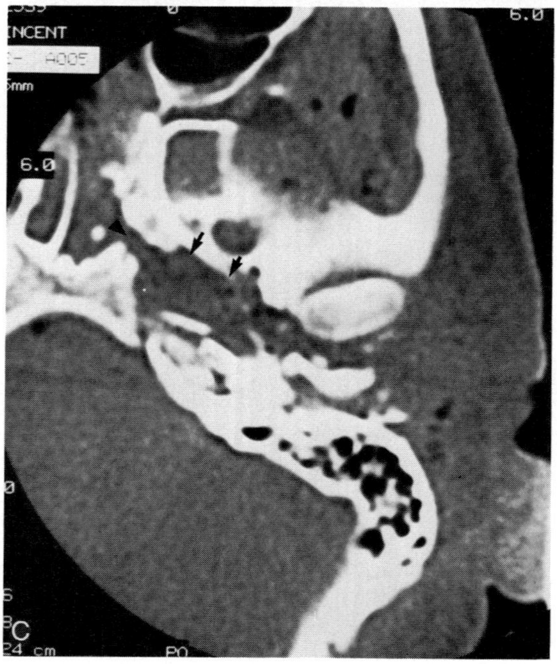

Figure 11–21. Longitudinal temporal bone fracture (10-year-old male).

A, Axial CT. A diastatic fracture *(arrow)* extends through the junction of the squamosal and petromastoid temporal bone.

B, C, Axial CT. The fracture extends along the external auditory canal *(bold arrow),* anterior to the vestibule *(open arrow)* and parallel to the course of the internal carotid artery *(small arrows),* toward the foramen lacerum *(curved arrow)* to the sphenoid sinus *(arrowhead).* The ossicles *(long arrow)* are dislocated.

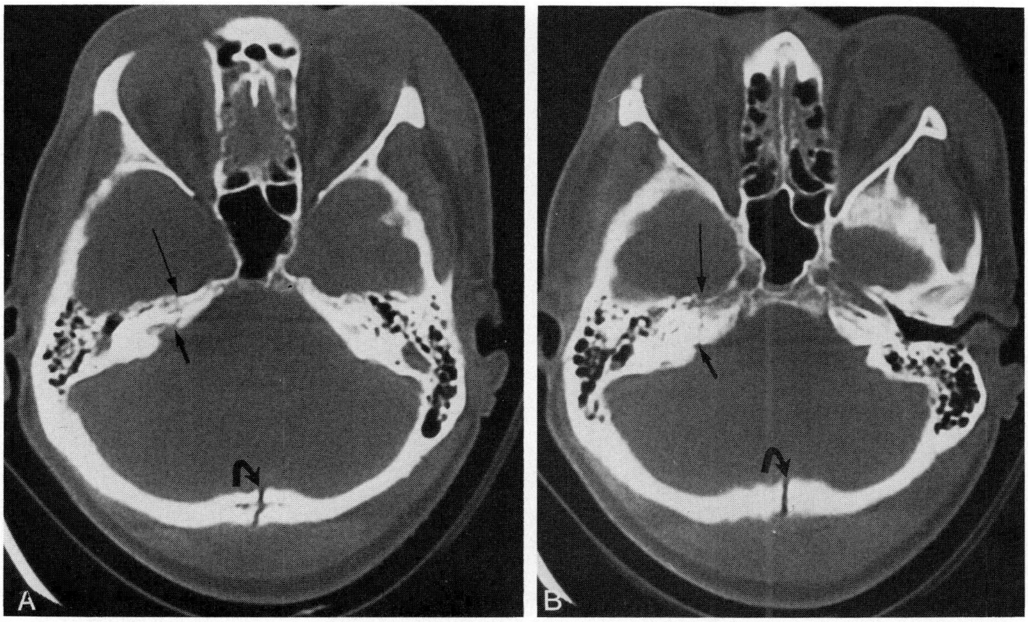

Figure 11–22. Transverse fracture of the temporal bone (44-year-old male).
A, B, Axial CT. A linear fracture *(long arrow)* extends from the medial IAC *(short arrow)* through the apex of the right petrous temporal bone. Also present is a slightly diastatic linear fracture *(curved arrow)* through the midline occipital bone.

both. Medial transverse fractures extend along the IAC to the fundus of the canal, medial to the otic capsule. Hearing is usually intact. Facial paralysis occurs in 40 to 50% of patients with transverse fractures. The paralysis is usually immediate and irreversible secondary to significant nerve injury.

Additional complications of temporal bone fractures include dural laceration with pneumocephalus and otorrhea or rhinorrhea.[36] Dural lacerations most commonly occur at the tegmen tympani[32] and may result in meningitis. Rarely, patients may present with abducens nerve (VI) or trigeminal nerve (V) dysfunction. Aseptic sigmoid sinus thrombosis may occur after temporal bone fracture.[37]

The primary CT sign of temporal bone fracture is visualization of a lucent fracture line. It may be necessary to obtain narrow collimated images (1 to 2 mm) to detect the fracture.[34] Secondary signs of fracture include fluid within the mastoid air cells or tympanic cavity,[33] intracranial gas, or disruption of the ossicular chain. Gas within the temporomandibular joint has been reported in 20% of patients with temporal bone fractures[38] (Fig. 11–23). Temporomandibular joint gas was the only indication of the temporal bone fracture in 12% of patients in this study.[38] The role of MRI in temporal bone fractures is limited. MRI is superior to CT in detecting the intracranial sequelae of trauma; however, MRI is able to detect only those fractures that are filled with blood or cerebrospinal fluid (CSF).[36]

Neoplasm

Glomus Tumors (Paragangliomas)

These soft tissue, locally infiltrative tumors arise from the small foci of paraganglionic tissue that are distributed along the course of Jacobson's nerve (tympanic branch of the glossopharyngeal nerve, IX) and Arnold's nerve (auricular branch of the vagus nerve, X).[39] The nerves have a variable course within the adventitia of the jugular bulb through the middle ear. Glomus jugulare tumors arise within the jugular bulb region; glomus tympanicum tumors arise within the tympanic cavity. These tumors are the most common neoplasms to affect the tympanic cavity and the second most common, after acoustic schwannomas, to affect the temporal bone.[40] The tumors are two to three times more common in females. Patients usually present in the fourth to fifth

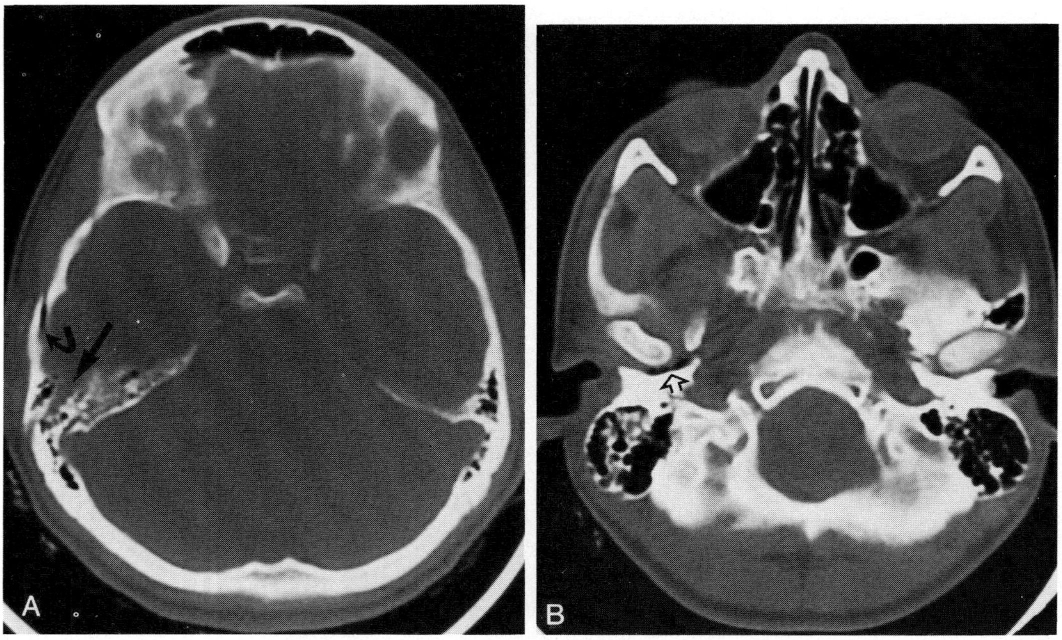

Figure 11–23. Longitudinal fracture of the temporal bone (37-year-old female).
A, Axial CT. A longitudinal fracture is present in the right temporal bone. Diastatic linear fractures extend through the squamosal temporal bone *(curved arrow)* and petromastoid temporal bone *(straight arrow)*.
B, Axial CT. Gas *(open arrow)* is present within the right temporal mandibular joint.

decade with symptoms that vary according to the origin and extension of the tumor.

Glomus jugulare tumors are three to five times more common than glomus tympanicum tumors. The lesions arise in the adventitia of the jugular bulb and are locally invasive, usually extending along pathways of least resistance.[41] The jugular and caroticojugular spines may be destroyed. The tumor may extend through the jugular plate into the hypotympanum or intracranially, as well as a variable distance along the vascular sheath, inferior to the skull base. Patients usually present with otalgia, symptoms of conductive hearing loss (63%), pulsatile tinnitus (56%), retrotympanic mass (40%), and cranial nerve involvement (37%).[40]

The CT findings of glomus jugulare tumor include an enhancing soft tissue mass in the jugular fossa with variable extension in all directions[42] (Fig. 11–24). The jugular fossa may be enlarged with a moth-eaten permeative pattern, the jugular and caroticojugular spine eroded, and the dura adjacent to the jugular bulb posteriorly displaced, indicating epidural tumor.[43] The tumor may be heterogeneous on MRI because of flow effects and hemoglobin degradation products. These lesions have been described as "salt and pepper" in appearance. The tumors usually enhance heterogeneously and markedly.

Glomus tympanicum tumors tend to present early with a conductive hearing loss (81%), tinnitus (72%), and retrotympanic mass (54%).[8, 40] Accordingly, these tumors tend to be smaller than jugular tumors at presentation. Rarely, bony changes are evident. These are most commonly located in the hypotympanum along the cochlear promontory.

CT depicts a small homogeneously enhancing mass along the cochlear promontory or lateral surface of the vertical carotid canal (Fig. 11–25). It is imperative to exclude an aberrant or laterally displaced carotid or dehiscent jugular bulb as the cause of the hypotympanic mass, as this cannot always be done clinically. MRI is slightly less useful in evaluating these lesions owing to their size and the signal void of adjacent bone and air. Enhanced MRI will, however, demonstrate small enhancing mass within the hypotympanum (Fig. 11–26).

The angiographic findings of these lesions include hypervascularity; early draining veins; and early, moderately sustained vascular

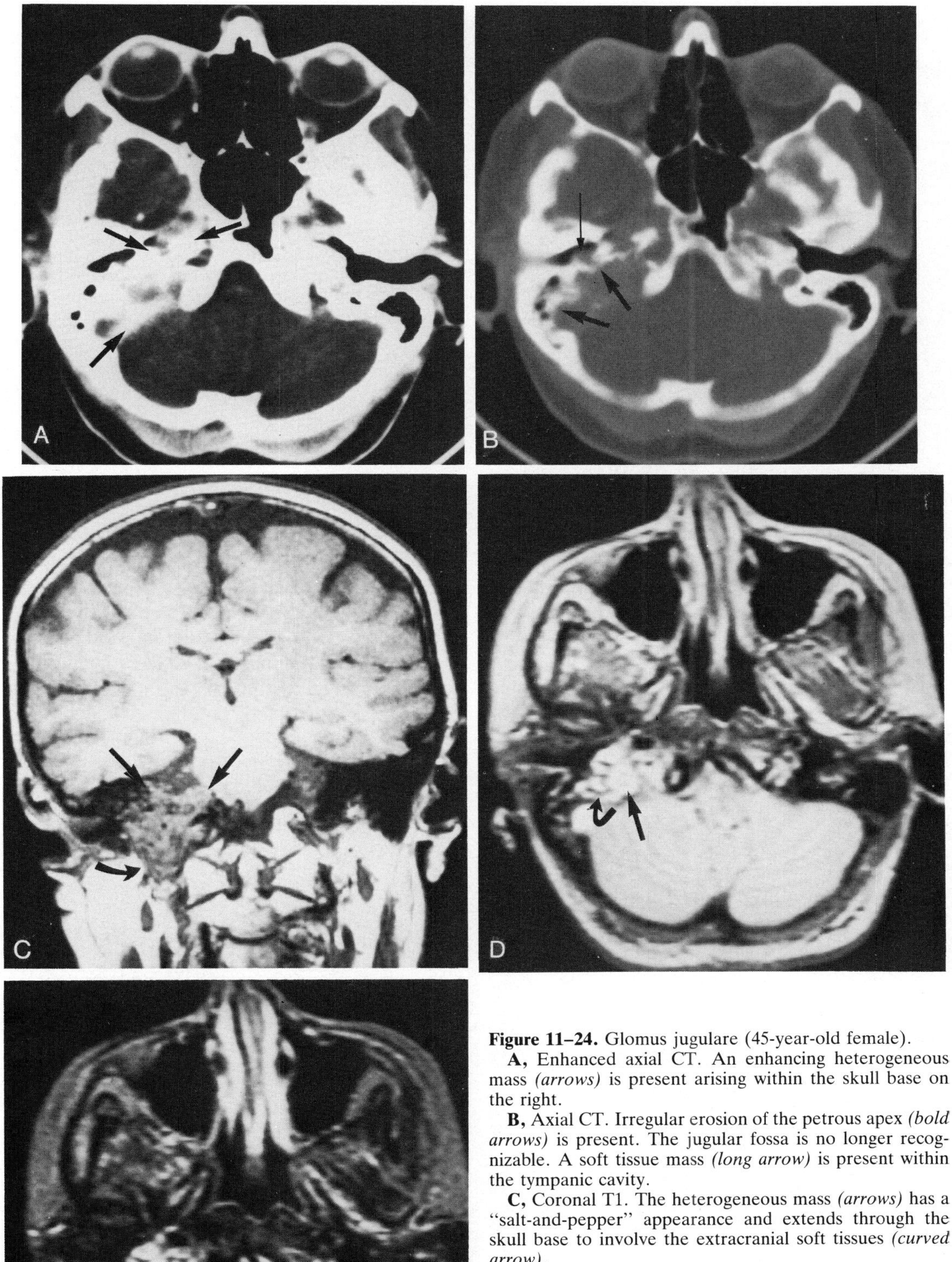

Figure 11–24. Glomus jugulare (45-year-old female).

A, Enhanced axial CT. An enhancing heterogeneous mass *(arrows)* is present arising within the skull base on the right.

B, Axial CT. Irregular erosion of the petrous apex *(bold arrows)* is present. The jugular fossa is no longer recognizable. A soft tissue mass *(long arrow)* is present within the tympanic cavity.

C, Coronal T1. The heterogeneous mass *(arrows)* has a "salt-and-pepper" appearance and extends through the skull base to involve the extracranial soft tissues *(curved arrow)*.

D, E, Axial SD and T2. The mass *(straight arrow)* is predominantly high signal, yet remains heterogeneous. Foci of diminished signal *(curved arrow)* are present, which may represent flow or hemoglobin breakdown products. (Lizak PF, and Woodruff WW: Posterior fossa neoplasms: multiplanar imaging. Semin Ultrasound CT MRI 1992; 13(3):182–206.)

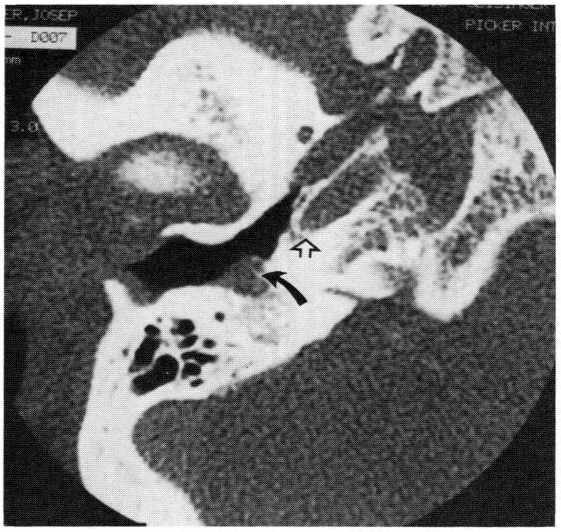

Figure 11–25. Glomus tympanicum (78-year-old male). Unenhanced axial CT; a soft tissue mass *(curved arrow)* can be seen in the hypotympanum. Note the normal appearance of the carotid canal and the carotid plate *(open arrow)*.

blush. Typically, the ascending pharyngeal artery is the dominant supply to these lesions followed by the posterior auricular, stylomastoid, and occipital arteries.

Nerve Sheath Tumor

Schwannomas of cranial nerves IX, X, and XI are rare, originating at the transition zone where Schwann cells replace the central oligodendroglial cells. The tumor begins in the jugular fossa and may remain localized or extend intracranially or extracranially.[44] These patients may have cerebellar signs if the lesion extends inward. Single cranial nerve deficits or jugular foramen syndrome may be present. It is impossible to distinguish the nerve of origin in most cases.

Planar imaging depicts a homogeneous, well-circumscribed soft tissue mass that en-

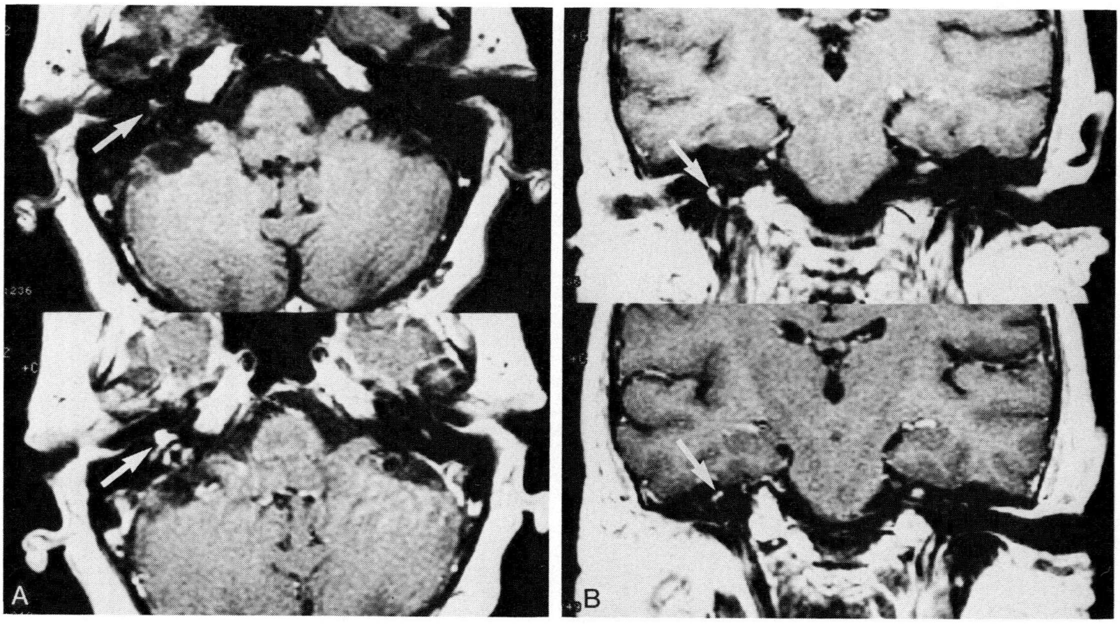

Figure 11–26. Glomus tympanicum.

A, Axial T1 (top unenhanced, bottom enhanced). An intermediate signal mass *(arrow)* is present within the hypotympanum. The mass *(arrow)* enhances vividly following contrast administration.

B, Enhanced coronal T1. The enhancing hypotympanic mass *(arrow)* is more clearly identified.

hances moderately. The mass is usually hypodense on CT, isointense to brain on T1, and hyperintense to brain on T2 (Figs. 11–27, 11–28). The mass may be localized to the jugular foramen or extend cephalad or caudad a variable distance. CT depicts sharply marginated, benign expansion of the jugular fossa and erosion of the jugular spine and possibly the jugular tubercle.[45] The main differential diagnosis for a lesion in this location is a glomus jugulare tumor. Distinguishing features include the heterogeneous "salt and pepper" appearance, the permeative bone destruction of the jugular foramen, and the angiographic hypervascularity of the glomus lesions in comparison to schwannoma.

Acoustic Schwannoma

Acoustic schwannomas represent more than 85% of CPA mass lesions and account for nearly 10% of intracranial tumors. The tumor originates at or within the lateral third of the IAC from Scarpa's ganglion in the superior vestibular division of cranial nerve VIII. Growing along the path of least resistance, the tumor extends through, often enlarging, the porus acusticus.

Clinically, patients present with sensorineural hearing loss, possibly accompanied by tinnitus. Women are affected twice as frequently as men. Patients vary widely in age, though usually they present in their fourth to seventh decade. Bilateral acoustic schwannomas more commonly occur in patients with neurofibromatosis II and typically occur by the third decade of life.

Planar imaging demonstrates a soft tissue mass in the IAC. The mass may be variable in size. Small (3- to 4-mm) intracanalicular cylindrical tumors may be detected (Fig. 11–29). Often the tumor extends into the CPA, forming a spheric mass 6 cm or more in greatest linear dimension. The mass is usually homogeneous and may be hypodense or isodense to brain on CT (Fig. 11–30). The mass is isointense to slightly hyperintense to brain on T1 and mildly hyperintense to brain on T2.[46] The lesions enhance moderately in a homogeneous fashion. Rarely, enhancement in the dura adjacent to the acoustic schwannoma may occur.[47] The larger lesions may be associated with cystic changes, increasing the heterogeneity of the lesion (Fig. 11–31). The hallmark of acoustic schwannoma is its origin in relationship to the IAC.[48] The tumor frequently causes flaring or widening of the porus acusticus; a 2- to 3-mm discrepancy in the diameter of the porus acusticus is abnormal. The brainstem and fourth ventricle may be displaced, with widening of the ipsilateral CPA, confirming the extra-axial nature of the tumor. Peri-

Text continued on page 419

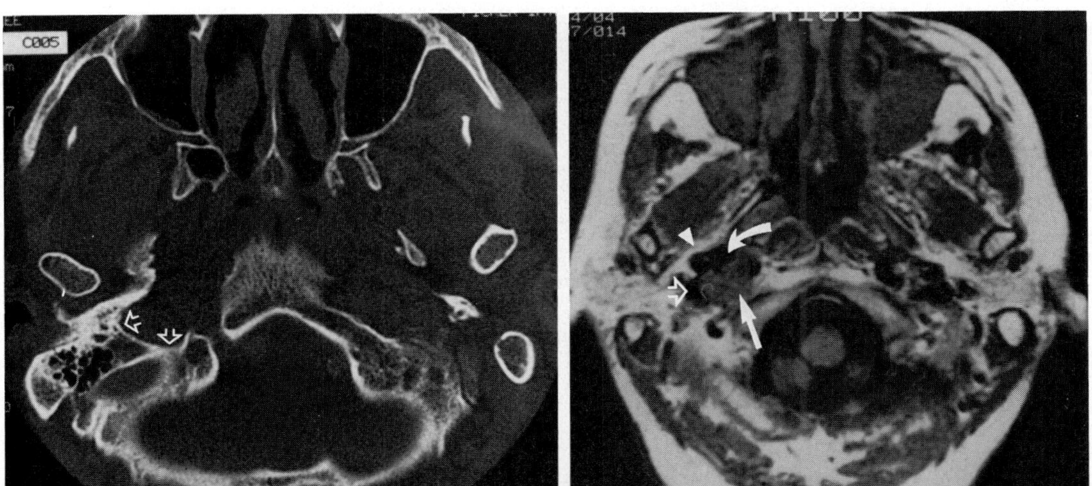

Figure 11–27. Vagus nerve schwannoma (46-year-old female).

A, Unenhanced CT. The right jugular foramen *(open arrows)* is enlarged. Benign bony erosive changes are evident.

B, Axial T1. A well-circumscribed, isointense-to-muscle mass *(arrow)* displaces a tortuous carotid artery *(curved arrow)* and jugular vein *(open arrow)*. The right buccopharyngeal fascia *(arrowhead)* is compressed.

Illustration continued on following page

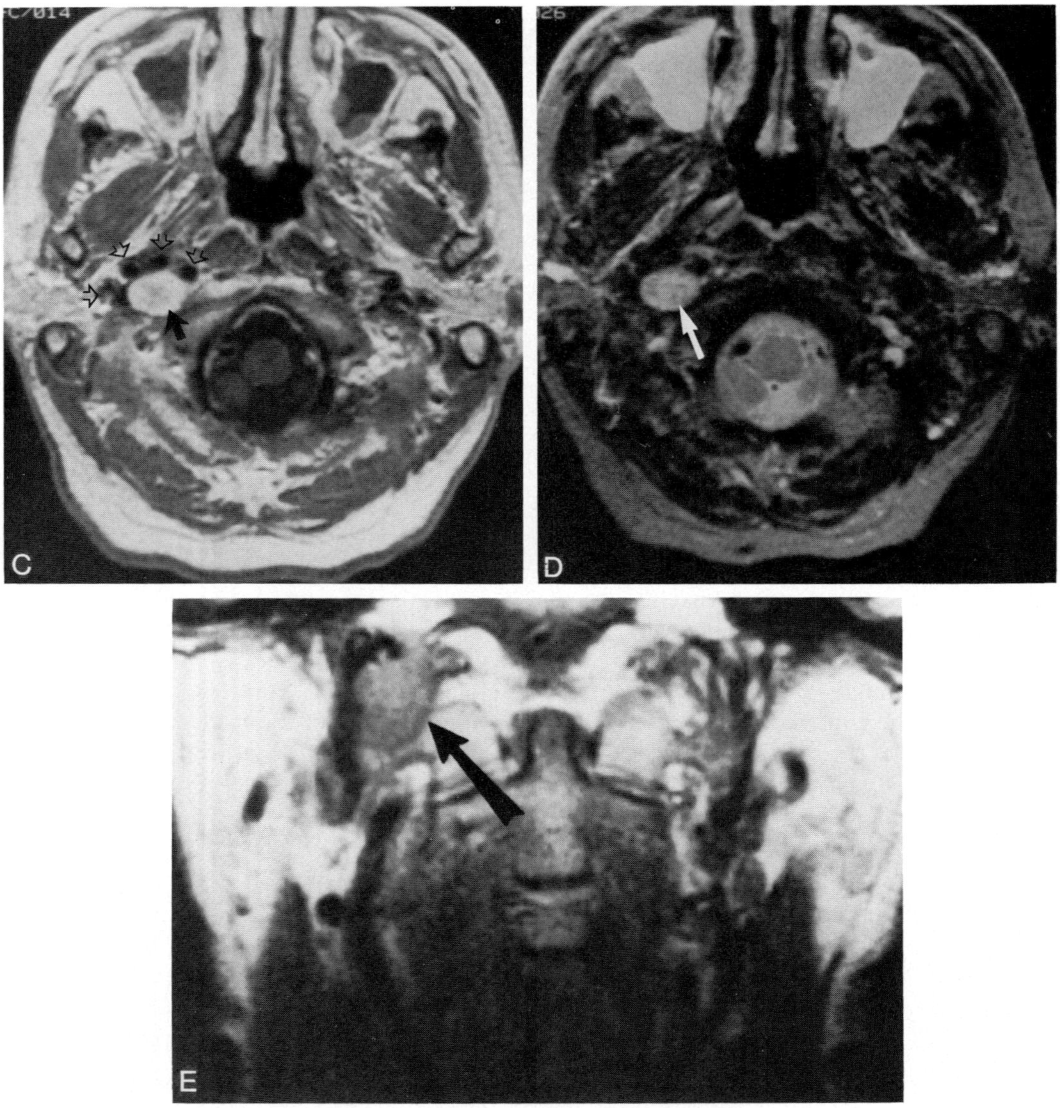

Figure 11–27 *Continued*

C, Enhanced axial T1. The mass *(arrow)* enhances homogeneously as its relationship with the adjacent vascular structures *(open arrows)* becomes more apparent.

D, Axial T2. The mass *(arrow)* is homogeneously high signal referable to surrounding structures.

E, Coronal T1. The mass *(arrow)* extends through the skull base to the C1 lateral mass.

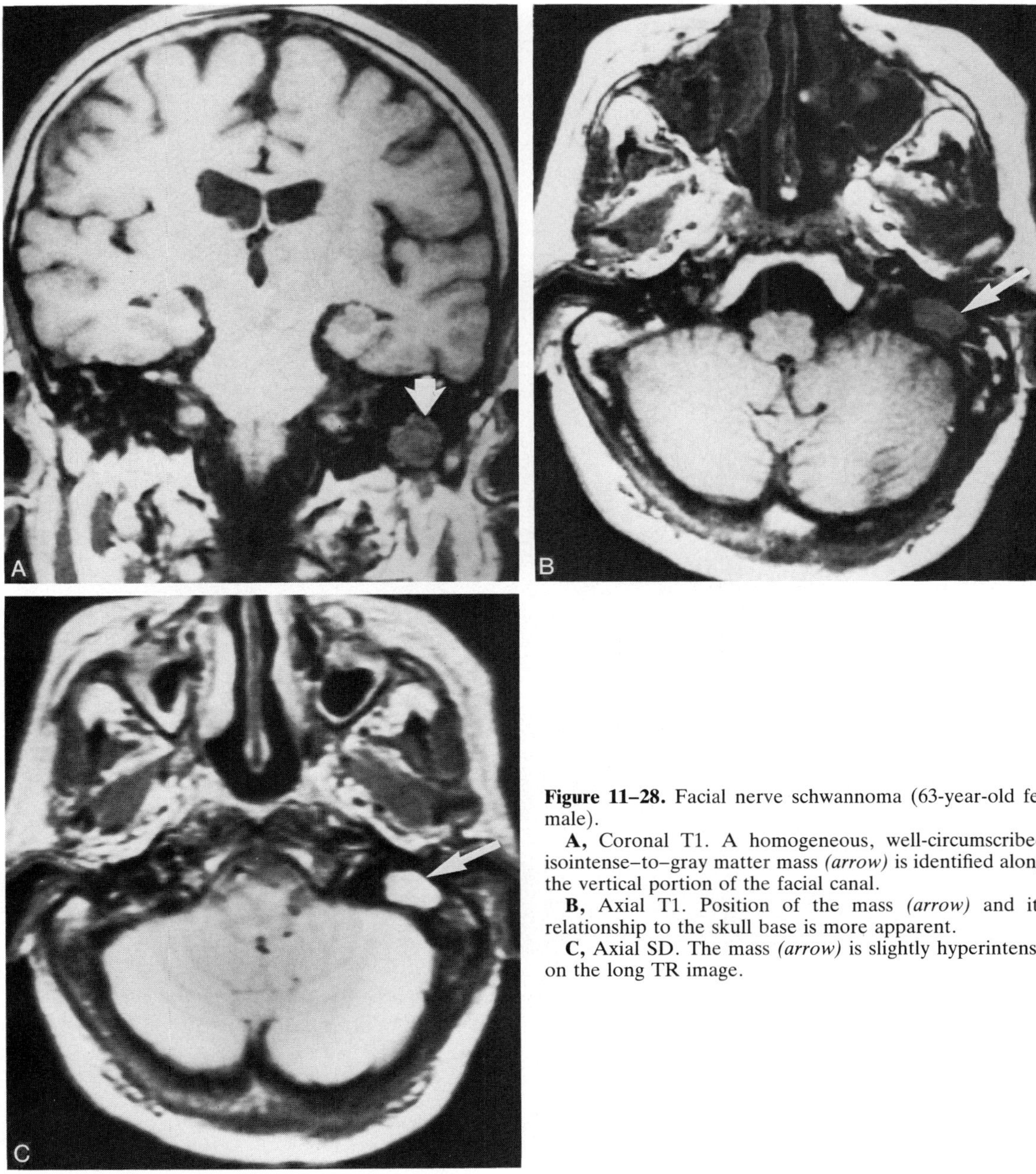

Figure 11–28. Facial nerve schwannoma (63-year-old female).

A, Coronal T1. A homogeneous, well-circumscribed isointense–to–gray matter mass *(arrow)* is identified along the vertical portion of the facial canal.

B, Axial T1. Position of the mass *(arrow)* and its relationship to the skull base is more apparent.

C, Axial SD. The mass *(arrow)* is slightly hyperintense on the long TR image.

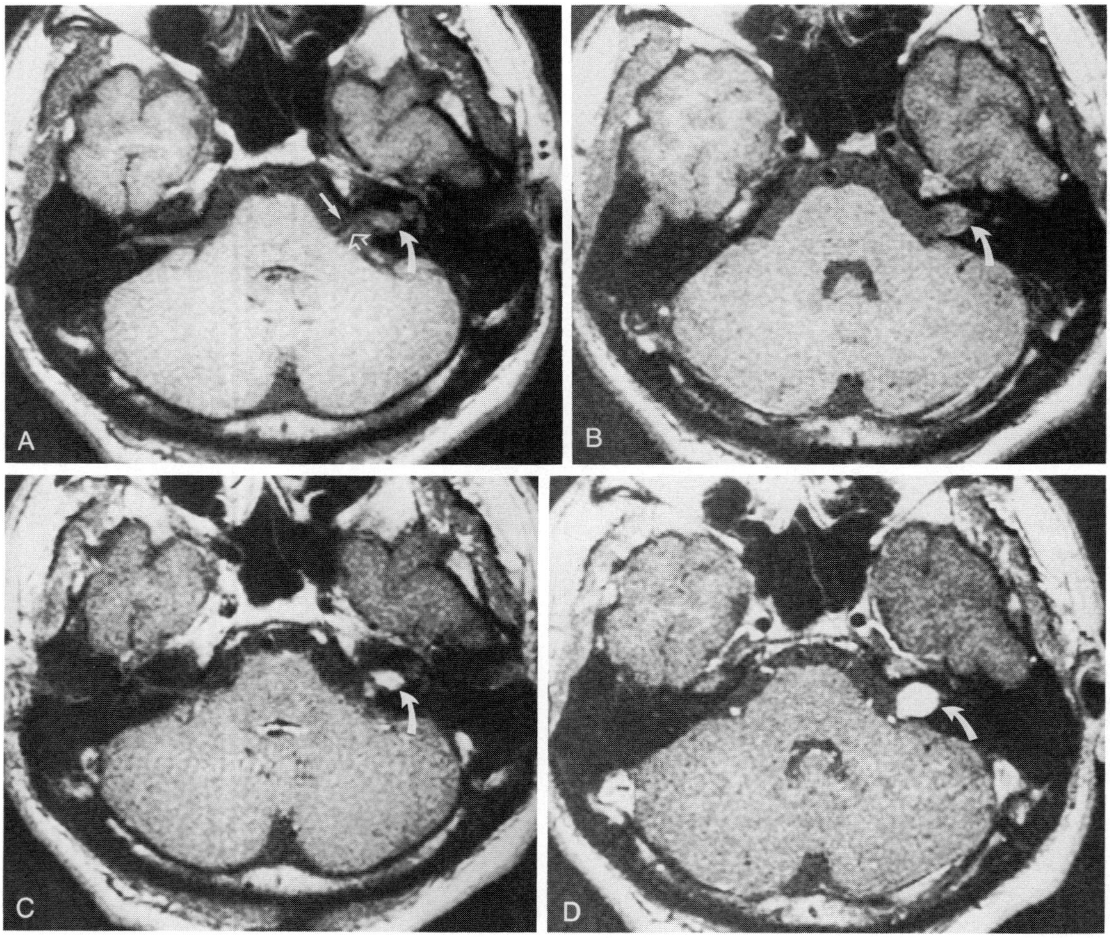

Figure 11–29. Acoustic schwannoma (25-year-old male).

A, B, Unenhanced axial T1. A left internal auditory canal mass *(curved arrow)* is identified. The internal auditory canal is enlarged. Proximal portion of the left seventh nerve *(closed arrow)* and eighth nerve *(open arrow)* within the cerebellopontine angle is normal.

C, D, Enhanced axial T1. The schwannoma *(curved arrow)* enhances homogeneously, more clearly delineating the size and extent of the tumor.

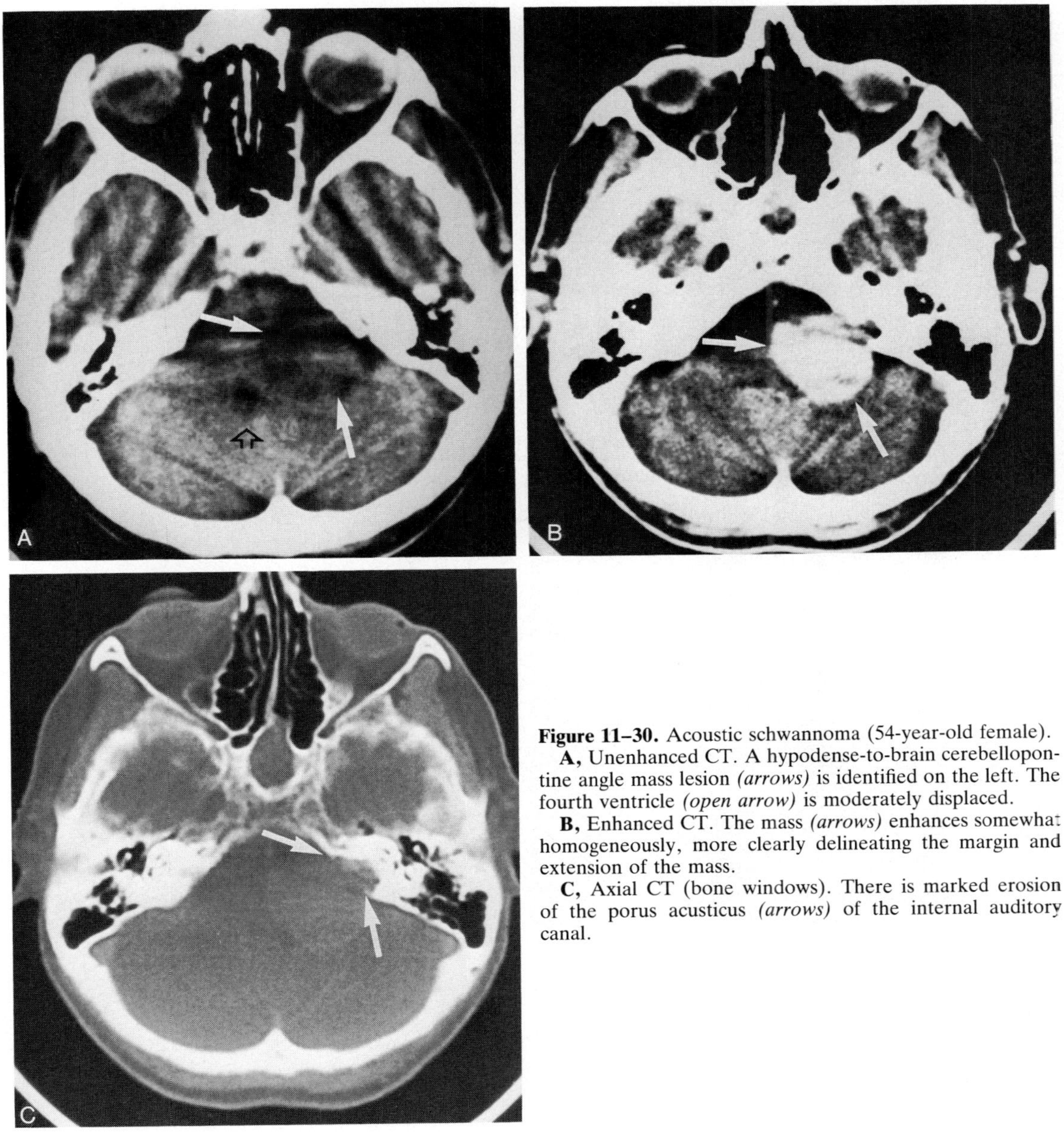

Figure 11–30. Acoustic schwannoma (54-year-old female).

A, Unenhanced CT. A hypodense-to-brain cerebellopontine angle mass lesion *(arrows)* is identified on the left. The fourth ventricle *(open arrow)* is moderately displaced.

B, Enhanced CT. The mass *(arrows)* enhances somewhat homogeneously, more clearly delineating the margin and extension of the mass.

C, Axial CT (bone windows). There is marked erosion of the porus acusticus *(arrows)* of the internal auditory canal.

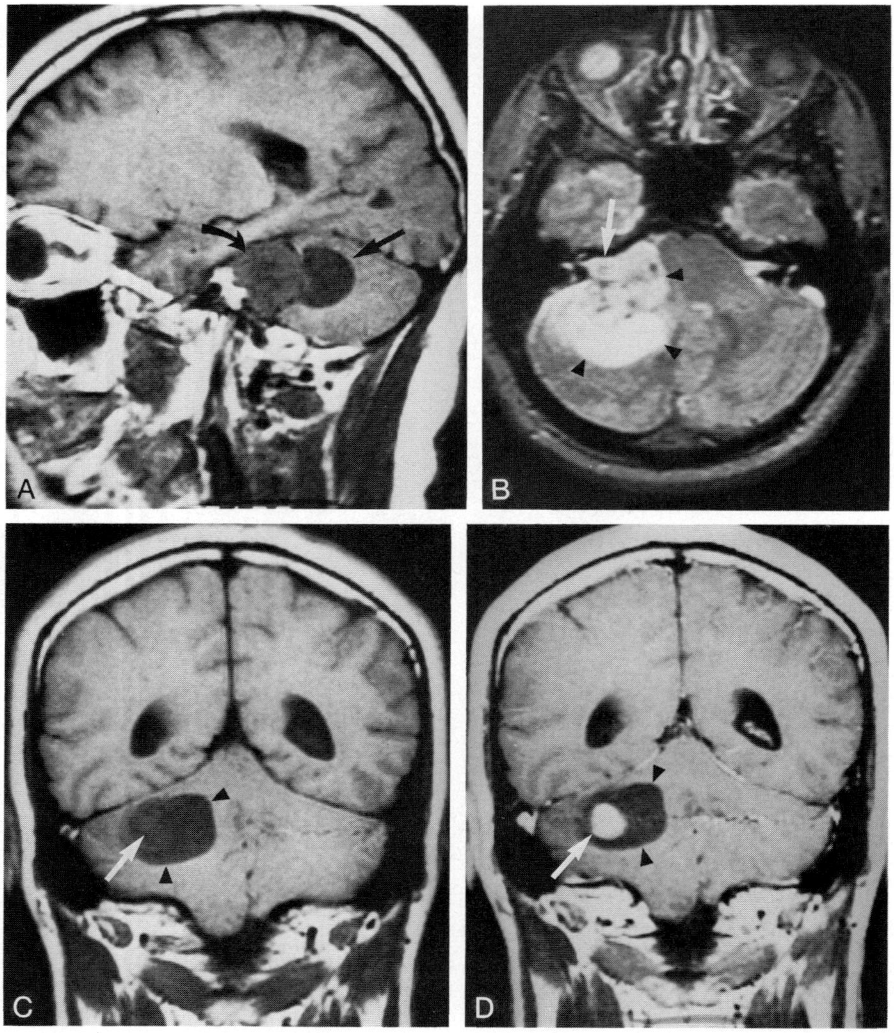

Figure 11–31. Acoustic schwannoma; atypical (43-year-old male).

A, Parasagittal T1. A complex, partially solid *(curved arrow),* partially cystic *(straight arrow)* mass rises from the right CPA.

B, Axial T2. The right IAC *(arrow)* is enlarged, and a complex, predominantly high-signal mass *(arrowheads)* is present.

C, Coronal T1. The posterior, cystic portion of the mass *(arrowheads)* is shown containing a focus of intermediate signal *(arrow).*

D, Enhanced coronal CT. The solid moiety *(arrow)* of the tumor enhances, surrounded by the nonenhancing cystic component *(arrowheads).*

tumoral edema is uncommon. Unenhanced T1 images must be performed to distinguish a small lipoma from an enhancing acoustic schwannoma on the enhanced examination (Fig. 11–32).

Meningioma

Meningiomas (discussed in more detail in Chapter 3) account for 20% of intracranial neoplasms and are the second most common CPA tumor, accounting for 7 to 10% of CPA lesions. These lesions arise from meningothelial cells located throughout the dura and may extend into the CPA from the posterior surface of the petrous ridge, the clivus, tentorium, or the foramen magnum. CPA meningiomas tend to be slightly larger than acoustic schwannomas at diagnosis because they grow for a longer time without symptoms.

Planar imaging demonstrates an exophytic or, less commonly, en plaque dural-based mass that typically is hyperdense to brain on CT owing to cellularity and the presence of psammomatous calcification. The lesion is isointense to brain on T1 and heterogeneous on T2 MRI. Meningiomas enhance in a homogeneous fashion (Fig. 11–33). The MRI signal characteristics and enhancement pattern of meningioma and acoustic schwannoma may overlap. The most helpful criteria to distinguish meningioma from acoustic schwannoma are the eccentricity of the meningioma to the IAC[48] (Fig. 11–34) and the lack of erosion of the porus acusticus.

Epidermoid Cyst

These congenital ectodermal inclusions (described in more detail in Chapter 3) are the third most common type of CPA lesions. The CPA is the most common intracranial location of epidermoid cysts; however, they also may occur within the petrous apex, the geniculate ganglion region, and in the tympanic cavity (congenital cholesteatoma).[22, 49] Patients usually present by the third to fourth decade. Patients with apex lesions exhibit trigeminal neuralgia; those with lesions of the CPA and geniculate ganglion present with facial paralysis. Patients with tympanic cavity cholesteatomas (epidermoids) have a conductive hearing loss secondary to ossicular dislocation.

The planar imaging appearance of epidermoid cysts has been presented previously. To review, these lesions are hypodense on CT, often with a lobulated surface, commensurate mass effect, and no edema or enhancement. T1 MRI images usually demonstrate a homogeneous mass of low signal similar to CSF (Fig. 11–35). Alternatively, these lesions may rarely be bright on T1-weighted images. These le-

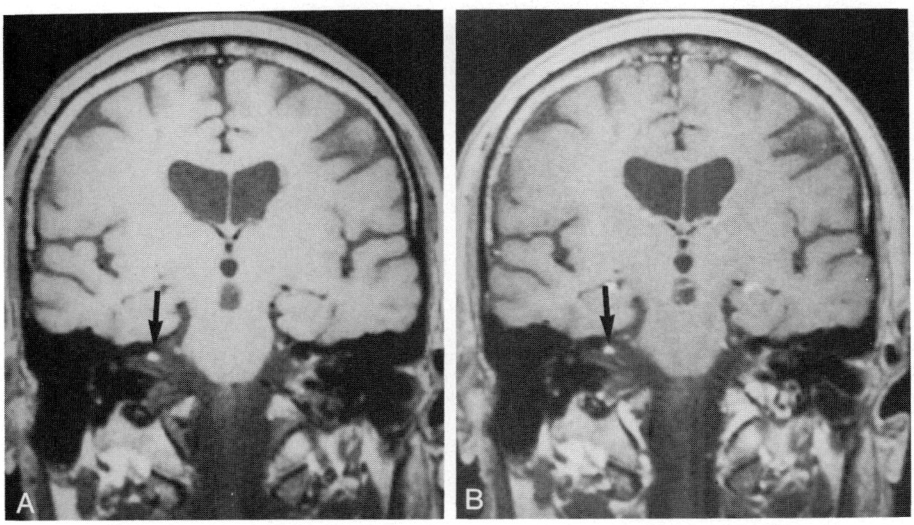

Figure 11–32. Lipoma (42-year-old male). A potential pitfall to omission of unenhanced T1-weighted sequence.
A, Coronal T1. A high-signal focus *(arrow)* is present in the proximal portion of the right IAC.
B, Enhanced coronal CT. There is no appreciable change in the appearance of this lipoma *(arrow)*. This is a potential pitfall when the IACs are evaluated solely with enhanced sequences.

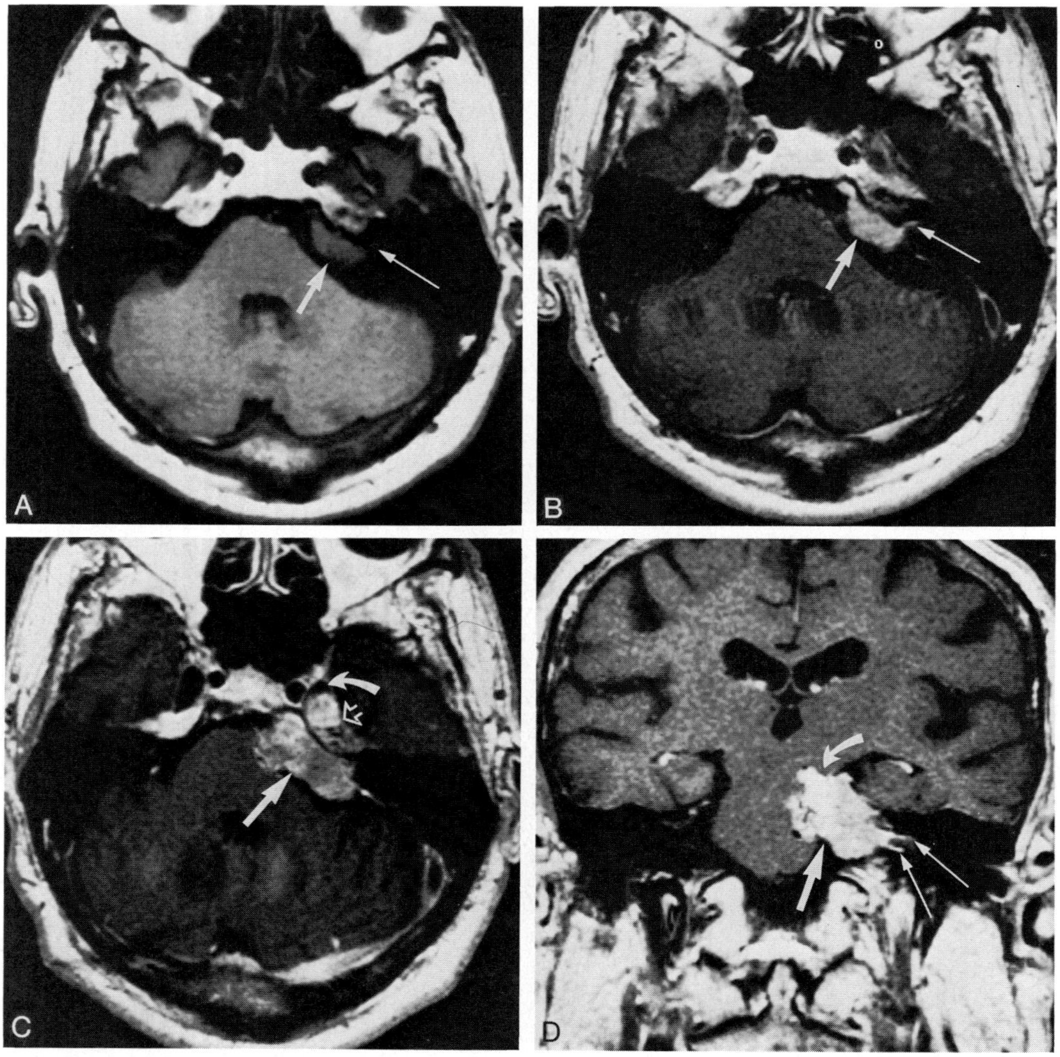

Figure 11–33. Meningioma (76-year-old male).

A, Unenhanced T1. An extra-axial dural-based mass *(bold arrow)* is located along the petrous apex, contiguous with the IAC *(thin arrow)*.

B, Enhanced axial T1. The mass *(bold arrow)* enhances homogeneously, as does a small focus *(thin arrow)* that has extended into the IAC.

C, Enhanced axial T1. The mass extends anteriorly to Meckel's cave *(open arrow)* compressing the gasserian ganglion *(curved arrow)*. The posterior fossa component *(arrow)* of the mass is well visualized.

D, Enhanced coronal T1. The supratentorial *(curved arrow)* and infratentorial *(bold arrow)* components of the mass enhance. There is also peripheral enhancement of the IAC *(thin arrows)*. (Lizak PF, and Woodruff WW: Posterior fossa neoplasms: multiplanar imaging. Semin Ultrasound CT MRI 1992; 13(3):182–206.)

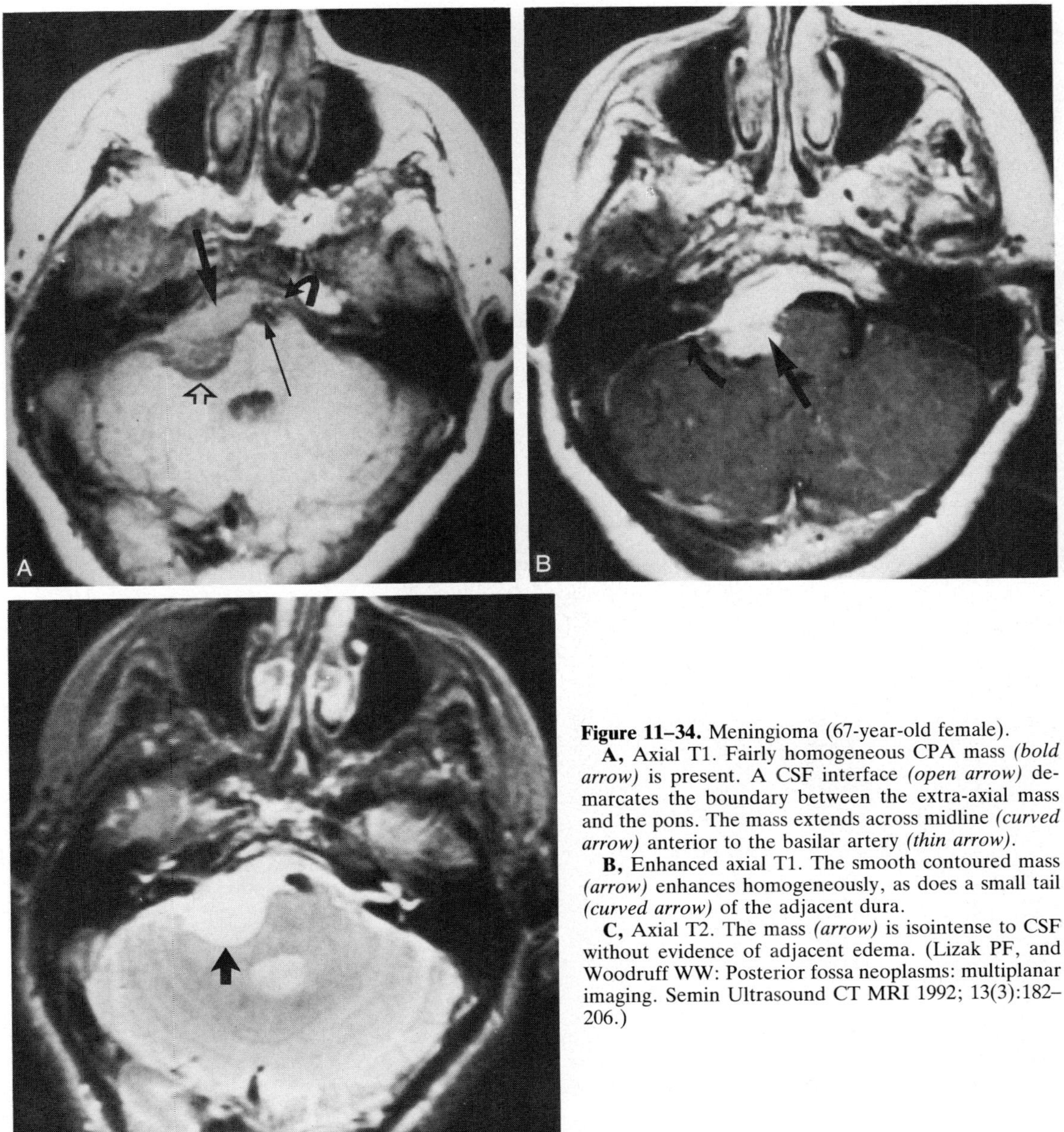

Figure 11–34. Meningioma (67-year-old female).

A, Axial T1. Fairly homogeneous CPA mass *(bold arrow)* is present. A CSF interface *(open arrow)* demarcates the boundary between the extra-axial mass and the pons. The mass extends across midline *(curved arrow)* anterior to the basilar artery *(thin arrow)*.

B, Enhanced axial T1. The smooth contoured mass *(arrow)* enhances homogeneously, as does a small tail *(curved arrow)* of the adjacent dura.

C, Axial T2. The mass *(arrow)* is isointense to CSF without evidence of adjacent edema. (Lizak PF, and Woodruff WW: Posterior fossa neoplasms: multiplanar imaging. Semin Ultrasound CT MRI 1992; 13(3):182–206.)

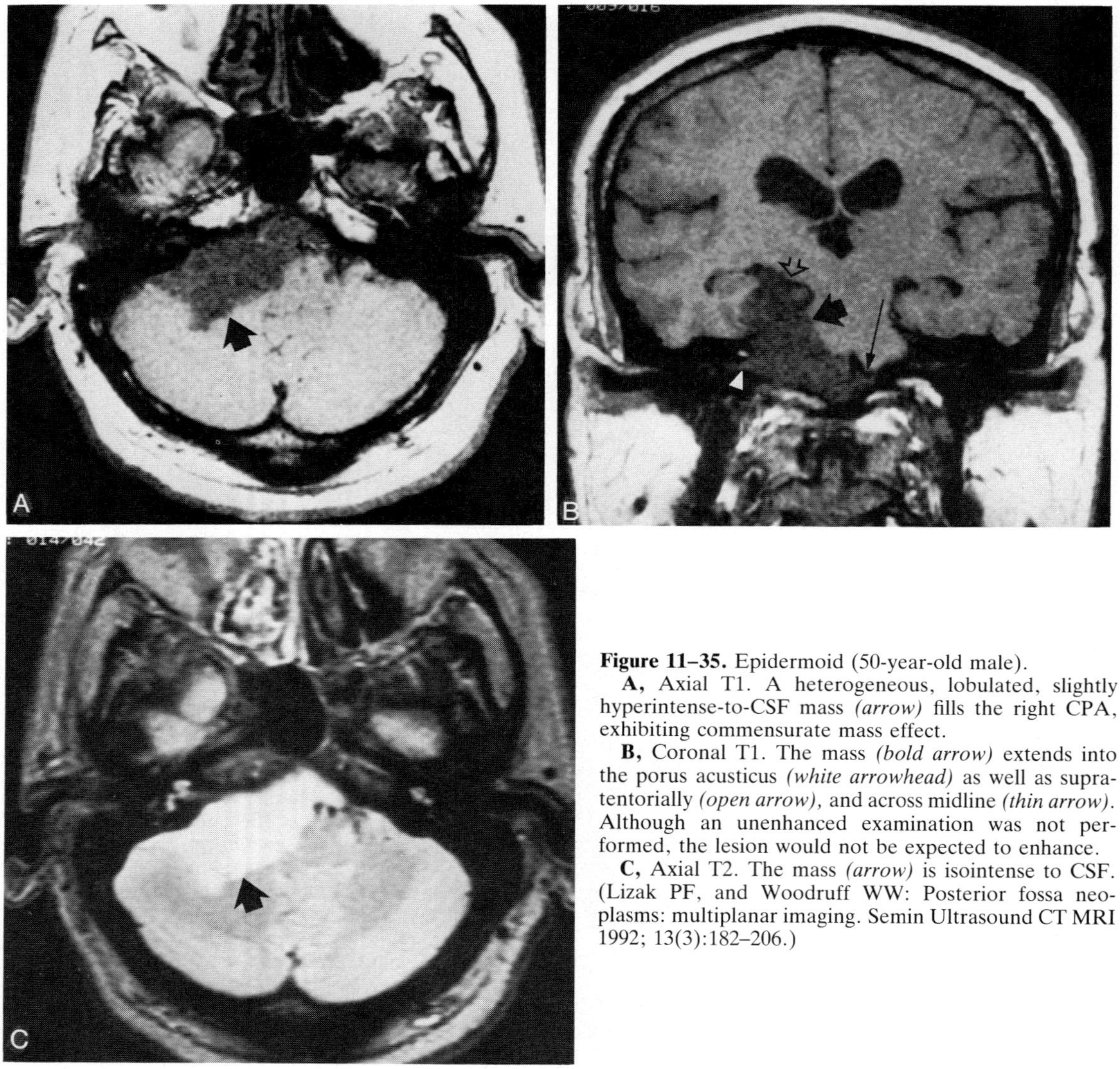

Figure 11–35. Epidermoid (50-year-old male).

A, Axial T1. A heterogeneous, lobulated, slightly hyperintense-to-CSF mass *(arrow)* fills the right CPA, exhibiting commensurate mass effect.

B, Coronal T1. The mass *(bold arrow)* extends into the porus acusticus *(white arrowhead)* as well as supratentorially *(open arrow),* and across midline *(thin arrow).* Although an unenhanced examination was not performed, the lesion would not be expected to enhance.

C, Axial T2. The mass *(arrow)* is isointense to CSF. (Lizak PF, and Woodruff WW: Posterior fossa neoplasms: multiplanar imaging. Semin Ultrasound CT MRI 1992; 13(3):182–206.)

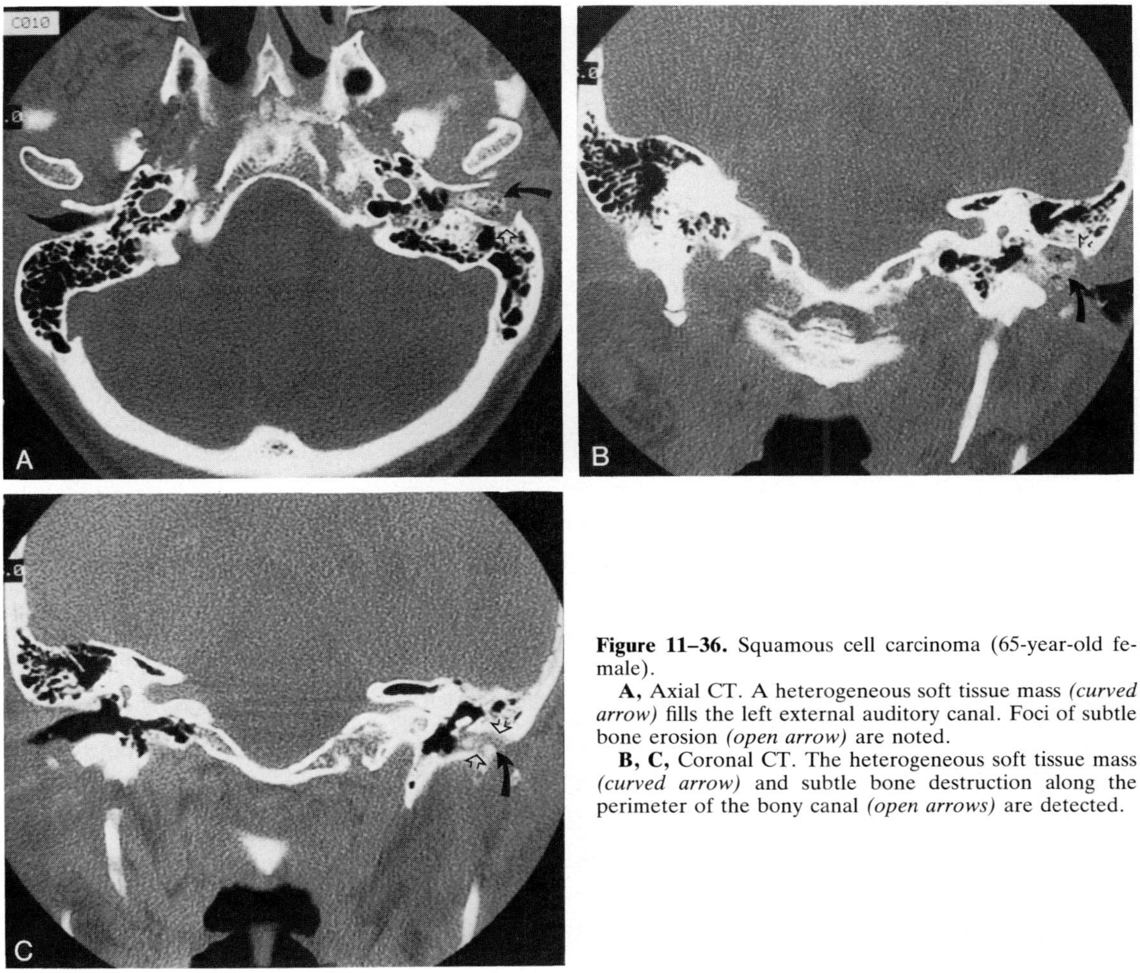

Figure 11–36. Squamous cell carcinoma (65-year-old female).

A, Axial CT. A heterogeneous soft tissue mass *(curved arrow)* fills the left external auditory canal. Foci of subtle bone erosion *(open arrow)* are noted.

B, C, Coronal CT. The heterogeneous soft tissue mass *(curved arrow)* and subtle bone destruction along the perimeter of the bony canal *(open arrows)* are detected.

sions are usually more heterogeneous on T2-weighted sequences and are usually higher than or equal to the signal intensity of CSF.

Squamous Cell Carcinoma

Squamous cell carcinoma is the most common malignant tumor of the temporal bone. The lesion usually occurs in the fifth to seventh decade in the setting of chronic middle ear infection. Patients may present with otalgia and bloody ear drainage. Later in the disease, patients may develop facial palsy, deafness, vertigo, and tinnitus.[50] The lesions are more common in women.

The mucosa of the external auditory canal is the most frequent temporal bone origin. These lesions may spread secondarily into the middle ear or externally through the external auditory meatus. Less commonly, the lesion begins in the tympanic cavity and extends either superiorly through the tegmen tympani, posteriorly to the mastoid air cells, or anteriorly along the eustachian tube to the nasopharynx. Involvement of the middle ear cavity has a significant impact on patient prognosis. The 5-year survival is 23% if the middle ear is involved. Alternatively, if the middle ear is free of disease, the 5-year survival is 59%.[30]

Planar imaging depicts a soft tissue mass and irregular bone destruction (Fig. 11–36). The squamosal temporal bone may be sclerotic, even though remote from the tumor.[50] MRI depicts an enhancing soft tissue mass. The adjacent dura may enhance if the tumor is in proximity.

References

1. *Gray's Anatomy.* Warwick R, Williams PL (eds). 35th ed, WB Saunders, Philadelphia, 1975.
2. Brogan M, Chakeres DW: Computed tomography and magnetic resonance imaging of the normal anatomy of the temporal bone. Semin Ultrasound CT MR 1989; 10:178–194.
3. Swartz JD: High-resolution computed tomography of the middle ear and mastoid. Radiology 1983; 148:449–454.
4. Daniels DL, Schenck JF, Foster T, et al: Magnetic resonance imaging at the jugular foramen. AJNR 1985; 6:699–703.
5. Lo WWM, Solti-Bohman LG: High-resolution CT of the jugular foramen: Anatomy and vascular variants and anomalies. Radiology 1984; 150:743–747.
6. Urman SM, Talbot JM: Otic capsule dysplasia: Clinical and CT findings. Radiographics 1990; 10:823–838.
7. Eelkema EA, Curtin HD: Congenital anomalies of the temporal bone. Semin Ultrasound CT MR 1989; 10:195–212.
8. Remley KB, Coit WE, Harnsberger HR, et al: Pulsatile tinnitus and the vascular tympanic membrane: CT, MR, and angiographic findings. Radiology 1990; 174:383–389.
9. Lo WWM, Solti-Bohman LG, McElveen JT: Aberrant carotid artery: Radiologic diagnosis with emphasis on high-resolution CT. Radiographics 1985; 5:985–993.
10. Sinnreich AI, Parisier SC, Cohen NC, et al: Arterial malformations of the middle ear. Otolaryngol Head Neck Surg 1984; 92:194–206.
11. Davis WL, Harnsberger HR: MR angiography of an aberrant internal carotid artery. AJNR 1991; 12:1225.
12. Overton SB, Ritter FN: A high placed jugular bulb in the middle ear: A clinical and temporal bone study. Laryngoscope 1973; 83:1986–1991.
13. Farrell FW, Hantz O: Protruding jugular bulb presenting as a middle ear mass: Case report and brief review. AJR 1977; 128:685–687.
14. Glassock ME, Dickins JRE, Jackson CG, et al: Vascular anomalies of the middle ear. Laryngoscope 1980; 90:77–88.
15. Holliday RA: Inflammatory diseases of the temporal bone: Evaluation with CT and MR. Semin Ultrasound CT MR 1989; 10:213–235.
16. Swartz JD, Goodmar RS, Russell KB, et al: High-resolution CT of the middle ear and mastoid. Radiology 1983; 148:455–459.
17. Martin N, Sterkers O, Nahum H: Chronic inflammatory disease of the middle ear cavities: Gd-DTPA-enhanced MR imaging. Radiology 1990; 176:399–405.
18. Martin N, Sterkers O, Mompoint D, et al: Cholesterol granulomas of the middle ear cavities: MR imaging. Radiology 1989; 172:521–525.
19. Johnson DW, Hinshaw DB, Hasso AN, et al: Computed tomography of local complications of temporal bone cholesteatomas. J Comput Assist Tomogr 1985; 9:519–523.
20. Swartz JD, Glazer AV, Faerber EN, et al: Congenital middle ear deafness: CT study. Radiology 1986; 159:187–190.
21. Ishii K, Takahashi S, Matsumoto K, et al: Middle ear cholesteatoma extending into the petrous apex: Evaluation by CT and MR imaging. AJNR 1991; 12:719–724.
22. Latack JT, Kartush JM, Kemink JL, et al: Epidermoidomas of the cerebellopontine angle and temporal bone: CT and MR aspects. Radiology 1985; 157:361–366.
23. Lo WWM, Solti-Bohman LG, Brackmann DE, et al: Cholesterol granuloma of the petrous apex: CT diagnosis. Radiology 1984; 153:705–711.
24. Gherini SG, Brackmann DE, Lo WWM, et al: Cholesterol granuloma of the petrous apex. Laryngoscope 1985; 95:659–664.
25. Greenberg JJ, Oot RF, Wismer GL, et al: Cholesterol granuloma of the petrous apex: MR and CT evaluation. AJNR 1988; 9:1205–1214.
26. Haynes RC, Amy JR: Asymmetric temporal bone pneumatization: An MR imaging pitfall. AJNR 1988; 9:803.
27. Tien R, Dillon WP, Jackler RK: Contrast-enhanced MR imaging of the facial nerve in 11 patients with Bell's palsy. AJNR 1990; 11:735–741.
28. Daniels DL, Czervionke LF, Pojunas KW, et al: Facial nerve enhancement in MR imaging. AJNR 1987; 8:605–607.
28a. Gebarski SS, Telian SA, Niparko JK: Enhancement along the normal facial nerve in the facial canal: MR imaging and anatomic correlation. Radiology 1992; 183:391–394.
29. Bird CR, Hasso AN, Stewart CE, et al: Malignant primary neoplasms of the ear and temporal bone studies by high-resolution CT. Radiology 1983; 149:171–174.
30. Curtin HD, Wolfe P, May M: Malignant external otitis: CT evaluation. Radiology 1982; 145:383–388.
31. Rubin J, Curtin HD, Yu VL, et al: Malignant external otitis: Utility of CT in diagnosis and follow-up. Radiology 1990; 174:391–394.
32. Schubiger O, Valavanis A, Stuckmann G, et al: Temporal bone fractures and their complications: Examination with high resolution CT. Neuroradiology 1986; 28:93–99.
33. Avrahami E, Chen Z, Solomon A: Modern high resolution CT diagnosis of longitudinal fractures of the petrous bone. Neuroradiology 1988; 30:166–168.
34. Holland BA, Brant-Zawadzki M: High-resolution CT of temporal bone trauma. AJNR 1984; 5:291–295.
35. Dolan KD: Temporal bone fractures. Semin Ultrasound CT MR 1989; 10:262–279.
36. Zimmerman RA, Bilaniuk LT, Hackney DB, et al: Magnetic resonance imaging in temporal bone fractures. Neuroradiology 1987; 29:246–251.
37. Ghorayeb BY, Yeakley JW, Hall JW, et al: Unusual complications to temporal bone fractures. Arch Otolaryngol Head Neck Surg 1987; 113:749–753.
38. Betz BW, Wiener MD: Air in the temporomandibular joint fossa: CT sign of temporal bone fracture. Radiology 1991; 180:463–466.
39. Burger PC, Vogel FS: *Surgical Pathology of the Nervous System and Its Coverings.* 2nd ed. New York: John Wiley & Sons, 1982.
40. Lo WWM, Solti-Bohman LG, Lambert PR: High-resolution CT in the evaluation of glomus tumors of the temporal bone. Radiology 1984; 150:737–742.
41. Spector GJ, Sobol S, Thawley SE, et al: Glomus jugulare tumors of the temporal bone. Patterns of invasion of the temporal bone. Laryngoscope 1979; 89:1628–1639.

42. Gratten-Smith JD, Doust BD, Fagan PA: High resolution CT in the evaluation of glomus tumours of the temporal bone. Australas Radiol 1988; 32:190–196.
43. Chakeres DW, LaMasters DL: Paragangliomas of the temporal bone: High-resolution CT studies. Radiology 1984; 150:749–753.
44. Müller-Forell W, Dei-Anang K, Perneczky A, et al: Neurinoma of the jugular foramen. Neuroradiology 1990; 32:244–246.
45. Pinto RS, Kricheff II: Neuroradiology of intracranial neuromas. Semin Roentgenol 1984; 19:44–52.
46. Mikhael MA, Ciric IS, Wolff AP: Differentiation of cerebellopontine angle neuromas and meningiomas with MR imaging. J Comput Assist Tomogr 1985; 9:852–856.
47. Paz-Fumagalli R, Daniels DL, Millen SJ, et al: Dural "tail" associated with an acoustic schwannoma in MR imaging with gadopentetate dimeglumine. AJNR 1991; 12:1206.
48. Gentry LR, Jacoby CG, Turski PA, et al: Cerebellopontine angle—petromastoid mass lesions: Comparative study of diagnoses with MR imaging and CT. Radiology 1987; 162:513–520.
49. Latack JT, Kartush JM, Kemink JL, et al: Epidermoidomas of the cerebellopontine angle and temporal bone: CT and MR aspects. Radiology 1985; 157:361–366.
50. Friedman DP, Rao VM: MR and CT of squamous cell carcinoma of the middle ear and mastoid complex. AJNR 1991; 12:872–874.

12

THE SPINE

After a brief review of the normal spinal anatomy, this chapter discusses the radiographic evaluation of the spine and its contents, as well as the advantages and limitations of each radiographic modality. The radiographic manifestations of common conditions that afflict the spinal axis are reviewed subsequently.

ANATOMY

The spine is divided into five segments. From cephalad to caudad, the cervical (C1–C7), thoracic (T1–T12), and lumbar (L1–L5) spine constitute the majority of the spinal axis. Caudal still, the sacrum is composed of five fused vertebral bodies and the coccyx is a composite of four small vertebral bodies. From the lateral view, the spine contains shallow lordotic curves in the cervical and lumbar regions and a gentle kyphosis in the thoracic and sacral regions.

Spine

The vertebrae are composed of an anterior vertebral body and the posterior elements, which form an arch that surrounds and protects the cord. The posterior elements are further divided into the pedicles, which extend from the posterolateral surface of the vertebral bodies to the lamina. The lamina, in turn, extends posteromedial to fuse at the midline posteriorly at the base of the spinous process. The transverse and spinous processes extend laterally and posteriorly, respectively, from the arch into the adjacent soft tissue. Each vertebra has a superior and an inferior articular facet arranged in a stepwise fashion to interlock and support the spinal column. The articular facets are located at or near the junction of the pedicle with the lamina. The pars interarticularis is the bony junction between the superior and inferior articular facets.

The cervical spine (C-spine) is the smallest and most delicate segment of the upper spine, consisting of seven separate vertebrae (Figs. 12–1, 12–2). The transverse processes are small and contain the transverse foramen. The vertebral arteries traverse the transverse foramen from the C6 level cephalad before piercing the dura above the posterior arch of C1 to enter the posterior fossa through the foramen magnum. The articular facets are nearly horizontally oriented. Unique to the C-spine are the uncinate processes. These small bony projections extend cephalad from the posterosuperior margin of the vertebral body to loosely articulate with a depression in the posteroinferior surface of the vertebral body above.

The atlas (C1) is a bony ring, the only vertebra that lacks a vertebral body. The anterior and posterior arch of C1 meet at the lateral masses. The lateral masses of C1 articulate with the occipital condyles above, and the superior articular facets of the axis (C2) below. The odontoid process (dens) is a bony process that extends cephalad from the body of C2 to articulate with the posterior surface of the anterior arch of C1. The spinal canal is contiguous with the foramen magnum.

The thoracic spine is composed of 12 separate vertebrae. In a caudal progression, the vertebrae become progressively larger and the articular facets more vertically oriented (Figs. 12–3, 12–4). As the height of the bodies increases, the pedicles migrate toward the cephalad portion of the vertebral body, arising adjacent to the superior endplate. Unique to the thoracic spine is the articulation for the thoracic ribs. The posterior sixth rib articulates with the costal facets of the fifth and sixth vertebral body and the transverse process of the T6 vertebra. The surrounding dense ligaments maintain this articulation, creating a supporting framework unique to the thoracic spine.

The five lumbar vertebrae become progressively larger caudally as the transverse area of the spinal canal increases to its maximum. The articular facets are vertically oriented (Figs. 12–5, 12–6). The transverse and spinous processes increase progressively in size.

The intervertebral foramina are present at each spinal level and form the conduit for the traversing spinal nerves. The foramen is encased superiorly and inferiorly by the pedicles of adjacent vertebrae. The anterior margin of the foramen is composed of the vertebral body superiorly and the disk inferiorly. The articular facets form the posterior bony margin of the foramen. In the C-spine the uncinate processes also form a portion of the anterior medial boundary of the foramen.

Text continued on page 433

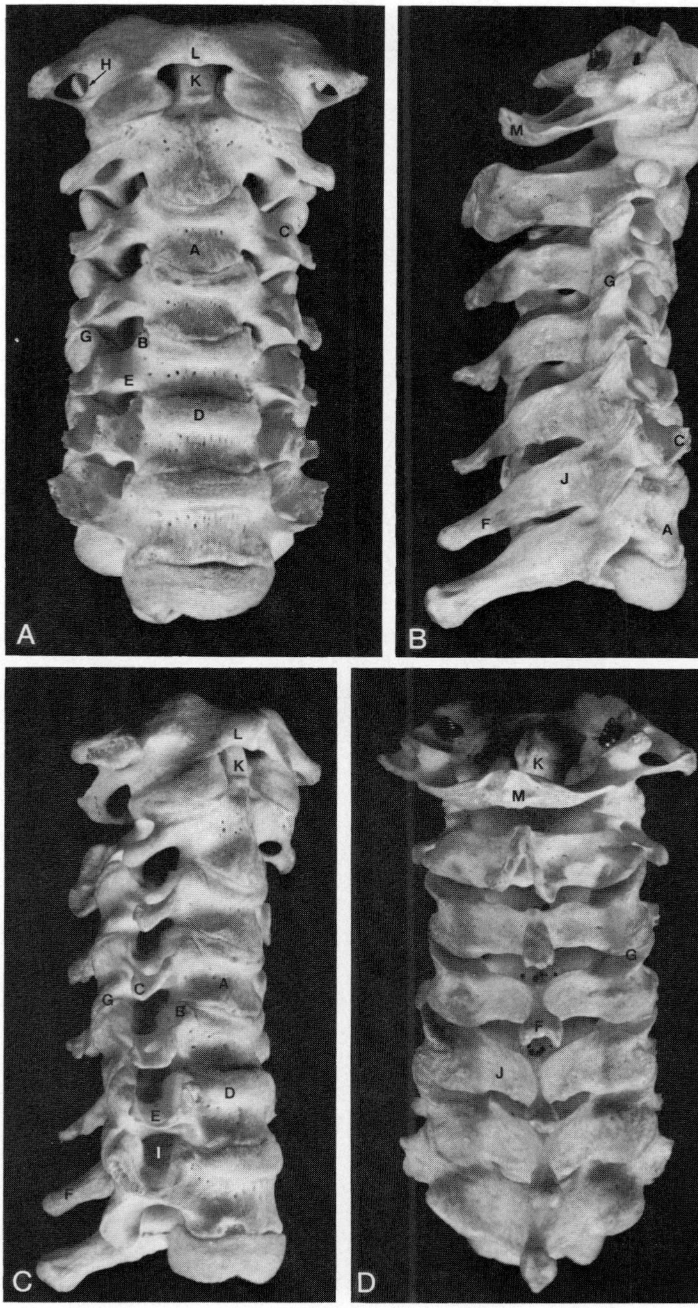

Figure 12–1. Photograph; cervical spine. **A,** Anterior; **B,** lateral; **C,** oblique; **D,** posterior.

(*A*) Vertebral body, (*B*) uncinate process, (*C*) transverse process, (*D*) disk space, (*E*) pedicle, (*F*) spinous process, (*G*) articular facet, (*H*) transverse foramen, (*I*) intervertebral foramen, (*J*) lamina, (*K*) odontoid, (*L*) anterior arch C1, (*M*) posterior arch C1.

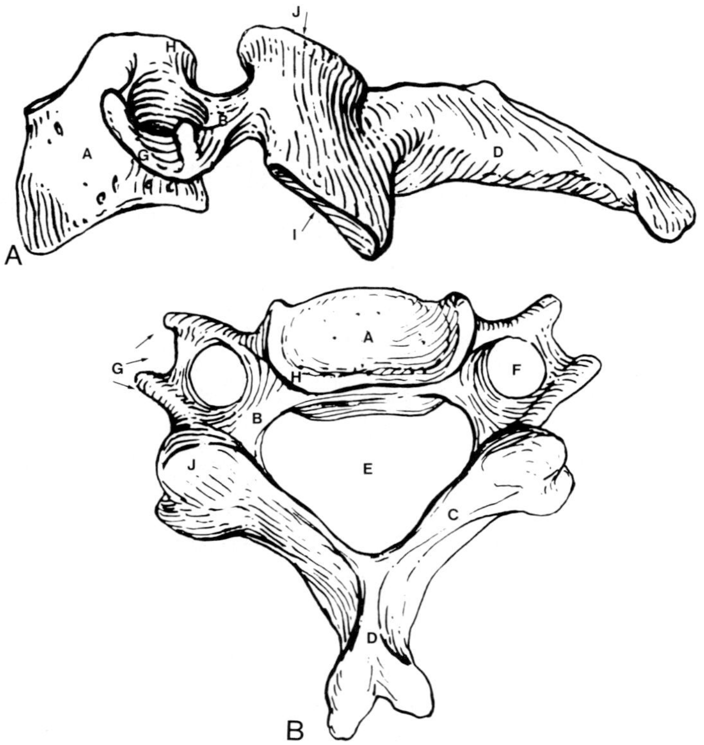

Figure 12–2. Drawing; cervical vertebra. **A,** Lateral view; **B,** cephalad view.

(*A*) Vertebral body, (*B*) pedicle, (*C*) lamina, (*D*) spinous process, (*E*) spinal canal, (*F*) transverse foramen, (*G*) transverse process, (*H*) uncinate process, (*I*) inferior articular facet, (*J*) superior articular facet.

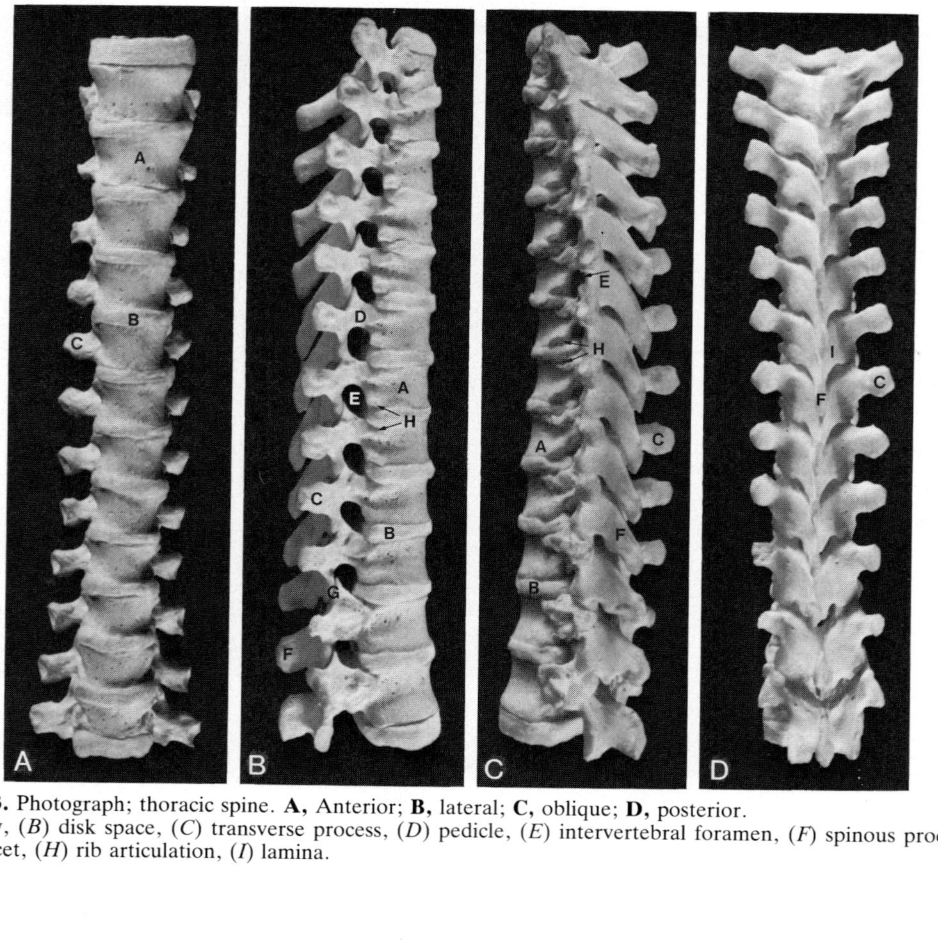

Figure 12–3. Photograph; thoracic spine. **A,** Anterior; **B,** lateral; **C,** oblique; **D,** posterior.

(*A*) Body, (*B*) disk space, (*C*) transverse process, (*D*) pedicle, (*E*) intervertebral foramen, (*F*) spinous process, (*G*) articular facet, (*H*) rib articulation, (*I*) lamina.

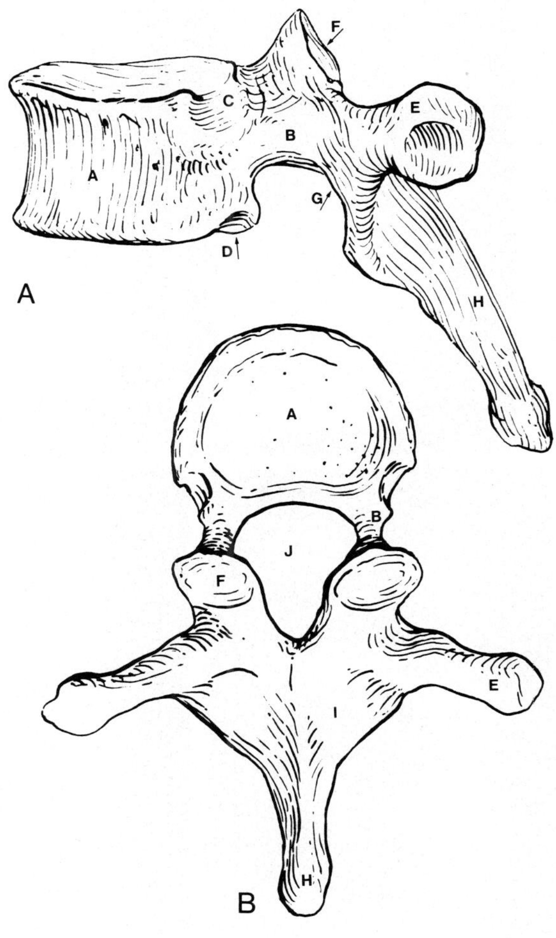

Figure 12–4. Drawing; thoracic vertebra. **A,** Lateral view; **B,** cephalad view.

(*A*) Body, (*B*) pedicle, (*C*) articulation for same level rib, (*D*) articulation for next lower rib, (*E*) transverse process, (*F*) superior articular facet, (*G*) inferior articular facet, (*H*) spinous process, (*I*) lamina, (*J*) spinal canal.

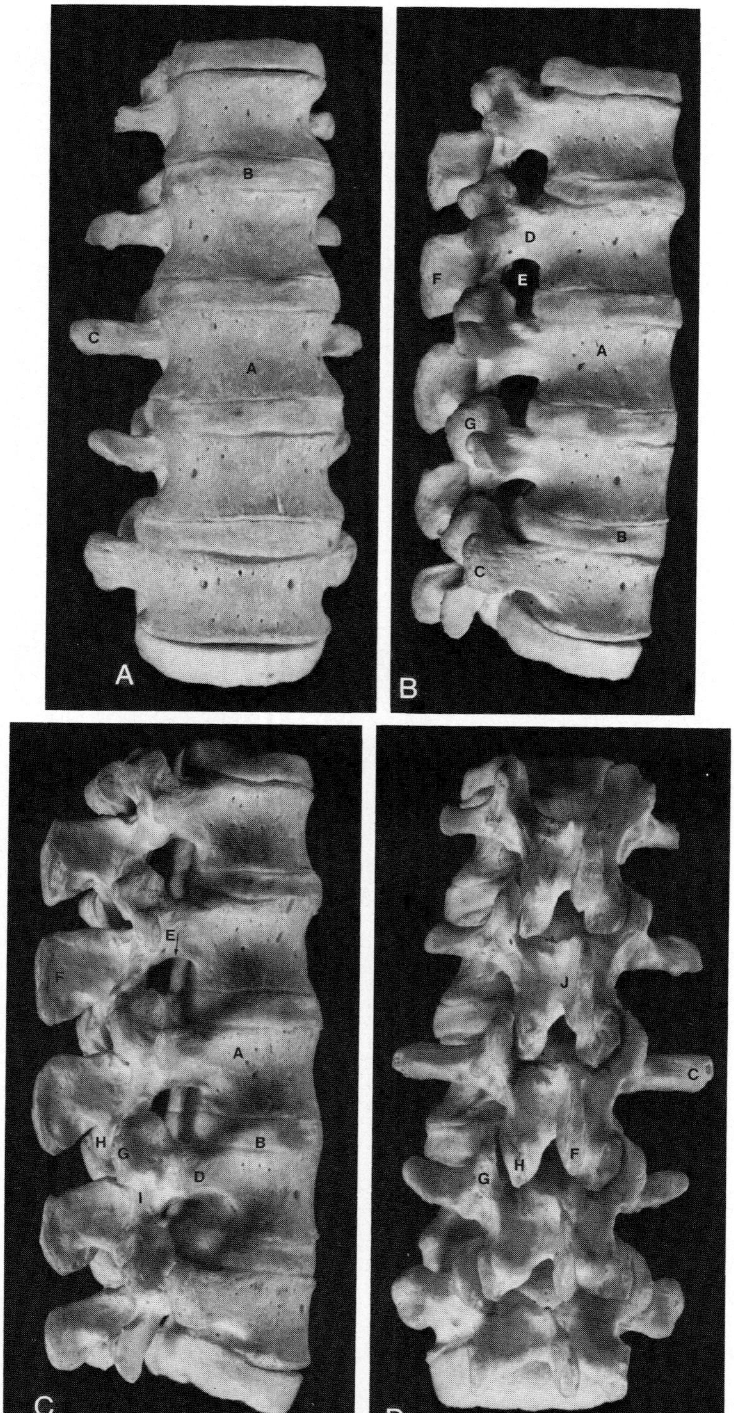

Figure 12–5. Photograph; lumbar spine. **A,** Anterior; **B,** lateral; **C,** oblique; **D,** posterior.

(*A*) Body, (*B*) disk space, (*C*) transverse process, (*D*) pedicle, (*E*) intervertebral foramen, (*F*) spinous process, (*G*) superior articular facet, (*H*) inferior articular facet, (*I*) pars interarticularis, (*J*) lamina.

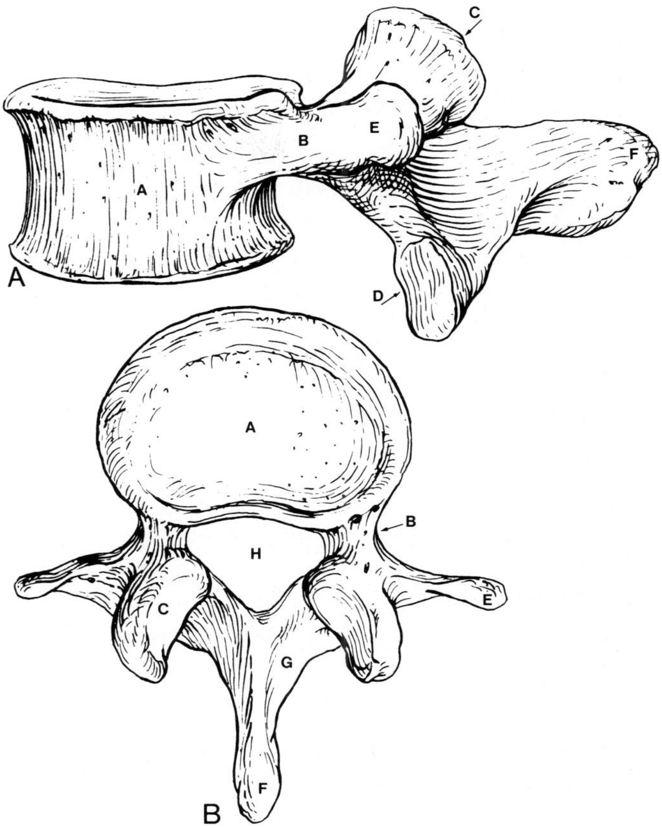

Figure 12–6. Drawing; lumbar vertebra. **A,** Lateral view; **B,** cephalad view.

(*A*) Body, (*B*) pedicle, (*C*) superior articular facet, (*D*) inferior articular facet, (*E*) transverse process, (*F*) spinous process, (*G*) lamina, (*H*) spinal canal.

Disk

The intervertebral disks are fibrocartilaginous structures juxtaposed between the vertebral bodies from C2 to the sacrum. The disks increase in size in the caudal progression and conform to the shape of the opposing vertebral body endplate. The disk is composed of a concentrically arranged fibrocartilaginous envelope (annulus fibrosus) that contains a central gelatinous material (nucleus pulposus). The cartilaginous endplate is the junctional zone between the disk and adjacent vertebral body endplate.

Ligaments

Myriad ligaments attach to and support the integrity of the spine. The anterior and posterior longitudinal ligaments (ALL, PLL) extend from the skull base to the sacrum, covering the anterior and posterior surface of each vertebral body, respectively. These ligaments attach to the margins of the vertebral bodies and the annulus fibrosus at each disk space level.

The vertebral arch is supported by the ligamentum flava, strong fibrous bands that extend from lamina to lamina, effectively enclosing the spinal canal. The interspinous ligament extends between the spinous processes. The supraspinous ligament fuses with the interspinal ligament and extends from the occiput to the sacrum. The ligamentum nuchae extends from the spinous processes of the cervical vertebrae to the external occipital protuberance and crest. Small capsular ligaments are present bilaterally at each level, supporting each articular capsule.

The craniocervical junction contains multiple ligaments unique to this region. The transverse alar ligament forms a sling from the anterior aspect of the lateral masses of C1, encompassing the odontoid process. This ligament maintains the close relationship between the odontoid process and the anterior arch of

C1. The lateral alar ligaments extend from the condyles of the occipital bone to the lateral odontoid surface. The cruciform ligament extends from the odontoid tip to the anterior margin of the foramen magnum (basion).

Cord

The spinal cord is a caudal extension of the medulla oblongata. The cord terminates in the conus medullaris, which is located just below the thoracolumbar junction in the adult. The cord is slightly flattened along the ventral and dorsal surfaces and enlarged in two regions—for the brachial plexus (C3 to T2) and the lumbar plexus (T9 to T12). The filum terminale extends from the tip of the conus to the coccyx. The cauda equina refers to the roots that extend caudal from the conus in the lumbar subarachnoid space.

In contradistinction to the brain, the gray matter of the cord is located internally, surrounded by white matter tracks. The proportion of gray to white matter increases in the cervical and lumbar regions of the cord. Dorsal (sensory) and ventral (motor) roots arise throughout the course of the cord, uniting to form the spinal nerves. A total of 31 paired spinal nerves exist, including eight paired cervical roots. In the C-spine, the roots traverse the intervertebral foramen above the respective pedicle; ergo, the seventh spinal nerve exits between the C6 and C7 pedicles. The eighth cervical root exits between the C7 and T1 pedicles. Twelve thoracic and five lumbar roots traverse the foramen, each below their corresponding pedicles. Five paired sacral roots and one paired coccygeal root are also present.

Dura

The three-layered meningeal investment of the brain is contiguous with the spinal canal. The pia mater adheres to the surface of the cord and invests the penetrating arteries. The pia also extends from the lateral surface of the cord to the dural membrane, forming the dentate ligaments. The arachnoid membrane is relatively closely applied to the outer dura mater with a potential subdural space between these layers. The subarachnoid space of the spine is filled with cerebrospinal fluid (CSF) and is contiguous with the intracranial subarachnoid compartment. The dura extends to the S2 level, forming the dural or thecal sac. The dural sac is surrounded by epidural fat filling the remaining volume of the spinal canal.

Vascular Supply

Arterial supply to the cord, although variable, can be divided into three major regions—the cervicothoracic, midthoracic, and thoracolumbar.[1] The cervicothoracic region is supplied by the anterior spinal artery, which descends from the intracranial vertebral artery to the C4 level. In addition, two to three branches from the cervical vertebral arteries and the costocervical trunk supply the lower cervical and upper thoracic regions. The midthoracic segment is supplied by a single spinal artery, usually situated at the T7 level. The thoracolumbar region is supplied by the large artery of Adamkiewicz that arises from a low thoracic intercostal or upper interlumbar artery usually on the left side.

MODALITIES

Plain Films

The plain film evaluation of the spine may be the initial imaging procedure. Plain films are obtained in orthogonal views—anteroposterior (AP) and lateral. Left anterior oblique (LAO) and right anterior oblique (RAO) films may be obtained to evaluate the intervertebral foramen or pars interarticularis or both. Plain films offer excellent means to evaluate alignment of the vertebral bodies, as well as presence or absence of degenerative bone disease. Gross evaluation of mineralization and soft tissue can be made from plain films. Contiguity of the cortex may be grossly evaluated. Although the bony perimeter of the canal and intervertebral foramen can be assessed, the contents of the spinal canal and intervertebral foramen cannot be evaluated.

Cervical Spine

The AP film of the normal cervical spine demonstrates alignment of the lateral masses and of the uncinate and spinous processes (Fig.

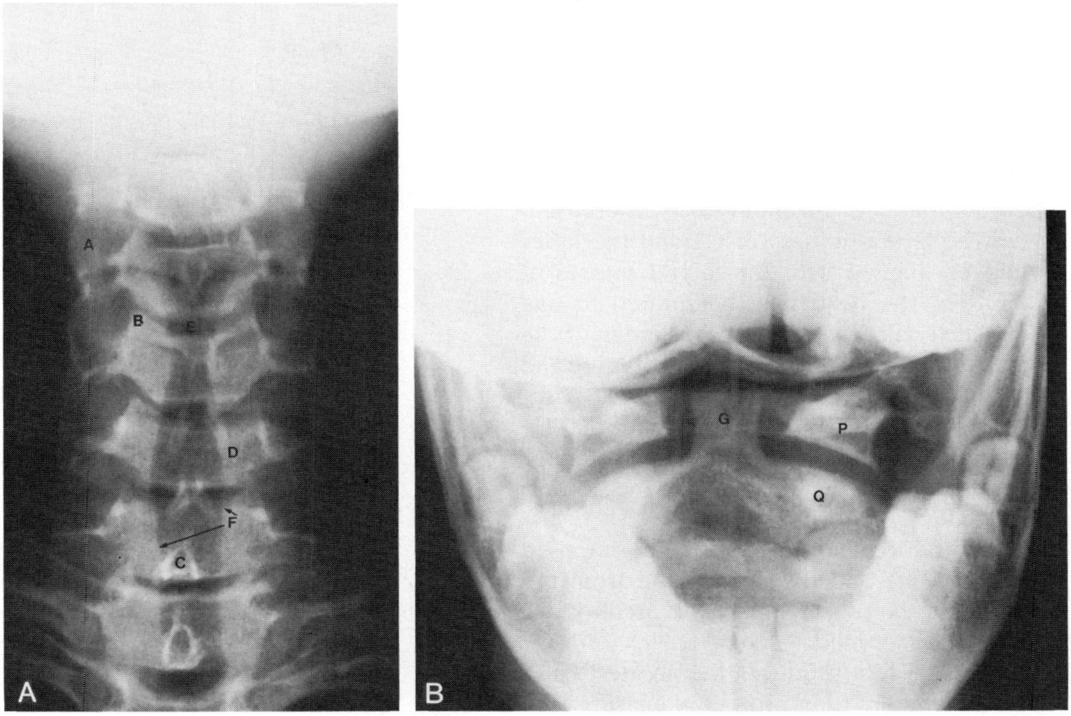

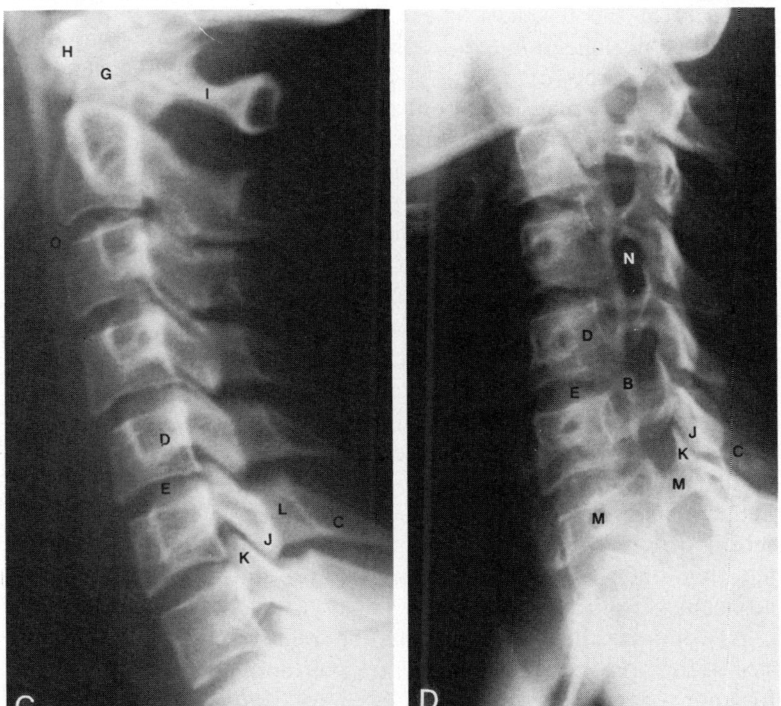

Figure 12–7. Normal C-spine. **A,** Anteroposterior (AP); **B,** open-mouth odontoid; **C,** lateral; **D,** oblique.

(*A*) Lateral mass, (*B*) uncinate process, (*C*) spinous process, (*D*) vertebral body, (*E*) disk space, (*F*) tracheal air column, (*G*) odontoid, (*H*) C1 anterior arch, (*I*) C1 posterior arch, (*J*) inferior articular facet, (*K*) superior articular facet, (*L*) lamina, (*M*) pedicle, (*N*) intervertebral foramen, (*O*) prevertebral soft tissue; (*P*) lateral mass C1; (*Q*) lateral mass C2.

12–7). The tracheal air column should be midline. The pedicles are not usually identified on the frontal film partly because of their oblique origin and course. The upper two to three vertebral bodies may be obscured by the density of the superimposed occiput and the mandible.

The AP open-mouth odontoid film demonstrates the relationship between C1 and C2. The odontoid process should be centered between the lateral masses of C1 and the latter should be aligned with the lateral masses of C2. Often, the head may be rotated to one side, which will result in foreshortening of the lateral mass toward the side of rotation and elongation of the opposite lateral mass. Also, the distance between the dens and the C1 lateral mass widens toward the side of rotation, with commensurate narrowing of the contralateral side.[2]

Spurious lucencies from the superimposed central incisors and the mock band from the inferior cortex of the posterior arch of C1 should be discounted.

The lateral film produces the greatest challenge and amount of information regarding the integrity of the C-spine. The C7-T1 junction should be visualized in every case, particularly if there is a history of trauma. A gentle lordosis of the cervical spine is present and should be persistent in four regions—the anterior and posterior margins of the vertebral bodies, the spinolaminar line (marking the posterior bony apex of the spinal canal), and the interspinous line (which connects the tip of each spinous process) (Fig. 12–8). The articular facets are arranged in a stepwise fashion. The dens should be closely applied to the anterior arch of C1. (The atlantodental interval [ADI] is the space between the C1 arch and the odontoid process. This should not exceed 3 mm in adults.) The disk space and vertebral body heights should be maintained. The prevertebral soft tissues cephalad to C4 should be less than one third of the AP dimension of the adjacent vertebral body.

AP oblique films demonstrate the relative size of the bony perimeter of the intervertebral foramen contralateral to the side of rotation (i.e., with the head turned to the right, the LAO film demonstrates the left foramen). The pedicles and vertebral body alignment are assessed. The stepwise relationship of the articular facets is demonstrated. Lateral flexion and extension films may be obtained to evaluate for ligamentous laxity. Also in trauma cases, trauma oblique views should be obtained to evaluate the lateral masses.

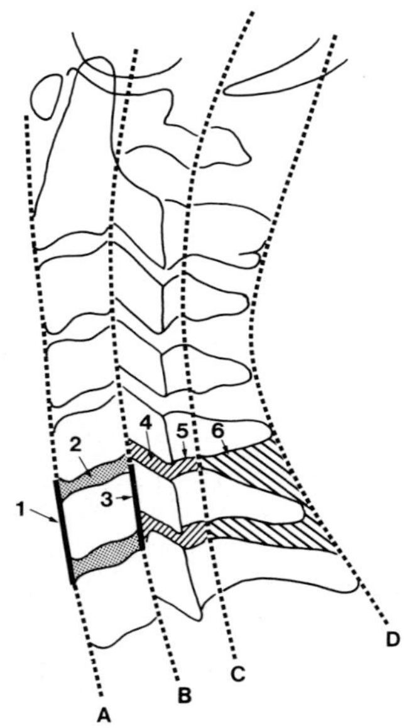

Figure 12–8. Diagram depicting alignment of the cervical spine on lateral film. (*A*) Anterior vertebral body, (*B*) posterior vertebral body, (*C*) spinolaminar line, (*D*) interspinous line, (*1*) anterior longitudinal ligament, (*2*) intervertebral disk, (*3*) posterior longitudinal ligament, (*4*) capsular ligaments, (*5*) ligamentum flavum, (*6*) interspinous ligament. (Medical illustration by Diane Blue.)

Thoracic and Lumbar Spine

AP and lateral films are obtained to evaluate for alignment, preservation of vertebral body, and disk space height (Fig. 12–9). The pedicles are identified on the frontal film, and the paravertebral soft tissues may be grossly evaluated. Oblique films may be obtained to evaluate the status of the intervertebral foramen.

Myelography

Myelography is the diagnostic evaluation of all or a portion of the spinal cord and the

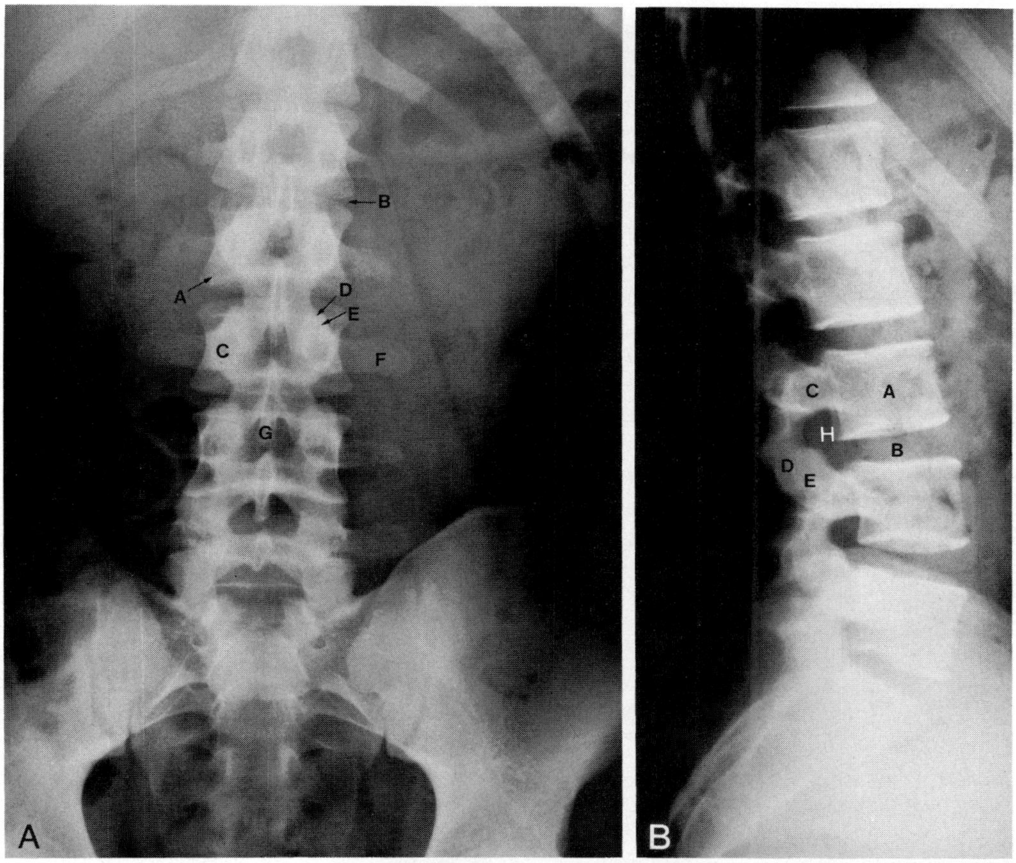

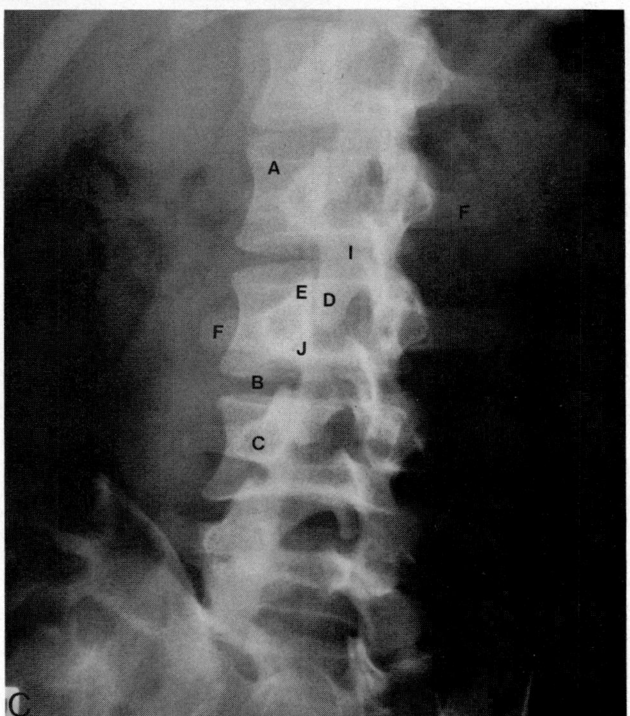

Figure 12–9. Normal lumbar spine. **A,** Frontal; **B,** lateral; **C,** oblique.

(*A*) Vertebral body, (*B*) disk space, (*C*) pedicle, (*D*) inferior articular facet, (*E*) superior articular facet, (*F*) transverse process, (*G*) spinous process, (*H*) intervertebral foramen, (*I*) lamina, (*J*) pars interarticularis.

proximal, intradural portion of the spinal nerve roots that necessitates intrathecal administration of iodinated contrast. Access to the thecal sac is usually at the lumbar level, though less commonly contrast material may be administered at the C1-C2 level or via a cisternal puncture. However, myelography is an invasive procedure and results in a multitude of predictable complications including headache, nausea, vomiting, meningitis, spinal CSF leak, and arachnoiditis.

Although myelography is still frequently performed in many institutions, our procedure of choice for evaluating the spinal contents is magnetic resonance imaging (MRI). We reserve myelography for patients with cardiac pacemakers in whom MRI is an absolute contraindication. Myelography is the initial procedure of choice in patients with metallic posterior spinal fusion rods, which will likely significantly degrade the MRI examination. Also, myelography is performed in that small subset of patients in whom the clinical symptoms and the C-spine MRI findings are discordant.

Myelography requires the examiner to position the subarachnoid contrast material appropriately in the clinically symptomatic region and obtain orthogonal images (AP and lateral) and, when indicated, oblique films to evaluate the spinal roots. The contents of the dural sac displace the contrast, resulting in predictable filling defects (Figs. 12–10, 12–11).

Water-soluble, non-ionic contrast is currently used for myelography. In general, high-volume low concentration (20 ml, 180 to 200

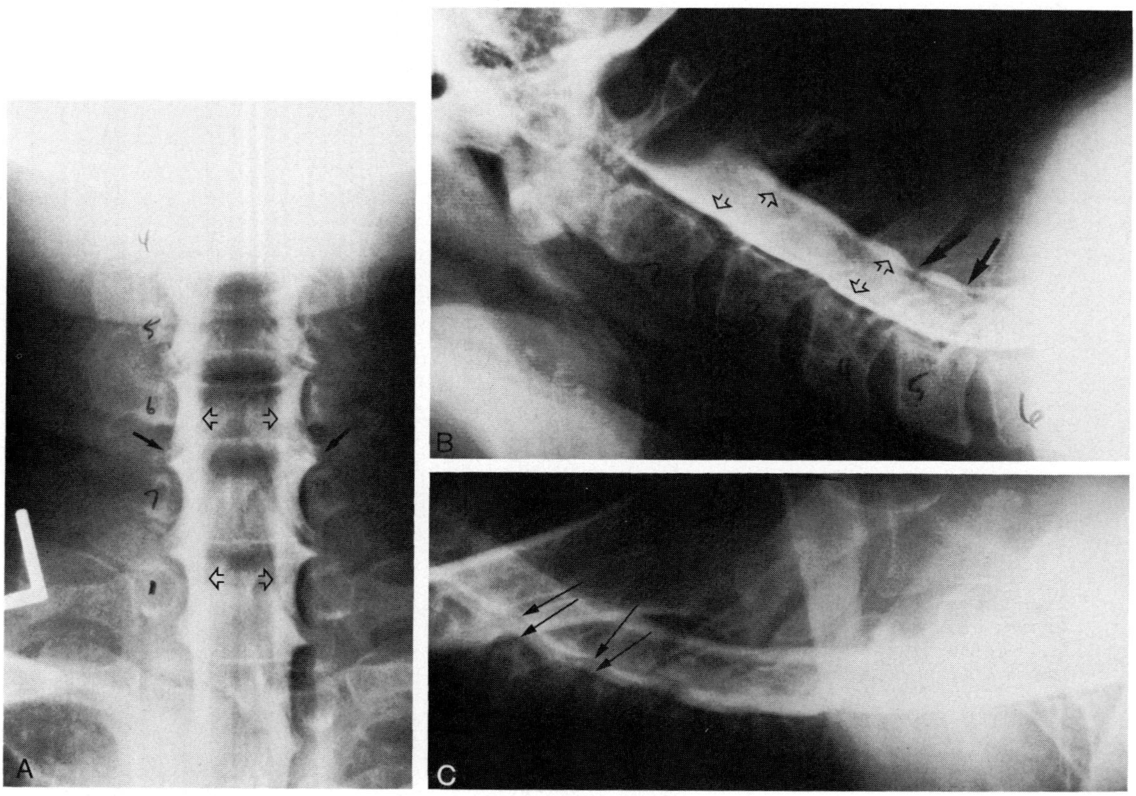

Figure 12–10. Cervical myelogram.

A, AP. There is symmetric filling of the nerve roots (*arrows*) and a normal size, smooth contoured filling defect (*open arrows*) from the cervical cord.

B, High lateral. The contrast-laden dural sac is normal, as is the central cord filling defect (*open arrows*). In extension, the ligamentum-flavum commonly buckles, resulting in focal dorsal extradural defects (*arrows*).

C, Swimmer's view. With one arm extended, a more homogeneous mass is produced, leading to better exposure and allowing accurate evaluation of the cervicothoracic junction. The double density noted at some midcervical disk spaces (*arrows*) is related to the slight obliquity in this patient.

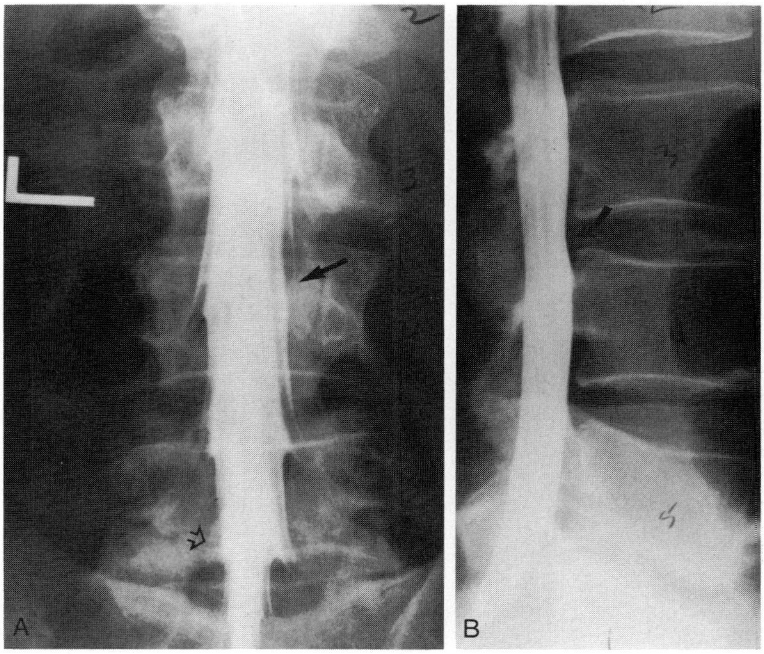

Figure 12–11. Normal lumbar myelogram.

A, B, AP and lateral. Mild underfilling of the right L4 root (*arrow*) and left S1 root (*open arrow*) is noted. This was transient. The roots filled on oblique films. A mild ventral extradural defect (*curved arrow*) is noted at the L3–4 disk space, secondary to minimal disk bulge.

mg%) is used for the thoracic and lumbar spine, whereas low-volume high concentration (10 cc, 300 mg%) is used for the C-spine examination. The relatively small size of the cervical subarachnoid space and dilution effects from lumbar puncture are responsible for this strategy.

Lumbar and cervical examinations are performed in the prone position to take advantage of the lordosis to collect contrast material. If the cervical examination is performed with a lumbar puncture, the patient is placed in a head-extended, head-down position to allow contrast material to opacify the cervical subarachnoid space. Once the contrast material fills the cervical region, the patient is returned to a horizontal position, and AP, lateral, and bilateral oblique spot films are obtained. A swimmer's view (one arm extended) is obtained in the C-spine to evaluate the cervicothoracic junction. Similar films are obtained in the lumbar examination with the supine conus film replacing the lateral swimmer's view film.

The lumbar puncture is performed with the patient in a prone position and one hip elevated from the tabletop 10 to 20 degrees. This positions the spine obliquely enough to avoid the spinous process while permitting the myelographer to advance the 22- to 20-gauge needle perpendicular to the tabletop through the ligamenta flava into the spinal canal (Fig. 12–12). Frequently, the needle will give way or "pop" when the dura is entered. The needle should be advanced 3 to 5 mm more and the transfer of fluids commenced. The initial installation of contrast should be monitored with fluoroscopy to ensure that contrast material readily flows away from the needle tip into the gravity-dependent subarachnoid space. Pooling of contrast material at the needle tip usually indicates a subdural or epidural injection.

The cervical puncture may be performed with the patient prone if lateral fluoroscopy is available. The patient must be placed in a true decubitus position if lateral fluoroscopy is not available. The spinal canal is divided into thirds and the puncture (18- to 20-gauge) performed at the junction of the middle and dorsal thirds at the C1-C2 level (Fig. 12–13). Once the dura is entered, the needle should be advanced 3 to 5 mm and fluid exchange initiated. Contrast material should immediately flow away from the needle toward the gravity-dependent subarachnoid space.

The thoracic spine myelogram is performed through a high lumbar puncture. Contrast material is instilled in a slight head-down position. When contrast administration is complete, the

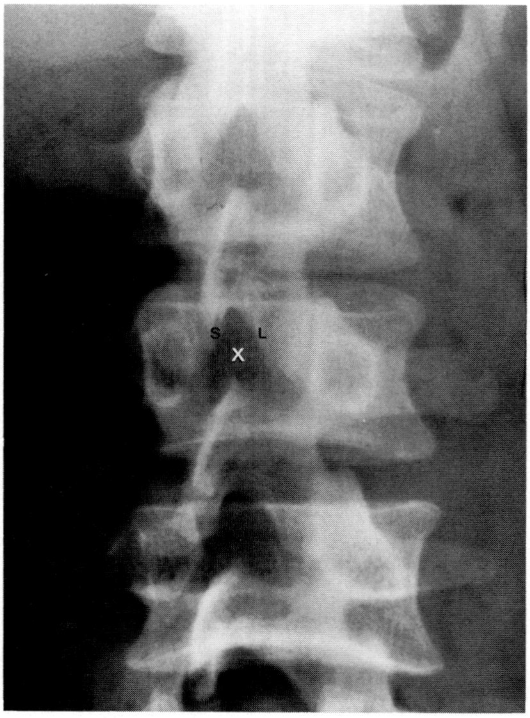

Figure 12–12. Positioning for lumbar puncture. A slight 10- to 20-degree obliquity projects the spinous process (*S*) off the intralaminar space (*X*). The puncture can be made with the needle perpendicular to tabletop, medial to the lamina of L2 (*L*), and the spinous process (*S*) directed toward the X.

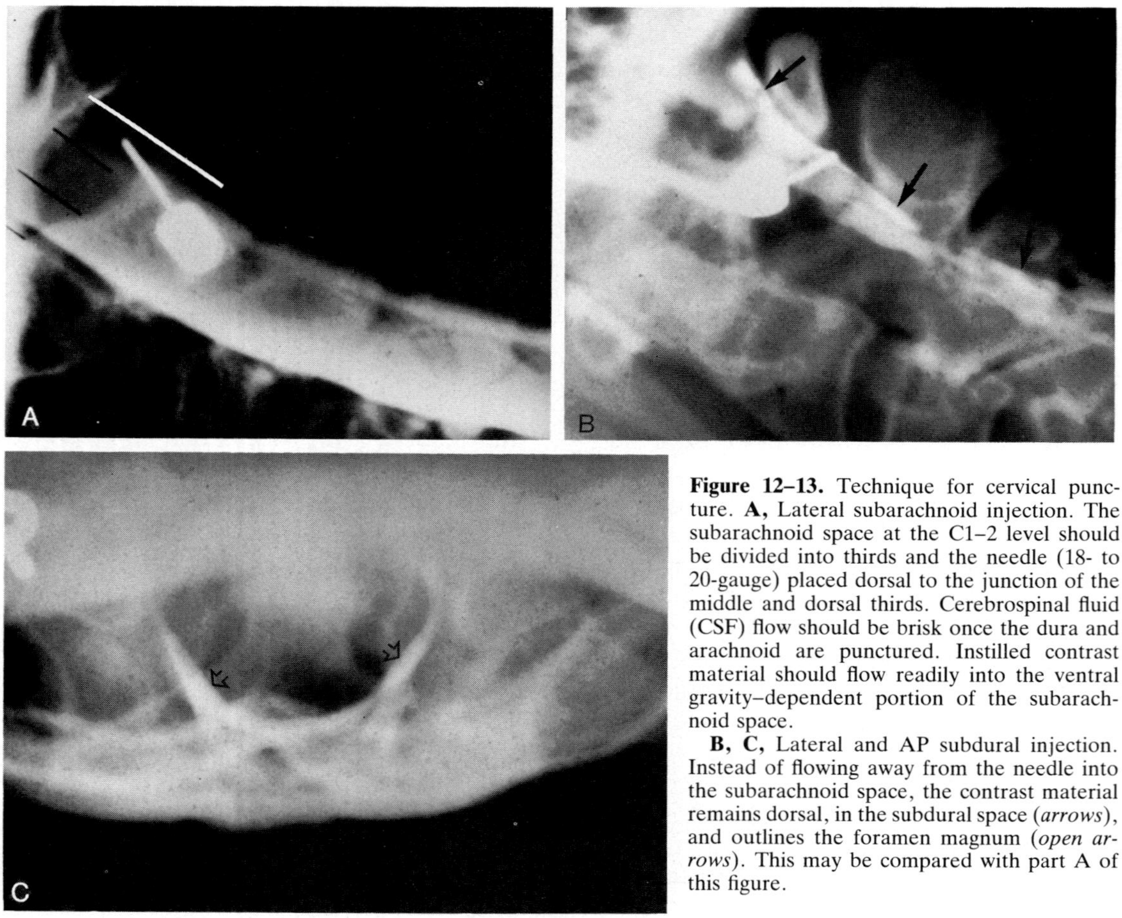

Figure 12–13. Technique for cervical puncture. **A,** Lateral subarachnoid injection. The subarachnoid space at the C1–2 level should be divided into thirds and the needle (18- to 20-gauge) placed dorsal to the junction of the middle and dorsal thirds. Cerebrospinal fluid (CSF) flow should be brisk once the dura and arachnoid are punctured. Instilled contrast material should flow readily into the ventral gravity–dependent portion of the subarachnoid space.

B, C, Lateral and AP subdural injection. Instead of flowing away from the needle into the subarachnoid space, the contrast material remains dorsal, in the subdural space (*arrows*), and outlines the foramen magnum (*open arrows*). This may be compared with part A of this figure.

patient is rolled into the supine position, to pool contrast material in the thoracic kyphosis, and the tabletop is returned to a horizontal position. Collimated overhead AP and high and low lateral films of the contrast column are obtained.

In patients with known or suspected metastasis or block to the spine, it is important to evaluate the entire spinal axis and, if a block is present, to define the upper and lower margins of the block, which may necessitate a C1-C2 puncture. Increasing the pressure below a block by injecting Ringer's lactate or room air may permit passage of contrast beyond the block.[3] It is of utmost importance not to remove CSF in a patient suspected of having a block, as this may alter the fluid dynamics of the canal, and result in further cord compression and exacerbation of symptoms. Progression of symptoms following lumbar puncture in patients with spinal block has been reported in as high as 16 to 24% of patients.[4]

As myelography was the first, time-honored means to evaluate the spinal axis, disease processes of the spine have been categorized into three distinct compartments (Fig. 12–14). Although most helpful with myelography, distinguishing these three regions is also useful in planar imaging. The most common diseases responsible for these lesions will be discussed and are presented in Table 12–1.

Lesions that arise within the cord proper are considered intramedullary. Intramedullary lesions expand the cord, tapering the contrast gutters, often symmetrically. The intramedullary lesion may result in a complete block. Orthogonal films must be obtained to confirm myelographic abnormalities, as the most common cause of apparent cord enlargement is a compressive extradural process (i.e., disk herniation or osteoarthritis).

Table 12–1. LESION BY LOCATION

Intramedullary	Intradural Extramedullary	Extradural
Neoplasm	Meningioma	Disk
Hydrosyringomyelia	Nerve sheath tumor	Osteophyte
Trauma	Metastasis	Tumor
AVM	Arachnoiditis	Trauma
Demyelinating disease	AVM	Infection
Transverse myelitis	Arachnoid cyst	
Radiation myelitis		

Lesions that arise within the dural sac, yet are extrinsic to the cord, are considered intradural extramedullary lesions. These lesions displace the cord, widening the ipsilateral contrast gutter, while commensurately narrowing the contralateral side. The mass is usually well marginated, as it is in direct contact with the contrast material. A meniscus defect may be detected.

Extradural lesions arise outside the dural sac, yet secondarily distort or compress the sac. Extradural processes displace the sac centripetally, away from the disk, ligaments, or bone that compose the perimeter of the spinal canal. Associated bony destructive or degenerative changes may be seen.

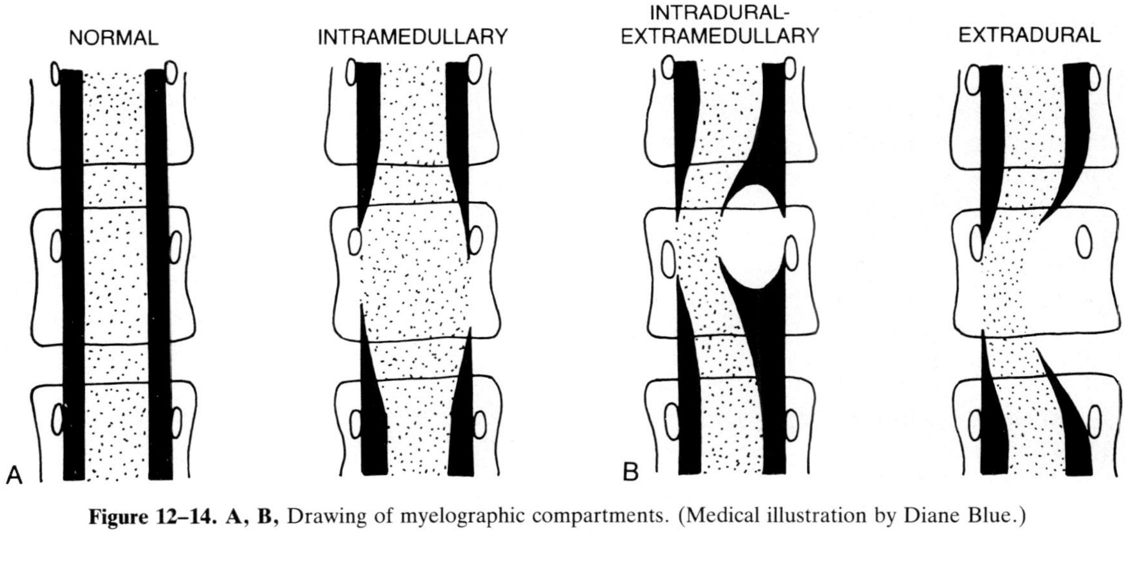

Figure 12–14. A, B, Drawing of myelographic compartments. (Medical illustration by Diane Blue.)

Computed Tomography (CT)

CT provides an improved means to evaluate the spinal axis, adroitly depicting the vertebral bodies and distinguishing the dense cortical bone from the medullary cavity of the vertebrae (Fig. 12–15). Although the bony anatomy of the spine is accurately depicted, the thick vertebral body camouflages the slight difference in intrinsic attenuation coefficient of the canal contents, often rendering them inseparable. The CSF is hypodense, and occasionally the cord and roots may be identified in the upper cervical spine. The ability to assess surrounding soft tissue is improved, yet CT is still unable to evaluate directly the parenchyma of the cord. The intervertebral disks are of muscle density on CT, juxtaposed between the vertebral bodies.

Contrast administration improves the sensitivity of the CT examination. In limited circumstances, intravenous (IV) contrast material may be used to opacify epidural veins within the cervical foramen to detect lateral disk disease. Intrathecal contrast material opacifies the subarachnoid space, permitting visualization of the cord, cauda equina, proximal nerve roots, and configuration of the thecal sac (Fig. 12–16). Gross evaluation of the size of the cord can be made, but intramedullary processes that do not enlarge the cord are not usually detected.

Our current technique for CT evaluation of degenerative disk disease (DDD) is 5-, 3-, and 2-mm contiguous axial images parallel to the lumbar, thoracic, and cervical spine disk spaces, respectively. Images are obtained from the pedicle above the disk space to the pedicle below.

Trauma patients are also evaluated with 5-mm images in the lumbar, 3-mm images in the thoracic, and 2-mm images in the cervical spine. Images are obtained perpendicular to the tabletop with a high-bone algorithm and reconstructed in the sagittal plane. It is imperative to evaluate the reconstructed images, as significant malalignment may not be apparent on the contiguous axial images.

Magnetic Resonance Imaging (MRI)

Application of MRI has dramatically changed the imaging algorithm of the spinal axis. In most circumstances, the invasive myelogram and CT evaluation have been replaced by MRI. The latter permits multiplanar imaging and superior tissue contrast to permit direct evaluation of the cord parenchyma, roots, and paravertebral soft tissues without the use of ionizing radiation (Figs. 12–17 through 12–19). MRI also allows unprecedented evaluation of the marrow of the spinal axis and superior contrast sensitivity.

In general, parasagittal spin echo T1, spin density (SD), and T2-weighted images are performed in the spine. In addition, gradient echo (GRE) pulse sequences[5, 6] may be performed in lieu of the T2 images. Using a short flip angle (less than 20 degrees), the "myelographic effect," with bright CSF and intermediate signal cord, can be achieved.

Motion reduction techniques have been applied with cardiac and respiratory gating to decrease vascular and CSF pulsations that would otherwise severely degrade the diagnostic quality of the examination. The GRE sequence can obtain images in less time, have less CSF flow artifact, and have greater signal to noise than spin echo images.

GRE images were judged superior or equal to comparable T2-weighted images in evaluating a variety of spinal pathology in 75% of cases.[5] The disadvantage of GRE images are increased magnetic susceptibility, increased artifact from patient motion, difficulty in staging hematomas, and a decreased number of slices available compared with T2-weighted images. Volume GRE acquisitions, which are available to image a slab of tissue, are particularly applicable to the C-spine evaluation. Contiguous 2-mm axial images can be obtained and reformatted in any plane without loss of imaging data.[7, 8]

The vertebral bodies contain high-signal marrow outlined by low-signal cortex on T1 sequences, which is due to the adipose within the marrow and the lack of mobile protons in the cortical bone. On T2 images, the signal intensity of the marrow decreases, minimizing the contrast between the cortical bone and the marrow cavity.

The disk is relatively low signal on T1 sequences. The disk blends with a low-signal vertebral body endplate via the cartilaginous endplate. This portion of the disk is even lower signal than the nucleus pulposus on T1 images.

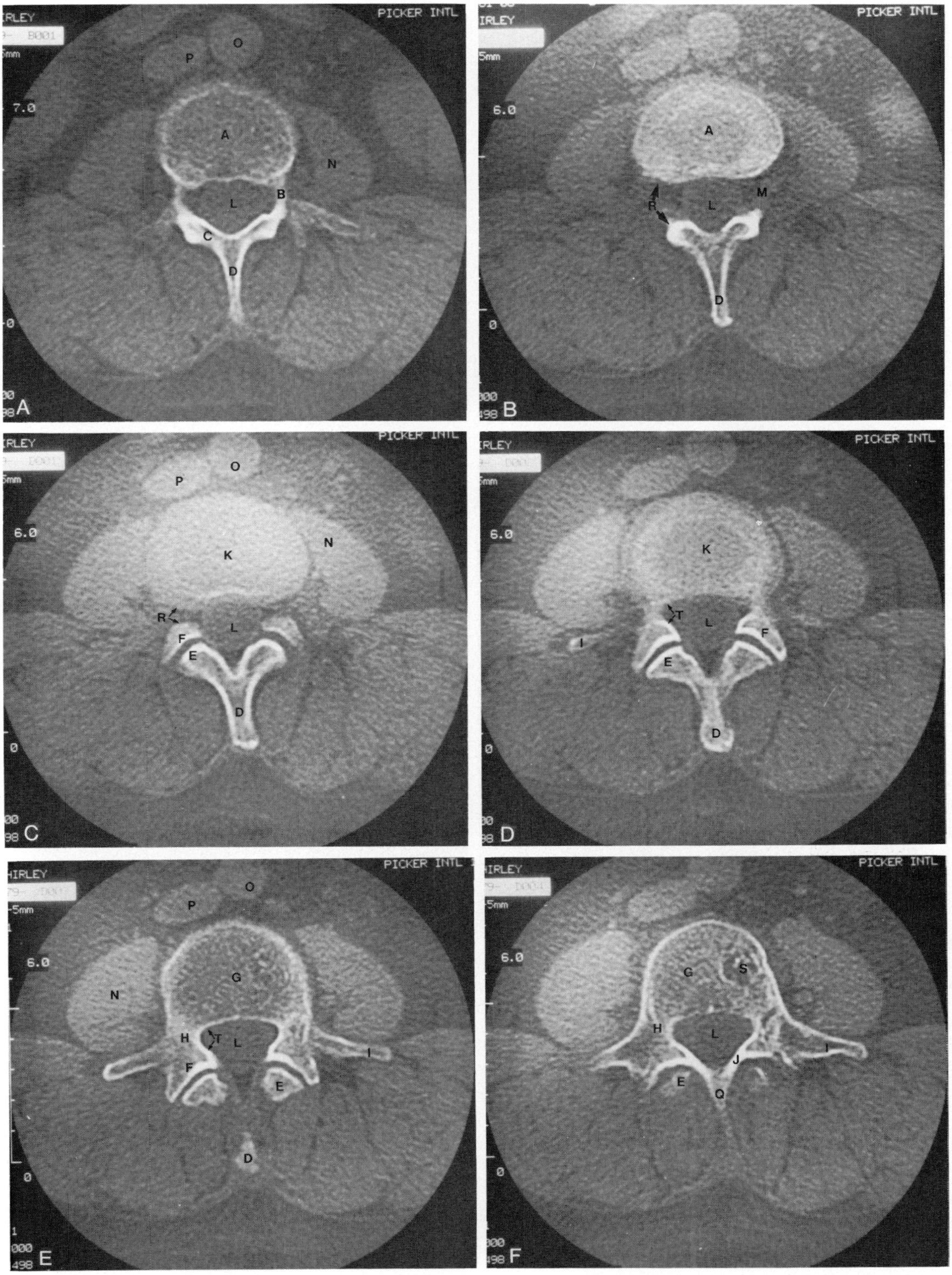

Figure 12–15. Normal unenhanced lumbar spine computed tomography (CT) (L2–3) cephalad to caudal (*A–F* axial 5-mm contiguous images).

(*A*) L2 vertebral body, (*B*) L2 pedicle, (*C*) L2 lamina, (*D*) spinous process L2, (*E*) inferior articular facet L2, (*F*) superior articular facet L3, (*G*) body L3, (*H*) pedicle L3, (*I*) transverse process L3, (*J*) lamina L3, (*K*) L2–3 disk, (*L*) thecal sac, (*M*) L2 root, (*N*) psoas muscle, (*O*) aorta, (*P*) inferior vena cava, (*Q*) base L3 spinous process, (*R*) L2–3 intervertebral foramen, (*S*) incidental hemangioma, (*T*) lateral recess L3.

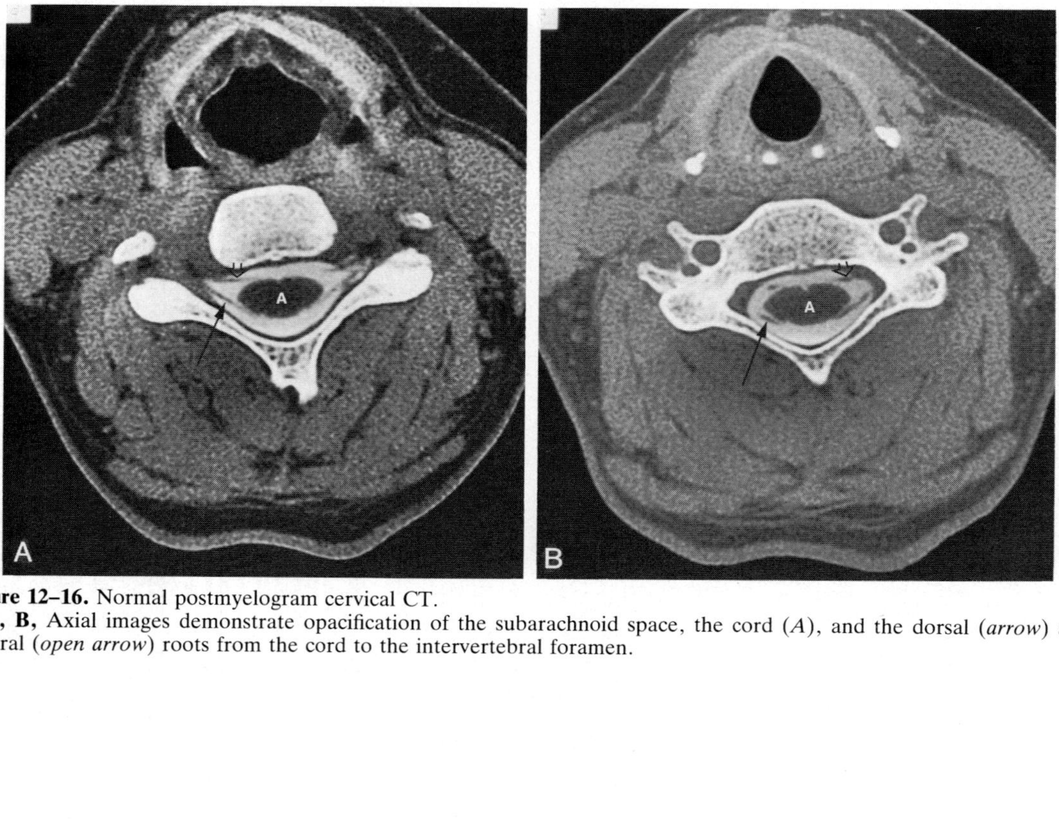

Figure 12–16. Normal postmyelogram cervical CT.

A, B, Axial images demonstrate opacification of the subarachnoid space, the cord (*A*), and the dorsal (*arrow*) and ventral (*open arrow*) roots from the cord to the intervertebral foramen.

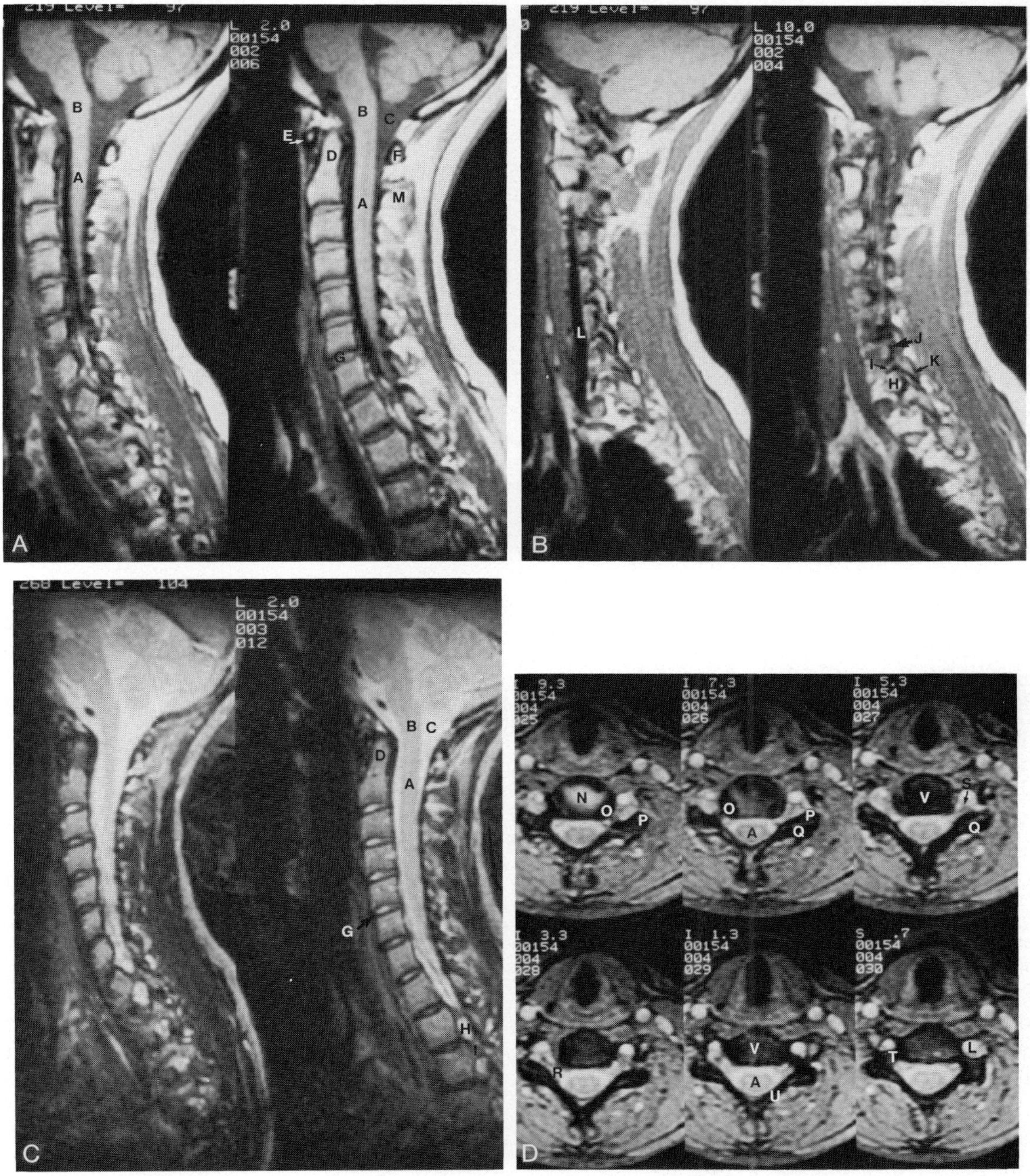

Figure 12–17. Normal cervical magnetic resonance imaging (MRI). **A, B,** Parasagittal T1; **C,** parasagittal T2; **D,** axial gradient echo volume (C5–6).

(*A*) Cervical cord, (*B*) cervicomedullary junction, (*C*) CSF, (*D*) odontoid, (*E*) anterior arch C1, (*F*) posterior arch C1, (*G*) intervertebral disk, (*H*) intervertebral foramen, (*I*) pedicle, (*J*) superior articular facet, (*K*) inferior articular facet, (*L*) vertebral artery, (*M*) spinous process, (*N*) C5–6 disk, (*O*) uncinate process C6, (*P*) superior articular facet C6, (*Q*) inferior articular facet C5, (*R*) C5–6 intervertebral foramen, (*S*) C6 root, (*T*) C5 pedicle, (*U*) C5 lamina, (*V*) C5 body.

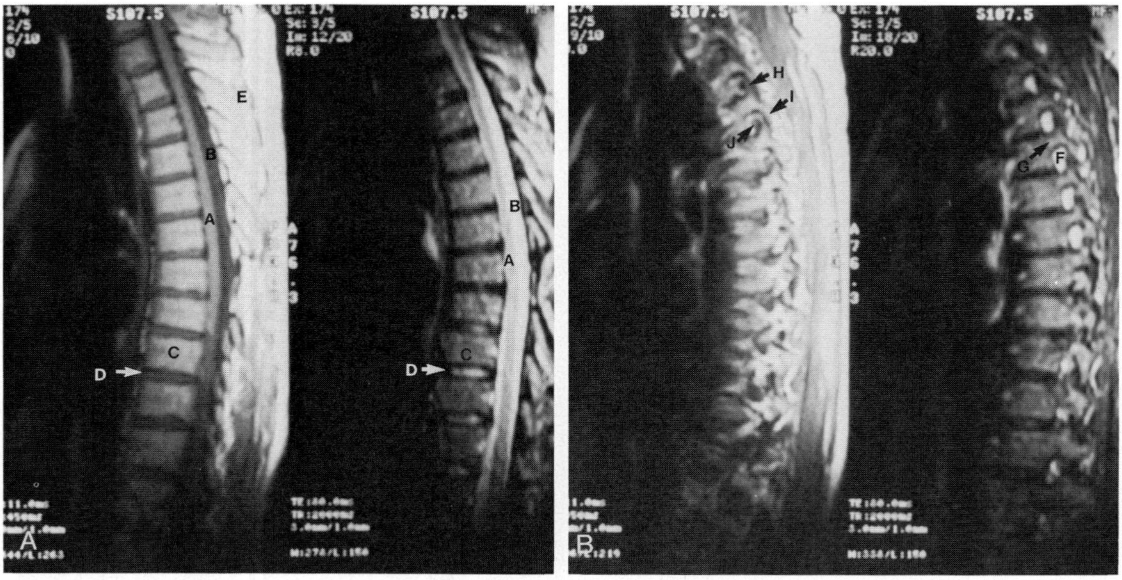

Figure 12–18. Normal thoracic MRI. **A, B,** Parasagittal (*left,* T1; *right,* T2).
(*A*) Thoracic cord, (*B*) CSF, (*C*) vertebral body, (*D*) intervertebral disk, (*E*) spinous process, (*F*) intervertebral foramen, (*G*) pedicle, (*H*) superior articular facet, (*I*) inferior articular facet, (*J*) nerve root.

T2 images demonstrate a high-signal gelatinous hydrated nucleus with a central low-signal band representing the intranuclear cleft.[9] The anterior and posterior longitudinal ligaments are decreased signal on T1 and T2 images, blending imperceptibly with the outer fibers of the disk annulus and the adjacent cortical bone. The ligamenta flava, which extend between lamina, are isointense to muscle on T1 images, intermediate in signal between the cortical bone and marrow.

The cord is intermediate signal on T1- and T2-weighted images, higher in signal than CSF on T1- and lower on T2-weighted images. The signal intensity of the nerve roots parallels the cord. The lumbar dorsal and ventral roots and the dorsal root ganglion appear as intermediate-signal structures in the proximal intervertebral foramen surrounded by high-signal epidural fat on T1 sequences.[10] Epidural fat is variably present throughout the spinal canal. It may be anterior, lateral, and/or posterior to the thecal sac. The epidural veins are variable in signal and on the T1-weighted images they may be low or high.

The role of gadolinium in evaluation of the spinal axis has been the subject of many investigators.[11–20] Normally, the epidural venous plexus and basivertebral veins enhance significantly. Mild enhancement may be detected in the marrow, ligamenta flava, muscle, fat, and disk material (annulus and nucleus). Owing to superior contrast sensitivity, the administration of contrast material is more applicable in MRI than in CT images of the spine. Gadolinium is most helpful for intradural extramedullary processes (tumor), intramedullary processes (tumor, hydrosyringomyelia), and, to a lesser degree, extradural processes (the major extradural application is differentiating scar from disk in the failed back syndrome).

LESIONS BY LOCATION

The major diseases are presented here based on a compartment approach, with emphasis on the distinguishing characteristics of each lesion.

Intramedullary (Table 12–2)

Neoplasm

Ependymoma

Ependymomas constitute 65% of cord neoplasms, occur slightly more commonly in men, and tend to manifest between 20 and 60 years of age. Three quarters of ependymomas arise within the conus or filum terminale.[21] The

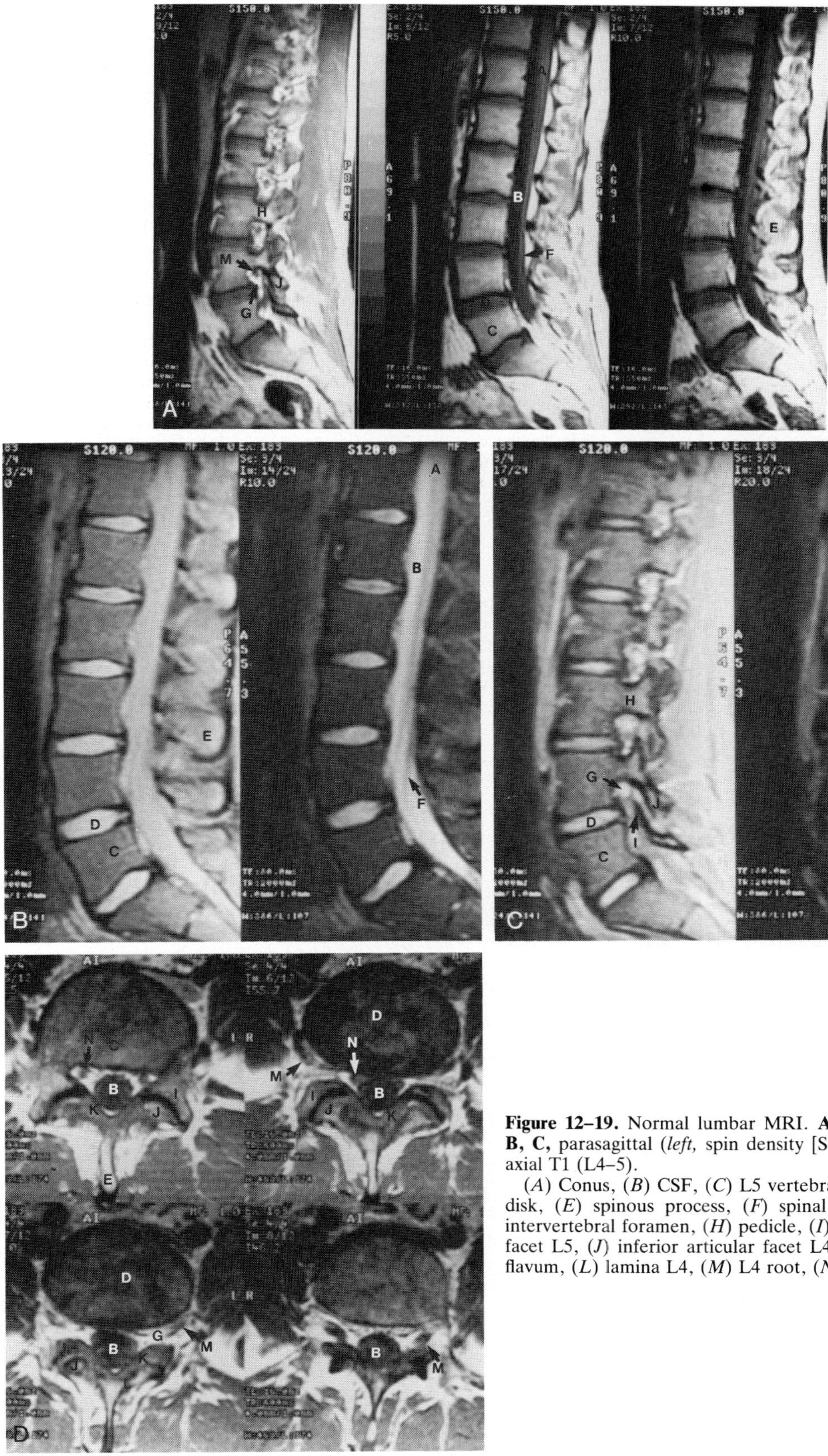

Figure 12–19. Normal lumbar MRI. **A,** Parasagittal T1; **B, C,** parasagittal (*left,* spin density [SD]; *right,* T1); **D,** axial T1 (L4–5).

(*A*) Conus, (*B*) CSF, (*C*) L5 vertebral body, (*D*) L4–5 disk, (*E*) spinous process, (*F*) spinal roots, (*G*) L4–5 intervertebral foramen, (*H*) pedicle, (*I*) superior articular facet L5, (*J*) inferior articular facet L4, (*K*) ligamentum flavum, (*L*) lamina L4, (*M*) L4 root, (*N*) L5 root.

Table 12–2. INTRAMEDULLARY DISEASE

Entity	Plain Film	Myelography and Postmyelographic CT	MRI	Comments
Ependymoma	Benign bone scalloping 15–33%	Cord enlargement	IM mass T1:→ ↓, T2: ↑ Homogeneous enhancement	65% cord gliomas 75% occur in conus or filum
Astrocytoma	Benign bone scalloping 50%	Cord enlargement	IM mass T1:→ ↓, T2: ↑ Heterogeneous enhancement	Intratumoral cysts 40%
Hemangioblastoma	—	Diffuse cord enlargement Vascular filling defects	IM mass T1:→ ↓, T2: ↑ Often large syrinx	Von Hippel-Lindau disease ± large syrinx with enhancing nidus
Hydrosyringomyelia	Charcot's joints	Diffuse cord enlargement Delayed cyst opacification	IM fluid cavity T1:→, T2:→	Evaluate foramen magnum for Chiari malformation Gd to exclude tumor
Trauma	± fracture/dislocation	Cord edematous or macerated Pseudomeningocele—avulsion	Blood: T1: ↑, T2: ↓ later ↑ Edema: T1:→ ↓, T2: ↑	MRI excels in evaluating trauma induced cord abnormalities
AVM	—	Serpentine filling defect; focal cord enlargement rare	Heterogeneous T2: ↓ Flow void in vessels	Spinal angiography to evaluate AVM
Demyelinating disease Transverse myelitis Radiation myelitis	—	Usually normal, rarely focal cord enlargement	T1:→ ↓, T2: ↑ Gd (acute phase) enhances	History

IM = intramedullary; Gd = gadolinium.

remainder may be found in the cervical or thoracic cord. Ependymomas of the cervical or thoracic cord are indistinguishable from astrocytomas; however, astrocytomas are much more common in the C-spine and slightly more common in the thoracic spine than are ependymomas.[20]

Ependymomas are histologically benign, growing by centrifugal extension into an oblong mass, with rare CSF seeding. These slow-growing lesions produce benign scalloping of the perimeter of the bony canal in 15 to 33% of cases.[20] The cervical or thoracic lesions may be associated with multilocular syringes or cavities at either the cephalad or the caudad pole.[17] The cord may be focally enlarged, with fluid-containing cysts.

The myelogram demonstrates an intramedullary lesion that may be focal or diffuse. The lesion may expand the cord enough to block contrast flow (Fig. 12–20). Cord enlargement can be confirmed on postmyelography CT.

MRI depicts a mass of variable size that is hypointense to isointense to cord on T1 and hyperintense on T2 (Fig. 12–21). Gadolinium enhancement will render the lesion more conspicuous.[14] Ependymomas generally enhance in a homogeneous, well-circumscribed pattern.

Astrocytoma

Astrocytomas represent one third of intramedullary tumors. These tumors may occur at any location along the cord. They are most common between 20 and 50 years of age and are slightly more common in men.[20] Seventy-five percent of these tumors are low grade (I–II). Benign pressure erosion of the canal is present with flattening of the medial pedicle surface reported in 50% of patients.[22] Intratumoral cysts have been reported in nearly 40% of tumors.

The myelographic and CT appearances of astrocytoma are similar to those of ependymoma. The mass may enlarge the cord focally or diffusely. The tumor is isointense to hypointense to cord on T1 and hyperintense on T2 (Fig. 12–22). Astrocytomas tend to enhance

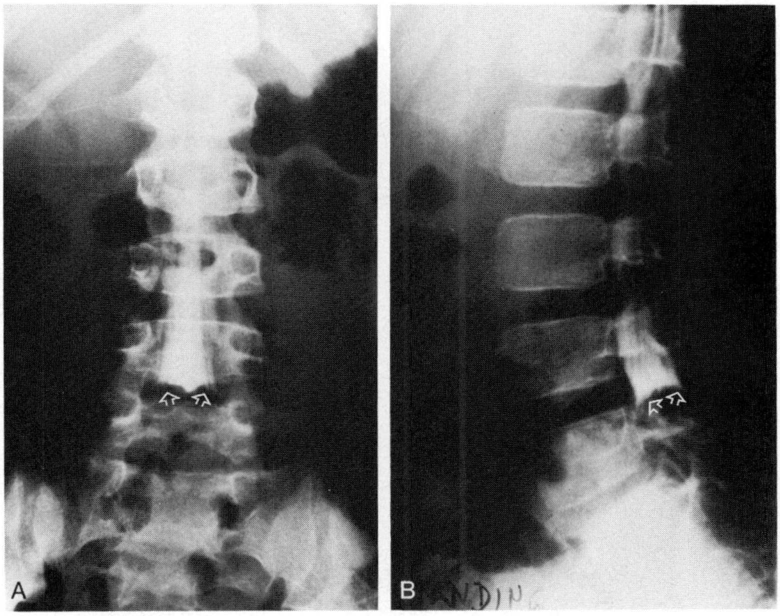

Figure 12–20. Ependymoma (4-year-old male).

A, B, AP and lateral lumbar myelogram. An intradural filling defect blocks flow of contrast material caudal to the L4–5 interspace. The well-defined meniscus (*open arrows*) is intradural, along the filum.

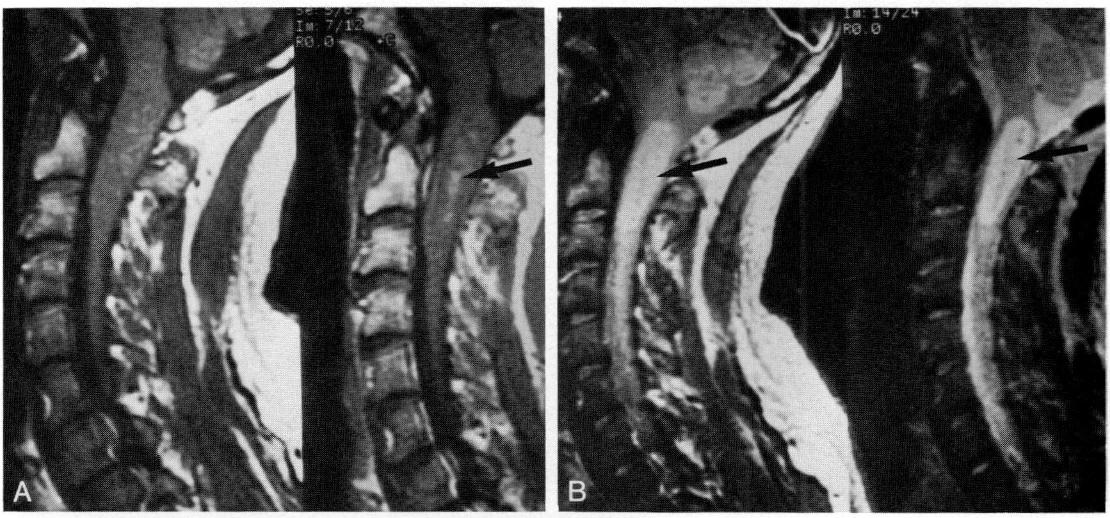

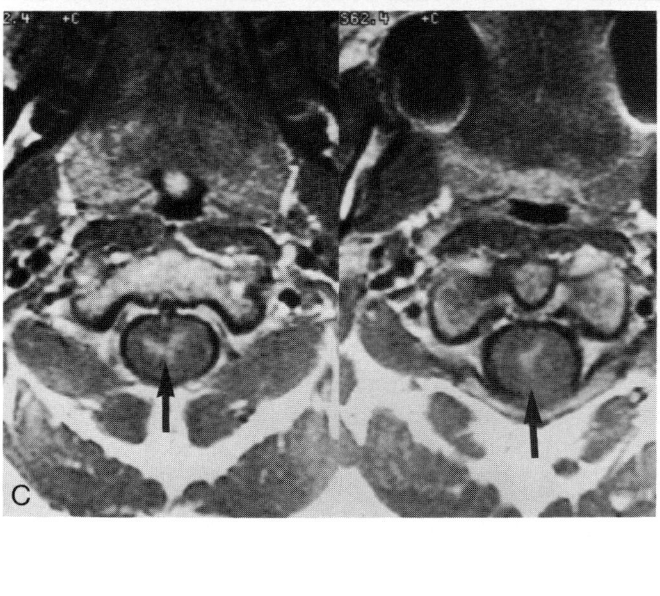

Figure 12–21. Ependymoma (24-year-old female).

A, Parasagittal T1 (*left,* unenhanced; *right,* enhanced). The cervical cord is enlarged from the craniocervical junction to C3. The signal intensity of the cord is homogeneous. The tumor enhances (*arrow*) centrally in a heterogeneous fashion.

B, Parasagittal (*left,* SD; *right,* T2). The focality of the high-signal intramedullary lesion (*arrow*) is depicted.

C, Enhanced axial T1. The heterogeneous pattern of enhancement (*arrow*) is noted within the enlarged cord.

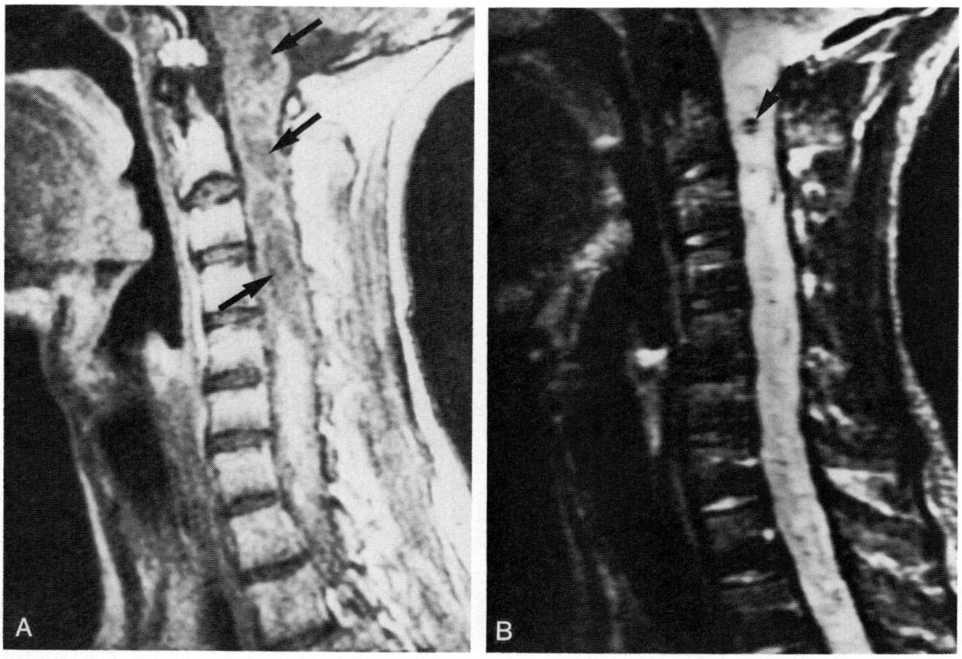

Figure 12–22. Astrocytoma (28-year-old male).
A, Parasagittal T1. The cord is diffusely enlarged from the medulla to the cervicothoracic junction. Multiple heterogeneous areas of decreased signal (*arrows*) are present.
B, Parasagittal T2. The cervical cord is heterogeneous and high signal, with focal regions of decreased signal (*arrow*) likely representing hemoglobin degradation products.

more heterogeneously than do ependymomas, partly because of the high incidence of intratumoral cysts.[17] Despite this, the enhancement of ependymomas and that of astrocytomas overlap considerably. Gadolinium may be administered to differentiate gross tumor from edema and cysts to aid in directing tumor biopsy.[15]

Hemangioblastoma

Hemangioblastomas represent 1.6 to 3.6% of cord tumors.[20] These tumors are most often associated with von Hippel-Lindau disease in middle-aged adults. The tumors are solitary in 80% of cases. There is no sexual predilection.

The tumors may arise in the cervical or thoracic cord, and may cause diffuse or focal widening of the cord. Myelography demonstrates cord enlargement associated with multiple serpentine filling defects caused by the arteries and veins associated with this relatively vascular tumor (Fig. 12–23). MRI demonstrates an enlarged infiltrated cord.[17] Half the lesions contain cysts with mural nodules (a common posterior fossa appearance). A sizable syrinx may accompany the lesion, corroborating the diagnosis.[17] Gadolinium enhancement is most useful to delineate the tumor nidus from reactive changes[13, 15, 17, 20] (Fig. 12–24).

Hydrosyringomyelia

Hydromyelia refers to dilatation of the central canal; the canal retains contact with the fourth ventricle and is lined with ependymal cells. Syringomyelia refers to any fluid cavity within the cord that is not lined by ependymal cells. The syrinx may or may not communicate with the central canal. In truth, hydromyelia and syringomyelia are usually radiographically indistinguishable. Fluid cavities within the cord are thus referred to as hydrosyringomyelia.[23]

Hydrosyringomyelia may be acquired or congenital. Congenital cases include developmental anomalies of the spine, foramen magnum, and posterior fossa (Chiari malforma-

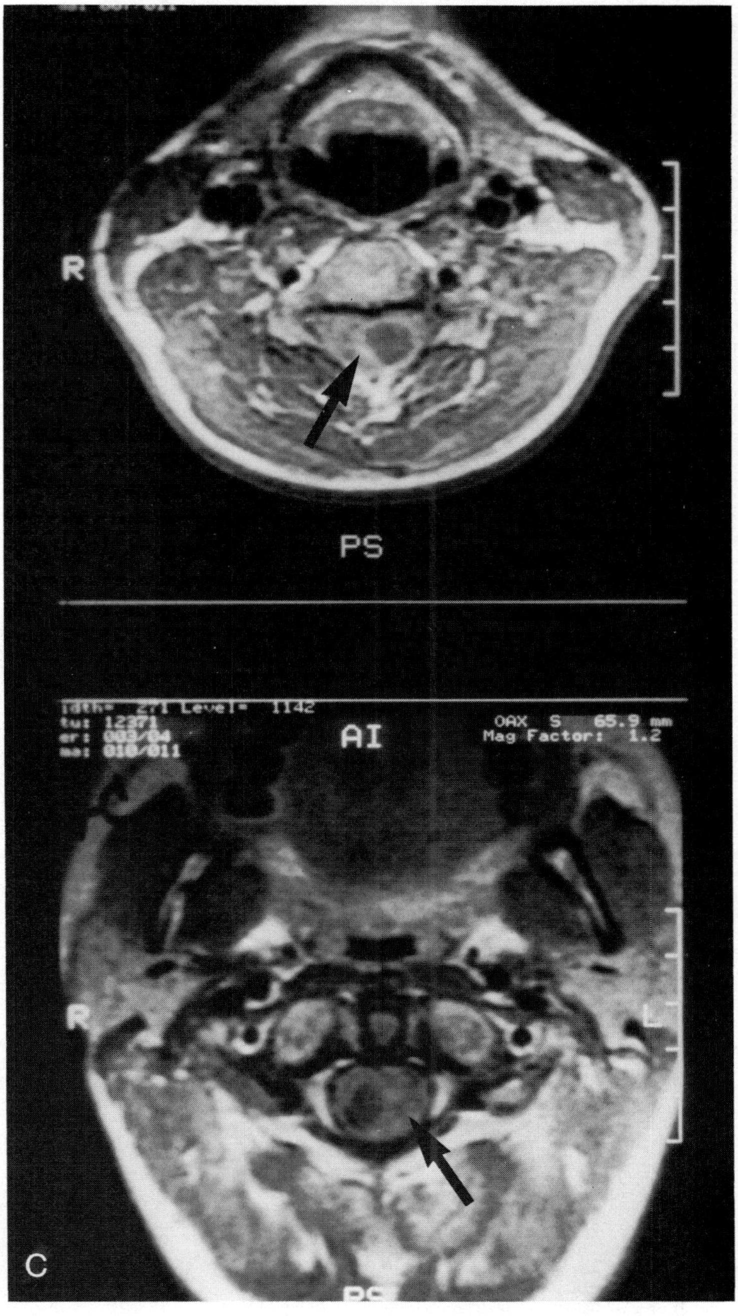

Figure 12–22 *Continued*
C, Axial T1. The heterogeneous nature and marked enlargement of the cord (*arrow*) are noted. The CSF that normally surrounds the cord is completely effaced.

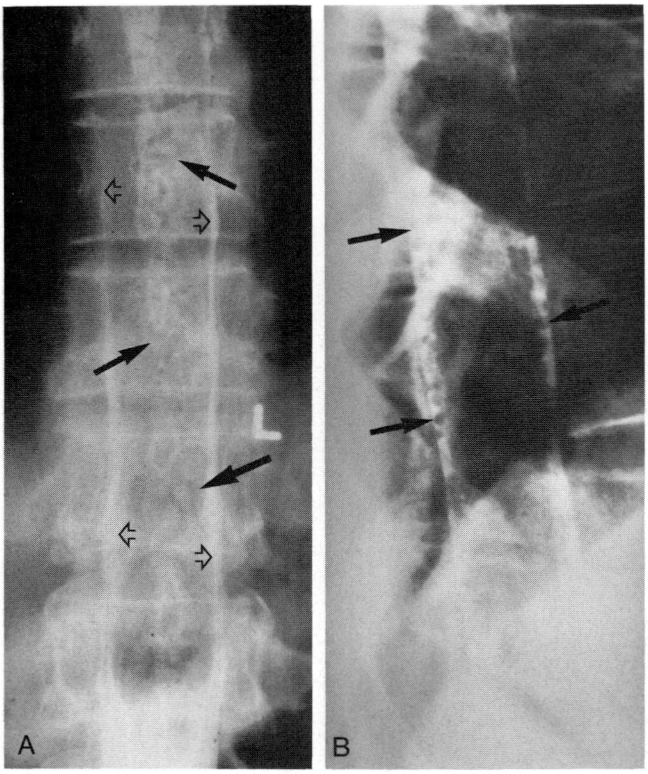

Figure 12–23. Hemangioblastoma (27-year-old male).

A, B, Myelography. Supine AP and lateral views. The CSF surrounding the cord is significantly attenuated secondary to diffuse cord enlargement (*open arrows*). Serpentine filling defects are noted overlying the cord on the AP film, as well as ventral and dorsal to the cord on the lateral film (*arrows*). Diffuse cord enlargement, in association with vascular hypertrophy, corroborates hemangioblastoma.

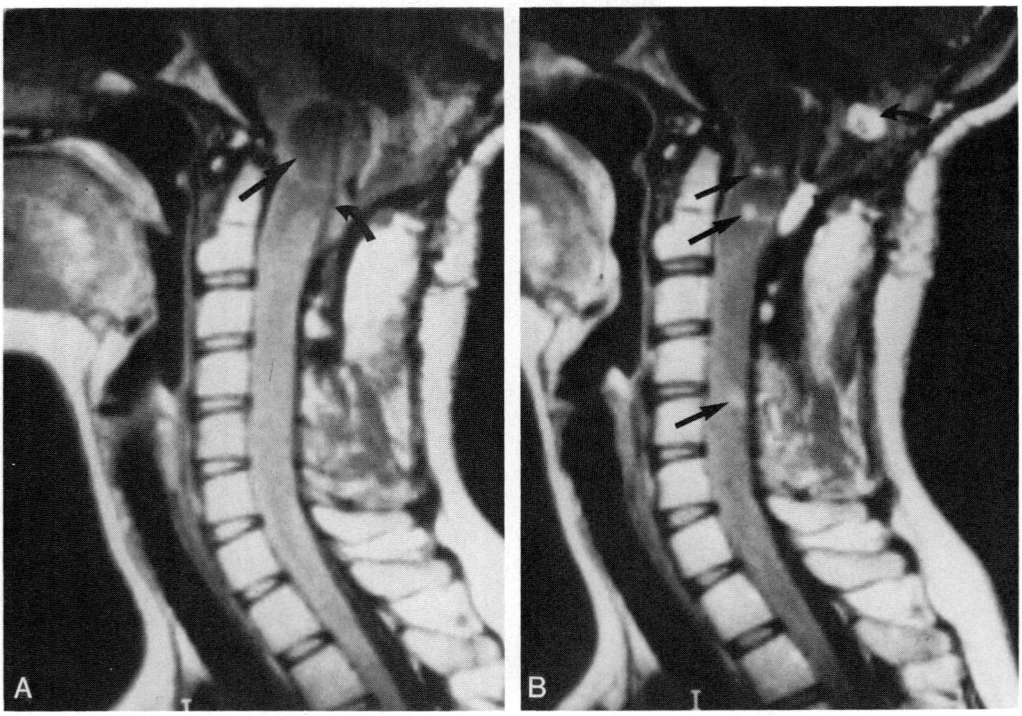

Figure 12–24. Hemangioblastoma (24-year-old male).

A, Parasagittal T1. The cord is diffusely enlarged and a cyst (*arrow*) is present in the cervicomedullary junction. A shunt catheter (*curved arrow*) drains the cyst. A remote bilateral laminectomy has been performed from the occiput to the C5 level.

B, Enhanced parasagittal T1. Multiple tumors enhance (*arrows*), including an inferior vermian lesion (*curved arrow*).

tion). Acquired causes may be related to tumor, vascular insufficiency, or postinflammatory or traumatic origins.[24] The latter category includes chronic cord compression in patients with severe spondylosis.

To explain the pathogenesis of hydrosyringomyelia, various theories have been proposed, related to defective CSF drainage, from either the fourth ventricle or the foramen magnum.[25–27] The enlarging cavity disrupts the decussating pain and temperature fibers, anterior horn cells, and pyramidal tracts. Accordingly, patients present with loss of pain and temperature sensation, trophic changes in the skin and joints, muscle weakness and wasting, spasticity, and abnormal plantar reflexes.[28] Charcot's joints occur in 25% of patients with hydrosyringomyelia, 80% of which are in the upper extremity. Clinical distinction between hydrosyringomyelia and tumor is difficult. Hydrosyringomyelia tends to occur at an earlier age (24 versus 34 years) and lasts longer (10 to 15 years); in hydrosyringomyelia, paresis, loss of sensation, and low CSF protein are more common than with neoplasm.[29]

The spinal cord is often diffusely enlarged, indistinguishable on myelography from tumor. The cavity may be decompressed depending on patient position, resulting in a small, atrophic cord. The postmyelography CT may demonstrate contrast within the cavity.[30] The contrast may enter directly from the spinal subarachnoid space or from a more circuitous pathway through the fourth ventricle.

As nearly 25% of all hydrosyringomyelias are related to tumor, MRI offers an ideal means to evaluate these lesions. The signal intensity of the benign cyst may be isointense to CSF on T1- and T2-weighted images (Fig. 12–25). The T2 study may demonstrate high signal adjacent to the cyst that represents gliosis in benign cases and tumor and edema in cases of neoplasm.[15] Hydrosyringomyelia secondary to benign, non-neoplastic causes may be associated with large, smoothly marginated cysts. Malignancy is suggested by con-

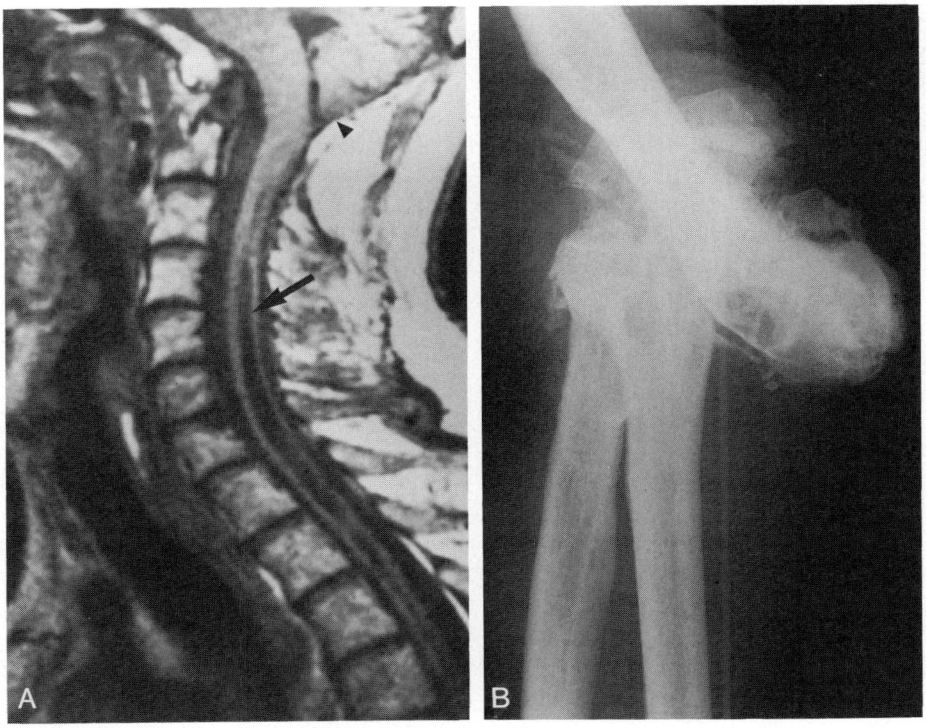

Figure 12–25. Hydrosyringomyelia; Chiari I (56-year-old female).

A, Parasagittal T1. The cerebellar tonsils (*arrowhead*) are ectopic. A fluid cavity (*arrow*) is present in the cord from the C2 level to at least the T4 level.

B, Lateral oblique film, left elbow. Bony sclerosis, destruction, and subluxation corroborate Charcot's joint.

trast enhancement; small, irregularly contoured eccentric cysts; and discordant signal intensity referable to CSF.

Trauma

Intramedullary hematoma (hematomyelia) or cord edema (concussion) may result from trauma. Associated vertebral body fractures, subluxation, traumatic disk herniation, ligamentous and soft tissue injury may be present (Fig. 12–26). CT excels in evaluation of the bony moiety of the trauma, detecting small fractures often missed by MRI.[31] MRI is, however, the modality of choice to evaluate the disk, paravertebral soft tissue, ligament integrity, and most importantly, the trauma-induced alterations of the cord. Edema is confirmed by increased T2 signal. Initially, hematomyelia is depicted as well-defined focus of decreased signal on T2 and gradient echo acquisition in a steady state (GRASS) images. After 8 days, deoxyhemoglobin is converted to methemoglobin and will appear bright on T1-weighted images. Hematomyelia correlates with significant initial injury and poor prognosis.[31] Significant neurologic defect is not seen without cord signal alterations.

Arteriovenous Malformation (AVM)

AVM may be located within the cord or along the dural surface. The intramedullary lesions occur four times more often in men than in women and present with symptoms often indistinguishable from other causes of cord dysfunction.[32] Patients present with progressive pain, weakness, sensory disturbance, and early disturbance in micturition. Patients may also present with subarachnoid hemorrhage or hematomyelia. The CSF protein is elevated in 75% of patients and mild pleocytosis is documented in 20%. The lesions are more commonly located caudal to the T7-T8 level along the dorsal portion of the cord.

Myelographic evaluation may demonstrate

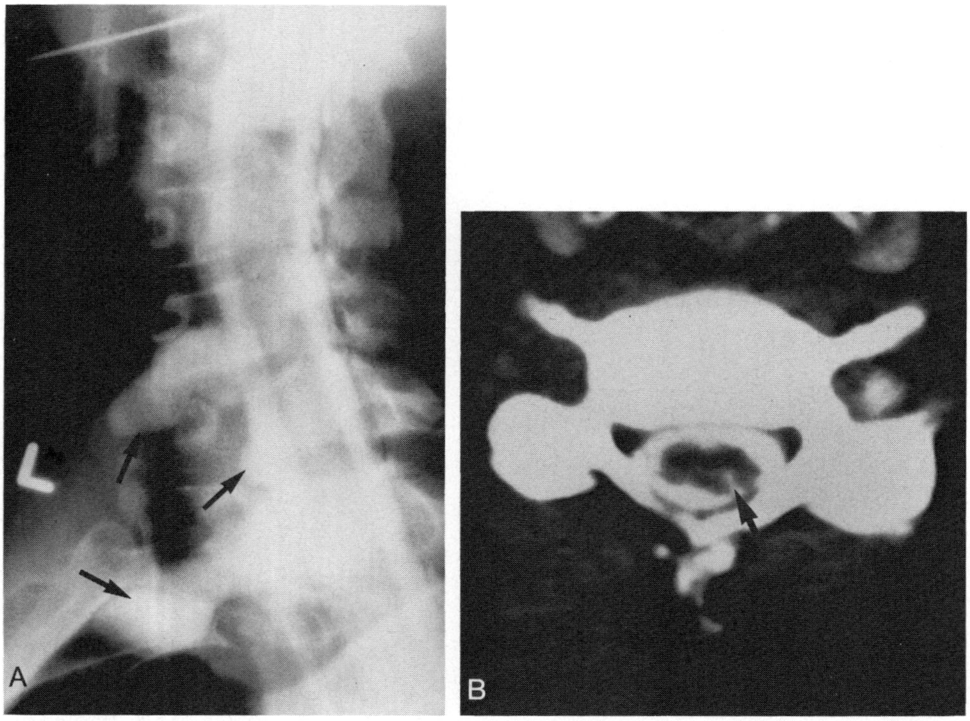

Figure 12–26. Trauma (21-year-old male).

A, Right anterior oblique (RAO) myelogram. Avulsion of left brachial plexus roots and disruption of the dura permitted formation of pseudomeningoceles (*arrows*). These fluid collections communicate with the subarachnoid space, filling readily with contrast material. Pseudomeningocele is in the differential diagnosis for an apical lung mass.

B, Postmyelogram CT. Demonstrates maceration of the cord that contains a post-traumatic dorsal cleft (*arrow*) secondary to a high-velocity injury.

serpentine filling defects in the contrast-laden CSF in 75 to 90% of cases.[32] The cord may be slightly widened. Postmyelographic CT confirms the intradural extramedullary serpentine vessels (Fig. 12–27). Spinal angiography should be performed to evaluate the nidus, arterial feeders, and venous drainage pattern.

Di Chiro[33] has proposed a classification of spinal cord AVMs based on the size and number of supplying vessels, as well as the transit time. Type I is the most common, consisting of only one to two arteries that supply a long, tortuous network of vessels on the dorsal cord surface. Transit time is long, with opacification of the venous side for 15 to 20 seconds. Type II, the least common AVM, is supplied by one to two arteries that supply a compact, tightly woven nidus on the dorsal cord surface. The flow in type II is slow. Type III is referred to as the juvenile type, has multiple feeders, has shunts with rapid transit time, and is usually located on the dorsal and ventral surface of the cord.

MRI demonstrates a decreased-signal intramedullary mass with variable cord enlargement and flow void on T1-weighted images. The flow void is best visualized on axial images.[34] The T2 images demonstrate more clearly the flow void of the draining veins and the heterogeneous intramedullary focus of decreased signal representing the nidus. In some cases, high T2 signal may be detected cephalad and caudad to the lesions, presumably representing gliosis rather than edema.[15]

Demyelinating Disease

The demyelinating lesions of multiple sclerosis (MS) frequently involve the white matter of the spinal cord. The most common location of involvement is the middle to upper cervical cord. The lesions tend to be focal, involving one or perhaps two vertebral body levels. The lesions result in focal cord enlargement in only 5% of cases,[21] a feature that may distinguish this from neoplasm. Infrequency of cord enlargement renders myelography and postmyelographic CT relatively ineffective means to evaluate this disease.

MRI demonstrates a heterogeneous slightly decreased-signal region on T1-weighted images. T2 images demonstrate focal increased signal. Gadolinium enhancement occurs in the acute setting and can be used to follow response to therapy[15, 16, 35] (Fig. 12–28). Peak enhancement is noted 45 to 60 minutes after contrast administration[35]—another feature to distinguish this from tumor, which typically enhances immediately. In the chronic disease state, the cord may be significantly atrophic (Fig. 12–29).

Transverse Myelitis

Acute transverse myelitis is an idiopathic inflammatory or demyelinating condition of the cord that is usually confined to a few segments. The disease occurs most commonly in young adults, who experience a relatively rapid onset of a spinal motor and sensory level in the absence of cord compression or other neurologic disease. Acute transverse myelitis may be the result of viral or postviral infection. Its relationship to MS is not clear. The disease is usually nonprogressive, stabilizing within 2 to 3 weeks. Rapid onset of symptoms and back pain at the onset of disease are signs of poor prognosis.[36] The cord may be focally enlarged on myelography, postmyelographic CT, and MRI. The T2 MRI sequence demonstrates high signal throughout the region of involvement. The acute lesion will enhance following gadolinium administration.[36]

Radiation Myelitis

Radiation myelitis is a rare condition that occurs an average of 9 to 15 months after spinal radiation therapy. Patients initially develop paresthesias and an inability to perceive pain and temperature. Usually within 6 months, the symptoms progress to involve all cord segments.[37] Pathologic review demonstrates marked hyaline thickening and thrombosis of the arterioles with necrosis of predominantly the white matter. The vascular changes may not, however, be of significant magnitude to cause the coagulative cord necrosis.[38]

Criteria for diagnosis of radiation myelitis are exclusion of primary cord tumor or metastasis and presence of neurodeficits that relate to the cord segment included in the radiation port. Higher radiation fraction size, shorter treatment time, increased total dose, and concomitant administration of specific chemotherapeutic agents are factors that place patients at a higher risk.

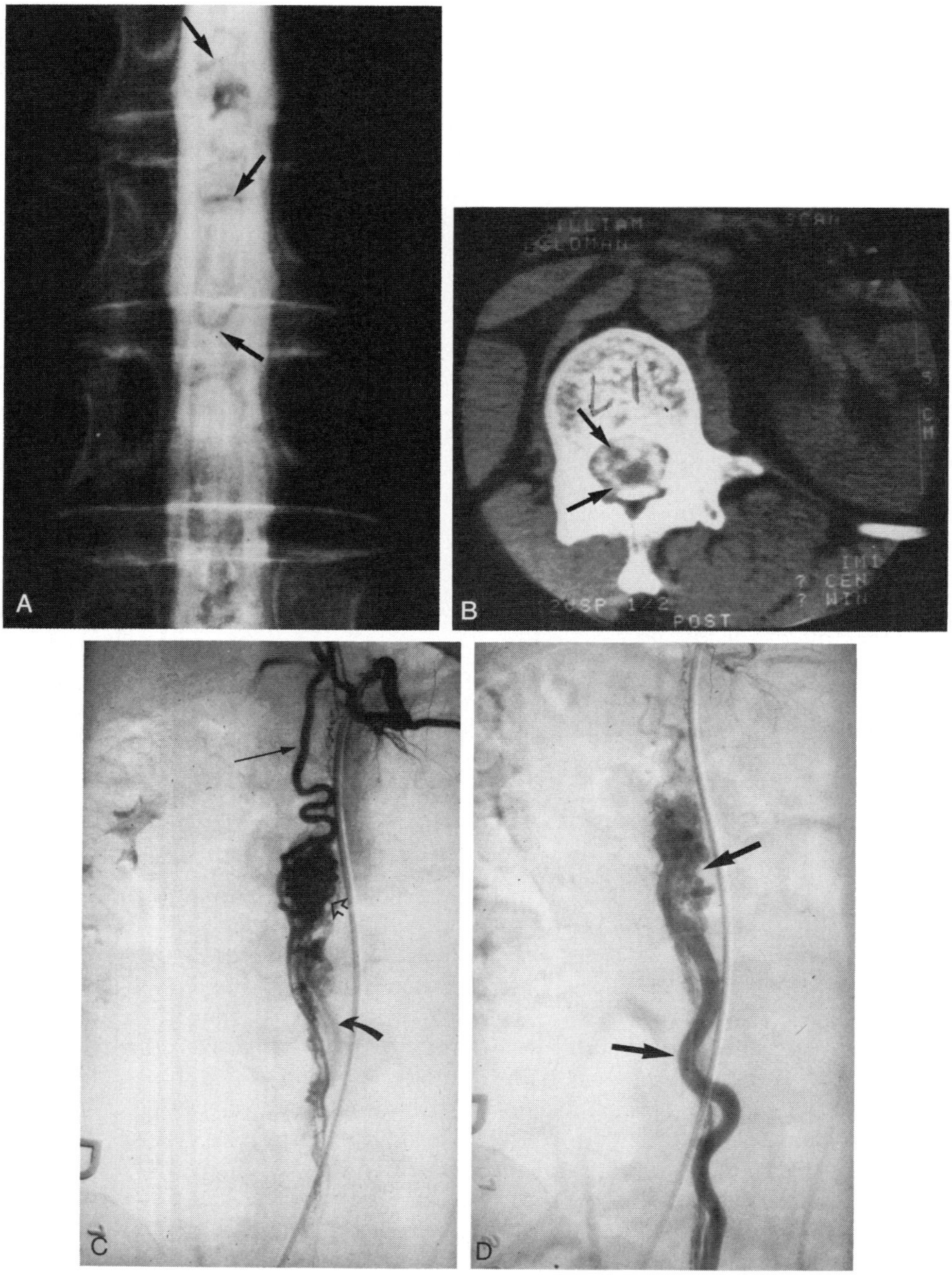

Figure 12–27. Arteriovenous malformation (AVM) (38-year-old male).

A, AP myelogram; thoracolumbar junction. The cord is of normal size. Multiple serpentine filling defects (*arrows*) are noted within the contrast column.

B, Postmyelogram CT (L1). Irregular filling defects (*arrows*) are present within the subarachnoid space.

C, AP spinal angiogram (arterial phase). The artery of Adamkiewicz (*arrow*) is markedly enlarged. A racemose vascular nidus (*open arrow*) is present with evidence of early venous opacification (*curved arrow*).

D, AP spinal angiogram (venous phase). Multiple hypertrophied veins (*arrows*) drain the cord AVM.

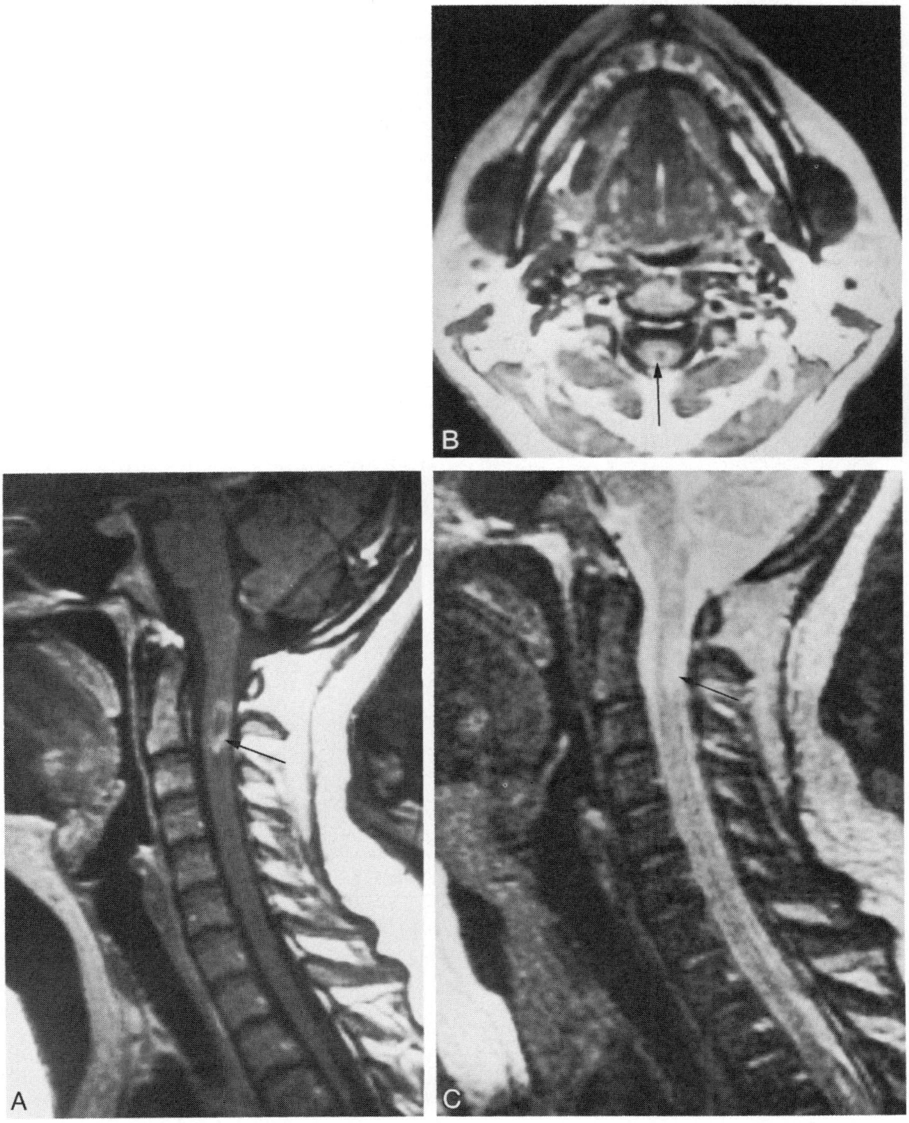

Figure 12–28. Acute multiple sclerosis (30-year-old female).

A, B, Enhanced parasagittal and axial T1. A 2-cm oblong intramedullary focus of ring enhancement (*arrow*) is present at the C2 level. Despite the enhancement, the cord remains of normal size.

C, Parasagittal T2. An ill-defined high-signal focus (*arrow*) correlates with the findings on the enhanced examination.

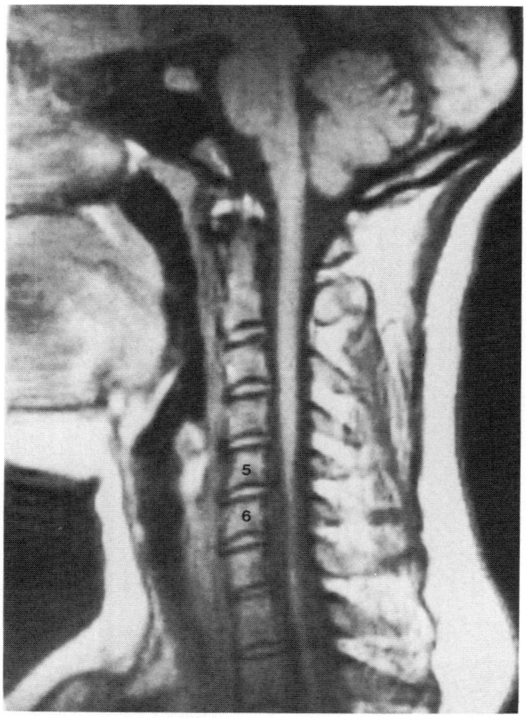

Figure 12–29. Chronic multiple sclerosis (36-year-old female). Parasagittal T1; the cord is diffusely atrophic secondary to chronic demyelination. This is most marked caudal to the C5–6 disk space.

Radiographically, the cord may be normal or diffusely enlarged. MRI demonstrates increased T2 signal in the involved region. The lesion will enhance on postgadolinium T1 sequences.

Intradural Extramedullary

(Table 12–3)

Meningioma

Meningiomas are benign tumors that occur at least four to eight times more frequently in women, usually in the fifth to sixth decade, and most commonly within the thoracic spine. The tumors usually arise anterolateral or posterolateral to the cord near the dentate ligament and dorsal root ganglia. The lesions are solitary in more than 95% of cases. Multiplicity implicates neurofibromatosis. Eighty-five percent of meningiomas are in the intradural extramedullary compartment. The remaining 15% are either extradural or both intradural and extradural.

Plain film findings demonstrate bone changes in less than 10% of patients. The medial aspect of the pedicle may be eroded,

Table 12–3. INTRADURAL EXTRAMEDULLARY DISEASE

Entity	Plain Film	Myelography and Postmyelographic CT	MRI	Comments
Meningioma	Benign bone erosion or hyperostosis 10%	Focal mass, ± calcification Cord displacement	T1:→ ↓ , T2: ↓ or ↑ Homogeneous enhancement	Female:male ratio 4–8:1 Thoracic most common location
Nerve sheath tumor	Benign bone scalloping Enlarged IV foramen	Focal mass(es) Cord displacement	T1:→, T2: ↑ Homogeneous enhancement	Anywhere along spinal axis Neurofibromatosis: Multiplicity Vertebral dysplasia Thoracic meningocele
Metastasis	—	Multiple filling defects within thecal sac	T1:→, T2: ↑ Homogeneous enhancement	Drop Mets from CNS primary tumors
Arachnoiditis	± prior surgical defects	Irregular root placement Underfilling of sac Focal mass	T1: Best to evaluate pattern of root abnormality Minimal enhancement	History of prior intervention Caudal to L3
Arachnoid cyst	Rarely benign bone erosion	Filling defect Mass effect Delayed opacification	T1:→, T2:→ T2 contingent on flow effects	Primary or acquired

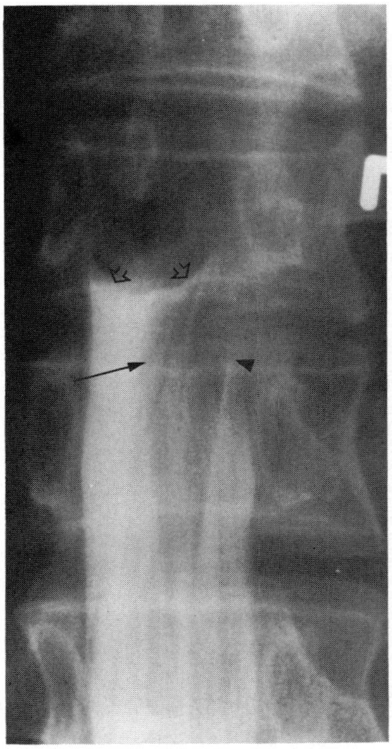

Figure 12–30. Meningioma (42-year-old female). Supine AP myelogram, lower thorax; a well-defined meniscus (*open arrows*) indicates that an intradural extramedullary mass is present. The cord (*arrow*) is displaced to the left with widening of the right CSF space and narrowing on the left (*arrowhead*).

or there may be hyperostosis of the arch, focal enlargement of the intervertebral foramen, or tumoral calcification. Myelography demonstrates an intradural extramedullary mass (Fig. 12–30). There may be a complete block at the level of the mass. CT demonstrates a soft tissue mass of slightly increased density that may be partially calcified. Bony erosive changes are more apparent on CT than on plain films. Postmyelographic CT demonstrates the mass as well as cord displacement. The MRI demonstrates an isointense-to-hypointense mass on T1 that is variable from slightly decreased to increased signal on T2.[17, 20, 39] As with myelography, on MRI the CSF forms a cap or meniscus at its junction with the lesion. The meningioma generally enhances homogeneously (Fig. 12–31).

Nerve Sheath Tumor

These tumors, which may be schwannomas or neurofibromas, are histologically similar lesions that arise from the Schwann cells covering the peripheral sensory nerves. Schwannomas do not incorporate the nerve root and tend to be solitary tumors. Neurofibromas, on the other hand, tend to contain fibroblasts and incorporate the nerve root within the tumor matrix and may be multiple.

Nerve sheath tumors may occur at any age, though most commonly in the 20- to 50-year age group, with no gender predilection. These tumors can arise anywhere along the spinal axis, but slightly more frequently within the thoracic spine. Two thirds of nerve sheath tumors are completely intradural. The location of the remainder is split equally between extradural and both intradural and extradural.[20]

Radiographic findings on plain films include benign bony erosion with enlargement of the intervertebral foramen. Myelography demonstrates the intradural extramedullary lesion, cord displacement, and possibly spinal block. The lesion may be multiple if neurofibromatosis is the underlying cause (Fig. 12–32); vertebral body dysplasia and thoracic meningocele may be present in these patients. CT demarcates a hypodense soft tissue mass. The paraspinal component of the mass can be evaluated. Bony changes are more accurately detected on CT. T1 MRI depicts an intraspinal mass that is isointense to the cord, surrounded by low-signal CSF (Fig. 12–33). The mass is hyperintense to cord on T2 images yet may be obscured in part or total by the high-signal CSF. Gadolinium-enhanced T1 MRI offers the most sensitive means to detect these homogeneously enhancing intraspinal tumors[17] (Fig. 12–34).

Metastatic Disease

Metastatic tumors to the spinal axis most commonly result from drop seed metastasis from intracranial primary tumors. Accordingly, these occur most frequently in children with primitive neuroectodermal tumor (PNET), ependymoma, or glioma.[20] Any high-grade intracranial malignancy may metastasize to the spinal axis. Less commonly, tumors extrinsic to the central nervous system (CNS) may metastasize via CSF pathways. This usually occurs late in the disease process and may accompany breast cancer, small and non–small cell lung cancer, melanoma, cancers of the

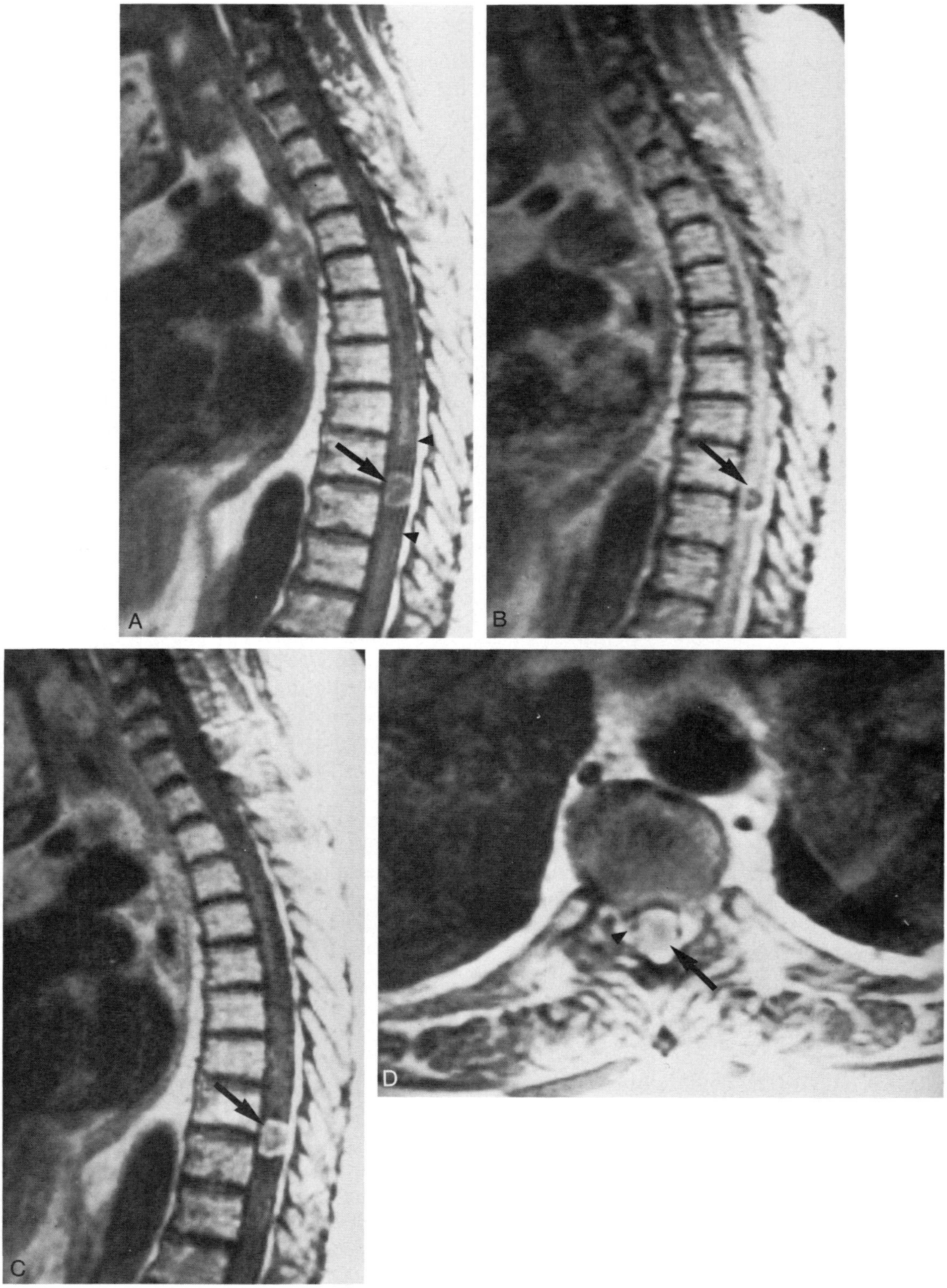

Figure 12–31. Thoracic meningioma (66-year-old female).

A, Parasagittal T1. A focal intraspinal mass (*arrow*) fills the dural space. The displaced cord (*arrowheads*) can be identified above and below the tumor.

B, Parasagittal T2. The mass (*arrow*) is moderately hypointense with a hyperintense periphery.

C, Enhanced parasagittal T1. The mass (*arrow*) enhances, somewhat more so along the periphery.

D, Enhanced axial T1. The mass (*arrow*) fills the canal, resulting in marked cord (*arrowhead*) compression.

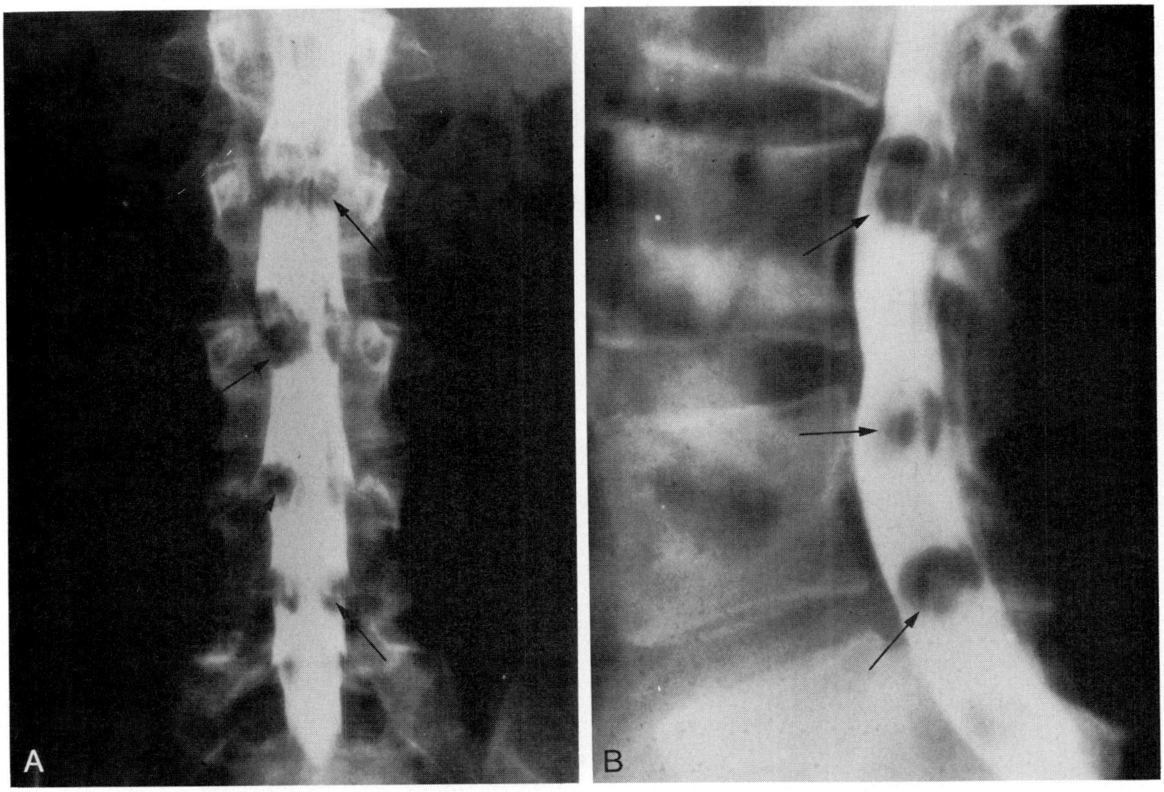

Figure 12–32. Neurofibromas (34-year-old male).
A, B, AP and lateral myelogram. Multiple intradural lesions (*arrows*) are noted. These appear bilaterally at each lumbar root level.

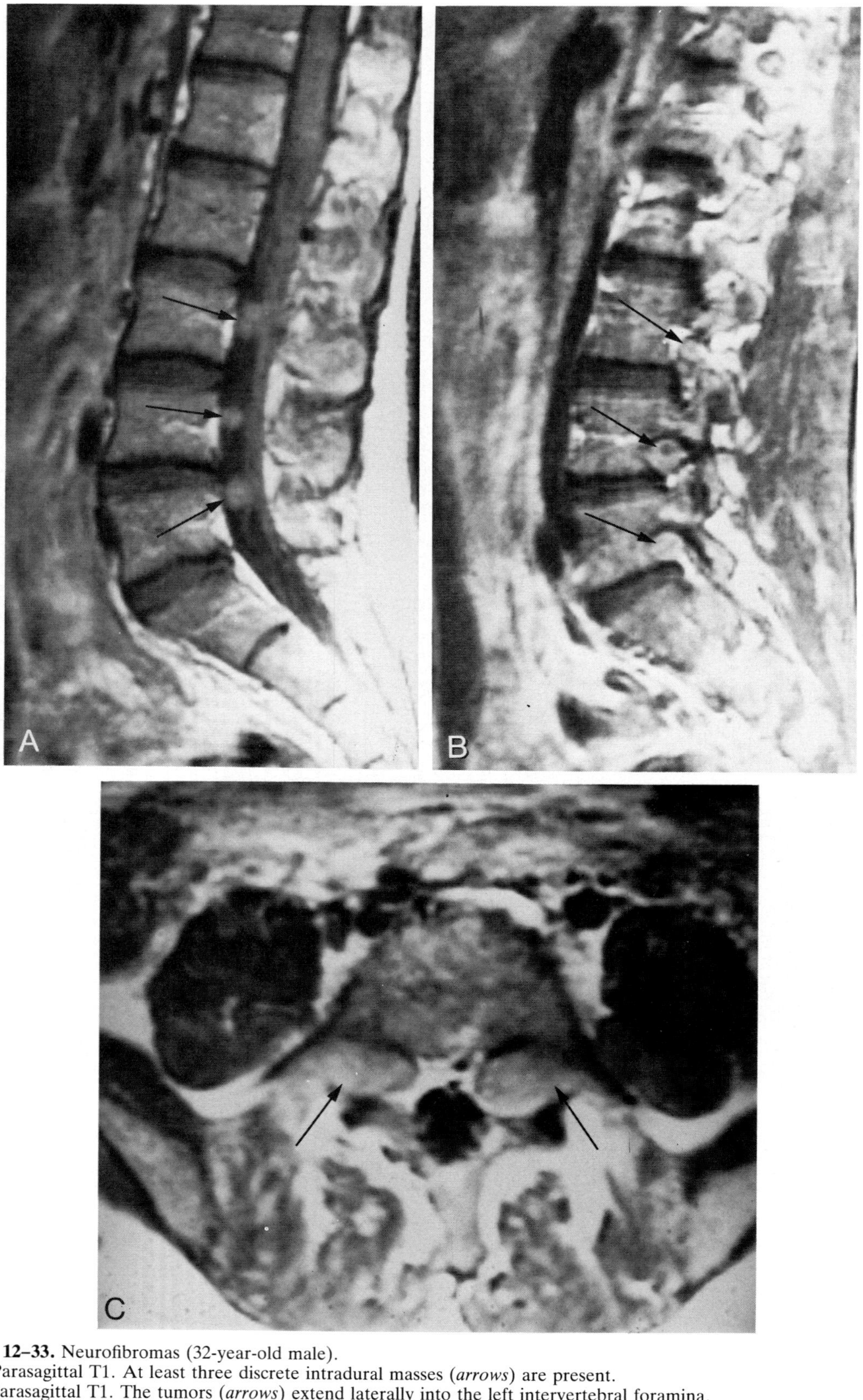

Figure 12–33. Neurofibromas (32-year-old male).
A, Parasagittal T1. At least three discrete intradural masses (*arrows*) are present.
B, Parasagittal T1. The tumors (*arrows*) extend laterally into the left intervertebral foramina.
C, Axial T1 (L5–S1). The neurofibromas (*arrows*) extend into the enlarged intervertebral foramen bilaterally.

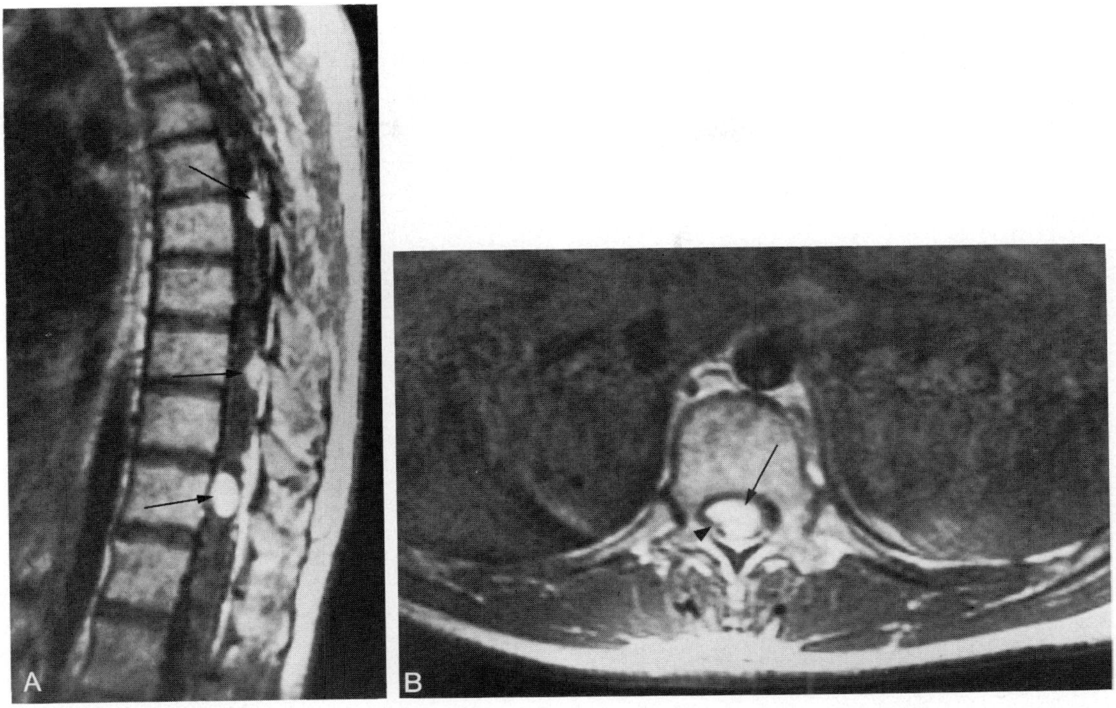

Figure 12–34. Neurofibromas (28-year-old female).

A, Enhanced parasagittal T1. Three homogeneously enhancing intradural tumors (*arrows*) are present. The neurofibromas were isointense to the cord on unenhanced images.

B, Enhanced axial T1. The cord (*arrowhead*) is markedly compressed by the enhancing neurofibroma (*arrow*), which occupies nearly the entire transverse area of the canal at this level.

gastrointestinal system, lymphoma, and leukemia.[18] Rarely, drop seed metastases may adhere to the surface of the cord and grow into the cord parenchyma, appearing as intramedullary masses.

The myelographic workup of these patients may reveal multiple filling defects of varying size (Fig. 12–35). The cauda equina may be studded with multiple small nodular metastases or adhere to one or more larger tumor deposits. The postmyelogram CT reveals the intradural filling defects and their relationship to the cord and cauda equina.

The MRI reveals multiple intermediate-signal masses along the cord, roots, or thecal sac on T1 images. High-signal CSF obscures the masses on T2 images.[40] Gadolinium-enhanced MRI is excellent for detection of leptomeningeal tumor[17] (Fig. 12–36). Routinely, 3-mm lesions can be detected within the dural sac.[19]

Arachnoiditis

Arachnoiditis is an inflammatory process of the arachnoid membrane and its contents, resulting from various causes including agents injected into the subarachnoid space (contrast material, anesthetics, steroids), infection, trauma, intradural or extradural surgery, or intrathecal hemorrhage. Initially, a fibrinous exudate coats the arachnoid and spinal roots. These surfaces adhere to one another, permitting proliferating fibroblast to collagenize these structures.[41] Arachnoiditis may lead to cord necrosis and cavitation caused by compromise of the pial arterial supply to the cord or by obstruction of venous drainage.[42]

Myelography demonstrates a spectrum of abnormalities from underfilling of one or more nerve root sleeves to a complete block of contrast (Figs. 12–37, 12–38). The roots may be adherent and thickened, and the thecal sac narrowed and foreshortened or featureless (the myelographic moulage sign). Additionally, discrete masses may be identified. Although arachnoiditis usually occurs caudal to the L3 level, the myelographic findings may appear otherwise indistinguishable from those of leptomeningeal tumor.

The MRI findings of arachnoiditis have been

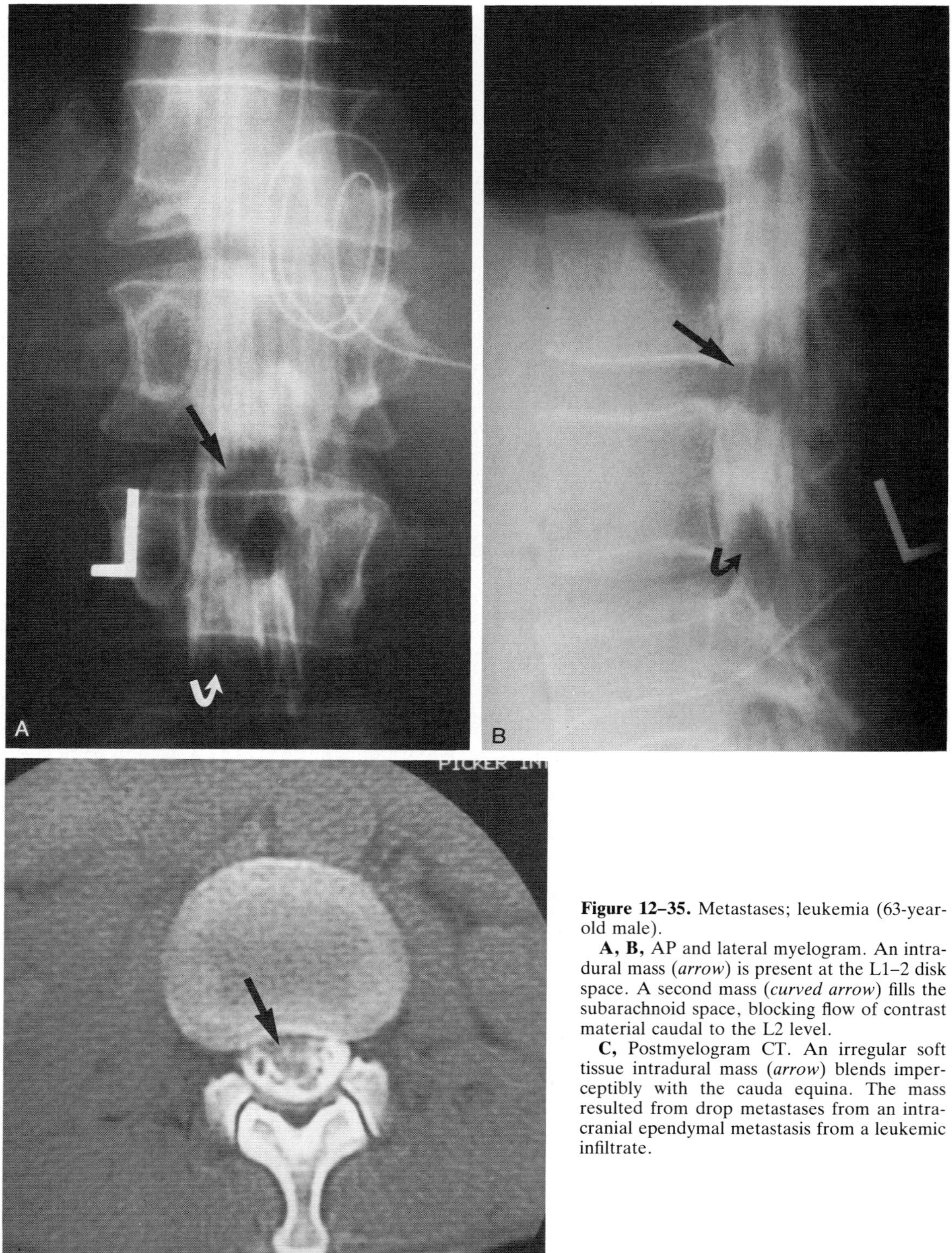

Figure 12–35. Metastases; leukemia (63-year-old male).

A, B, AP and lateral myelogram. An intradural mass (*arrow*) is present at the L1–2 disk space. A second mass (*curved arrow*) fills the subarachnoid space, blocking flow of contrast material caudal to the L2 level.

C, Postmyelogram CT. An irregular soft tissue intradural mass (*arrow*) blends imperceptibly with the cauda equina. The mass resulted from drop metastases from an intracranial ependymal metastasis from a leukemic infiltrate.

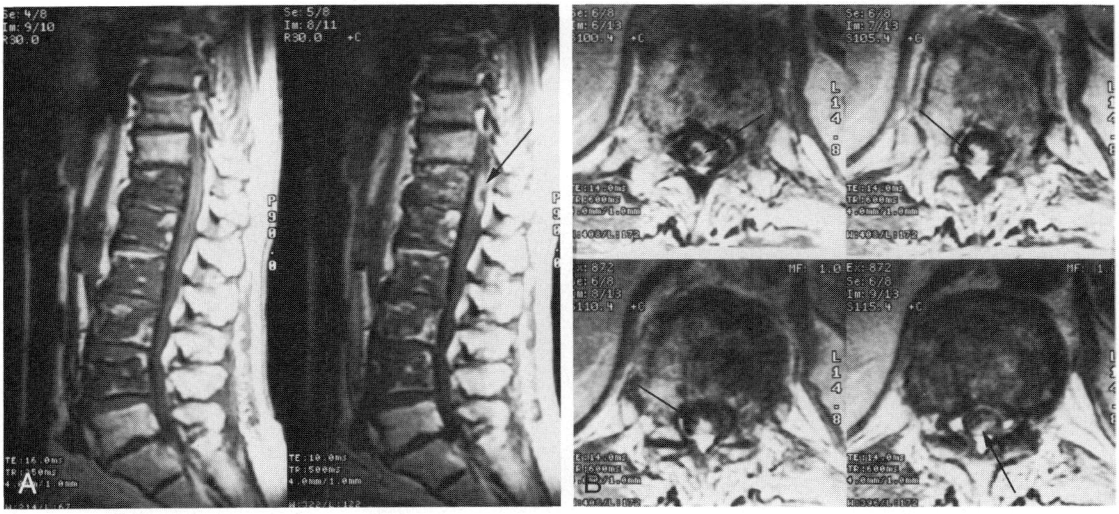

Figure 12–36. Lung metastases (65-year-old male).

A, Parasagittal T1 (*left,* unenhanced; *right,* enhanced). Infiltrative osseous metastases replace the high-signal marrow from T12 to L4 inclusive. After administration of the contrast material, an intradural mass (*arrow*) becomes apparent.

B, Enhanced axial T1. The enhancing intradural mass (*arrow*) is corroborated.

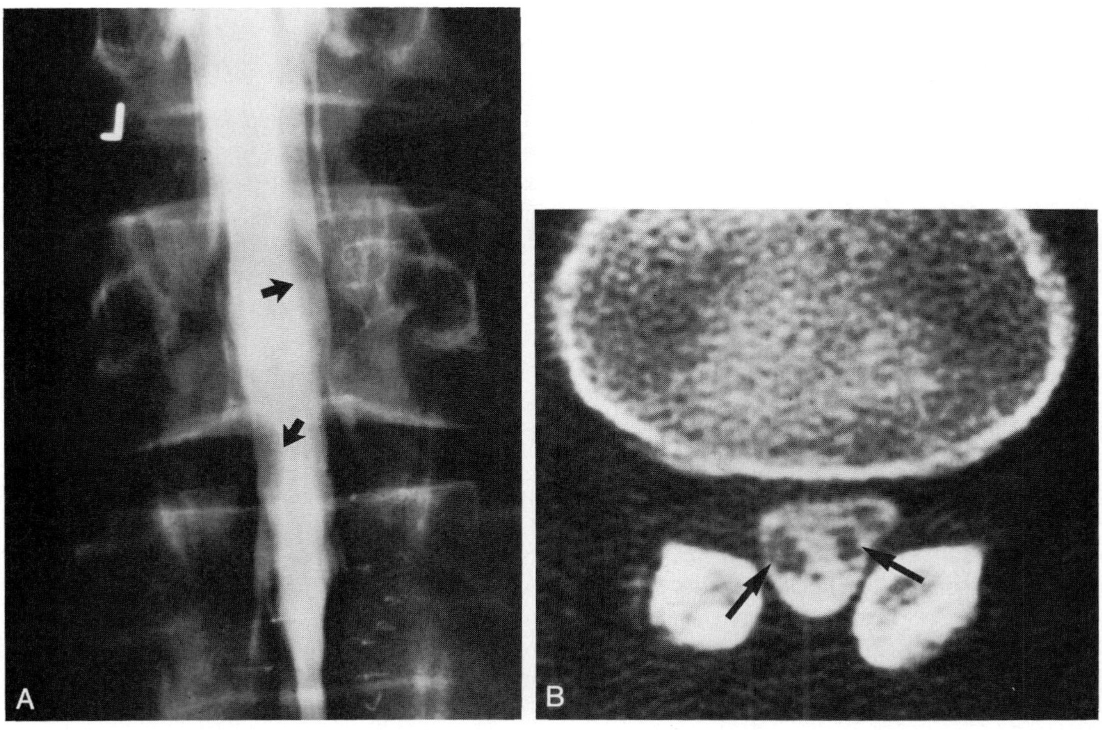

Figure 12–37. Arachnoiditis (43-year-old male).

A, AP myelogram. The thecal sac caudal to mid-L3 is abnormally attenuated. The cauda equina is markedly abnormal with adherent scarred roots (*arrows*). Laminectomy and sutures corroborate prior surgery.

B, Postmyelogram CT. The thickened, clumped roots (*arrows*) are demonstrated. Bilateral laminectomy defects are present.

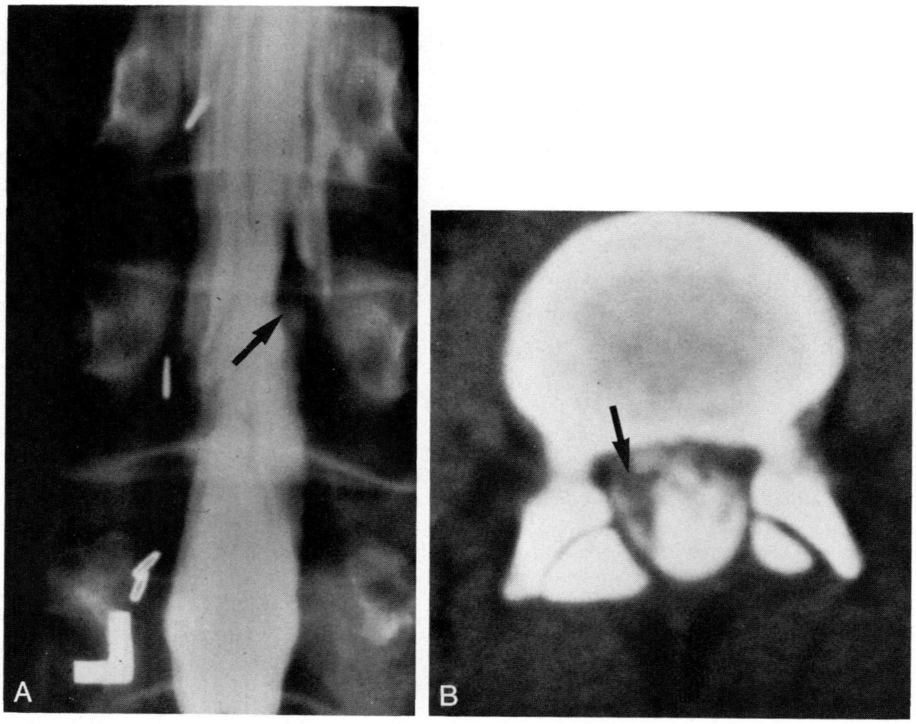

Figure 12–38. Arachnoiditis (42-year-old male).
A, AP myelogram. The distal thecal sac is featureless; an irregular filling defect (*arrow*) is noted on the right.
B, Postmyelogram CT. Thickened adherent fibrotic roots (*arrow*) are noted within the canal.

grouped[43] in three categories: group 1, central conglomeration of cauda; group 2, roots adherent to the thecal sac ("empty sac"); and group 3, soft tissue mass that replaces the subarachnoid space. These findings are best demonstrated on axial T1-weighted images. A relatively good correlation exists between moderate to severe arachnoiditis on myelography and the extent of MRI findings.

The role of gadolinium in arachnoiditis is limited.[41] Enhancement is variable and only moderate at best. Rarely, the gadolinium-enhanced examination offers information not available on the unenhanced T1 image. The correlation between chronicity and severity of patient symptoms and the contrast-enhanced MRI findings is poor. The paucity of enhancement may be useful to exclude leptomeningeal CSF metastasis from the differential diagnosis.

Arachnoid Cyst

Arachnoid cysts may be primary or acquired. Primary arachnoid cysts are congenital lesions that result from a separation of the arachnoid membrane and accumulation of CSF within the arachnoid membrane. Secondary arachnoid cysts are referred to as subarachnoid cysts and result from chronic inflammation, trauma, intrathecal contrast material, or subarachnoid blood, or may be a late complication of spinal epidural anesthesia.[42] Granulation material forms in the subarachnoid space, resulting in constricting bands that trap CSF and subsequently enlarge, possibly because of a ball-valve mechanism.[44]

Myelography demonstrates an intradural extramedullary mass that may block the cephalad CSF flow. The cyst remains of CSF density on immediate postmyelography CT, yet may fill with contrast material on delayed CT examination. MRI usually demonstrates an isointense-to-CSF collection. Although a discrete mass may not be identified, mass effect may be detected (Fig. 12–39). The cord may be focally compressed or contain cysts with evidence of myelomalacia. The T2 appearance of these lesions varies, depending on the CSF motion within the cyst.

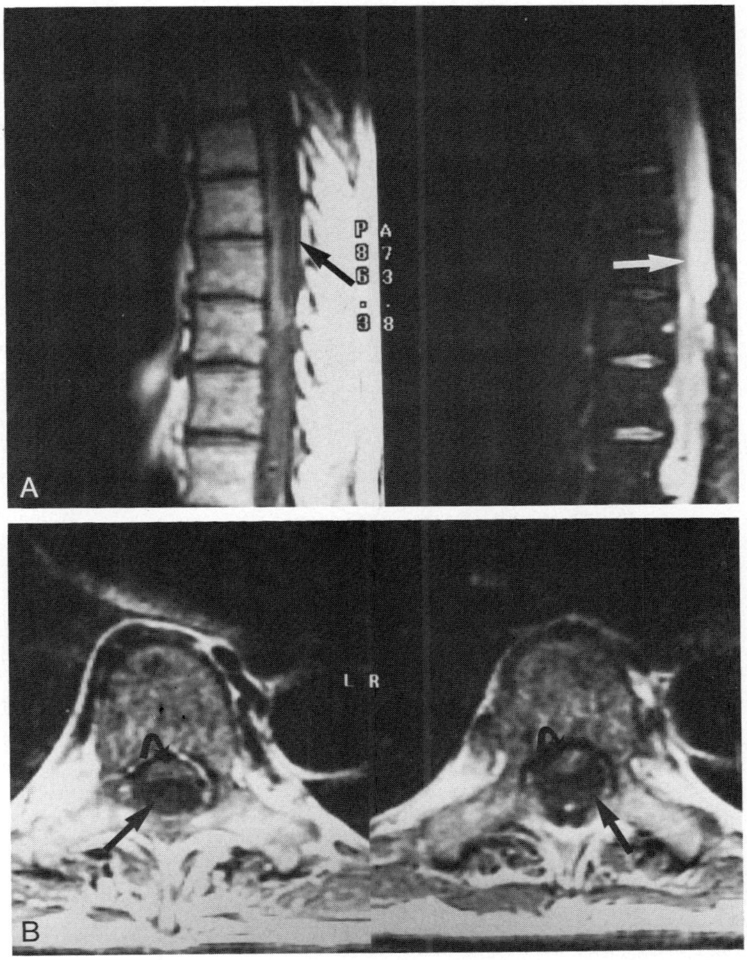

Figure 12–39. Arachnoid cyst (62-year-old male).

A, Parasagittal (*left,* T1; *right,* T2). An isointense-to-CSF "mass" (*arrow*) displaces the cord ventrally in the mid-thoracic spine.

B, Axial T1. The deformity and displacement of the cord (*curved arrow*) are better demonstrated. The dorsal CSF intensity collection (*arrow*) is an arachnoid cyst.

Extradural (Table 12–4)

Degenerative Disease

This is the most common disease process to affect the extradural compartment. As the disk degenerates and the vertical dimension of the disk diminishes, the spinal axis becomes malaligned. The altered mechanical stresses on the facet joints and ligaments result in a compensatory hypertrophy of these structures and the cartilaginous endplates.[21]

Degenerative Disk Disease (DDD)

DDD is a continuum that begins in the early teens and continues throughout life. The process begins with biochemical alterations that lead to thinning of the cartilaginous endplates, weakening of the annulus fibrosis, and dehydration of the nucleus pulposus. The annulus may tear, resulting in varying degrees of annular bulge or herniation.[45]

Disk bulges result in concentric, centrifugal displacement of the weakened annulus. The annulus extends beyond the margins of the opposing vertebral bodies and the disk height is commensurately diminished. Plain films may demonstrate mild disk space narrowing. The bulging annulus may be detected on CT examinations. A focal ventral extradural defect at the disk space may be demonstrated on myelography. The disk bulge, unless severe, does not produce any significant effect on the spinal roots that exit above or descend through the disk space level.

Owing to the dehydration that often accompanies a bulge, the T2 signal of the disk may

Table 12–4. EXTRADURAL DISEASE

Entity	Plain Film	Myelography and Postmyelographic CT	MRI	Comments
Disk	↓ Height of disk space	Deviation, amputation, dilatation of nerve root Soft tissue mass at or near disk space	ED soft tissue mass Parallels disk signal	Generally contiguous with disk space
Osteophyte	Sclerosis with osteophyte on appropriate oblique film	ED defect similar to disk Postmyelographic CT confirms osteophyte	ED mass Parallels signal intensity of bone	Predictable locations: Uncinate process Articular facets Vertebral body endplates
Tumor	Bone destruction—pedicle Soft tissue mass	ED mass(es) presence of block(s) CT to evaluate extent of soft tissue mass and bone destruction	Infiltration and replacement of vertebral marrow Associated intraspinal and extraspinal mass Assessing degree of cord compression Evaluating occult or myelographically inaccessible regions	Gd may mask osseous metastasis
Trauma	Fracture/dislocation	ED defect CT confirms bone vs soft tissue CT demonstrated fracture	MRI excels with alignment, distinguishing disk from hematoma, and assessing degree of cord compression	History
Infection	Irregular destruction and sclerosis of opposing endplate Loss of disk space height	ED mass initially at disk space CT demonstrates extent of bony destruction and inflammatory mass	T1: disk space indistinguishable ↓ signal adjacent endplates T2: ↑ signal disk and endplates Gd: Inflammatory mass and intraspinal abscess	MRI most sensitive to demonstrate inflammatory changes Myelography may result in meningitis

ED = extradural; Gd = gadolinium.

be diminished (Fig. 12–40). Minute regions of increased T2 signal intensity may be seen in the annulus, indicating presence of contained annular tears. These foci often enhance on gadolinium T1 images due to invasion of reparative granulation tissue.[46, 47]

Disk protrusion refers to a more severe, though focal, disruption of the inner annulus. The outer fibers of the annulus remain intact and contain a focal extension of the nuclear material to, but not through, the outer annular fibers. The disk protrusion is also contained by the posterior longitudinal ligament, and its effect on the thecal sac and adjacent roots may be minimal (Fig. 12–41).

Disk extrusion occurs when a full-thickness disruption of the annular fibers is present and the nucleus pulposus extends through and beyond the disrupted annulus. The nuclear material may be contained by the PLL (subligamentous extrusion) or extend through the PLL into the epidural space. The nucleus may remain midline or lateralize but maintains its contiguity with the parent disk. The thecal sac and adjacent roots are commensurately displaced (Figs. 12–42 through 12–44).

When the herniated nuclear material loses contiguity with the parent disk, it is termed a free fragment or sequestered disk. The fragment may migrate in any direction and extends by equal incidence cephalad or caudad to the disk space.[48] Most frequently the disk is lodged in the anterior epidural space, either to the left or right of midline. Infrequently the disk will migrate to the lateral aspect of the spinal canal.

The spinal roots exit below the pedicles into the intervertebral foramen. Ergo, posterior

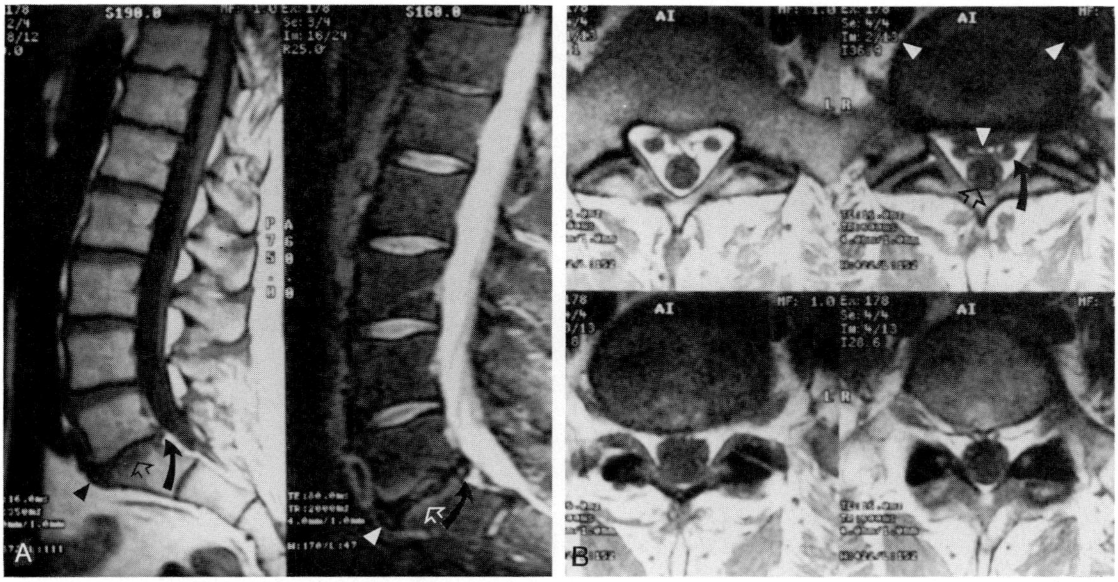

Figure 12–40. Disk bulge (49-year-old male).

A, Parasagittal (*left,* T1; *right,* T2). The L5–S1 disk height is decreased and the signal intensity of the disk diminished on T2 sequence. The disk bulges anteriorly (*arrowhead*) and posteriorly (*curved arrow*). Type I degenerative changes (low-signal T1, high-signal T2) are noted at the opposing L5 and S1 endplates (*open arrow*).

B, Axial T1. The disk bulges circumferentially (*arrowheads*) and is in contact with the S1 root (*curved arrow*) but does not distort the thecal sac (*open arrow*).

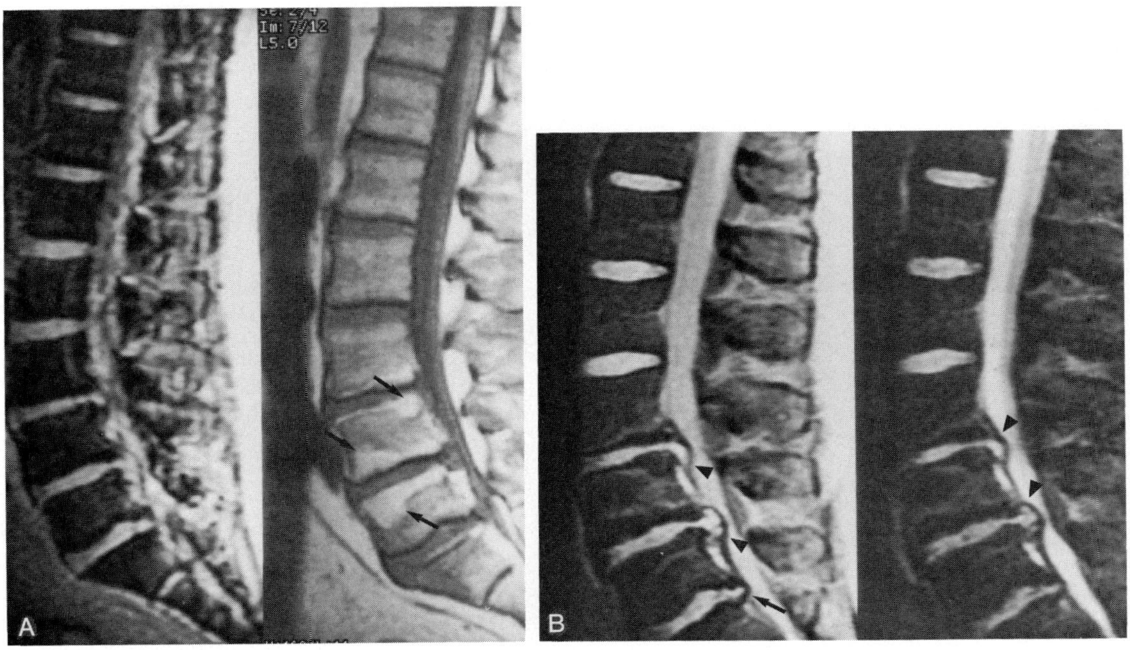

Figure 12–41. Degenerative disk disease (57-year-old male).

A, Parasagittal (*left,* gradient echo (GRE) localizer; *right,* T1). Three-level disk disease is noted at the caudal three lumbar disk spaces. Type II degenerative bone changes (*arrows*) are present at the L3–4 and, to a greater degree, the L4–5 disk spaces.

B, Parasagittal (*left,* SD; *right,* T2). Disk extrusion is detected at L3–4 and L4–5 (*arrowheads*). The nucleus has not violated the posterior annulus at L5–S1, confirming the presence of a disk protrusion (*arrow*).

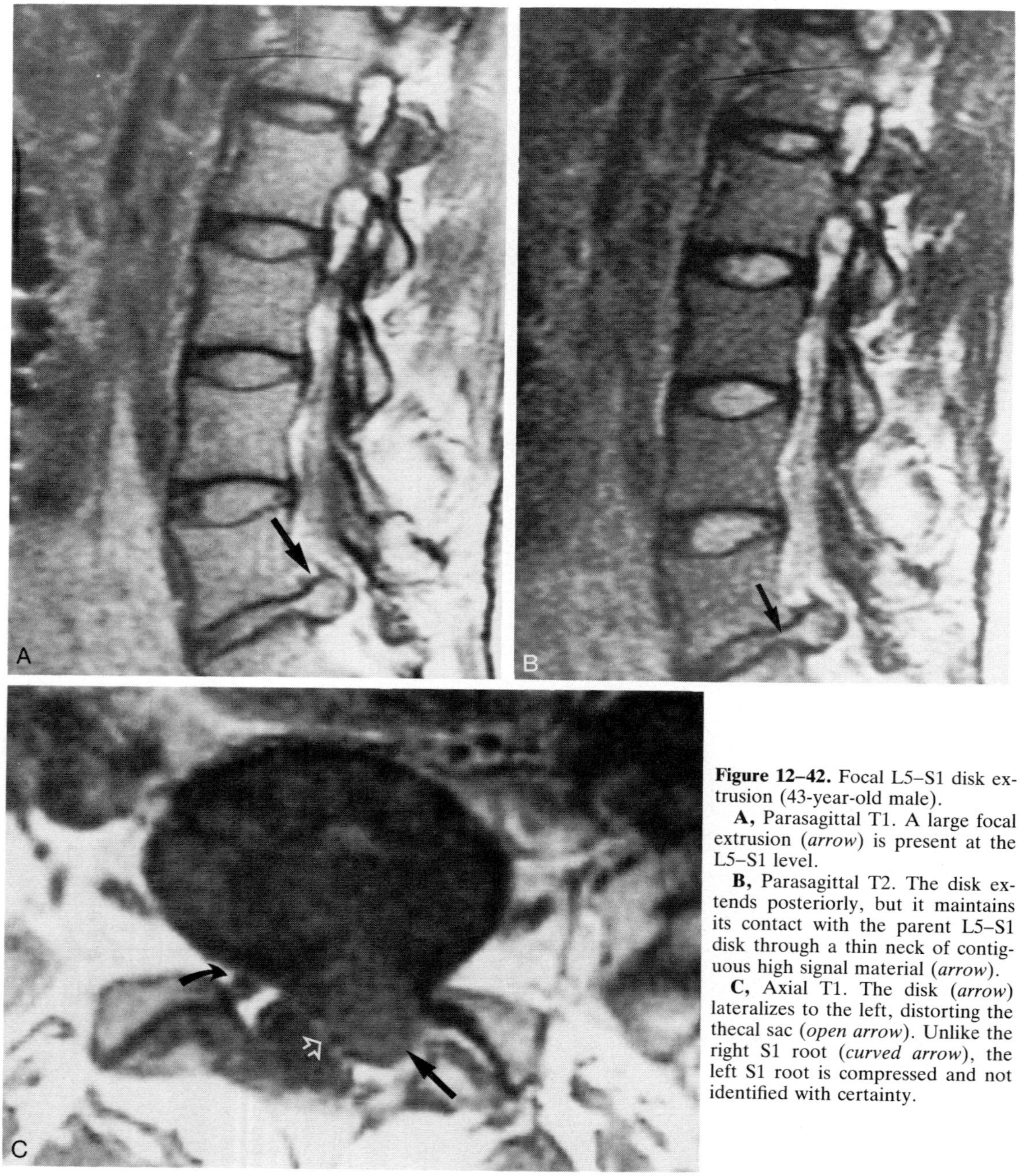

Figure 12–42. Focal L5–S1 disk extrusion (43-year-old male).

A, Parasagittal T1. A large focal extrusion (*arrow*) is present at the L5–S1 level.

B, Parasagittal T2. The disk extends posteriorly, but it maintains its contact with the parent L5–S1 disk through a thin neck of contiguous high signal material (*arrow*).

C, Axial T1. The disk (*arrow*) lateralizes to the left, distorting the thecal sac (*open arrow*). Unlike the right S1 root (*curved arrow*), the left S1 root is compressed and not identified with certainty.

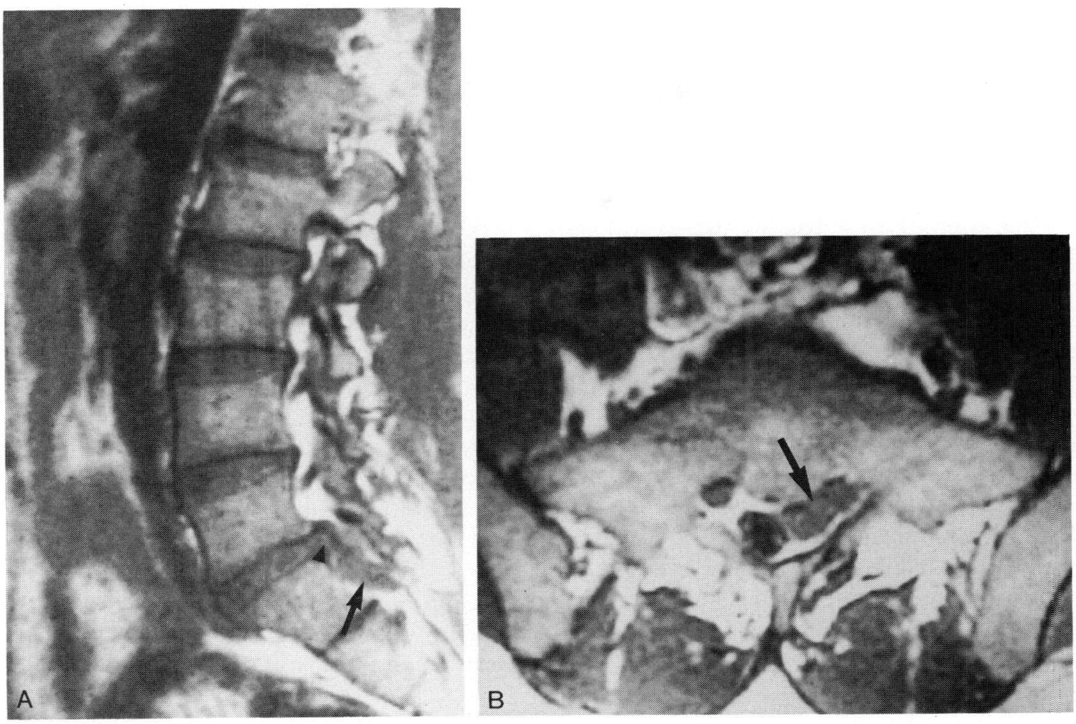

Figure 12–43. Disk extrusion with caudal migration (33-year-old male).

A, Parasagittal T1. The L5–S1 nucleus (*arrow*) has extruded through the annulus (*arrowhead*) and migrated caudally. The herniated disk remains contiguous with the parent L5–S1 disk.

B, Axial T1. A large disk fragment (*arrow*) distorts the distal thecal sac. The left S1 root is not identified.

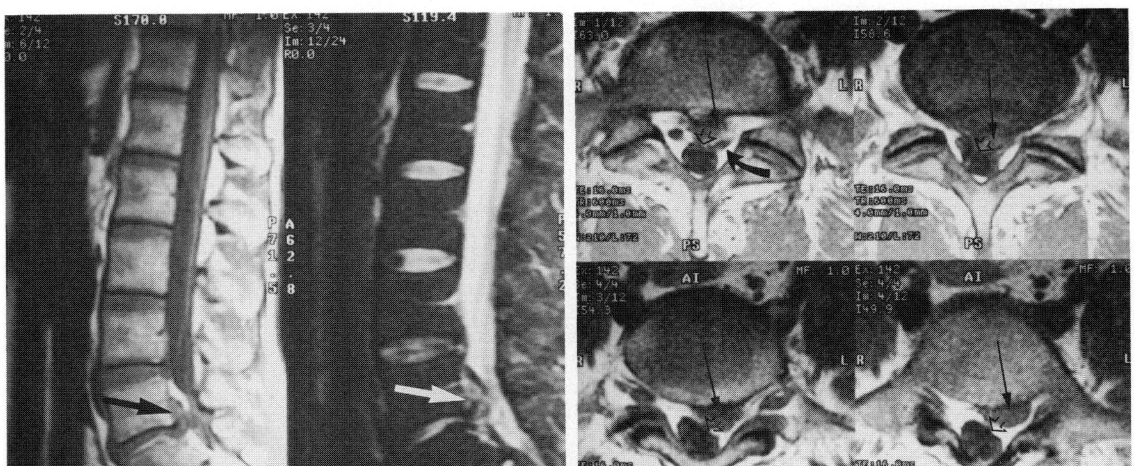

Figure 12–44. Disk extrusion (cephalad migration) (35-year-old male).

A, Parasagittal (*left,* T1; *right,* T2). The L5–S1 disk space is narrowed and disk material (*arrow*) has migrated cephalad to the disk space.

B, Axial T1. The large disk herniation (*arrow*) deforms the thecal sac (*open arrow*) and displaces the left S1 root (*curved arrow*).

herniations in the thoracic and lumbar spine will compress the roots that descend along the disk space to the subjacent level. A posterior L4-L5 disk will likely compress the L5 roots that descend dorsal to the disk space. However, a lateral disk herniation at the L4-L5 level will compress the L4 root as it traverses the intervertebral foramen beneath the pedicle. This lateral L4-L5 disk herniation will not affect the L5 roots, which descend within the spinal canal dorsal to the disk space.

Because of the diminished height of the cervical vertebral bodies, proximity of the disk space to the pedicles, and the horizontal course of the nerve roots from the cord to the intervertebral foramen, the posterolateral disk at C6-C7 will compress the root that exits under the C6 pedicle (the C7 root).

Radiographic evaluation of disk herniation is designed to detect the extradural mass. Plain films may document decreased height of the involved disk space. Myelographic findings of extruded disks consist of dilatation, deviation, and amputation of the affected nerve root (Figs. 12–45, 12–46). The lesion is usually focal at the disk space level unless the fragment has migrated. The unenhanced CT may demonstrate the herniated disk as a focal soft tissue density mass that extends beyond the normal margin of the vertebral body. The accuracy of CT in the lumbar region exceeds that for the cervical and thoracic regions, in part owing to the overall size of the disk and the presence of epidural fat, a natural contrast substance found in the lumbar epidural space. The postmyelographic CT is especially sensitive at detecting extruded disks at all levels of the spinal axis (Fig. 12–47). A ventral extradural mass with distortion of the contour of the thecal sac may be detected at the disk space level within the spinal canal or laterally in the intervertebral foramen.

MRI of the spine has dramatically changed our approach to the diagnosis of disk disease. The T1-weighted examination offers little contrast among the disk, posterior longitudinal

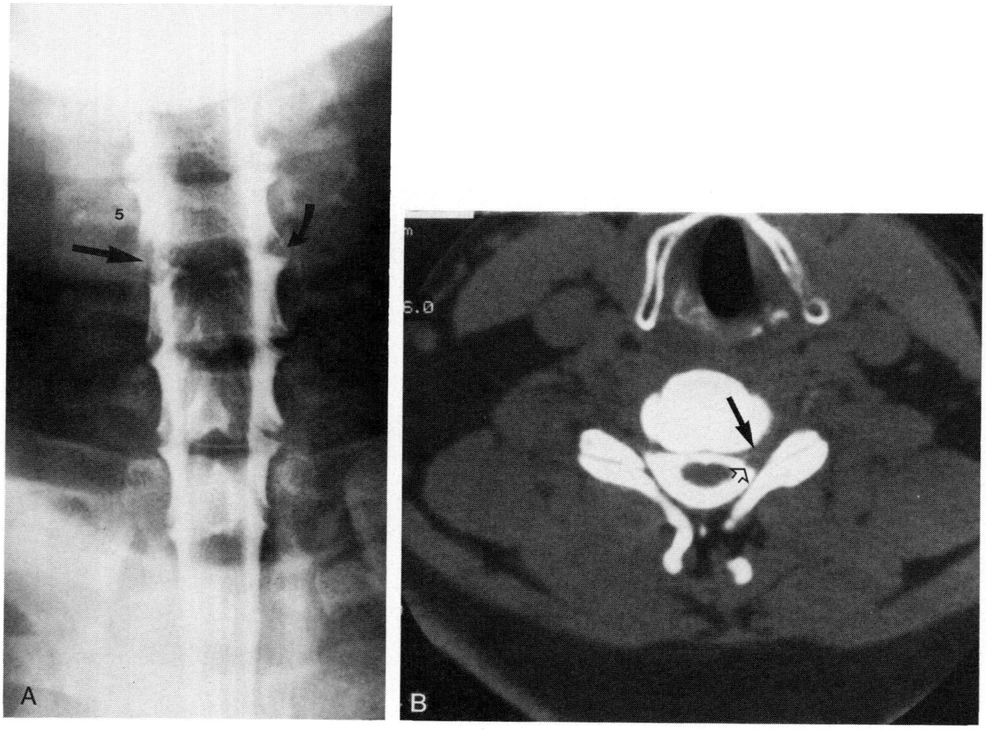

Figure 12–45. Cervical disk herniation (38-year-old male).
A, AP myelogram. The left C6 root (*arrow*) is underfilled compared with its counterpart (*curved arrow*).
B, Postmyelogram CT. CT corroborates a soft tissue mass (*arrow*) that fills the C5–6 foramen and distorts the exiting root sleeve (*open arrow*).

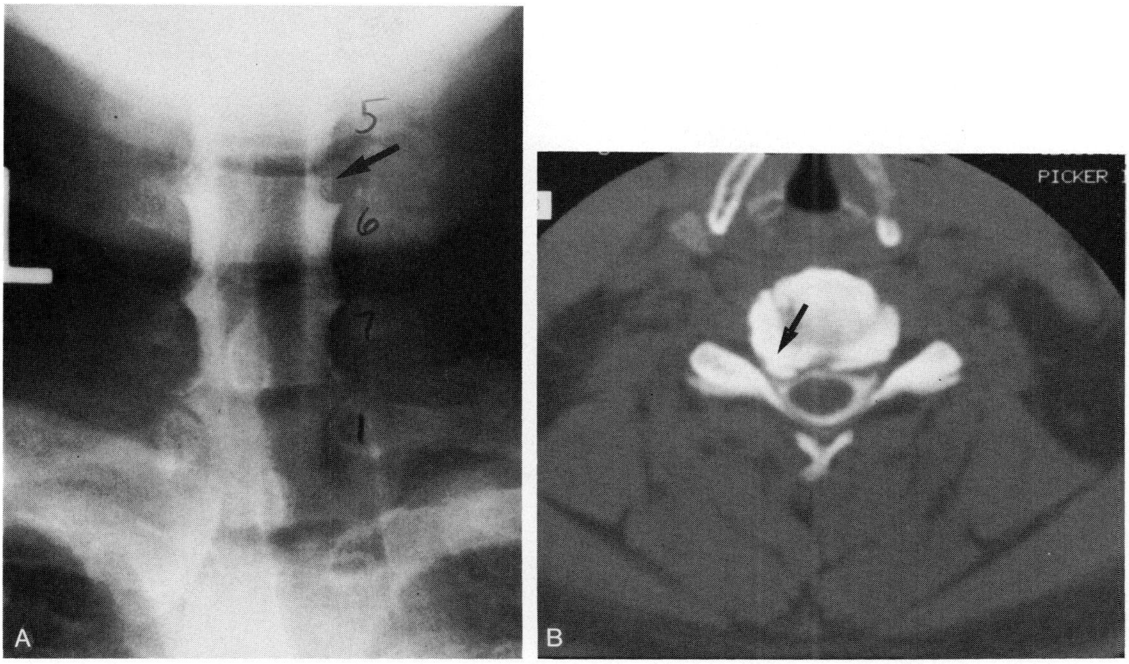

Figure 12–46. Cervical osteoarthritis (46-year-old male).
A, AP myelogram. The right C6 root (*arrow*) is underfilled.
B, Postmyelogram CT. Extensive osteophytes from the right C6 uncinate process (*arrow*) are responsible for the intervertebral foraminal stenosis, resulting in compression of the right C6 root.

ligament, and thecal sac; however, the improved signal to noise and explicit anatomic detail secure this sequence in the imaging protocol. Epidural fat, when present, improves the sensitivity of the T1 sequence.

The T2 examination demonstrates the distortion of the thecal sac because of the extruded fragment. The signal intensity of the extruded disk parallels that of the disk of origin. However, free or sequestered fragments are often higher in signal on T2 than the parent disk,[49] likely owing to the local edema. Also, the fragments that remain near the disk space tend to be rounded, whereas those that migrate away from the disk space tend to be irregular or oblong. In the lumbar spine one investigator[50] reported the axial GRE images were more sensitive at detecting disk prolapse and less sensitive at detecting disk extrusion than were spin density and T2 spin echo sequences.

Thoracic disk herniation occurs commonly in the middle and lower thoracic spine, usually between the T6 and T9 levels (Fig. 12–48). In addition to the aforementioned findings of disk herniation, the "nuclear trail sign" has been described.[51] A cleft or fissure in the vertebral body endplate or centrally within the disk extending to the herniating disk material may be detected. This is thought to represent the pathway of the herniated material and has been reported in 46% of CT and 44% of MRI examinations associated with thoracic disk herniation, occurring even more frequently in herniations of middle and lower thoracic spine. CT reveals a straight or curvilinear region of reactive bone sclerosis that is directed toward the herniated disk. On MRI, this finding is most apparent on the gradient echo sequence because of the contrast between the high signal of the disk and the low signal of the adjacent bone. Spin echo images, although less sensitive, may also demonstrate this abnormality.

MRI evaluation of cervical disk disease has been less successful than in the lumbar spine. This is related to the relatively small size of the cervical disk, the relatively thick (3- to 5-mm) spin echo or gradient echo images, and the interslice gap. A variety of imaging sequences have been used to evaluate the C-spine, including gradient echo imaging,[5] GRASS,[52] and three-dimensional (3-D) gra-

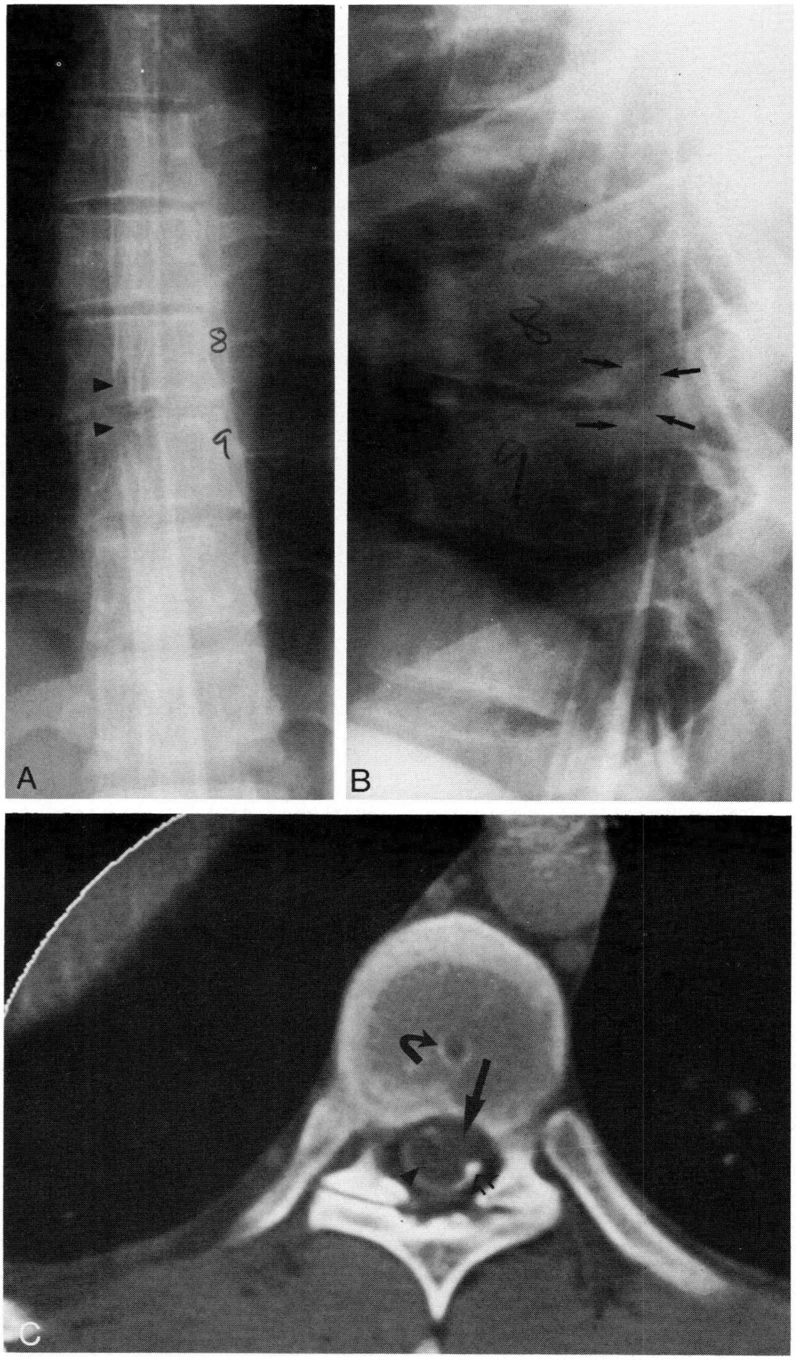

Figure 12–47. Thoracic disk (24-year-old male).

A, Supine AP myelogram. The cord is displaced slightly to the right with narrowing of the right CSF space (*arrowheads*). A mild focal scoliosis is present at this level.

B, Lateral myelogram. A double density (*arrows*) is detected in the contrast column at the disk space.

C, Postmyelogram CT. A left-sided ventral extradural mass (*arrow*) displaces the cord (*arrowhead*) and enlarges the ipsilateral CSF space (*open arrow*). The sclerotic deformity of the endplate (*curved arrow*) may be related to simultaneous herniation into the vertebral body—the "nuclear trail sign."

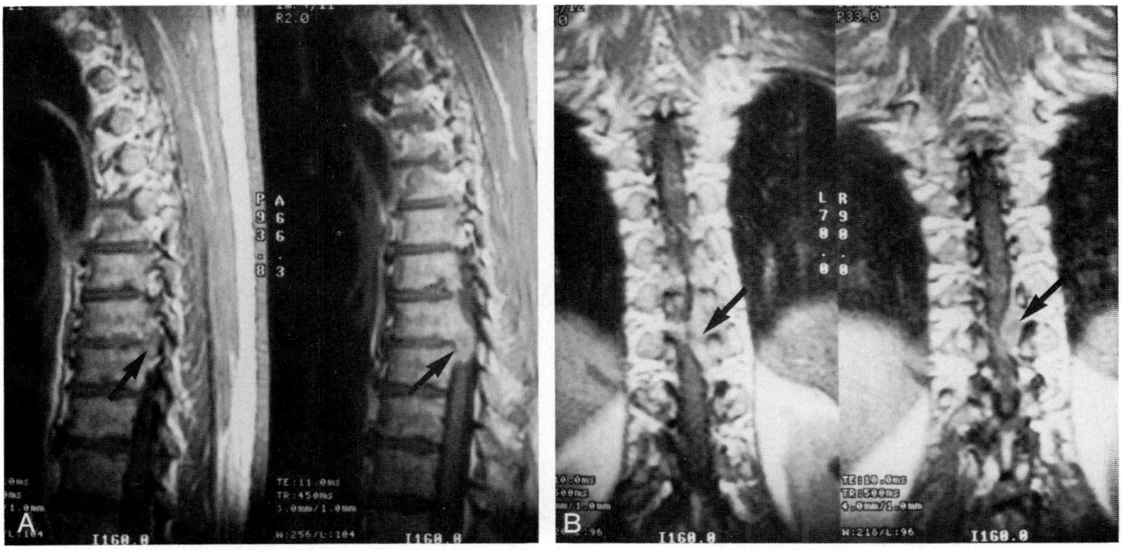

Figure 12–48. Thoracic disk (60-year-old male).
A, Enhanced parasagittal T1. A peripherally enhancing extradural mass (*arrow*) is contiguous with the disk space.
B, Enhanced coronal T1. The extradural nature of this peripherally enhancing mass (*arrow*) is confirmed.

dient echo volume.[7, 8] Even though two-dimensional (2-D) gradient echo images have improved signal to noise over spin echo, the volume acquisition allows for 1- to 2-mm contiguous images that may be reformatted in any plane. High-signal disks may be distinguished from low-signal osteophytes on the gradient echo sequences (Fig. 12–49).

A significant degree of cervical DDD exists in the asymptomatic population. This increases with age to involve 57% of patients older than 64 years of age.[53] Actual cord impingement was present in 16% of patients under age 64 and in 26% of patients over 64.

Failed Back Syndrome

This syndrome is the condition in which there is no relief of symptoms after surgery. The failed back syndrome has received a great deal of attention in the literature,[54–62] and has a significant socioeconomic impact on our workforce. In the lumbar region this can occur in 8 to 25% of patients,[61] and causes may include recurrent or residual disk, scar, lateral or central canal stenosis, adhesive arachnoiditis, nerve injury, pseudarthrosis, or surgery that was performed on the wrong side or wrong level. Although women tend to have a significantly better response than men to reoperation, the main prognisticator regarding favorable response to reoperation is the presence of an extradural mass.[61] Thus, it is imperative to evaluate the source of this mass and to distinguish disk from scar, as reoperation is contraindicated in the latter.[61]

The accuracy of CT to differentiate disk from scar is 43% and 74% when performed without and with IV contrast, respectively.[55] Multiple criteria to distinguish disk from scar have been offered. The CT criteria to corroborate scar as the source of an extradural mass include a homogeneous soft tissue mass which may be remote from the disk space along the operative route, lack of mass effect, retraction of the thecal sac toward the scar, and homogeneous enhancement. Disk is often more focal, adjacent to the disk space, nonenhancing, and associated with mass effect.

MRI has significantly improved our ability to differentiate disk from scar and has become the procedure of choice in routine evaluation of the patient with failed back syndrome. Even prior to the commercial availability of gadolinium, unenhanced MRI showed improved differentiation of disk from scar when compared to contrast-enhanced CT.[54, 60] Relative to the parent annulus, scar was most often hyperintense and recurrent disk most often hypointense to isointense to annulus on T2 sequences.

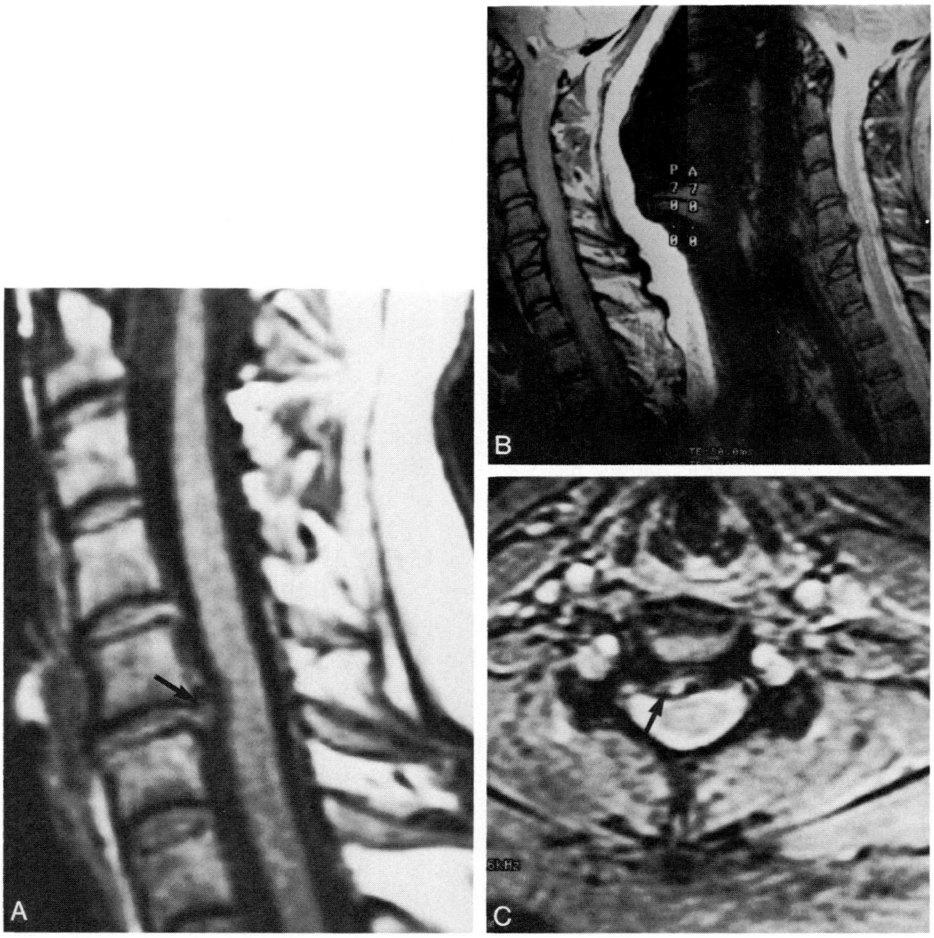

Figure 12–49. Cervical disk herniation (43-year-old female).

A, Parasagittal T1. A disk extrusion (*arrow*) is present at the C5–6 level. Mild focal indentation of the ventral surface of the cord is noted.

B, Parasagittal (*left,* SD; *right,* T2). A C5–6 disk herniation (*arrow*) is present. The disk is in contact with the cord.

C, Axial GRE volume. The intrinsic high signal corroborates disk herniation (*arrow*). Osteophyte or calcified disk would be dark, isointense to bone on this sequence.

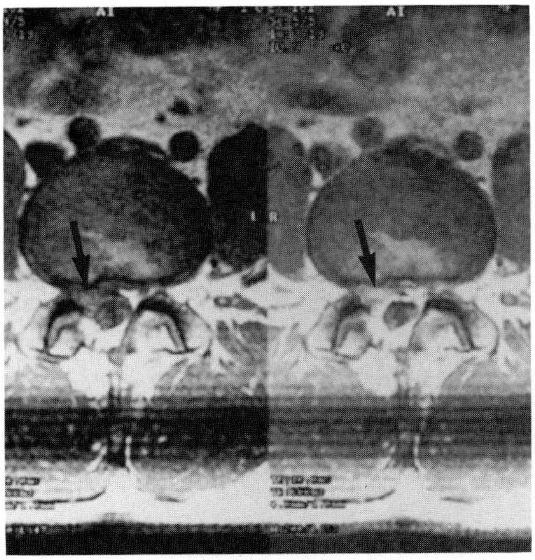

Figure 12–50. Postoperative scar (26-year-old male). Axial T1 (*left,* unenhanced; *right,* enhanced). An isointense-to-muscle soft tissue mass (*arrow*) is present in the right posterolateral position. The mass (*arrow*) enhances homogeneously following contrast material administration, corroborating cicatrix.

Sequestered disks may, however, be high signal on T2.

Accuracy rates of 96% have been reported using gadolinium to differentiate scar from disk.[59] Gadolinium rapidly diffuses through the intracellular junctions and incompetent endothelium into the extravascular space of the epidural scar, resulting in maximum enhancement within 5 minutes after contrast administration.[56, 57] The scar usually enhances homogeneously (Fig. 12–50). Chronic disk herniation may also enhance, owing to surrounding granulation tissue, though it usually does so in a peripheral fashion (Fig. 12–51).

Finally, Pantopaque, once the mainstay of myelographic contrast media and a frequent cause of arachnoiditis, is often identified in follow-up spine MRI. The contrast material is oil-based, accounting for the high T1 signal and intermediate T2 signal characteristics (Fig. 12–52). The contrast may be loculated into varying-sized collections or form fluid levels in the gravity-dependent subarachnoid space.

Associated Conditions

Synovial Cyst. Synovial cysts usually arise from the articular facets of the lower lumbar spine and are most common at the L4-L5 level (61%), the L3-L4 level (17%), and the L5-S1 level (13%).[63, 64] These cysts are degenerative or post-traumatic in origin, occurring in association with focal degeneration of the articular facets, usually after age 50.[65] On CT the lesions are cystic, adjacent to the facet, and may be peripherally calcified. The MRI signal intensity of the cysts varies, though usually decreased signal on T1 and increased to decreased signal on T2 (Fig. 12–53). A peripheral rim of diminished signal may signify the presence of calcium or hemosiderin.[63]

Vertebral Body Endplate Changes. MRI detectable bony degenerative endplate and marrow changes frequently accompany DDD. Initially the disrupted fissured endplates are invaded and replaced by fibrous vascular tissue. The T1 signal decreases and the T2 signal increases. This has been termed type I degenerative change (Fig. 12–54).[66] Type I changes will enhance following gadolinium administration on the T1 sequences, becoming nearly isointense to normal marrow. Type II degenerative changes occur when the yellow marrow replaces fibrous vascular tissue, resulting in an increased T1 and an isointense-to-slightly-hyperintense T2 signal[66] (Fig. 21–55).

Spinal Stenosis. Spinal stenosis may be primary or acquired. Spondylosis and osteoarthritis are the most common causes of acquired canal stenosis. Progressive degenerative disease of the disk, bone, and ligament results in narrowing of the spinal canal and lateral recesses. The normal AP dimension of the canal is 13 mm. Bulging or herniated disks, redundant ligamentum flavum, and osteoarthritic changes of the facets result in central canal stenosis. This will result in compression of the contents of the canal at the level of involvement (Fig. 12–56).

Classically, patients with lumbar stenosis present with neurogenic claudication. This may resemble true vascular claudication except that the pain may or may not be related to activity, is exacerbated in the upright position, and is ameliorated in the recumbent position.

The lateral recess is the space between the posterior vertebral body and the same level superior articular facet. The lateral recess is the proximal pathway that the spinal nerve traverses toward the intervertebral foramen. Osteoarthritic overgrowth of the superior ar-

Text continued on page 482

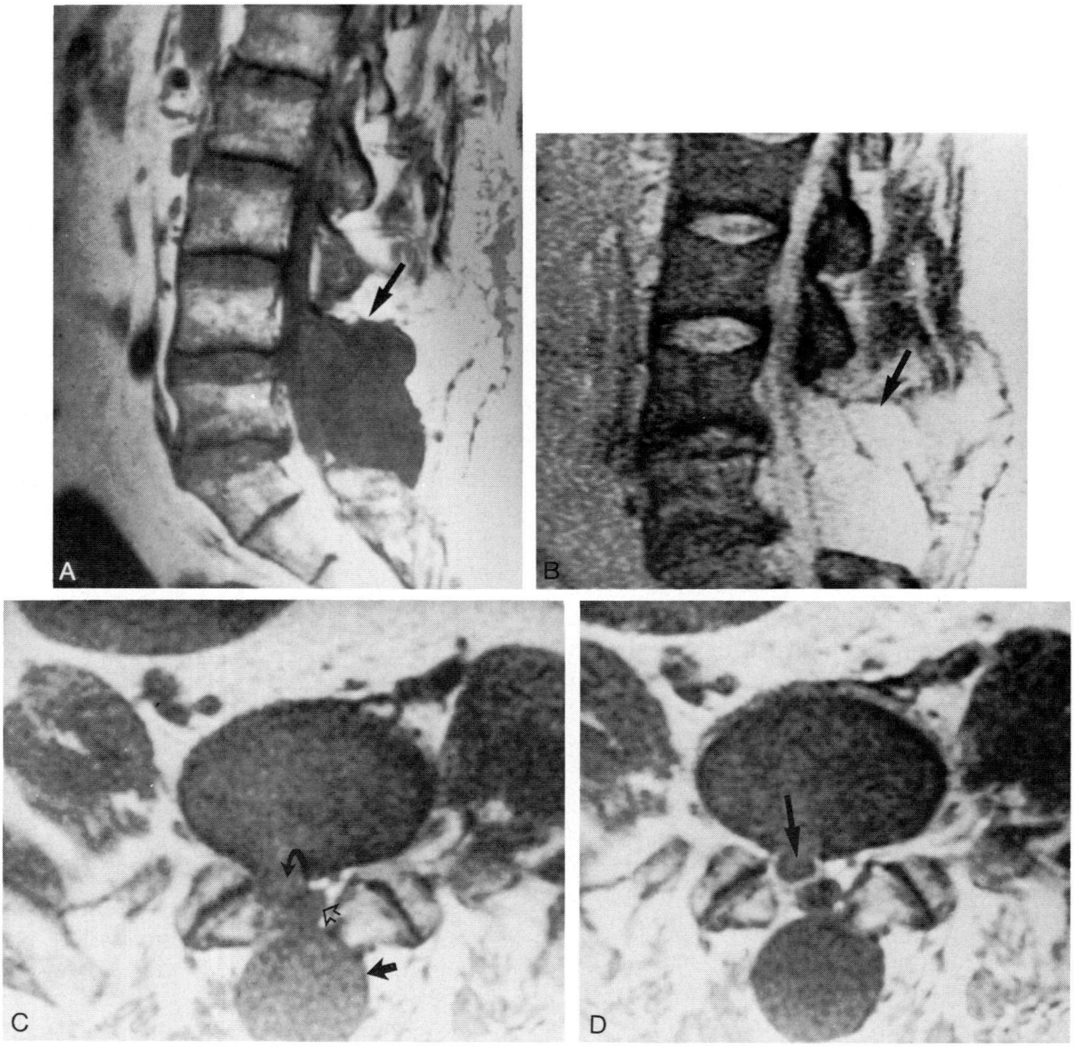

Figure 12–51. Failed back syndrome (39-year-old male).

A, B, Parasagittal T1 and T2. A large CSF signal abnormality (*arrow*) represents a postoperative pseudomeningocele.

C, Axial T1. The relationship of the pseudomeningocele (*arrow*) and thecal sac (*open arrow*) is apparent. Also, a soft tissue mass (*curved arrow*) is present between the sac and the disk space.

D, Enhanced axial T1. Peripheral enhancement denotes granulation tissue that surrounds a chronic recurrent disk herniation (*arrow*).

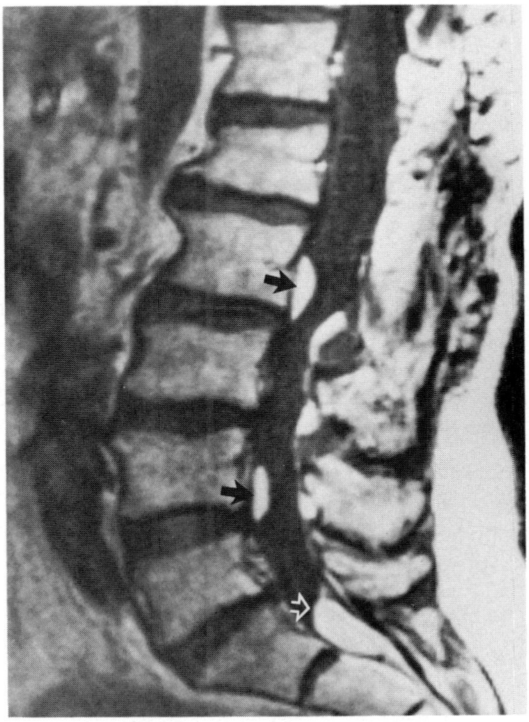

Figure 12–52. Pantopaque (68-year-old male). Parasagittal T1; multiple foci of high signal are noted within the thecal sac. Some material is loculated ventrally (*arrows*), and some layers in the gravity-dependent thecal sac (*open arrow*).

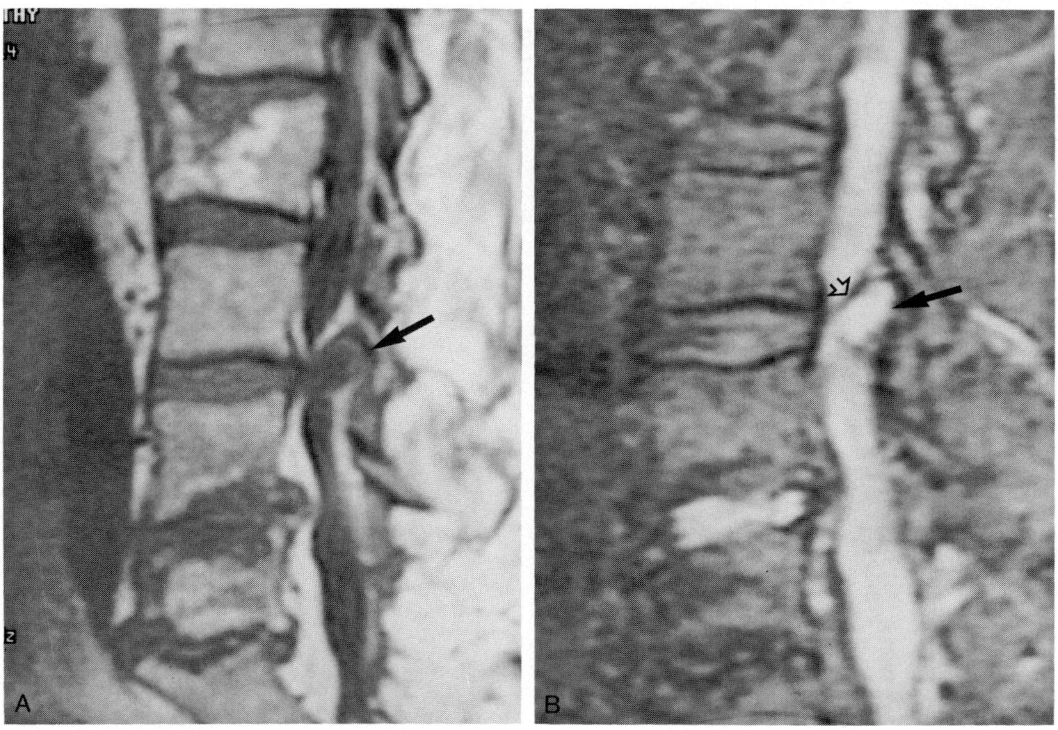

Figure 12–53. Synovial cyst (85-year-old female).

A, Parasagittal T1. An intermediate-signal mass (*arrow*) is present in the dorsal aspect of the spinal canal.

B, Parasagittal T2. The mass (*arrow*) is high signal on the long TR sequence, with a rim of diminished signal (*open arrow*).

Illustration continued on following page

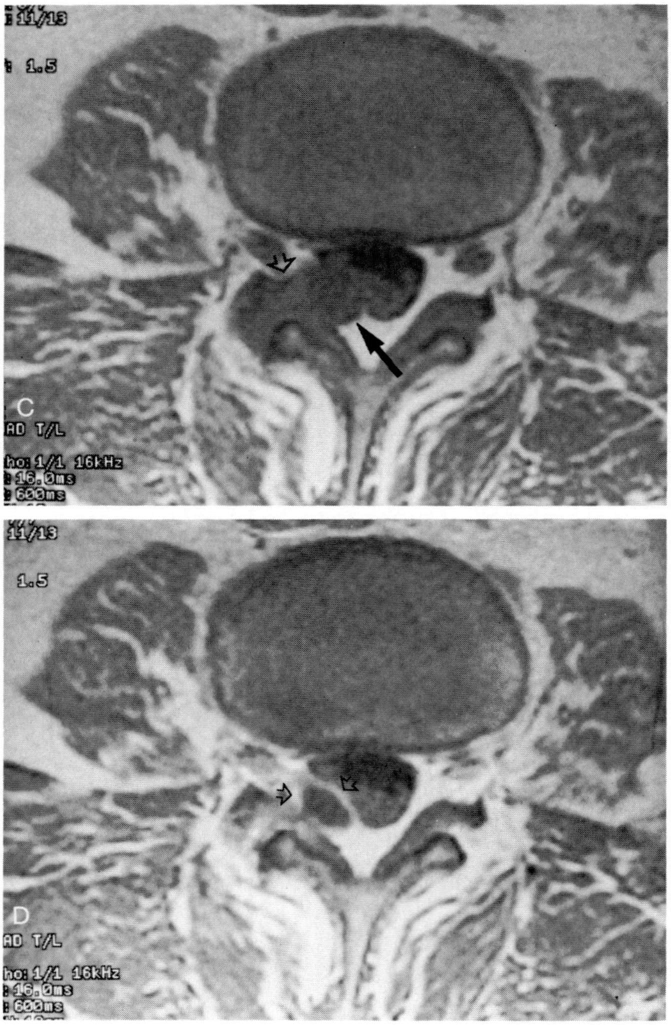

Figure 12–53 *Continued*

C, Axial T1. The relationship between the mass (*arrow*) and the markedly degenerated facet joint (*open arrow*) is noted.

D, Enhanced axial T1. The cyst enhances along the periphery (*open arrows*), most likely because of chronic granulation tissue. The relationship of the cyst and the thecal sac is more apparent.

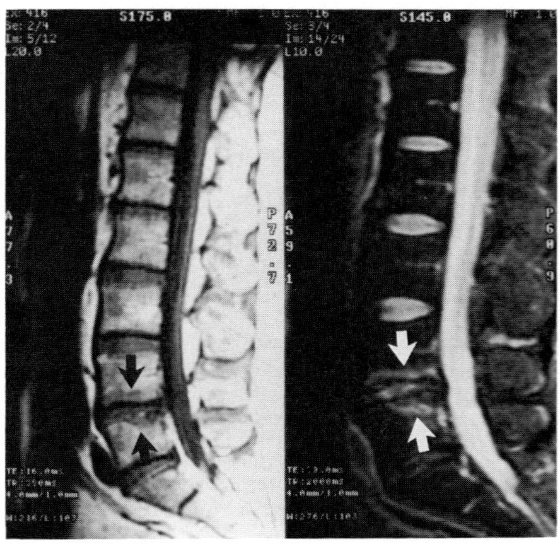

Figure 12–54. Type I degenerative endplate changes (43-year-old male). Parasagittal (*left,* T1; *right,* T2); heterogeneous low signal (*arrows*) is present in the opposing endplates of L4 and L5. The disk space height and T2 signal are diminished. High-signal changes (*arrows*) are present on the T2 sequence. Signal alterations are secondary to infiltration of fibrous vascularized tissue.

Figure 12–55 is on the right and its caption on the left.

Figure 12–55. Type II degenerative endplate changes (45-year-old male). Parasagittal (*left,* T1; *right,* T2); homogeneous high signal (*arrows*) is present along the opposing endplates of L5 and S1. There are subtle regions of decrease in signal on the T2-weighted sequence (*arrows*). The changes are ascribed to replacement of vascularized fibrous tissue with yellow marrow.

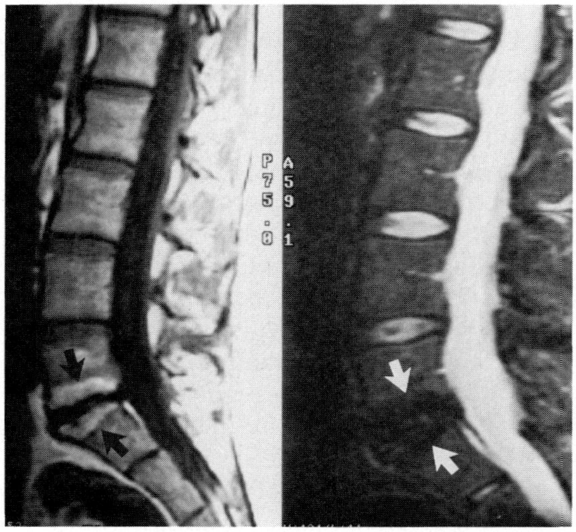

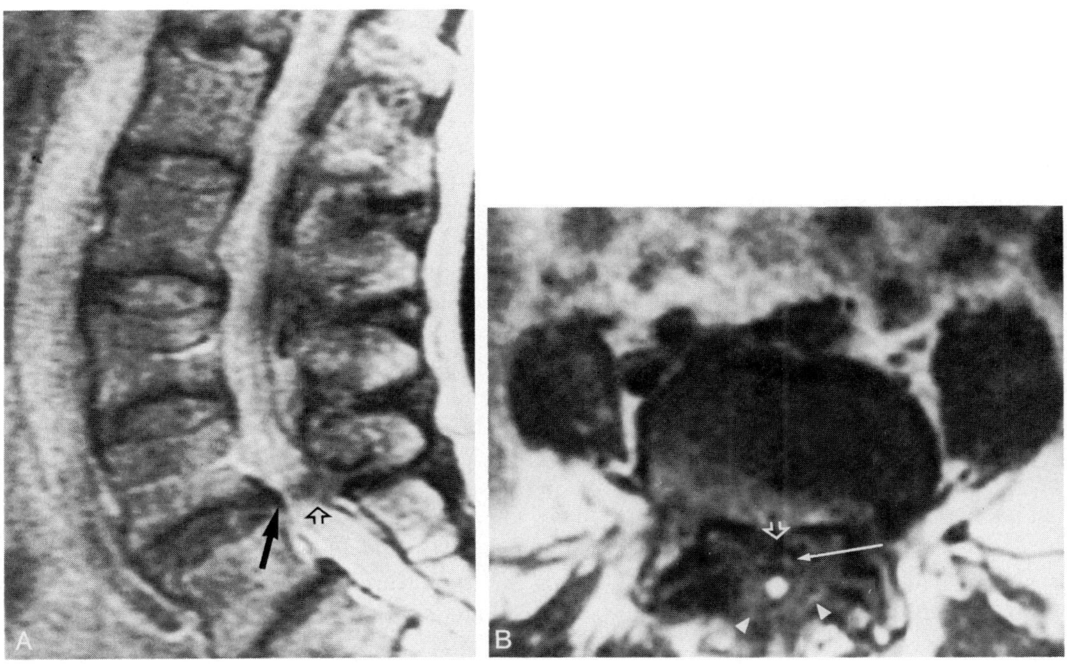

Figure 12–56. Spinal stenosis (59-year-old male).

A, Parasagittal T2. A bulging disk (*arrow*) is present at the L4–5 level. There is marked redundancy of the ligamentum flavum (*open arrow*), which buckles into the spinal canal, resulting in severe stenosis.

B, Axial T1. In concert, the bulging disk (*open arrow*) and redundant ligamentum flavum (*arrowheads*) significantly compress the thecal sac (*arrow*).

ticular facet and osteophytes from the adjacent vertebral body will alone or in concert narrow this region. The lateral recess should normally exceed 4 to 5 mm. Recess stenosis is most common in the lumbar spine and compresses the same level root producing a radiculopathy.

Ossification of the Posterior Longitudinal Ligament (OPLL). Although relatively uncommon in the United States, OPLL leads to canal stenosis and cord compression in 2.4% of the Japanese population.[67] In the United States, OPLL is associated with diffuse idiopathic skeletal hyperostosis in 50% of cases. Membranous bone formation occurs in the PLL, which may appear segmental or continuous. The density may be detected on plain films or CT. MRI depicts a low-signal band between the vertebral body and the cord, and also provides information regarding cord compression, edema, or myelomalacia, which may accompany OPLL (Fig. 12–57).

Spondylolisthesis. This refers to a malalignment of the vertebral bodies in which one body is displaced (usually forward) referable to the subjacent body. This condition may result from spondylolysis (defect in pars interarticularis), degenerative disease (apophyseal joint laxity), or trauma (fracture of posterior arch with malalignment).

Spondylolysis causes varying degrees of anterolisthesis of the body at the affected level. The pars defect may be unilateral or bilateral. Bilaterality is associated with more severe anterolisthesis. True disk extrusion at the level of spondylolysis is uncommon. The "pseudo disk" results from the slippage of the disk in attempts to bridge the malaligned vertebral bodies.

Planar imaging demonstrates elongation of the AP dimension of the canal at the anterolisthesis, sclerotic pars defects, and proportional narrowing of the intervertebral foramen (Fig. 12–58). Parasagittal images often demonstrate the pars defect, related anterolisthesis, and foraminal stenosis.

Neoplasm

Neoplasms to the bony spinal axis may be primary or much more commonly metastatic from a variety of primary neoplasms.

Metastasis

Metastases to the spine most frequently involve the thoracic (66%) and lumbar spine (20%), followed by the C-spine and sacrum.[20] There is a tendency for breast and lung malignancies to metastasize to the thoracic spine, and for rectal and colon malignancies to metastasize to the lumbar spine. Nearly 40% of all bone metastases affect the spine.[68] Tumors may arrive at the spinal axis by a hematogenous route or direct extension from a paravertebral source. Prostate or pelvic malignancies may ascend along the valveless Batson's venous plexus to any level of the spine or skull.[69] The metastases extend to the marrow, which is more concentrated in the body, pedicles, and lamina. Neoplasms generally respect the disk space, which is avascular and acts as a relative barrier to the contiguous spread of tumor.

Metastasis may be primarily lytic (kidney and thyroid), blastic (breast and prostate), or both. Lytic tumors present at a smaller size owing to pain from associated microfractures. In 66 to 90% of patients with spine metastasis, back pain,[20] bowel and bladder dysfunction, and paraplegia secondary to cord compression are present.

Plain film findings are markedly less sensitive than CT, bone scintigraphy, or MRI at detecting osseous metastasis. In order to detect metastasis on plain films, cortical disruption or replacement of more than 1 cm of marrow must be present.[20] Erosion or destruction of a pedicle may be noted. The myelographic findings of tumor extension into the canal are extradural defects that may arise in any location along the circumference of the bony canal (Figs. 12–59, 12–60). Cephalad or caudad flow of contrast material may be blocked at any level. CT detects similar changes, though earlier than detected on plain films; grossly evaluates the paraspinal mass; and, with application of intrathecal contrast material, effectively evaluates the canal disease.

MRI is more specific than bone scintigraphy in evaluation of metastatic spinal disease. The normal marrow is a good marker for vertebral body health. Infiltrative tumor replaces the marrow, resulting in decreased T1 signal[13, 16, 70] with a less conspicuous increase in the T2 signal (Figs. 12–61 to 12–63). MRI is particu-

Text continued on page 487

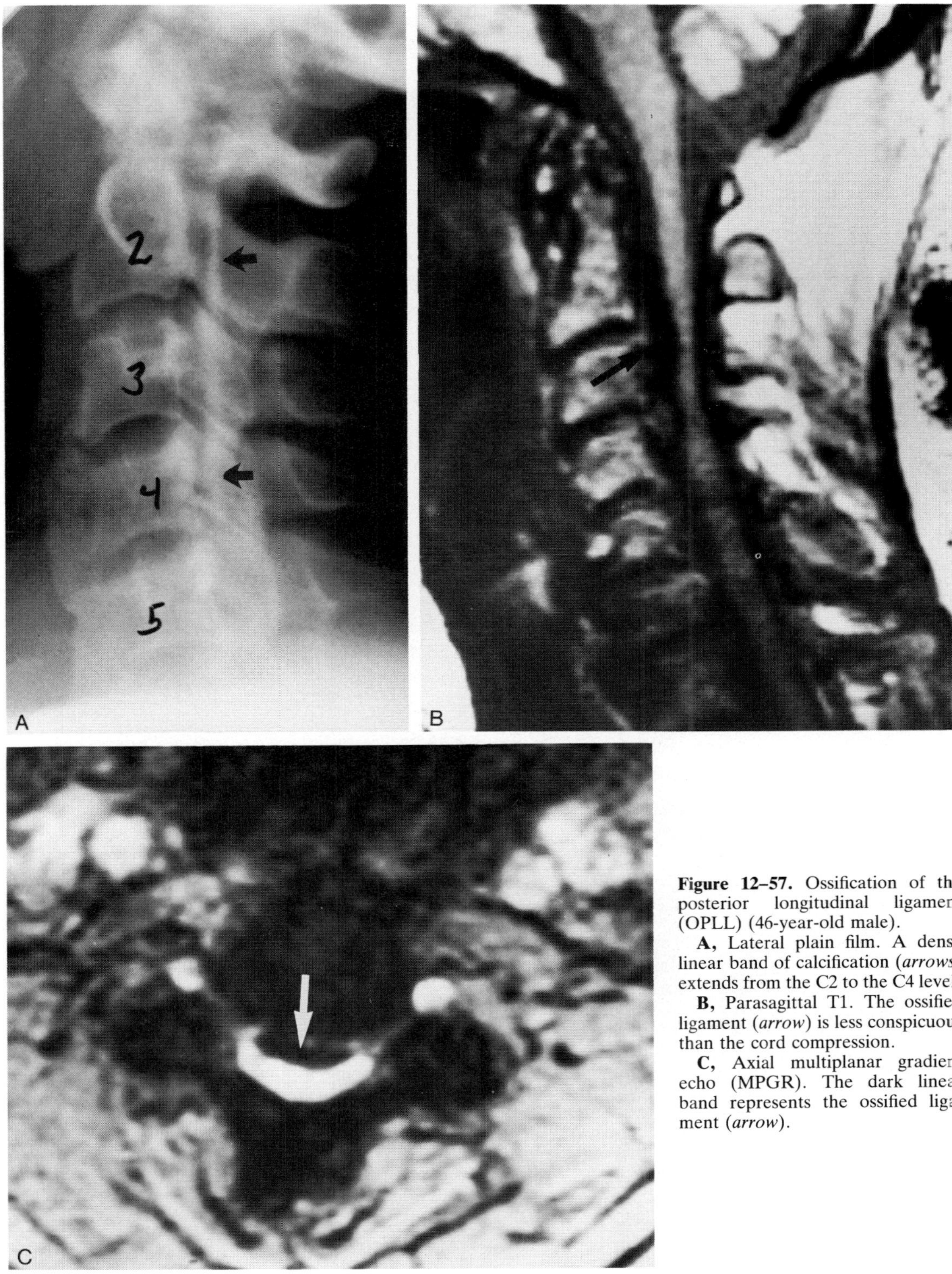

Figure 12–57. Ossification of the posterior longitudinal ligament (OPLL) (46-year-old male).

A, Lateral plain film. A dense linear band of calcification (*arrows*) extends from the C2 to the C4 level.

B, Parasagittal T1. The ossified ligament (*arrow*) is less conspicuous than the cord compression.

C, Axial multiplanar gradient echo (MPGR). The dark linear band represents the ossified ligament (*arrow*).

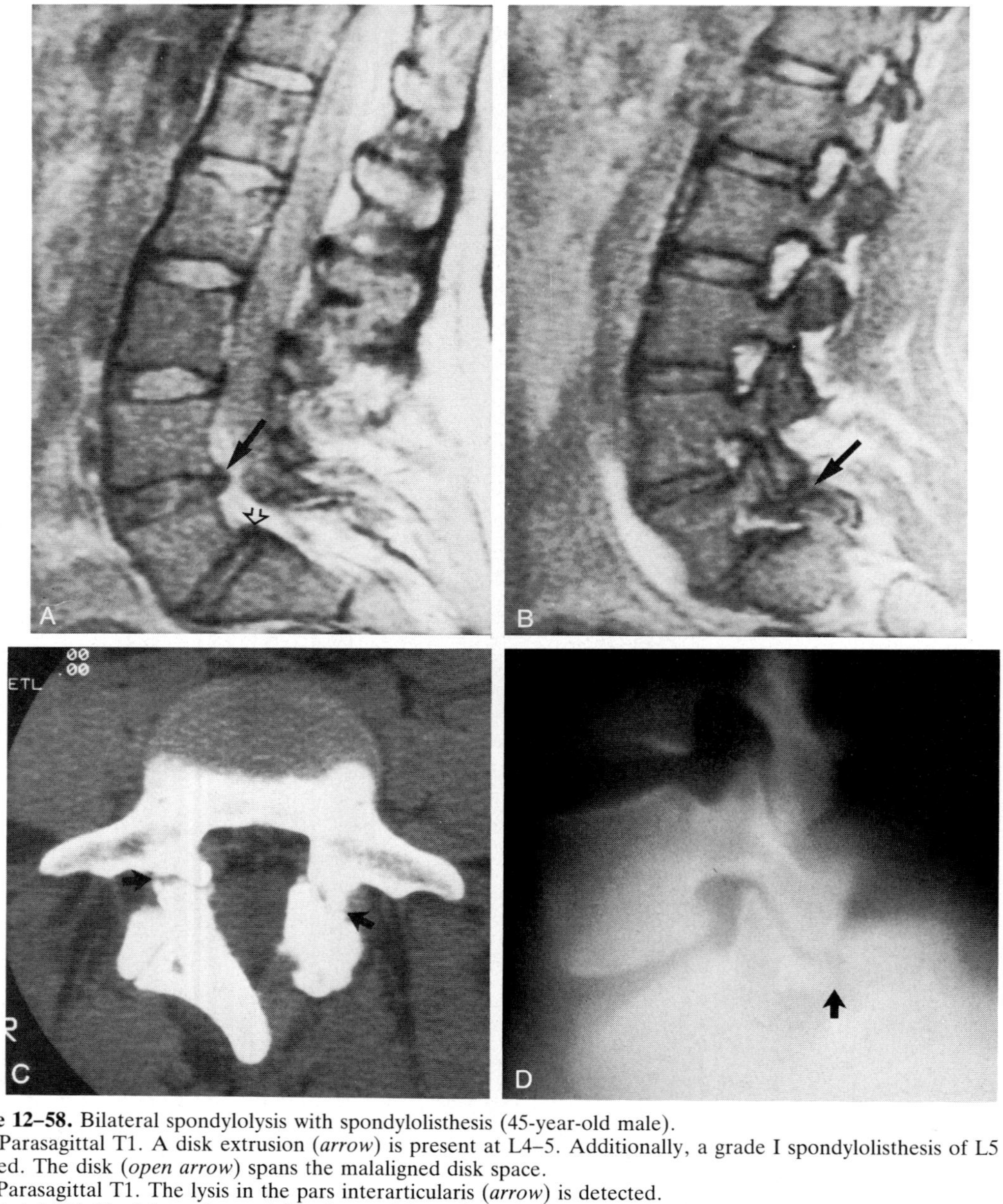

Figure 12–58. Bilateral spondylolysis with spondylolisthesis (45-year-old male).

A, Parasagittal T1. A disk extrusion (*arrow*) is present at L4–5. Additionally, a grade I spondylolisthesis of L5 on S1 is noted. The disk (*open arrow*) spans the malaligned disk space.

B, Parasagittal T1. The lysis in the pars interarticularis (*arrow*) is detected.

C, Axial CT. The bilateral pars defect (*arrows*) is confirmed. This frequently results in elongation of the AP dimension of the canal, as well as varying degrees of intervertebral foraminal stenosis.

D, Lateral tomogram. The pars defect (*arrow*) and the anterolisthesis, can be identified.

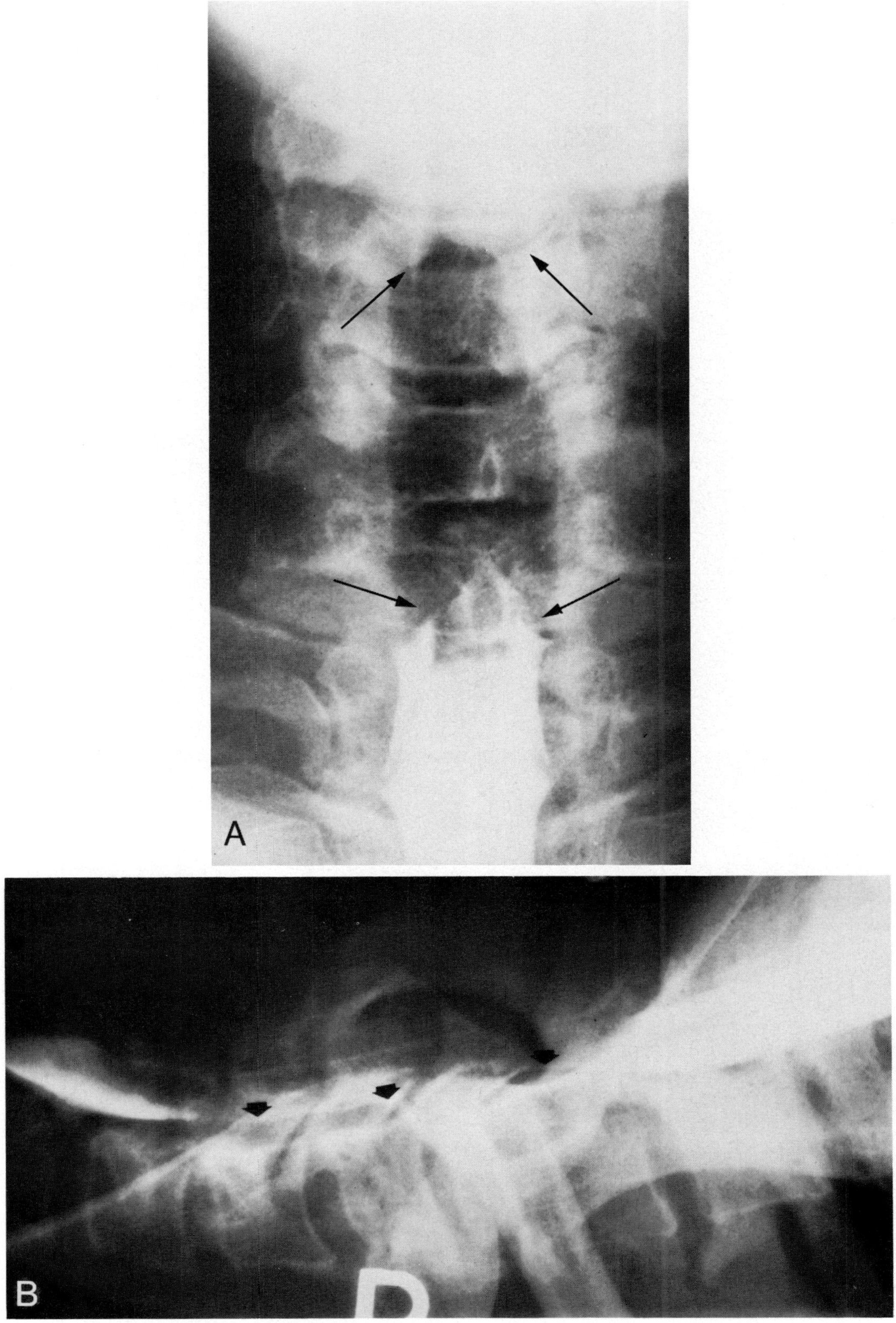

Figure 12–59. Epidural tumor; lung (55-year-old male).

A, AP myelogram. There is abrupt attenuation of the thecal sac (*arrows*) from C3 to C7 inclusive.

B, Lateral myelogram. The contrast-laden thecal sac is displaced dorsally (*arrows*) by epidural tumor within the ventral spinal canal.

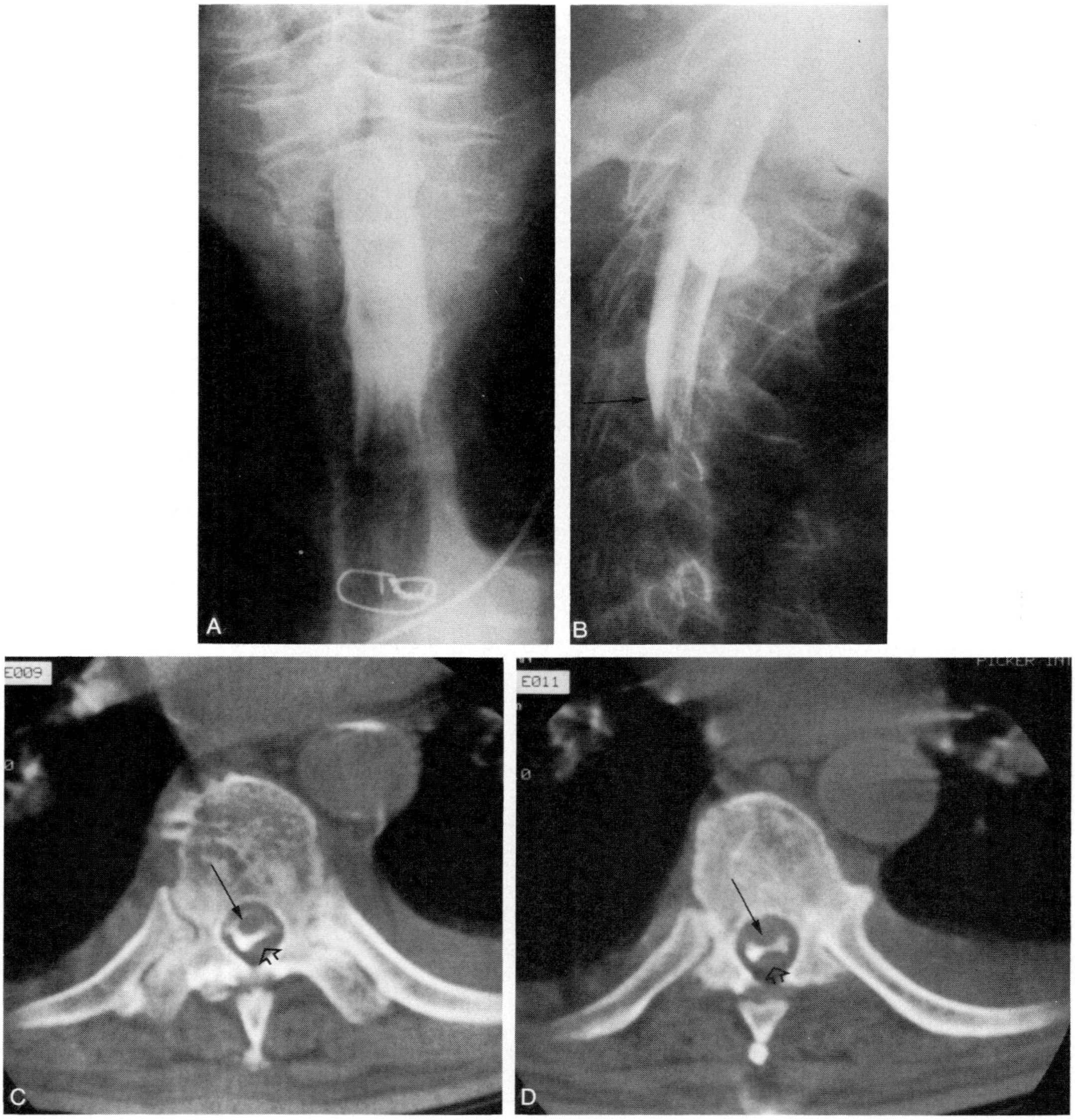

Figure 12–60. Epidural tumor; lung (71-year-old male).

A, Supine AP myelogram. The caudal flow of contrast material ceases at the T6 level. It may be difficult to compartmentalize a lesion when a complete block is present.

B, Lateral myelogram. Ventral displacement of the contrast material from the bony perimeter of the canal (*arrow*) confirms the dorsal extradural nature of this mass.

C, D, Postmyelogram CT. The cord (*arrow*) is displaced anteriorly by the dorsal epidural tumor (*open arrow*).

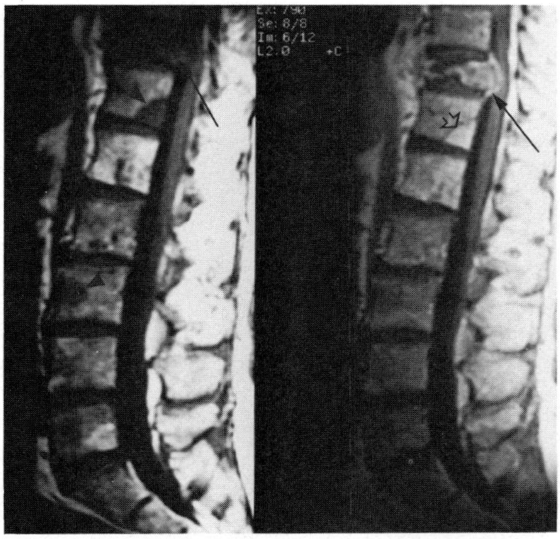

Figure 12–61. Osseous lung metastases (64-year-old female). Parasagittal T1 (*left,* unenhanced; *right,* enhanced); multiple vertebral body metastases (*arrowheads*) are present. The T11 vertebral body (*arrow*) is pathologically fractured and a fragment retropulsed into the canal. Contrast material renders some of the occult osseous metastases (*open arrow*) less apparent.

larly useful in evaluating the clinically occult concomitant metastasis and the spinal axis between myelographic blocks, notoriously a limitation of myelography.[71]

Once vertebral body fractures occur, criteria exist to help differentiate benign from malignant causes. It is not possible in all cases to distinguish the cause of the fracture, in which case a repeat examination should be obtained within 1 to 2 months or sooner, as clinically indicated. Factors that corroborate malignancy include complete or nearly complete marrow replacement of vertebral bodies and posterior elements, multilevel involvement, and paravertebral masses (60%).[68, 72] Benignancy is supported by normal preserved marrow signal within the entire body or along the posterior third, the "posterior band" sign,[68] or a horizontal band of decreased signal representing type I marrow changes at the endplate. The use of gadolinium for evaluation of osseous metastasis is limited, as the pathologic vertebral body may enhance to become isointense to normal marrow.[73] Gadolinium enhancement is useful to evaluate the extent of intraspinal soft tissue tumor.

Primary Neoplasms

Primary neoplasms of the spine are relatively rare, and may be benign or malignant.

Benign

Osteoid Osteoma. Night pain relieved by aspirin in patients younger than 30 years old is a typical clinical presentation of osteoid osteoma. The lesion consists of a central lucent nidus surrounded by sclerosis. The lesion occurs most frequently in the femur and tibia, though it may occur in the spinal arch and articular facets, promoting adjacent sclerosis. The nidus may be intramedullary or intracortical.

Osteoblastoma. Osteoblastoma is often an expansile lesion of the posterior arch (spinous and transverse processes) that usually occurs in patients in their second to fourth decades. The vertebral body may be secondarily involved. The cord may be compressed and a palpable mass detected.

Giant Cell. These tumors uncommonly affect the spine, and when they do so, the sacrum is the most common location of origin. Patients present in the third to fourth decade with an expansile lesion, lacking new bone formation or periosteal reaction. The mass is peripherally calcified. The relationship of this tumor to aneurysmal bone cysts remains controversial (Fig. 12–64).

Hemangioma. Cavernous hemangiomas are relatively common lesions incidentally found on MR spinal exams. The lesions may rarely result in compression or expansion of the vertebral body with subsequent cord compression.

Plain films demonstrate coarse thickened vertical trabeculae in the involved vertebral body. This is readily confirmed with CT. MRI demonstrates increased T1 and T2 signal in the involved body, thought secondary to blood and adipose tissue (Fig. 12–65).

Malignant

Primary malignant bone tumors of the spine are rare lesions.

Chordoma. These notochordal remnant tumors occur most frequently in the sacrum in elderly patients. This destructive tumor usually occurs at the extremes of the spinal axis, but less commonly may arise anywhere along the spinal axis. CT demonstrates an infiltrative soft tissue mass that may contain calcification. MRI demonstrates a high-signal T2 mass that often contains septa. The mass is of intermediate signal on T1, or less commonly hypointense (Figs. 12–66, 12–67).

Multiple Myeloma. Multiple myeloma is the

Text continued on page 492

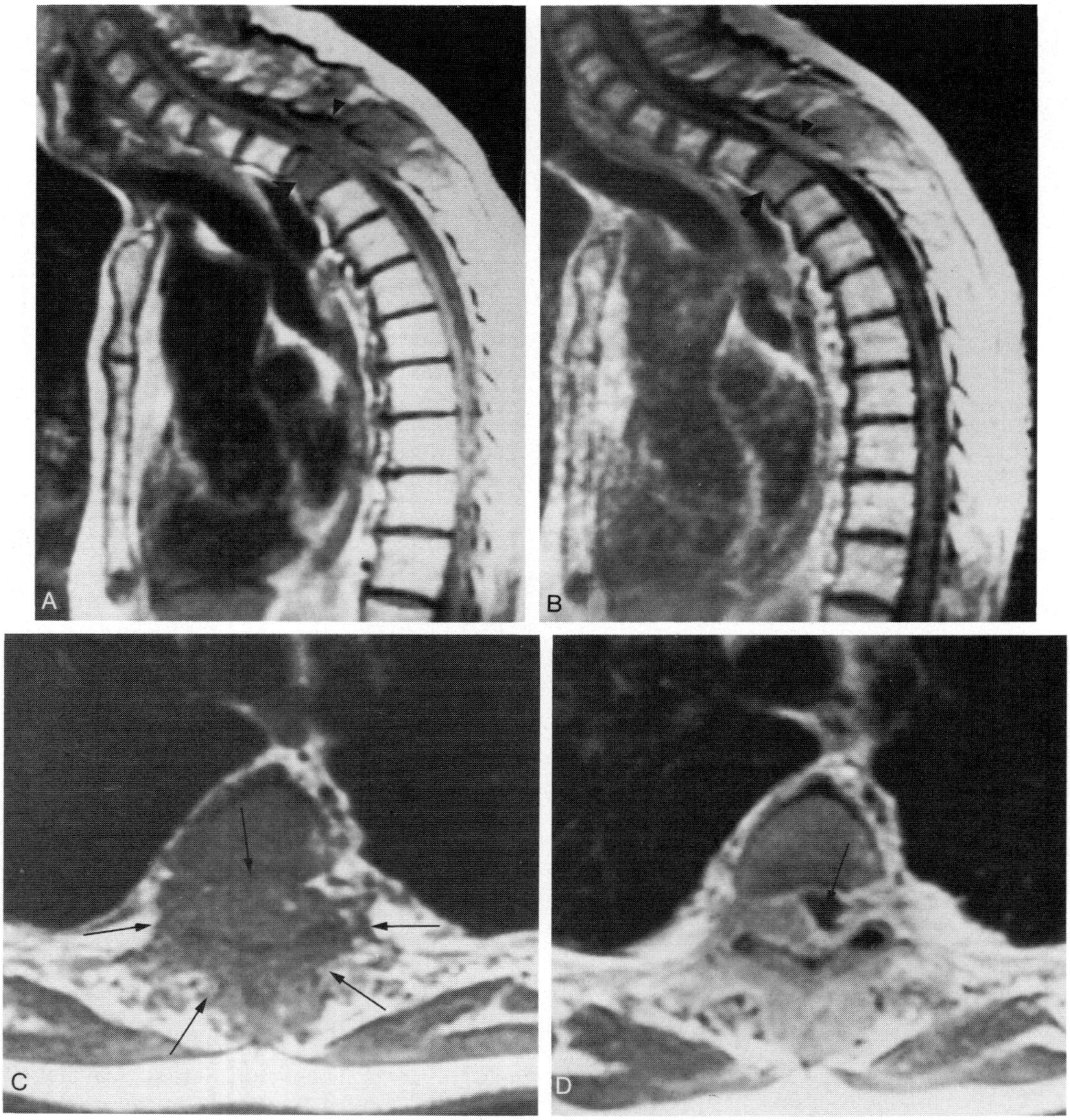

Figure 12–62. Osseous renal metastasis (85-year-old male).

A, Parasagittal T1. The T2 vertebral body (*arrow*) is of normal height but markedly decreased in signal secondary to infiltrative renal cell. A dorsal intraspinal mass (*arrowhead*) is present but is inseparable from the cord.

B, Enhanced parasagittal T1. Although the vertebral body (*arrow*) signal enhances to near normal, masking the metastasis, the intraspinal mass (*arrowhead*) has become better defined.

C, Axial T1. The accompanying infiltrative mass (*arrows*) fills the spinal canal and is indistinguishable from the normal canal contents.

D, Enhanced axial T1. The enhancing mass outlines the dura and compressed cord (*arrow*).

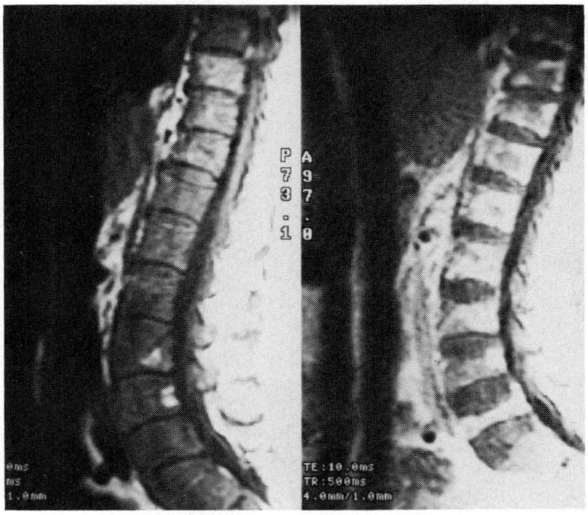

Figure 12–63. Lymphoma (79-year-old female). Parasagittal T1 (*left,* unenhanced; *right,* enhanced); there is diffuse infiltration of tumor throughout the lumbar spine, which results in dramatic signal loss of the normal marrow. The vertebral bodies are partly indistinguishable from the disk. After contrast material administration, the vertebrae enhance to the normal marrow signal.

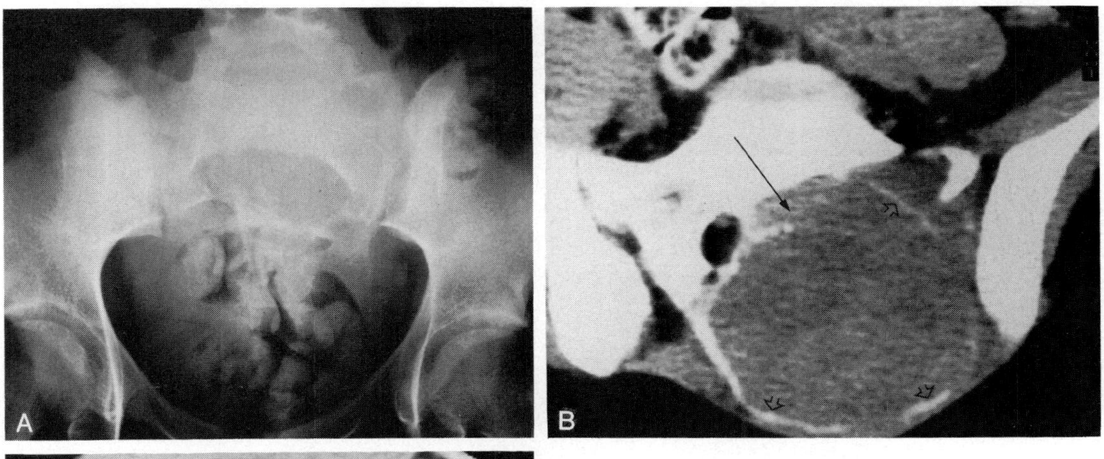

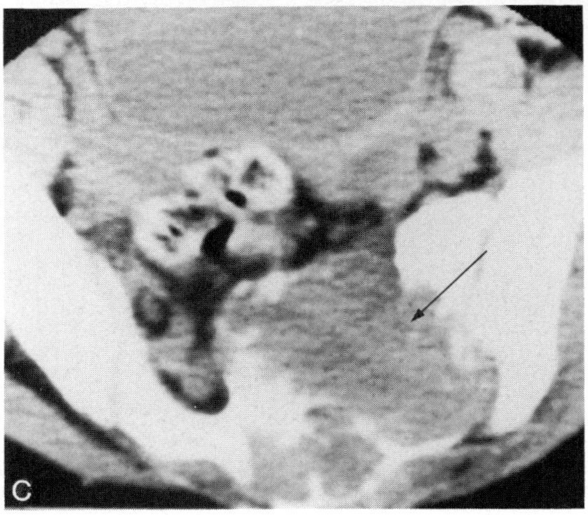

Figure 12–64. Giant cell tumor; sacrum (14-year-old female).

A, AP pelvis. The alar ridges of the sacrum on the left are absent and the bony architecture of the sacrum is grossly abnormal.

B, C, Axial CT. A homogeneous soft tissue mass (*arrow*) has infiltrated the sacrum. The mass is, in part, peripherally calcified (*open arrows*).

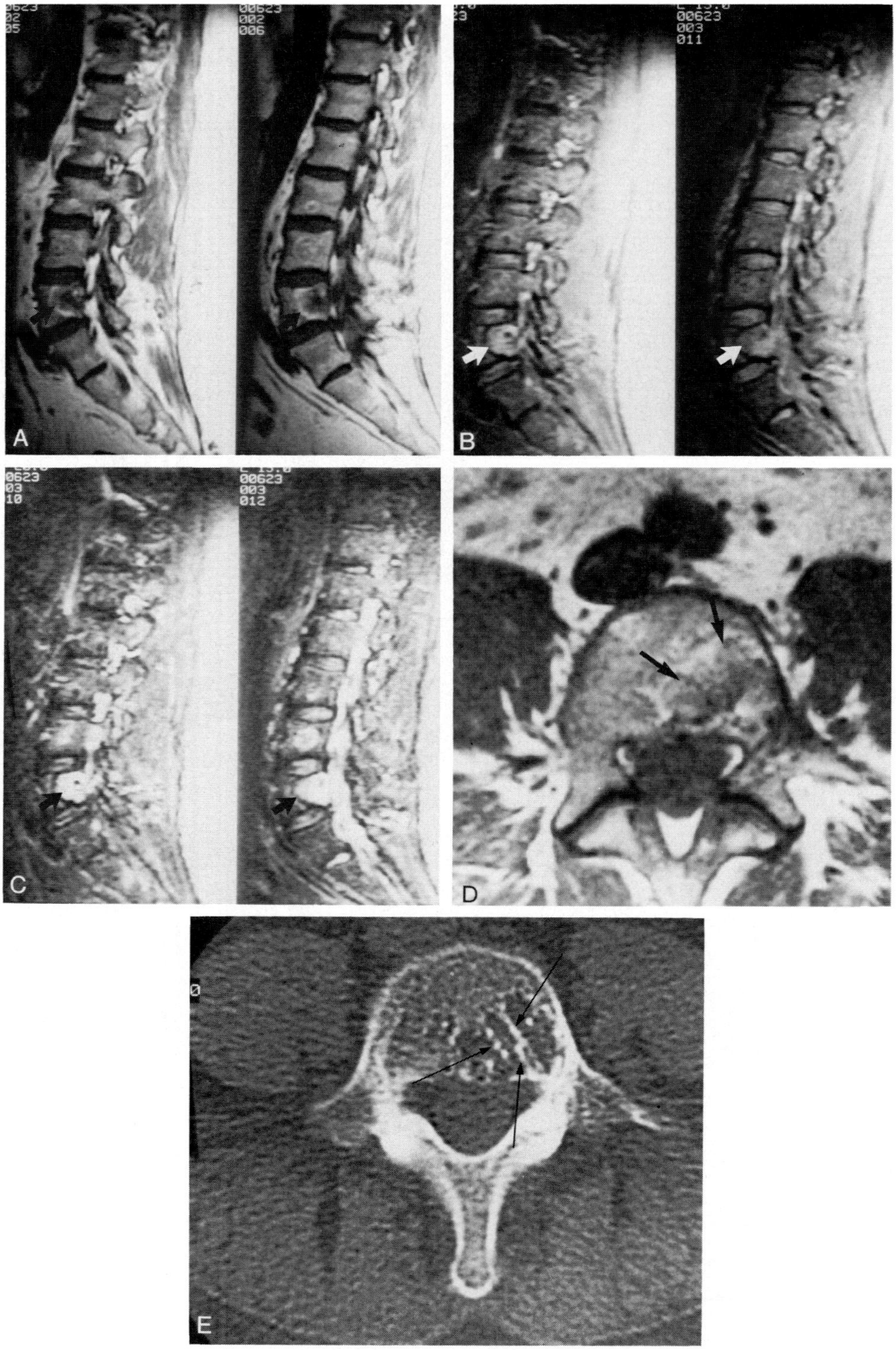

Figure 12–65. Hemangioma (23-year-old female).

A, Parasagittal T1. A central, slightly hypointense, peripherally hyperintense mass (*arrow*) is noted in the L5 vertebral body.

B, C, Parasagittal SD and T2. The mass (*arrow*) is more homogeneous and hyperintense on the long TR sequence and becomes higher in signal on the more heavily T2-weighted series.

D, Axial T1. The mass (*arrows*) is located in the posterior lateral portion of the body and is slightly hypointense to adjacent marrow, with a ring of high signal.

E, Axial CT. The coarse thickened trabeculae (*arrows*) corroborate the diagnosis of hemangioma.

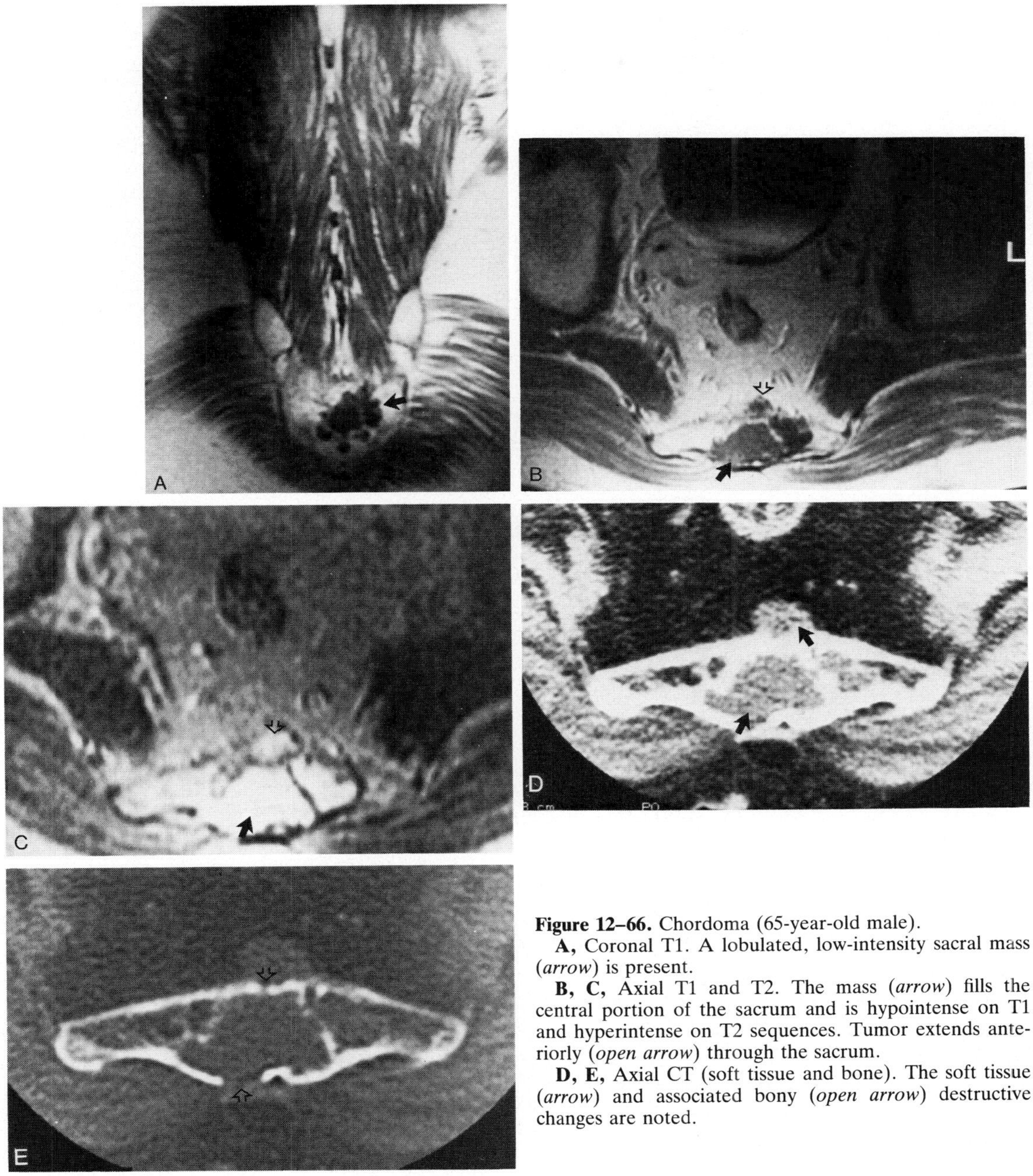

Figure 12–66. Chordoma (65-year-old male).

A, Coronal T1. A lobulated, low-intensity sacral mass (*arrow*) is present.

B, C, Axial T1 and T2. The mass (*arrow*) fills the central portion of the sacrum and is hypointense on T1 and hyperintense on T2 sequences. Tumor extends anteriorly (*open arrow*) through the sacrum.

D, E, Axial CT (soft tissue and bone). The soft tissue (*arrow*) and associated bony (*open arrow*) destructive changes are noted.

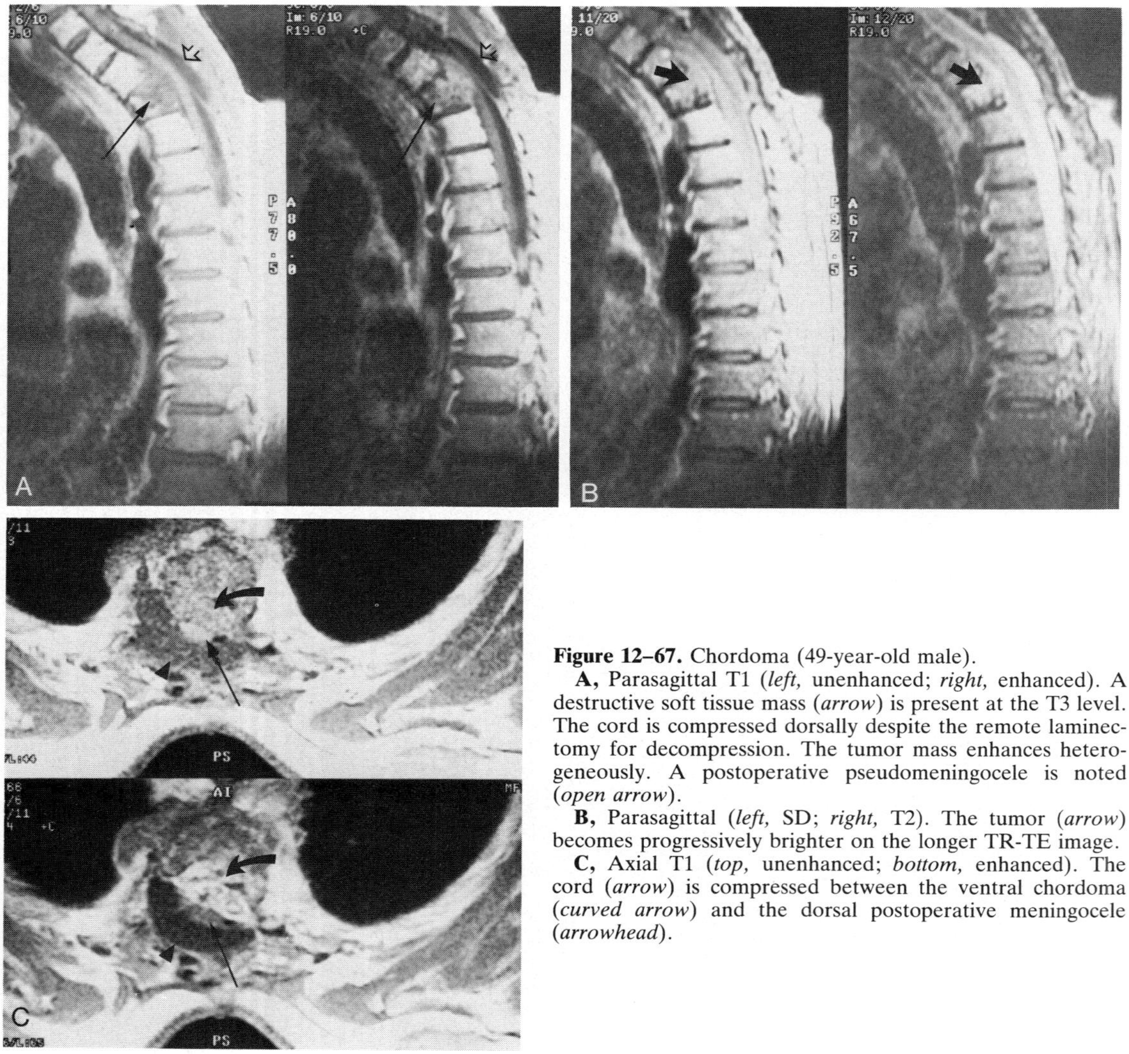

Figure 12–67. Chordoma (49-year-old male).

A, Parasagittal T1 (*left,* unenhanced; *right,* enhanced). A destructive soft tissue mass (*arrow*) is present at the T3 level. The cord is compressed dorsally despite the remote laminectomy for decompression. The tumor mass enhances heterogeneously. A postoperative pseudomeningocele is noted (*open arrow*).

B, Parasagittal (*left,* SD; *right,* T2). The tumor (*arrow*) becomes progressively brighter on the longer TR-TE image.

C, Axial T1 (*top,* unenhanced; *bottom,* enhanced). The cord (*arrow*) is compressed between the ventral chordoma (*curved arrow*) and the dorsal postoperative meningocele (*arrowhead*).

most common primary malignancy of bone and results from proliferation of a plasma cell–like primitive stem cell. The tumor affects men twice as commonly as women, usually in the sixth to eighth decade. The spine is commonly involved and may produce loss of bone density on the plain film examination. Focal "punched-out" lesions, although common in the skull, are rare in the spine. The vertebral bodies may be compressed.

MRI of multiple myeloma demonstrates infiltration of the red marrow. This is usually diffuse, involving many or all vertebral bodies, and in the early stages may be difficult to differentiate from osteopenic or degenerative marrow changes. Myeloma may also be focal, found in a solitary body (Fig. 12–68). Vertebral body fracture and cord compression are readily diagnosed.

Inflammatory

Inflammatory disease to the spine most often results from hematogenous spread. There is increased risk of acquiring this disease in the immunocompromised, chronically ill, and IV drug abuser populations. Although *Staphylococcus aureus* is the most common causative organism, a wide variety of organisms may be responsible. In children, the organism seeds the vascularized disk; the endplate is often seeded in adults. As the organism multiplies and inflammatory material accumulates, the

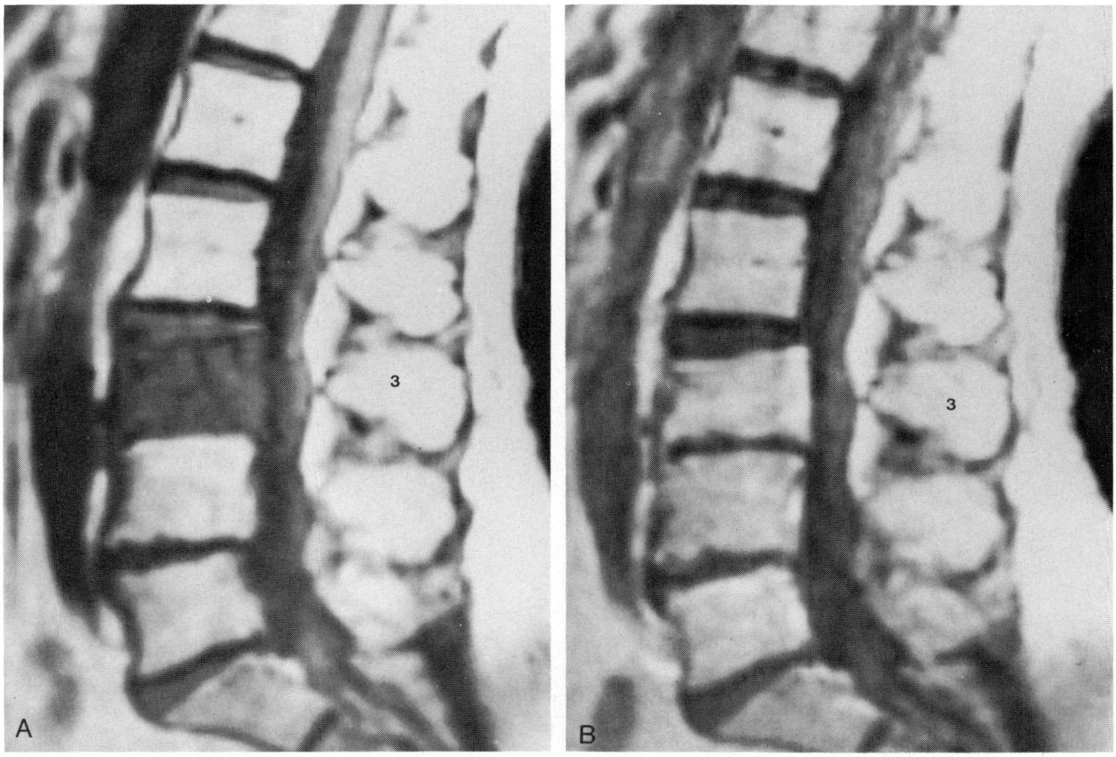

Figure 12–68. Multiple myeloma (63-year-old male).
A, Parasagittal T1. The L3 vertebral body marrow is replaced in total by infiltrative tumor.
B, Enhanced parasagittal T1. The L3 vertebral body becomes isointense to the adjacent normal bodies, masking the disease.

disk and vertebral bodies become secondarily involved, producing the characteristic disk space narrowing and endplate destruction that occurs late (8 to 10 days) in the disease on plain films[74] (Fig. 12–69). CT excels in detecting destruction, grossly evaluating paravertebral masses and, with the aid of intrathecal contrast, evaluating the extent of intraspinal soft tissue. Myelography must be performed with caution, as iatrogenic meningitis may result from inadvertent puncture of an abscess and seeding of the CSF.[21]

MRI affords a 96% sensitivity and 92% specificity when evaluating for vertebral osteomyelitis.[75] The overall accuracy of MRI (94%) surpasses those of plain films (73%) and bone scintigraphy (86%), and equals that of combined bone scintigraphy and gallium-imaging (94%) in evaluating vertebral osteomyelitis.[75] The characteristic T1 findings include confluent decreased signal in the opposing vertebral body endplates and marrow spaces, decreased disk height, inability to distinguish the disk, and a soft tissue mass of variable size. On T2, the signal intensity of the disk, opposing endplates, and adjacent centrum is high, and the intranuclear cleft may be inapparent. Gadolinium enhancement will highlight areas of inflammation in the disk, vertebral body, and paraspinal tissues (Fig. 12–70).

An intraspinal inflammatory mass is usually isointense to hypointense to cord on T1 and hyperintense to cord on T2. The mass may enhance homogeneously or peripherally (Fig. 12–71). The latter would support abscess formation.[76] Rarely, inflammatory masses will not enhance.

Tuberculous spondylitis and osteomyelitis differs from bacterial osteomyelitis and may resemble tumor with relative preservation of the disk space, involvement of the posterior elements and vertebral body, and a prominent paraspinal soft tissue mass.[77] Although the disk may be affected in children, tuberculosis (TB) lacks a proteolytic enzyme to destroy the disk. TB is typically insidious at onset and occurs

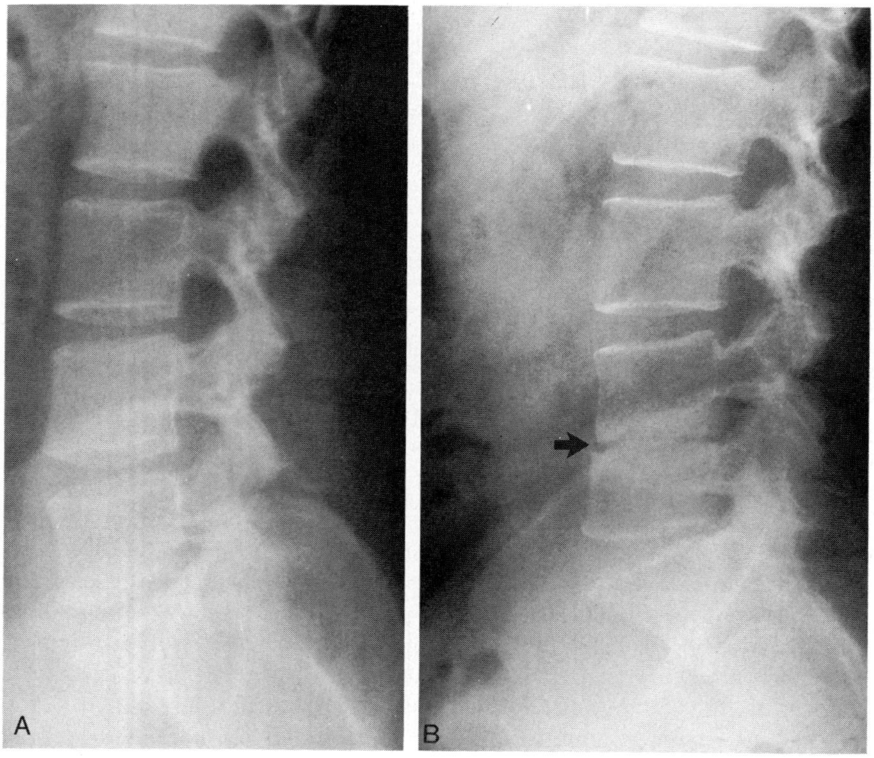

Figure 12–69. Discitis (33-year-old male).
A, Lateral film. Interpreted as normal.
B, Lateral film (3 weeks after **A**). The L4–5 disk space is almost completely compressed (*arrow*) with destruction and sclerosis of the opposing vertebral body endplates.

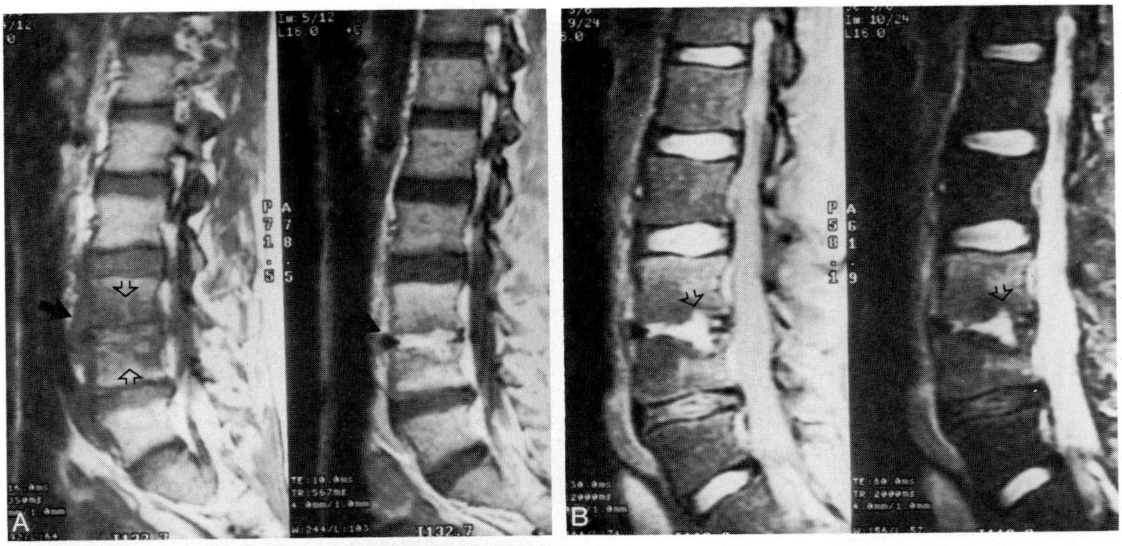

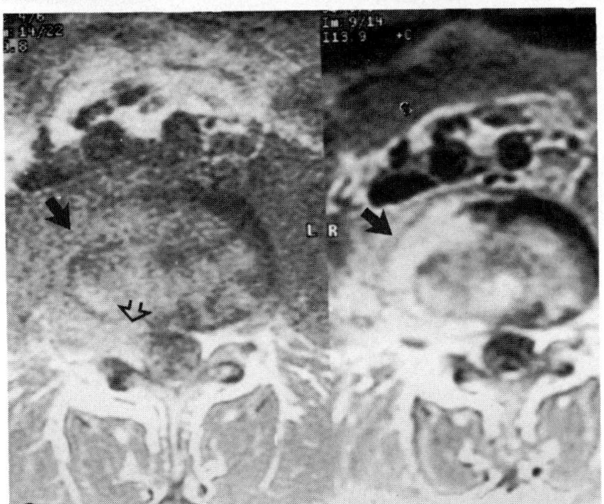

Figure 12–70. Discitis (20-year-old male).

A, Parasagittal T1 (*left,* unenhanced; *right,* enhanced). The L3–4 disk space is narrowed; a prevertebral soft tissue mass (*arrow*) is present. The markedly hypointense vertebral bodies (*open arrows*) merge with the abnormal disk. The disk enhances vividly with enhancement into the upper L4 vertebral body.

B, Parasagittal (*left,* SD; *right,* T2). The disk (*open arrow*) is abnormal in signal. The intranuclear cleft is absent.

C, Axial T1 (*left,* unenhanced; *right,* enhanced). An enhancing infiltrative inflammatory mass (*arrow*) is present in the right paravertebral region with extension into the intervertebral foramen (*open arrow*).

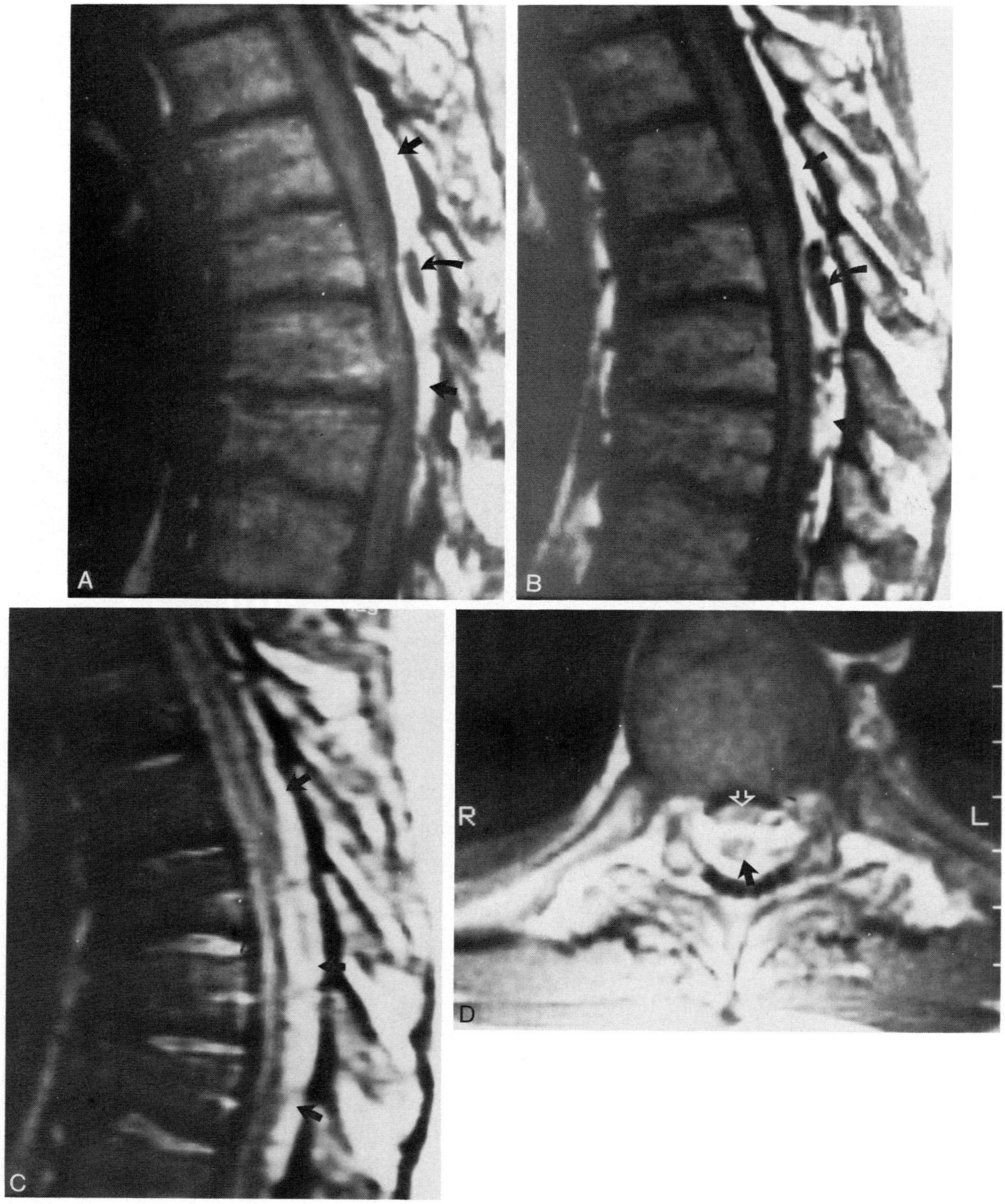

Figure 12–71. Intraspinal abscess (43-year-old male).

A, B, Enhanced parasagittal T1. An enhancing dorsal extradural mass (*arrows*) extends throughout the midthoracic spine. A central nonenhancing focus (*curved arrow*) indicates the presence of a multiloculated abscess.

C, Parasagittal T2. The mass (*arrows*) is heterogeneous, though predominantly high signal. The cord is displaced ventrally.

D, Enhanced axial T1. The enhancing abscess (*arrow*) significantly compresses the cord (*open arrow*).

over several months to several years compared with the acute onset of bacterial infection. Also, TB tends to occur in young and middle-aged adults, whereas pyogenic infection occurs more frequently in those in their sixth to seventh decade.

TRAUMA

Cervical Spine

C-spine trauma may be separated into conditions caused by hyperextension, hyperflexion, and those resulting from axial-loading injuries. In general, the hyperflexion injuries will narrow the anterior column of the spine and distract the posterior column. This results in narrowing of the disk space anteriorly and/or compression of the anterior vertebral body and disruption of the posterior ligamentous complex (Fig. 12–72). Extension injuries may fracture the posterior arches and disrupt the anterior longitudinal ligament or annulus, or both (Fig. 12–73). Avulsion fractures of the vertebral body may be present with extension injuries. Stability implies integrity of the osseous and ligamentous anatomy, with low likelihood of aggravating an existing cord or root compression with physiologic head and neck mobility.

Hyperflexion

Wedge Fracture. These fractures are the result of a hyperflexion injury that occurs usually in the middle to lower C-spine. The anterior margin of the vertebral body is narrowed and the posterior margin of the vertebral body maintained. The posterior ligamentous complex, though stretched, is intact. This is considered a stable fracture.

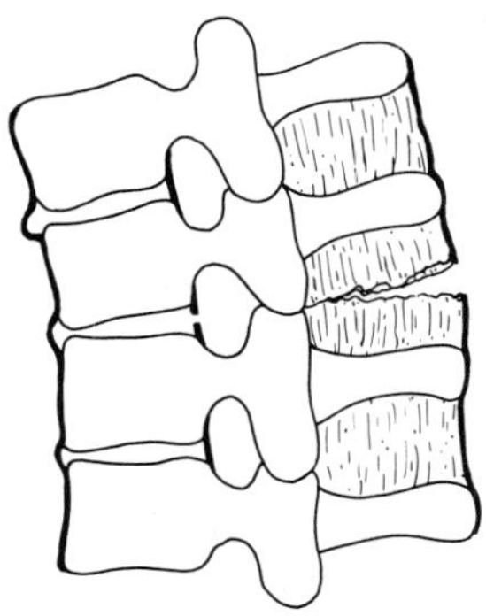

Figure 12–72. Schematic hyperflexion injuries. Hyperflexion results in narrowing of the height of the disk space anteriorly at the expense of widening the interspinous distance. The degree of flexion may be sufficient to tear the posterior ligaments and compress the anterior aspect of the vertebral bodies. (Medical illustration by Diane Blue.)

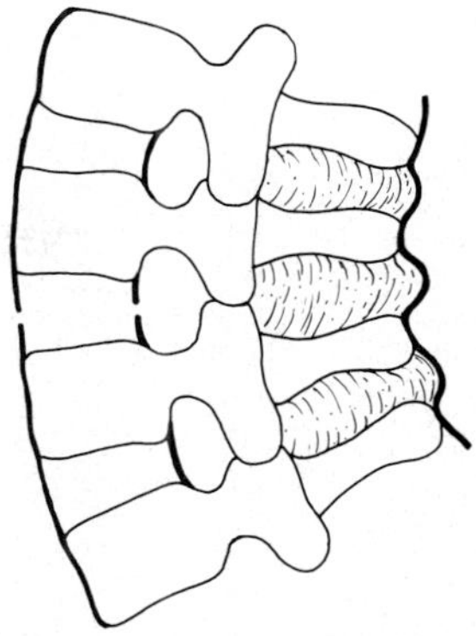

Figure 12–73. Schematic hyperextension injuries. Hyperextension results in narrowing the interspinous distance with commensurate widening of the anterior disk space. The ALL, disk, and PLL may rupture. An avulsion fracture of the anterior inferior vertebral body may occur. (Medical illustration by Diane Blue.)

Radiographs demonstrate loss of anterior vertebral body height and prevertebral soft tissue swelling. A burst fracture can be excluded if a vertical lucency is absent on the AP films. With the exception of a slight focal kyphosis, the C-spine is normally aligned.

Dens Fracture. The transverse alar ligament remains intact, with extreme flexion of the head, shearing the dens from its union with the body of C2. Three types of odontoid fractures have been described.[78] Type 1 is an uncommon avulsion of the odontoid tip. Type 2 results from a fracture at the base of the dens and the junction of the vertebral body. Type 3 fracture extends into the body of C2. Types 2 and 3 may be accompanied by varying degrees of atlantoaxial dislocation.

Plain films may demonstrate malalignment of the dens and the body of C2 as well as prevertebral soft tissue swelling. The AP films may demonstrate the lucent fracture line and slight tilting of the odontoid process[78] (Figs. 12–74, 12–75).

Facet Dislocation. Facet dislocations may be unilateral (stable) or bilateral (unstable) in more severe cases. The bilateral dislocation is associated with complete disruption of the posterior ligamentous complex, the PLL, and often the ALL with anterior dislocation of the

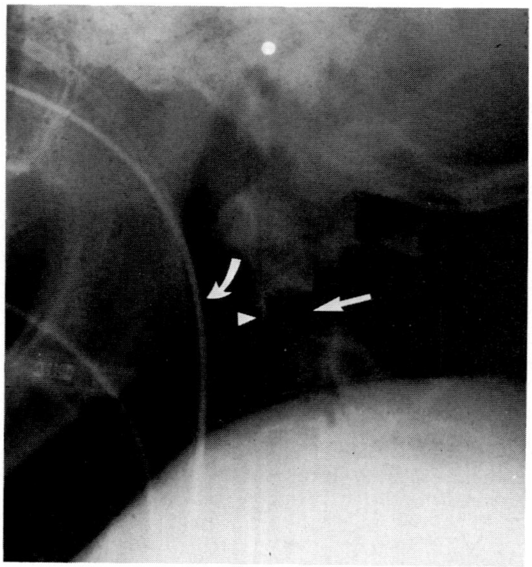

Figure 12–74. Type II odontoid fracture (anterior displacement) (28-year-old male). Lateral; the odontoid is fractured and distracted (*arrow*) from the body of C2. A small anterior chip of the C2 body (*arrowhead*) remains attached to the dens. The prevertebral soft tissue is thickened, causing the nasogastric (NG) tube (*curved arrow*) to be significantly displaced from the spine.

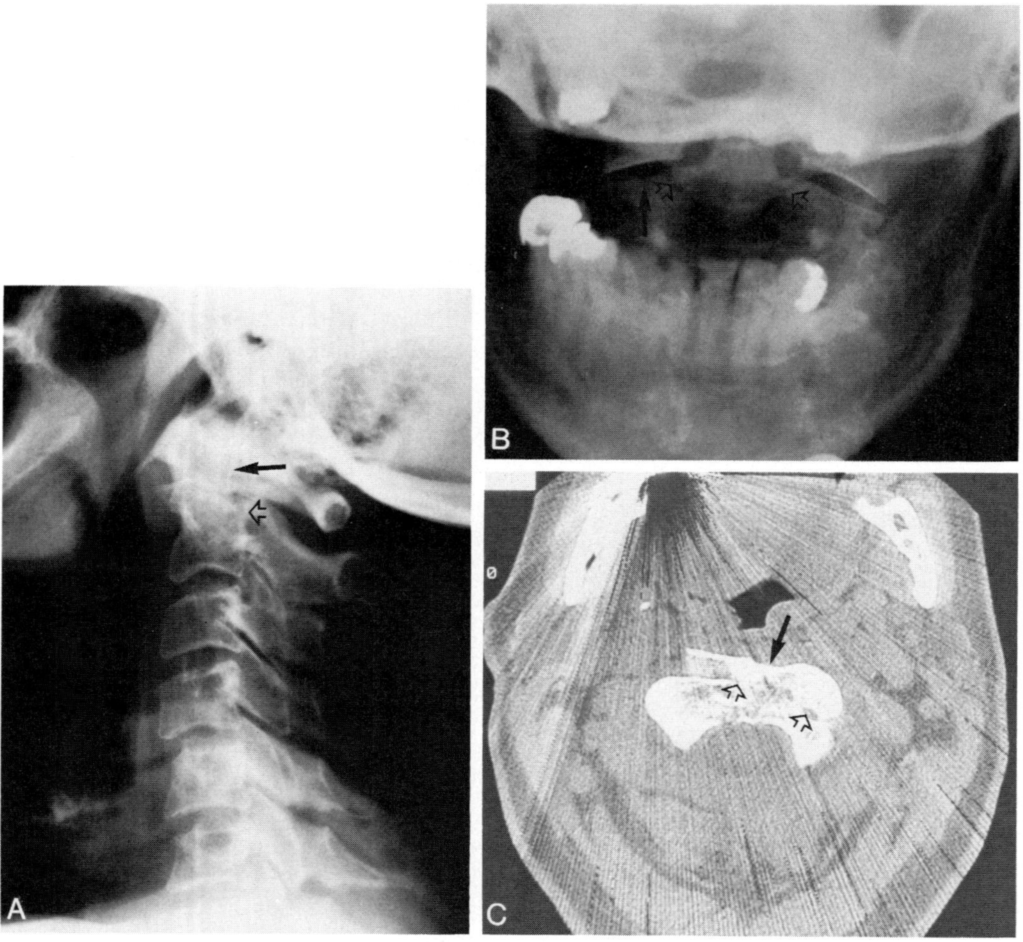

Figure 12–75. Type III odontoid fracture (65-year-old male).

A, Lateral. There is anterior displacement of the odontoid and upper body of C2 (*arrow*) referable to the body of C2 (*open arrow*).

B, Open-mouth odontoid. A subtle lucency (*open arrows*) extends through the upper body of the axis. There is also subtle compression (*arrow*) of the right lateral mass of C2.

C, Axial CT. The anteriorly displaced cephalad component of the axis (*arrow*) is separated by an irregular fracture line (*open arrows*) from the body of C2.

inferior facets of the cephalad vertebra into the neural foramina. Frequently, this may be associated with a fracture of either facet at the level of the disk location. Unilateral dislocation is a stable injury in which only a single facet is dislocated. The inferior facet is dislocated into the intervertebral foramen, locked in place by the intact ligaments. Posterior ligaments and capsular ligaments are disrupted. The PLL and annular ligaments are often intact.

The radiographic findings of bilateral dislocation include anterolisthesis of the vertebral body by greater than or equal to one-half the AP dimension of the body (Fig. 12–76). A small facet fracture may be detected. The prevertebral soft tissues are excessive. The AP film may be normal.

Unilateral facet dislocation involves anterolisthesis of less than one-half the AP dimension of the vertebral body and abrupt oblique orientation of the vertebral bodies above the level of injury. Prevertebral soft tissues are abnormal. The AP film demonstrates displacement of the spinous processes above the level of injury toward the side of the dislocation.

Flexion Teardrop. Flexion teardrop fractures result from a combination of flexion and axial loading, which may occur from a diving accident. The anterior portion of the vertebral body is compressed and displaced forward. More significantly, there is retrolisthesis of the posterior fragment with varying degrees of cord compression. Degree of retrolisthesis determines the patient's clinical status from neurologically normal to quadriplegic. This is an unstable injury involving all of the anterior and posterior ligaments.

The lateral film demonstrates retrolisthesis, focal kyphosis at the level of injury, excess prevertebral soft tissue swelling, an anterior or anterior-inferior vertebral body fracture resembling a teardrop, and subjacent disk space narrowing (Fig. 12–77). Frontal film demonstrates a vertical lucency in the vertebral body that may be midline or lateralized and a possible wedge fracture that may lateralize to one side of the vertebral body.[79]

Hyperflexion Sprain. Hyperflexion sprain injuries result in disruption of all the posterior ligaments and partial disruption of the disk. The ALL is intact. The patient may experience neck pain without neurologic deficit.

The radiographs demonstrate kyphotic an-

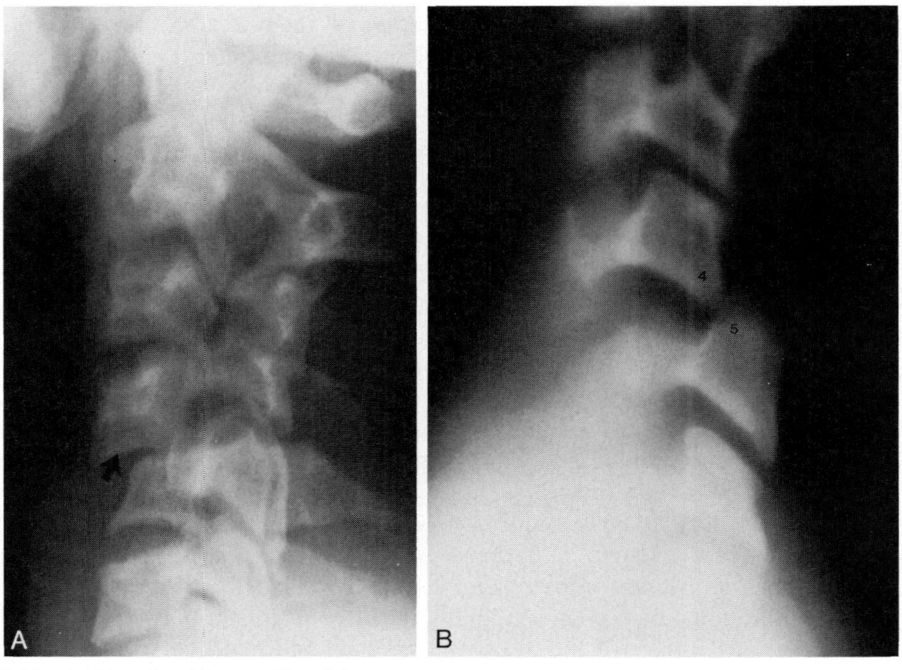

Figure 12–76. Facet dislocation (8-year-old male).

A, Lateral. The C4 vertebral body (*arrow*) is anterolisthesed 60 to 70% of the AP dimension of the vertebral body. The C4 facets override the C5 facets.

B, Lateral linear tomography. Confirms the anterior displacement of the inferior facet of C4, referable to the superior facet of C5.

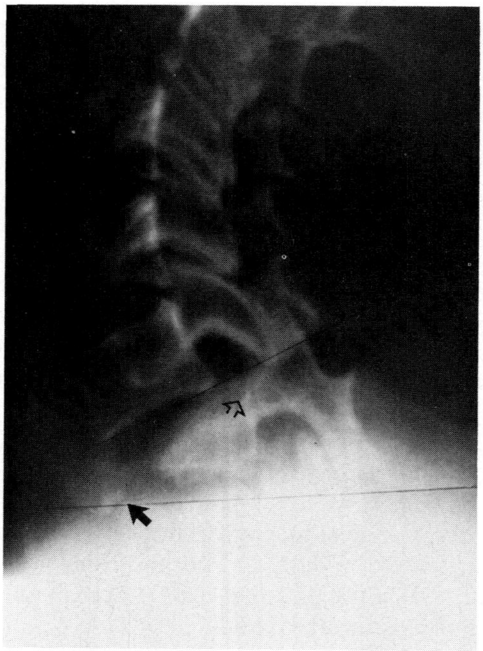

Figure 12–77. Flexion teardrop (24-year-old male). An anterior compression deformity of C6 is present. A small anterior fragment (*arrow*) is present. The deformed C6 vertebral body (*open arrow*) is retrolisthesed into the canal.

gulation, widening of the interspinous space, and narrowing of the anterior disk space that may coexist with mild subluxation. The angulation may be inapparent on cross-table films, often requiring an upright examination for detection. Extension will reduce the subluxation. Delayed instability occurs in 20 to 50% of patients with this injury.

Hyperextension Injuries

Hyperextension Fracture Dislocation with Fractured Articular Pillar. Hyperextension and axial compression result in compression and a comminuted fracture of the unilateral pedicle and lamina. In this unstable injury, the ALL may be disrupted or remain intact.

Lateral film demonstrates minimal anterolisthesis, the disk space is narrow, and the vertebral body is slightly rotated above the level of injury. Oblique films demonstrate the disruption of the bony perimeter of the intervertebral foramen.

Traumatic Spondylolisthesis of the Axis (Hangman's Fracture). This fracture is due to hyperextension of the cranium at an instant of abrupt deceleration and results in bilateral C2 pedicle fractures. Plain films demonstrate varying degrees of anterolisthesis of C2 on C3, diastasis, kyphosis, and soft tissue swelling (Fig. 12–78). This unstable fracture may result in neurologic deficit although most frequently it does not.

Hyperextension Sprain. The hyperextension forces the articular and spinous processes together, acting as a fulcrum. The ALL and the disk are torn. The vertebral bodies above the level are temporarily forced posteriorly, crushing the cord between the retrolisthesis body above and the lamina below. The dislocation is transient, with spontaneous reduction. Patients present with severe neurologic deficit but may have near-normal plain films. The paraspinal soft tissues and anterior disk space may be widened, with small vertebral body avulsion fractures present at the disk space.

Axial Loading

Jefferson Fracture. This type of fracture results from a vector force transmitted from the occipital condyles to the lateral masses of the atlas. The lateral masses are compressed between the occiput and C2, leading to fractures of the C1 arch. The fractures may be bilateral or unilateral and involve the anterior or the posterior ring.

Lateral film may demonstrate a widening of the atlantodental interval if there is a fracture of one or more of the anterior arches. The open-mouth odontoid film demonstrates lateral displacement of one or both lateral masses of C1 referable to C2. CT readily demonstrates the C1 ring fractures, relationship of the dens to C1, and degree of fragment diastasis (Fig. 12–79).

Atlanto-occipital Dislocation. Atlanto-occipital dislocation usually, but not always, results from anterior displacement of the calverium from the C-spine. The patients present with severe neurologic findings yet rarely may survive intraoperative fusion without neurologic sequelae.[80] The cervicomedullary junction is compressed between the opisthion and the odontoid process, with more severe anterior displacement. Associated soft tissue and, less commonly, bony injuries are variably present (Fig. 12–80).

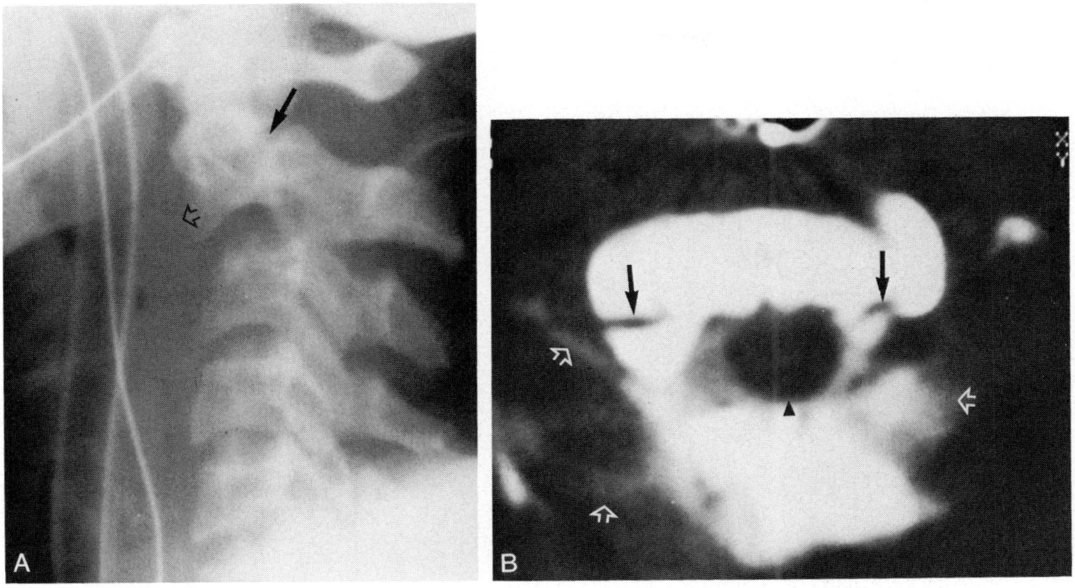

Figure 12–78. Hangman's fracture (18-year-old female).

A, Lateral. Bilateral pedicle fractures at C2 (*arrow*) are present allowing anterolisthesis and kyphosis at the C2–3 interval. The prevertebral soft tissues (*open arrow*) are excessive.

B, Axial postmyelogram CT. The bilateral pedicle fractures (*arrows*) are detected. The cord (*arrowhead*) is enlarged, and contrast material leaks into the surrounding tissues (*open arrows*) from a dural tear.

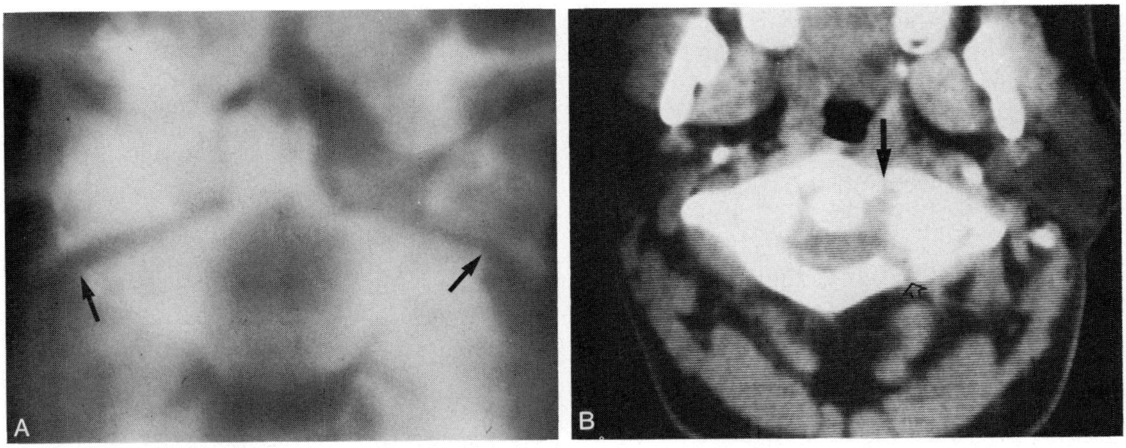

Figure 12–79. Jefferson fracture (32-year-old male).

A, AP linear tomography. Displacement of both lateral masses (*arrows*) of C1 is present, greater on the left.

B, Axial CT. Fractures through the anterior (*arrow*) and posterior (*open arrow*) arch of C1 are noted. Although the odontoid is in good apposition with the anterior arch of C1, the transverse ligament attaches on C1 lateral to the fracture site and must be disrupted.

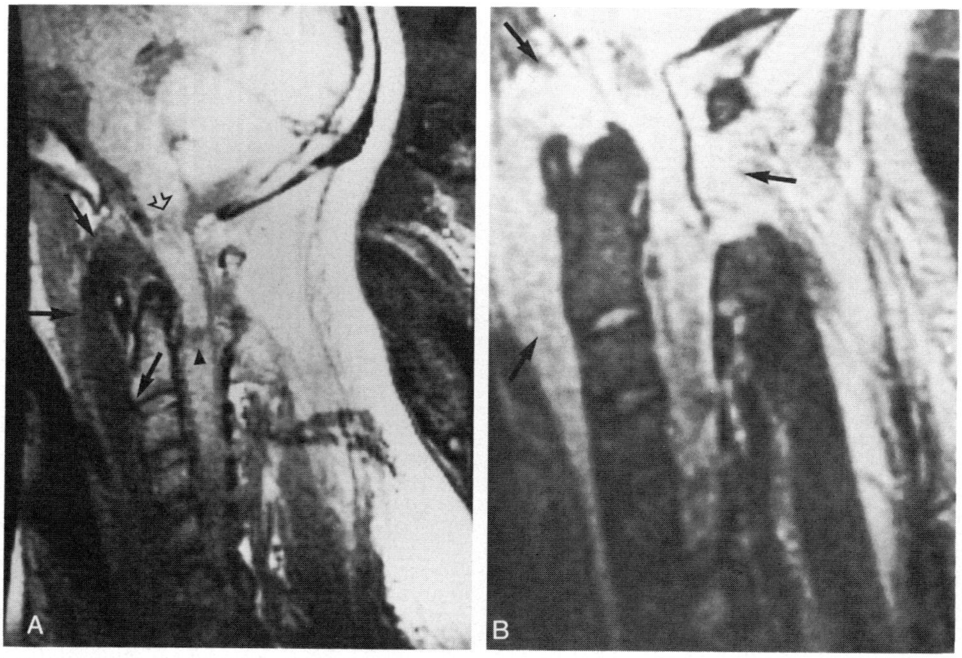

Figure 12–80. Atlanto-occipital dislocation (22-year-old male).

A, Parasagittal T1. The skull has been anteriorly displaced and distracted from the spine. Excessive soft tissue edema (*arrows*) is juxtaposed between the skull and spine as well as the prevertebral space. The cord has been traumatized at the craniocervical junction (*open arrow*) and the mid-C2 level (*arrowhead*).

B, Parasagittal T2. Marked soft tissue edema (*arrows*) is noted. The cord is markedly high in signal from the craniocervical junction to the C3 level.

Thoracic and Lumbar Spine

Compression Fracture. These fractures result from a combination of vertical loading and flexion, causing an anterior wedge deformity of the vertebral body, which is located most frequently in the lower thoracic and lumbar spine. Plain films demonstrate the fracture deformity, which can be confirmed by planar imaging (Fig. 12–81).

Chance Fracture. Chance[81] originally described this fracture, also known as the seat belt injury, nearly 40 years before use of seat belts became mandatory. The fracture results from abrupt flexion of the upper spine over a restrained lower segment. Although little anterior compression of the vertebral body is noted, the horizontal fracture involves all of the posterior elements and a portion of the posterior vertebral body. The fracture characteristically extends anteriorly into the cephalad endplate of the vertebral body, just anterior to the intervertebral foramen. This injury causes no major ligament damage.

Burst Fracture. The burst fracture results from axial compression forces that herniate the nucleus pulposus through the inferior endplate into the vertebral body above. In this unstable injury, the vertebral body fractures into multiple fragments, resulting in anterior-

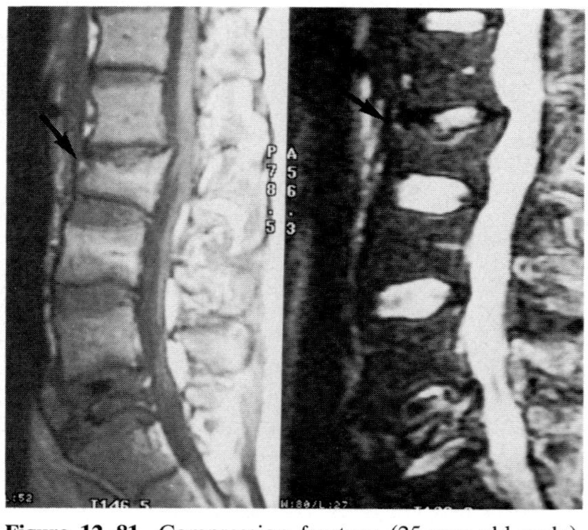

Figure 12–81. Compression fracture (25-year-old male). Parasagittal (*left,* T1; *right,* T2); a compression fracture is present at the L2 level (*arrows*). This involves the anterior vertebral body with relative sparing of the posterior body. Mild anterolisthesis of L1 on L2 is noted. A burst fracture is noted at L5.

wedge deformity and retropulsion of the superoposterior margin of the vertebral body into the spinal canal. Acute neurologic deficit occurs in 65% of patients.[82] Burst fractures may extend to one or both laminae, the interpediculate distance increases, and a vertical fracture is detected in the vertebral body.

Plain films demonstrate the fracture deformity of the body, retropulsion of the posterior superior margin, widened interpediculate distance, and vertical vertebral body fracture line. CT and MRI more clearly demonstrate fractures of the body and posterior elements and the extent of canal compromise (Figs. 12–82, 12–83).

CONGENITAL ANOMALIES OF THE SPINE

Spinal dysraphism refers to incomplete or aberrant fusion of the dorsal midline neural, osseous, and mesenchymal elements. Dysraphic lesions may be placed in one of two groups, contingent on whether the spinal contents herniate through the defect. In spina bifida cystica the contents of the spinal canal have herniated through the midline defect. The skin may or may not be absent. Spina bifida cystica lesions include meningocele, meningomyelocele, and lipomyelomeningocele. If the midline defect is covered with skin and the spinal contents remain within the canal, the lesion falls into the spina bifida occulta category, which includes spinal lipoma, hydrosyringomyelia, tethered cord, diastematomyelia, and split notochord.

MRI is an ideal means to evaluate spinal dysraphic lesions. Multiplanar imaging can be performed without the use of invasive lumbar punctures, which may be technically quite difficult and hazardous in these patients.

Meningocele

This is the rarest type of spina bifida cystica lesion, consisting of a herniation of dura mater and arachnoid through a midline osseous defect. The lesion is usually covered with skin, occurs with equal frequency in males and females, and may occur anywhere along the

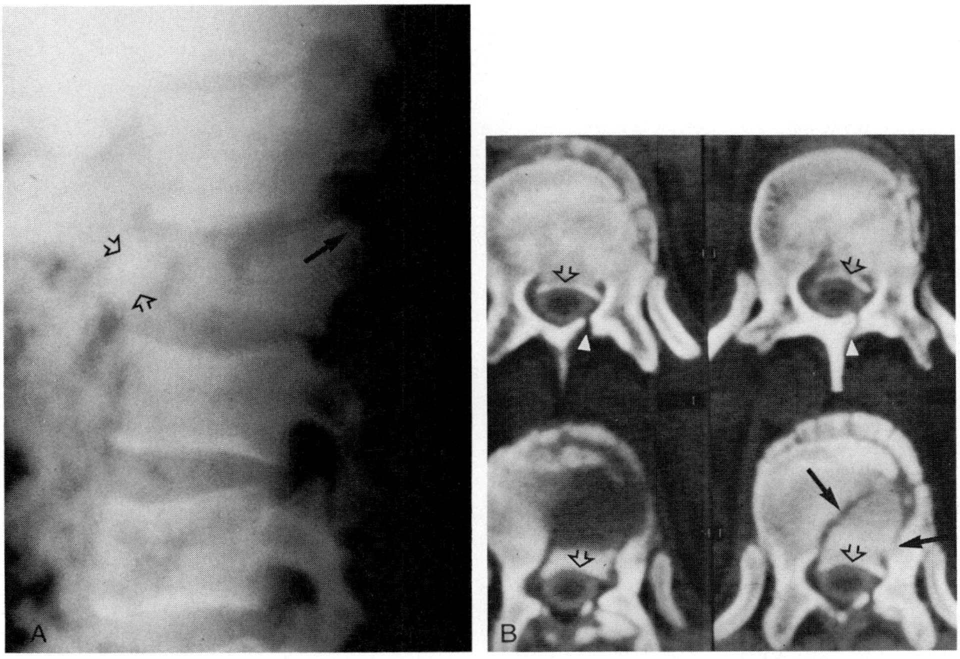

Figure 12–82. Burst fracture (29-year-old male).

A, Lateral. A burst fracture is noted at the T11 level. There is retropulsion of the superior-posterior margin of the vertebral body (*arrow*) into the canal. The anterior margin of the body (*open arrows*) is fractured and anteriorly displaced.

B, Axial postmyelogram CT. A comminuted fracture through the body (*arrows*) and left lamina (*arrowhead*) is present. The posterior-superior vertebral body margin (*open arrow*) is retrolisthesed, narrowing the canal without cord compression.

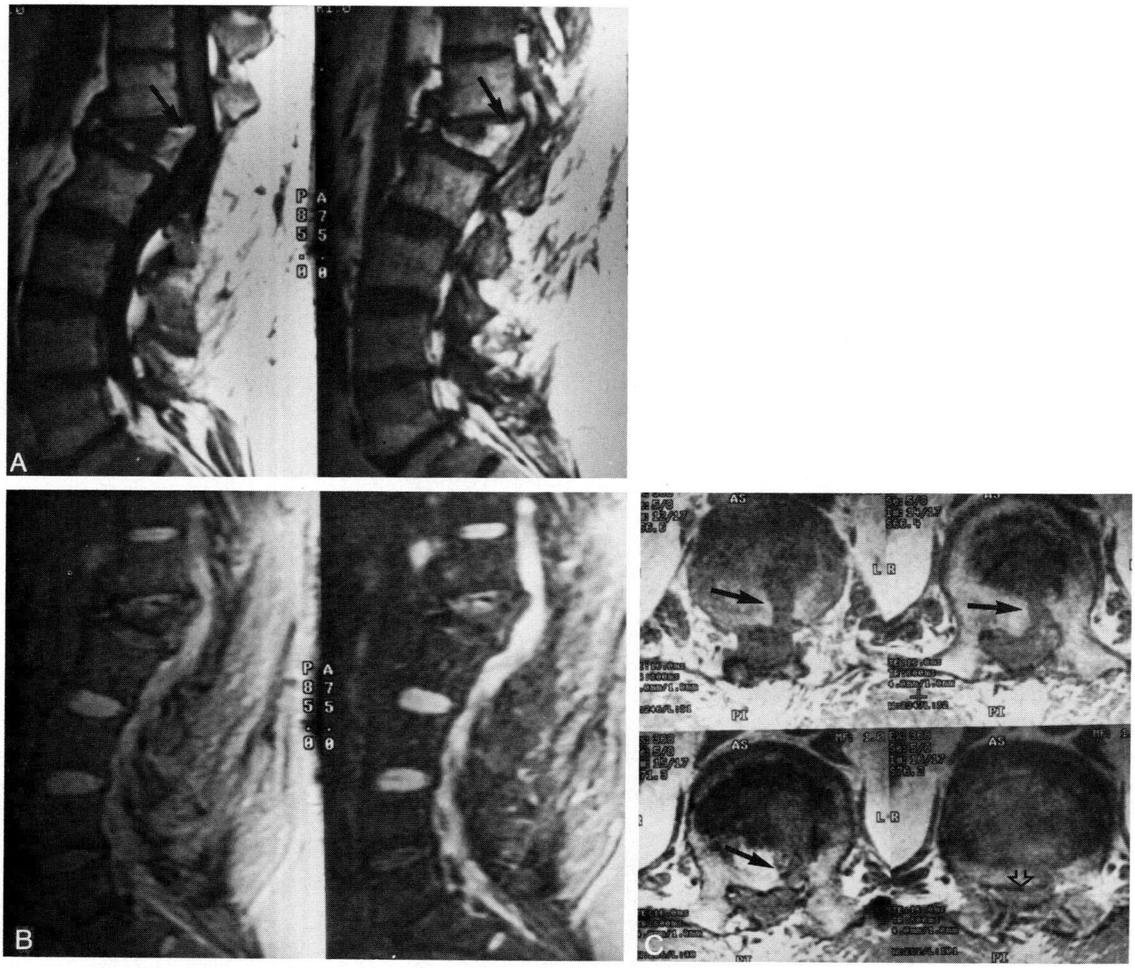

Figure 12–83. Burst fracture (20-year-old male).

A, Parasagittal T1. A burst fracture of T12 is present with retrolisthesis of the posterior-superior margin of the body (*arrow*) and anterior wedging of the body.

B, Parasagittal (*left,* SD; *right,* T2). The extent of the ventral extradural defect is noted.

C, Axial T1. The severely comminuted body fracture (*arrow*) and retrolisthesis with cord compression (*open arrow*) are noted.

spinal axis but most commonly in the lumbar spine.

Myelomeningocele

Myelomeningocele, the most common spina bifida cystica lesion, consists of exposed neural elements (neural placode) that may be level with the surface of the back (myelocele) or elevated above the paraspinal soft tissues by ectatic caudal subarachnoid space (myelomeningocele). Myelomeningoceles are almost invariably associated with Chiari II malformations and less frequently with hydrosyringomyelia, diastematomyelia, or lipomas, often at the filum (Fig. 12–84).

Lipomyelomeningocele

Lipomyelomeningocele may occur as an occult or cystic lesion and is four times less common than myelomeningocele.[83] The lesion consists of a partial split of the dorsal surface of the cord in association with a dural deficiency and infiltration of adipose material a variable distance into the defect and toward the placode.[84] The subarachnoid space is ectatic, forming an associated meningocele (Fig. 12–85).

Spinal Lipoma

In this anomaly, small collections of ectopic adipose material and fibrous tissue may be

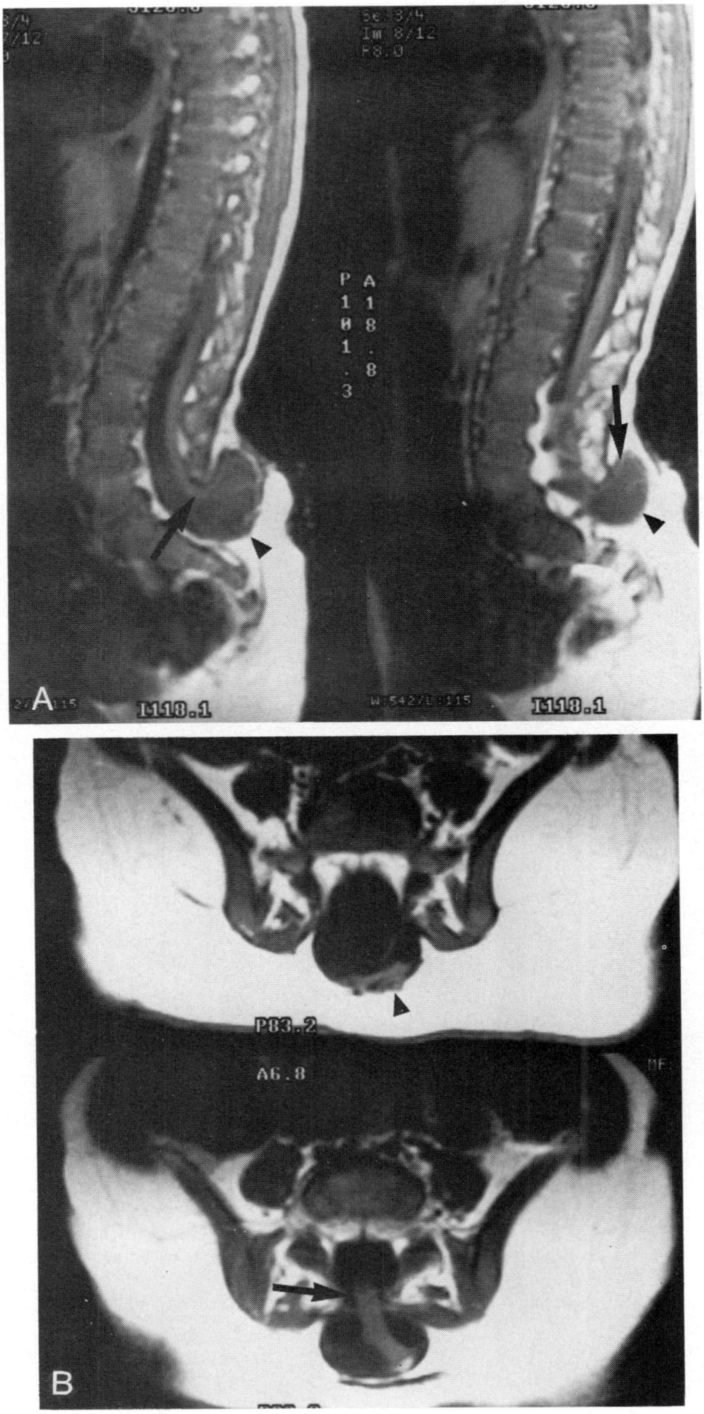

Figure 12–84. Myelomeningocele (3-week-old male).

A, Parasagittal T1. The cord extends to a low lumbar myelomeningocele (*arrowhead*). Neural elements (*arrow*) herniate into the dural ectasia.

B, Axial T1. The neural placode (*arrowhead*) is tethered to the dural surface. The distal cord (*arrow*) extends through the dysraphic spinal canal.

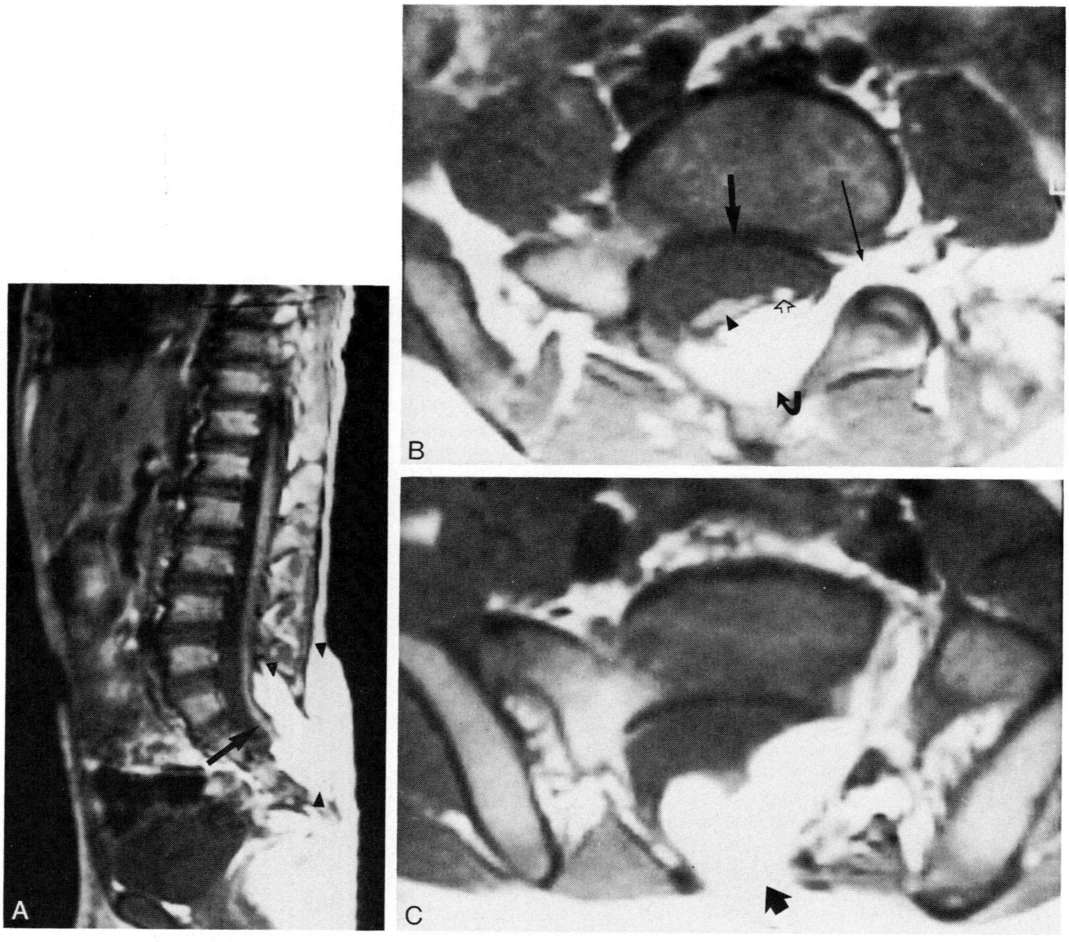

Figure 12–85. Lipomyelomeningocele (5-month-old male).

A, Parasagittal T1. The cord (*arrow*) is tethered posteriorly to an ectatic thecal sac. A large subcutaneous lipoma (*arrowheads*) has extended through the dysraphic posterior elements into the extradural and intradural compartments.

B, Axial T1. The neural placode (*arrowhead*), ectatic thecal sac (*arrow*), and intraspinal lipoma (*curved arrow*) are noted. Intradural fat (*open arrow*) is present. In addition, the adipose tissue has extended through the L5–S1 intervertebral foramen (*long arrow*).

C, Axial T1. Adipose tissue extends into the canal through dysraphic posterior elements (*arrow*).

found within the dura, associated with the filum, conus, or cauda equina. Alternatively, the lipoma may be extradural or, in some instances, both intradural and extradural. The lipoma may be associated with cord tethering (Fig. 12–86).

Tethered Cord

As the axial skeleton matures and elongates, the cord effectively ascends. The cord may be tethered by a thickened filum, resulting in increased tension on the cord as the axial skeleton grows. The normal conus should be above the L3 level in children younger than 6 years of age and above the L2-L3 disk space in patients older than 12. This condition is associated with most of the spina bifida cystica and occulta lesions (Fig. 12–87).

Diastematomyelia

This anomaly, which may be associated with lipomyelomeningocele and tethered cord, refers to a split in the spinal cord. The split is usually segmental, occurring most commonly caudal to the middle thoracic spine. Each half of the cord gives rise to the ipsilateral, dorsal, and ventral nerve roots. The cord is united above and below the cleft. A bony or fibrous septum may be present. The dural sac remains undivided in 50% of cases. Vertebral body anomalies are frequent, consisting of butterfly vertebrae, hemivertebrae, and block vertebrae (Figs. 12–88, 12–89).

Split Notochord

A spectrum of anomalies exists that relate to splitting of the notochord and the surrounding germ cell layers. These may result in communication of the gut and the skin over the dorsal spine. This may cause a dorsal enteric fistula in which bowel contents empty on the back after extending through the vertebral body, spinal canal, and cord. Remnant tracks are termed neurenteric cysts. These cysts may be located anywhere along the track, including within the spinal canal.

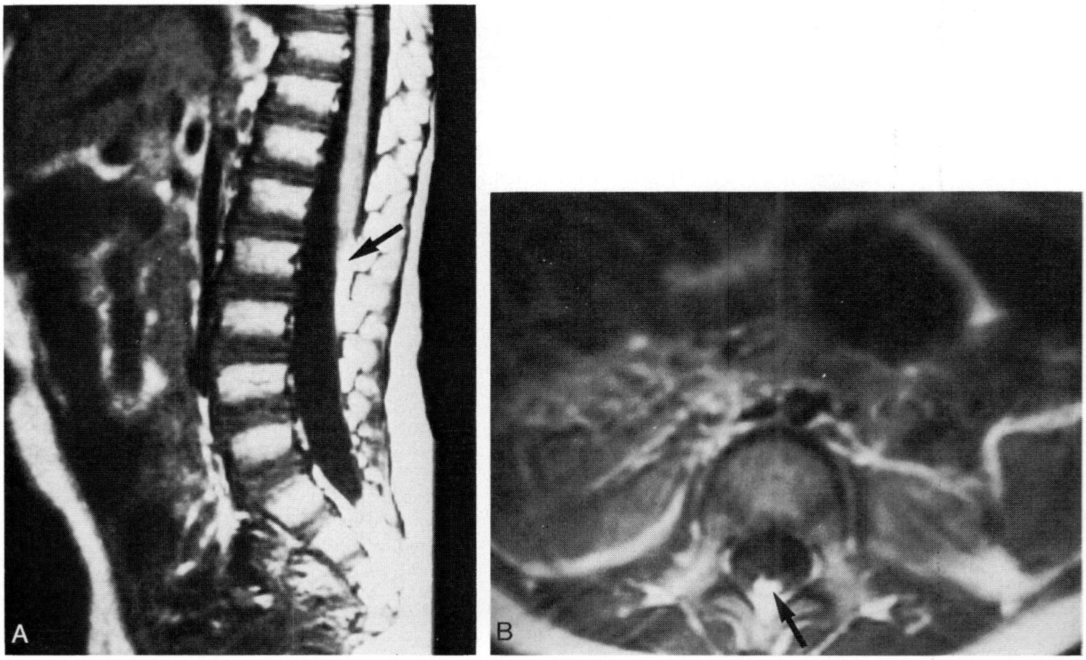

Figure 12–86. Intraspinal lipoma (2-year-old male).
A, Parasagittal T1. An intradural lipoma (*arrow*) tapers caudally from the conus. The cord is not tethered.
B, Axial T1. The lipoma (*arrow*) is positioned along the dorsal thecal sac.

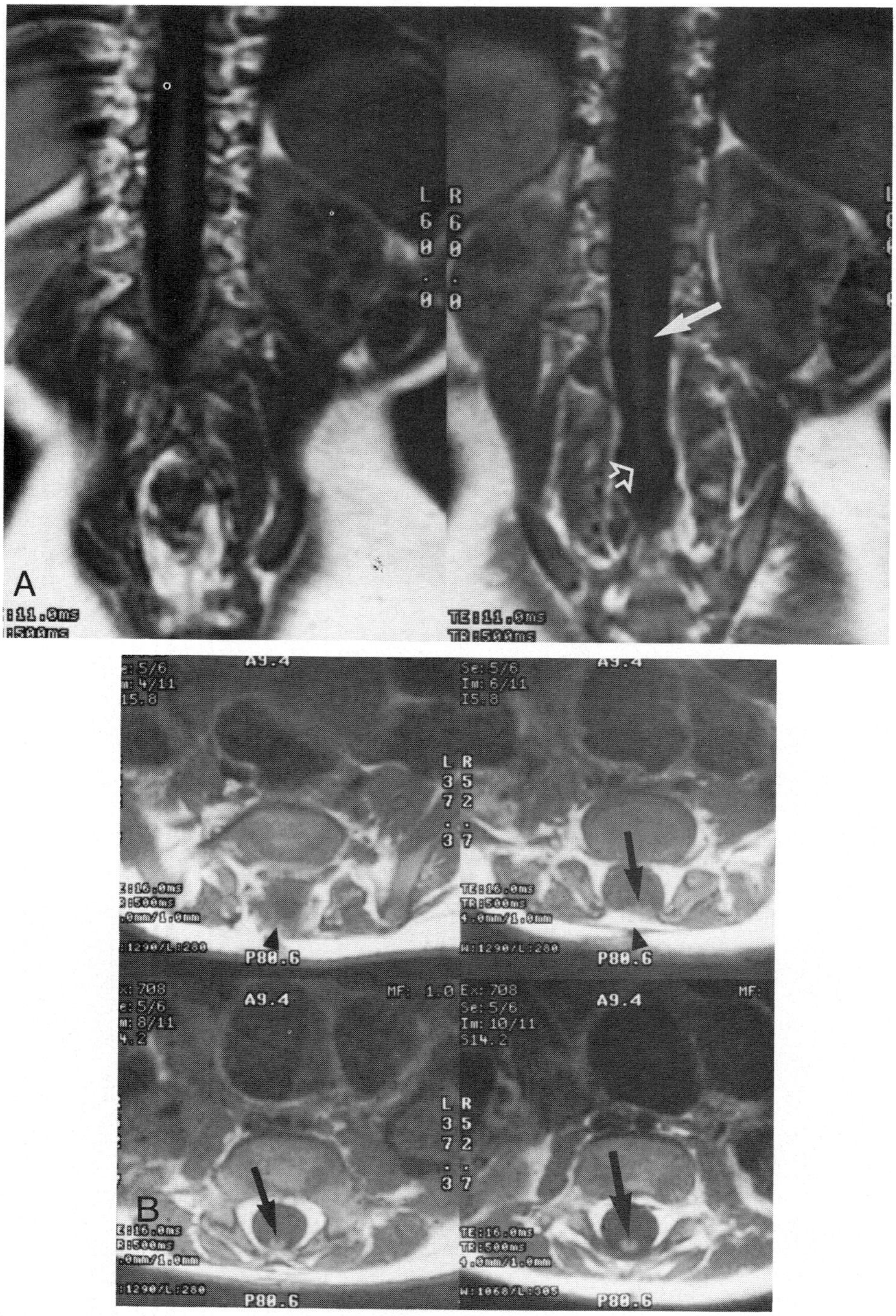

Figure 12–87. Tethered cord (3-year-old female).

A, Coronal T1. The cord (*arrow*) is tethered to the distal dorsal thecal sac (*open arrow*).

B, Axial T1. The cord (*arrow*) extends into the ectatic thecal sac and to, but not through, the dysraphic dorsal spine (*arrowhead*).

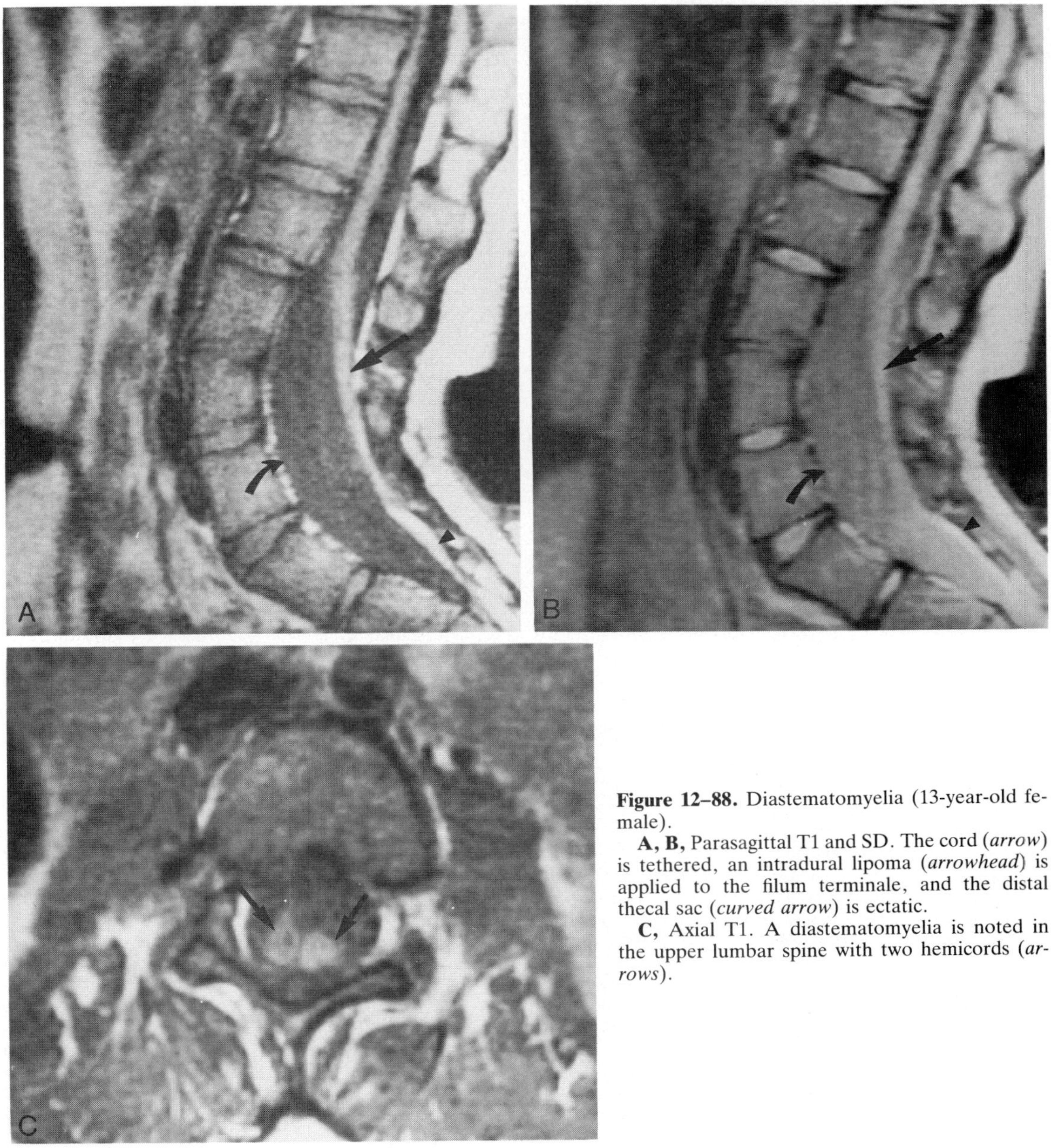

Figure 12–88. Diastematomyelia (13-year-old female).

A, B, Parasagittal T1 and SD. The cord (*arrow*) is tethered, an intradural lipoma (*arrowhead*) is applied to the filum terminale, and the distal thecal sac (*curved arrow*) is ectatic.

C, Axial T1. A diastematomyelia is noted in the upper lumbar spine with two hemicords (*arrows*).

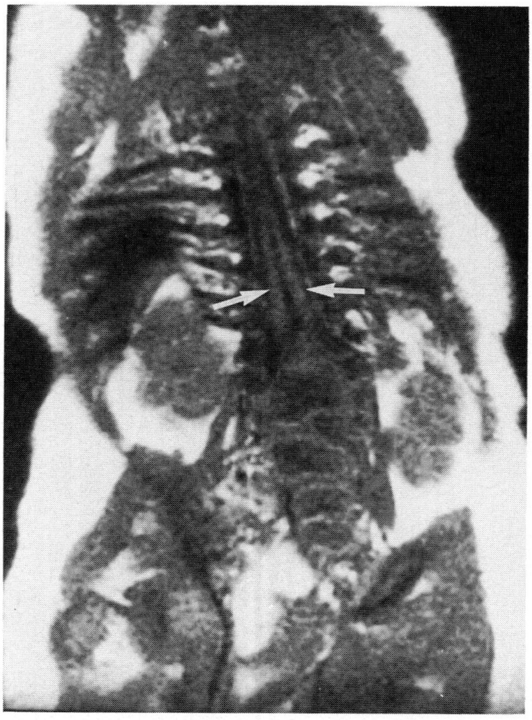

Figure 12–89. Diastematomyelia (2-day-old male). Coronal T1; the cord (*arrows*) is split from the midthoracic region to the tethered conus. The lower spine is markedly dysraphic with multiple segmentation anomalies.

References

1. Lazorthes G, Gouaze A, Zadeh JO, et al: Arterial vascularization of the spinal cord: Recent studies of the anastomotic substitution pathways. J Neurosurg 1971; 35:253–262.
2. Wortzman G, Dewar FP: Rotary fixation of the atlantoaxial joint: Rotational atlantoaxial subluxation. Radiology 1968; 90:479–487.
3. Lee YY, Glass JP, Wallace S: Myelography in cancer patients: Modified technique. AJNR 1985; 6:617–621.
4. Hollis PH, Malis LI, Zappulla RA: Neurological deterioration after lumbar puncture below complete spinal subarachnoid block. J Neurosurg 1986; 6:253–256.
5. Katz BH, Quencer RM, Hinks RS: Comparison of gradient-recalled-echo and T2-weighted spin-echo pulse sequences in intramedullary spinal lesions. AJNR 1989; 10:815–822.
6. Czervionke LF, Daniels DL: Cervical spine anatomy and pathologic processes: Applications of new MR imaging techniques. Radiol Clin North Am 1988; 26:921–947.
7. Yousem DM, Atlas SW, Goldberg HI, et al: Degenerative narrowing of the cervical spine neural foramina: Evaluation with high-resolution 3DFT gradient-echo MR imaging. AJNR 1991; 12:229–236.
8. Tsuruda JS, Norman D, Dillon W, et al: 3-Dimensional gradient-recalled MR imaging as a screening tool for the diagnosis of cervical radiculopathy. AJNR 1989; 10:1263–1271.
9. Aguila IA, Piraino DW, Modic MT, et al: The intranuclear cleft of the intravertebral disk: Magnetic resonance imaging. Radiology 1985; 155:155–158.
10. Kostelic JK, Haughton VM, Sether LA: Lumbar spinal nerves in the neural foramen: MR appearance. Radiology 1991; 178:837–839.
11. Nguyen CM, Ho KC, Yu S, et al: An experimental model to study contrast enhancement in MR imaging of the intervertebral disk. AJNR 1989; 10:811–814.
12. Sze G, Stimac GK, Bartlett C, et al: Multicenter study of gadopentetate dimeglumine as an MR contrast agent: Evaluation in patients with spinal tumors. AJNR 1990; 11:967–974.
13. Sze G: Gadolinium-DTPA in spinal disease. Radiol Clin North Am 1988; 26:1009–1024.
14. Breger RK, Williams AL, Daniels DL, et al: Contrast enhancement in spinal MR imaging. AJNR 1989; 10:633–637.
15. Sze G, Krol G, Zimmerman RD, et al: Intramedullary disease of the spine: Diagnosis using gadolinium-DTPA-enhanced MR imaging. AJNR 1988; 9:847–858.
16. Stimac GK, Porter BA, Olson DO, et al: Gadolinium-DTPA-enhanced MR imaging of spinal neoplasms: Preliminary investigation and comparison with unenhanced spin-echo and STIR sequences. AJNR 1988; 9:839–846.
17. Parizl PM, Balériaux D, Rodesch G, et al: GD-DTPA-enhanced MR imaging of spinal tumors. AJNR 1989; 10:249–258.
18. Lim V, Sobel DF, Zyroff J: Spinal cord pial metastases: MR imaging with gadopentetate dimeglumine. AJNR 1990; 11:975–982.
19. Sze G, Abramson A, Krol G, et al: Gadolinium-DTPA in the evaluation of intradural extramedullary spinal disease. AJNR 1988; 9:153–163.
20. Zimmerman RA, Bilaniuk LT: Imaging of tumors of the spinal canal and cord. Radiol Clin North Am 1988; 26:965–1007.
21. Miller GM, Forbes GS, Onofrio BM: Magnetic resonance imaging of the spine. Mayo Clin Proc 1989; 64:986–1004.
22. Lee SH, Coleman PE, Hahn FJ: Magnetic resonance imaging of degenerative disk disease of the spine. Radiol Clin North Am 1988; 26:949–964.
23. Sigal R, Denys A, Halimi P, et al: Ventriculus terminalis of the conus medullaris: MR imaging in four patients with congenital dilatation. AJNR 1991; 12:733–737.
24. Banna M: Syringomyelia in association with posterior fossa cyst. AJNR 1988; 9:867–873.
25. Gardner WJ: Hydrodynamic mechanism of syringomyelia: Its relationship to myelocele. J Neurol Neurosurg Psychiatry 1965; 28:247–259.
26. Williams B: Pathogenesis of syringomyelia. Lancet 1970; 1:142–143.
27. Ball MJ, Dayan AD: Pathogenesis of syringomyelia. Lancet 1972; 2:799–801.
28. Batnitzky S, Price HI, Gaughan MJ, et al: The radiology of syringohydromyelia. Radiographics 1983; 3:585–611.
29. Pinto I, Ibarburen C, Castello J: CT findings in cystic intramedullary oligodendroglioma. AJNR 1988; 9:213–214.
30. Kan S, Fox AJ, Vinúela F: Delayed metrizamide CT enhancement of syringomyelia: Postoperative observations. AJNR 1985; 6:613–616.
31. Flanders AE, Schaefer DM, Doan HT, et al: Acute cervical spine trauma: Correlation of MR imaging

findings with degree of neurologic deficit. Radiology 1990; 177:25–33.
32. Tobin WD, Layton DD: The diagnosis and natural history of spinal cord arteriovenous malformations. Mayo Clin Proc 1976; 51:637–646.
33. Di Chiro G, Doppman J, Ommaya AK: Selective arteriography of arteriovenous aneurysms of spinal cord. Radiology 1967; 88:1065–1085.
34. Dormont D, Gelbert F, Assouline E, et al: MR imaging of spinal cord arteriovenous malformations at 0.5 T: Study of 34 cases. AJNR 1988; 9:833–838.
35. Larsson E-M, Holtas S, Nilsson O: GD-DTPA-enhanced MR of suspected spinal multiple sclerosis. AJNR 1989; 10:1071–1076.
36. Sanders KA, Khandji AG, Mohr JP: Gadolinium-MRI in acute transverse myelopathy. Neurology 1990; 40:1614–1616.
37. Zweig G, Russell EJ: Radiation myelopathy of the cervical spinal cord: MR findings. AJNR 1990; 11:1188–1190.
38. Burns RJ, Jones AN, Robertson JS: Pathology of radiation myelopathy. J Neurol Neurosurg Psychiatry 1972; 35:888–898.
39. Sze G, Bravo S, Krol G: Spinal lesions: Quantitative and qualitative temporal evolution of gadopentetate dimeglumine enhancement in MR imaging. Radiology 1989; 170:849–856.
40. Barloon TJ, Yuh WTC, Calvin Yang CJ, et al: Spinal subarachnoid tumor seeding from intracranial metastases: MR findings. J Comput Assist Tomogr 1987; 11:242–244.
41. Johnson CE, Sze G: Benign lumbar arachnoiditis: MR imaging with gadopentetate dimeglumine. AJNR 1990; 11:763–770.
42. Sklar EML, Quencer RM, Green BA, et al: Complications of epidural anesthesia: MR appearance of abnormalities. Radiology 1991; 181:549–554.
43. Ross JS, Masaryk TJ, Modic MT, et al: MR imaging of lumbar arachnoiditis. AJNR 1987; 8:885–892.
44. Sklar E, Quencer RM, Green BA, et al: Acquired spinal subarachnoid cyst: Evaluation with MR, CT, myelography and intraoperative sonography. AJNR 1989; 10:1097–1104.
45. Yu S, Haughton VM, Sether LA, et al: Criteria for classifying normal and degenerated lumbar intervertebral disks. Radiology 1989; 170:523–526.
46. Ross JS, Modic MT, Masaryk TJ: Tears of the anulus fibrosus: Assessment with GD-DTPA-enhanced MR imaging. AJNR 1989; 10:1251–1254.
47. Ross JS, Modic MT, Masaryk TJ, et al: Assessment of extradural degenerative disease with GD-DTPA-enhanced MR imaging: Correlation with surgical and pathological findings. AJNR 1989; 10:1243–1249.
48. Schellinger D, Manz HJ, Vidic B, et al: Disk fragment migration. Radiology 1990; 175:831–836.
49. Masaryk TJ, Ross JS, Modic MT, et al: High resolution MR imaging of sequestered lumbar intervertebral disks. AJNR 1988; 9:351–358.
50. Murayama S, Namaguchi Y, Robinson AE: The diagnosis of herniated intervertebral disks with MR imaging. A comparison of gradient-refocused-echo and spin-echo pulse sequences. AJNR 1990; 11:17–22.
51. Awwad EE, Martin DS, Smith KR: The nuclear trail sign in thoracic herniated disks. AJNR 1992; 13:137–143.
52. Hedberg MC, Drayer BP, Flom RA, et al: Gradient echo (GRASS) MR imaging in cervical radiculopathy. AJNR 1988; 9:145–151.
53. Teresi LM, Lufkin RB, Reicher MA, et al: Asymptomatic degenerative disk disease and spondylosis of the cervical spine: MR imaging. Radiology 1987; 164:83–88.
54. Sotiropoulos S, Chafetz NI, Lang P, et al: Differentiation between postoperative scar and recurrent disk herniation: Prospective comparison of MR, CT and contrast enhanced CT. AJNR 1989; 10:639–643.
55. Braun IF, Hoffman JC, Davis PC, et al: Contrast enhancement in CT differentiation between recurrent disk herniation and postoperative scar: Prospective study. AJNR 1985; 6:607–612.
56. Ross JS, Delamarter R, Hueftle MG, et al: Gadolinium-DTPA-enhanced imaging of the postoperative lumbar spine: Time course and mechanism of enhancement. AJNR 1989; 10:37–46.
57. Bundschuh CV, Stein L, Slusser JH, et al: Distinguishing between scar and recurrent herniated disk in postoperative patients: Value of contrast-enhanced CT and MR imaging. AJNR 1990; 11:949–958.
58. Ross JS, Blaser S, Masaryk TJ, et al: GD-DTPA-enhancement of postoperative epidural scar: An experimental model. AJNR 1989; 10:1083–1088.
59. Ross JS, Masaryk TJ, Schrader M, et al: MR imaging of the postoperative lumbar spine: Assessment with gadopentetate dimeglumine. AJNR 1990; 11:771–776.
60. Bundschuh CV, Modic MT, Ross JS, et al: Epidural fibrosis and recurrent disk herniation in the lumbar spine: MR imaging assessment. AJNR 1988; 9:169–178.
61. Law JD, Lehman RAW, Kirsch WM: Reoperation after lumbar intervertebral disk surgery. J Neurosurg 1978; 48:259–263.
62. Hueftle MG, Modic MT, Ross JS, et al: Lumbar spine: Postoperative MR imaging with GD-DTPA. Radiology 1988; 167:817–824.
63. Liu SS, Williams KD, Drayer BP, et al: Synovial cysts of the lumbosacral spine: Diagnosis by MR imaging. AJNR 1989; 10:1239–1242.
64. Gorey MT, Hyman RA, Black KS, et al: Lumbar synovial cysts eroding bone. AJNR 1992; 13:161–163.
65. Silbergleit R, Gebarski SS, Brunberg JA, et al: Lumbar synovial cysts: Correlation of myelographic, CT, MR, and pathologic findings. AJNR 1990; 11:777–779.
66. Modic MT, Steinberg PM, Ross JS, et al: Degenerative disk disease: Assessment of changes in vertebral body marrow with MR imaging. Radiology 1988; 166:193–199.
67. Yamashita Y, Takahashi M, Matsuno Y, et al: Spinal cord compression due to ossification of ligaments: MR imaging. Radiology 1990; 175:843–848.
68. Yuh WTC, Zachar CK, Barloon TJ, et al: Vertebral compression fractures: Distinction between benign and malignant causes with MR imaging. Radiology 1989; 172:215–218.
69. Batson OV: The vertebral vein system as a mechanism for the spread of metastases. AJR 1942; 48:715–718.
70. Baker LL, Goodman SB, Perkash I, et al: Benign versus pathologic compression fractures of vertebral bodies: Assessment with conventional spin-echo, chemical-shift, and STIR MR imaging. Radiology 1990; 174:495–502.
71. Smoker WRK, Godersky JC, Knutzon RK, et al: The role of MR imaging in evaluating metastatic spinal disease. AJNR 1987; 8:901–908.
72. Horowitz SW, Fine M, Azar-Kia B: Differentiation of benign versus metastatic vertebral body compression fractures. Neuroradiology 1991; 33:114–116.

73. Sze G, Krol G, Zimmerman RD, et al: Malignant extradural spinal tumors: MR imaging with Gd-DTPA. Radiology 1988; 167:217–223.
74. Thrush A, Enzmann D: MR imaging of infectious spondylitis. AJNR 1990; 11:1171–1180.
75. Modic MT, Feiglin DH, Piraino DW, et al: Vertebral osteomyelitis: Assessment using MR. Radiology 1985; 157:157–166.
76. Sandhu FS, Dillon WP: Spinal epidural abscess: Evaluation with contrast-enhanced MR imaging. AJNR 1991; 12:1087–1093.
77. Smith AS, Weinstein MA, Mizushima A, et al: MR imaging characteristics of tuberculous spondylitis versus vertebral osteomyelitis. AJNR 1989; 10:619–625.
78. Thomeier WC, Brown DC, Mirvis SE: The laterally tilted dens: A sign of subtle odontoid fracture on plain radiography. AJNR 1990; 11:605–608.
79. Gehweiler JA, Clark WM, Schaaf RE, et al: Cervical spine trauma: The common combined conditions. Radiology 1979; 130:77–86.
80. Powers B, Miller MD, Kramer RS, et al: Traumatic anterior atlanto-occipital dislocation. Neurosurgery 1979; 4:12–17.
81. Chance GQ: Note on a type of flexion fracture of the spine. Br J Radiol 1948; 21:452–453.
82. Atlas SW, Regenbogen V, Rogers LF, et al: The radiographic characterization of burst fractures of the spine. AJNR 1986; 7:675–682.
83. Brunberg JA, Latchaw RE, Kanal E, et al: Magnetic resonance imaging of spinal dysraphism. Radiol Clin North Am 1988; 26:181–205.
84. Naidich TP, McLone DG, Mutluer S: New understanding of dorsal dysraphism with lipoma (lipomyeloschisis): Radiologic evaluation and surgical correlation. AJR 1983; 140:1065–1078.

13

PEDIATRIC NEUROIMAGING

CONGENITAL MALFORMATIONS

The common congenital malformations will be presented in four separate categories based upon a classification scheme proposed by van der Knapp and Valk.[1] Multiplanar imaging capabilities and increased tissue contrast render magnetic resonance imaging (MRI) the ideal modality to evaluate these anomalies.

Dorsal Induction

Dorsal induction takes place between the third and fourth gestational weeks. The notochordal process extends from the primitive knot to the cranial pole of the embryo, inducing the formation of the neural plate. The neural plate gives rise to the neural tube, the precursor of the brain and spinal cord. Failure of dorsal induction encompasses the neural tube defects, which include anencephaly, Chiari malformations, encephalocele, and various spinal dysraphic conditions previously discussed (see Chapter 12) (Table 13–1).

Chiari Malformations

Chiari I

The Chiari I malformation results in caudal displacement of the cerebellar tonsils more than 5 mm below the foramen magnum. Typ-

Table 13–1. DORSAL INDUCTION (3–4 WEEKS)

	Radiographic Findings	Comments
Chiari I malformation	Cerebellar tonsillar ectopia (>5 mm below foramen magnum) 4th ventricle—normal position, may be small	Hydromyelia Hydrocephalus Craniocervical junction anomalies
Chiari II malformation	Cerebellum—dysplastic, tonsillar and vermian ectopia 4th ventricle—caudally displaced, small or absent Mesencephalon—elongated Tectal plate—dysplastic Aqueduct—stenotic Falx cerebri—hypoplastic, fenestrated Tentorium—hypoplastic Lateral ventricles—dysmorphic	Myelomeningocele Corpus callosum dysgenic (1/3) Lückenschädel—transient
Encephalocele	Skull defect—occipital, parietal, frontal, basal Contains herniated meninges and brain parenchyma	Chiari III—occipital encephalocele that contains dysplastic cerebellum

ically, the fourth ventricle is in normal position but may be attenuated in shape. Patients may be asymptomatic until early adulthood, at which time they show clinical evidence of a foramen magnum lesion. Frequently, the Chiari I malformation is detected as an incidental finding on MRI.

Patients have hydrocephalus (35%), hydromyelia (30 to 70%), and anterior angulation or mild kinking of the cervical medullary junction. Craniocervical junction abnormalities may include basilar impression, occipitalization of C1, and Klippel-Feil syndrome.[2]

Cerebellar ectopia and hydromyelia are best detected on MRI (Fig. 13–1). Myelography may be used in conjunction with postmyelographic computed tomography (CT) to document tonsilar ectopia and hydromyelia.

Chiari II

The Chiari II malformation involves a constellation of abnormalities affecting the cerebellum, brainstem, posterior fossa, and craniocervical junction. The volume of the posterior fossa is decreased and there is caudal herniation of the cerebellar tonsils and the vermis through the foramen magnum a variable distance into the dorsal aspect of the cervical spinal canal (Fig. 13–2). The cervicomedullary

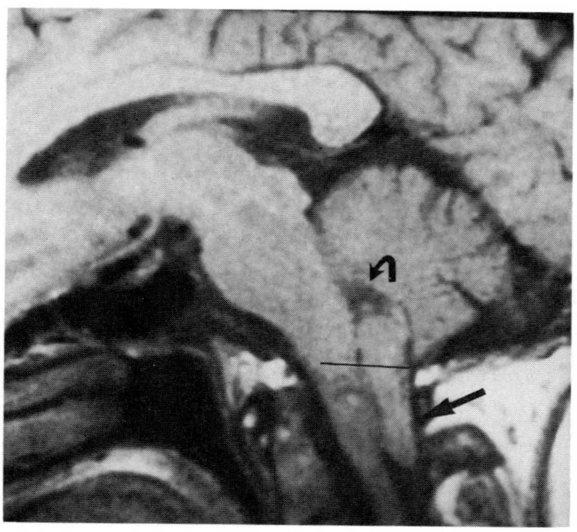

Figure 13–1. Chiari I malformation (40-year-old male). Parasagittal T1. The cerebellar tonsils (*arrow*) are ectopic, extending 2.5 cm below the foramen magnum (*black line*). The fourth ventricle (*curved arrow*) is caudally displaced and moderately attenuated.

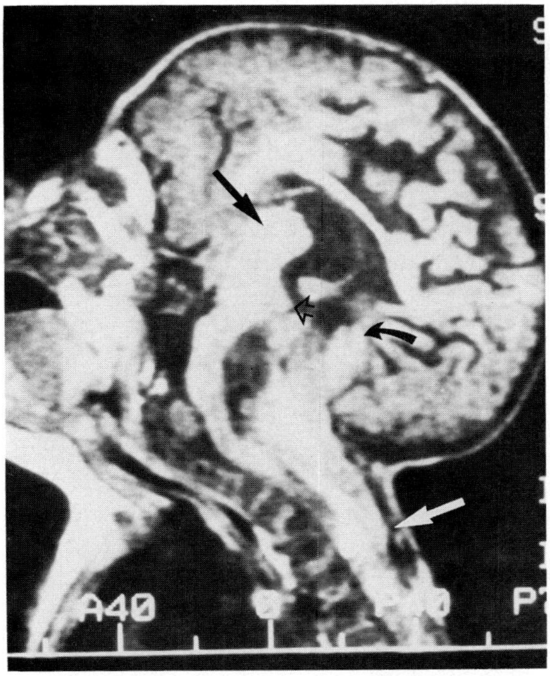

Figure 13–2. Chiari II malformation (6-month-old male). Parasagittal T1. The cerebellum is markedly dysmorphic, extending through an enlarged foramen magnum dorsal to the cervical cord to the lower cervical spine (*white arrow*). The dysplastic cerebellum also extends above the hypoplastic tentorium (*curved arrow*). The brainstem is elongated and the tectal plate (*open arrow*) beaked dorsally. The massa intermedia (*black arrow*) is markedly prominent.

junction is frequently kinked and may be partially compressed because of the excessive tissue within the enlarged foramen magnum. The fourth ventricle is caudally displaced and may be small or inapparent. The petrous ridges may be scalloped and the internal auditory canal foreshortened owing to the deformity caused by the contents of the small posterior fossa.[3] The straight sinus may be vertically oriented with a low insertion near the foramen magnum.[4] The tentorial leaves are hypoplastic, creating a prominent or widened tentorial incisura[3] (Fig. 13–3).

A towering cerebellum has been described,[2, 5, 6] in which the cephalad surface of the cerebellum ascends through the widened incisura. Varying degrees of cerebellar dysplasia may also be present.[6] The cerebellum may be small in up to 75% of cases, allowing the supratentorial parenchyma to herniate downward through the incisura,[4] and flattening the superior surface of the cerebellum.

The falx cerebri is hypoplastic or fenestrated in all cases; this is most marked anteriorly.[3] Interdigitation of gyri of the inner hemispheric fissure corroborates the falx hypoplasia.

A spectrum of midbrain anomalies may exist. The midbrain may range from normal in appearance to severely dysplastic with fusion of the tectal plate and beaking or dorsal pointing of the midbrain.[5] The cerebellum may overgrow the midbrain anterolaterally, effacing the cerebellopontine angle (CPA).[2, 5] The mesencephalon is elongated, resulting in an increased mammillopontine distance (the distance between the mammillary bodies and the upper surface of the pons). Normal mammillopontine distance is 1.2 cm; however, it ranges between 1.3 and 3 cm in patients with Chiari II malformation.[4]

The lateral ventricles are dysmorphic, the extent of which may not be apparent until after the patient has been shunted. The caudate nucleus is prominent, resulting in inferior pointing of the frontal horns. The superolateral surfaces of the frontal horns are flattened.[7] The septum pellucidum is absent in approximately 40% of patients.[2] The atria and occipital horns are asymmetrically enlarged with less cerebral mantle over the occipital lobes.

The third ventricle may be normal in size to mildly dilated and may maintain an hourglass configuration owing to the enlarged massa intermedia that is present in more than two thirds of patients.[6] The aqueduct may be stenotic in nearly 50% of patients because of the midbrain deformity.[4]

The posterior corpus callosum is dysgenic in one third of patients.[6] The radiographic findings of dysgenesis of the corpus callosum are presented at the end of this section.

The typical skull changes are presented in Chapter 1 and consist of irregular honeycombed ridges along the inner table. This mesenchymal developmental anomaly is transient, generally seen in only the first year of life.

Nearly all patients with Chiari II malformation present with myelomeningocele, most commonly located in the lumbar region. The more cephalad the origin of the myelomeningocele, the greater the neurologic sequelae. Hydrocephalus, present in up to 90% of patients, may not develop until after the repair

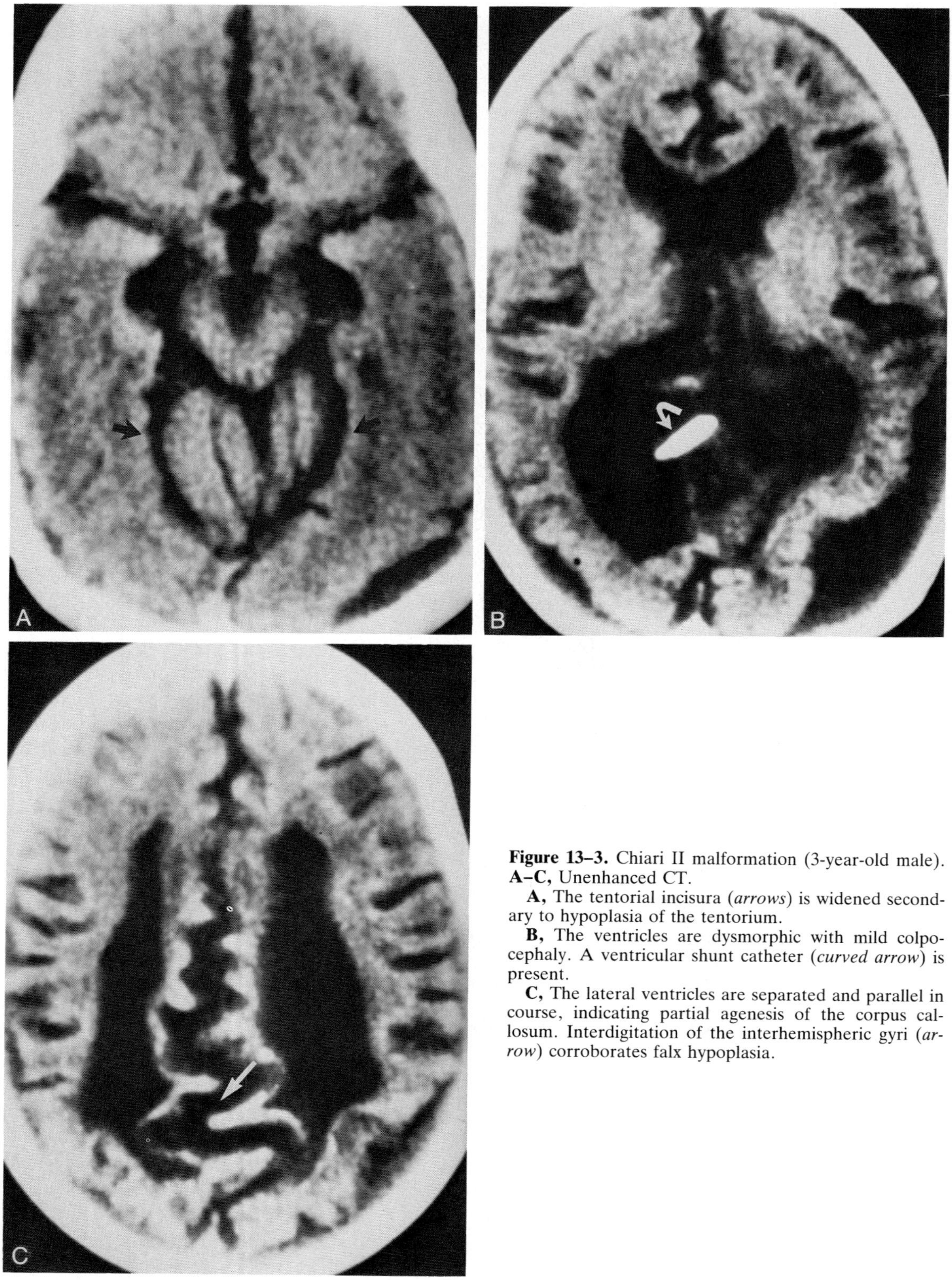

Figure 13–3. Chiari II malformation (3-year-old male). **A–C,** Unenhanced CT.

A, The tentorial incisura (*arrows*) is widened secondary to hypoplasia of the tentorium.

B, The ventricles are dysmorphic with mild colpocephaly. A ventricular shunt catheter (*curved arrow*) is present.

C, The lateral ventricles are separated and parallel in course, indicating partial agenesis of the corpus callosum. Interdigitation of the interhemispheric gyri (*arrow*) corroborates falx hypoplasia.

of the myelomeningocele. Hydromyelia occurs in 20 to 80% of pathologic reports yet is detected by MRI in only 5% of patients.[4]

Encephalocele

Encephaloceles, which result from herniation of brain or meninges, or both, through a skull defect, occur in approximately 1 in 4000 to 5000 deliveries. Encephaloceles most commonly occur in the occipital region followed by the parietal, frontal, and basal regions.

Encephaloceles associated with herniated dysplastic posterior fossa contents are designated Chiari III malformations. In addition to the encephalocele, radiographic findings similar to those of Chiari II are present.[8] The midbrain is deformed in all patients, the corpus callosum is partially or completely dysgenic (77%), the petrous temporal bone and clivus are scalloped (56%), the tonsils are herniated (43%), and hydrocephalus and hydromyelia are present in 22% and 30% of patients, respectively. The contents of the encephalocele vary in size and degree of dysplasia (Figs. 13–4, 13–5). At least a portion of the cerebellum herniates in all patients, and in one third of patients this portion may be accompanied by a variable amount of the occipital lobe. Aberrant deep veins and venous sinuses are frequently found traversing the encephalocele. A dysmorphic ventricle may be trapped within the encephalocele.

Ventral Induction

Ventral induction, which occurs during the fifth to 10th week of gestation, is the series of events that result in formation of the brain and face. The primitive brain forms from the prosencephalon (forebrain), mesencephalon (midbrain), and rhombencephalon (hindbrain). The prosencephalon forms the bulk of the supratentorial brain parenchyma and further subdivides into the telencephalon (cerebral hemispheres and lateral ventricles) and the diencephalon (thalamus, hypothalamus). The rhombencephalon divides into the myelen-

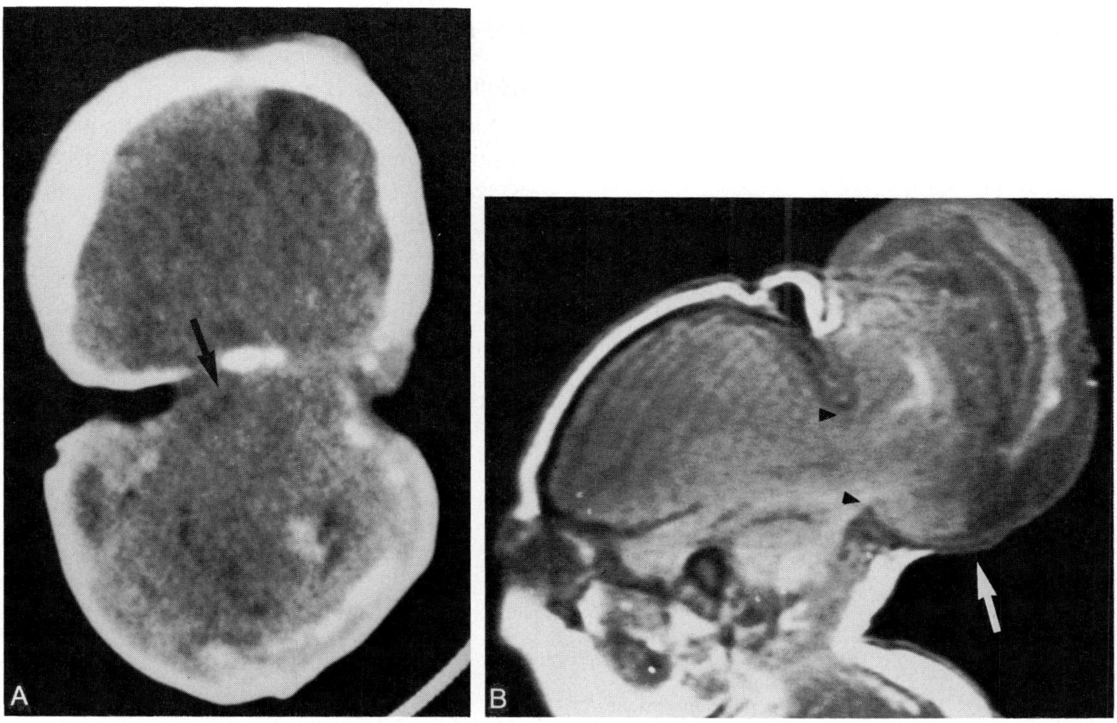

Figure 13–4. Chiari III malformation (newborn male).

A, Axial CT. The skull is small, and a significant proportion of the intracranial contents are within an encephalocele (*arrow*).

B, Parasagittal T1. A large skull defect (*arrowheads*) permits herniation of dysplastic brain into the large encephalocele (*arrow*).

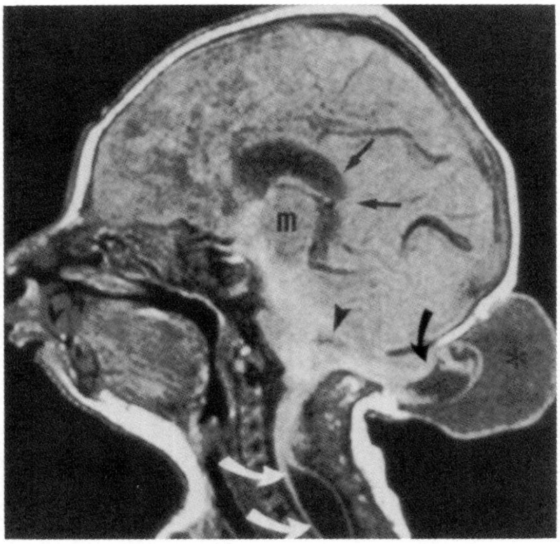

Figure 13–5. Chiari III malformation (newborn). Parasagittal T1. The massa intermedia (*M*) is prominent and the tectal plate deformed and nonrecognizable. The fourth ventricle (*arrowhead*) is deformed and the posterior corpus callosum (*arrows*) dysmorphic. The dysplastic cerebellum (*curved arrow*) herniates through a skull defect into the cerebrospinal fluid (CSF)–filled encephalocele. A syringomyelia (*curved white arrows*) is noted in the middle to lower cervical cord. (From Castillo M, Quencer RM, Dominguez R: Chiari III malformation: Imaging Features. AJNR 13:107–113, 1992, © by American Society of Neuroradiology.)

cephalon (medulla) and the metencephalon (pons, cerebellum, and upper fourth ventricle). Disorders of ventral induction result in holoprosencephaly, septo-optic dysplasia, and Dandy-Walker syndrome (Table 13–2).

Holoprosencephaly

Holoprosencephaly results in incomplete diverticulation of the forebrain. A spectrum of severity ranges from the most severe alobar form to the less severe semilobar form to the least severe lobar form. Because of the intimate relationship between the developing face and brain, the more severe forms are associated with midline facial anomalies including hypotelorism, micro-ophthalmia, micrognathia, cleft lip and palate, cyclopia, and trigonocephaly.

Alobar

Alobar holoprosencephaly results in an enlarged horseshoe-shaped monoventricle. A

Table 13–2. VENTRAL INDUCTION (5–8 WEEKS)

	Radiographic Findings	Comments
Holoprosencephaly		
Alobar	Horseshoe-shaped monoventricle Dorsal cyst Absent falx, tentorium, corpus callosum, septum pellucidum and interhemispheric fissure Fused thalami	Facial anomalies: cyclopia, hypotelorism, microphthalmia, micrognathia
Semilobar	Monoventricle smaller, partial differentiation into frontal temporal, occipital horns Septum pellucidum and corpus callosum absent Falx and interhemispheric fissure partially developed posteriorly	Facial anomalies less severe and less frequent
Lobar	Shallow, incomplete interhemispheric fissure anteriorly Septum pellucidum absent	Facial anomalies uncommon
Septo-optic Dysplasia	Absent to hypoplastic septum pellucidum Optic nerves hypoplastic	Schizencephaly Pituitary axis dysfunction
Dandy-Walker Syndrome	Posterior fossa cyst Hypoplastic vermis	Hydrocephalus Dysgenesis of corpus callosum Variant form more common

thin rim of cerebral mantle is present, separating the anterior portion of the monoventricle from the skull (Fig. 13–6). The posterior portion of the ventricle may be deformed by an enlarged dorsal cyst. The residual parenchyma is featureless with absence of the sylvian fissure and the opercular cortex, as well as the interhemispheric fissure, falx, tentorium, and corpus callosum.[2] Aplasia of the falx and tentorium are accompanied by absence of the internal cerebral vein, vein of Galen, inferior sagittal sinus, and superior sagittal sinus. The thalami are fused at the base of the monoventricle.

Semilobar

In this form the monoventricle persists, but it is smaller with early differentiation into occipital, temporal, and frontal horns. Septum pellucidum and corpus callosum are absent. The falx and interhemispheric fissure are partially present posteriorly. The cerebral mantle increases significantly in volume (Figs. 13–7, 13–8).

Lobar

Excluding incomplete separation of the anterior-most cerebral hemisphere, the brain parenchyma may be normal. A shallow interhemispheric fissure is noted anteriorly. The septum pellucidum is absent and there may or may not be dysgenesis of the corpus callosum.

Septo-optic Dysplasia (SOD)

SOD is an anterior midline developmental anomaly of the forebrain thought to represent a mild form of holoprosencephaly. The ocular findings are presented in Chapter 9. The septum pellucidum is completely or partially absent and the optic nerves are hypoplastic (Fig. 13–9). In one study[9] nearly half of the patients with SOD had associated schizencephaly. The subset of patients with schizencephaly had normal-sized ventricles, a remnant of the septum pellucidum, and normal optic radiations, and they presented with visual symptoms or seizures. Patients with isolated SOD had white matter hypoplasia resulting in ventricular dilatation and complete absence of the septum pellucidum, and they had signs and symptoms of hypothalamic pituitary axis dysfunction. In 50 to 67% of patients, diabetes insipidus exists.[2, 9]

Dandy-Walker Syndrome

Dandy-Walker syndrome results in partial or complete vermian aplasia and a large posterior fossa cyst that displaces the cerebellum and replaces the fourth ventricle. The anomaly may be caused by atresia of the foramen of Magendie and foramina of Luschka of the fourth ventricle, with resultant cystic ventricular dilatation and displacement of the adjacent cerebellum. The noncommunicating hydrocephalus leads to megalocephaly. The posterior fossa cyst does not communicate with the subarachnoid space.

The Dandy-Walker variant, a more common form of this anomaly, results in partial dysgenesis of the vermis and a remnant fourth ventricle that communicates with a retrocerebellar cyst (Fig. 13–10). The supratentorial ventricular system is not usually obstructed.

A multitude of central nervous system (CNS) anomalies coexist with the Dandy-Walker syndrome, the most common of which is dysgenesis of the corpus callosum.

Neuronal Proliferation, Differentiation, and Histogenesis

The end result of this developmental process, the organization of cells into specific tissues, occurs between the second and fourth gestational months. Disorders of proliferation, differentiation, and histogenesis result in neoplastic and vascular malformations (Table 13–3). Phakomatoses are a result of abnormal histogenesis.

Phacomatoses

The phacomatoses are a group of hereditary disorders that involve dysplasias of one or more organ systems. Commonly, the lesions have cutaneous and CNS involvement. Most phacomatoses are autosomal dominant with a high spontaneous mutation rate and variable expressivity and penetrance.

Neurofibromatosis

Neurofibromatosis Type I (NF I) (von Recklinghausen's Disease). NF I is the most com-

Text continued on page 524

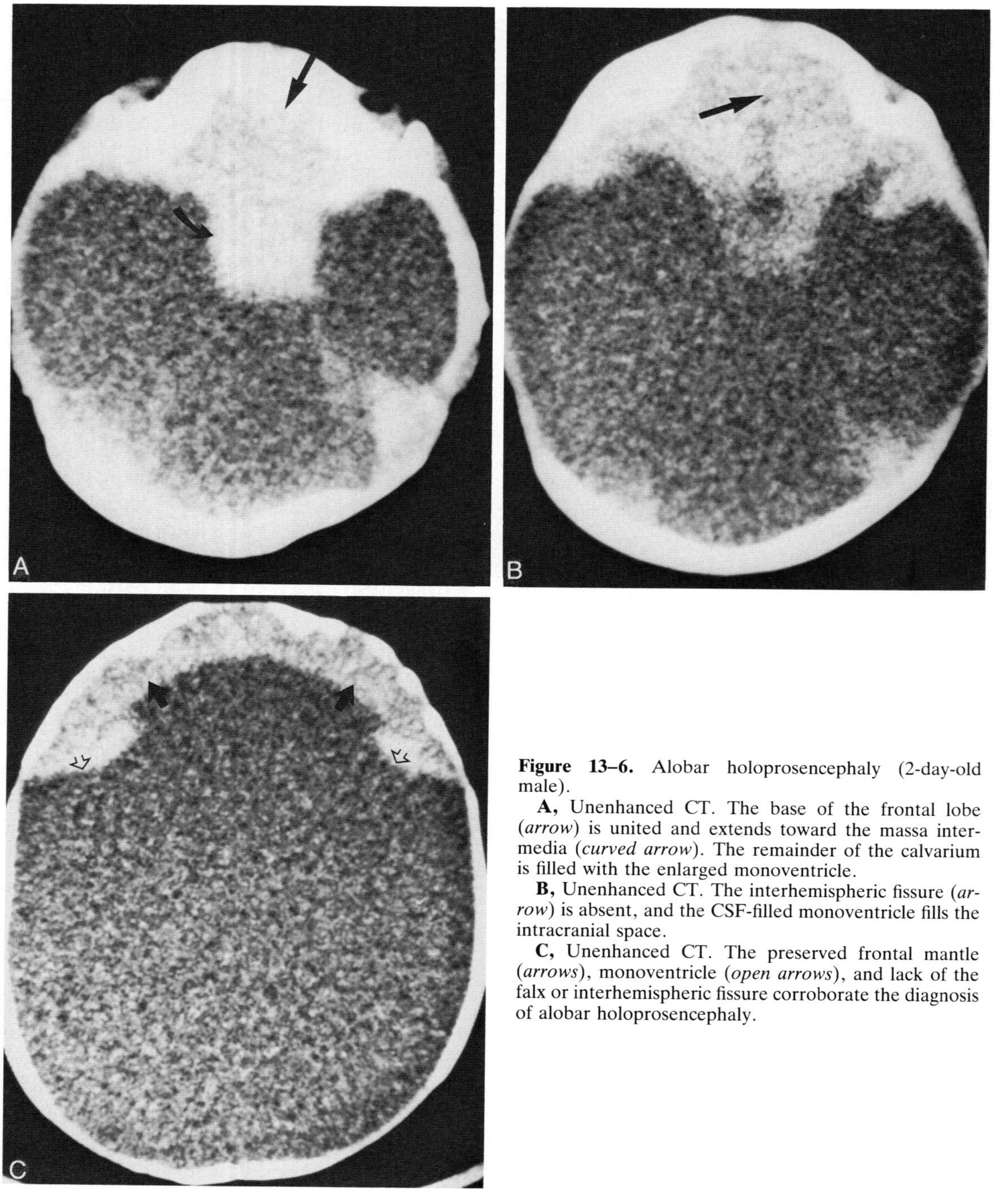

Figure 13–6. Alobar holoprosencephaly (2-day-old male).

A, Unenhanced CT. The base of the frontal lobe (*arrow*) is united and extends toward the massa intermedia (*curved arrow*). The remainder of the calvarium is filled with the enlarged monoventricle.

B, Unenhanced CT. The interhemispheric fissure (*arrow*) is absent, and the CSF-filled monoventricle fills the intracranial space.

C, Unenhanced CT. The preserved frontal mantle (*arrows*), monoventricle (*open arrows*), and lack of the falx or interhemispheric fissure corroborate the diagnosis of alobar holoprosencephaly.

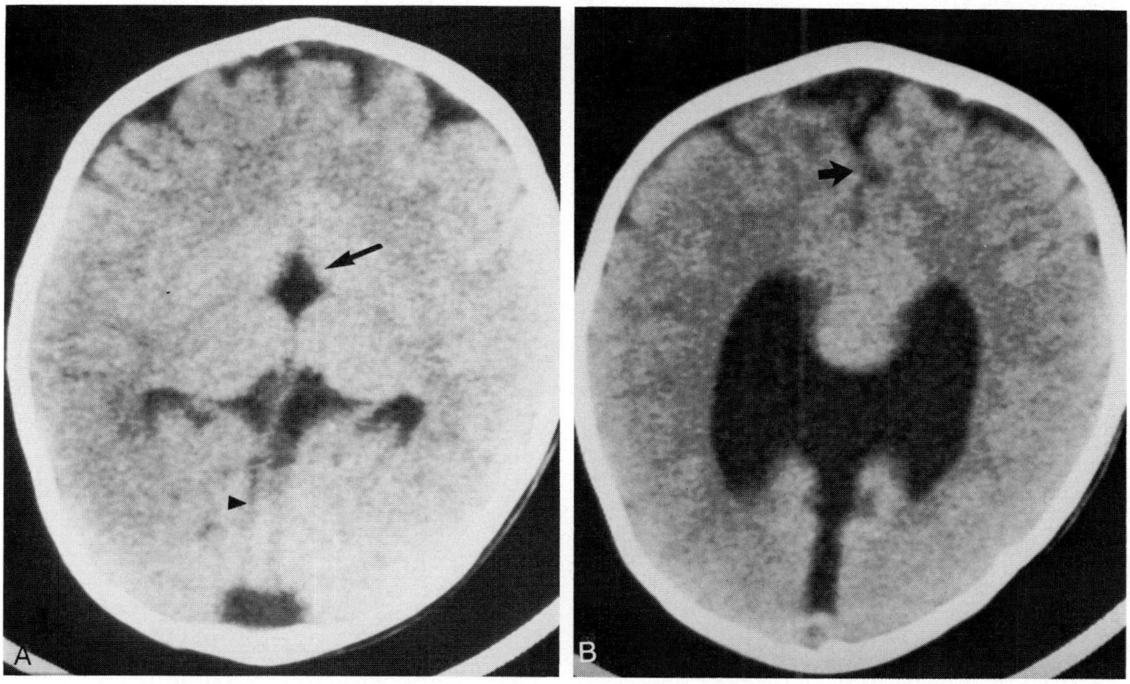

Figure 13–7. Semilobar holoprosencephaly (1-year-old male).

A, Unenhanced CT. A rudimentary third ventricle (*arrow*) is present. The anterior interhemispheric fissure is absent but is prominent posteriorly (*arrowhead*). The frontal lobes are fused.

B, Unenhanced CT. The monoventricle is present with a rudimentary interhemispheric fissure (*arrow*).

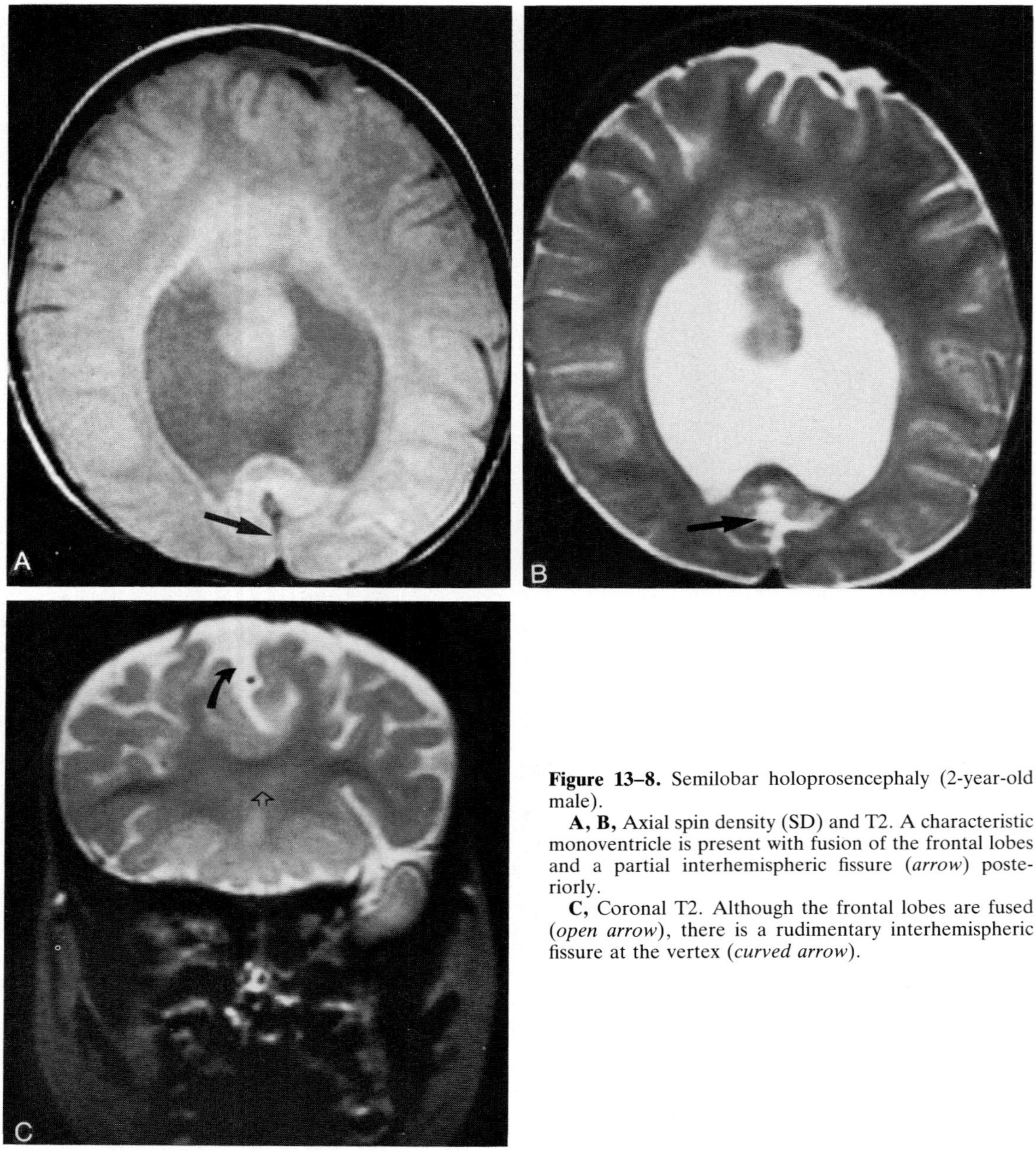

Figure 13–8. Semilobar holoprosencephaly (2-year-old male).

A, B, Axial spin density (SD) and T2. A characteristic monoventricle is present with fusion of the frontal lobes and a partial interhemispheric fissure (*arrow*) posteriorly.

C, Coronal T2. Although the frontal lobes are fused (*open arrow*), there is a rudimentary interhemispheric fissure at the vertex (*curved arrow*).

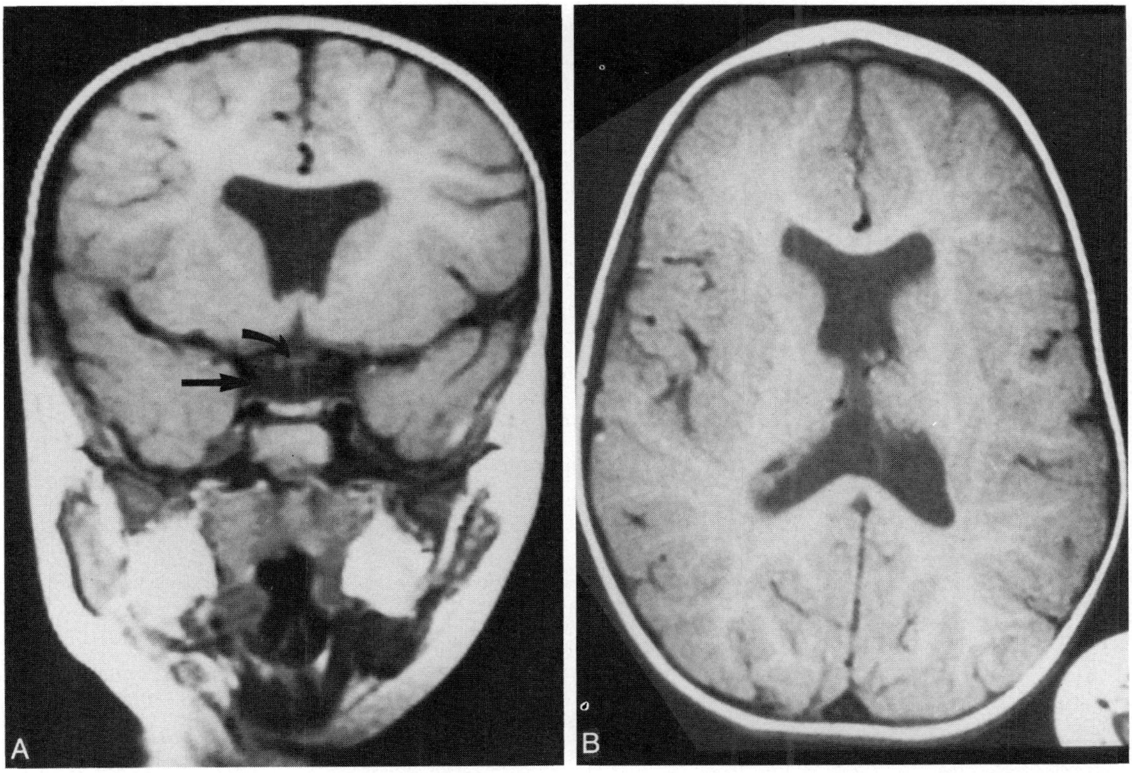

Figure 13–9. Septo-optic dysplasia (2-year-old female).

A, Coronal T1. The septum pellucidum is absent. The optic chiasm (*curved arrow*) is hypoplastic, and the suprasellar cistern (*arrow*) is prominent.

B, Axial T1. The frontal horns of the lateral ventricle communicate owing to absence of the midline septum pellucidum.

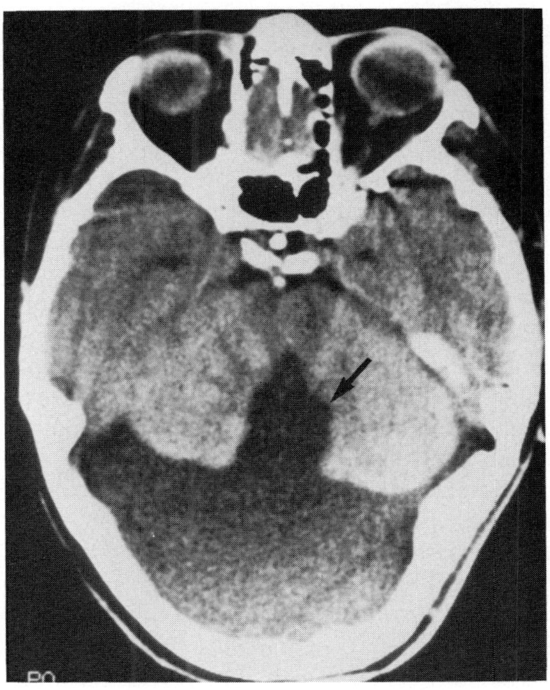

Figure 13–10. Dandy-Walker variant (61-year-old female). Enhanced CT; the vermis is hypoplastic, permitting direct communication between the rudimentary fourth ventricle (*arrow*) and the posterior fossa cyst. The cerebellar hemispheres are dysplastic.

Table 13–3. NEURONAL PROLIFERATION, DIFFERENTIATION, HISTOGENESIS (8–16 WEEKS)

	Radiographic Findings	Comments
Neurofibromatosis I	Optic nerve gliomas Gliomas of brain and spine High-signal T2 lesions in globus pallidus, brainstem, cerebellum, thalamus	1/4000 Chromosome 17 Tumors of glial origin Café-au-lait spots Lisch nodules Sphenoid dysplasia
Neurofibromatosis II	Multiple cranial nerve schwannomas and/or meningiomas	1/50,000 Chromosome 22 Tumors of brain covering
Tuberous Sclerosis	Subependymal nodules (calcified) Hamartomas (cortical, subcortical) Giant cell astrocytoma (foramen of Monro) White matter abnormalities	1/10,000–500,000 Chromosome 9? Facial angiofibroma, seizures, mental deficiency Cardiac rhabdomyosarcoma Retinal and renal hamartomas
Von Hippel–Lindau Disease	Cerebellar or cord hemangioblastomas	CNS hemangioblastomas Renal cell carcinoma Pheochromocytoma Cystic disease of liver, pancreas, kidney
Sturge-Weber Syndrome	Leptomeningeal venous angioma Parenchymal atrophy Calcified subjacent cortex Enlarged vascular choroid	Seizures, hemiplegia, mental retardation
Hydranencephaly	Anterior circulation parenchyma infarcted Posterior circulation parenchyma intact	In utero internal carotid artery occlusion Falx intact

mon of the phacomatoses, occurring in 1 in 4000 births. It is an autosomal dominant condition that has been traced to chromosome 17. Spontaneous mutation accounts for 50% of cases.

A multitude of CNS tumors occur with increased frequency in patients with NF I. The most common is optic nerve glioma, occurring in 10 to 70% of these patients.[10] Optic nerve gliomas most commonly present in the first decade, are relatively benign, and are of juvenile pilocystic histology. Bilaterality occurs in 25% of patients with NF I.[2] Multicentricity of visual pathway gliomas is pathognomonic for NF I. Tumors may extend to the optic chiasm, along the optic tracts, and to the optic radiations. Patients with NF I are also at risk for developing gliomas elsewhere within the brain and spinal cord.

Patients may have one or more neurofibromas or plexiform neurofibromas, the latter being pathognomonic for neurofibromatosis. Plexiform neurofibromas, although nonmetastasizing, are locally aggressive and tend to grow centripetally toward the brain.

Lisch nodules, which are small hamartomas or low-grade malignancies on the anterior surface of the iris, are associated conditions present in 90% of patients. Cutaneous manifestations include café-au-lait spots that may occur in the axilla. The greater wing of the sphenoid bone may be dysplastic or hypoplastic, permitting the temporal lobe to herniate into the orbit and producing pulsatile exophthalmos. A focal lucent defect in the left mid-lambdoid suture may be present. The dura may be ectatic and a thoracic meningocele may be present.

The radiographic workup of these patients is directed toward evaluating the multicentric mass lesions associated with the disease (Figs. 13–11 to 13–13). The orbital lesions are variable in size and may extend along the posterior visual apparatus; they have been discussed in Chapter 9.

The multifocal, high–T2 signal lesions discovered with MRI have received considerable attention.[10–15] The lesions are located in the globus pallidus, brainstem, cerebellum, and, less frequently, thalamus and internal capsule. The brainstem lesions tend to be more confluent and those elsewhere more discrete. These are clinically occult lesions[13–15] and do not correlate with CT findings, brainstem au-

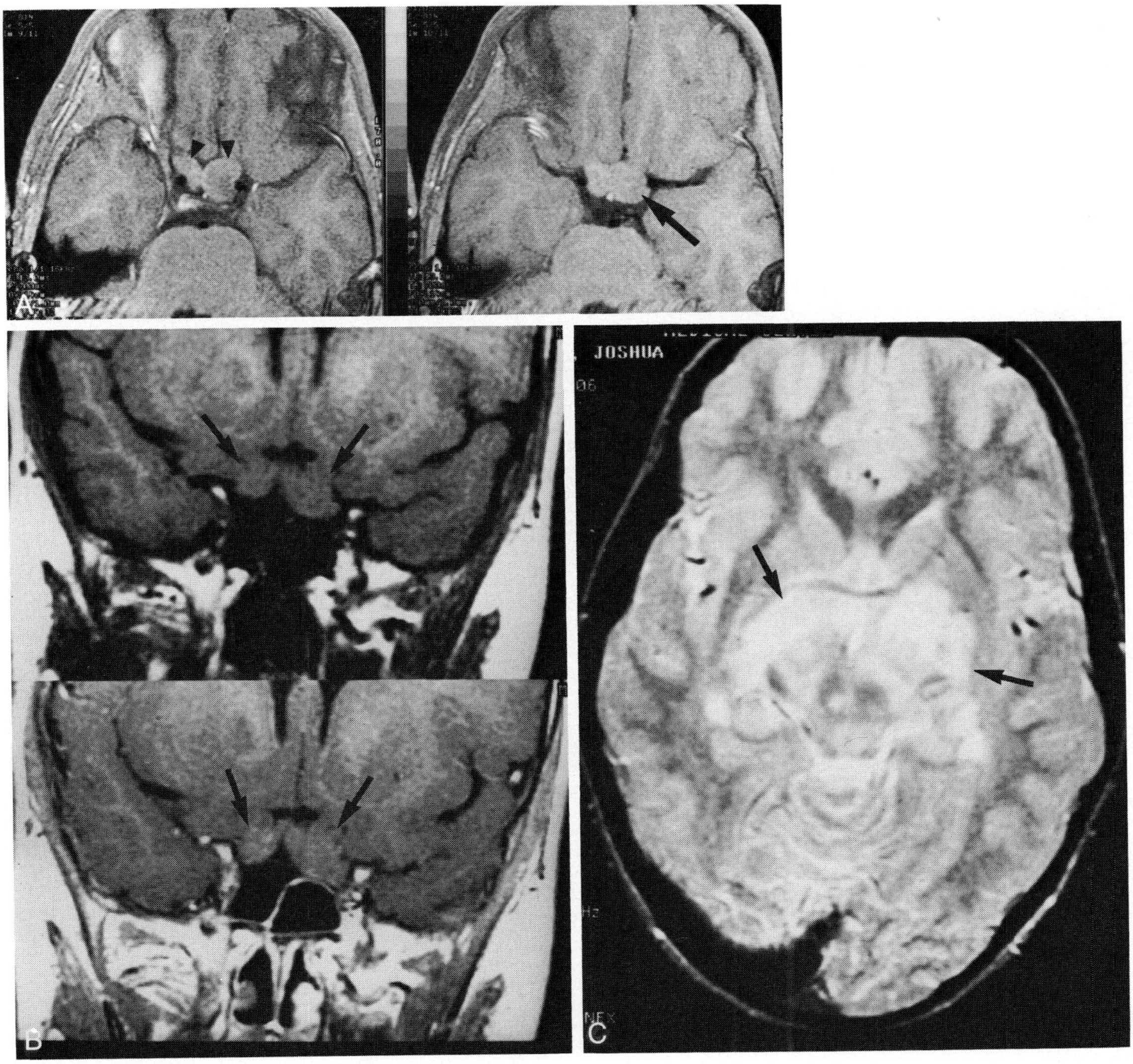

Figure 13–11. Neurofibromatosis (NF I) (6-year-old male).

A, Enhanced fat-saturated T1. A nonenhancing chiasmal mass (*arrow*) extends to the proximal optic nerves (*arrowheads*) bilaterally.

B, Coronal T1 (*top,* unenhanced; *bottom,* enhanced). The optic nerve tumors (*arrows*) extend into the optic canals bilaterally. There is no evidence of significant enhancement.

C, Axial T2. Multiple confluent high-signal foci (*arrows*) are present in the basal ganglia and midbrain bilaterally.

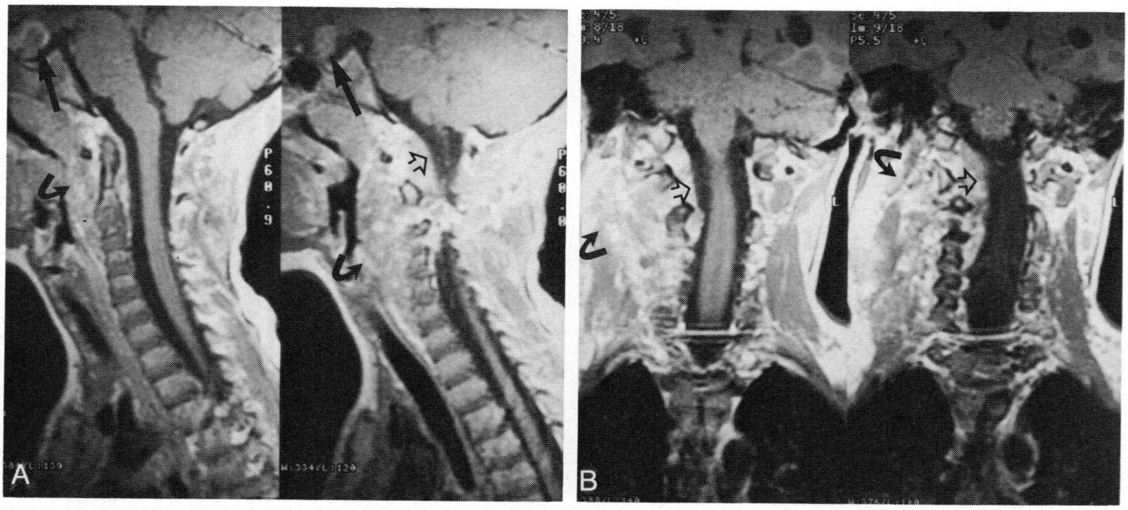

Figure 13–12. Neurofibromatosis (NF I) (12-year-old female).

A, Enhanced parasagittal T1. In addition to the heterogeneous enhancing optic nerve glioma (*arrow*), a heterogeneously enhancing plexiform neurofibroma infiltrates the paraspinal region, widening the prevertebral soft tissues (*curved arrow*) and extending into the spinal canal (*open arrow*).

B, Enhanced coronal T1. The paraspinal (*curved arrow*) and intraspinal (*open arrow*) moieties of the lesion are better depicted.

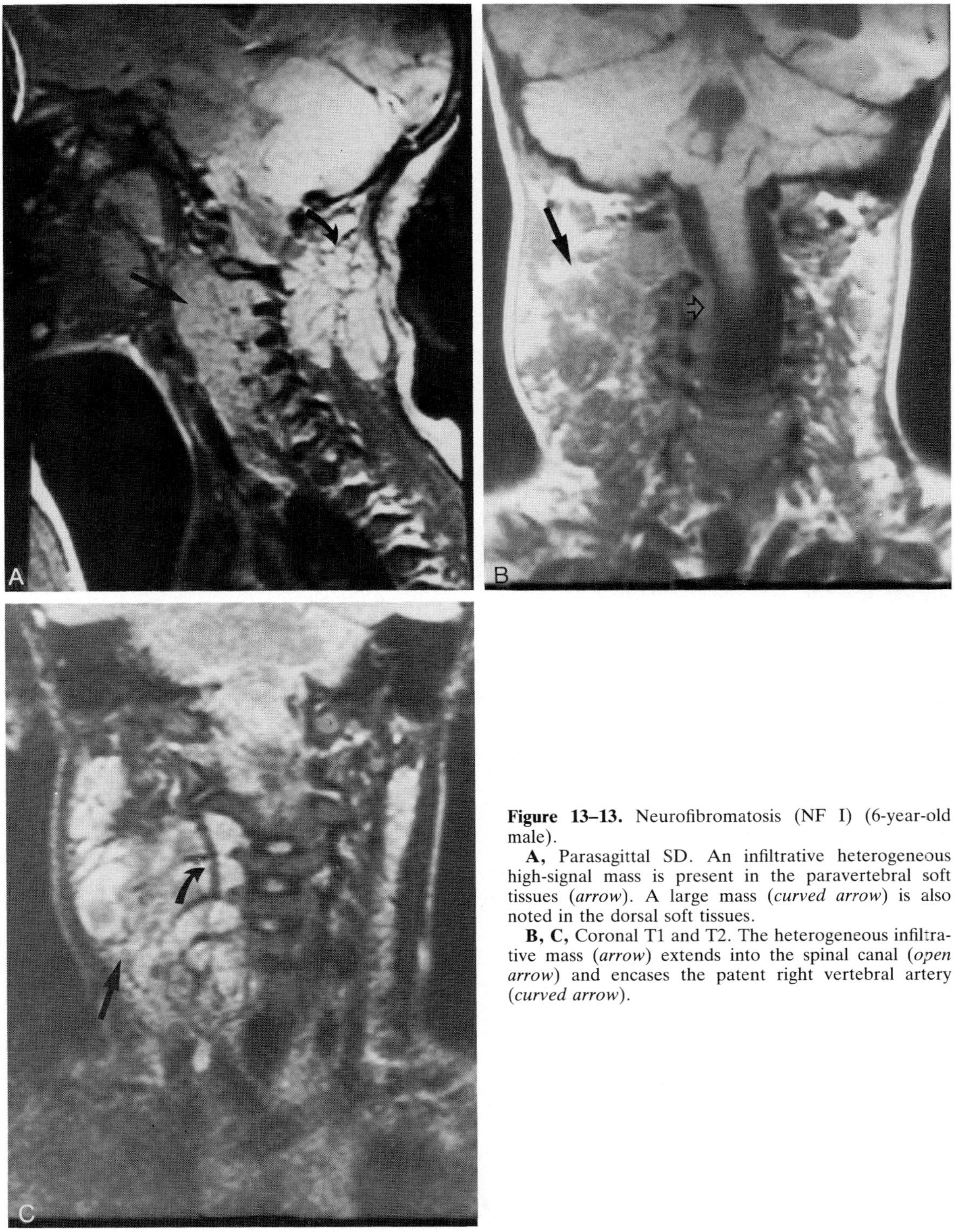

Figure 13–13. Neurofibromatosis (NF I) (6-year-old male).

A, Parasagittal SD. An infiltrative heterogeneous high-signal mass is present in the paravertebral soft tissues (*arrow*). A large mass (*curved arrow*) is also noted in the dorsal soft tissues.

B, C, Coronal T1 and T2. The heterogeneous infiltrative mass (*arrow*) extends into the spinal canal (*open arrow*) and encases the patent right vertebral artery (*curved arrow*).

ditory evoked response (BAER), electroencephalogram (EEG), school performance, or neurologic examination. The etiology and significance of these lesions remain speculative. Most commonly, the high-signal changes have been ascribed to hamartomas, heterotopias, or dysplastic tissue. These tend to be more common in younger patients and in those who have optic nerve gliomas.[12] Globus pallidus lesions are slightly different in that they tend to be larger than the others and uniquely hyperintense on T1-weighted images.

Neurofibromatosis Type II (NF II). NF II is an autosomal dominant condition that occurs in 1 in 50,000 individuals. NF II involves chromosome 22 and is associated with tumors of the covering of the brain.[12] Patients have multiple cranial nerve schwannomas and meningiomas. Bilateral eighth nerve schwannomas are strongly suggestive of NF II. The next most common cranial nerve to develop a schwannoma is the trigeminal nerve (Fig. 13–14).

The meningiomas may be multiple,[11] and in one series[12] nearly half the meningiomas were intraventricular. Use of intravenous (IV) contrast is imperative in evaluating extradural lesions that occur in patients with NF II.[12]

Recently, one investigator[16] reported a 63% incidence of intracranial calcifications in patients with NF II. Six calcifications were located on the choroid plexus, four in the cerebellar hemisphere, and one on the surface of the cerebral hemisphere. The proposed etiology of the intracranial calcification is calcium deposits within hamartomatous lesions.

Tuberous Sclerosis

Tuberous sclerosis is an autosomal dominant disease consisting of hamartomatous malformations of the brain, skin, heart, and kidney. Spontaneous mutation accounts for a high percentage (50 to 80%) of patients with this disease. The incidence is 1 in 500,000, with less severe forms found in up to 1 in 10,000 patients. The long arm of chromosome 9 has been implicated as the gene locus. There is no sexual or racial predilection. Patients may present at birth or between 2 and 6 years of age.[17]

The typical clinical triad consists of facial adenoma sebaceum (angiofibromas), seizures, and mental deficiency. In addition, patients may have subungual fibromas, cardiac rhabdomyosarcomas, and retinal and renal hamartomas. Intracranial involvement is characterized by subependymal nodules, cortical and subcortical hamartomas, giant cell astrocytomas, and white matter abnormalities.

Subependymal nodules are present on CT in up to 96% of patients.[18] The soft tissue masses are isodense to gray matter, less than 1.5 cm in greatest linear dimension, and variably located in the subependymal region, extending into the lateral ventricle. The nodules originate most often from the surface of the caudate nucleus or elsewhere along the lateral ventricle. It is very uncommon to see the nodules elsewhere within the ventricular system. CT detects calcification in these nodules in up to 88% of patients[18] (Fig. 13–15).

The subependymal nodules are variable in signal intensity and best seen with T1 sequences,[19] yet T2 spin echo more accurately detects the calcification. Gradient echo techniques are more sensitive than spin echo at detecting these periventricular calcified nodules.[20] The majority of subependymal nodules do not enhance; however, ringlike or nodular enhancement has been reported with MRI in up to 31% of lesions.[21] This enhancement appears to be field strength dependent, occurring in 10% and 57% of lesions imaged on a 0.3-T and 1.5-T unit, respectively.[21]

Parenchymal hamartomas may be located in the cortical or subcortical region and are more common in the frontal lobe, followed by the parietal, occipital, and temporal lobes.[21] These lesions are variable in size and shape and are generally hypointense to parenchyma on T1 and hyperintense on T2 (Fig. 13–16). MRI-documented incidence of hamartomas in patients with tuberous sclerosis is 94%.[18] The hamartomas are less apparent on CT (62%), appearing as subtle regions of hypodensity. The hamartomas are not associated with edema or a significant degree of mass effects. Nodular or homogeneous enhancement has been reported in 34% of lesions on MRI.[21]

Giant cell astrocytomas are low-grade neoplasms derived from giant astrocytes found within the subependymal nodules. Although malignant degeneration into a giant cell has been reported everywhere along the ventricular surface, the most common location is at the foramen of Monro. The giant cell tumors

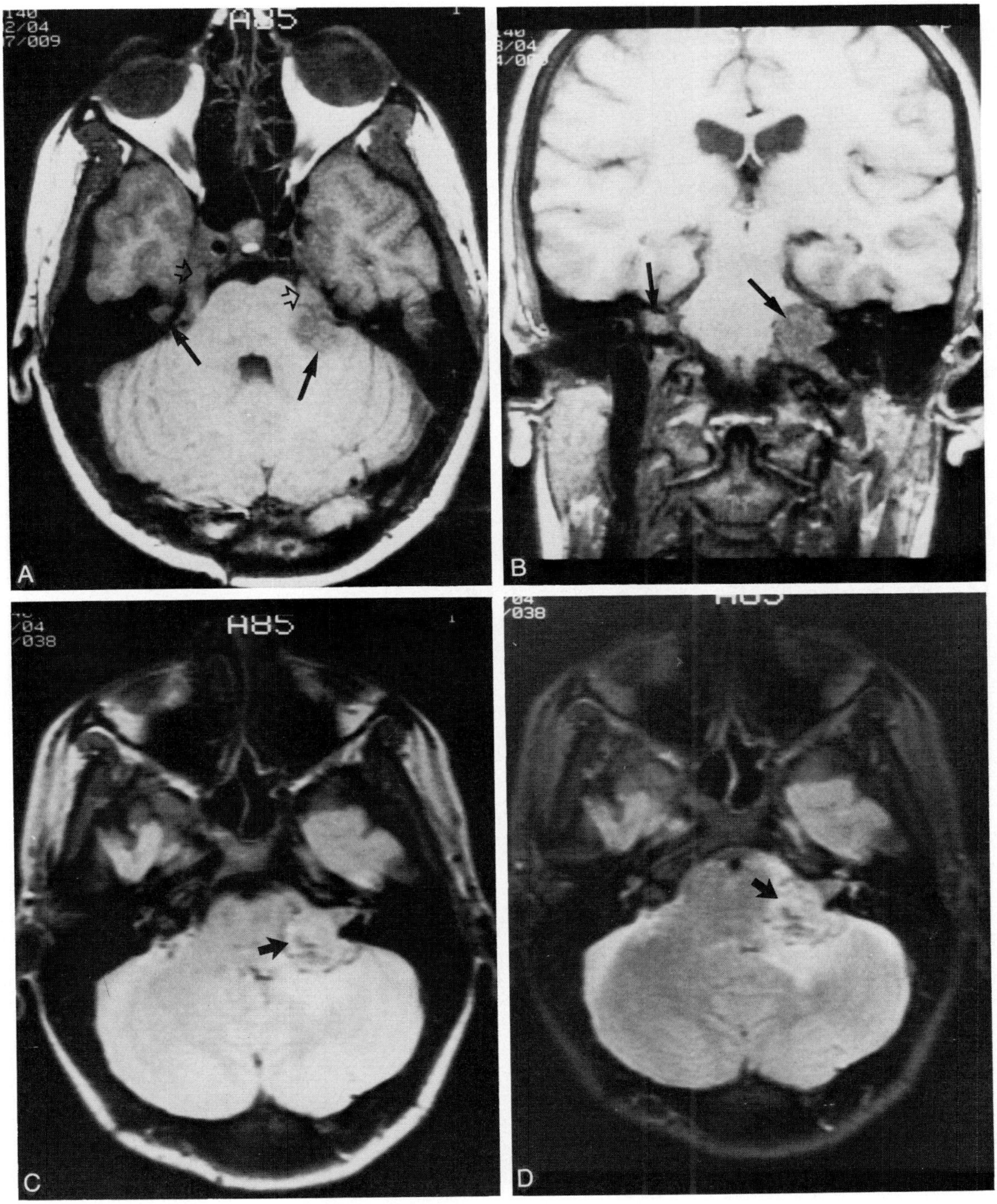

Figure 13–14. Neurofibromatosis (NF II) (17-year-old male).
A, Axial T1. Bilateral eighth nerve (*arrows*) and fifth nerve (*open arrows*) tumors are present.
B, Coronal T1. Bilateral eighth nerve (*arrows*) tumors are noted.
C, D, Axial SD and T2. The left eighth nerve tumor (*arrow*) is larger and more heterogeneous than its counterpart.

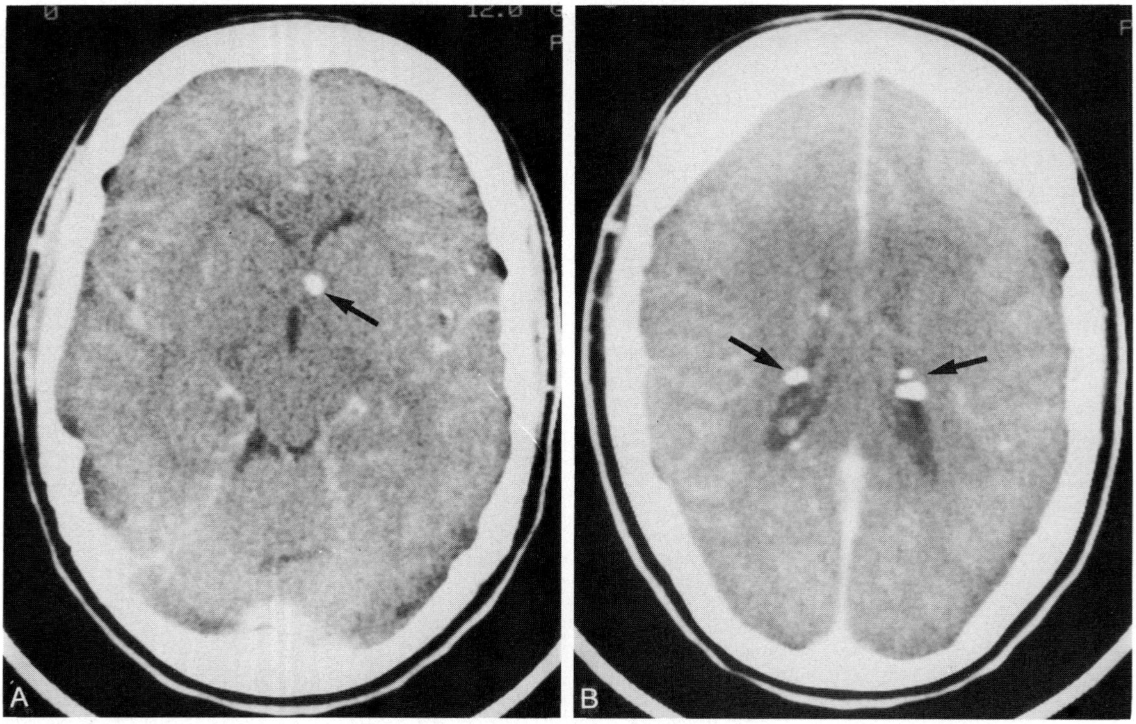

Figure 13–15. Tuberous sclerosis (25-year-old male).

A, B, Enhanced CT. Multiple subependymal periventricular calcifications (*arrows*) are present, which extend into the bodies of both lateral ventricles.

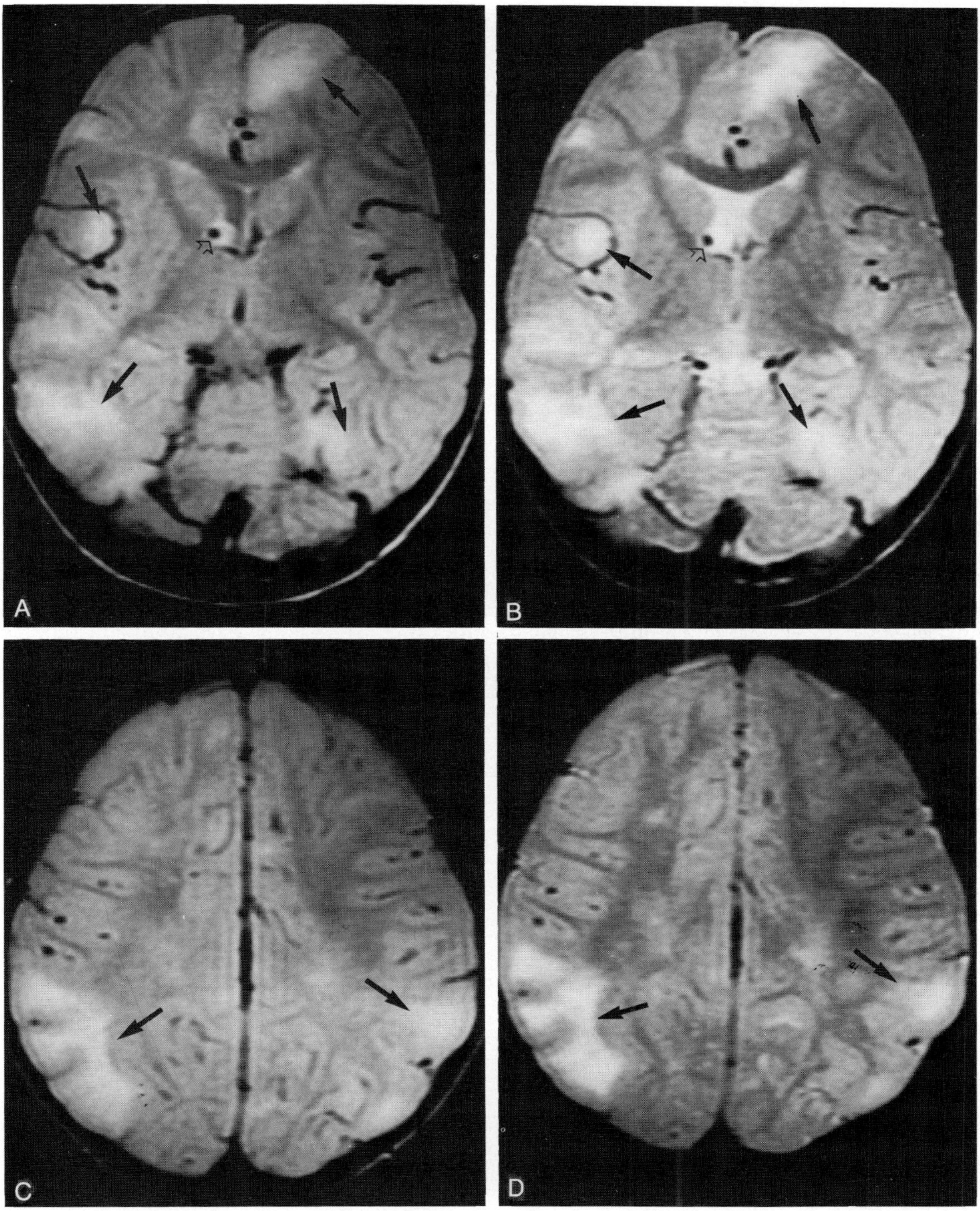

Figure 13–16. Tuberous sclerosis (9-year-old male).

A, B, Axial SD and T2. Multiple high-signal subcortical hamartomas (*arrows*) are present. A subependymal mass (*open arrow*) is noted that contains a focus of decreased signal (calcification) surrounded by a higher-signal soft tissue nodule.

C, D, Axial SD and T2. The subcortical hamartomas (*arrows*) are present throughout the supratentorial parenchyma.

tend to be larger (2 to 5 cm) than other subependymal nodules, enhance homogeneously, and may occlude the foramen of Monro leading to a noncommunicating hydrocephalus[21] (Fig. 13–17). Patients with giant cell astrocytomas present on average at 13 years of age; however, these tumors have been reported at birth.[22] The tumor, although most commonly seen with tuberous sclerosis, may occur in an isolated form.

White matter abnormalities have been reported in 93% of patients with tuberous sclerosis.[21] Straight or curvilinear white matter abnormalities extending from the ventricle to the subependymal nodule have been reported.[23] The tracts are hyperintense on T2- and hypointense on T1-weighted images. The T2-weighted sequence is approximately twice as sensitive as T1 at detecting this tract. CT may demonstrate subtle linear regions of high density. In addition, wedge-shaped or confluent foci of high T2 signal may be seen juxtaposed between the ventricular surface and the cortical tuber. The etiology is not clear, but demyelination, dysmyelination, hypomyelination, or lines of migrational disorder have been proposed.[23]

Von Hippel-Lindau Disease

Von Hippel-Lindau disease is an autosomal dominant condition in which patients are afflicted with CNS hemangioblastomas associated with renal cell carcinomas, pheochromocytomas, and cystic disease of the kidney, pancreas, and liver. There is no sexual predilection.

The CNS hemangioblastomas most commonly originate within the cerebellum and retina, with less frequent involvement of the medulla or spinal cord. Multiple hemangioblastomas are pathognomonic for von Hippel-Lindau disease. Patients with this disease present in their early 30s, 10 to 20 years earlier than patients with isolated hemangioblastomas.[10] The tumor may be cystic with a mural nodule, solid, or solid with small cysts. Tumors often contain a vascular nidus that is usually in contact with the pial surface, and a cyst of variable size.

MRI depicts the vascular nidus as isointense to hypointense to parenchyma on T1 and hyperintense on T2. The cyst usually contains a greater protein concentration than CSF and may accordingly be hyperintense to CSF on T1 and spin density images and isointense to hyperintense on T2 (Figs. 13–18, 13–19). The gadolinium-enhanced MRI examination is the most sensitive means of tumor detection.

Sturge-Weber Syndrome

Sturge-Weber syndrome is a congenital abnormality of vascular development that affects the face, brain, and orbit. The mechanism of inheritance has been attributed to autosomal dominant and autosomal recessive patterns, as well as being sporadic.[24] Patients have a port wine vascular nevus in the distribution of one or more branches of the trigeminal nerve (V). Clinically, the patients may present with seizures, hemiplegia, and mental retardation.[25]

A leptomeningeal venous angioma is located within the pia overlying the parietal and/or occipital lobes ipsilateral to the facial vascular nevus. Rarely, the lesion may be contralateral or multiple, or both. The pial angiomatosis alters the parenchymal blood flow, resulting in chronic hypoxia, which leads to focal cerebral atrophy and serpentine calcification within the second and fourth layers of the hypoxic cortex underlying the pial angioma.[24, 26] There is commensurate thickening of the calvarium overlying the atrophic cortex and shunting of blood into a prominent deep venous system. The choroid plexus is enlarged with angiomatous changes. Scleral angiomatosis is present in 30% of patients[27] and is often ipsilateral to the facial nevus.

Radiographically, the characteristic tram-track pattern of calcification may be evident on plain films after the patient reaches 2 to 3 years of age. Planar imaging detects the cerebral atrophy, skull changes, cortical calcification, enlarged choroid, and prominent deep venous system (Fig. 13–20). MRI more accurately identifies the ocular findings and the prominent venous system.[28] The calcifications are more apparent on gradient echo than on spin echo MRI sequences.[26] The gadolinium-enhanced MRI examination depicts the enhancing pial angioma (Fig. 13–21).

Hydranencephaly

Hydranencephaly is a destructive process of the cerebral hemisphere that most likely results

Text continued on page 537

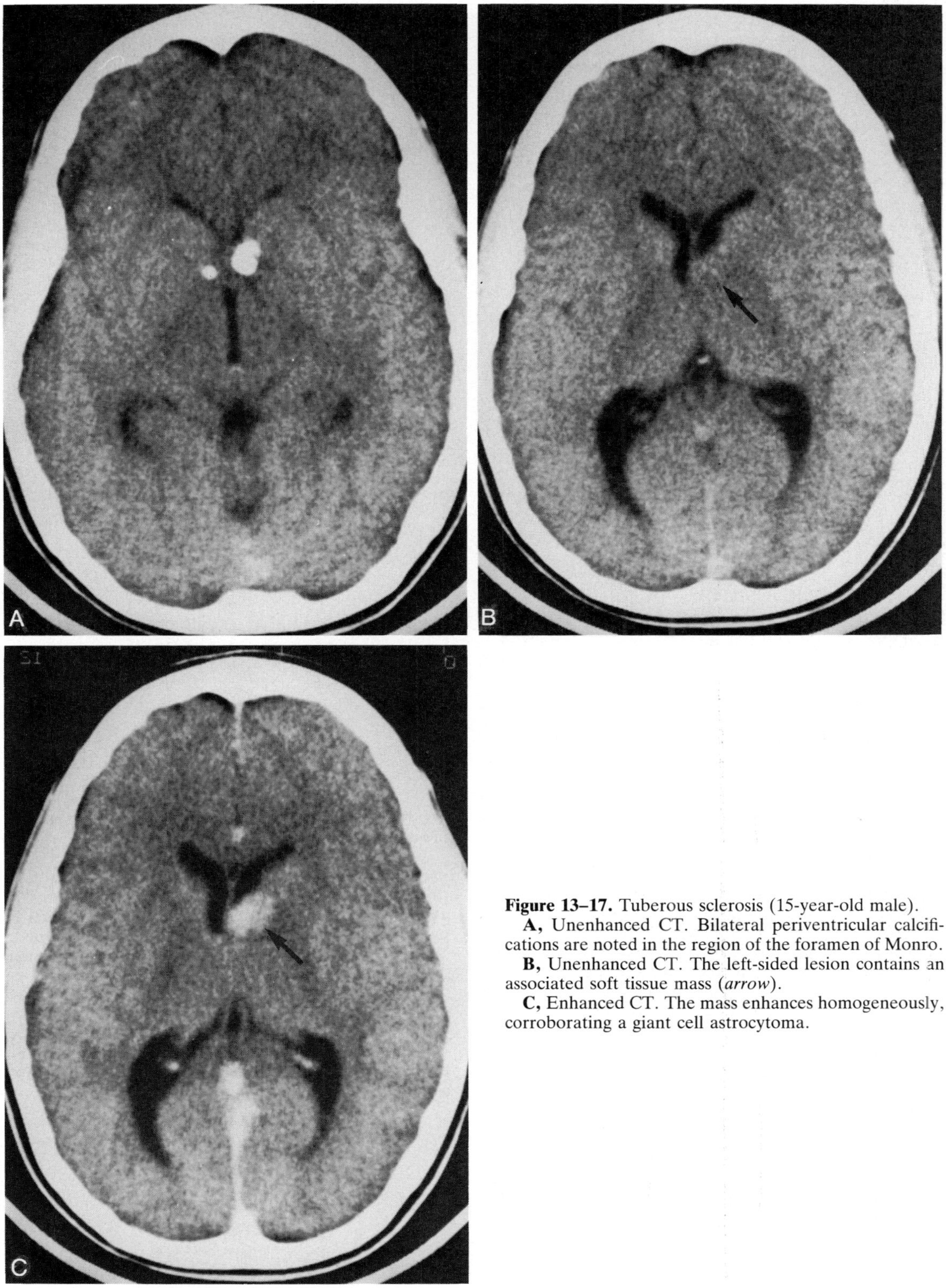

Figure 13–17. Tuberous sclerosis (15-year-old male).

A, Unenhanced CT. Bilateral periventricular calcifications are noted in the region of the foramen of Monro.

B, Unenhanced CT. The left-sided lesion contains an associated soft tissue mass (*arrow*).

C, Enhanced CT. The mass enhances homogeneously, corroborating a giant cell astrocytoma.

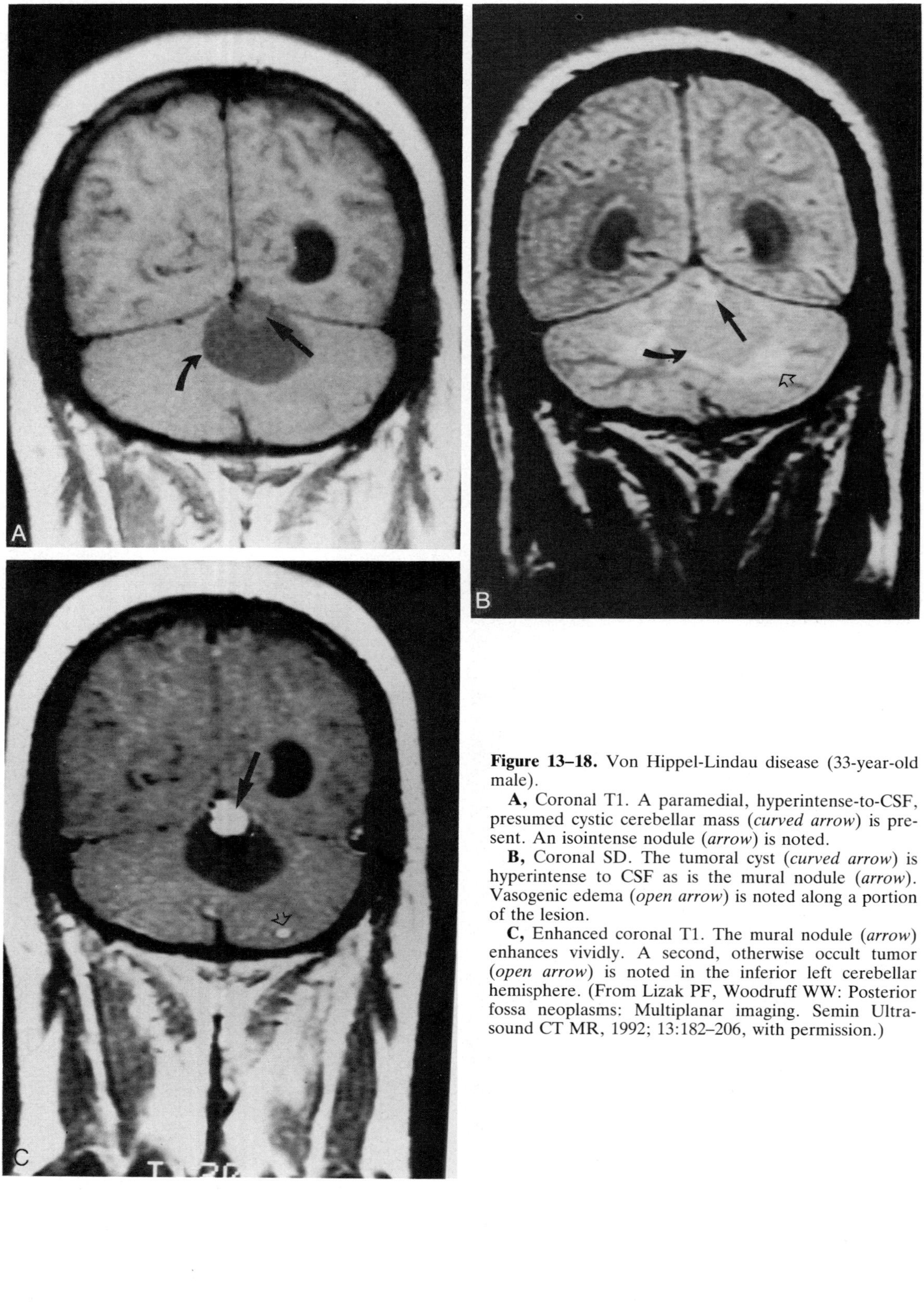

Figure 13–18. Von Hippel-Lindau disease (33-year-old male).

A, Coronal T1. A paramedial, hyperintense-to-CSF, presumed cystic cerebellar mass (*curved arrow*) is present. An isointense nodule (*arrow*) is noted.

B, Coronal SD. The tumoral cyst (*curved arrow*) is hyperintense to CSF as is the mural nodule (*arrow*). Vasogenic edema (*open arrow*) is noted along a portion of the lesion.

C, Enhanced coronal T1. The mural nodule (*arrow*) enhances vividly. A second, otherwise occult tumor (*open arrow*) is noted in the inferior left cerebellar hemisphere. (From Lizak PF, Woodruff WW: Posterior fossa neoplasms: Multiplanar imaging. Semin Ultrasound CT MR, 1992; 13:182–206, with permission.)

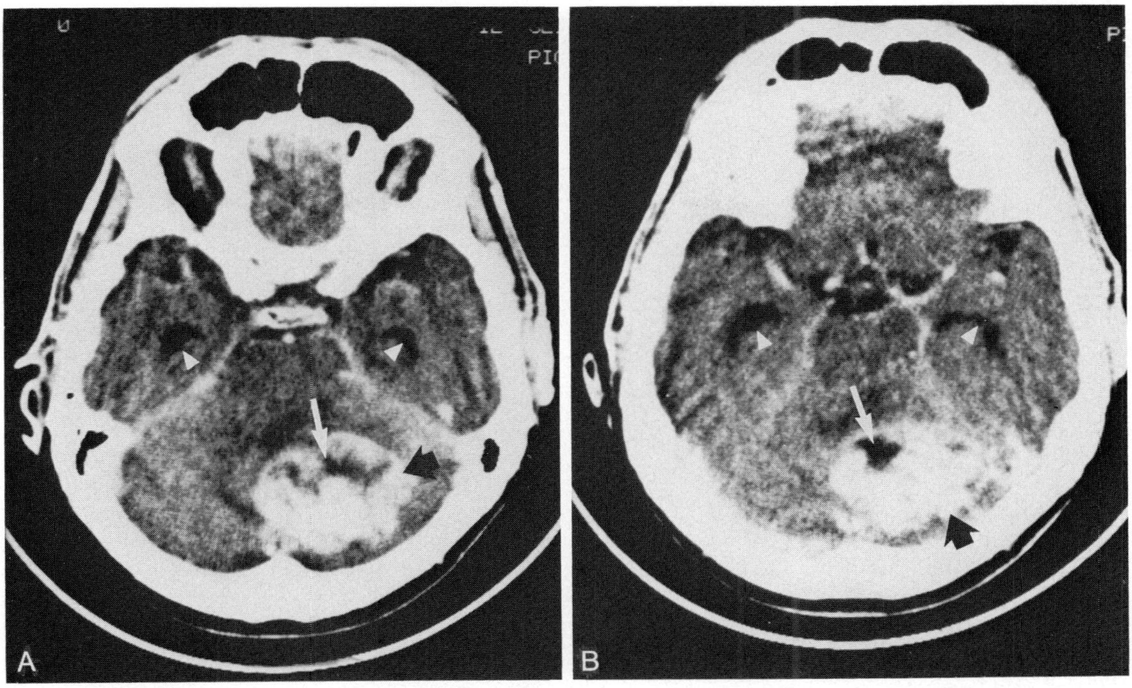

Figure 13–19. Von Hippel-Lindau disease (36-year-old male).

A, B, Enhanced CT. A heterogeneous, peripherally enhancing cerebellar mass (*black arrow*) is noted. The intratumoral cyst or necrosis (*white arrow*) does not enhance. The temporal horns (*arrowheads*) are enlarged, indicating early obstructive hydrocephalus.

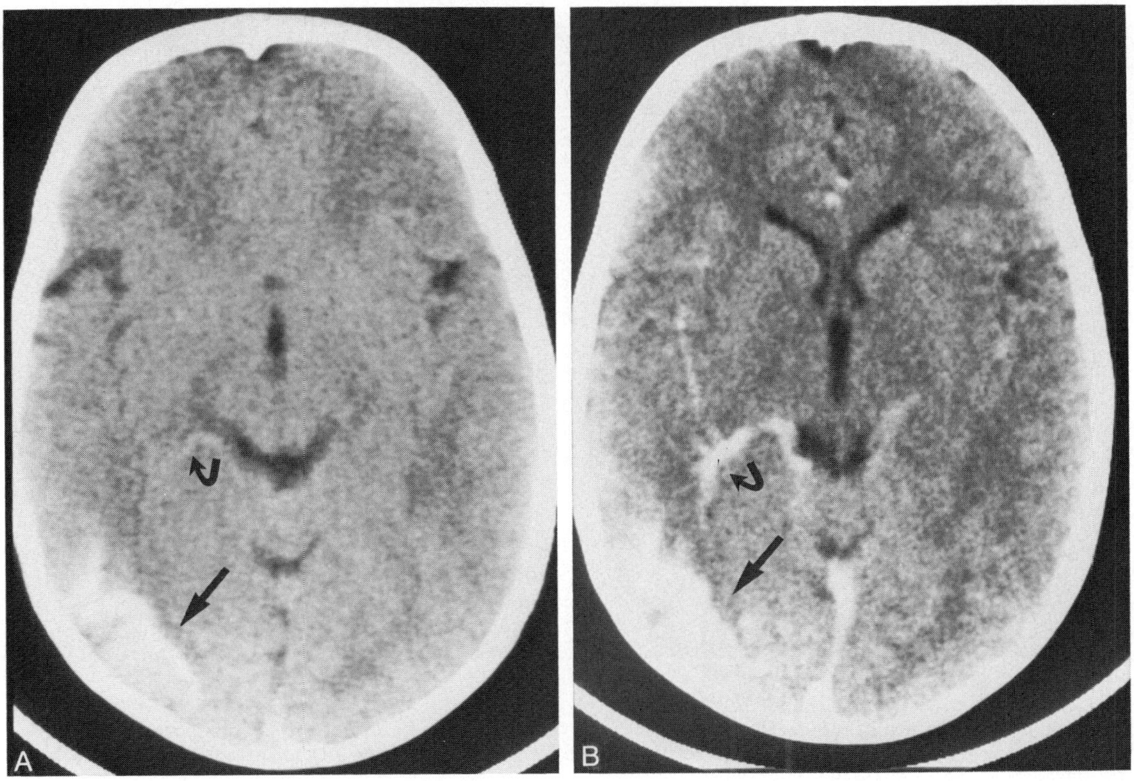

Figure 13–20. Sturge-Weber syndrome (2-year-old male).

A, Unenhanced CT. A serpentine calcification (*arrow*) is present in the right parietal occipital region. An intrinsically dense vessel (*curved arrow*) is noted near the quadrigeminal plate cistern.

B, Enhanced CT. The calcified cortex (*arrow*) enhances minimally. The choroid plexus angioma (*curved arrow*) also enhances.

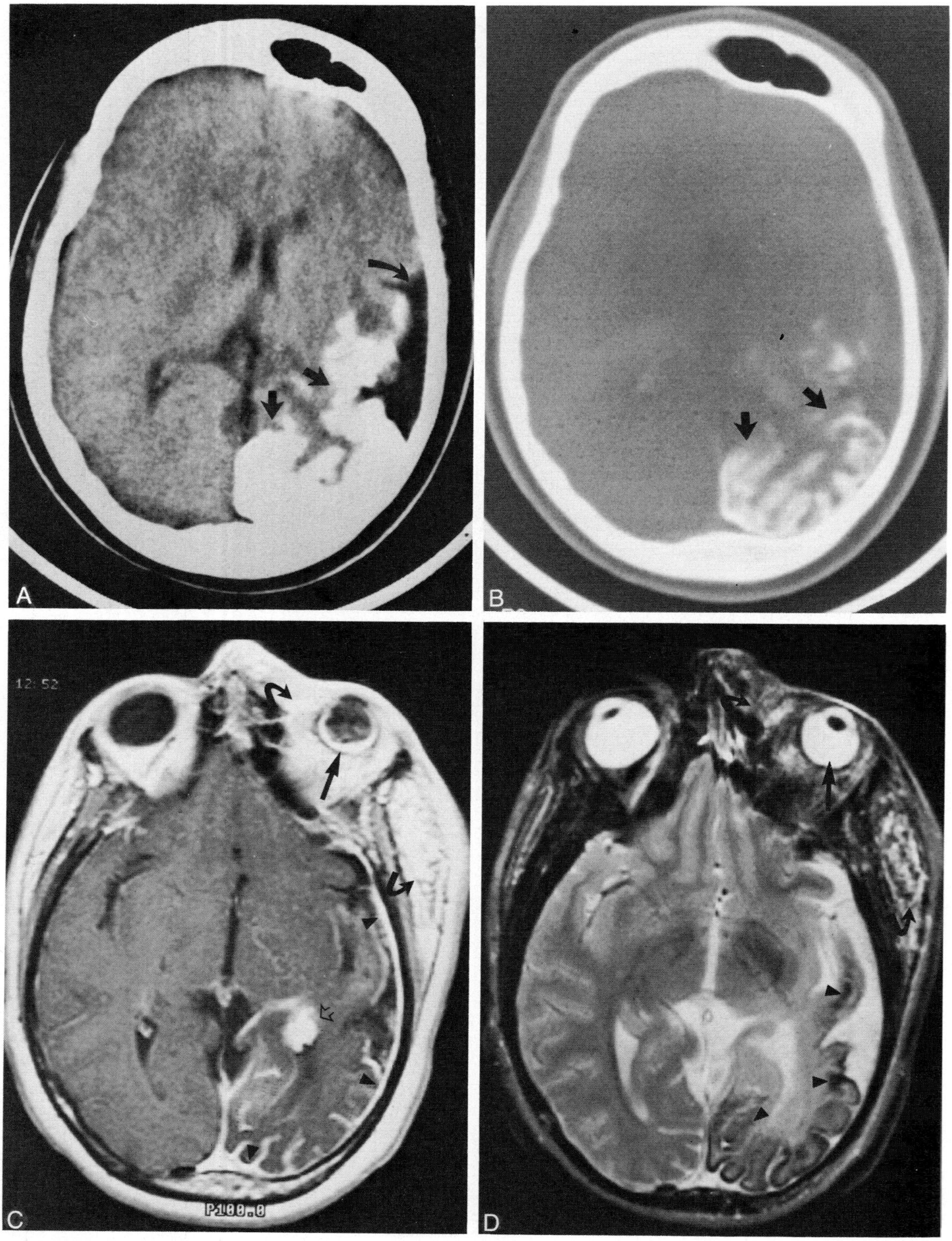

Figure 13–21. Sturge-Weber syndrome (13-year-old male).

A, Unenhanced CT. A thick rind of calcification (*arrows*) overlies the atrophic cortex of the left parietal and occipital lobes. Volume loss is manifest as focal enlargement of the CSF space (*curved arrow*) over the parietal cortex.

B, Unenhanced CT. Bone windows reveal the serpentine gyral distribution of the parieto-occipital calcification (*arrows*).

C, Enhanced axial T1. There is marked linear enhancement of the pial angioma (*arrowheads*), left glomus (*open arrow*), facial hemangioma (*curved arrows*), and left retinal angioma (*arrow*).

D, Axial T2. The serpentine cortical calcification (*arrowheads*) is decreased signal. The extracranial hemangioma (*curved arrows*) is markedly heterogeneous. The left globe (*arrow*) is small.

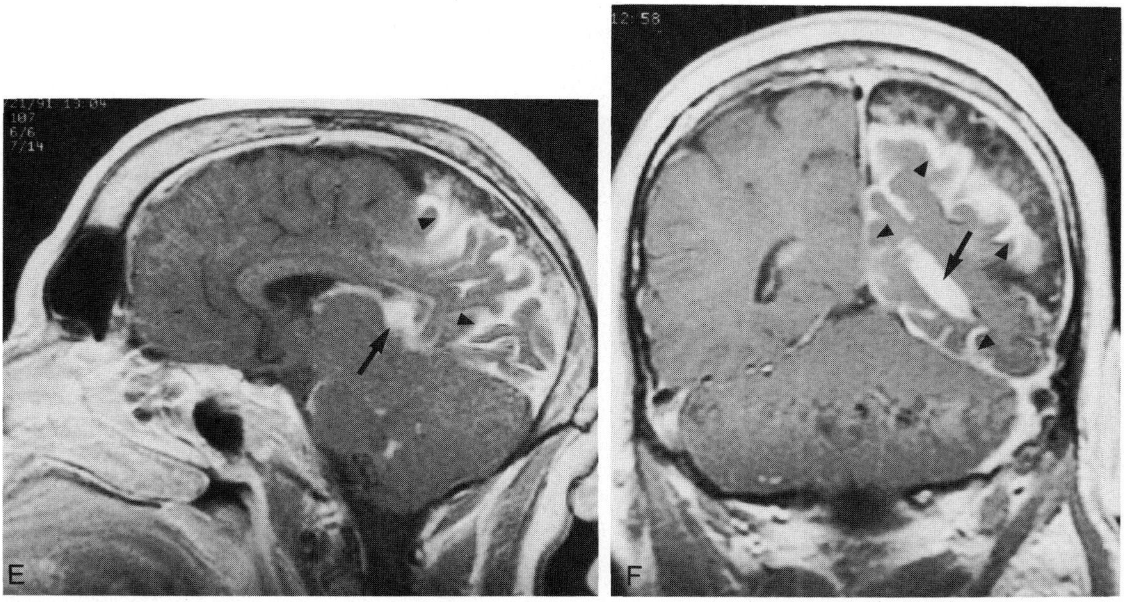

Figure 13–21 *Continued*
E, F, Enhanced parasagittal and coronal T1. The serpentine angioma (*arrowheads*) and vascular left choroid plexus (*arrow*) enhance markedly.

from an in utero occlusion of the internal carotid arteries after the normal development of the cerebral hemispheres is complete.[29] Clinically, the patient may be normal until developmental delay becomes apparent by 7 to 8 weeks of age.[29]

The components of the cerebral hemisphere supplied by the anterior circulation are replaced by a fluid-filled membranous sac. The brain parenchyma supplied by the posterior circulation (posterior fossa, thalami, hypothalamus, occipital lobes and basitemporal lobes) is intact. The falx is midline or slightly deviated, but it is present.

Angiographic findings include absence of the supraclinoid internal carotid arteries. The external carotid arteries and posterior circulation are normal.[30] Planar imaging reveals cerebrospinal fluid (CSF) density or intensity fluid collections in place of the supratentorial parenchyma (Fig. 13–22). The thalami are normal and not fused. The falx is intact. Remnant temporal and occipital lobes may be identified.[30, 31] Absence of the anterior cerebral mantle and facial anomalies, presence of the falx, and normal appearance of the thalami distinguish this from alobar holoprosencephaly.

Migration

Between 2 and 5 months' gestation, the proliferating neurons in the germinal matrix migrate from the periventricular region to the superficial cortex and deep nuclei of the brain. Disorders of neuronal migration result in schizencephaly, an abnormal gyral pattern, heterotopic gray matter, and dysgenesis of the corpus callosum (Table 13–4).

Schizencephaly

Schizencephaly results from delayed, incomplete, or abnormal migration of neurons from the germinal matrix to the cortex. Accordingly, a pia-covered, gray matter–lined cleft extends from the ventricular surface to the superficial gray matter. The gray matter margins of the cleft are thickened[32] and histologically polymicrogyric.[33–36] The cleft is most commonly located in the parasylvian region and is usually bilateral and symmetric. In type I schizencephaly, the cleft is closed and the margins apposed; this is also called fused lip schizencephaly. In type II schizencephaly, the lips of the cleft are open to some degree, separated by CSF.

The clinical presentation of patients corre-

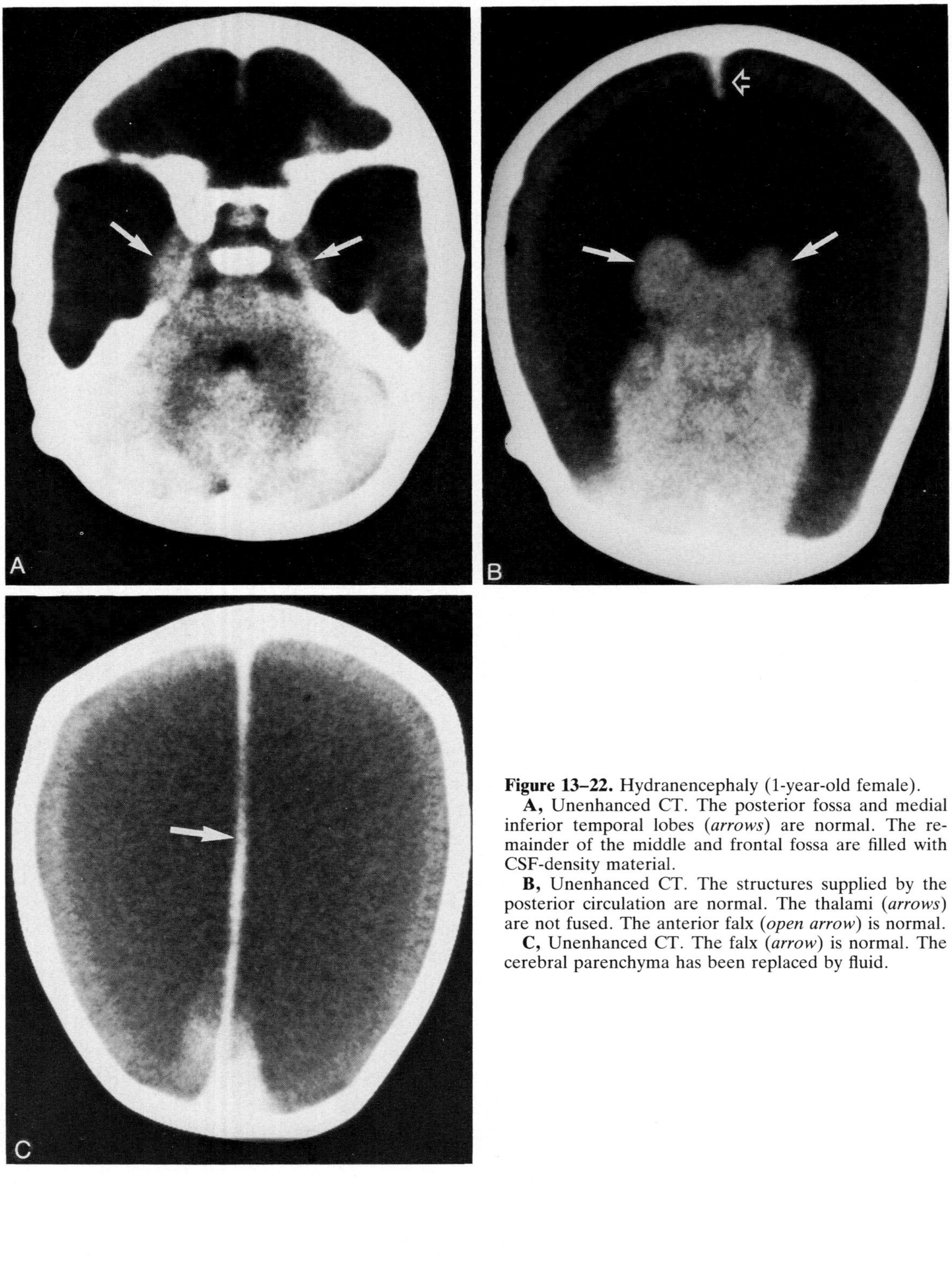

Figure 13–22. Hydranencephaly (1-year-old female).

A, Unenhanced CT. The posterior fossa and medial inferior temporal lobes (*arrows*) are normal. The remainder of the middle and frontal fossa are filled with CSF-density material.

B, Unenhanced CT. The structures supplied by the posterior circulation are normal. The thalami (*arrows*) are not fused. The anterior falx (*open arrow*) is normal.

C, Unenhanced CT. The falx (*arrow*) is normal. The cerebral parenchyma has been replaced by fluid.

Table 13–4. MIGRATION (2–5 MONTHS)

	Radiographic Findings	Comments
Schizencephaly	Gray matter lined cleft from ventricle to cortex	Type I closed lip Type II open lip (most common) Usually bilateral and symmetric
Agyria/Pachygyria	Thickened gray matter Poor sulcation and gray-white interdigitation ± ventricular dilatation	Usually focal Associated with many conditions including Dandy-Walker syndrome and dysgenesis of the corpus callosum
Heterotopia	Ectopic gray matter: Nodular Laminar Bandlike	Associated with agyria/pachygyria, schizencephaly, polymicrogyria, and dysgenesis of the corpus callosum
Dysgenesis of Corpus Callosum	Separation of lateral ventricles Viking horn deformity lateral ventricles (Probst bundle–cingulate gyrus) Third ventricle elevated Gyri of interhemispheric fissure radiate from the 3rd ventricle	Partial or complete; associated with Dandy-Walker syndrome, Chiari malformation, holoprosencephaly, lipoma

lates with the size and location of the cleft. The larger clefts are associated with greater motor and intellectual deficits than are smaller clefts. Frontal lobe involvement is associated with a greater likelihood of motor dysfunction.[35] Type I schizencephaly is less common than type II,[34] and patients usually present in late infancy or early childhood with seizures, delayed development, failure to thrive, and mental retardation.[33] Patients afflicted with type II schizencephaly present as newborns or infants with hydrocephalus, macrocephaly, and seizures. Patients with type II schizencephaly may die as a result of failure to thrive, chronic infection, or respiratory problems.

Type II schizencephaly is readily detected with both CT and MRI (Figs. 13–23 to 13–25). CSF density-intensity collections extend from the ventricle to the superficial CSF spaces. The gray matter lining the cleft is most apparent on MRI. Multiplanar imaging and increased tissue contrast permit MRI identification of some type I schizencephalies that are not apparent on CT.

Agyria and Pachygyria

Agyria, or lissencephaly, refers to lack of cortical gyri, resulting in a smooth brain surface. Agyria is more frequently partial, although complete forms do exist. Pachygyria refers to thickened, broad-based gyri. In both agyria and pachygyria, the abnormal cortex is only four cell layers thick.[36] Polymicrogyria results in multiple small gyri and is indistinguishable from agyria on planar imaging; the distinction is based on histologic review.

Complete agyria results in an hourglass or "figure-8" configuration of the brain on axial planar imaging[2, 37, 38] owing to incomplete or lack of opercularization of the insula that leads to sylvian grooves. In both agyria and pachygyria, the cortex is thickened with commensurate decrease in the amount of white matter, and the gray-white interdigitation is replaced with a smooth interface (Fig. 13–26). Secondary findings of agyria include ventricular dilatation and colpocephaly (disproportionate enlargement of the atria and occipital horns), dysgenesis of the corpus callosum, and/or Dandy-Walker syndrome.[38]

The pachygyric brain may be an isolated finding or associated with fused lip (type I) schizencephaly or heterotopia, or both. The pachygyric patient is usually retarded but may live until adulthood. These patients may present in infancy or young adulthood with developmental delay, seizures, and failure to thrive.

Gray Matter Heterotopias

Heterotopic gray matter results from incomplete migration of neurons from the germinal matrix along the radially aligned glial cells, which guide these neurons to their respective distant position. Accordingly, neurons may be located between the ventricular surface and the cortex and have been described as appearing nodular, laminar, or bandlike. Heteroto-

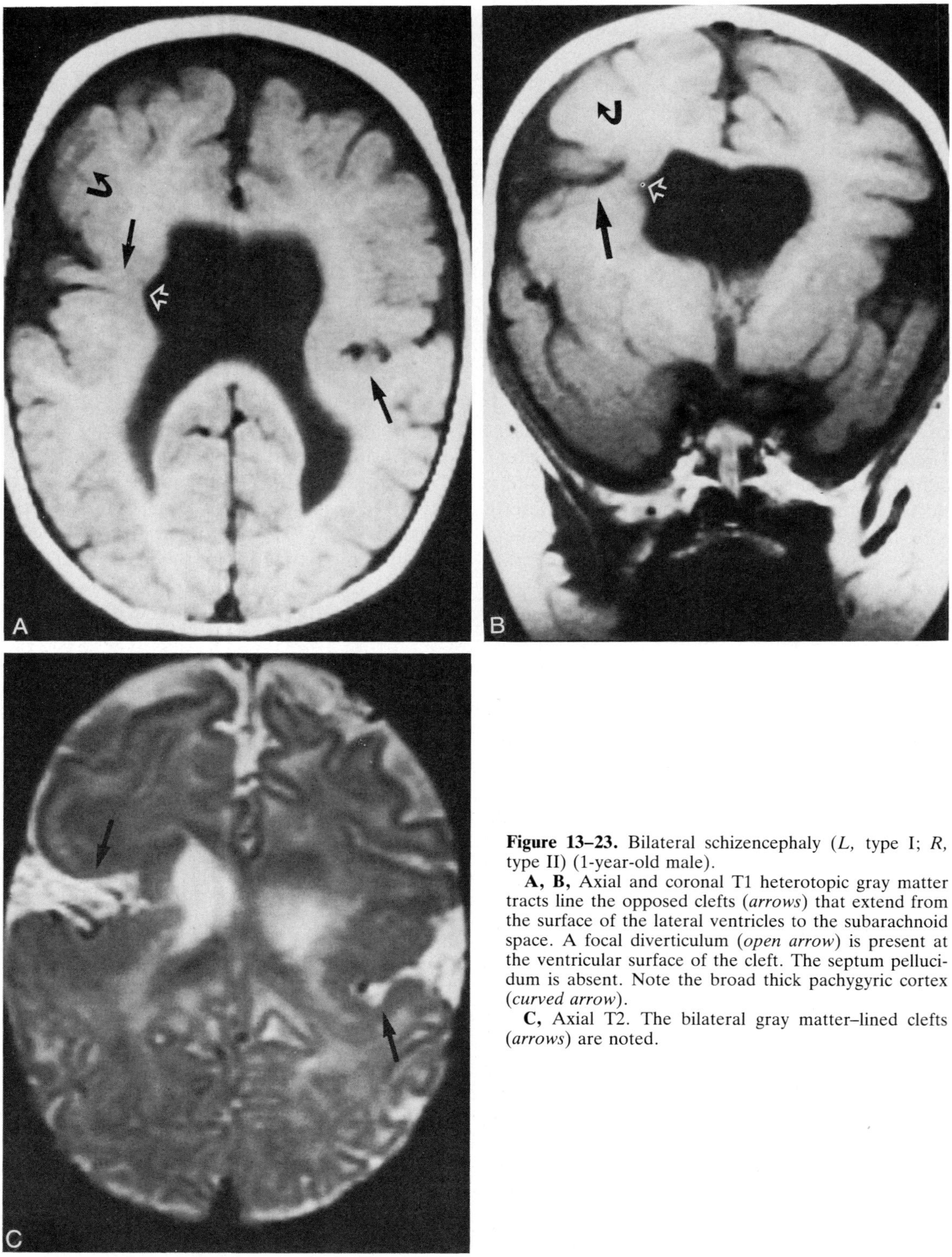

Figure 13–23. Bilateral schizencephaly (*L,* type I; *R,* type II) (1-year-old male).

A, B, Axial and coronal T1 heterotopic gray matter tracts line the opposed clefts (*arrows*) that extend from the surface of the lateral ventricles to the subarachnoid space. A focal diverticulum (*open arrow*) is present at the ventricular surface of the cleft. The septum pellucidum is absent. Note the broad thick pachygyric cortex (*curved arrow*).

C, Axial T2. The bilateral gray matter–lined clefts (*arrows*) are noted.

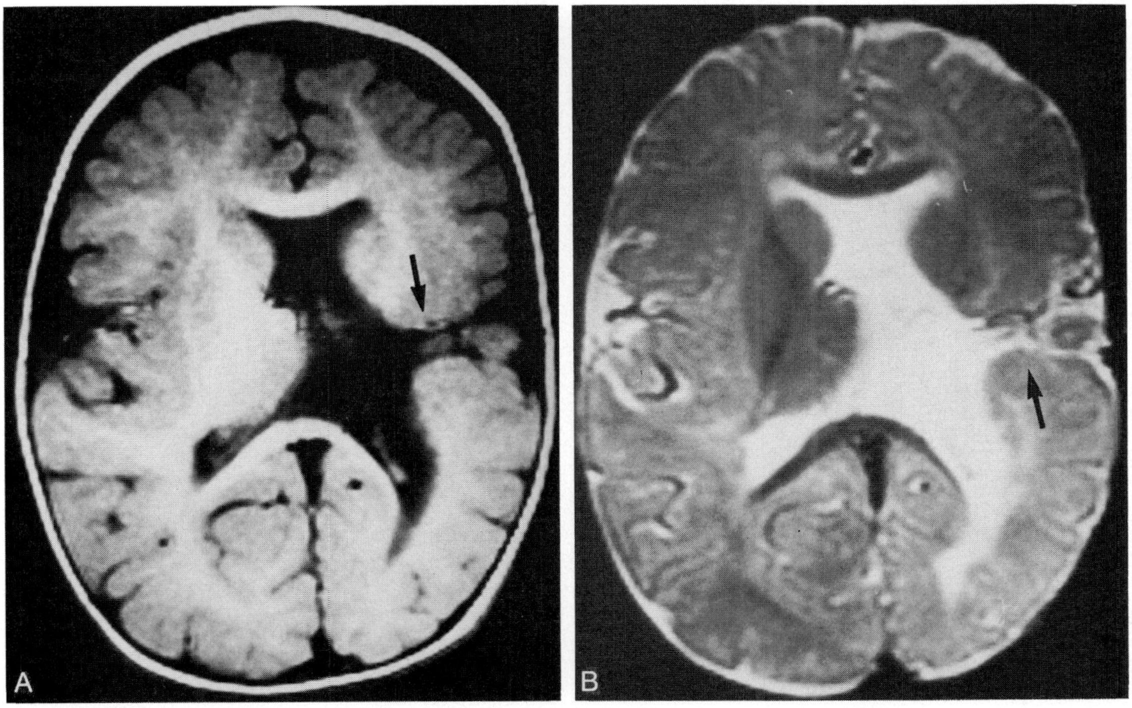

Figure 13–24. Unilateral schizencephaly (type II) (10-month-old male).
A, B, Axial T1 and T2. A gray matter–lined cleft (*arrow*) is present. The CSF within the lateral ventricle communicates freely with the subarachnoid space. The septum pellucidum is absent.

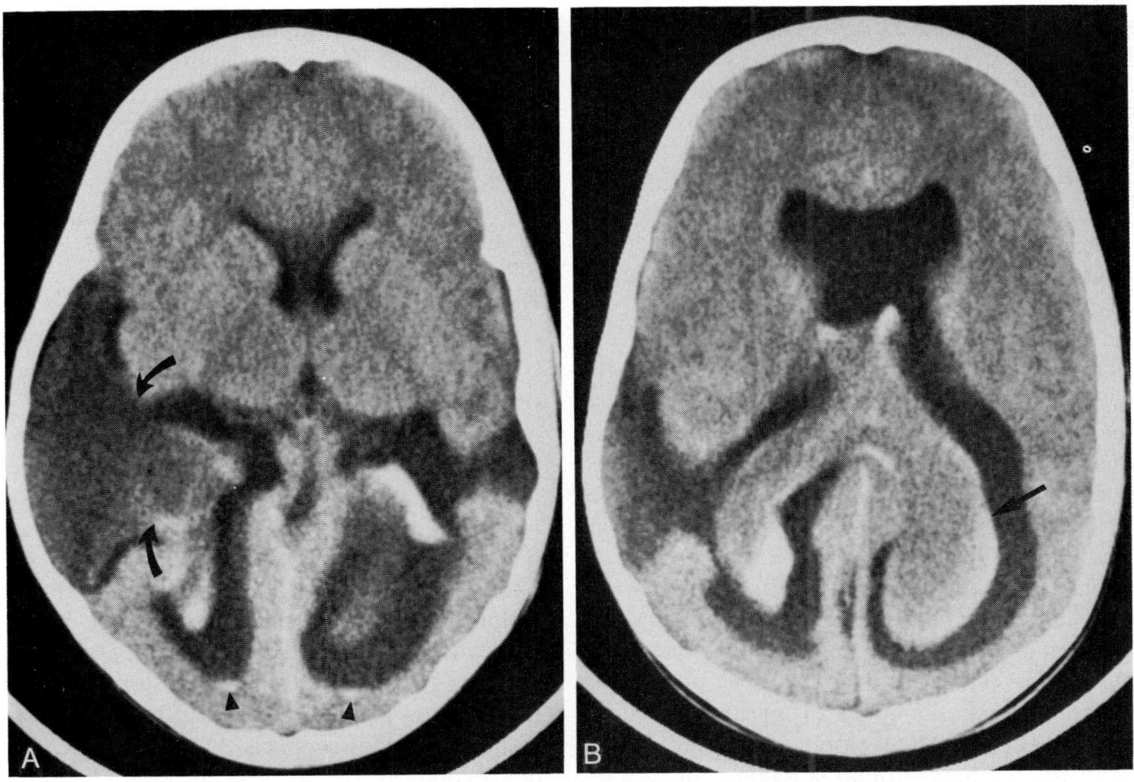

Figure 13–25. Bilateral schizencephaly (type II) with intraventricular hemorrhage (3-year-old female).
A, B, Unenhanced CT. An intraventricular clot forms a cast (*arrow*) of the ventricles. The blood communicates with the subarachnoid space (*curved arrows*). Minimal blood products (*arrowheads*) layer in the gravity-dependent occipital horns.

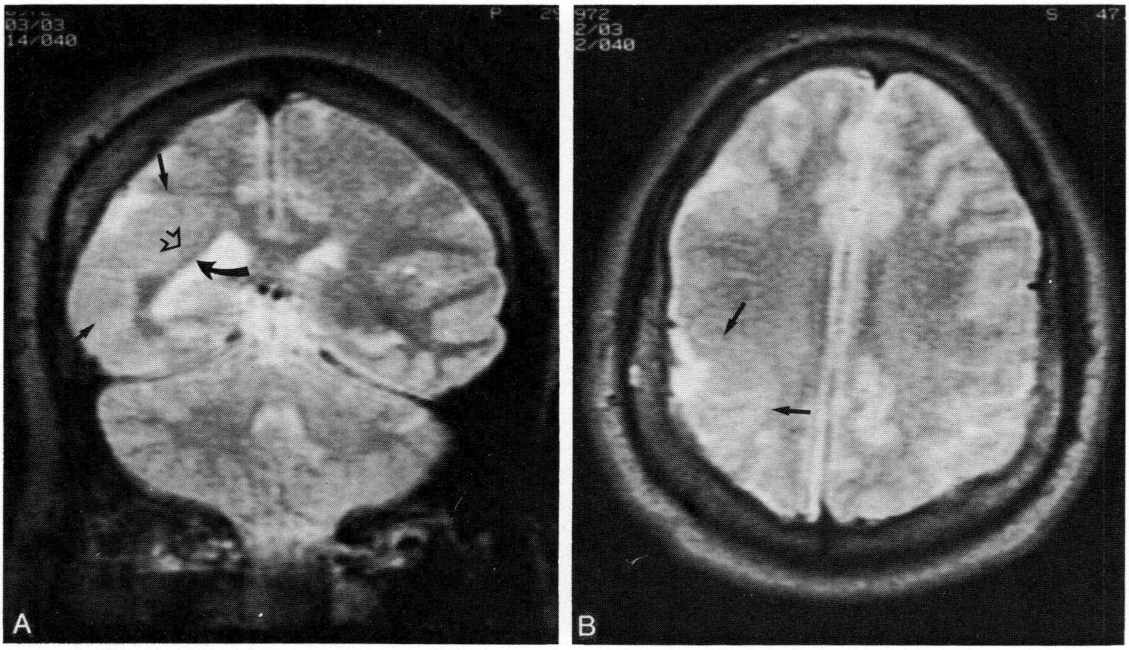

Figure 13–26. Pachygyria (20-year-old male).
A, B, Coronal and axial T2. A thick band of gray matter (*arrows*) is present in the right posterior parietal lobe. There is a relatively smooth interface of the gray white junction (*open arrow*) and marked focal decrease in the amount of white matter (*curved arrow*).

pias may be isolated or associated with other developmental brain anomalies including agyria, pachygyria, schizencephaly, polymicrogyria, and dysgenesis of the corpus callosum.

Nodular heterotopias appear as small round masses of gray matter within the subependymal region of the lateral ventricle or within the subcortical white matter. The islands of gray matter are 0.5 to 3 cm in greatest linear dimension[33] (Fig. 13–27). Subependymal heterotopias may be indistinguishable from the subependymal nodules associated with tuberous sclerosis.[32] If isolated, these lesions may be asymptomatic. Infrequently, these lesions may result in seizures.

Laminar heterotopias are linear collections of gray matter separated from the ventricle and cortex by white matter. Laminar heterotopias are less common than the nodular variety.[39] The thicker the heterotopic plate, the greater the degree of motor dysfunction.[40] Also, the thicker the heterotopic plate, the greater the likelihood of an overlying cortical anomaly as well as developmental delay. Large gray matter heterotopias affecting the posterior frontal lobe are frequently associated with contralateral hemiparesis.[40]

In band heterotopias, the least common form of heterotopic gray matter, a thick continuous band of gray matter is present between the lateral ventricles and the cortex. Patients present with intractable seizures and developmental delay.[41] The margins of the heterotopic gray matter are smooth and do not parallel the gray-white interdigitation.

Dysgenesis of the Corpus Callosum

The embryogenesis of the corpus callosum is complex. This midline commissural fiber tract develops from the massa commissuralis, which arises from the anterior wall of the telencephalon, the lamina terminalis. Induction of the decussating callosal fibers must be maintained to permit the complete development of the corpus callosum[42] between the 12th and 20th weeks of gestation. The corpus callosum develops from front to back beginning with the genu, body, splenium, and finally the small rostrum extending posteriorly from the inferior genu. An interruption of growth results in partial agenesis that affects the caudal segment of the corpus callosum. Complete agenesis of the corpus callosum results from an insult that occurs before the initial induction

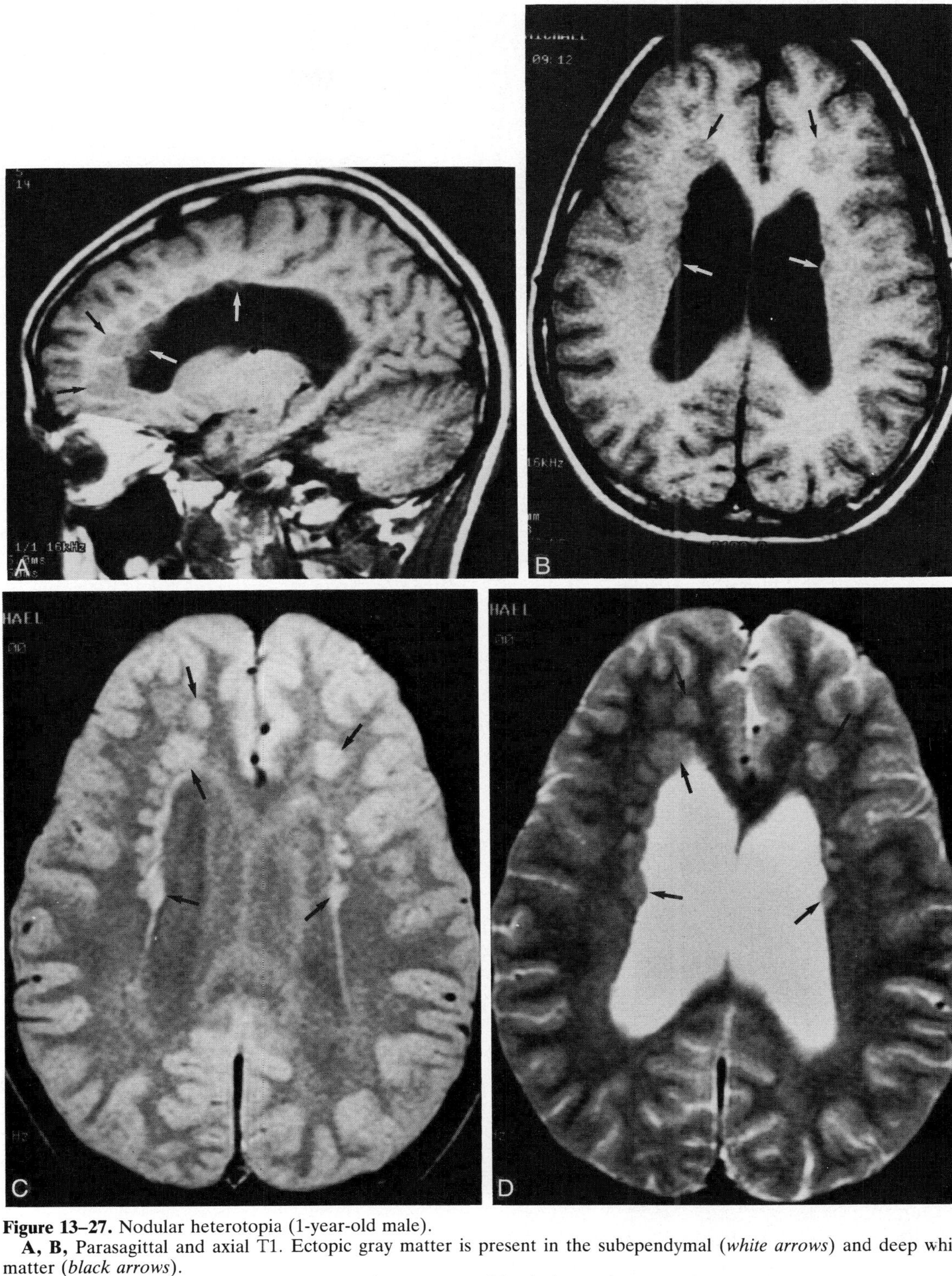

Figure 13–27. Nodular heterotopia (1-year-old male).

A, B, Parasagittal and axial T1. Ectopic gray matter is present in the subependymal (*white arrows*) and deep white matter (*black arrows*).

C, D, Axial SD and T2. Nodular heterotopic gray matter islands (*arrows*) are noted.

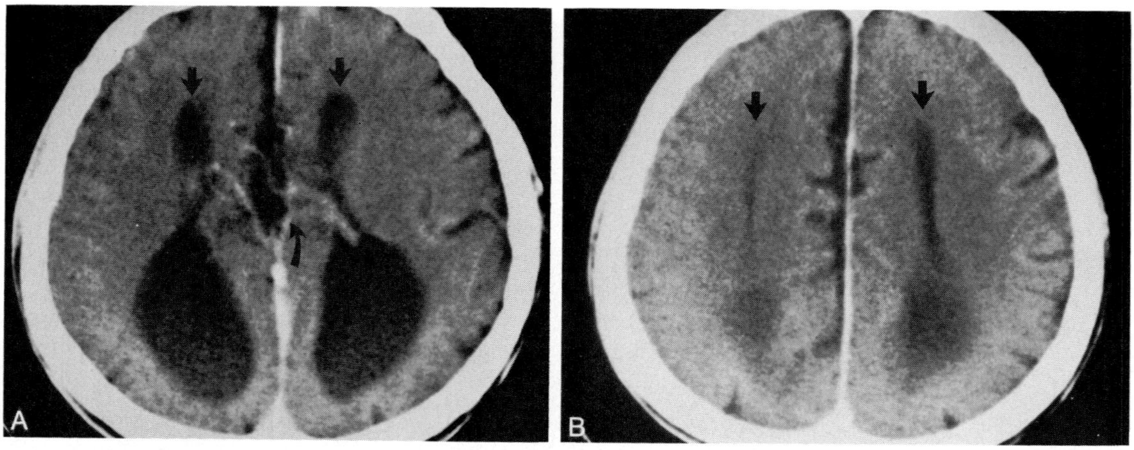

Figure 13–28. Dysgenesis of the corpus callosum (81-year-old male).
A, B, Enhanced axial CT. The lateral ventricles (*arrows*) are separated and their long axes are parallel. The third ventricle (*curved arrow*) is high riding.

at 12 weeks[42] and is associated in 80 to 90% of cases with other CNS anomalies including Dandy-Walker, Chiari I, Chiari II, holoprosencephaly, and midline lipoma.[2]

Absence of the corpus callosum results in separation of the lateral ventricles and elevation at the third ventricle (Fig. 13–28). The third ventricle may be dilated, causing separation of the thalami. Coronal images demonstrate inferior pointing of the frontal horns and the "viking-horn" deformity of the lateral ventricles resulting from the Probst bundle–cingulate gyrus complex that runs parallel to the interhemispheric fissure in the medial wall of the lateral ventricle.

Parasagittal images demonstrate gyri radiating perpendicular to the third ventricle with failure of the normal convergence of the calcarine and parieto-occipital sulci (Figs. 13–29, 13–30). The cingulate gyrus is rotated inferior and lateral and is not identified on parasagittal images.[2]

Development of the limbic system and corpus callosum are intimately related. Accord-

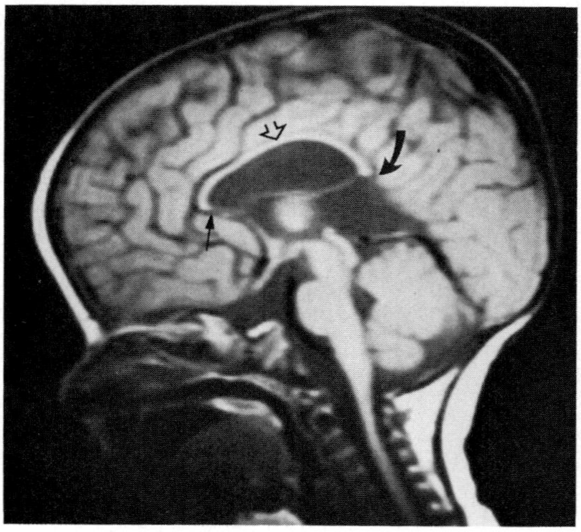

Figure 13–29. Dysgenesis of the corpus callosum (4-month-old male). Parasagittal T1; the corpus callosum (*open arrow*) is thinned and incomplete. The splenium (*curved arrow*) and rostrum (*arrow*) are hypoplastic.

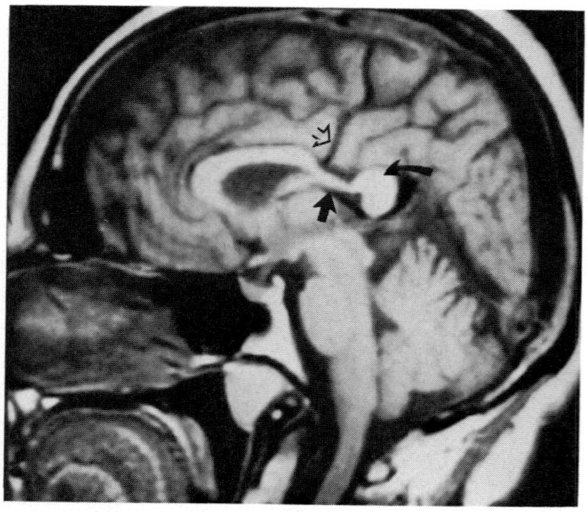

Figure 13–30. Dysgenesis of the corpus callosum (32-year-old male). Parasagittal T1; the corpus callosum is focally dysgenic (*arrow*). The splenium (*curved arrow*) is normal, indicating the insult responsible for this focal defect occurred after the corpus callosum was fully developed at 20 weeks' gestation. Note the focal loss of the cingulate gyrus and radiation of the gyri perpendicular (*open arrow*) to the surface of the corpus callosum.

ingly, the fornix and septum pellucidum may be hypoplastic. Hypoplasia of the hippocampus leads to a patulous or keyhole deformity of the temporal horn.[2] Colpocephaly is a frequent finding.

CHILD ABUSE

The incidence of nonaccidental brain injury in children is increasing. In excess of 400,000 cases are reported yearly, the majority (81%) occurring in children under age 2.[43] Child abuse is a common cause of intellectual, psychologic, and motor developmental delay. The neuroimager may be the first member of the medical team to suggest child abuse as a cause of intracranial injury, as the clinical history is intentionally obfuscated in such cases. Recognition of this injury is of paramount importance in initiating the legal removal of the child from the hostile home environment. Up to 50% of patients will be subject to repeat injury.

The most common pattern of CNS injury in child abuse results from a to-and-fro shaking of the child by the shoulders. The neck muscles are expectedly weak and the head disproportionately large in the infant and young child. This results in a repeated acceleration-deceleration whiplash injury.[44]

The most common radiographic abnormality in these patients is a posterior interhemispheric hyperdensity (Fig. 13–31). Although one investigator[43] equates this to subarachnoid hemorrhage, another attributes this hyperdensity to subdural hematoma.[45] In truth, it is likely to be a combination of the two and has been reported in 58 to 73% of patients with CT-documented abnormalities. Regardless of location, the pathophysiology relates to the stretching and interruption of cortical vessels that drain the cerebral cortex into the superior sagittal sinus. The resultant hemorrhage is most apparent in the interhemispheric fissure.

Diffuse supratentorial cytotoxic edema occurs in a high percentage (65%) of patients.[43] This post-traumatic edema results in obscuration of the gray-white junction and diffuse attenuation of the CSF spaces, including the ventricles. The cytotoxic edema results in parenchymal hypodensity that may accentuate the interhemispheric hemorrhage. Edema may be so severe as to create a "reversal sign" in which the gray matter has lower attenuation than the white matter. Generally, the thalamus, brainstem, and cerebellum are spared. This particular injury results in severe neurologic consequences.[43]

Parenchymal contusions and hemorrhage may result from a direct blow to the calvarium. Such an insult may be associated also with a scalp hematoma and skull fracture. Skull fractures are reported in 13 to 30% of child abuse cases.[43, 45] This number is relatively low compared with numbers of patients having similar intracranial injuries unrelated to child abuse.

One type of hemorrhage that is relatively specific for child abuse has been described in patients under 5 months of age.[44] This consists of contusional slitlike tears in the white matter of the frontal and occipital lobes. The typical cortical parenchymal contusions seen in older patients are not present in infants, partly because of the relatively smooth surface of the inner table. The contusional tears are lined with large reactive astrocytes that are hemosiderin stained. There may be evidence of acute and chronic hemorrhage. Parietal bone fractures are common in such injuries.

Follow-up CT on patients with interhemispheric hemorrhages demonstrates atrophy in 100% and focal parenchymal infarcts in 50%.[45] The parenchyma may undergo cystic encephalomalacia resulting in marked parenchymal volume loss (Figs. 13–32, 13–33). These patients experience devastating neurologic consequences.

The role of MRI in the evaluation of child abuse is increasing. Clearly, CT is adequate to evaluate for surgically amenable disease; however, MRI is more sensitive than CT at detecting small subdural hematomas, cortical contusions, and shearing or axonal injuries.[46, 47] Accordingly, MRI should be performed in all children suspected of being victims of child abuse with normal CT examinations.

Secondary signs of child abuse can be demonstrated with plain film series of the ribs and long bones. Multiple fractures of varying chronicity may be present. Funduscopic examination reveals subretinal hemorrhages, which are relatively specific for the shaken infant.

Text continued on page 551

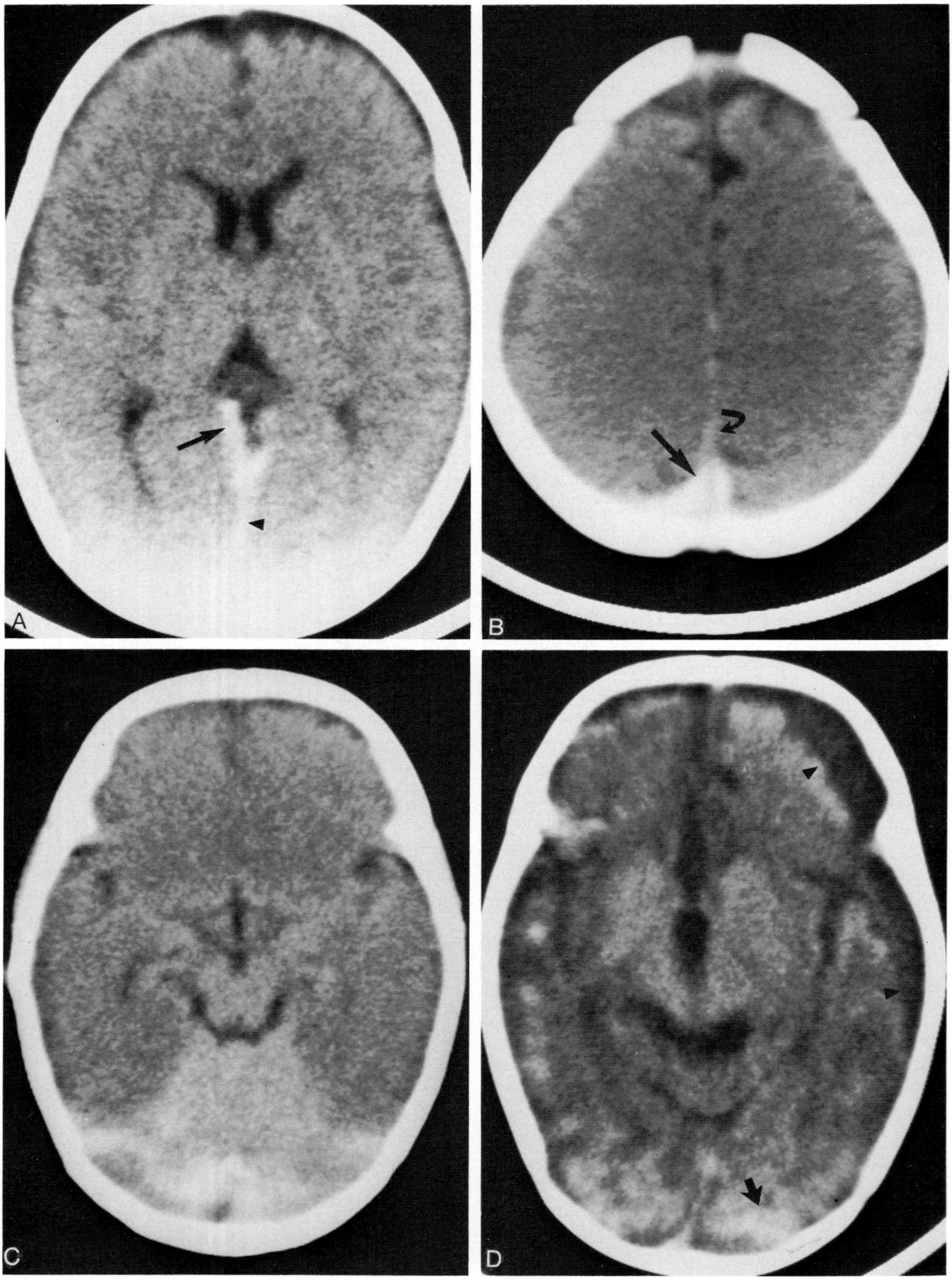

Figure 13–31 *See legend on opposite page*

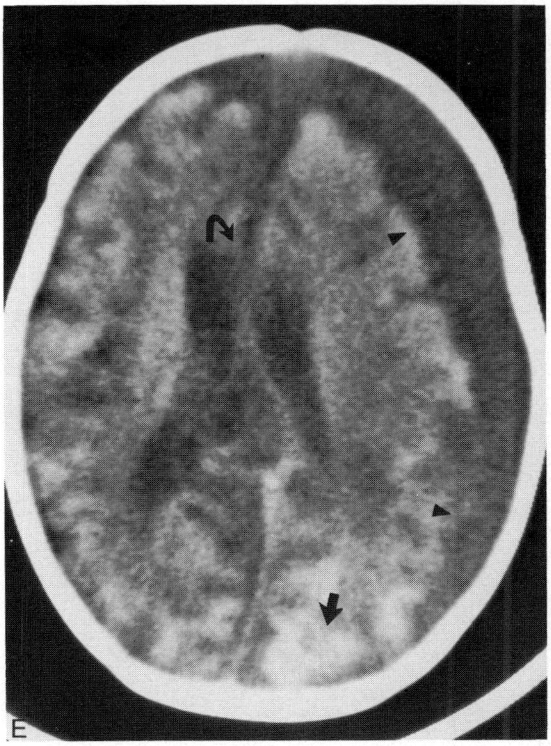

Figure 13–31. Child abuse (2-year-old female).

A, Unenhanced CT (at 12 hours). The tentorium (*arrow*) and posterior falx (*arrowhead*) are dense. The cortical sulci are attenuated.

B, Unenhanced CT. The posterior falx (*arrow*) is dense secondary to subdural hematoma. Subarachnoid blood (*curved arrow*) is present in the interhemispheric fissure. The cortical sulci are in part effaced secondary to early cytotoxic edema.

C, Unenhanced CT (at 4 days). Progressive cytotoxic edema has decreased the density of the supratentorial parenchyma referable to the posterior fossa parenchyma and brainstem.

D, E, Unenhanced CT (at 22 days). The supratentorial parenchyma is diffusely abnormal, exhibiting global encephalomalacia. The ventricles have enlarged to compensate for the parenchymal volume loss. Parenchymal hemorrhage (*arrow*) is noted in the left occipital lobe. A left-sided chronic subdural hematoma (*arrowheads*) causes subfalcial herniation (*curved arrow*).

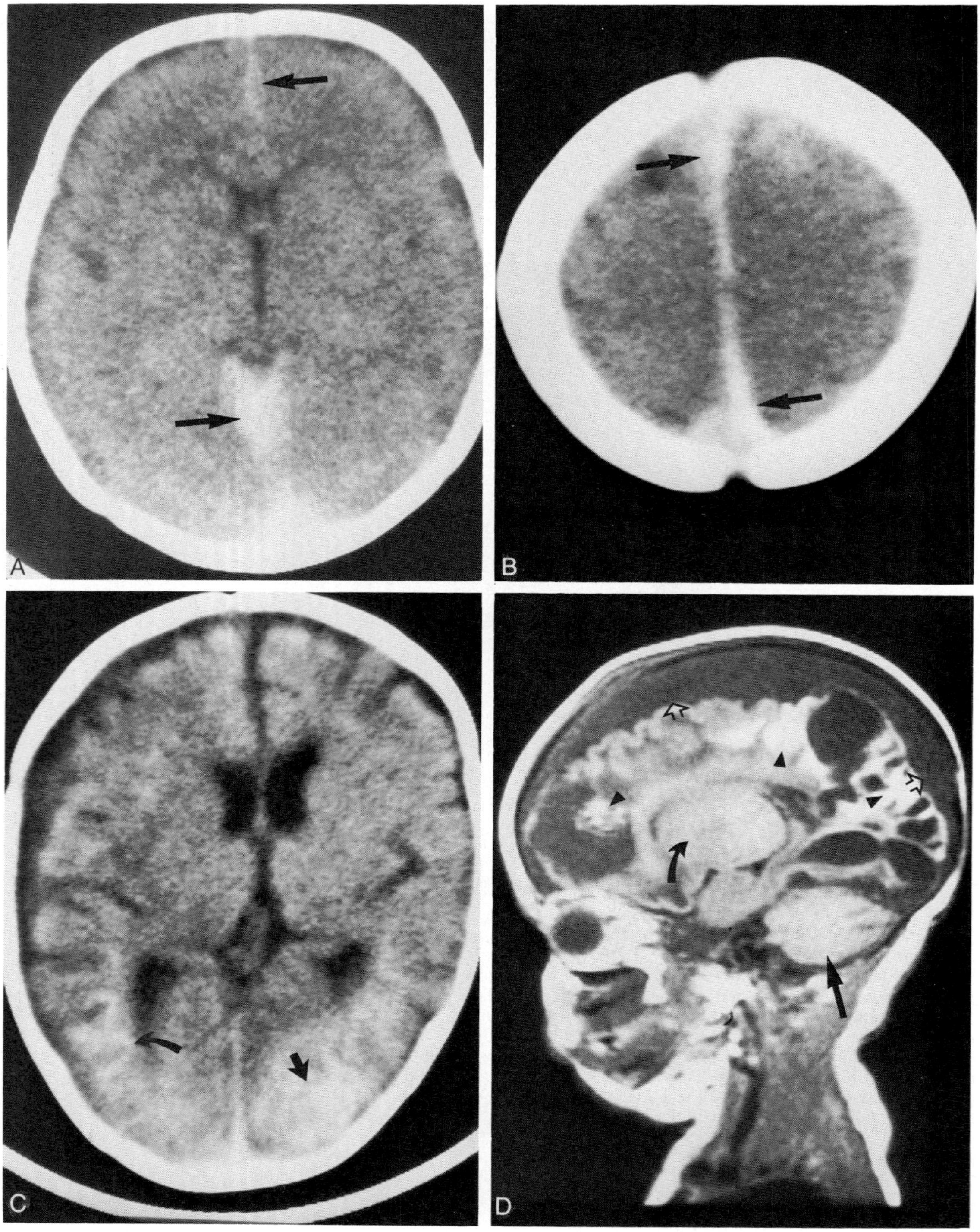

Figure 13–32. Child abuse (6-year-old male).

A, B, Unenhanced CT (at 1 day). The falx and interhemispheric fissure (*arrows*) are dense secondary to subdural and subarachnoid hemorrhage.

C, Unenhanced CT (at 10 days). The CSF spaces have enlarged, indicating diffuse supratentorial atrophy. Parenchymal hemorrhage is present in the left occipital (*arrow*) and right posterior parietal lobes (*curved arrow*).

D, Parasagittal T1 (at 4 months). Marked volume loss is present, with cystic encephalomalacic changes throughout the supratentorial parenchyma. Remote parenchymal hemorrhage (*arrowheads*) and a subdural hygroma (*open arrows*) are present. Note relative preservation of the posterior fossa (*arrow*) and basal ganglia (*curved arrow*).

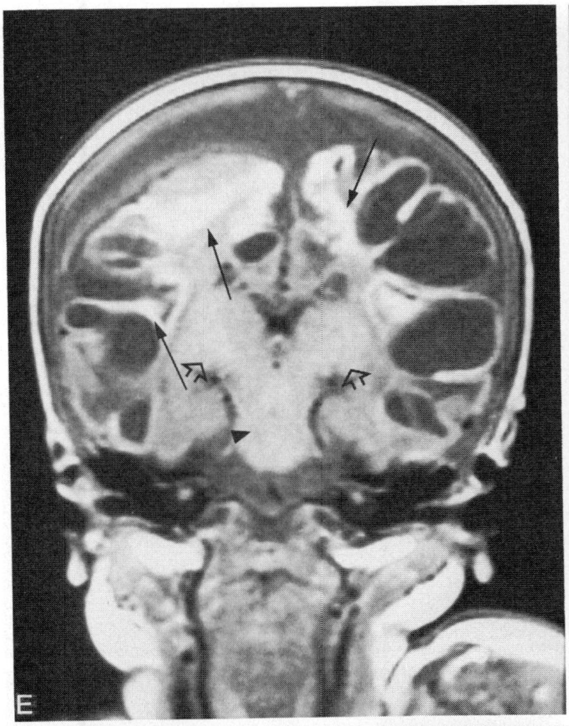

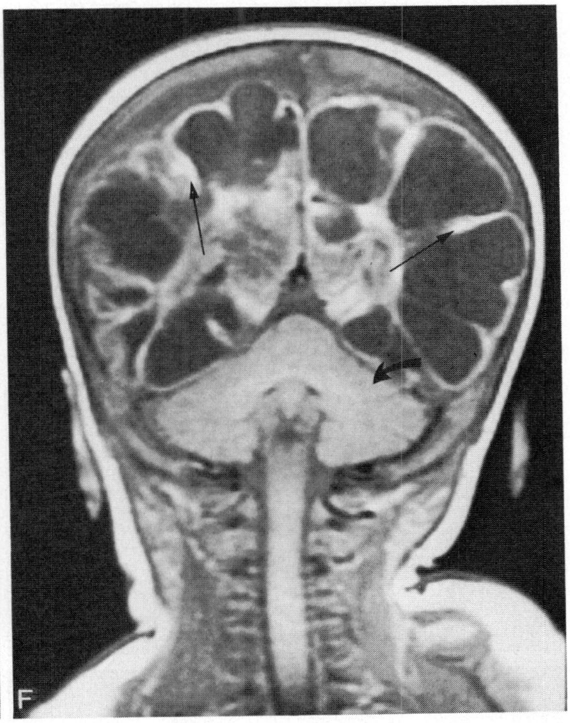

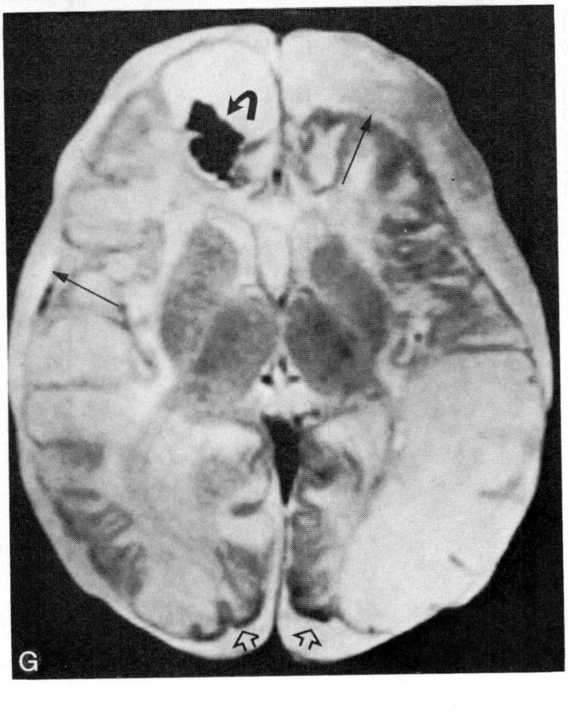

Figure 13–32 *Continued*

E, F, Coronal T1. Many of the encephalomalacic cavities are surrounded by hemorrhage (*arrows*). The brainstem (*arrowhead*), basal ganglia (*open arrows*), and posterior fossa parenchyma (*curved arrow*) appear normal.

G, Axial T2. Subdural collections (*arrows*) remain isointense to CSF. Hemosiderin is noted along the pial surface (*open arrows*) and within a cystic cavity of the right frontal lobe (*curved arrow*).

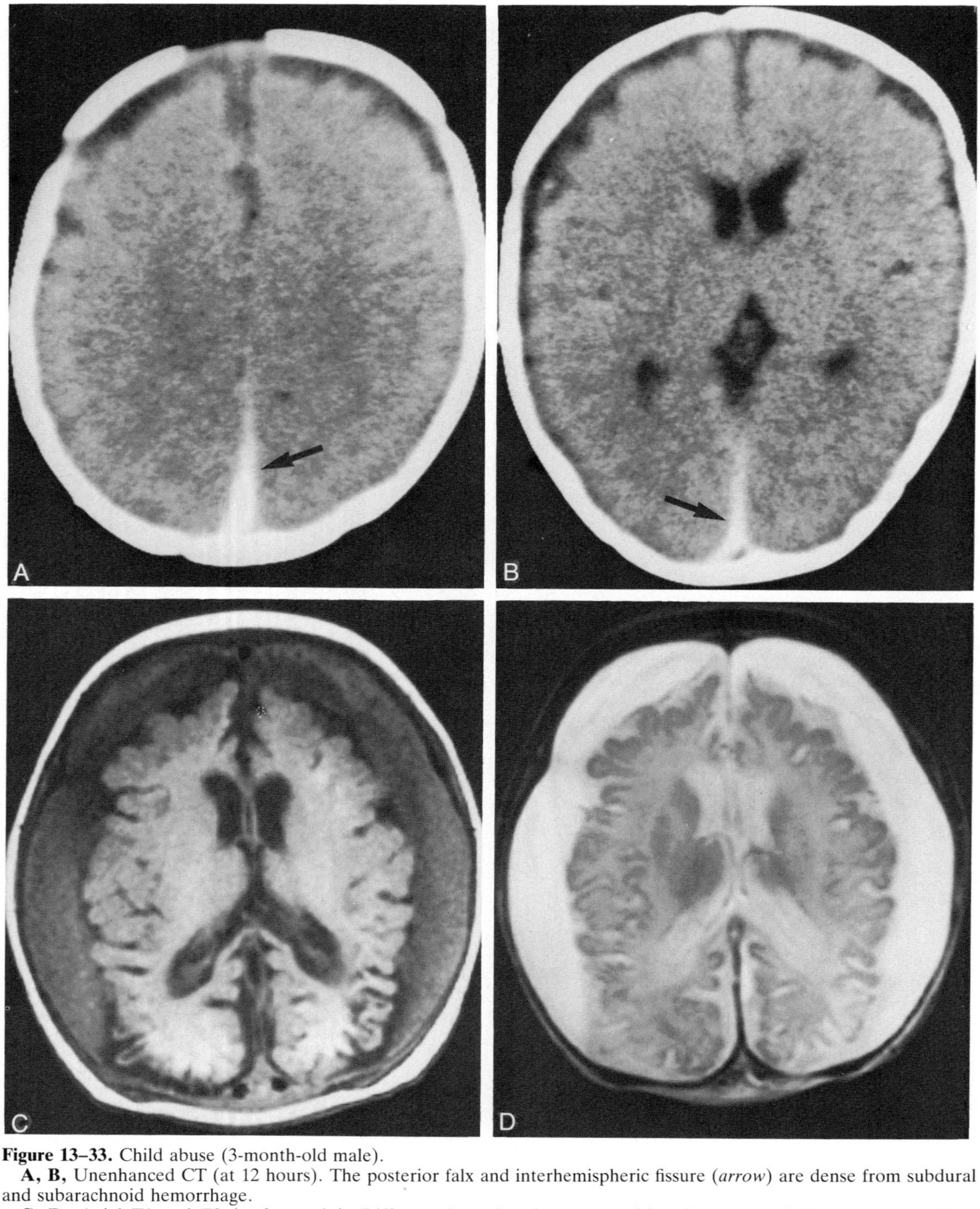

Figure 13–33. Child abuse (3-month-old male).

A, B, Unenhanced CT (at 12 hours). The posterior falx and interhemispheric fissure (*arrow*) are dense from subdural and subarachnoid hemorrhage.

C, D, Axial T1 and T2 (at 3 months). Diffuse volume loss is present with enlargement of the lateral ventricles. Bilateral subdural hemorrhages have developed in the 3-month interval since initial presentation.

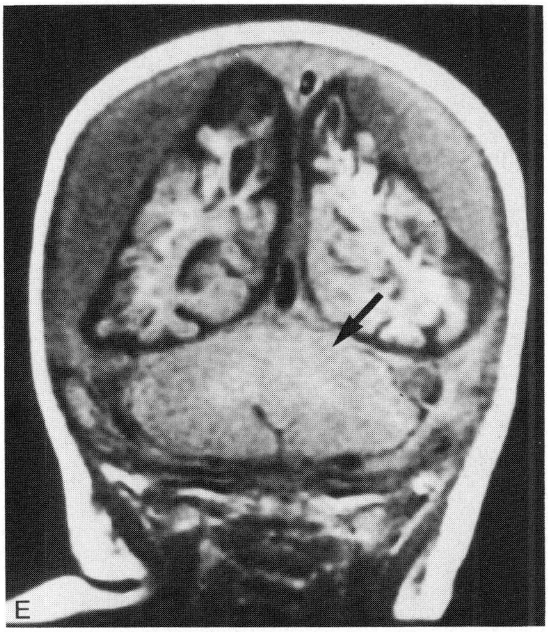

Figure 13–33 *Continued*
E, Coronal T1. The cerebellum (*arrow*) appears grossly normal despite the significant encephalomalacic changes of the supratentorial parenchyma.

NEOPLASMS

Brain tumors represent the second most common group of tumors in childhood, after leukemia. In the neonate (less than 2 months old) supratentorial tumors are three times more common than infratentorial tumors,[48] a prevalence that persists until 2 to 3 years of age. Common supratentorial tumors identified in this age group include astrocytomas,[49] choroid plexus papilloma,[48] and teratoma. Between the ages of 4 and 11 years, tumors are more frequently infratentorial[50] (Table 13–5).

Infratentorial

Pontine Glioma

Pontine gliomas represent 20 to 30% of posterior fossa neoplasms in children. The peak age of diagnosis is between 4 and 13 years of age, with 80% of tumors occurring before age 20. Males are affected equally or slightly more than are females.[50, 51] Most tumors of the brainstem occur in the pons, although they may affect the medulla or midbrain primarily or by contiguous extension from the pons.

Clinically, patients present with cranial nerve neuropathy that is often multiple and bilateral. Cranial nerves VI and VII are most frequently involved.[51] As the tumor enlarges, long track signs, ataxia, paraparesis, gaze disorders, and hemisensory syndromes may develop. In 30% of patients signs and symptoms of hydrocephalus are present.

Histologically, two subgroups exist.[51] The most common (80%) consists of diffuse fibrillary astrocytes. There is histologic evidence of anaplastic transformation, with resultant necrosis and hemorrhage. Foci of anaplasia compatible with glioblastoma are present. Pilocytic astrocytes represent only 20% of the pontine gliomas seen in children. There is no evidence of anaplasia despite mild necrosis. The growth rate is substantially slower and prognosis substantially better than with fibrillary astrocytes.

CT depicts enlargement of the pons and an ill-defined isodense-to-hypodense pontine mass. The mass enlarges the pons, compressing the prepontine and CPA cisterns. The fourth ventricle is displaced posteriorly. The tumor may grow exophytically through the parenchyma into the adjacent cisterns. The basilar artery may be encased by tumor and paradox-

Table 13–5. PEDIATRIC POSTERIOR FOSSA NEOPLASMS

				CT			MRI			
	Age	**Sex**	**Location**	***Density****	***Ca²⁺***	***Margins***	***T1†***	***T2†***	***Enhancement***	**Comments**
Medulloblastoma (PNET)	75% 1st decade	M:F, 2:1	Anterior vermis, lateralizing with age	→ ↑	15%	Usually well defined	↓ →	→ ↑	Marked, heterogeneous	May fill 4th ventricle, ± cleavage plane with floor of 4th ventricle High incidence of CSF metastasis Most common CNS tumor to metastasize outside of CNS
Cerebellar astrocytoma	60% 1st decade	M = F	Vermis, paramedian cerebellar hemisphere	Cyst/solid ↓/→	20%	Cyst well defined	Cyst → ↑ Solid → ↓	→ ↑ → ↑	Moderate	Varied morphology: Solid Solid with small cyst Cyst with mural nodule
Ependymoma	Bimodal: <5, 30s	Male slightly greater than female	4th ventricle	Variable ↑ ↓	50%	Poorly defined	→ ↓	↑	Marked heterogeneous	Fills the enlarged 4th ventricle, extending through exit foramina into CSF spaces
Pontine glioma	1st decade: 80% by 20 years	M ≥ F	Pons	↓	Rare	Poorly defined	→ ↓	↑	Minimal heterogeneous	Centrifugal expansion of pons, displacement of adjacent structures ± exophytic moiety

*Density referrable to pons.
†Intensity referrable to pons.

ically displaced from the clivus by the exophytic tumor.[50] Rarely, pontine gliomas will undergo CT-detectable hemorrhage or contain calcification. Enhancement is only minimal and is heterogeneous in 50% of pontine gliomas. The exophytic component of the tumor is more likely to enhance than the parenchymal moiety.[51]

MRI is more sensitive than CT at detection and defining extension of pontine gliomas.[52–54] The tumors are isointense to hypointense on T1 and dramatically hyperintense on spin density and T2 images (Fig. 13–34). Tumoral cysts are slightly hyperintense to CSF on T1 and T2 sequences. MRI may be effectively used to evaluate response to therapy.[51]

Medulloblastoma

Medulloblastomas are highly malignant tumors that arise from embryonal cells originating in the germinative zone of the posterior medullary velum. The cells migrate superolateral to form the external granular layer of the cerebellum.[55] Medulloblastomas are considered by some[56] to be a subset of the small round cell tumors called primitive neuroectodermal tumors (PNET) which also includes ependymoblastoma, pineoblastoma, and retinoblastoma. Medulloblastomas are the most common posterior fossa neoplasm in pediatric patients,[57] accounting for 50% of cerebellar neoplasms.[58] Medulloblastomas are twice as common in males, and 75% of these tumors present in the first decade.

As medulloblastomas are rapidly growing tumors, affected patients are diagnosed approximately 1 month after onset of symptoms of increased intracranial pressure (headaches, nausea, and vomiting). Patients less than 1 year old present with increasing circumference from hydrocephalus. Patients older than age 1 often have truncal ataxia.

The tumor may infiltrate the surrounding parenchyma and traverse the foramen of the fourth ventricle to gain access to the CSF cisterns. Medulloblastoma is one of the most common tumors to spread to the CSF. The frequency of CSF metastases to the spine (12 to 43%)[50] warrants evaluation of the entire spinal axis in all patients. In addition, medulloblastoma is the most common primary CNS tumor to metastasize outside of the CNS. The most common location for metastases are bone (86%), peritoneum through shunt catheters

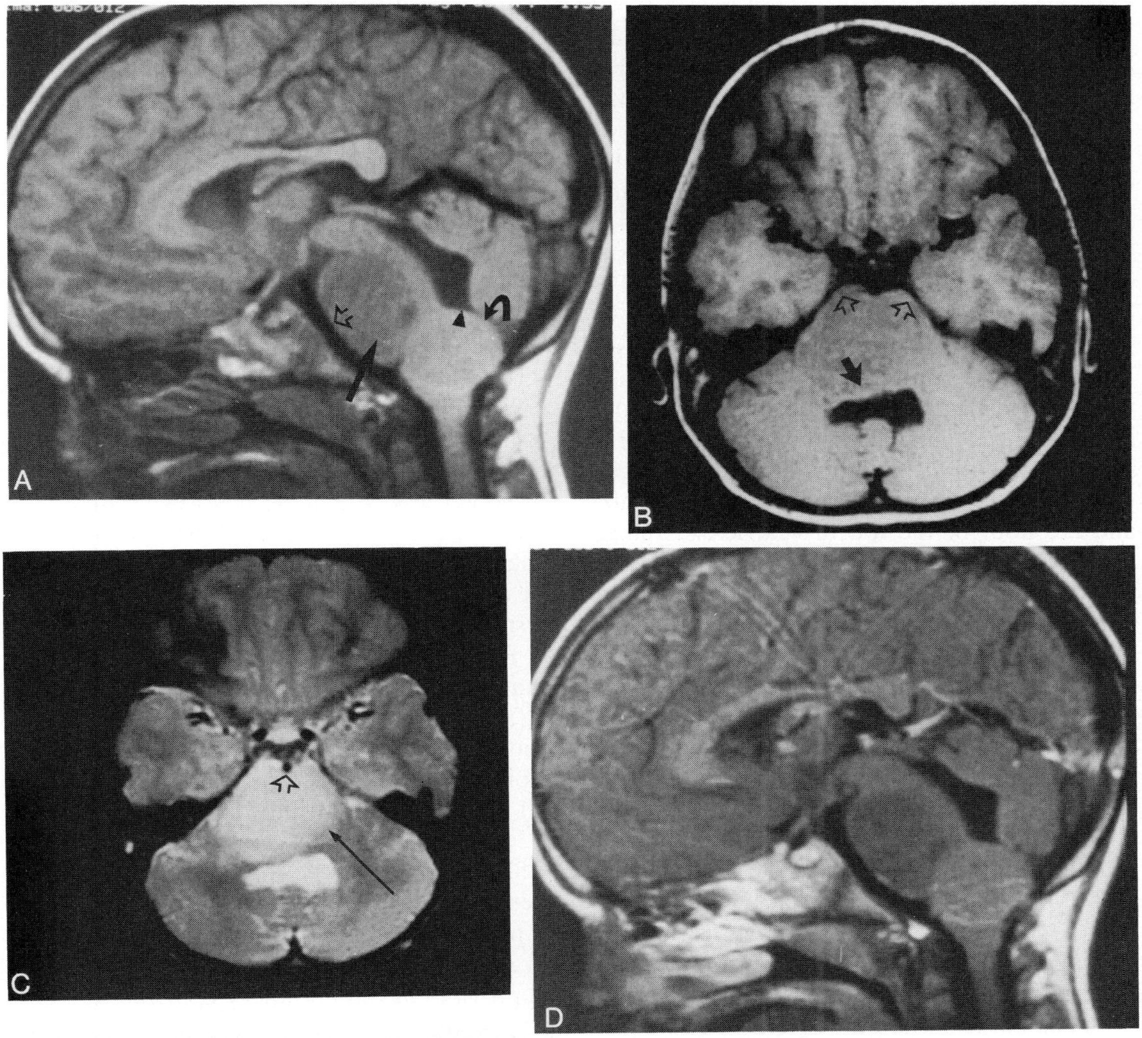

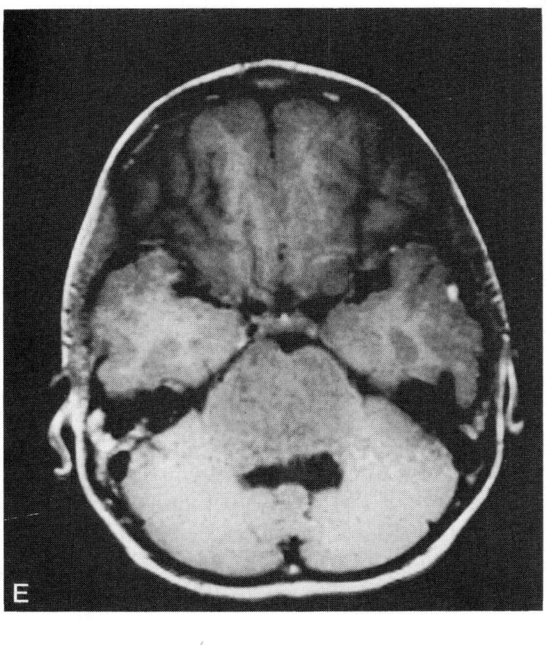

Figure 13–34. Pontine glioma (5-year-old male).

A, Parasagittal T1. A slightly hypointense mass enlarges the pons (*arrow*) at the expense of the prepontine cistern (*open arrow*). An isointense mass enlarges the medulla (*curved arrow*), deforming the caudal fourth ventricle (*arrowhead*).

B, Axial T1. The pons is diffusely enlarged, with distortion of the fourth ventricle (*arrow*) and prepontine cistern (*open arrows*).

C, Axial T2. The tumor is now more apparent as a homogeneous focus of high signal (*arrow*). The basilar artery (*arrowhead*) is in part surrounded by tumor.

D, E, Enhanced parasagittal and axial T1. There is no appreciable enhancement of the pontine glioma. (From Lizak PF, Woodruff WW: Posterior fossa neoplasms: Multiplanar imaging. Semin Ultrasound CT MR, 1992; 13:182–206, with permission.)

(43%), lymph nodes (30%), and lung (7%).[50] Factors that adversely affect the prognosis are diagnosis at less than 4 years of age, tumor dissemination, and tumor size greater than 3 cm.[57]

CT depicts a well-defined hyperdense midline vermian mass that enhances uniformly. The mass tends to lateralize with increasing age of diagnosis.[55] Hydrocephalus is present in 95% of patients.[57] Cysts and necrosis are usually rare. Calcification is present in 4 to 15% of patients.[50, 57]

MRI more accurately defines the isointense-to-hypointense tumor on T1 which is isointense to hyperintense on T2. The tumor usually enhances homogeneously unless cysts are present (Figs. 13–35, 13–36). Parasagittal images may detect a cleavage plane between the tumor and the floor of the fourth ventricle. Administration of gadolinium is particularly useful in documenting CSF spread of tumor.[59] Gadolinium-enhanced MRI is the procedure of choice in evaluating for intracranial or intraspinal metastases, as a lumbar puncture may yield positive cytology in only 15 to 60% of patients with CSF metastasis.[59]

Gadolinium-enhanced evaluation of the spinal axis should be performed more than 2 weeks after surgery, to avoid false-positive examination results that may be caused by surgery-related occult subarachnoid hemorrhage. Postoperative hemorrhage results in meningeal irritation and leakage of contrast material into the CSF.[60] A baseline evaluation of the spinal axis should be performed before surgery whenever PNET is a likely diagnosis.

Tumor may recur locally (56%) or in the CSF space and leptomeninges (39%).[61] Nodular leptomeningeal, dural, or ependymal enhancement corroborates metastasis[62] (Fig. 13–37). Mild focal or diffuse enhancement occurs normally in patients who have undergone biopsy, craniotomy, or ventricular shunt placement. Recurrent tumor does not enhance in all cases (33%), and not all enhancement is related to recurrent tumor (22%).[63] Radiation therapy may result in local mass effect and enhancement between 3 and 9 months after therapy.

Cerebellar Astrocytoma

Cerebellar astrocytomas are the second most common posterior fossa neoplasm in the pediatric population and account for approximately 40% of cerebellar neoplasms. The peak incidence of tumor is in the first decade. The tumors are comparatively benign and may be quite large (often greater than 5 cm) at presentation. Also, patients may have symptoms up to 3 years before diagnosis is established.[57] Symptoms are secondary to increased intracranial pressure.

The tumors may be one of two histologic subtypes. Juvenile pilocytic astrocytomas account for 75 to 85% of tumors. These carry a 25-year survival of 94%. Histologically the remaining tumors are diffusely fibrillary, with a 40% 25-year survival.[57]

The tumor usually arises from the vermis, although less commonly it arises in a paramedian location or completely within the hemisphere.[50] The tumor morphology varies: it may be cystic with a mural nodule (50%), solid with a small cyst (40%), or completely solid (10%).[57]

Planar imaging demonstrates a sharply demarcated, smoothly marginated mass (Fig. 13–38). The solid moiety is isodense to brain and the cyst hypodense on CT. MRI depicts an isointense-to-hypointense solid component on T1 that correlates with a high-signal focus on T2. The cyst is isointense to hyperintense to CSF on T1 and hyperintense to CSF on spin density and T2.[63, 64] Calcification, although not a prevalent feature of this tumor, does occur in 20% of patients. This calcification may vary, appearing on the periphery or within the central portion of the tumor. The solid tumor and mural nodule enhance vividly after contrast administration (Figs. 13–39, 13–40).

Ependymoma

Ependymomas are the third most common tumor of the posterior fossa, representing less than 10% of primary CNS neoplasms in children.[57] Males are affected slightly more commonly than females. A bimodal age peak is noted, with patients affected before 5 years of age and in the mid 30s.

Location of 60 to 70% of ependymomas is infratentorial. Tumors arise from the ependymal lining, usually in the floor of the fourth ventricle. Tumor growth is restricted to the fourth ventricle in 80% of patients.[50] Alternatively, the tumor may extend through the fourth ventricular foramen into the CSF spaces

Text continued on page 565

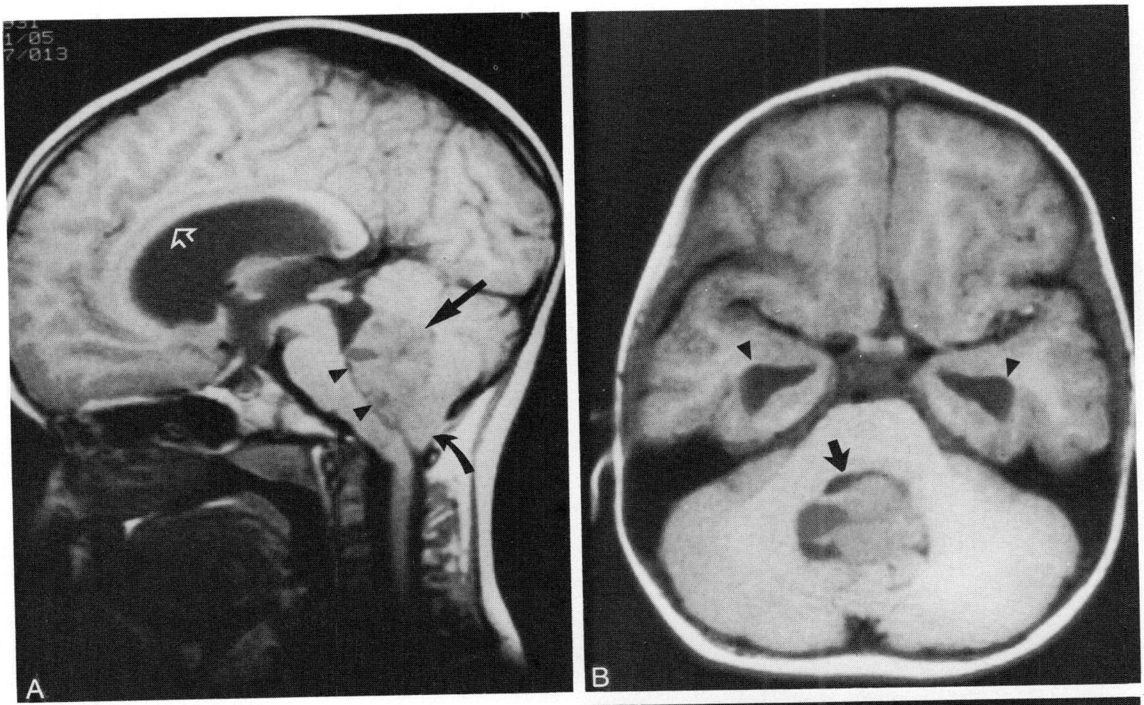

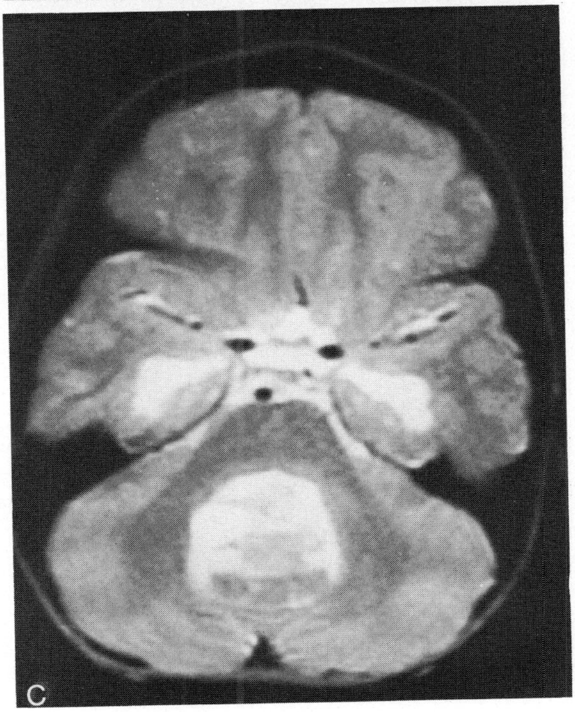

Figure 13–35. PNET; medulloblastoma (5-year-old male).

A, Parasagittal T1. A heterogeneous mass (*arrow*) fills the caudal fourth ventricle. The mass distorts the cephalad fourth ventricle and causes obstructive hydrocephalus (*open arrow*). The cerebellar tonsils (*curved arrow*) have herniated through the foramen magnum owing to the mass effect. The mass maintains a cleavage plane (*arrowhead*) with the fourth ventricle yet is inseparable from the inferior vermis.

B, Axial T1. The heterogeneity of the mass is confirmed. The fourth ventricle (*arrow*) is distorted and the temporal horns (*arrowheads*) enlarged because of obstructive hydrocephalus.

C, Axial T2. The mass is both high- and intermediate-signal intensity and does not appear to be macroscopically invasive.

Illustration continued on following page

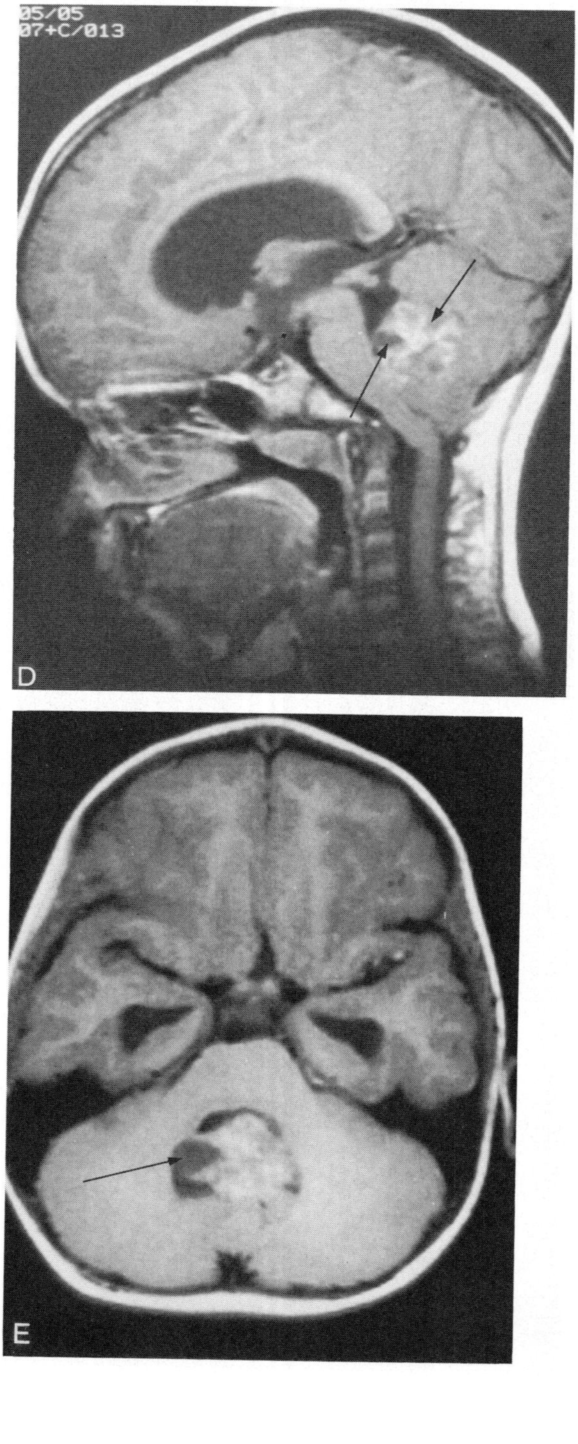

Figure 13–35 *Continued*
D, E, Enhanced parasagittal and axial T1. The mass enhances heterogeneously, revealing nonenhancing moieties (*arrows*) that represent cysts or necrosis. (From Lizak PF, Woodruff WW: Posterior fossa neoplasms: Multiplanar imaging. Semin Ultrasound CT MR, 1992; 13:182–206, with permission.)

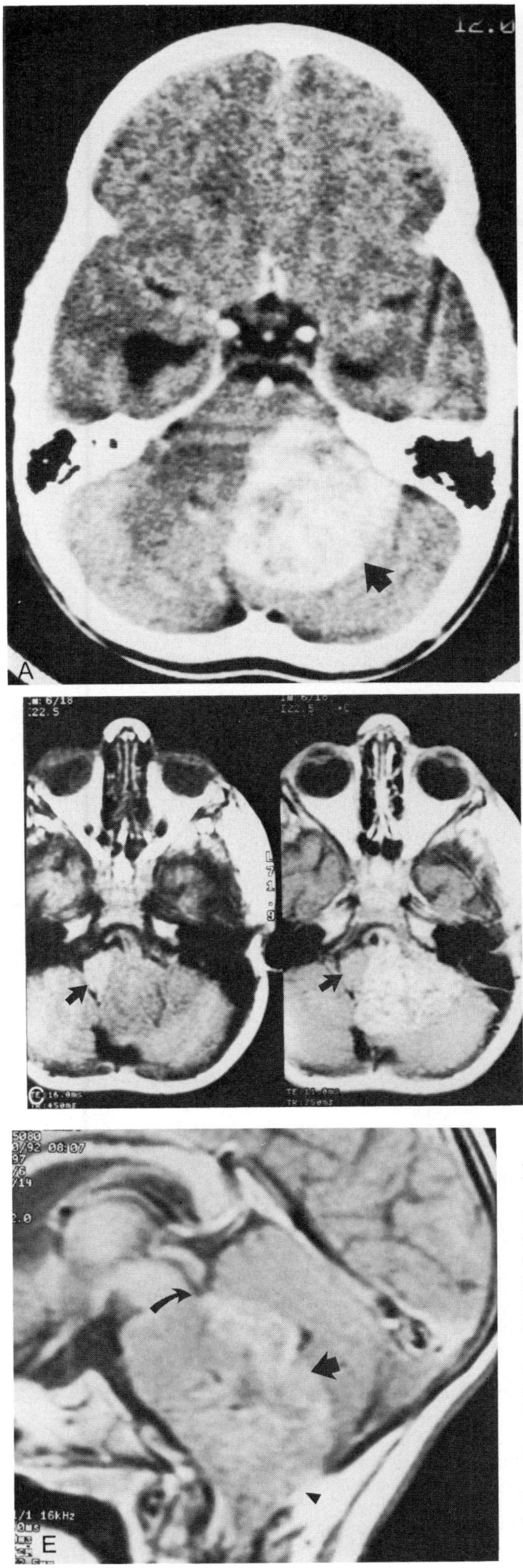

Figure 13–36. PNET (medulloblastoma) (2-year-old female).

A, B, Enhanced CT. A heterogeneously enhancing mass (*arrow*) is present in the left paramedian posterior fossa. A cystic or necrotic focus (*open arrow*) is noted. The mass has extended through the lateral recess of the fourth ventricle to gain access to the left cerebellopontine angle (CPA). The temporal horns (*arrowhead*) are enlarged owing to obstructive hydrocephalus.

C, Axial T1 (*left,* unenhanced; *right,* enhanced). The mass distorts the medulla (*arrow*) and has infiltrated the caudal surface of the left cerebellar hemisphere. The mass enhances heterogeneously.

D, Axial (*left,* SD; *right,* T2). The tumor (*arrows*) is heterogeneously hyperintense.

E, Enhanced parasagittal T1. The tumor (*arrow*) fills the fourth ventricle, extending to the caudal aqueduct (*curved arrow*) and through the foramen magnum (*arrowhead*).

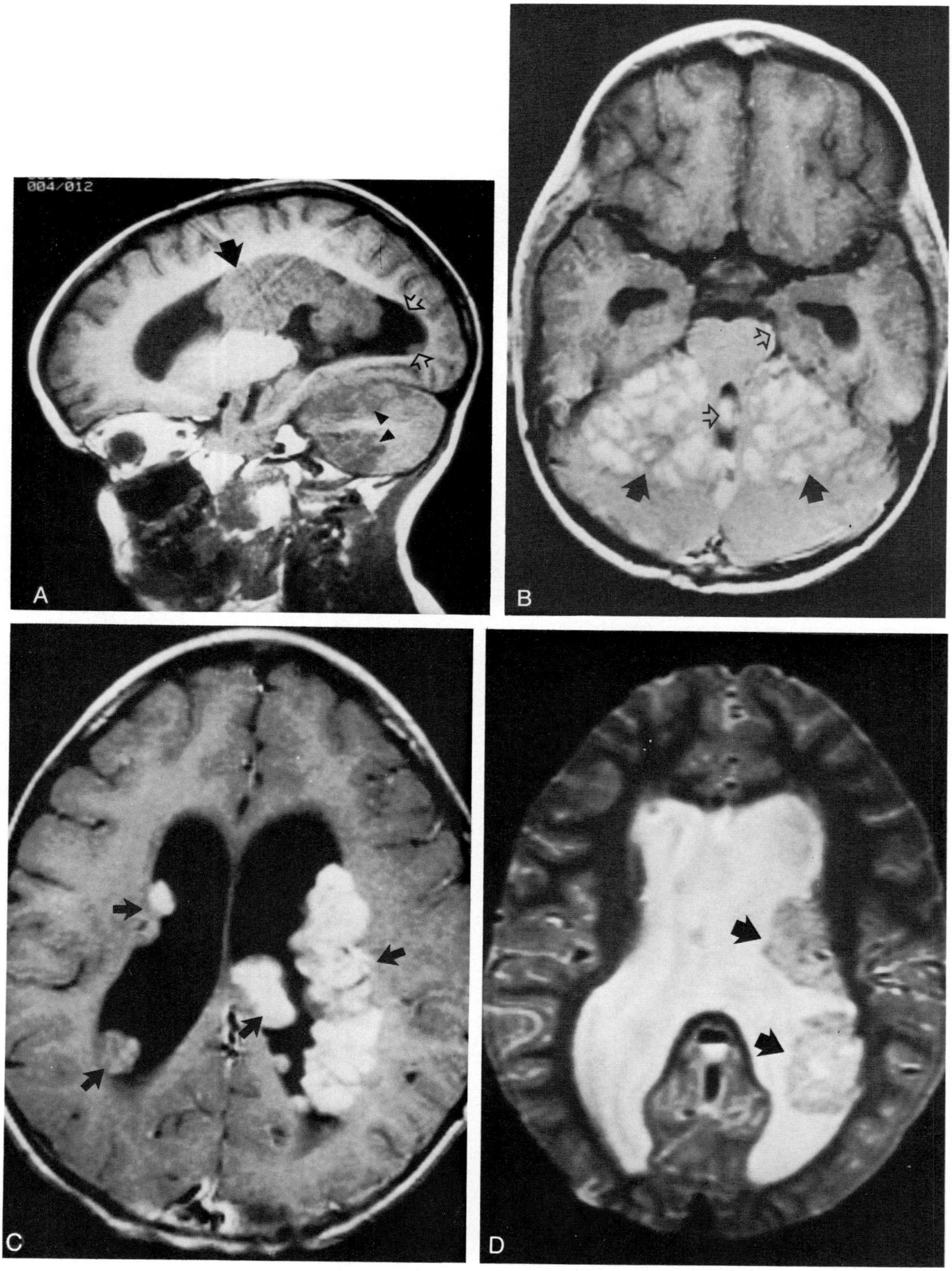

Figure 13–37. Medulloblastoma, metastatic (6-year-old male, 6 months following resection).

A, Parasagittal T1. A large exophytic mass (*arrow*) fills the enlarged left lateral ventricle. Small ependymal nodules (*open arrows*) are also detected. The cerebellum is markedly hypointense to normal parenchyma.

B, Enhanced axial T1. Multiple foci of enhancement corroborate parenchymal (*arrows*) and CSF (*open arrows*) metastases.

C, Enhanced axial T1. Multiple intraventricular masses (*arrows*) are present owing to CSF metastases.

D, Axial T2. The tumors (*arrows*) are heterogeneous and nearly isointense to gray matter. (From Lizak PF, Woodruff WW: Posterior fossa neoplasms: Multiplanar imaging. Semin Ultrasound CT MR, 1992; 13:182–206, with permission.)

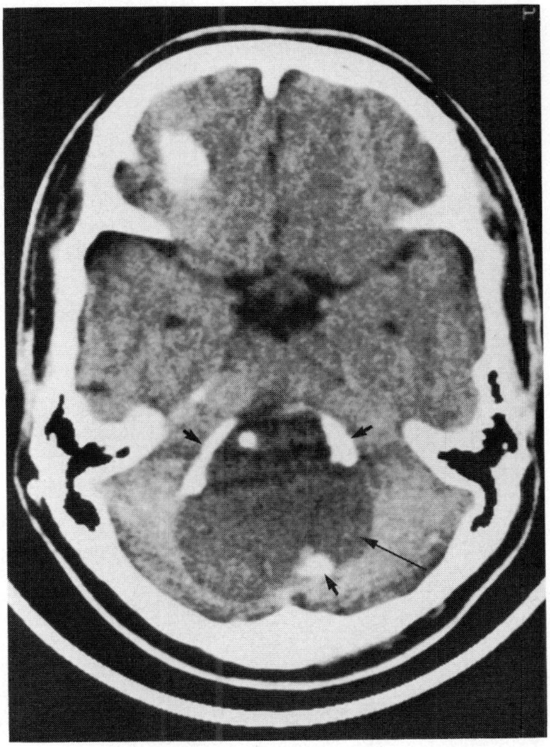

Figure 13–38. Cystic cerebellar astrocytoma (10-year-old male). Unenhanced CT; a large midline cystic tumor (*long arrow*) is present in the posterior fossa. The tumor is partially calcified (*short arrows*).

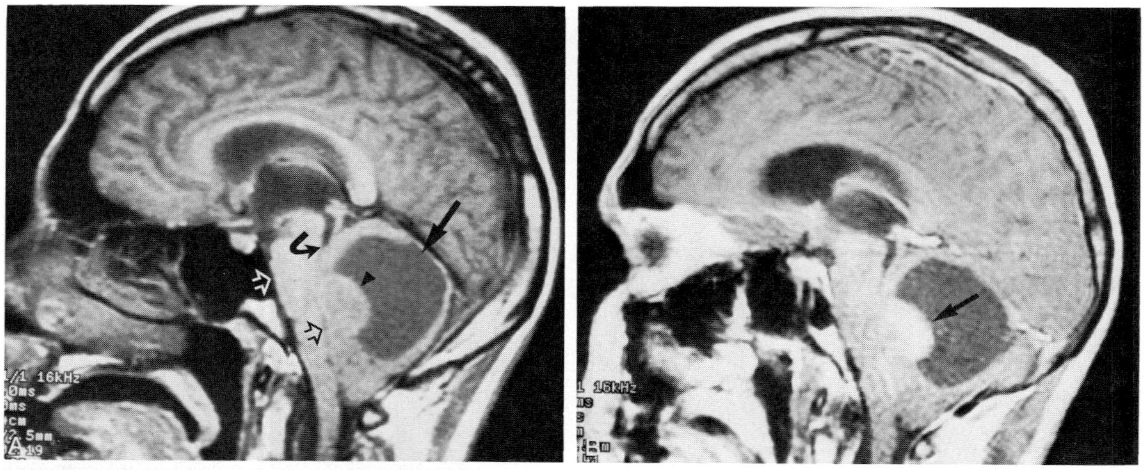

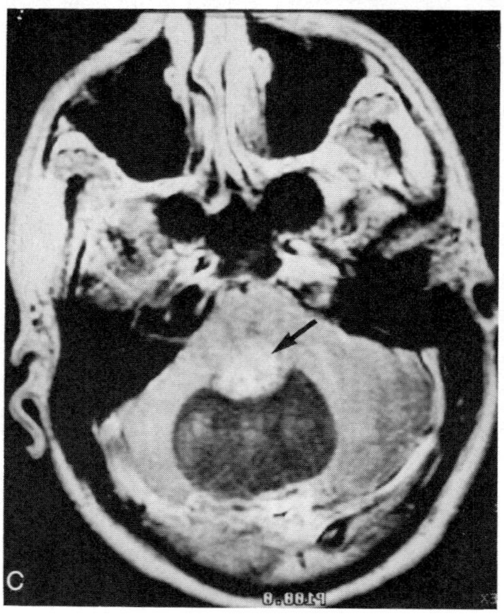

Figure 13–39. Cystic cerebellar astrocytoma (12-year-old male).
A, Parasagittal T1. A midline posterior fossa tumor is present containing a large dorsal cyst (*arrow*) and a smaller ventral solid moiety (*arrowhead*). The fourth ventricle (*open black arrow*) is compressed and the caudal aqueduct (*curved arrow*) deformed. The pons is compressed against the clivus (*open white arrow*).
B, C, Enhanced parasagittal and axial T1. The solid moiety (*arrow*) enhances homogeneously.

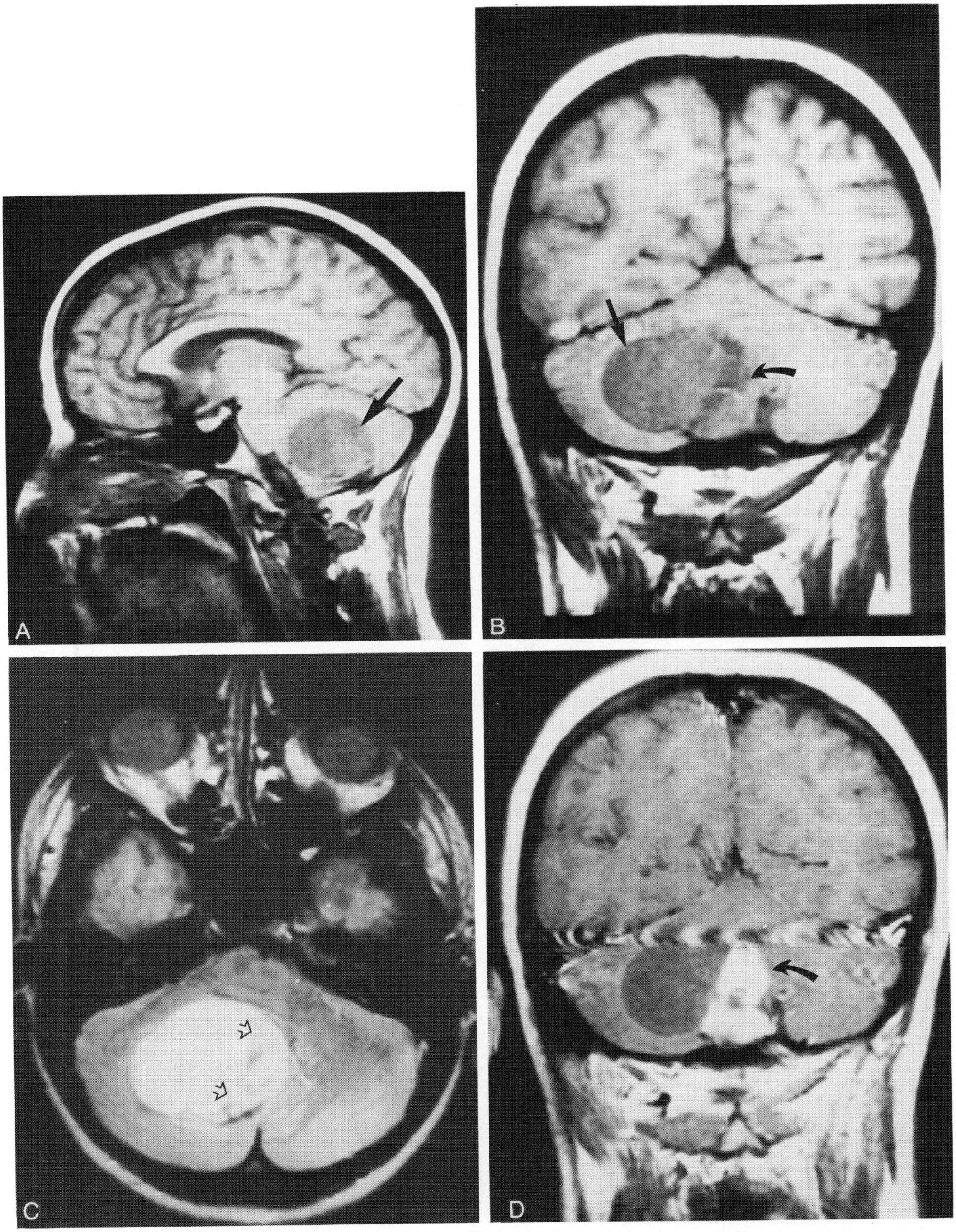

Figure 13–40. Cystic cerebellar astrocytoma (22-year-old male).

A, Parasagittal T1. A circular hypointense cerebellar mass (*arrow*) is present. The adjacent CSF spaces are attenuated. The ventricles are not obstructed.

B, Coronal T1. The well-demarcated, presumed cystic moiety of the mass (*arrow*) is lateral to a less well-demarcated, solid component (*curved arrow*).

C, Axial SD. The solid tumor (*open arrows*) can be distinguished from cyst. There is no significant vasogenic edema surrounding this mass.

D, Enhanced coronal T1. The medial solid component (*curved arrow*) enhances with better distinction between tumor and normal parenchyma. (From Lizak PF, Woodruff WW: Posterior fossa neoplasms: Multiplanar imaging. Semin Ultrasound CT MR, 1992; 13:182–206, with permission.)

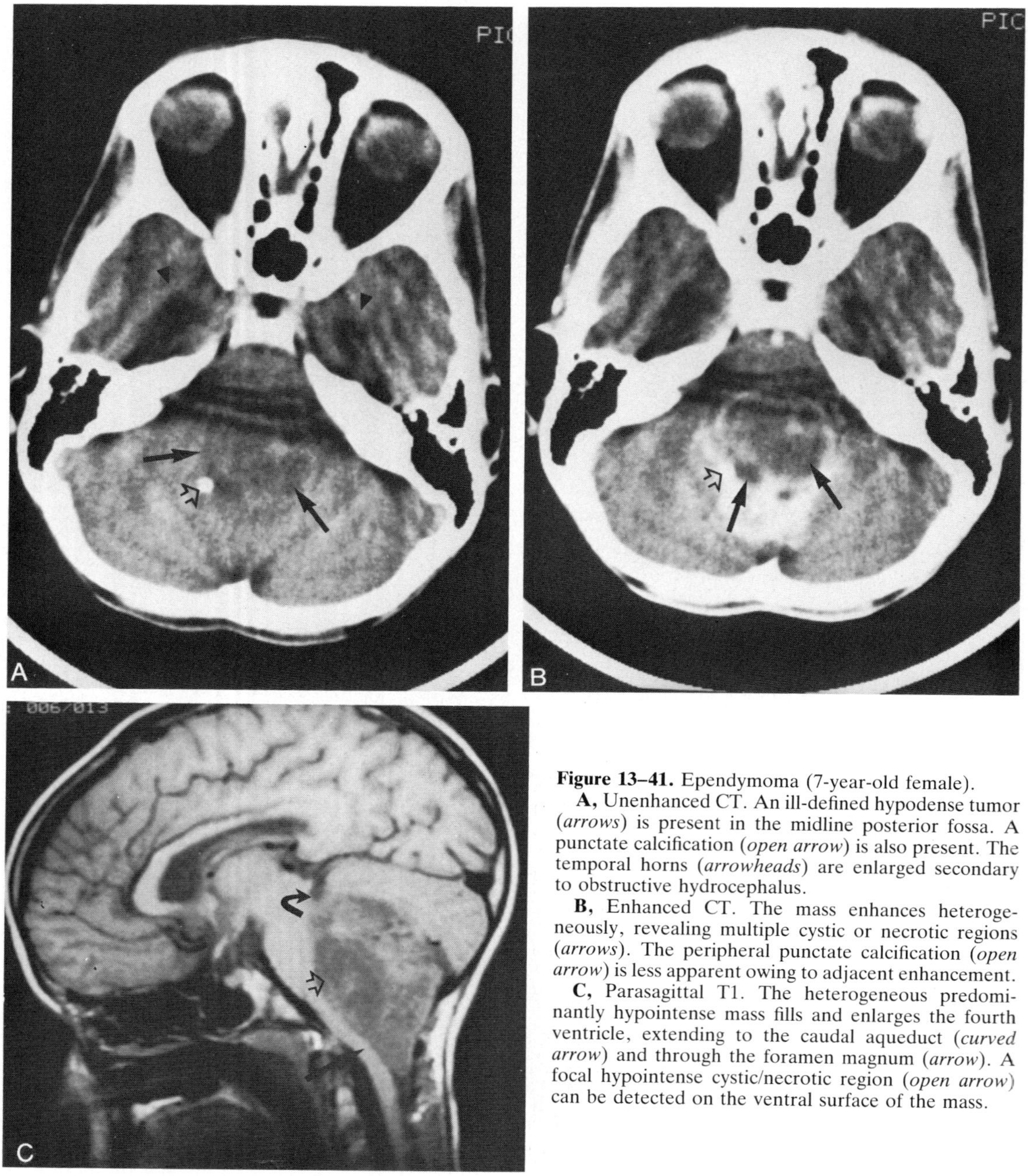

Figure 13–41. Ependymoma (7-year-old female).

A, Unenhanced CT. An ill-defined hypodense tumor (*arrows*) is present in the midline posterior fossa. A punctate calcification (*open arrow*) is also present. The temporal horns (*arrowheads*) are enlarged secondary to obstructive hydrocephalus.

B, Enhanced CT. The mass enhances heterogeneously, revealing multiple cystic or necrotic regions (*arrows*). The peripheral punctate calcification (*open arrow*) is less apparent owing to adjacent enhancement.

C, Parasagittal T1. The heterogeneous predominantly hypointense mass fills and enlarges the fourth ventricle, extending to the caudal aqueduct (*curved arrow*) and through the foramen magnum (*arrow*). A focal hypointense cystic/necrotic region (*open arrow*) can be detected on the ventral surface of the mass.

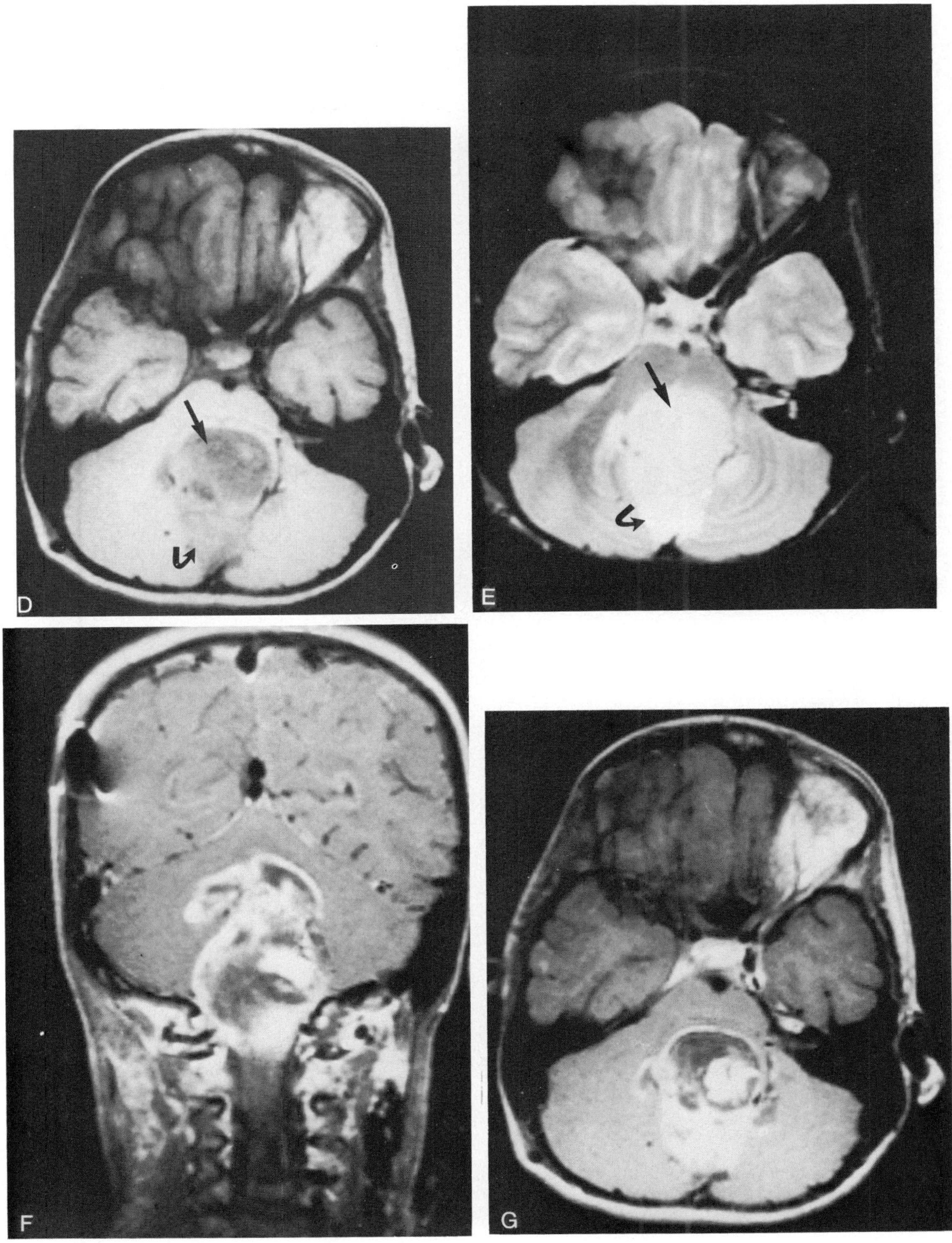

Figure 13–41 *Continued*

D, E, Axial T1 and T2. The heterogeneity of the mass is noted. Cystic/necrotic (*arrow*) and solid tumor (*curved arrow*) regions are present.

F, G, Enhanced coronal and axial T1. Tumor extension is more apparent, as is the heterogeneity of the mass. (From Lizak PF, Woodruff WW: Posterior fossa neoplasms: Multiplanar imaging. Semin Ultrasound CT MR, 1992; 13:182–206, with permission.)

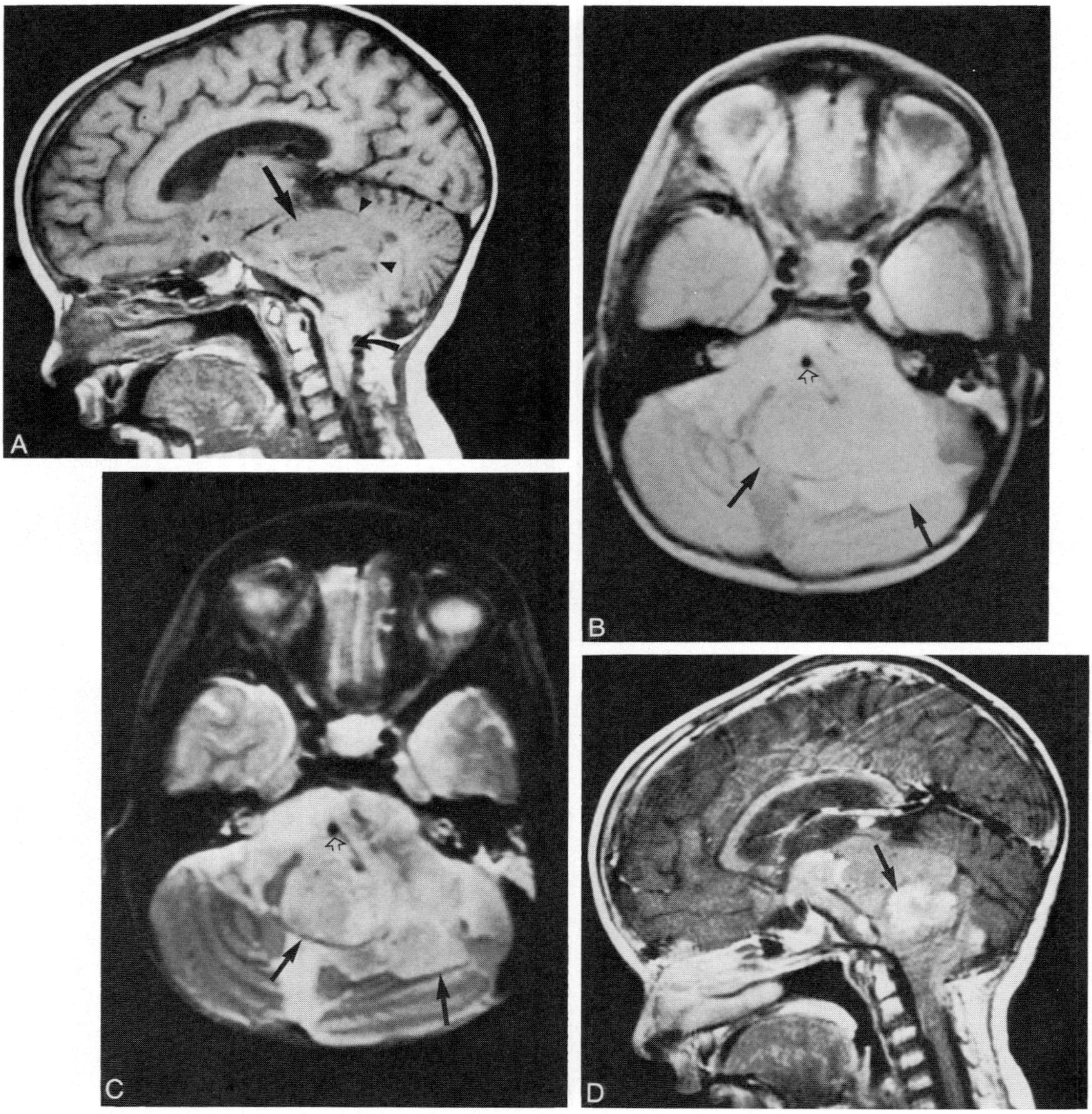

Figure 13–42. Ependymoma (5-year-old male).

A, Parasagittal T1. A heterogeneous mixed-intensity mass (*arrow*) is present in the anterior portion of the posterior fossa. The mass has a cleavage plane with the vermis (*arrowheads*) and extends into the cervical spinal canal (*curved arrow*).

B, C, SD and T2. The diffusely infiltrative mass (*arrows*) has extended throughout the cerebellum and fills the cisterna magnum and prepontine cisterns. The basilar artery (*open arrow*) is encased with exophytic tumor.

D, Enhanced parasagittal T1 (7 months later). Residual posterior fossa tumor (*arrow*) is present.

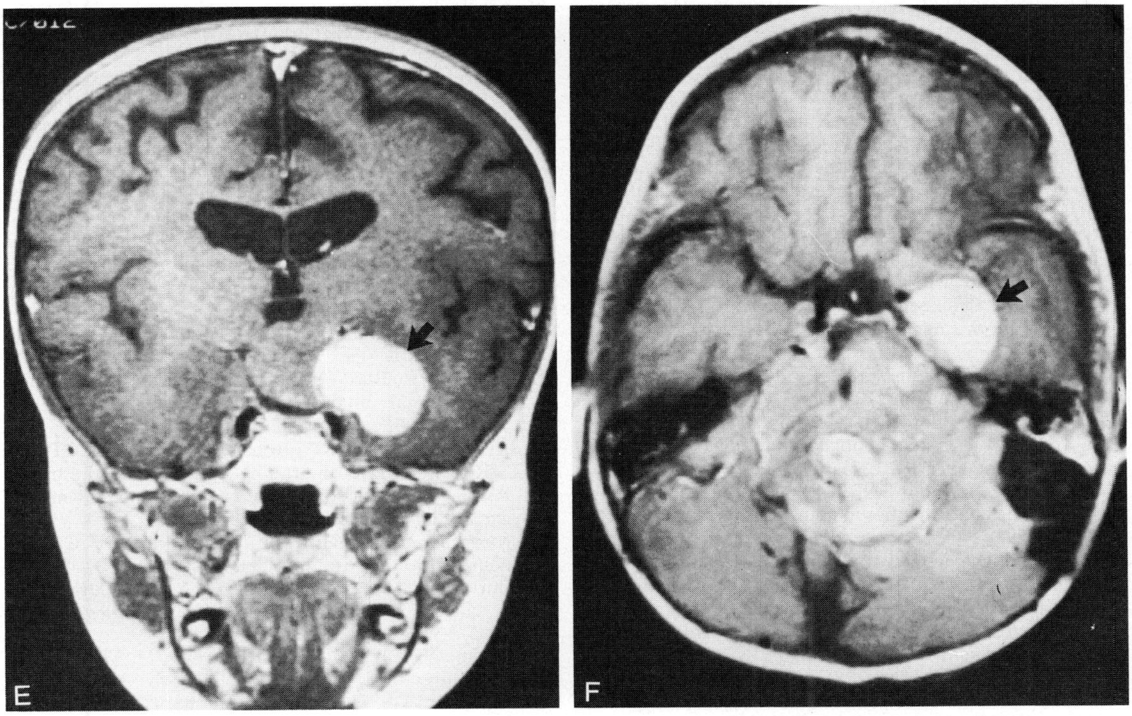

Figure 13–42 *Continued*
E, F, Enhanced coronal and axial T1. Reveals a large supratentorial metastasis (*arrow*) to the medial left temporal lobe.

or extend directly into the cerebellar or pontine parenchyma.

The CT characteristics of ependymoma are variable: the tumor may be hypodense to hyperdense; it may be calcified and/or contain cysts in 50% of patients. Moderate contrast enhancement occurs within the solid tumor moiety (Fig. 13–41).

MRI reveals a heterogeneous mass that fills the fourth ventricle. A cleavage plane between the mass and the fourth ventricular roof may be detected. The solid mass is isointense to hypointense on T1- and hyperintense on T2-weighted images (Fig. 13–42). The cysts are hyperintense to CSF on T1 and isointense to hyperintense to CSF on T2. Enhancement increases the heterogeneity of the tumor.

Supratentorial

As previously mentioned, supratentorial tumors are more common in children below the age of 4 and above age 11. These tumors have been discussed in appropriate sections elsewhere. In general, these tumors may arise within the parenchyma, ventricle, pineal gland, suprasellar region, or orbit.

Parenchymal tumors include glioma (most commonly astrocytoma), ganglioglioma, and PNET. Intraventricular tumors are most commonly choroid plexus papilloma and, less frequently, ependymomas. Pineal region tumors include those originating in germ cell lines such as germinoma, teratoma, choriocarcinoma, embryonal cell carcinoma and those originating in the pineal stem cell such as pineocytoma and pineoblastoma. The suprasellar tumors are most commonly chiasmatic or hypothalamic gliomas or craniopharyngiomas. Orbital tumors include the retinoblastoma and rhabdomyosarcoma.

References

1. van der Knapp MS, Valk J: Classification of congenital abnormalities of the CNS. AJNR 1988; 9:315–326.
2. Poe LB, Coleman LL, Mahmud F: Congenital central nervous system anomalies. Radiographics 1989; 9:801–826.
3. Naidich TP, Pudlowski RM, Naidich JB, et al: Computed tomographic signs of the Chiari II malforma-

tion. Part I: Skull and dural partitions. Radiology 1980; 134:65–71.
4. El Gammal T, Mark EK, Brooks BS: MR imaging of Chiari II malformation. AJNR 1987; 8:1037–1044.
5. Naidich TP, Pudlowski RM, Naidich JB: Computed tomographic signs of Chiari II malformation. II: Midbrain and cerebellum. Radiology 1980; 134:391–398.
6. Wolpert SM, Anderson M, Scott RM, et al: Chiari II malformation: MR imaging evaluation. AJNR 1987; 8:783–792.
7. Naidich TP, Pudlowski RM, Naidich JB: Computed tomographic signs of the Chiari II malformation. III: Ventricles and cisterns. Radiology 1980; 134:657–663.
8. Castillo M, Quencer RM, Dominguez R: Chiari III malformation: Imaging features. AJNR 1992; 13:107–113.
9. Barkovich AJ, Fram EK, Norman D: Septo-optic dysplasia: MR imaging. Radiology 1989; 171:189–192.
10. Braffman BH, Bilaniuk LT, Zimmerman RA: MR of central nervous system neoplasia of the phakomatoses. Semin Roentgenol 1990; 25:198–217.
11. Hurst RW, Newman SA, Cail WS: Multifocal intracranial MR abnormalities in neurofibromatosis. AJNR 1988; 9:293–296.
12. Aoki S, Barkovich AJ, Nishimura K, et al: Neurofibromatosis Types I and II: Cranial MR findings. Radiology 1989; 172:527–534.
13. Bognanno JR, Edwards MK, Lee TA, et al: Cranial MR imaging in neurofibromatosis. AJNR 1988; 9:461–468.
14. Duffner PK, Cohen ME, Seidel FG, et al: The significance of MR abnormalities in children with neurofibromatosis. Neurology 1989; 39:373–378.
15. Goldstein SM, Curless RG, Donovan Post MJ, et al: A new sign of neurofibromatosis on magnetic resonance imaging of children. Arch Neurol 1989; 46:1222–1224.
16. Mayfrank L, Mohadjer M, Wullich B: Intracranial calcified deposits in neurofibromatosis Type II, a CT study of 11 cases. Neuroradiology 1990; 32:33–37.
17. Vaghi M, Visciani A, Testa D, et al: Cerebral MR findings in tuberous sclerosis. J Comput Assist Tomogr 1987; 11:403–406.
18. Altman NR, Purser RK, Donovan Post MJ: Tuberous sclerosis: Characteristics at CT and MR imaging. Radiology 1988; 167:527–532.
19. Nixon JR, Houser OW, Gomez MR, et al: Tuberous sclerosis: MR imaging. Radiology 1989; 170:869–873.
20. Berns DH, Masaryk TJ, Weisman B, et al: Tuberous sclerosis: Increased MR detection using gradient echo technique. J Comput Assist Tomogr 1989; 13:896–898.
21. Braffman BH, Bilaniuk LT, Naidich TP, et al: MR imaging of tuberous sclerosis: Pathogenesis of this phakomatosis, use of gadopentetate dimeglumine, and literature review. Radiology 1992; 183:227–238.
22. Tien RD, Hesselink JR, Duberg A: Rare subependymal giant-cell astrocytoma in a neonate with tuberous sclerosis. AJNR 1990; 11:1251–1252.
23. Iwasaki S, Nakagawa H, Kichikawa K, et al: MR and CT of tuberous sclerosis: Linear abnormalites in the cerebral white matter. AJNR 1990; 11:1029–1034.
24. Chamberlain MC, Press GA, Hesselink JR: MR imaging and CT in three cases of Sturge-Weber syndrome: Prospective comparison. AJNR 1989; 10:491–496.
25. Elster AD, Chen MYM: MR imaging of Sturge-Weber syndrome: Role of gadopentetate dimeglumine and gradient echo technique. AJNR 1990; 11:685–689.
26. Lipski S, Brunelle F, Aicardi J, et al: GD-DTPA-enhanced MR imaging in two cases of Sturge-Weber syndrome. AJNR 1990; 11:690–692.
27. Smirniotopoulos JG, Murphy FM: Phakomatoses. AJNR 1992; 13:725–746.
28. Wasenko JJ, Rosenbloom SA, Duchesneau PM, et al: The Sturge-Weber syndrome: Comparison of MR and CT characteristics. AJNR 1990; 11:131–134.
29. Crome L: Hydranencephaly. Dev Med Child Neurol 1972; 14:224–234.
30. Dublin AB, French BN: Diagnostic image evaluation of hydranencephaly and pictorially similar entities, with emphasis on computed tomography. Radiology 1980; 137:81–91.
31. Poe LB, Coleman L: MR of hydranencephaly. AJNR 1989; 10:S61.
32. Osborn RE, Byrd SE, Naidich TP, et al: MR imaging of neuronal migrational disorders. AJNR 1988; 9:1101–1106.
33. Byrd SE, Osborn RE, Bohan TP, et al: The CT and MR evaluation of migrational disorders of the brain. Part II: Schizencephaly, heterotopia and polymicrogyria. Pediatr Radiol 1989; 19:219–222.
34. Bird CR, Gilles FH: Type I schizencephaly: CT and neuropathologic findings. AJNR 1987; 8:451–454.
35. Barkovich AJ, Kjos BO: Schizencephaly: Correlation of clinical findings with MR characteristics. AJNR 1992; 13:85–94.
36. Barkovich AJ, Chuang SH, Norman D: MR of neuronal migration anomalies. AJNR 1987; 8:1009–1017.
37. Titelbaum DS, Hayward JC, Zimmerman RA: Pachygyriclike changes: Topographic appearance at MR imaging and CT and correlation with neurologic status. Radiology 1989; 173:663–667.
38. Byrd SE, Osborn RE, Bohan TP, et al: The CT and MR evaluation of migrational disorders of the brain. Part I: Lissencephaly and pachygyria. Pediatr Radiol 1989; 19:151–156.
39. Gallucci M, Bozzao A, Curatolo P, et al: MR imaging of incomplete band heterotopia. AJNR 1991; 12:701–702.
40. Barkovich AJ, Kjos BO: Gray matter heterotopias: MR characteristics and correlation with developmental and neurologic manifestations. Radiology 1992; 182:493–499.
41. Barkovich AJ, Jackson DE, Boyer RS: Band heterotopias: A newly recognized neuronal migrational anomaly. Radiology 1989; 171:455–458.
42. Jinkins JR, Whittemore AR, Bradley WG: MR imaging of corticocallosal dysgenesis. AJNR 1989; 10:339–344.
43. Cohen RA, Kaufman RA, Myers PA, et al: Cranial computed tomography in the abused child with head injury. AJR 1986; 146:97–102.
44. Calder IM, Hill I, Scholtz CL: Primary brain trauma in non-accidental injury. J Clin Pathol 1984; 37:1095–1100.
45. Zimmerman RA, Bilaniuk LT, Bruce D, et al: Computed tomography of craniocerebral injury in the abused child. Radiology 1979; 130:687–690.
46. Sato Y, Yuh WTC, Smith WL, et al: Head injury in child abuse: Evaluation with MR imaging. Radiology 1989; 173:653–657.
47. Alexander RC, Schor DP, Smith WL: Magnetic resonance imaging of intracranial injuries from child abuse. J Pediatr 1986; 109:975–979.
48. Radkowski MA, Naidich TP, Tomita T, et al: Neonatal brain tumors: CT and MR findings. J Comput Assist Tomogr 1988; 12:10–20.

49. Ambrosino MM, Hernanz-Schulman M, Genieser NB, et al: Brain tumors in infants less than one year of age. Pediatr Radiol 1988; 19:6–8.
50. Naidich TP, Zimmerman RA: Primary brain tumors in children. Seminars in Roentgenology 1984; 19:100–114.
51. Smith RR: Brain stem tumors. Seminars in Roentgenology 1990; 25:249–262.
52. Hueftle MG, Han JS, Kaufman B, et al: MR imaging of brain stem gliomas. J Comput Assist Tomogr 1985; 9:263–267.
53. Lee BCP, Kneeland JB, Walker RW, et al: MR imaging of brain stem tumors. AJNR 1985; 6:159–163.
54. Kucharczyk W, Brant-Zawadzki M, Sobel D, et al: Central nervous system tumors in children. Detection by magnetic resonance imaging. Radiology 1985; 155:131–136.
55. Zimmerman RA, Bilaniuk LT, Pahlajani H: Spectrum of medulloblastomas demonstrated by computed tomography. Radiology 1978; 126:137–141.
56. Rorke LB: The cerebellar medulloblastoma and its relationship to primitive neuroectodermal tumors. J Neuropathol Exp Neurol 1983; 42:1–15.
57. Gusnard DA: Cerebellar neoplasms in children. Seminars in Roentgenology 1990; 25:263–278.
58. Lizak PF, Woodruff WW: Posterior fossa neoplasms: Multiplanar imaging. Seminars in Ultrasound CT and MR 1992; 13:182–206.
59. Rippe DJ, Boyko OB, Friedman HS, et al: GD-DTPA-enhanced MR imaging of leptomeningeal spread of primary intracranial CNS tumor in children. AJNR 1990; 11:329–332.
60. Wiener MD, Boyko OB, Friedman HS, et al: False-positive spinal MR findings for subarachnoid spread of primary CNS tumor in postoperative pediatric patients. AJNR 1990; 11:1100–1103.
61. Lee YY, Glass JP, van Eys J, et al: Medulloblastoma in infants and children: Computed tomographic follow-up after treatment. Radiology 1985; 154:677–682.
62. Hudgins PA, Davis PC, Hoffman JC: Gadopentetate dimeglumine—enhanced MR imaging in children following surgery for brain tumor: Spectrum of meningeal findings. AJNR 1991; 12:301–307.
63. Rollins N, Mendelsohn D, Mulne A, et al: Recurrent medulloblastoma: Frequency of tumor enhancement on GD-DTPA MR imaging. AJNR 1990; 11:583–587.
64. Lee YY, van Tassel P, Bruner JM, et al: Juvenile pilocytic astrocytomas: CT and MR characteristics. AJNR 1989; 10:363–370.

INDEX

Note: Page numbers followed by an i indicate illustrations; those followed by a t indicate tables.

S

T

U

V

W

ISBN 0-7216-3717-5

90038

9 780721 637174